GUIDE TO THE ESSENTIALS IN
EMERGENCY MEDICINE
SECOND EDITION

Edited by
Shirley Ooi
Peter Manning

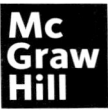

Mc
Graw
Hill

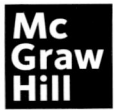

Guide to the Essentials in Emergency Medicine
Second Edition

10 9 8 7 6
20 19
SLP

When ordering this title, use **ISBN 978-9-814-74258-0** or **MHID 9-814-74258-9**

Printed in Singapore

To:

God, for so graciously blessing and strengthening me. All I have achieved is by your grace and grace alone. To God be all glory!

My husband, Andrew, for your generosity in allowing me to contribute my best towards my vocation. Without your support, I would not have been able to be where I am today.

My 3 children, Samuel, Joshua and Janice, who have helped me keep a healthy work life balance.

All my students, past and present, for being the fuel that has kept my flame for teaching and mentoring alive! Without you all, I would have 'shrivelled up' a long time ago!

Shirley Ooi

I dedicate my offerings in this edition to my wife Margret who continues to put up with my strange hours and utterings, and, who probably feels at times that she is number two in my life after Emergency Medicine.

Peter Manning

It was a pleasure to review the second edition of this handy tome. The *Guide To The Essentials In Emergency Medicine* has already won a place on the bookshelves of many GPs and the pocket coats of medical students and residents. Here, in a major upgrade, Prof Ooi and her team has scoured for the latest in the emergency medicine literature, and incorporated them into easily referenced chapters. Concise yet thorough, it makes for easy reading for the person who needs quick information at the bedside of an ill patient. Especially worthwhile reading are the 'tips for GPs', which emphasize the pitfalls and red flags that could trip up the unwary GP or Medical Officer. Gems include the sections on dealing with infectious disease outbreaks, haematologic/oncologic emergencies, and a timely updates on geriatric emergencies. Recommended also for Advanced Practise Nurses and Advanced Diploma Nursing Courses

Dr Goh Siang Hiong, *Clinical Professor (NUS-YLL School of Medicine), Deputy Chairman Medical Board, (Ambulatory Division and Medical Education), Changi General Hospital*

All of the relevant conditions are covered in just the right level of detail for practising clinicians who are seeking definitive, clear guidance on what to lock for, how to manage the condition here and now and when and how to refer. The use of flowcharts and information boxes makes the text easy to access with the maximum of information.

Professor Colin Robertson, *Professor of Emergency Medicine, University of Edinburgh, Scotland*

This 2nd edition not only contains updates in the essentials of emergency medicine management but also nicely categorizes specific conditions into various headings for easy reference. It is a comprehensive survival guide to the novice and quick reference for the experts.

Dr Ho Hiu-fai, *President Hong Kong College of Emergency Medicine, Deputy Hospital Chief Executive (Professional Service), Queen Elizabeth Hospital, HK*

Ten years is a long time but it is worth the wait! The second edition of Professor Shirley Ooi's *Guide to the Essentials in Emergency Medicine* is an excellent compact companion to any doctor who deals with emergency conditions either in the emergency department or even clinic. I notice the topics have been rearranged accordingly with better subheadings making it simpler for users to get quickly to the information they seek. New chapters have been added like *Emergency Ultrasound, Common Emergency Procedures, & Chikungunya* and will make this book more valuable. I'm sure all students either from the residency program or the undergraduate program and doctors working in the ED will love this second edition of the book. Congratulations and well done to Prof Shirley and colleagues!

Professor Ismail Mohd Saiboon, *Head and Senior Consultant Emergency Medicine, Department of Emergency Medicine, Universiti Kebangsaan Malaysia Medical Centre (UKMMC)*

Emergent conditions require a cool head armed with the essential information to do the right thing at the right time. This edition of *Guide to the Essentials in Emergency Medicine* continues to provide the reader with a storehouse of succinct exposition of caveats, GPs tips, management approach and up to date survival information that were hallmarks of the previous edition. There are now 143 chapters compared to the 127 chapters in the 2004 edition. References and chapter content have been updated, some chapters extensively, and new chapters added. This book should be within reach at any time of the fingertips of all doctors who have to deal with emergencies in their work.

Associate Professor Goh Lee Gan, *Professorial Fellow, Associate Program Director, Family Medicine Residency, & Senior Consultant, Division of Family Medicine, University Medicine Cluster, National University Health System*

Contents

Foreword (*Professor Amal Mattu*)   xi

Foreword (*Associate Professor Yeoh Khay Guan*)   xiii

Preface   xv

Contributors   xix

Abbreviations   xxiii

Part 1   Common Presentations In Adult Patients

1	Altered Mental State	2
2	Bleeding, Gastrointestinal Tract (GIT)	6
3	Bleeding, Vaginal, Abnormal	11
4	Blurring of Vision	16
5	Breathlessness, Acute	20
6	Diarrhoea and Vomiting	23
7	Fever	26
8	Giddiness	30
9	Haemoptysis	38
10	Headache	41
11	Hyperventilation	45
12	Lower Limb Swelling	47
13	Pain, Abdominal	51
14	Pain, Chest, Acute	58
15	Pain, Joint, Peripheral	66
16	Pain, Low Back	72
17	Pain, Scrotal and Penile	76
18	Palpitations	85
19	Poisoning, General Principles	107
20	Red Eye	122
21	Seizure	126
22	Shock/Hypoperfusion States	131
23	Stridor	142
24	Syncope	147
25	Trauma Multiple, Initial Management	154
26	Urinary Retention, Acute	165
27	Violent and Psychotic Patients	168

Part 2   Specific Conditions
Part 2A   Airway and Resuscitation
28   Airway Management/Rapid Sequence Intubation   172
29   Allergic Reactions/Anaphylaxis   186
30   Cardiac Arrest Algorithms   193
31   Cardiogenic Shock   211
32   Neurogenic Shock   214
33   Sepsis/Septic Shock   216

Part 2B   Cardiovascular Emergencies
34   Aortic Emergencies   221
35   Bradysrhythmias   229
36   Coronary Syndromes, Acute   239
37   Other Heart Conditions (Pericarditis, Myocarditis, Infective Endocarditis, and   250
     Cardiomyophathy)
38   Heart Failure, Acute   261
39   Hypertensive Crises   270
40   Acute Limb Ischaemia   286
41   Pulmonary Embolism   289
42   Venous Emergencies   297
43   Tachydysrhythmias   303

Part 2C   Respiratory Emergencies
44   Asthma   316
45   Chronic Obstructive Pulmonary Disease (COPD)   322
46   Pneumonia, Community Acquired (CAP)   327
47   Pneumothorax   334
48   Respiratory Failure, Acute   339

Part 2D   Gastrointestinal Emergencies
49   Appendicitis, Acute   345
50   Hepatic Encephalopathy, Acute   350
51   Hepatobiliary Emergencies   354
52   Intestinal Obstruction   361
53   Ischaemic Bowel/Mesenteric Ischaemia   364
54   Pancreatitis, Acute   368
55   Peptic Ulcer Disease/Dyspepsia   373
56   Perianal Conditions   376

Part 2E   Endocrine/Metabolic Emergencies
57   Acid Base Emergencies   382
58   Adrenal Insufficiency, Acute   392
59   Fluid and Electrolyte Disorders   395
60   Diabetic Ketoacidosis (DKA) and Hyperosmolar Hyperglycaemic State (HHS)   403
61   Hypoglycaemia   409
62   Thyroid Emergencies – Thyroid Crisis and Myxoedema   416

Part 2F   Renal and Genitourinary Emergencies
63 Renal Emergencies   422
64 Urinary Tract Infections   430
65 Urolithiasis   433

Part 2G   Neurologic Emergencies
66 Meningitis   436
67 Migraine and Cluster Headache   442
68 Stroke   449
69 Subarachnoid Haemorrhage (SAH)   456
70 Temporal Arteritis   460
71 Transient Ischaemic Attack   462

Part 2H   Infectious Diseases
72 Coping with Emerging Infectious Diseases of the 21st Century in the Emergency   465
    Department – A New Norm
73 Dengue Fever and Chikungunya   470
74 Malaria   477
75 Needlestick/Body Fluid Exposure   481
76 Tetanus   484

Part 2I   Haematologic/Oncologic Emergencies
77 Administration of Blood Products in the Emergency Department   486
78 Oncology Emergencies   491
79 Overwarfarinization   500

Part 2J   Dermatologic Emergencies
80 Dermatology in Emergency Care   504

Part 2K   Geriatric Emergencies
81 Geriatric Emergencies   533

Part 2L   Toxicology
82 Alcohol Intoxication and Poisoning with Other Alcohols   539
83 Poisoning, Benzodiazepine   549
84 Poisoning, Carbon Monoxide   551
85 Poisoning, Cyclic Anti-depressants   557
86 Poisoning, Digoxin   564
87 Poisoning, Organophosphates   571
88 Poisoning, Paracetamol   576
89 Poisoning, Salicylates   581

Part 2M   Toxicology (Including Bites)
90 Bites, Mammalian and Human   585
91 Bites, Snake   592

Part 2N   Surgical & Orthopaedic Trauma/Infectious Emergencies

92	Crush Syndrome	598
93	Trauma, Abdominal	600
94	Trauma, Chest	606
95	Trauma, Head	616
96	Trauma and Infections, Hand	624
97	Trauma, Lower Extremity	637
98	Trauma, Maxillofacial	649
99	Trauma, Paediatric (refer to Chapter 137)	659
100	Trauma, Pelvic	660
101	Trauma in Pregnancy	662
102	Trauma, Spinal Cord and Cervical Spine Clearance	667
103	Trauma, Upper Extremity	675
104	Wound Care and Management	693

Part 2O   ENT Emergencies

105	Common Ear, Nose and Throat Emergencies	703

Part 2P   Eye Emergencies

106	Refer to Chapter 4, *Blurring of Vision* and Chapter 20, *Red Eye*	714

Part 2Q   Psychiatric Emergencies

107	Assault (non-sexual)	715

Part 2R   Obstetric and Gynaecologic Emergencies

108	Eclampsia	717
109	Ectopic Pregnancy	721
110	Emergency Delivery of the Newborn	725
111	Pelvic Inflammatory Disease (PID)	731

Part 2S   Environmental Emergencies

112	Burns, Major	733
113	Burns, Minor	739
114	Diving Emergencies	746
115	Electrical and Lightning Injuries	749
116	Hyperthermia	755
117	Submersion Injuries	759

Part 2T   Imaging

118	Emergency Ultrasound	762
119	Views of X-rays to Order	774

Part 2U   Pharmacology

120	Commonly Used Emergency Drugs in Adults	780
121	List of Drugs to Avoid in G6PD Deficiency	805
122	Prescribing in Pregnancy	807

Part 2V   Paediatric Emergencies

123   Child, Abdominal Pain   810
124   Child with Breathlessness   815
125   Child/Baby, Crying   819
126   Child with Diarrhoea   821
127   Child with Fever   825
128   Child, Fitting   831
129   Child, Vomiting   835
130   Paediatric Asthma   838
131   Bronchiolitis   842
132   Febrile Fit   845
133   Fluid Replacement in Paediatrics   848
134   Newborn Resuscitation in the Emergency Department   850
135   Non-accidental Injury in Paediatrics   853
136   Paediatric Drugs and Equipment   857
137   Trauma, Paediatric   867

Part 2W   Miscellaneous Useful Information

138   Commonly Used Scoring Systems   872
139   Common Emergency Procedures   876
140   Pain Management   887
141   Procedural Sedation   902
142   Simple Statistics   908
143   Useful Formulae   915

Index

920

Foreword

The practice of emergency medicine is not easy to define. It encompasses everything from acute care and resuscitation of the critically ill to subacute care and occasional chronic care of patients with mild illnesses. Emergency care providers must be able to care for every type of patient, of any age, with any co-morbidity or complaint, at any stage of the illness. The competent emergency care provider must be prepared to care for the acute illnesses of every specialty in medicine. For these reasons we often have difficulty defining not just the scope, but the *limits* of this specialty as well.

With this challenge in mind, one understands the complexity involved in trying to create a textbook that focuses on the specialty of emergency medicine. Such a textbook could easily encompass thousands of pages and still be incomplete in its attempt to be comprehensive. Alternatively, the textbook could be briefer and simply focus on acute resuscitation, ignoring the vast majority of cases that one encounters on a daily basis in the emergency department. Editors of medical textbooks must constantly deal with these challenges – if they create a textbook that is too comprehensive it will be judged as too unwieldy and undoubtedly be relegated to the bookshelves only to collect dust and quickly become outdated. However, if they create a textbook that is too concise it will be judged to be too shallow in depth to be useful in clinical practice. Finding the middle ground is the great challenge.

Fortunately for students and practitioners of emergency medicine, Drs Shirley Ooi and Peter Manning seem to have succeeded in finding this ideal middle ground. In this second edition of *Guide to the Essentials in Emergency Medicine*, they have assembled a talented group of clinician authors with a clear understanding of what is useful in an emergency medicine textbook. They have created a textbook that is succinct enough to be read cover-to-cover and used in real-time clinical practice, but is still comprehensive enough to avoid leaving gaps in knowledge of key points.

Part 1 focuses on common presenting symptoms and signs in emergency medicine. This section is somewhat unique to emergency medicine textbooks in its recognition that most patients present with undifferentiated complaints. In other words, patients do not complain of a heart attack, stroke, pneumonia, etc.; instead, they present with chest pain, weakness or dyspnoea. These chapters address presentations in sufficient detail such that the reader knows exactly what the 'can't-miss' differential diagnoses are and how to approach these patients in terms of evaluation and workup. This section represents the most important portion of the book and will likely be used by the student and junior physician more than any other. These 27 chapters alone could constitute an incredibly useful handbook or guide for students and trainees in emergency medicine, and I recommend this section as a must-read for all students and junior physicians in emergency medicine.

Part 2 constitutes the majority of this textbook and addresses specific diseases and emergency conditions. These are organized into organ systems for ease of reference. Once again, the authors perfectly address these conditions with appropriate depth and relevance to emergency medicine. They avoid overly lengthy pathophysiological explanations of disease states that may appear in an internal medicine or pathology text, but still address the underlying processes in sufficient depth for the reader to understand the concepts underlying the workup and treatment. These chapters can be accessed and read quickly so the book can be used in real-time in the emergency department. The recommendations for workup and management are up-to-date and referenced appropriately so that the reader knows where to seek more in-depth knowledge when desired.

This textbook can serve appropriately as a Board Examination review book as well. National and international guidelines and standards of care are addressed nicely, and key points that commonly appear in examinations are emphasized and repeated. Personally, being very involved in teaching US physicians at Written Board Examination Courses, I can attest to the fact that this textbook would be a very suitable syllabus that would assure success in any written examination in virtually any country.

My kudos go to Dr Ooi, Dr Manning and their talented group of authors for producing a truly outstanding textbook. Readers will find this a valuable addition to emergency medicine literature. Students and physicians that take the time to read this textbook will be rewarded with a marked increase in clinical knowledge, and most importantly their patients will benefit from it directly as well. I certainly am looking forward to seeing this textbook continue to progress alongside our specialty in future editions for many years to come.

Amal Mattu, MD, FAAEM, FACEP
Professor and Vice Chair
Director, Emergency Cardiology Fellowship
Director, Faculty Development Fellowship
Department of Emergency Medicine
University of Maryland School of Medicine
Baltimore, Maryland, USA

Foreword

Drs Shirley Ooi and Peter Manning and all the authors are to be congratulated on the second edition of the *Guide to the Essentials in Emergency Medicine*. This handbook is a compilation of the authors' extensive practical experience and management protocols used in the Emergency Department at the National University Hospital in Singapore. The first edition was an overwhelming success, having been reprinted nine times with more than 16,000 copies sold in eight countries including Singapore, Malaysia, Hong Kong and Taiwan.

What has made their book such a success is its unique approach and innovative features. The book is at once very clear and concise, yet comprehensive in its coverage, earning its place as a quick reference in the emergency room or the clinic of a family physician. The first section in the book focuses on the common presentations of patients in the Emergency Department. This is invaluable and practical, as of course real patients present to the ED with symptoms like drowsiness, breathlessness or weakness, and not by neat diagnoses. This section of the book gives guidance on evaluation, management, key tips and what not to miss. The second section describes various specific conditions organized by organ systems and aetiology.

Throughout the book the clinical management advocated is founded on an evidence-based approach and on international guidelines which are well-referenced. Having served as Chair of the Evidenced-based medicine (EBM) education committee at the National University Hospital in Singapore for many years, Dr Shirley Ooi is an accomplished teacher in EBM methodologies and this strength has certainly benefited the text.

The first edition of this book has been widely used in the Asia Pacific region and I am proud that this is an indigenous textbook born from local needs, yet its popular use internationally speaks of its special strengths and wide appeal. While its evidence-based approach, practical information and its conciseness wins many fans internationally, it also covers diseases seen in our region such as dengue fever, chikungunya and malaria which may not be covered well in occidental texts.

From my vantage point as an experienced clinician, teacher and academic, I feel certain that all readers will benefit immensely and that the high quality instruction and information will in turn lead to high quality and safe care for their patients. From the point of view of a resident or student preparing for exams, the book is easily readable from cover to cover and not overly long, while its evidence-based approach and pithy information explains the rationale for sound management. Family physicians too are well advised by the sections on 'Special Tips to GPs'. In short I am fully confident that this second edition of the *Guide to the Essentials in Emergency Medicine* will find even more readers and fans than did the very successful first edition.

Khay Guan Yeoh MBBS, MMed (Int Med), FRCP, FRCP (Glasg)
Dean, Yong Loo Lin School of Medicine, National University of Singapore
Deputy Chief Executive, National University Health System
Senior Consultant, Division of Gastroenterology & Hepatology
National University Hospital, Singapore

Preface

The first edition of this book was published in 2004. The original contents of this book were developed from the National University Hospital's Emergency Medicine Department (NUHEMD) Clinical Guidelines to ensure a uniform standard of medical care for our patients. The authors are mainly our current and past doctors of NUHEMD with a few 'guest contributors'. What was surprising and most fulfilling for us was that over the past decade there have been nine reprints of the book with more than 16,000 copies sold internationally! What is even more surprising is that over 50 per cent of the sales of this book are from outside of Singapore!

Readers will find once again that the hallmark succinct yet comprehensive style of our book makes it easy to use in the bedside care of a patient. The very popular sections of *Caveats* and *Special Tips for GPs* have also been retained. We have endeavoured to put together a thoroughly revised 2nd edition taking into account the feedback we have received so as to make this book even more useful. All chapters have been painstakingly revised to reflect the latest evidence. The book is now more vibrant as colour has been added to the individual pages to enhance reading. New illustrations, colour photographs, additional electrocardiograms and x-rays, CT scans, and ultrasound images have also been added. Included among the other new features are the following:

Part 1: Common Presentations in Adult Patients

This section is one of the key strengths of this book. Emergency patients present in a myriad of ways. Mastery in the approach to different presenting complaints is one of the core skills of an emergency doctor and this book places a lot of emphasis in this area as can be seen by the 27 chapters in this section.

All the chapters in the 1st edition in relation to common symptom presentation in adults have been retained.

A new chapter entitled *Pain, Joint, Peripheral* has been added (Chapter 15).

The paediatric symptom presentation has been shifted to Part 2V under *Paediatric Emergencies*.

Part 2: Specific Conditions

This section is now organized into 23 different subsections to facilitate learning and revision for examinations.

Related topics in the 1st edition have been consolidated into single chapters in this edition for ease of reference. These include *Coronary Syndromes, Acute* and *Myocardial Infarction, Acute* which have been merged into Chapter 36, *Coronary Syndromes, Acute*. Similarly, *Diabetic Ketoacidosis*

(DKA) and *Hyperosmolar Hyperglycaemic State* (HHS) have been consolidated into Chapter 60, *DKA and HHS*. *Heart Failure* and *Pulmonary Oedema, Cardiogenic,* have been merged as Chapter 38, *Heart Failure, Acute*. *Spinal Cord Injury* and *Cervical Spine Clearance* have been consolidated into Chapter 102, *Trauma, Spinal Cord and Cervical Spine Clearance*.

The 19 new chapters in this section include the following:

- Chapter 31 *Cardiogenic Shock*
- Chapter 32 *Neurogenic Shock*
- Chapter 35 *Bradydysrhythmias*
- Chapter 37 *Other Heart Conditions*
- Chapter 40 *Acute Limb Ischaemia*
- Chapter 42 *Venous Emergencies*
- Chapter 43 *Tachydysrhythmias*
- Chapter 59 *Fluid and Electrolyte Disorders*
- Chapter 64 *Urinary Tract Infection*
- Chapter 67 *Migraine and Cluster Headache*
- Chapter 71 *Transient Ischaemic Attack*
- Chapter 72 *Coping with Emerging Infectious Diseases of the 21st Century in the Emergency Department – A New Norm*
- Chapter 79 *Overwarfarinization*
- Chapter 86 *Poisoning, Digoxin*
- Chapter 110 *Emergency Delivery of the Newborn*
- Chapter 118 *Emergency Ultrasound*
- Chapter 120 *Commonly Used Emergency Drugs in Adults*
- Chapter 134 *Newborn Resuscitation in the Emergency Department*
- Chapter 139 *Common Emergency Procedures*

Myxoedema has been added to Chapter 62, *Thyroid Emergencies – Thyroid Crisis and Myxoedema*. *Chikungunya* has been added to Chapter 73, *Dengue Fever and Chikungunya*.

This book is meant for:

- *Junior Doctors serving their EM rotations and Emergency Nurses*. This will be a quick reference for at least 90–95% of the most commonly encountered conditions in their daily practice. The section on *Caveats* is especially useful to help prevent fatal and costly errors in patient management.

- *Emergency Medicine Residents preparing for the postgraduate exams*. This is a book that can be easily read from cover to cover as it is written in point form with key words highlighted. The contents are evidence-based and follow international guidelines. Pertinent information to explain the rationale of certain points in the management is given without the cumbersome details of the pathophysiology. This is one book that if you master the contents, you can almost be certain of being able to handle any international exams!

- *Medical Students doing their ED rotations.* This book details virtually all the common conditions they may encounter during their EM posting. Part 1 is practical, focused and concise, and students should be able to finish reading it within their 4-week posting.

- *Junior Doctors serving their rotations outside of ED.* This book will assist them in managing multidisciplinary emergencies as these can arise unexpectedly in the course of their work. It will help them to manage the patient in the first half-hour while awaiting additional help.

- *General Practitioners.* This book will guide them on how to treat multidisciplinary emergencies within the first half-hour while arrangements are made to send their patients to the ED. Of particular interest will be the *Special Tips for GPs* section.

- *Paramedics and Prehospital Care Personnel.* Part 1 and *Special Tips for GPs* will be very useful in guiding them in the symptom-based approach to emergency conditions.

This book would not have been possible without the invaluable help of our numerous contributors. We wish to thank Dr Chong Chew Lan, Ms Rebecca Long, Dr Swati Jain and Ms Sandra Han for so willingly assisting us with the illustrations in this book. We also wish to specially acknowledge the tireless and dedicated efforts of our department secretary, Ms Neo Yen Yen, who has assisted us in countless ways from start to finish. Without her, this book would not have been possible. We are greatly indebted to

- Professor Amal Mattu of the University of Maryland School of Medicine, USA, who has reviewed this book, given his most useful comments, and graciously written a Foreword for us;

- Associate Professor Yeoh Khay Guan, Deputy Chief Executive of the National University Health System (NUHS) and Dean of the Yong Loo Lin School of Medicine, National University of Singapore for writing a Foreword;

- Professor Colin Robertson from the University of Edinburgh, Scotland;

- Clinical Professor Goh Siang Hiong, Senior Consultant Changi General Hospital Department of Emergency Medicine and former President of the Society for Emergency Medicine in Singapore;

- Associate Professor Goh Lee Gan, Professorial Fellow, Associate Program Director, Family Medicine Residency, and Senior Consultant, Division of Family Medicine, University Medicine Cluster, NUHS;

- Dr Paul Ho, President of the Hong Kong College of Emergency Medicine; and

- Professor Ismail Saiboon, Head, Department of Emergency Medicine, University Kebangsaan Malaysia,

for writing the endorsements for our book.

We wish to thank our EM Chief Resident, Dr Chua Mui Teng for collating the list of contributors for this book. Last but not the least, we would like to thank Ms Sarah Han and Mr Gerald Bok from McGraw-Hill Education Asia for their help in publishing this book.

We hope you will find this edition an even more pleasant and useful book to read and would welcome your feedback. You can e-mail your feedback to Neo Yen Yen at nuh_emd@nuhs.edu.sg

Associate Professor Shirley Ooi
MBBS (S'pore), FRCSEd (A&E), FAMS (Emerg Med)
Senior Consultant
Designated Institutional Official
NUHS Residency Programme

Associate Professor Peter George Manning
MBBS (London), FACEP, FAMS (Emerg Med)
Emeritus Consultant
Vice-Chairman Medical Board
(Medicolegal and Risk Management)

Singapore, May 2014

Contributors

Emergency Medicine Department, National University Health System (NUHS), Singapore

Dr Chan Wai Han, Gene
MBBS (S'pore), MRCSEd (A&E), MMed
(Emerg Med)
Consultant

Dr Chiu Liqi
MBBS (S'pore), MCEM, MMed
(Emerg Med)
Registrar

Dr Ho Weng Hoe, Keith
MBBS (S'pore), MRCS Ed (A&E), MMed
(Emerg Med), EMDM
Consultant

Dr Ian Mathews
MBBS (S'pore), MCEM, MMed
(Emerg Med)
Senior Resident

Dr Irwani Ibrahim
MBBS (S'pore), FRCS (A&E) (Edin)
Consultant

Dr Koh Chi Ping, Brandon
MB ChB (Manchester), MRCSEd (UK)
Consultant

Asst Prof Kuan Win Sen
MBBS (S'pore), MRCS (A&E) (Edin), MCI
(NUS)
Consultant

Dr Lau Thian Phey
MB ChB (Auckland), MCEM, MMed
(Emerg Med)
Associate Consultant

Dr Lee Sock Koon
MBBS (S'pore), MRCSEd (A&E), MMed
(Emerg Med)
Senior Consultant

Dr Leong Sieu-Hon, Benjamin
MBBS (S'pore), MRCSEd (A&E), MMed
(Emerg Med)
Senior Consultant

Dr Lim Er Luen
MBBS (S'pore), MRCSEd (A&E)
Consultant

A/Prof Malcolm Mahadevan
MBBS (S'pore), MRCP(UK), FRCP (Edin),
FRCSEd (A&E), FAMS (Emerg Med)
Head & Senior Consultant

A/Prof Peter G. Manning
MBBS (London), FACEP, FAMS
(Emerg Med)
Emeritus Consultant
Vice-Chairman Medical Board
(Medicolegal and Risk Management)

Dr Ong Pei Yuin
MBBS (S'pore), MMed (Emerg Med),
MRCSEd
Consultant

Dr Ong Yeok Kein, Victor
MBBS (Singapore), FRCS Edin (A&E)
Senior Consultant

A/Prof Ooi Beng Suat, Shirley
MBBS (S'pore), FRCSEd (A&E), FAMS
(Emerg Med)
Senior Consultant
Designated Institutional Official
NUHS Residency Programme

Asst Prof Peng Li Lee
MBBS (S'pore), FRCSEd (A&E), FAMS
Senior Consultant

A/Prof Pillai, Suresh
MBBS (S'pore), FRCS Ed(A&E), PBM
Senior Consultant

Dr Rakhee Yash Pal
MBBS (S'pore), MMed (Emerg Med)
Consultant

Asst Prof Sim Tiong Beng
MBBS (S'pore), MRCS (A&E)
Senior Consultant

Dr Zulkarnain Ab Hamid
MBBS (S'pore), MMed (Emerg Med)
Associate Consultant

Guest Contributors

Dr Chong Chew Lan
MBBS (S'pore), MRCSEd (A&E)
Executive Director Medical Research
Celerion Inc

Dr Quek Lit Sin
MBBS (S'pore), MRCS (A&E) (Edin), MMed
(Emerg Med)
Head and Senior Consultant
Department of Emergency Medicine
Ng Teng Fong General Hospital (NTFGH),
Jurong Health Services (JHS), Singapore

Dr Goh Ee Ling
MBBS (S'pore), MRCS (A&E) (Edin), MMed
(Emerg Med)
Consultant
Department of Emergency Medicine
NTFGH, JHS, Singapore

Dr Amila Punyadasa
MB BCh, BAO (Belfast), MRCS (A&E)
(Edin), MMed (Emerg Med), FCEM Ad
Eundem, FAMS (Emerg Med)
Consultant
NTFGH, JHS, Singapore

Asst Prof Lee Yin Mei
MBChB (Dundee), MRCP (UK), SAB
(Gastroenterology, Singapore)
Senior Consultant
Division of Gastroenterology & Hepatology
University Medicine Cluster
NUHS

Prof Lim Seng Gee
MBBS (Hons)(Monash), FRACP, MD
(Monash), FAMS(Gastroenterology), FRCP
(London), Cert Immunology (King's College)
Senior Consultant
Division of Gastroenterology & Hepatology.
University Medicine Cluster
NUHS

Dr Andrea Rajnakova
MD (Hons.) (Slovakia), MMed (Hons.)
(Slovakia), PhD (S'pore), MRCP (UK), FAMS
(Gastroenterology)
Consultant
Andrea's Digestive, Colon, Liver and
Gallbladder Clinic Pte Ltd
Mount Elizabeth Medical Centre, Singapore

Dr Citra N Mattar
MBBS, MRANZCOG, MMed (O&G)
Associate Consultant
Department of Obstetrics and Gynaecology
NUHS

Dr Lee Chun Yue, Francis
MBBS (S'pore), FRCSEd (A&E), FAMS
Head and Senior Consultant
Acute & Emergency Care Department
Khoo Teck Puat Hospital (KTPH), Singapore

Dr Seet Chong Meng
MBBS (S'pore), FRCSEd (A&E),
MRCP (UK)
Senior Consultant
Acute & Emergency Care Department
KTPH, Singapore

Dr Toh Hong Chuen
MBBS (S'pore), MRCSEd (A&E)
Consultant
Acute & Emergency Care Department
KTPH, Sngapore

Adj A/Prof Charles Bih-Shiou Tsang
MBBS (S'pore), MMed (Surgery),
MS (Exp Surgery), FRCS (Edinburgh),
FRCS (Glasgow), FAMS (Surgery)
Senior Consultant
Director of Colorectal Clinic Associates
(Mt Elizabeth Novena Hospital, Gleneagles
Hospital, Mt Alvernia Hospital, Parkway East
Hospital), Singapore

Dr Emily Gan Yiping
MBBS (Honours), MRCP (UK), MMed
(Int Med)
Senior Resident
National Skin Centre, Singapore

A/Prof Lee Jiun
MBBS (S'pore), MMed (Paeds)
Head & Senior Consultant
Department of Neonatology
NUHS

Dr Darryl Lim
MBBS, MRCPCH (UK), FAMS
Consultant
Kinder Clinic Pte Ltd (Mt Alvernia),
Singapore

Dr Elizabeth Khor
MBBS (S'pore), MMed (Paeds), FAMS
Senior Consultant
Elizabeth Kids Clinic, Singapore

Dr Wong Chin Khoon
MBBS (S'pore), MMed (Paeds), FAMS
Consultant Paediatrician
SBCC baby and child clinic, Singapore

A/Prof Ng Kee Chong
MBBS, MMed (Paeds)
Head and Senior Consultant
Children's Emergency
KK Women's and Children's Hospital
(KKWCH), Singapore

Dr Angeline Ang
MBBS, MRCP (Paeds) (UK)
Senior Consultant
Children's Emergency
KKWCH, Singapore

Dr Petrina Wong
MBBS (Singapore), MRCPCH (Paed)(UK)
Associate Consultant
Department of Paediatric Medicine
KKWCH, Singapore

Dr Saumya Shekhar Jamuar
MBBS, MRCPCH (UK)
Associate Consultant
Department of Paediatric Medicine
KKWCH, Singapore

Abbreviations

AAA	abdominal aortic aneurysm	COPD	chronic obstructive pulmonary disease
ABC	airway, breathing, circulation		
ABG	arterial blood gas	CONSB	carbon monoxide neuropsychological screening battery
AIS	Abbreviated Injury Scale		
ALP	alkaline phosphatase		
ALT	alanine transaminase	CRAO	central retinal artery occlusion
AMI	acute myocardial infarction	CRVO	central retinal vein occlusion
ANOVA	analysis of variance	CSF	cerebrospinal fluid
AP	anteroposterior	CSM	carotid sinus massage
ARDS	Adult Respiratory Distress Syndrome	CT	computed tomography
		CVA	cerebrovascular accident
AST	aspartate transaminase	CVS	cardiovascular system
AXR	abdominal x-ray	CXR	chest x-ray
BBB	bundle branch block	D_5W	5% dextrose-water
BCI	blunt cardiac injury	DBP	diastolic blood pressure
BCU	body cooling unit	DCI	decompression illness
bd	twice daily	DIPJ	distal interphalangeal joint
BIPAP	biphasic positive airway pressure	DIVC	disseminated intravascular coagulation
BP	blood pressure		
BVM	bag-valve-mask	DKA	diabetic ketoacidosis
BW	body weight	DL	direct laryngoscopy
BZD	benzodiazepine	DM	diabetes mellitus
		DPL	diagnostic peritoneal lavage
C&S	culture and sensitivity	DVT	deep vein thrombosis
Ca	calcium		
CAGE	cerebral arterial gas embolism	ECG	electrocardiogram
CAP	community acquired pneumonia	ECM	external cardiac massage
CAPD	continuous abdominal peritoneal dialysis	ESRF	end stage renal failure
		ETT	endotracheal tubes
CCF	congestive cardiac failure		
CCU	Coronary Care Unit	FAST	focused assessment using sonography in trauma
CK	creatine kinase		
CNS	central nervous system	FB	foreign body
CO	carbon monoxide	FBC	full blood count
CO_2	carbon dioxide	FDP	flexor digitorum profundus
COHB	carboxyhaemoglobin	FDS	flexor digitorum superficialis

FFP	fresh frozen plasma		LFT	liver function test
FRC	functional residual capacity		LOC	loss of consciousness
			LOV	loss of vision
g	gram			
GA	general anaesthesia		M&R	manipulation and reduction
GCS	Glasgow coma scale		MAP	mean arterial pressure
GE	gastroenteritis		MCPJ	metacarpophalangeal joint
GGT	gamma glutamyl transferase		mg	milligram
GI	gastrointestinal		Mg	magnesium
GOLD	global initiative for chronic obstructive lung disease		ml	millilitre
			MMR	measles, mumps, rubella
GTN	glyceryl trinitrate		MRI	magnetic resonance imaging
GXM	group and cross match		MRI-A	magnetic resonance imaging with angiogram
HA	hyperventilation attack		MSP	Munchausen Syndrome by Proxy
Hb	haemoglobin			
HCG	human chorionic gonadotrophin		Na^+	sodium
HCW	health care worker		NAI	non-accidental injury
HD	high dependency		NBM	nil by mouth
H,E,E,N,T	head, eyes, ear, nose and throat		NG	nasogastric
HHNK	hyperosmolar hyperglycaemic non-ketotic state		NIV	non-invasive ventilation
			NS	normal saline
HHS	hyperosmolar hyperglycaemic state		NSAIDs	non-steroidal antiinflammatory drugs
I&D	incision and drainage		NWB	non-weight-bearing
IV	intravenous			
ICH	intracerebral haemorrhage		O_2	oxygen
ICU	intensive care unit		om	every morning
IDL	indirect laryngoscopy		ORIF	open reduction and internal fixation
IHD	ischaemic heart disease			
IPPV	intermittent positive pressure ventilation		PA	posteroanterior
			PCP	phencyclidine
IS	ischaemic stroke		PEEP	peak end-expiratory pressure
ISDN	isosorbide dinitrate		PID	pelvic inflammatory disease
ISS	Injury Severity Score		PIPJ	proximal interphalangeal joint
IVC	inferior vena cava		PO_4	phosphate
			PPV	positive pressure ventilation
K^+	potassium		PR	pulse rate
KUB	kidney, ureter and bladder x-ray		PSA	procedural sedation and analgesia
			PT	prothrombin time
l	litre		PT/PTT	prothrombin time/partial thromboplastin time (coagulation profile)
LBBB	left bundle branch block			
LBP	low back pain			
LDH	lactate dehydrogenase			

PUD	peptic ulcer disease	SOC	specialist outpatient clinic
PUO	pyrexia of unknown origin	SP	special precautions
qds	four times daily	SVT	supraventricular tachycardia
		SXR	skull x-ray
RBBB	right bundle branch block	SYNC	synchronization
RBCs	red blood cells		
RHC	right hypochondrial pain	T&S	toilet and suture
RICE	rest, ice, compression and	TCA	tricyclic antidepressant
	elevation	TCM	traditional Chinese medicine
RLQ	right lower quadrant	tds	three times daily
RSI	rapid sequence intubation	TEE	transoesophageal
RTA	road traffic accidents		echocardiography
rtPA	recombinant tissue plasminogen	TIA	transient ischaemic attack
	activator	TWC	total white count
RTS	Revised Trauma Score		
		u	units
SAH	subarachnoid haemorrhage	UC9	urine dipstick
SBI	serious bacterial infection	URTI	upper respiratory tract infection
SBP	systolic blood pressure	UTI	urinary tract infection
SC	subcutaneous		
SIRS	systemic inflammatory response	V/Q	ventilation-perfusion
	syndrome	VBI	vertebrobasilar insufficiency
SK	streptokinase	VF	ventricular fibrillation
SL	sublingual	VT	ventricular tachycardia
SLE	systemic lupus erythematosus	VZV	varicella zoster virus
SOB	shortness of breath	WBCs	leucocytes

PART 1
COMMON PRESENTATIONS IN ADULT PATIENTS

1 Altered Mental State

Peter Manning • Goh Ee Ling

CAVEATS

The primary focus of the ED evaluation of a patient with altered mental state (AMS) is as follows:

- To address easily reversible causes, e.g. hypoxaemia, hypercarbia, and hypoglycaemia.
- To differentiate structural from toxic-metabolic causes since the former require emergent central nervous system imaging, whereas the latter are usually more readily identified by laboratory studies.

Refer to Chapter 138 *Commonly Used Scoring System* under Glasgow Coma Scale for a definition of coma.

> ⇨ **SPECIAL TIP FOR GPs**
> - Always consider reversible causes of AMS that you can initiate treatment for in your office: e.g. hypoglycaemia (oral sugar or IV Dextrose 50%), hypoxaemia (supplemental oxygen), or heat stroke (cooling measures and IV normal saline), before sending the patient to the ED by ambulance.

MANAGEMENT

Initial priorities

- See Figure 1 for approach to differential diagnosis of altered mental state.
- The patient should be managed initially in the critical care area.
- If a promptly reversible cause of AMS is found, then the patient can be downgraded to the intermediate acuity area.
- **Positive airway control/C-spine immobilization**.
  1. Open the airway and search for foreign bodies.
  2. Insert oral or nasopharyngeal airway.
  3. Apply stiff collar or manual immobilization if history does not exclude trauma.
  4. Definitive airway if patient is comatose: intubation with/without rapid sequence intubation **or** perform surgical airway such as emergency cricothyrotomy.
- **Oxygenation/ventilation.**
  1. Provide supplemental high-flow oxygen.
  2. Institute hyperventilation in moderation to achieve a PCO_2 between 30–35 mmHg if there are indications of raised intracranial pressure. In general, the PCO_2 level should be between 35–40 mmHg.

FIGURE 1   Approach to differential diagnosis of altered mental state

Altered mental state

Airway
Breathing
Circulation
} Check SpO$_2$
Give 100% O$_2$
Check pulse

Vital signs/temperature
ECG monitor
Bedside glucose

Targeted history and physical examination
Head injury
Neck stiffness
Respiration rate and pupil size
Focal neurological signs[1]
Chronic organ failure signs

Structural causes

Toxic/metabolic causes

Head trauma
Intracranial
  haemorrhage

Non-head trauma
Intracranial
  haemorrhage
Subarachnoid
  haemorrhage[2]
Brainstem stroke
Cerebellar stroke
Cerebral tumour

Febrile
Cerebral abscess
Meningitis
Encephalitis
Cerebral malaria
Bacteraemia
Septicaemia
UTI in elderly
Heat stroke
Thyroid crisis

Afebrile
Poisons
Drug overdosage:
  Opioids, BZD, barbiturate, TCA,
    ketamine, ecstasy
  Alcohol intoxication
  Wernicke's encephalopathy
  Carbon monoxide
Metabolic
Hypoglycaemia, cerebral hypoperfusion,
  hypercarbia, diabetic coma,
  myxoedema coma, hypothermia,
  dehydration, electrolyte and
  acid-base abnormalities
Organ failure
Uraemia, hepatic, respiratory, cardiac
Post-ictal state
Psychiatric
Psychogenic stupor[3], dementia

Notes:
[1] Structural causes usually have focal neurological signs whereas the toxic and metabolic causes do not.
[2] Subarachnoid haemorrhage (SAH) usually does not have focal neurological signs. SAH and some of the toxic and metabolic causes may be accompanied by fever.
[3] Psychogenic stupor is a dissociative state in which the patient is apparently fully conscious but makes no spontaneous movement and shows little response to external stimuli. It is usually related to major stressful events and the onset is sudden. Patient often has 'flickering' of eyelids. It is a diagnosis of exclusion.

- **Cardiac output.**
  1. Check that there is a major pulse; if not, start CPR!
  2. Obvious external haemorrhage should be stopped with direct pressure only.
- **Do stat capillary blood sugar.**
- Monitoring: ECG, pulse oximetry, vital signs q5–15 minutes.
- Start peripheral IV at a slow rate (unless hypoperfusion present) with isotonic crystalloid.
- Labs: mandatory for FBC, urea/electrolytes/creatinine, ABG (look for metabolic acidosis and hypercarbia).

NOTE: CO_2 narcosis does not necessarily present with respiratory distress; they are usually in respiratory depression. Consider serum calcium, drug screen, serum ethanol, carboxyhaemoglobin level, and GXM.

- **AMS cocktail**: consider its use in part or whole.
  1. $D_{50}W$ 40 ml IV if patient is hypoglycaemic, followed by **infusion** of $D_{10}W$ over 3–4 hours.
  2. Naloxone (Narcan®) 0.8–2.0 mg IV bolus.
  3. Thiamine 100 mg IV bolus in alcoholics or malnourished patients.
  4. Flumazenil (Anexate®) 0.5 mg IV bolus.
     a. Can be repeated within 5 minutes if necessary.
     b. Do not use empirically unless the history is **strongly against a mixed OD**. If the patient has been taking cyclic antidepressants or is taking chronic benzodiazepines for fits, unnecessary use of flumazenil may produce intractable fits.
  5. **X-ray cross-table lateral film of C-spine** if trauma cannot be excluded.

TABLE 1　Clues from history and physical examination pointing to causes of AMS

Non-structural causes	Structural causes
Empty pill containers	Complained of headache to family/friends prior to AMS
Medical diseases, e.g. epilepsy, liver disease, diabetes, etc	History of brain tumour
Possible CO exposure	Trauma
Absence of focal neurological signs	Presence of focal neurological signs
Signs of metabolic acidosis	Head trauma
Anticholinergic signs	

- **Clinical evaluation**: the focus is on differentiating structural from toxic-metabolic causes of AMS (Table 1).

- **History**: rarely clear-cut; look for clues from patient's family, friends, belongings, and information scene from paramedic/ambulance officer.
- **Examination**: brief external assessment of patient searching for stigmata of numerous disease processes. While a head-to-toe examination is important, in AMS pay most attention to a **focused neurological examination**.

AMS due to suspected structural causes

- Give supplemental oxygen to maintain SpO_2 of at least 95%.
- Start IV at a slow rate.
- Perform head CT scan.
- **Lower intracranial pressure** if indicated.
  1. Controlled ventilation: works fastest. See Chapter 5, *Breathlessness, Acute*, for details.
  2. **IV mannitol** is useful in conjunction with neurosurgical consult. Dose is 1 g/kg body weight (BW), i.e. BW × 5 mls/kg BW of 20% mannitol solution.
  3. Steroids are debatable.

AMS due to suspected toxic-metabolic causes

- Do gastric lavage; to be performed with airway protection if required.
- Use activated charcoal in suspected drug overdoses. Refer to Chapter 19, *Poisoning, General Principles*.
- Check rectal temperature and consider heat stroke if temp >40°C and taking anticholinergics.
- If meningitis is suspected, consider early lumbar puncture (after CT head scan). **Start empiric antibiotics before either of the tests** together with a neurological consult. Refer to Chapter 66, *Meningitis*.

Disposition

- Admit all cases of AMS. Admit to ICU those who are intubated or exhibiting haemodynamic instability.

References/Further Reading

1. Hamilton GC. Altered mental status: Depressed level of consciousness. In: Hamilton GC, ed., *Presenting Signs and Symptoms in the Emergency Department: Evaluation and Treatment*. Baltimore: Lippincott Williams & Wilkins; 1993: 528–536.
2. Huff JS. Confusion. In: Marx JA, Hockberger RS, Walls RM, et al., eds. *Rosen's Emergency Medicine: Concepts and Clinical Practice*. 7th ed. Philadelphia: Mosby Elsevier; 2010: 101–105.
3. Cooke JL. Depressed consciousness and coma. In: Marx JA, Hockberger RS, Walls RM, et al., eds. *Rosen's Emergency Medicine: Concepts and Clinical Practice*. 7th ed. Philadelphia: Mosby Elsevier; 2010: 106–112.

2　Bleeding, Gastrointestinal Tract (GIT)

Lim Er Luen • Sim Tiong Beng • Peter Manning

CAVEATS

- Syncope or near-syncope, dyspepsia, or epigastric pain may be the presenting symptoms for bleeding gastrointestinal tract (GIT) and pose diagnostic issues. Patients with a history of haematemesis, melaena, or haematochezia are more clear-cut.

- The **management** of GIT bleeding is essentially as follows:
  1. To identify shock and resuscitate: correct fluid losses and restore blood pressure/perfusion.
  2. To identify potentially reversible causes of the bleeding (both systemic, e.g. over-anticoagulation, and local).
  3. To identify physiologic derangements resulting from blood loss (cardiac ischaemia, acute kidney injury, or symptomatic anaemia requiring blood transfusion).

- Assess for the source of bleeding. Bear in mind the possibility of non-GI sources, e.g. haemoptysis or bleeding from the oropharynx. The corollary is that GI bleeding may still be present despite a non-GI source being found.

- Always be aware that **aortic aneurysm** (aortoenteric fistula) may present as GIT bleeding.

- Always do a **rectal examination** to establish whether frank melaena is present, or if it is due to local bleeding from the anal canal/perianal area.

- Black stools due to iron treatment are differentiated from melaena by the greenish tinge.

- **Common causes** of GI bleeding are given in Table 1.

TABLE 1　Common causes of GI bleeding (from Rosen's Emergency Medicine, 7th ed.)

Upper GI bleeding	Lower GI bleeding
Peptic ulcer	Diverticular disease
Gastric erosions	Angiodysplasia
Oesophageal varices	Upper GI bleeding
Mallory–Weiss tear	Cancer/polyps
Oesophagitis	Rectal disease
Duodenitis	Inflammatory bowel disease

⇨ **SPECIAL TIPS FOR GPs**

- Assess if shock is present (tachycardia and/or hypotension). If it is, call for an ambulance and transfer to the nearest ED. Set up IV line(s) and infuse saline in the first instance.
- If the patient is vomiting blood and conscious, place him in the recovery position and establish IV lines.
- Examine the abdomen for tenderness and do a rectal examination to confirm melaena.
- Establish the risk factors for peptic ulcer disease (PUD): alcohol abuse, non-steroidal anti-inflammatory drugs (NSAIDs)/steroids including traditional Chinese medicine (TCM), chronic renal failure, age, and anticoagulation treatment.
- Always bear in mind abdominal pulsation and aortic aneurysm.
- Advise the patient to stay nil by mouth (NBM).
- Consider dengue haemorrhagic fever in patients with bleeding GIT and fever or myalgia.
- There is a strong association of *Helicobacter pylori* infection with duodenal ulcers; eradication reduces the risk of both recurrent ulcers and recurrent haemorrhage.

MANAGEMENT

Supportive measures

Haemodynamically unstable patients

- Patients must be managed in the critical care area.
- Maintain airway. Consider intubation if haematemesis is copious and the patient is unable to protect his own airway, e.g. depressed mental status from previous cerebrovascular accident (CVA).
- Provide supplemental high-flow oxygen to maintain SpO_2 at >94%.
- Monitoring: ECG, vital signs every 5 minutes, and pulse oximetry.
- Perform 12-lead ECG to exclude cardiac ischaemia.
- Establish two or more large-bore peripheral IV lines (14/16G).
- **Labs**:
  1. GXM for at least four units.
  2. FBC, urea/electrolytes/creatinine, coagulation profile.
  3. Order liver function tests if the patient is jaundiced.
  4. Order cardiac enzymes if there is ECG evidence of myocardial ischaemia/injury.
- Infuse 1 L normal saline rapidly and reassess parameters. Arrange for blood transfusion if there is no significant improvement after the initial fluid challenge.
- Insert a nasogastric (NG) tube to free drainage for diagnostic purposes (and to prevent aspiration if the patient vomits). **Do not** insert a nasogastric tube if oesophageal varices are suspected.

NOTE: NG tube insertion is controversial as studies have failed to demonstrate a benefit with regard to clinical outcomes.

- Insert a urinary catheter to monitor urine output.
- Administer **IV esomeprazole** 80 mg bolus. This should be followed by 8 mg/h infusion if there is ongoing blood loss such as patient in hypovolaemic shock, if endoscopy shows stigmata of recent haemorrhage (Forrest Class I and II).
- Arrange for emergency oesophagogastroduodenoscopy (OGD).

Haemodynamically normal patients
- The patient can be managed in the intermediate care area though it must be remembered that the patient may decompensate after his first evaluation due to continued blood loss.
- Provide supplemental oxygen to maintain SpO_2 at >94%.
- Monitor vital signs every 10–15 minutes and pulse oximetry. Establish at least one peripheral IV (14/16G).
- Perform 12-lead ECG.
- **Labs**:
  1. GXM for two units.
  2. FBC, urea/electrolytes/creatinine, coagulation profile.
  3. Liver function tests and cardiac enzymes (see earlier).
- Start normal saline infusion 500 ml over 1–2 hours.
- Insert a nasogastric tube to free drainage for diagnostic purposes (and to prevent aspiration if the patient vomits).
- Give IV **esomeprazole** 80 mg. Note that infusion is not required for haemodynamically stable patients with no overt signs of bleeding.
- Upgrade to the critical care area if instability develops.

Specific measures

Oesophageal varices
- Do not insert a nasogastric tube as it may worsen the bleeding!
- Start IV **somatostatin** 250 µg bolus, followed by an IV infusion of 250 µg/h (successful in up to 85–90% of cases). If somatostatin is unsuccessful in stopping the bleeding, and there is the risk of the patient exsanguinating before endoscopy can be arranged, then the insertion of a **Sengstaken–Blakemore tube** should be considered. This should be inserted only by an experienced operator.
- Administer **IV antibiotic prophylaxis** with **ceftriaxone** or **ciprofloxacin** to prevent spontaneous bacterial peritonitis.

Others
- Look for scar of previous abdominal aortic aneurysm surgery: this episode of GIT bleeding may represent an **aortoenteric fistula**, which is a dire emergency. If this is suspected, consult the general surgical registrar and cardiothoracic registrar.

Disposition

Stable low-risk patients

- Patients with small amounts of GI bleeding may be admitted to the **observation unit** for further treatment/endoscopy provided the following conditions are met:
  1. **For upper GI bleeding:**
     a. Age <65 years.
     b. No significant comorbidities.
     c. No hypotension (systolic blood pressure >110 mmHg), postural hypotension or tachycardia.
     d. Haemoglobin (Hb) >11 g/dL for males or >10 g/dL for females.
     e. No overt GI bleeding, e.g. haematemesis or fresh melaena.
     f. The patient is reliable.
     g. No stigmata of recent haemorrhage on endoscopy.
  2. **For lower GI bleeding:**
     a. Directly visualized haemorrhoidal bleeding clinically assessed to be self-limited.
     b. An otherwise healthy individual with normal vital signs.
     c. No comorbidities.
- For all other patients, consultations for admission to either General Surgery or Gastroenterology depending on institutional practice.
- The **Glasgow-Blatchford bleeding score (GBS)**, which is based on simple clinical and laboratory variables, has been developed to identify patients presenting with upper GI bleeding to the EMD who can be **safely discharged** and managed safely as outpatients without urgent need for endoscopy or monitoring. Patients must fulfil the following criteria:
  1. Blood urea <6.5 mmol/L.
  2. Hb >13 g/dL for men, >12 g/dL for women.
  3. Systolic blood pressure >110 mmHg.
  4. Pulse <100/min.
  5. No melaena or syncope.
  6. No hepatic disease or cardiac failure.

NOTE: For prediction of need for intervention or death, the GBS was superior to the full **Rockall score** (ROC of 0.90 versus 0.81). GBS scoring reduces admissions for this condition, allowing more appropriate use of inpatient resources. Rockall scoring incorporates endoscopic diagnosis which limits its use in EMD as emergency endoscopy is usually indicated for patients with major bleeding.

Intermediate or high-risk patients

- Consultations for admission to either General Surgery or Gastroenterology depending on institutional practice.

References/Further Reading

1. Lau JY, Sung JJ, Lee KK, et al. Effect of intravenous omeprazole on recurrent bleeding after endoscopic treatment of bleeding peptic ulcers. *N Engl J Med.* 2000; 343(5): 310–316.

2. Westhoff J, Holt KR. Gastrointestinal bleeding: An evidence-based ED approach to risk stratification. *Emerg Med Pract.* 2004; 6(3): 1–18.

3. British Society of Gastroenterology Endoscopy Committee. Non-variceal upper gastrointestinal haemorrhage Guidelines. *Gut.* 2002; 51(SuppIV): iv 1–iv 6.

4. Habib A, Sanyaj AJ. Acute variceal hemorrhage. *Gastrointest Endosc Clin N Am.* 2007; 17: 223–252.

5. Stanley AJ, Ashley D, Dalton HR, et al. Outpatient management of patients with low-risk upper-gastrointestinal haemorrhage: Multicentre validation and prospective evaluation. *Lancet.* 2009; 373: 42–47.

6. Pallin DJ, Saltzman JR. Is nasogastric tube lavage in patients with acute upper GI bleeding indicated or antiquated? *Gastrointest Endosc.* 2011 Nov; 74(5): 981–4.

3　Bleeding, Vaginal, Abnormal

Citra N Mattar • Lau Thian Phey

CAVEATS

- For the majority of women this presentation is indicative of a menstrual disturbance which can be adequately controlled with simple outpatient treatment prior to a gynaecological review.
- Unexpected bleeding may be a complication in early pregnancy, while a minority of women encountering vigorous or prolonged bleeding may already be haemodynamically compromised at the point of consultation.
- The preliminary assessment should focus on recognizing the woman who requires resuscitation, identifying the source of bleeding (and determining the pregnancy status), and initiating the appropriate management.

CLINICAL ASSESSMENT

Assessment of patient with abnormal vaginal bleeding

- Age: reproductive age group, perimenopausal or postmenopausal.
- Medical history: previously diagnosed pelvic inflammatory disease or sexually transmitted infections (in particular, gonorrhoea and chlamydia), use of anticoagulants, coagulopathy, unopposed oestrogens, postmenopausal hormone therapy, or tamoxifen.
- Surgical history: recent hysterectomy, or vaginal or other pelvic surgery.
- Significant drug history: warfarin or other anticoagulants.
- **Gynaecological symptoms:**
  1. Parity and obstetric history.
  2. Menstrual cycle: regularity, date of last normal menstrual period.
  3. Contraceptive use: combined oral contraceptive pill, progesterone-only implant or injections, intrauterine device, and if the patient is on hormonal contraception whether she has deviated from her schedule.
  4. Bleeding characteristics: number of episodes, duration, volume, and previous treatment.
  5. Abdominal or pelvic pain.
  6. Symptoms of early pregnancy.
  7. Symptoms of chronic anaemia.

Physical examination

- Haemodynamic instability.
- **Abdominal examination** (for evidence of intraperitoneal bleeding): abdominal tenderness with/without rebound tenderness and guarding; pelviabdominal mass (suggestive of gravid uterus).

- **Pelvic examination**:
  1. Speculum examination (to identify the source and magnitude of bleeding): from the uterus (blood discharged through the cervical canal), cervix (from local lesions or tumours), vagina and vulva (trauma or lesions), or extragenital bleeding from the urethra/anus.
  2. Bimanual examination: external cervical os (opened or closed); uterine size, mobility, and tenderness; adnexal masses and tenderness (possible ectopic pregnancy).

Diagnostic investigations

The following are usually performed by the gynaecologist:

- Pelvic ultrasonography (transvaginal, TVUS; or transabdominal, TAUS).
- Endometrial biopsy where indicated.

⇨ **SPECIAL TIPS FOR GPs**
- Perform a urine pregnancy test (UPT) for all women in the reproductive/premenopausal age group, regardless of menstrual pattern or the reported last menstrual period.
- Perform GXM if the patient is likely to require an urgent transfusion.
- Check FBC and coagulation profile.

MANAGEMENT

See Figure 1 for an overview of the management of abnormal vaginal bleeding.

Haemodynamically unstable patients

- Consult the gynaecologist immediately.
- Secure venous access and initiate fluid resuscitation.
- Perform a UPT to confirm pregnancy.
- Consider in-dwelling catheter for fluid monitoring.
- Investigations: FBC, GXM, and coagulation profile (optional).

If the patient is **pregnant**:

- A **ruptured** or **bleeding ectopic pregnancy** must be excluded. The gynaecologist will perform a TVUS to determine if there is an intrauterine gestational sac, fluid in the peritoneal cavity, and/or an adnexal mass suggestive of a haemorrhaging ectopic pregnancy. When this is confirmed the patient needs to be admitted and prepared for emergency surgery.
- Differential diagnosis: haemorrhage from a miscarried intrauterine pregnancy.

FIGURE 1   Management of abnormal vaginal bleeding

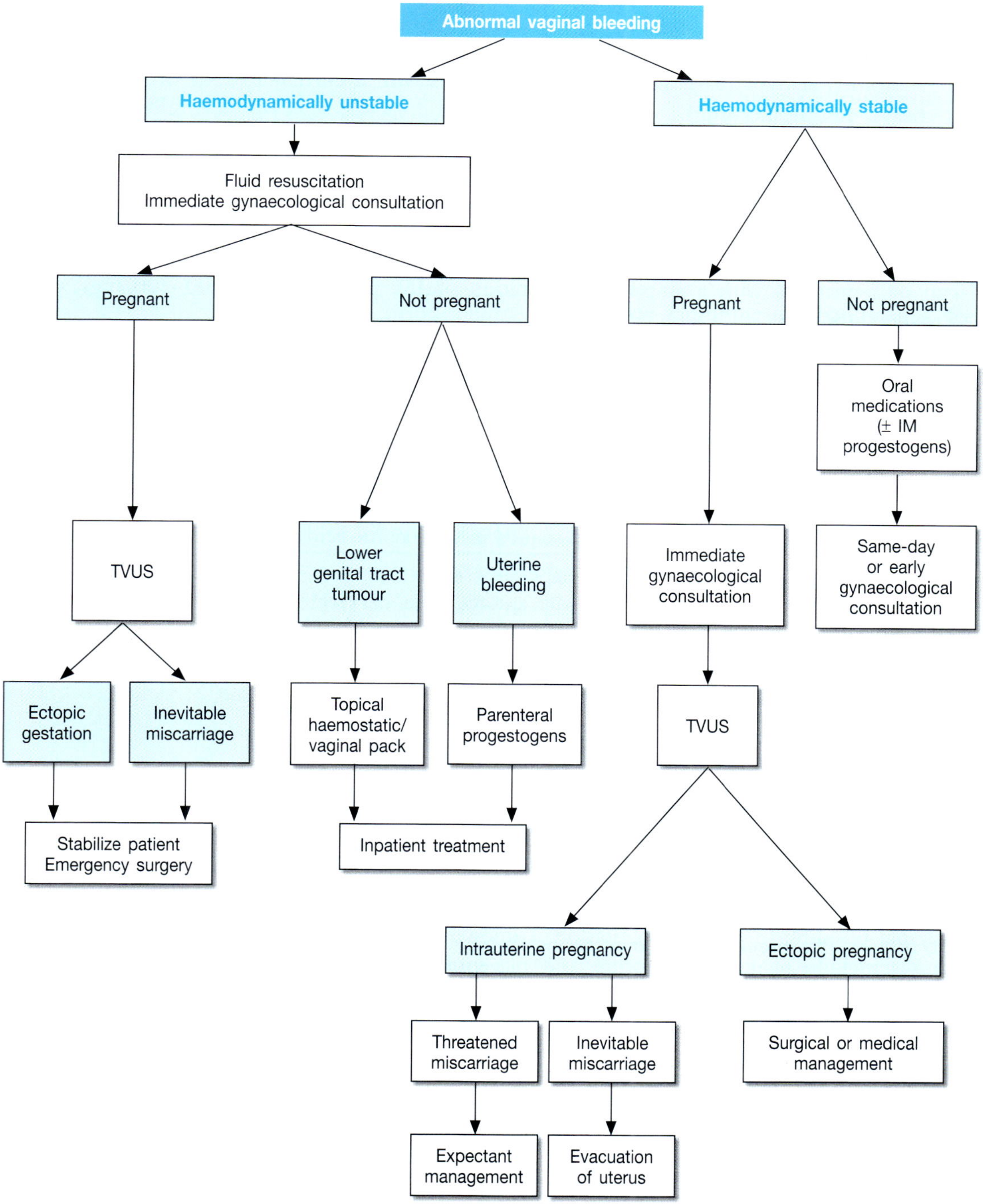

If the patient is **not pregnant**:
- Differential diagnoses:
  1. Menstrual disorders
  2. Endometrial hyperplasia (e.g. anovulatory cycles with a current episode of prolonged and heavy uterine bleeding)
  3. Lower genital tract malignancy (commonly cervical or endometrial tumours).
  4. Genital tract trauma (e.g. postcoital vaginal laceration, cervical cone biopsy).

Acute management is cause-specific:
- Once pregnancy and a lower genital tract lesion are excluded, abnormal uterine bleeding can be controlled with a single administration of **IM progesterone** (100–200 mg), or **IM Provera** (150 mg).
- **Local bleeding** from a cervical tumour or cone biopsy site can be controlled with the topical application of a haemostatic agent, such as Monsel's solution (ferric subsulphate, usually available as a paste and applied with a Q-tip), a painless and effective means of achieving haemostasis.
- **Small bleeders** on the **surface** of the **cervix** can be accurately cauterized using silver nitrate (available as a solid pencil to facilitate topical application). Alternatively, a vaginal pack (lubricated with saline and with the tip soaked in tranexamic acid) may be applied to tamponade the bleeding.
- If there is **vigorous bleeding** from the surface of a **cervical tumour**, consider the use of **IV tranexamic acid** as a slow bolus (500–1000 mg).
- The patient should be stabilized, admitted, and investigated adequately before definitive treatment is administered.

Haemodynamically stable patients

If the patient is pregnant:
- Bleeding in the first trimester may be caused by an ectopic pregnancy; this must be excluded by TVUS. Other possible causes of early gestational bleeding include a threatened or inevitable miscarriage.
- Vaginal bleeding in advanced gestation is known as **antepartum haemorrhage** and common causes include placental abruption and placenta praevia. In any situation, initially modest bleeding may quickly escalate in volume and vigour, leading to haemodynamic compromise. Thus, serial monitoring and immediate or same-day gynaecological review is important.

If the patient is not pregnant:
- These common conditions should be considered:
  1. Menstrual disorders (e.g. menorrhagia, polymenorrhoea, anovulatory cycles with prolonged menstrual bleeding).
  2. Endometrial hyperplasia.

3. Genital tract lesions (e.g. cervical or endometrial malignancies) or trauma.

4. Postmenopausal bleeding due to atrophic endometritis/cervicitis/vaginitis.

- **Cervical tumours** are identified on speculum examination. Local bleeding can be controlled with the application of haemostatic agents or a vaginal pack (as described earlier). A same-day gynaecological review should be arranged.

- If the patient has **recently** had uterine, cervical, or vaginal **surgery** and the bleeding is suspected to originate from the operative site, immediate gynaecological review should be arranged.

- An episode of **heavy uterine bleeding** can be controlled with the administration of IM progesterone (100–200 mg) or IM Depo-Provera (150 mg) followed by oral norethisterone (10 mg three times daily) continuously until the patient is reviewed by the gynaecologist.

- If the **bleeding** episode is **moderate** the patient may be started on oral medications directly. The options include tranexamic acid (1000 mg two to four times daily), non-steroidal anti-inflammatory medications, e.g. mefenamic acid (500 mg three times daily), or progestogens (e.g. norethisterone 10 mg three times daily). An early gynaecological referral should be arranged for a complete assessment before definitive treatment is offered. Medications are to be continued until the patient is reviewed.

References/Further Reading

1. National Institute for Health and Clinical Excellence. Heavy menstrual bleeding. *NICE Clinical Guideline 44.* 2007.

2. Royal College of Obstetricians and Gynaecologists. The management of tubal pregnancy. *Green-top Guideline No. 21.* 2004.

3. Jetmore AB, Heryer JW, Conner WE. Monsel's solution: A kinder, gentler hemostatic. *Dis Colon Rectum.* 1993; 36(9): 866–867.

4. Grimes DA, Hubacher D, Lopez LM, Schulz KF. Non-steroidal anti-inflammatory drugs for heavy bleeding or pain associated with intrauterine-device use. *Cochrane Database Syst Rev.* 2006(4): CD006034.

5. Lethaby A, Augood C, Duckitt K, Farquhar C. Nonsteroidal anti-inflammatory drugs for heavy menstrual bleeding. *Cochrane Database Syst Rev.* 2007(4): CD000400.

5. Lethaby A, Irvine G, Cameron I. Cyclical progestogens for heavy menstrual bleeding. *Cochrane Database Syst Rev.* 2000(2): CD001016.

7. Coulter A, Kelland J, Peto V, Rees MC. Treating menorrhagia in primary care. An overview of drug trials and a survey of prescribing practice. *Int J Technol Assess Health Care.* 1995; 11(3): 456–471.

4   Blurring of Vision

Toh Hong Chuen • Peter Manning

CAVEATS

- Blurring of vision is a subjective complaint that may mean anything, from blurred vision in one visual field in one eye, to total blindness.
- The role of the emergency physician is to perform a systematic and thorough examination of the eye, with the intent of **identifying potentially reversible or vision-threatening conditions**.

> ⇨ **SPECIAL TIPS FOR GPs**
> - Assume the complaint of visual loss is genuine till proven otherwise. Send the patient to hospital for ophthalmological review.
> - In cases of corrosive injury to the eye, institute immediate eye irrigation with normal saline before arrival of ambulance to take the patient to the hospital.

CLINICAL ASSESSMENT AND MANAGEMENT

History

- A pertinent history includes the following:
  1. Unilateral or bilateral involvement; onset (sudden or gradual) and associated eye pain.
  2. Inciting events such as trauma, chemical injury, or exposure to foreign body (contact lens in particular).
  3. Past medical history (e.g. multiple sclerosis, previous retinal detachment, migraine with visual symptoms).
  4. Medication (e.g. corticosteroids, which are associated with cataracts, glaucoma, and keratitis due to HSV; anti-TB medication ethambutol; antimalarial agent hydroxychloroquine).
  5. Previous similar episodes.
  6. Family history (e.g. of glaucoma, macular degeneration).
  7. Occupational history (e.g., whether the patient has worked as a welder).

Examination

See Chapter 20, *Red Eye*.

Differentials and respective management

See Tables 1–3.

TABLE 1   Differential diagnosis of gradual vision loss

Unilateral, painless		Bilateral, painless	
Common	Rare	Common	Exceedingly rare
Cataract	Slowly progressive inflammatory or neoplastic processes (e.g. optic granuloma, optic neuroma)	Cataract	Chronic inflammatory process (e.g. collagen vascular disease, sarcoidosis)
Age-related macular degeneration		Age-related macular degeneration	
Slowly compressing lesions involving the orbit or intracranial space		Ocular toxicity (e.g. hydroxychloroquine, ethambutol)	

TABLE 2   Differential diagnosis of acute vision loss[1]

Unilateral, painless	Unilateral, painful	Bilateral, painless[2]	Bilateral, painful[2]
Usually from posterior segment; requires urgent ophthalmologic consultation	Usually from anterior segment, and may be associated with red eye	Usually from acute refractive exacerbation, such as from swelling of lens	Usually accompanying trauma to the anterior segment
Vitreous haemorrhage	Corneal abrasion	Diabetes mellitus (DM) poor control	Chemical exposure
Retinal haemorrhage	Corneal ulcers		Ultraviolet radiation exposure (welder)
Retinal detachment	Uveitis	Medication, e.g. anticholinergics/ steroids	
Central retinal vein occlusion (CRVO)	Traumatic hyphaema		
Central retinal artery occlusion (CRAO)	Acute glaucoma		
	Orbital cellulitis		
	Keratitis		
	Optic neuritis[3]		
	Temporal arteritis[4]		
	Migraine[5]		

Notes:
[1] Suddenly *perceived* unilateral painless loss of vision: slowly progressive conditions (such as refractive errors, cataracts, age-related macular degeneration without haemorrhage), usually affecting the non-dominant eye, may present with a 'sudden onset' when the *unaffected eye is inadvertently covered*.
[2] Acute unilateral eye conditions may sometimes present bilaterally, ranging from rare occasions such as bilateral acute glaucoma, to around 50% of the time in scleritis.
[3] White eye, not red.
[4] White eye, not red.
[5] Eye may be red or white.

TABLE 3   Specific entities presenting as loss of vision

	History	Examination findings	EMD management
Acute angle-closure glaucoma[1]	Unilateral frontal headache with ocular pain; nausea and vomiting; decreased vision; haloes around light (due to corneal oedema). Bilateral involvement can infrequently occur, in particular due to medications	Diffusely reddened congested eye; decreased visual acuity (VA); hazy cornea; pupil mid-dilated (4–6 mm), not reactive; positive oblique flash light test; shallow anterior chamber	Stat eye consultation. Decrease aqueous production (with **IV acetazolamide** 500 mg and **timolol eyedrop:** one drop stat and second drop in 10 minutes) and increase aqueous flow (with **4% pilocarpine eyedrop:** one drop every 15 minutes for 1 hour, then four drops hourly)
CRAO	Unilateral, painless loss of vision (LOV); ± previous amaurosis fugax	Reduced VA; afferent pupillary defect; pale oedematous retina; markedly reduced vasculature; cherry red spot (intact fuveal blood supply)	Intermittent globe massage; paper bag rebreathing; stat eye consultation
CRVO	Unilateral LOV	Reduced VA; engorged tortuous retinal veins without physiological pulsations	Stat eye consultation
Vitreous haemorrhage	Varies from a few floaters to profound, painless LOV	Reduced VA; vitreous floaters on fundoscopy	Place patient in upright position; stat eye consultation
Temporal arteritis (Refer to Chapter 70, *Temporal Arteritis*)	Elderly patient; unilateral headache; jaw claudication and muscle aches	Tender temporal artery with decreased pulse	Send ESR. Stat eye consultation. High-dose prednisolone if diagnosis confirmed
Optic neuritis[2]	Unilateral LOV over hours to days; pain for a few days, increased by eye movements. Visual loss commences as pain improves	Reduced VA and painful; relative afferent pupillary defect (RAPD); papillitis[3]	Stat eye consultation, with admission for intravenous methylprednisolone
Retinal detachment	Acute LOV; usually total, with preceding streaks or flashes of light common	Fundoscopy shows grey, billowed, or folded area of retina with overlying vessels having an undulating course	Stat eye consultation
Retinal haemorrhage	Painless, acute focal or generalized LOV	Focal or generalized reduction in VA; fundoscopy shows retinal haemorrhage	Stat eye consultation
Migraine	Headache consistent with migraine; scintillating scotoma	Fundus usually normal; extraocular muscle (EOM) paralysis; pupillary dilation	Stat eye/neurology consultation

TABLE 3 Specific entities presenting as loss of vision *(cont'd)*

	History	Examination findings	EMD management
Hysteria	Often total bilateral LOV	Normal optokinetic nystagmus; variable responses to different techniques of testing VA	Stat eye/psychiatry consultation
Corrosive burn	Sudden pain with LOV; tearing	Ulcerations of cornea, especially with alkali burns; pain++; photophobia with tearing	Stat eye consultation. Immediate irrigation with NS to pH neutral using pink/blue litmus paper[4]
Scleritis[5]	Severe, boring pain, worse with eye movement; progresses insidiously over weeks. Blurring of vision; teary, red[6] eye. Headache	Dilation of the deep episcleral vessels, thinning of sclera resulting in a bluish discoloration. Impaired VA (16% of patients). Tender globe unlike in episcleritis. Bilateral in 50%	Initiate oral NSAIDs and stat eye consultation
Uveitis	Sudden painful red eye, worse with eye movement or accommodation; photophobia, conjunctival injection and sometimes blurred vision	Perilimbal injection.[7] Watery, non-purulent discharge. A helpful distinguishing feature of anterior uveitis is consensual photophobia (pain on affected eye when light is shone into the non-affected eye). Hypopyon may be seen	Stat eye consultation
Keratitis	Photophobia, foreign body sensation, tearing, and exquisite pain[8]	Perilimbal injection. Cells and flare in the anterior chamber on slit-lamp exam; hypopyon in more severe cases	Stat eye consultation

Notes:
[1] Optic nerve atrophy and permanent visual loss can occur within hours if the condition is not adequately treated. Exercise caution with use of timolol in patients with chronic obstructive lung disease or congestive cardiac failure. Acetazolamide is contraindicated in patients with sulpha allergy.
[2] 35 percent of patients with optic neuritis, an inflammatory demyelination of optic nerve, develop multiple sclerosis.
[3] Looks like papilloedema but is unilateral and has greater loss of VA.
[4] The normal pH of tears is 6.5–7.0.
[5] Associated with rheumatic conditions 50% of the time.
[6] The radial configuration of the superficial scleral plexus is disrupted by the congested scleral plexus.
[7] Contrast with conjunctivitis which tends to spare the limbal area.
[8] Due to rich sensory innervation from the ophthalmic division of the trigeminal nerve.

References/Further Reading

1. Shingleton BJ, O'Donoghue MW. Blurred vision. *N Engl J Med.* 2000; 343: 556–562.

2. Sharma R, Brunette DD. Ophthalmology. In: Marx JA, Hockberger RS, Walls RM, eds. *Rosen's Emergency Medicine: Concepts and Clinical Practice.* 7th ed. Philadelphia: Mosby Elsevier; 2010: 877–887.

3. Wightman JM, Hamilton GC. Red and painful eye. In: Marx JA, Hockberger RS, Walls RM, et al, eds. *Rosen's Emergency Medicine: Concepts and Clinical Practice.* 6th ed. Philadelphia: Mosby Elsevier; 2006: 283–298.

5   Breathlessness, Acute

Goh Ee Ling

DEFINITIONS

- **Dyspnoea** is a subjective feeling of difficulty in breathing.
- **Hyperventilation** is a sensation of dyspnoea associated with excessive breathing.

CAVEATS

- Not all cases of dyspnoea are caused by cardiorespiratory pathology. Always exclude metabolic causes, especially in patients without lung findings.
- It may be the only presenting symptom of acute coronary syndrome, especially in the elderly, hence ECG should be performed early.
- The **common causes** of acute breathlessness are shown in Table 1.

TABLE 1   Common causes of acute breathlessness

Cardiac	Acute pulmonary oedema* (refer to Chapter 38)
	Heart failure* (refer to Chapter 38)
	Cardiac tamponade
	Acute coronary syndrome* (refer to Chapter 36)
	Pericarditis* (refer to Chapter 37)
	Aortic dissection* (refer to Chapter 34)
	Cardiac dysrhythmias* (refer to Chapters 18, 35 and 43)
Respiratory	Upper airway obstruction, e.g. angioedema, foreign body inhalation
	Asthma* (refer to Chapter 44)
	Chronic obstructive pulmonary disease (COPD)* (refer to Chapter 45)
	Pneumonia, including aspiration pneumonia* (refer to Chapter 46)
	Pulmonary embolism* (refer to Chapter 41)
	Pneumothorax, both tension and simple* (refer to Chapter 47)
	Chest trauma*, e.g. tension pneumothorax, haemothorax, pulmonary contusion, flail chest (refer to Chapter 94)
	Near drowning* (refer to Chapter 117)
	Pleural effusion
	Lung collapse
Others	Metabolic acidosis, e.g. diabetic ketoacidosis (DKA)*, uraemia*, poisoning (salicylates*, methyl alcohol, ethylene glycol), lactic acidosis
	Adult respiratory distress syndrome (ARDS), e.g. near drowning
	Fever* (refer to Chapter 7)
	Anaphylaxis* (refer to Chapter 29)
	Anaemia
	Diaphragmatic splinting
	Hyperventilation syndrome (diagnosis of exclusion)* (refer to Chapter 11, *Hyperventilation*)

*Please refer to the individual chapters for further details.

CLINICAL ASSESSMENT

History

- Associated symptoms, e.g. cough, chest pain, fever, lower limb swelling.
- Exacerbating and relieving factors.
- Exposure to allergens or poisons, e.g. poisoning or anaphylaxis.
- Past medical history, e.g. asthma, congestive cardiac failure (CCF).
- Medication history.
- Recent trauma.

Physical examination

- General appearance of patient: cyanosis, confusion, drowsiness, tachypnoea, pallor.

NOTE: Hypercarbia usually results in drowsiness while hypoxia leads to agitation and confusion.

- Cardiovascular: evidence of heart failure (raised jugular venous pressure [JVP]), pedal oedema, lung crepitations), equality of pulses (in aortic dissection).
- Respiratory: lung crepitations, air entry good and equal.
- Others, e.g. skin: urticaria, severe dehydration in patients with diabetic ketoacidosis, evidence of trauma.

Investigations

Investigations will be guided by the history and physical examination, and may include the following:

- **Arterial blood gas**: useful and important to determine metabolic and/or respiratory cause of dyspnoea.
- **ECG**: especially in elderly patients who usually present atypically with dyspnoea in acute coronary syndrome.
- **Bedside glucose level**: should be obtained in cases of metabolic acidosis.
- **Chest X-ray (CXR)**: generally indicated to detect for cardiorespiratory pathology.
- Others: FBC, renal panel, drug screen.

⇨ **SPECIAL TIPS FOR GPs**

- Give oxygen and obtain intravenous access for breathless patients who need referral to the ED.
- Obtain stat capillary blood glucose level if metabolic acidosis is suspected.
- Obtain an ECG, especially in elderly patients, to rule out cardiac pathology.
- Send the patient by ambulance if a serious pathology is suspected.

MANAGEMENT

The principles of management of patients presenting with dyspnoea include the following:

- Resuscitation and stabilization of the following life-threatening conditions that must be treated within seconds or minutes:
  1. Acute upper airway obstruction.
  2. Tension pneumothorax.
  3. Acute respiratory failure (refer to Chapter 48, *Respiratory Failure, Acute*).
- Supportive treatment.
- Treat the underlying cause of the dyspnoea.

Treatment

- Supportive measures:
  1. The patient should be placed in a monitored area.
  2. Monitoring: ECG, pulse oximetry, and vital signs.

  NOTE: Respiratory rate and oxygen saturation may suggest underlying respiratory failure (refer to Chapter 48, *Respiratory Failure, Acute*).

  3. Secure airway if needed.
  4. Supplemental oxygen.
  5. Obtain IV access and administer fluids depending on the diagnosis and patient's haemodynamics.
- Treatment of the identified cause of acute breathlessness.
- Disposition of the patient would depend upon the diagnosis and the clinical state of the patient.

References/Further Reading

1. Tai DYH. Acute breathlessness. In: Tai DYH, Lew TWK, Loo S, eds. *Bedside ICU Handbook*. 2nd ed. Singapore: Armour Publishing; 2007: 33–36.

2. Wyatt JP, Illingworth RN, Graham CA, et al., eds. *Oxford Handbook of Accident and Emergency Medicine*. 3rd ed. Oxford: Oxford University Press; 2006: 98.

3. Sarko J, Stapczynski JS. Respiratory Distress. In: Tintinalli JE, Stapczynski JS, Ma OJ, et al., eds. *Tintinalli's Emergency Medicine: A Comprehensive Study Guide*. 7th ed. New York, NY: McGraw-Hill; 2011: 465–472.

6   Diarrhoea and Vomiting

Peng Li Lee

CAVEATS

- Diarrhoea and vomiting are common complaints seen in the ED, and in the majority of cases, they are due to food-borne toxigenic diarrhoea, which is self-limiting and requires only symptomatic treatment and rehydration therapy.
- The **most disastrous misdiagnosis** in the differential diagnosis of acute diarrhoeal illness is that of a **missed surgical abdomen**, e.g. appendicitis, intestinal obstruction, or ectopic pregnancy.
- In the **paediatric** population, vomiting and diarrhoea may be a non-specific presentation for **varied illnesses** including otitis media, urinary tract infection, metabolic acidosis, raised intracranial pressure, toxins/drugs, intussusception, and malrotation.
- In the **elderly**, be wary of the possibility of **ischaemic colitis**, which is associated with high mortality.
- When vomiting occurs without diarrhoea, a search should be performed for a non-infective and extraintestinal cause.
- In the clinical assessment, the general state of hydration and nutrition should be noted. Having excluded a surgical abdomen and an extraintestinal cause for the diarrhoea/vomiting, the patient can then be treated symptomatically.

> ⇨ **SPECIAL TIPS FOR GPs**
> - For travellers going to endemic areas where they may be prone to **travellers' diarrhoea**, the suggested empiric regime is a fluoroquinolone (ciprofloxacin 500 mg or norfloxacin 400 mg or ofloxacin 300 mg) bd for three days + loperamide when diarrhoea develops.
> - In children do not forget to perform a focused hydration history and physical examination. Refer to Chapter 129, *Child, Vomiting*, and Chapter 126, *Child with Diarrhoea*.

MANAGEMENT

Symptomatic treatment

- See Table 1 for symptomatic treatment of diarrhoea and vomiting.
- **Rehydration therapy:**
  1. **IV rehydration:**
     a. Indicated in the following: moderate to severe intractable vomiting; moderate to severe dehydration; altered mental state and ileus.
     b. Should be considered in patients with mild dehydration who are unable to tolerate oral fluids. They will usually feel symptomatically better after IV hydration of 1–1.5 L

TABLE 1   Drugs used in symptomatic treatment of diarrhoea and vomiting

Medication	Route	Dosage	Remarks
Antiemetic			
Maxolon® (metoclopramide)	IM/IV Tab	10 mg 10 mg 8H	Useful in the symptomatic relief of nausea and vomiting
Stemetil® (prochlorperazine)	IM Tab	12.5 mg 5–10 mg 8H	Caution in the paediatric population as it is associated with increased incidence of extra pyramidal side effects
Phenergan® (promethazine)	IM IM/PO	25 mg (adult) 0.25–1.0 mg/kg (>2 years)	
Antidiarrhoeal			
Lomotil® (diphenoxylate)	PO	2 tab tds	Used to decrease frequency of diarrhoeal stools Not recommended in children <9 years of age
Imodium® (loperamide)	PO	2 mg tds	
Activated charcoal	PO	1–2 tab tds/prn	**Note:** The use of antidiarrhoeal agents is generally not recommended for invasive enteritis as they may increase the risk of bowel invasion by the organism. Avoid also bismuth in patients with aspirin sensitivity
Bismuth subsalicylate	PO	*Adult* 2 tab or 30 ml q 1 h prn up to 8 doses in 24 h	
	PO	*Children* [9–12 years] 1 tab or 15 ml q 1 h prn up to 8 doses in 24 h [6–9 years] 2/3 tab or 10 ml q 1 h prn up to 8 doses in 24 h [3–6 years] 1/3 tab or 5 ml q 1 h prn up to 8 doses in 24 h	
Antispasmodic/motility			
Buscopan® (hyoscine-N-butylbromide)	IM PO	20–40 mg 10 mg tds/prn	For symptomatic relief of abdominal colic associated with diarrhoea Generally contraindicated in invasive enteritis

of Hartmann's solution over a period of 1–4 hours. In children, see Chapter 133, *Fluid Replacement in Paediatrics.*

   c. Clinical assessment to guide therapy: other than clinical signs, the **presence of ketonuria** and **elevated urine specific gravity (SG)** on urine dipstick are useful indicators of dehydration.

NOTE: Normal urine SG is 1.002–1.030.

2. **Oral rehydration:**

   a. It is as effective as IV rehydration in patients who can tolerate oral fluids.

   b. Administer in small amounts repeatedly.

c. **Principle:** water and sodium enter the intestinal cell via the linking (coupling) of one organic molecule, e.g. glucose. Hence the oral fluids should contain glucose to stimulate the absorption of water and electrolytes across the small intestines. This sodium glucose coupled with active absorption mechanisms is largely unaffected by enteric toxins. Servidrat, Pedialyte, and Gastrolyte are examples of useful oral rehydration agents.

Investigation at EMD

- This is generally not required unless clinical dehydration and a prolonged course of illness warrant a check for urea/electrolytes.

Use of antibiotics

- Most cases of food-borne toxigenic diarrhoea do not require antibiotics.
- The duration of travellers' diarrhoea (*E. coli, Shigella*) can be shortened by half with the use of ciprofloxacin or Bactrim®.
- **Indications:** invasive diarrhoea characterized by fever and toxicity ± bloody diarrhoea, i.e. presumed bacterial diarrhoea.
- **Choice:**
  1. **Ciprofloxacin** is the drug of choice when used empirically. Dosage: 500 mg bd. Duration: three days. Not suitable for the paediatric age group (<18 years old). An alternative for patients allergic to fluoroquinolones, pregnant, on warfarin or phenytoin, or travelling in Thailand where there is a high incidence of quinolone-resistant *Campylobacter* is **azithromycin** 1 g single dose.
  2. **Metronidazole (Flagyl®)**. Dosage: 800 mg tds. Duration: 5 days. Indicated when protozoan infection (giardiasis or amoebiasis) or *Clostridium difficile* (due to recent antibiotic usage) is suspected.

Indications for admission

- Invasive diarrhoea requiring stool investigations.
- Inability to retain oral fluids.
- Uncertain diagnosis requiring further evaluation.
- Management of complications: severe dehydration, electrolyte abnormality.

References/Further Reading

1. Hals GD. The traveler in the ED: Common presentations. *Emerg Med Rep.* 2008; 29(22).
2. Kahler J. Acute infectious diarrhoea. *Emerg Med Rep.* 2007; 28(21).
3. Gilbert DN, Moellering RC, Sande MA, Eliopoulos GM. *The Sanford Guide to Antimicrobial Therapy 2007.* Sperryville, VA: Antimicrobial Therapy; 2007.
4. Ooi SBS, Koh-Tai BC, Aw TC, et al. Assessment of dehydration in adults using hematologic and biochemical tests. *Acad Emerg Med.* 1997; 4(8): 840–844.

7 Fever

Goh Ee Ling

DEFINITIONS

- **Fever** is an increase in the body core temperature due to elevation of the hypothalamic set point. It should be differentiated from **hyperthermia**, which results from overwhelming of the body's thermoregulatory mechanisms without elevation of the hypothalamic set point.
- **Fever of unknown origin (FUO)** is a fever >38.3°C on several occasions over a period longer than 3 weeks with an uncertain diagnosis after 1 week of evaluation in the hospital.

CAVEATS

- A temperature of 37.5°C constitutes a fever in adults but this may be lower or even absent in immunocompromised patients, e.g. the elderly, cancer patients on chemotherapy, and IV drug abusers.
- The magnitude of temperature and response to antipyretics do not correlate with the severity of illness.
- There are many causes of fever but infections remain the most common cause. See Table 1.

TABLE 1 Causes of fever

Causes	Types
Infections	Viral Bacterial Fungal Parasitic
Neoplasms	Solid tumours Leukaemia Lymphoma
Collagen-vascular diseases	Systemic lupus erythematosus Rheumatoid arthritis Polyarteritis nodosa Giant cell arteritis
Central nervous system lesions	Stroke Intracranial bleeding Subarachnoid haemorrhage
Drugs	Antibiotics, e.g. penicillins, sulphonamides Anticonvulsants, e.g. carbamazepine, phenytoin NSAIDs, e.g. salicylates, ibuprofen Anticancer drugs, e.g. bleomycin Others, e.g. barbiturates, cimetidine

CLINICAL ASSESSMENT

History

- Duration of fever.
- Associated symptoms, e.g. cough, dysuria, vomiting/diarrhoea.
- Past medical history, especially immunocompromised states.
- Recent procedures, e.g. urinary catheterization, IV cannula insertion.
- Travel history/recent febrile contacts.
- Vaccination history (especially in children).
- Previous treatments for current illness.
- Medication history.

Physical examination

- General appearance, including mental status and hydration status.
- **Vital signs.** (*NOTE:* The pulse should increase by 10 beats/min for every 1°C increase in temperature.) Look for the following:
  1. **Pulse-temperature dissociation**: may be present in typhoid and malaria.
  2. **Tachycardia out of proportion to fever**: suggestive of early septic shock or myocarditis.
- **Systematic examination** often guided by history.
  1. Skin: rashes, ulcers, cellulitis, necrotizing soft-tissue infections, needle-track marks.
  2. Head and neck: otitis media, otitis externa, conjunctivitis.
  3. Cardiovascular: murmurs, pericardial rub.
  4. Respiratory: lung crepitations, tonsillitis, sinusitis, pharyngitis.
  5. Abdomen: renal punch, intra-abdominal sepsis, e.g. cholecystitis, appendicitis.
  6. Central nervous system: neck stiffness, other signs of meningism, e.g. Kernig's sign.
  7. Lines and tubes: urinary catheter, permanent catheter, Tenckhoff catheter site, arteriovenous fistula (AVF), ventriculoperitoneal (VP) shunt.

Investigations

Clinical judgement via history and physical examination guides the need for diagnostic studies. They may include the following:

- Blood investigations:
  1. **Full blood count**: increased neutrophil count/band forms indicate acute inflammation.
  2. **Blood cultures**: both aerobic and anaerobic bottles with a minimum of 7.5 ml of blood per bottle.
  3. **C-reactive protein**: an acute-phase reactant that rises in acute inflammation and shows marked increase in the presence of infections.

4. **Lactate**: an indicator of tissue hypoperfusion that can help in identifying patients with occult shock (i.e. stable vital signs). (Refer to Chapter 33, *Septic Shock*.)

5. **Arterial blood gas**: may pick up hypoxaemia in patients with severe pneumonia.

6. Others: renal panel, liver panel, blood film for malarial parasites.

- Stat **capillary blood sugar** to look out for associated hyperglycaemic complications like diabetic ketoacidosis, especially in all toxic-appearing febrile patients and even in the absence of a prior history of diabetes mellitus.

- **Radiographs:** chest, abdomen, extremities.

- **Ultrasound** and/or **CT abdomen/pelvis**: to look for the source of intra-abdominal sepsis, e.g. enlarged gallbladder with thickening of walls and gallstones suggestive of cholecystitis, pelvic abscesses.

- Others: urine, peritoneal fluid, wound swab.

⇨ **SPECIAL TIPS FOR GPs**
- Antibiotics should not be prescribed indiscriminately for non-specific viral fevers or upper respiratory tract infection.
- It is important to refer febrile septic patients to hospital immediately for evaluation and management.

MANAGEMENT

The principles of management of patients with fever are as follows:

- Early resuscitation and stabilization of patients in septic shock (refer to Chapter 33, *Septic Shock*).

- Evaluate the cause of fever through history, physical examination, and relevant investigations.

- Isolate patients as appropriate, e.g. pneumonia, meningococcaemia.

- Early and appropriate choice of **antibiotics** for patients with sepsis ± septic shock, e.g. IV gentamicin and IV ceftazidime for neutropenic sepsis, IV metronidazole and IV ceftriaxone for intra-abdominal sepsis, IV ceftriaxone empirically for sepsis of unknown source.

- Symptomatic treatment as needed.

- Appropriate **disposition** based on diagnosis and clinical status of the patients.

  1. Admit the unstable febrile patient to the medical department (high dependency unit or intensive care unit).

  2. If there is a potential surgical cause of intra-abdominal sepsis, the patient should be admitted to the surgical department.

  3. Patients with neutropenic sepsis should be admitted to the oncology department with reverse barrier nursing.

  4. Refer suspected dengue cases to the medical SOC for repeat FBC (see Chapter 73, *Dengue Fever*).

References/Further Reading

1. Jui J. Septic shock. In: Tintinalli J, Stapczynski JS, Ma OJ, et al., eds. *Tintinalli's Emergency Medicine: A Comprehensive Study Guide.* 7th ed. New York: McGraw-Hill; 2011: 1003–1013.

2. Eilbert W. Febrile adults. In: Hamilton GC, ed. *Emergency Medicine: An Approach to Clinical Problem-Solving.* 2nd ed. Philadelphia: Saunders; 2003: 235–256.

3. Lamb RP, Birnbaumer DM. Fever. In: Markovchick VJ, Pons PT, eds. *Emergency Medicine Secrets.* 3rd ed. Philadelphia: Hanley & Belfus; 2003: 46–49.

4. Blum FC. Fever in the adult patient. In: Marx JA, Hockberger RS, Walls RM, et al., eds. *Rosen's Emergency Medicine: Concepts and Clinical Practice.* 7th ed. Philadelphia: Mosby Elsevier; 2010: 83–86.

8   Giddiness

Francis Lee • Kuan Win Sen • Shirley Ooi

CAVEATS

- Although a clear distinction between vertigo and non-specific giddiness or lightheadedness is useful in pinpointing a diagnosis, many patients are unable to accurately describe the sensation they are feeling.
- The patient's description is most critical for establishing the aetiology of giddiness and physical examination generally confirms but does not make the diagnosis.
- **Vertigo** tends to point to an **otological** or **brainstem problem** while non-specific giddiness has many other causes (Table 1).
- **Lightheadedness** as a symptom is often **more sinister** and the approach should be that of syncope/presyncope.
- It is important, on first encounter, to ensure that the patient does not have a significant **life-threatening disease**, such as the following:
  1. Ischaemic heart disease, e.g. acute coronary syndrome.
  2. Cardiac failure.
  3. Cardiac dysrhythmias.
  4. Stroke/vertebrobasilar insufficiency (VBI).
  5. Sources of hypovolaemia, e.g. GIT bleeding.
  6. Gynaecological problems, e.g. ectopic pregnancy/vaginal bleeding.
  7. Hypoglycaemia.
- Evaluation in the elderly is even more complex as chronic problems such as failure of eyesight and gait instability could be interpreted as giddiness.

TABLE 1   Types of giddiness

Vertigo	An illusion of motion, which is frequently rotatory, but may be rocking, swaying, or a sense of linear propulsion and can be of varying degrees of intensity and persistence. It is indicative of vestibular dysfunction, whether peripheral or central. Not all patients will be able to describe vertigo in vivid terms.
Presyncope	A sensation that fainting is about to occur. During the episode, the patient often senses his vision growing dark or dim. There may be nausea, vomiting, weakness, dyspnoea, and anxiety. It is transient in nature.
Non-specific giddiness	Vague giddiness symptoms that do not fit into the above.

FIGURE 1   General approach to giddiness/dizziness

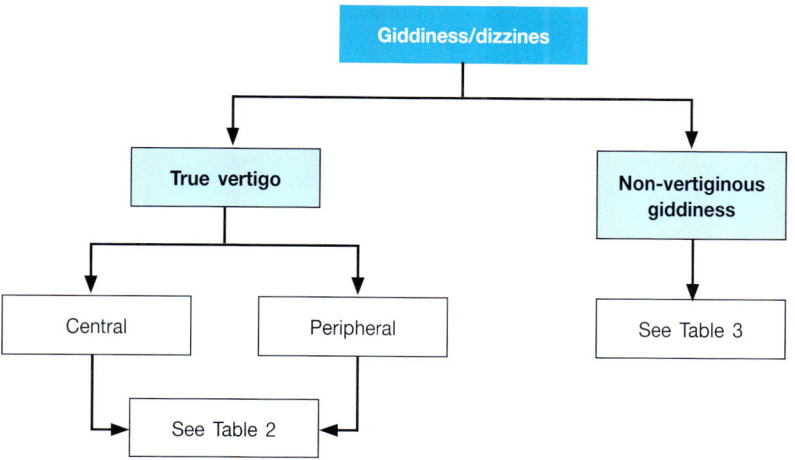

MANAGEMENT

Initial management

- Patients with significant giddiness and unsteadiness should be managed in the intermediate care area.
- The ABCs of patients should be addressed.
- Low-flow supplemental oxygen should be administered.
- Patients should be placed on cardiac monitoring.
- Vitals should be taken and patients should be upgraded to critical care area status if they are found to be abnormal.
- Postural parameters should be taken. **Definition of postural hypotension**: a decrease in systolic blood pressure of >20 mmHg on standing and an increase in pulse rate of >20/min upon standing may indicate significant volume loss. This has added significance in combination with **postural symptoms**. It may be a cause of giddiness in up to 30% of elderly patients. Polypharmacy has been an attributing factor, especially with antihypertensive and antidepressant medications.

TABLE 2   **Characteristics of peripheral and central vertigo**

Characteristics	Peripheral	Central
Onset	Abrupt	Gradual
Intensity	Moderate to intense	Mild to moderate
Temporal pattern	Brief, episodic, lasts <1 min, fatigues with repetition	Chronic, continuous, lasts >1 min, does not fatigue
Nystagmus	Rotatory/unidirectional/ horizontal Suppressed by visual fixation	Any kind/multidirectional including bizarre/vertical Not suppressed by visual fixation
Head motion	Aggravation of symptoms	Little aggravation of symptoms
CNS symptoms and signs (e.g. dysarthria, diplopia, ataxia, cranial nerve palsies)	Rare	Common
Imbalance	Mild to moderate, patient can usually walk	Severe. Patient has great difficulty walking
Risk factors for vascular disease	May be present or absent	Commonly present
Tinnitus	Characteristic	Uncommon
Hearing loss	Characteristic. May be present in otosclerosis, Meniere's disease	Uncommon. May occur in labyrinth infarctions.
Nausea/vomiting	Common	Uncommon
Differential diagnosis	Vestibular neuronitis Benign positional vertigo Meniere's disease Middle ear infection Cholesteatoma	Vertebrobasilar insufficiency Brainstem infarct Tumour (acoustic neuroma) Haemorrhage (cerebellar) Multiple sclerosis

TABLE 3 Common important causes of non-vertiginous giddiness

System	Examples
Cardiac	Acute myocardial infarction or any condition that causes decreased cardiac output Dysrhythmias Valvular heart disease Congestive heart failure
Orthostatic hypotension	Blood loss, e.g. GIT bleeding, ruptured ectopic pregnancy Dehydration Drugs (see Table 4)
Metabolic	Hypoxia Hypoglycaemia Hyperventilation Drugs Uraemia Hepatic failure
Haematologic	Anaemia Hyperviscosity syndromes

TABLE 4 Medications associated with giddiness

Alcohol	Anti-inflammatory agents, e.g. salicylates
Antibiotics, e.g. aminoglycosides	Antiparkinson agents
Antidysrhythmics	Diuretics
Anticonvulsants, e.g. phenytoin	Hypoglycaemic agents
Antidepressants	Phenothiazines
Antihistamines	Sedatives
Antihypertensives	

Investigations

- **Stat capillary glucose** should be considered (mandatory for all diabetics).
- Stat **ECG** for patients with the following:
  1. Risk factors:
     a. Age >40 years.
     b. History of coronary artery disease.
     c. History of diabetes mellitus.
     d. History of hypertension.
     e. History of dyslipidaemia.
     f. Smoker.
  2. Unstable vital signs.

- **Special attention** should be paid to the following:
    1. Evidence of anaemia.
    2. Evidence of hypovolaemia: blood loss or dehydration.
    3. Cardiovascular system: dysrhythmia, cardiac murmur, e.g. aortic stenosis.
    4. Neurological system: nystagmus, focal neurological deficits, cerebellar signs.
    5. Abdomen: sepsis or bleeding. Do rectal examination if there is postural hypotension.
- After excluding the above, the doctor could use the general approach shown in Figure 1 to evaluate the cause of giddiness.

SPECIFIC MANAGEMENT

Vertigo

- Symptomatic treatment:
    1. IV/IM prochlorperazine (Stemetil®) 12.5 mg or IV/IM promethazine (Phenergan®) 12.5–25 mg.
    2. PO diazepam (Valium®) 2 mg.
- IV hydration if vomiting is severe.
- Distinguish between peripheral and central vertigo (Table 2).
- The **Dix–Hallpike test** is the definitive diagnostic test for benign paroxysmal positional vertigo (BPPV):
    1. Bring the patient from a sitting to a supine position, with the head turned 45 degrees to the side.
    2. Extend the head 20 degrees backward.
    3. Observe the eyes for about 30 seconds.
    4. If no nystagmus ensues, the patient is brought back to the sitting position and the other side is tested after 30 seconds.

    A positive Dix–Hallpike test consists of a burst of nystagmus.
- The **Epley manoeuvre** can be used to treat BPPV:
    1. Bring the patient from a sitting to a supine position, with the head turned 45 degrees to the side where the vertigo is worse. Extend the head 20 degrees backward. Remain up to 5 minutes in this position.
    2. Turn the head 90 degrees to the other side (i.e. 45 degrees facing the opposite side). Remain up to 5 minutes in this position.
    3. Roll the patient's body onto the side in the direction he/she is facing, with the body and head moving as one. The head will be now pointing nose down. Remain up to 5 minutes in this position.
    4. Sit the patient back up, again with the body and head moving as one. Remain up to 30 seconds in this position.

The entire procedure should be repeated for a total of 3 times. Warn the patient that he/she may experience vertigo during this manoeuvre albeit with decreasing severity with subsequent attempts if the diagnosis is correct and the treatment is working.

- **Disposition**: Can **discharge** if the patient shows the following:
  1. Has true peripheral vertigo.
  2. Has no neurological deficits.
  3. Has no symptoms to suggest an episode of VBI, i.e. no diplopia or visual blurring, dysarthria, dysphagia, drop attacks, or focal neurological deficits (weakness).
  4. Is well and self-ambulatory after observation.
  5. Has no significant medical history.
  6. Has good home support (for the elderly).

Presyncope

Refer to Chapter 24, *Syncope*.

Non-specific giddiness

- Exclude, if possible, obvious neurological problems such as VBI, multiple sclerosis, brainstem or cerebello-pontine infarction/haemorrhage or trauma, or Parkinson's disease.
- Recommend bed rest.
- Symptomatic treatment if giddiness is severe:
  1. IM prochlorperazine.
  2. Admit the patient if he shows no improvement.
- **Disposition**: **Discharge** the patient if:
  1. Cerebrovascular disease or VBI has been excluded.
  2. The following significant diseases have been excluded:
     a. Ischaemic heart disease.
     b. Dysrhythmias.
     c. Pneumonia/infection.
     d. Bleeding or dehydration.
  3. The patient has no significant risk factors:
     a. Ischaemic heart disease.
     b. Diabetes mellitus.
     c. Hypertension.
  4. The patient is well after observation:
     a. Alert and attentive.
     b. No significant giddiness.
     c. Able to retain orally.

5. Good home care is available (for elderly patients).
6. General discharge advice should include the following. **Do not**:
   a. Drive a motor vehicle.
   b. Ride a bicycle or motorcycle.
   c. Climb heights.
   d. Operate heavy machinery.
   e. Drink alcoholic beverages.
   f. Swim.

Ischaemic heart disease

- Giddiness can be the presenting complaint in acute coronary syndrome (ACS), acute heart failure, and dysrhythmias.
- Diagnosis is based on cardiac risk factors, symptomatology, and ECG changes.
- Patients should be managed as for ACS, with a view to early myocardial salvage, e.g thrombolysis or percutaneous coronary intervention (PCI).
- Such patients should be admitted to the coronary care unit (CCU) for evaluation.

Cardiac failure

- Chronic heart failure can present with giddiness if cardiac output is insufficient to meet the demands of daily activities.
- Refer to Chapter 38, *Heart Failure, Acute*.

Cardiac dysrhythmias

- Either fast or slow heart rhythms can cause giddiness.
- This is detectable on the cardiac monitor and 12-lead ECG.
- The management depends on the cause.
- **Significant rhythms** that should receive immediate management and subsequent CCU placement include the following:
   1. Significant or unexplained bradycardias.
   2. Second- and third-degree heart blocks.
   3. Ventricular tachydysrhythmias.
   4. Supraventricular tachycardias with haemodynamic instability.
   5. Atrial fibrillation with rapid ventricular response and haemodynamic instability.

Stroke

- Giddiness, either non-specific giddiness or vertiginous forms, could be a sign of a transient ischaemic attack (TIA) or impending stroke.

- Patients tend to be middle-aged and above and many of them will have hypertension.
- The patient should be examined for evidence of brainstem signs and neurological deficits.
- Refer to Chapter 68, *Stroke*.

Hypovolaemia

- Any sources of bleeding or fluid loss producing hypovolaemia can cause symptoms of giddiness. In mild cases, persistent or recurrent non-specific giddiness may be felt. In severe cases, there may be a sensation of **blacking-out** or frank syncope.
- All patients should be screened for common sources of **bleeding**, e.g. GIT bleeding or in the case of a female, vaginal bleeding.
- Patients should be asked whether **severe vomiting** or **diarrhoea** has occurred.
- Take blood for FBC and electrolyte assessment.

Gynaecological conditions

- Women of childbearing age should be screened for evidence of vaginal bleeding or lower abdominal pain that may suggest **ectopic pregnancy**.

Hypoglycaemia

- Hypoglycaemia may be an important cause of giddiness in both healthy patients as well as diabetics.

References/Further Reading

1. Hauser SL, Josephson SA, Harrison TR, et al. *Harrison's Neurology in Clinical Medicine.* New York: McGraw-Hill Professional; 2006.

2. Bronstein AM, Lempert T. *Dizziness: A Practical Approach to Diagnosis and Management.* Cambridge: Cambridge University Press; 2007.

3. Macleod D, McAuley D. Vertigo: Clinical assessment and diagnosis. *Br J Hosp Med (Lond).* 2008; 69(6): 330–334.

9 Haemoptysis

Irwani Ibrahim

DEFINITION

- Haemoptysis is **defined** as the expectoration of blood or blood-stained sputum that originates from below the vocal cords or that has been aspirated into the bronchial tree.
- Haemoptysis can be **classified** as the following:
  1. Mild: <5 ml of blood in 24 hours.
  2. Massive: 50 ml in a single expectoration or >600 ml of blood in 24 hours. This accounts for 5% of all cases of haemoptysis.

CAVEATS

- Haemoptysis may be confused with haematemesis (Table 1).
- Physical examination is useful in determining the severity of haemoptysis, but is **unreliable** in localizing the site of bleeding.
- Massive haemoptysis is life-threatening because **asphyxiation**, rather than exsanguination, is the leading cause of death.
- Bleeding that results in respiratory distress and altered gas exchange is life-threatening, regardless of the amount of blood.
- The commonest cause of mild haemoptysis is upper respiratory tract infection (URTI) bronchitis (Table 2).

TABLE 1 **Differential points between haemoptysis and haematemesis**

Differential points	Haemoptysis	Haematemesis
History	Coughing	GI symptoms
Sputum colour	Bright red	Dark red
pH	Alkaline	Acidic
Character	Frothy	Smooth, non-frothy

TABLE 2   **Common causes of haemoptysis**

Respiratory	Bronchitis
	Tuberculosis
	Pulmonary neoplasms
	Bronchiectasis
	Pneumonia
	Aspirated blood from epistaxis
	Pulmonary embolism
	Sinusitis
Cardiovascular	Pulmonary oedema
	Mitral stenosis
	Aortobronchial fistula
Coagulation disorder	Bleeding dyscrasias (congenital or acquired)
Others	Foreign body aspiration
	Protracted cough
	Catamenial haemoptysis (associated with menstruation)

⇨ **SPECIAL TIPS FOR GPs**
- It is advisable to refer all cases of haemoptysis unless CXR can be done in the clinic.
- Insert 2 large-bore intravenous cannulae before transferring patients with massive haemoptysis.

MANAGEMENT OF MASSIVE HAEMOPTYSIS

- Transfer patient to the resuscitation area.
- The main objective is to **prevent asphyxiation**. Protect the airway and administer oxygen. Patients who have a depressed level of consciousness or who are in imminent danger of asphyxiation should be intubated with a large-diameter (8 mm or larger) endotracheal tube.
- Set up 2 large-bore IV lines and fluid resuscitate.
- **Labs:**
  1. FBC.
  2. Urea/electrolytes/creatinine.
  3. Coagulation profile.
  4. GXM four to six units of blood.
  5. ABG.
- Continuous monitoring.

- **Chest X-ray** is **mandatory** in all patients with haemoptysis.
- It is recommended that patients with ongoing haemoptysis from one lung (if known) be positioned with the bleeding lung dependent, to minimize soiling of the contralateral lung.
- The most effective non-surgical treatment for massive haemoptysis is **bronchial artery embolization**; hence an interventional radiologist should be contacted. Consider a consultation with a cardiothoracic surgeon as well.
- The use of **tranexamic acid**, though successful in published case reports, did not show benefits in randomized controlled trials.
- **Disposition**:
  1. Patients with **mild haemoptysis** can usually be sent home with rest and a cough suppressant.
  2. Refer to respiratory medicine specialist outpatient clinics for early follow-up unless the case is due to sinusitis or epistaxis, in which case patients should be in the ear, nose, and throat (ENT) specialist clinics.
  3. Consider admission in all other patients. Those with massive haemoptysis require admission to the intensive care unit.

References/Further Reading

1. Jean-Baptiste E. Clinical assessment and management of massive hemoptysis. *Crit Care Med.* 2000; 28(5): 1642–1647.

2. Bidwell JL, Pachner RW. Hemoptysis: Diagnosis and management. *Am Fam Physician.* 2005; 72(7): 1253–1260.

3. Tsoumakidou M, Chrysofakis G, Tsiligianni I, et al. A prospective analysis of 184 hemoptysis cases: Diagnostic impact of chest X-ray, computed tomography, bronchoscopy. *Respiration.* 2006; 73(6): 808–814.

4. Tscheikuna J, Chvaychoo B, Naruman C, Maranetra N. Tranexamic acid in patients with hemoptysis. *J Med Assoc Thai.* 2002; 85(4): 399–404.

5. Young WF, Jr. Hemoptysis. In: Tintinalli JE, Stapczynski JS, Ma OJ, et al., eds. *Tintinalli's Emergency Medicine: A Comprehensive Study Guide.* 7th ed. New York: McGraw-Hill; 2011: 473–476.

10   Headache

Sim Tiong Beng

CAVEATS

- Differentiate life-threatening/vision-threatening headaches from reversible/benign secondary or primary headaches (see Table 1).

TABLE 1   Secondary headaches

Life-threatening headache	Vision-threatening headache	Reversible benign headache
Subarachnoid haemorrhage (SAH) (refer to Chapter 69, *Subarachnoid Haemorrhage*),	Temporal arteritis (refer to Chapter 70, *Temporal Arteritis*)	Sinusitis
Extradural haemorrhage	Glaucoma (refer to Chapter 20, *Red Eye*)	Post-traumatic headache
Subdural haemorrhage		Chronic headache after whiplash injury
Intracerebral haemorrhage		Temporomandibular Joint (TMJ) disorder
Meningoencephalitis		Cervicogenic
Space-occupying lesion, e.g. neoplasm, abscess		
Cardiac cephalgia, e.g. acute myocardial ischaemia		
Others, e.g. cerebral venous thrombosis, carbon monoxide poisoning, toxins, idiopathic intracranial hypertension		

- The presence of **red flags** will warrant emergent head CT. These include the following:
  1. Severe sudden 'thunderclap' headache or 'worst' headache, e.g. SAH, or change in nature of the headache (increased frequency or severity).
  2. Early morning headache which is worsened by coughing/straining (raised intracranial pressure [ICP]).
  3. Syncope (SAH) or vomiting (raised ICP), although vomiting is also commonly seen in migraine attacks.
  4. Altered mental status or seizure.
  5. Fever or neck pain (meningism from SAH or meningitis).

6. Focal neurological deficits.

7. Visual disturbances, e.g. eye pain (glaucoma).

8. When the patient's age is >55 years with new-onset headache, it carries a higher risk of intracranial space-occupying lesions.

9. HIV/immunocompromised (toxoplasmosis/cryptococcosis).

10. Malignancy.

11. Patients on anticoagulants are at increased risk of intracranial bleeds.

12. Previous VP shunt.

13. Head injury.

- Hypertension is an overstated cause of headaches. **Do not** attribute a headache to elevated blood pressure unless the systolic pressure is >160 mmHg and the diastolic pressure exceeds 120 mmHg; the headache resolves within 1 hour after normalization of blood pressure.

- Headaches may be classified as primary (benign) or secondary headaches.

1. **Primary headaches** (those with no underlying pathology) include tension-type headache, migraine with or without aura, and cluster headache (see Chapter 67, *Migraine and Cluster Headache*).

2. **Secondary headaches** include life-threatening/vision-threatening causes or reversible (generally benign) causes, e.g. rhinosinusitis, temporomandibular joint disorder, chronic post-traumatic headache, chronic headache attributed to whiplash injury (Table 1).

ESSENTIAL FEATURES OF A FOCUSED EXAMINATION

- Review of vital signs (especially temperature and blood pressure).

- Fundoscopy.

- Pupils, visual fields, long tract signs, cranial nerves, and cerebellar examination for focal abnormalities.

- Gait.

⇨ **SPECIAL TIPS FOR GPs**

- A patient presenting with a sudden-onset thunderclap headache is presumed to have **SAH** until proven otherwise, even if there is good relief with analgesia. The CNS examination can be completely normal!

- Consider **meningoencephalitis** in a febrile and drowsy/confused patient with headache.

- Rule out **glaucoma** if eye pain/redness and blurred vision with headache is present (suggested by hazy cornea and semi-dilated pupil).

- Do **not** diagnose **migraine** if the **first** episode of severe headache occurs after the age of 50 years.

FIGURE 1   Approach to headaches in the ED

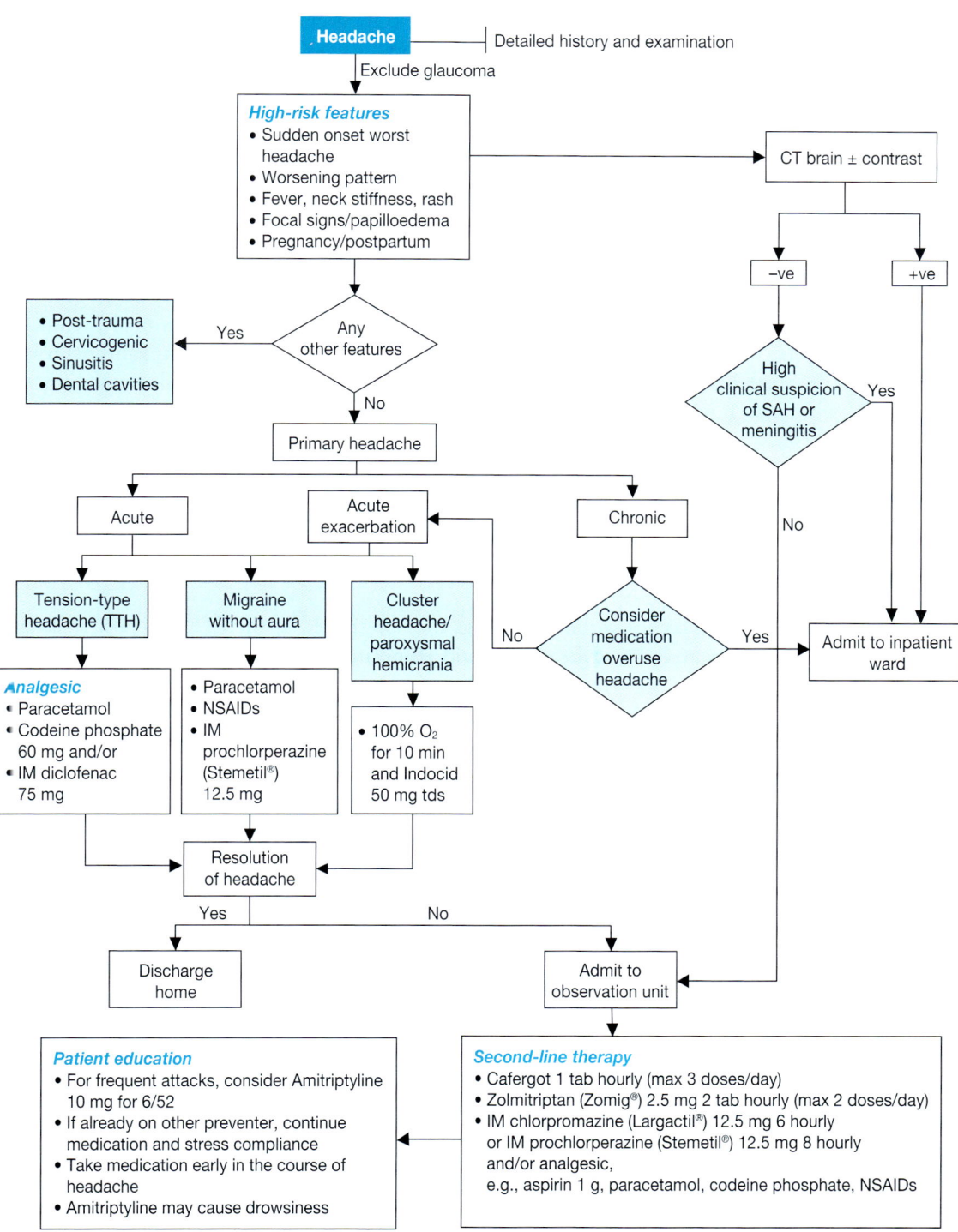

MANAGEMENT

- Monitoring of vital signs, and Glasgow Coma Scale (GCS) charting.
- CT head scan +/− lumbar puncture (LP) for high-risk patients.
- Labs: FBC, urea/electrolytes/creatinine, coagulation profile, GXM, and erythrocyte sedimentation rate (ESR) (if temporal arteritis is suspected).
- ECG and CXR, if indicated.
- Refer to Chapter 140, *Pain Management*, for symptomatic relief of headache.

Disposition

See Figure 1. Admit the following:

- All patients with life- and vision-threatening causes of headache. Traditionally, clinically suspected SAH with a normal CT brain will warrant an LP to rule out xanthochromia. However, in a recent study[4], the sensitivity for SAH using modern third generation CT to scan within 6 hours of headache onset was 100% (97.0%–100%), specifically 100% (99.5%–100%).
- Complicated migraine headaches of new onset.
- Abnormal CT head scans.

NOTE: 1. **Primary headaches** treated successfully at the ED may be discharged back to the primary care doctor for follow-up.

2. **Secondary headaches** without red flags may be treated at the ED, e.g. post-traumatic headache, nitrate-induced headache, and rhinosinusitis.

Consider the **observation unit** for the following:

- Treatment of clinically benign primary/secondary headache, but in which the severity may render the patient not ready for discharge from the ED yet.
- Evaluation of the patient who is deemed low-risk for serious causes of headache, but whose symptoms cannot be explained by any other disease process, e.g. viral infection. A period of observation and symptomatic treatment would make the diagnosis more definitive.

References/Further Reading

1. Field AG, Wang E. Evaluation of the patient with nontraumatic headache: An evidence based approach. *Emerg Med Clin North Am.* 1999; 17(1): 127–152.

2. Byyny RL, Mower WR, Shum N, et al. Sensitivity of noncontrast computed tomography for the emergency department diagnosis of subarachnoid hemorrhage. *Ann Emerg Med.* 2008; 51(6): 697–703.

3. American College of Emergency Physicians. Clinical policy: Critical issues in the evaluation and management of patients presenting to the emergency department with acute headache. *Ann Emerg Med.* 2002; 39(1): 108–122.

4. Perry JJ, Stiell IG, Sivilotti ML, et al. Sensitivity of computed tomography performed within six hours of onset of headache for diagnosis of subarachnoid haemorrhage: prospective cohort study. BMJ. 2011 Jul 18; 343: d4277. doi: 10.1136/bmj.d4277.

11 Hyperventilation

Seet Chong Meng • Peter Manning • Shirley Ooi

CAVEATS

- Although common and benign, hyperventilation attack (HA) or hyperventilation syndrome is a **diagnosis of exclusion** which can be achieved principally on historical and physical findings without extensive investigations.
- A typical episode involves a precipitating stressful event with a past history of similar occurrences.
- Common associated symptoms include numbness and/or cramping of hands and feet, perioral tingling, non-specific dizziness, chest tightness, a sensation of suffocation, and near-syncope.
- Do not diagnose a patient with HA if the SpO_2 on room air is below 97%.
- Table 1 shows the differential diagnosis of hyperventilation.

TABLE 1   Differential diagnosis of hyperventilation

Respiratory system	• Severe asthma (with silent chest)
	• Pulmonary embolism
	• Tension pneumothorax
	• Primary pulmonary hypertension
Cardiovascular system	• Cardiac tamponade
Metabolic causes	• Diabetic ketoacidosis
	• Chronic renal failure
	• Lactic acidosis from severe sepsis or shock of any cause
	• Poisoning, especially by salicylates
Neurological system	• Central neurogenic hyperventilation
Gastrointestinal system	• Abdominal distension from various causes with splinting of diaphragm
Hyperventilation attack/ syndrome	

> ⇨ **SPECIAL TIP FOR GPs**
> - It is important to exclude more serious medical conditions such as metabolic acidosis, e.g. diabetic ketoacidosis, before diagnosing HA.

MANAGEMENT

- Patient should be managed in the intermediate acuity area. However, if significant altered mental state exists or there is haemodynamic instability, then this patient probably does not have HA but some other significant disease process requiring management in the critical care area.
- Do a stat SpO_2 measurement for every patient before diagnosing HA.
- Provide reassurance.
- Advise on breathing technique.

NOTE: Rebreathing into a bag has been found to be potentially harmful as it causes significant hypoxaemia. It has also been shown to be ineffective in bringing up the pCO_2 level to a significant level.

- Monitoring: most cases require a pulse oximeter only.

NOTE: A patient with true HA is likely to have a normal SpO_2.

- Labs:
  1. Mandatory: **capillary blood glucose** estimation to exclude a hyperglycaemic state.
  2. Optional: **ABG** will show respiratory alkalosis in HA. Alternatively, this test may reveal underlying metabolic acidosis.
- **Chest X-ray**: to investigate such entities as pneumothorax, pneumonia, or pulmonary embolism.
- **ECG** (especially age >40 years): to investigate possible pulmonary embolism, pericarditis, or ischaemia. May sometimes show prolonged QT interval from hypocalcaemia due to hyperventilation.
- **Drug therapy** (for those patients who do not respond to rest and reassurance):
  1. **Valium® (diazepam)**: Dosage: 5 mg PO.
  2. **Dormicum® (midazolam)**: Dosage: 2.5 mg IV (rarely required).
- **Disposition:** Most cases can be discharged. If this is a recurrent problem in this patient, then he/she should be referred to Psychiatry for outpatient therapy. The occasional patient may benefit from being given a prescription for one to two doses of oral alprazolam (Xanax®).

References/Further reading

1. Phillipson EA, Duffin J. Hypoventilation and hyperventilation syndromes. In: Mason RJ, Murray JF, Broaddus CV, Nadel JA, eds. *Murray & Nadel's Textbook of Respiratory Medicine.* 4th ed. St. Louis: WB Saunders; 2005: Chapter 73.

2. Saisch SG, Wessely S, Gardner WN. Patients with acute hyperventilation presenting to an inner-city emergency department. *Chest.* 1996; 110(4): 952–957.

3. Callaham M. Hypoxic hazards of traditional paper bag rebreathing in hyperventilating patients. *Ann Emerg Med.* 1989; 18(6): 622–628.

12 Lower Limb Swelling

Quek Lit Sin • Shirley Ooi

CAVEATS

- Lower limb swelling is a common complaint among patients and will present frequently with associated non-specific signs and symptoms. Table 1 shows the important causes of lower limb swelling.
- As with all consultations, a good history will be able to reduce the number of differentials.

PREGNANCY WITH PRE-ECLAMPSIA

- All pregnant women will have lower limb swelling. As lower limb swelling is an early sign of pre-eclampsia, a high index of suspicion is necessary.
- The diagnosis of pre-eclampsia is an emergency and the patient must be treated in the hospital. Refer to Chapter 108, *Eclampsia*.

TABLE 1   Important causes of lower limb swelling

System	Examples	Unilateral/Bilateral
Cardiac	• Heart failure (refer to Chapter 38, *Heart Failure, Acute*)	Bilateral
Renal	• Acute/chronic renal failure with fluid overload (refer to Chapter 63, *Renal Emergencies*) • Nephrotic/nephritic syndrome	Bilateral
Pregnancy	• Pre-eclampsia (refer to Chapter 108, *Eclampsia*)	Bilateral
Hepatobiliary	• Liver failure (refer to Chapter 50, *Hepatic Encephalopathy, Acute*)	Bilateral
Veins/lymphatics	• Deep vein thrombosis (DVT) • Varicose veins • Lymphoedema	Unilateral Unilateral/bilateral Unilateral/bilateral
Infection	• Lymphangitis • Cellulitis	Unilateral
Orthopaedic causes	• Trauma • Compartment syndrome • Arthritis/gout • Ruptured Baker's cyst • Tumour: bone or soft tissue	Unilateral

VEINS AND LYMPHATICS

- **Deep vein thrombosis** (refer to Chapter 42, *Venous Emergencies*)
- **Varicose veins** are accompanied by skin pigmentation in chronic cases. Superficial thrombophlebitis of the varicose veins results in lower limb swelling. Unilateral varicose veins and swelling require more careful thought as they may indicate a sinister pathology in the pelviabdominal area.
- Lymphatic obstruction will result in oedema of the lower extremities. Secondary **lymphoedema** follows damage and obstruction to the lymphatic pathways by malignant disease involving the lymph nodes, by filariasis, and may be iatrogenic from surgical block dissection.

INFECTIONS: LYMPHANGITIS/CELLULITIS

- The infection spreads along the lymphatics causing **lymphangitis** and they become visible as thin, red, tender streaks on the skin, often with slight oedema of the overlying skin. When the infection gets into the oedema, **cellulitis** ensues.
- **Indications for admission**:
  1. Recurrent fever and chills.
  2. Increasing local pain.
  3. Spreading erythema.
  4. Elderly patients, as they become septicaemic easily.

ORTHOPAEDIC CAUSES: COMPARTMENT SYNDROME

Orthopaedic causes have a definite history and a good physical examination will usually clinch the diagnosis. It is important to exclude **compartment syndrome**, which is an orthopaedic emergency in all traumatic injuries to the lower limbs!

Clinical features

- Severe pain that gets worse, pain on passive stretch of the muscles, pallor, paraesthesia, pulselessness, and paralysis are the 6 classic signs of muscle ischaemia.
- The presence of **pain** with **passive range of motion of the muscles** is the **earliest clinical sign**. Others include delayed capillary refill and loss of two-point discrimination.
- Palpation of the affected muscles of that compartment will be tense and tenderness will be produced.

Common causes

- Lower limb: fracture of the tibia or fibula.
- Upper limb: supracondylar fracture of the humerus.
- High-voltage electrical burn injuries involving muscles.

Complications

- Severe myoglobinuria, renal failure, hyperkalaemia, and death.
- Volkmann's ischaemic contracture and loss of limb function.

OTHER RARER CAUSES OF LIMB OEDEMA

- Primary lymphoedema (congenital lymphoedema, lymphoedema praecox, lymphoedema tarda).
- Congenital venous malformations.
- May–Thurner syndrome (iliac vein compression syndrome).
- Protein-losing enteropathy, malnutrition, malabsorption.
- Restrictive cardiomyopathy.
- Beriberi.
- Myxoedema.
- Restrictive pericarditis.

⇨ **SPECIAL TIPS FOR GPs**
- A high index of suspicion is necessary to avoid missing important causes of lower limb swelling.
- The three most likely causes of bilateral lower limb swelling are **congestive cardiac failure**, **renal failure** with fluid overload, and **hypoalbuminaemia** (from liver failure or diabetic nephropathy).

GENERAL MANAGEMENT

- Ensure the vital signs are stable and that there is no acute coronary event that led to the lower limb swelling. Unstable patients must be managed in the critical care area.
- Labs:
  1. **Mandatory**:
     a. Urine dipstick for proteinuria.
     b. ECG for myocardial injury.
     c. CXR for heart failure/fluid overload.
  2. **Optional**: If no obvious cause is found after the mandatory investigations or if specific diagnoses are suspected, do the following:
     a. Liver function test (to rule out hypoalbuminaemia).
     b. Urea/electrolytes/creatinine (if renal failure is suspected).
     c. Cardiac enzymes/troponin T (if a cardiac cause is suspected).

    d. If DVT is suspected, do D-dimer, international normalized ratio (INR) (to guide treatment), colour-flow duplex scanning (regardless of the pretest probability), and GXM.

NOTE: A normal D-dimer in a patient with no risk factors for thrombosis makes proximal DVT extremely unlikely. FBC is not useful as the leucocyte count cannot distinguish between DVT and cellulitis and is neither sensitive nor specific for either condition.

    e. Blood culture and sensitivity (C&S) for **infective** causes before starting antibiotics.

- For **compartment syndrome**: call an orthopaedic surgeon early for fasciotomy.

NOTE: If elevated pressure is not relieved after approximately 8 hours, irreversible injury to entrapped muscles and nerves will occur.

- Treatment of lower limb swelling depends on the primary cause and this is discussed in the relevant chapters.
- **Disposition**: admit the following causes:
  1. Cardiac causes.
  2. Renal failure.
  3. DVT (although some critical pathways now emphasize outpatient management when appropriate).
  4. Pregnancy with pre-eclampsia.
  5. Infection.
  6. Liver failure.
  7. Compartment syndrome.
  8. Suspected bone tumours.

  The first 7 causes should have treatment started in the ED. Refer the remaining cause to the relevant outpatient clinic for further investigations and follow-up.

References/Further reading

1. Nandi PL, Li WS, Leung R, et al. Deep vein thrombosis and pulmonary embolism in the Chinese population. *Hong Kong Med J.* 1998; 4(3): 305–310.
2. Lumley JSP. *Hamilton Bailey's Demonstration of Physical Signs in Clinical Surgery.* 18th ed. Oxford: Butterworth Heinemann; 1997.
3. Braunwald E, Fauci AS, Kasper DL, et al., eds. *Harrison's Principles of Internal Medicine.* 15th ed. New York: McGraw-Hill; 2001: 850–981.
4. Skinner DV, Swain A, Peyton R, et al., eds. *Cambridge Textbook of Accident and Emergency Medicine.* Cambridge: Cambridge University Press; 1997: 866–897, 1003–1014.
5. Rose BD. Approach to the adult with edema. Available from UpToDate.com.
6. Young JR. The swollen leg. Clinical significance and differential diagnosis. *Cardiol Clin.* 1991; 9: 443–456.
7. Topham EJ, Mortimer PS. Chronic lower limb oedema. *Clin Med.* 2002; 2: 28–31.

13 Pain, Abdominal

Peter Manning • Sim Tiong Beng • Shirley Ooi

CAVEATS

- The role of the emergency physician is to identify patients with acute abdomen.
- Identify those patients with significant posturing, e.g. lying perfectly still (perforation/peritonitis) or rolling around in agony (bowel/ureteric colic).
- Always consider the **potentially life-threatening aetiologies** presented in Table 1.
- Always consider the possibility of ectopic gestation in pregnancy-capable females.
- A male patient with pain in the right iliac fossa has appendicitis until proven otherwise.
- Elderly patients often have vague, non-specific complaints and atypical presentations leading to time-consuming work-ups.
- Nowadays, because of the wide availability of imaging in the ED, care often does not involve surgical consultation. Frequently, surgeons are involved after the results of laboratory and imaging studies are made available.

TABLE 1   Potentially life-threatening causes of abdominal pain

Intra-abdominal	• Perforated peptic ulcer
	• Intestinal obstruction
	• AAA/aortic dissection
	• Appendicitis
	• Pancreatitis
	• Ectopic pregnancy
	• Ischaemic bowel
	• Peritonitis: spontaneous bacterial peritonitis in liver cirrhosis, peritoneal dialysis related
	• Hepatobiliary sepsis
Extra-abdominal	• Acute myocardial infarction (AMI)
	• Lower-lobe pneumonia
	• Basal pulmonary embolism
	• Diabetic ketoacidosis
	• Systemic lupus erythematosus (SLE) vasculitis

- In diagnosing patients with undifferentiated acute abdominal pain, multiple studies done have come to the following conclusions:
  1. **Abdominal CT imaging** performs uniformly better than plain abdominal X-rays (AXR).
  2. Thus, in patients with acute abdominal or flank pain, in whom CT scans are likely to be obtained, there is minimal to no additional benefit from performing AXR.

3. A non-contrast CT has sufficiently high sensitivity, specificity, and accuracy to make it a useful imaging, thus avoiding the risks of allergic reactions and contrast-induced nephropathy although further studies may be required to compare contrast and non-contrast studies in order to minimize the iatrogenic effects of IV contrasts.

- There are 3 reasons for doing an **abdominal X-ray** in emergency medicine:
  1. To identify '**free' air** (perforated viscus).
  2. To identify **air-fluid interfaces** (intestinal obstruction).
  3. To identify **ectopic calcification** (urolithiasis, hepatobiliary calculi, pancreatitis, abdominal aortic aneurysm (AAA)).

- The **chest X-ray** is utilized to identify the following:
  1. Subdiaphragmatic air.
  2. Basal consolidation.
  3. Pulmonary embolism (ruling out other lung pathologies).

NOTE: If a **perforated peptic ulcer** is suspected and the CXR shows no obvious subdiaphragmatic air, the instillation of 200 ml air into the stomach via a nasogastric tube may show 'free' air on X-ray. This practice should be considered in light of local custom/preference since it is controversial: in the presence of signs of perforation, instilling air does nothing to change the management (i.e. to operate), and can worsen spillage of bowel contents into the peritoneal cavity. Moreover, with the wide availability of CT scan in the ED, the role of gastric insufflation is now quite limited.

⇨ **SPECIAL TIPS FOR GPs**
- The site and nature of the abdominal pain will give the best clue as to what is causing it.
- Always suspect **ectopic pregnancy** in women of child-bearing age.
- Always suspect **appendicitis** in any man with lower abdominal pain.
- Do not forget to feel for epigastric pulsation and check all pulses to look for AAA and aortic dissection respectively.
- Myocardial infarction may give upper abdominal pain. Perform an ECG.

MANAGEMENT

Haemodynamically unstable patient

- The patient must be managed in the critical care area.
- Maintain the airway and give supplemental high-flow oxygen.
- Monitoring: ECG, vital signs q5 minutes, and pulse oximetry.

- Establish 2 large-bore peripheral IVs (14–16 g); fluid challenge of 1–2 L of crystalloid (if AMI is not suspected). Reassess parameters.
- Labs:
    1. Mandatory: capillary blood sugar; GXM 2 to 4 units; FBC; urea/electrolytes/creatinine; liver function tests (LFTs); serum amylase; urine pregnancy test (where relevant); and first blood and urine cultures (if sepsis is suspected).
    2. Optional: urinalysis, cardiac enzymes, LFTs, and coagulation profile.
- **IV antibiotics** in cases of intra-abdominal sepsis, e.g. ceftriaxone 1 g and metronidazole 500 mg. Depending on local practice, other antibiotics to cover Gram-negative and anaerobic organisms can be used.

NOTE: Aminoglycosides are best avoided if the patient has, or is at risk of, renal impairment.

- X-rays: CXR and kidneys, ureters, bladder (KUB) X-ray.
- ECG to identify AMI or as preparation for anticipated surgery in suitable age groups.
- Insert a urinary catheter.
- Keep the patient nil by mouth.
- Early consultations with, e.g. the following:
    1. General surgery registrar.
    2. Obstetrics and gynaecology registrar for suspected ectopic pregnancy.
    3. Cardiothoracic registrar for suspected abdominal aortic aneurysm.
    4. Medical or cardiology registrar for suspected basilar pneumonia or myocardial infarction.

Haemodynamically stable patient

(See next section for specific diagnostic entities.)

- This patient can be managed in the intermediate acuity area.
- Keep the patient nil by mouth till disposition has been decided.
- Consider a precautionary intravenous plug.
- Labs should be based on clinical suspicion of the possible causes of abdominal pain in a particular patient.
- Consider KUB, CXR, and ECG.
- Evaluate for signs of acute abdomen with frequent abdominal examinations.
- At one time it was believed that analgesia interferes with the assessment of patients with abdominal pain. Many studies have disproved this idea; patients with abdominal pain should be treated judiciously with appropriate analgesics.

DIFFERENTIAL DIAGNOSIS OF RIGHT HYPOCHONDRIAL (RHC) PAIN

Febrile patient

- Consider the following:
  1. Cholecystitis (refer to Chapter 51, *Hepatobiliary Emergencies*).
  2. Cholangitis (refer to Chapter 51, *Hepatobiliary Emergencies*).
  3. Liver abscess.
  4. Subdiaphragmatic abscess.
  5. Hepatitis.
  6. Pyelonephritis.
  7. Right-sided basilar pneumonia (refer to Chapter 46, *Pneumonia, Community Acquired*).
  8. Diverticulitis.
- Evaluate for acute abdomen.
- Establish a peripheral intravenous line.
- Administer crystalloids at the maintenance rate.
- Labs: FBC; urea/electrolytes/creatinine; serum amylase; urinalysis; liver panel and hepatitis markers (optional); first blood and urine cultures if patient is septic.
- KUB; consider CXR and ECG.
- Analgesia: NSAIDs or antispasmodics.
- Keep the patient nil by mouth.
- **Disposition**: admit to General Surgery. Inform the GS medical officer or registrar if any delay is anticipated in the admission process.

Afebrile patient

- Bear in mind that the elderly patient with a surgical abdomen may not be able to mount a febrile response.
- Consider the following:
  1. Biliary colic (refer to Chapter 51, *Hepatobiliary Emergencies*).
  2. Referred pain from chest conditions.
  3. Hepatitis.
- Evaluate for acute abdomen.
- Labs: FBC; urea/electrolytes/creatinine; serum amylase; urinalysis; liver panel and hepatitis markers (optional).
- KUB; consider CXR and ECG.
- Analgesia: NSAIDs or antispasmodics IM.
- **Disposition**: can be discharged to follow-up in General Surgery if pain settles and abdomen remains benign; otherwise admit to General Surgery. If hepatitis is suspected, the patient can be referred to Gastroenterology.

DIFFERENTIAL DIAGNOSIS OF FLANK PAIN

- Consider the following:
  1. Pyelonephritis.
  2. Ureteric calculi with or without obstruction (refer to Chapter 64, *Urolithiasis*).
- Consider **abdominal aortic aneurysm (AAA)** if the patient is >50 years, or aortic dissection in patients with risk factors (refer to Chapter 34, *Aortic Emergencies*).

NOTE: Classically, an AAA presents with central abdominal pain penetrating to the back. However, a number of atypical presentations exist for ruptured AAA, contributing to a misdiagnosis rate of up to 30%. AAAs can rupture into the retroperitoneum where they may tamponade, enabling the patient to remain normotensive initially. Abdominal aortic dissection can cause haematuria, leading to potential misdiagnosis as nephrolithiasis.

Febrile patient

- Labs: FBC; urea/electrolytes/creatinine; blood cultures (at least 7.5 ml blood per bottle); urine cultures if urosepsis is suspected.
- KUB.
- Consider CXR and ECG.
- Intravenous antibiotics: coverage for Gram-negative organisms and for anaerobic organisms if a hepatobiliary or enteric source is suspected.
- Analgesics: NSAIDs or narcotics.
- **Disposition**:
  1. Admit to Urology for all complicated urolithiasis.
  2. Admit to General Medicine or Urology (depending on institutional practice) for acute pyelonephritis.

Afebrile patient

- Labs: urinalysis, looking for blood and/or white blood cells and positive nitrites.
- KUB to locate the ectopic calcification of a calculus and to assess kidney size.
- Analgesics: NSAIDs or narcotics.
- **Disposition**:
  1. Admit if there is inadequate pain relief in the ED **or** any hint of ureteric obstruction with infection. Inform the urology in-house team if any delay is anticipated in the admission process.
  2. Can be discharged to follow-up in Urology if the patient becomes pain-free and remains afebrile in the ED. Advise to return if the following occur:
     a. Fever develops.
     b. Gross haematuria appears.
     c. Urine output decreases.

DIFFERENTIAL DIAGNOSIS OF LOWER ABDOMINAL PAIN

- Always consider appendicitis (refer to Chapter 49, *Appendicitis Acute*) and ectopic pregnancy (refer to Chapter 109, *Ectopic Pregnancy*) as possibilities. Differentials include ovarian torsion and ruptured ovarian cyst in females.
- Rectal examination is useful in both men and women since, in the latter, the cervix and adnexae can be palpated without the stress of a vaginal examination.
- Labs:
  1. Mandatory: urine human chorionic gonadotrophin (HCG) in pregnancy-capable females, and urine dipstick testing.
  2. Optional: FBC, urea/electrolytes/creatinine.

DIFFERENTIAL DIAGNOSIS OF EPIGASTRIC PAIN

- Consider both abdominal and extra-abdominal causes. Suspect abdominal aortic aneurysm in patients >50 years old, especially if the pain radiates to the lower back or one flank.
  1. Other **intra-abdominal** causes include the following:
     a. Perforated peptic ulcer/acute exacerbation of peptic ulcer disease (refer to Chapter 55, *Peptic Ulcer Disease/Dyspepsia*).
     b. Reflux oesophagitis.
     c. Hepatobiliary sepsis. Patients may just present with epigastric discomfort with dyspepsia symptoms. Systemic symptoms like fever, chills, and vomiting may be absent if presentation is early.
     d. Penetrating posterior peptic ulcer.
     e. Pancreatitis (refer to Chapter 54, *Pancreatitis*).
     f. Aortic dissection/ruptured AAA (refer to Chapter 34, *Aortic Emergencies*).
     The latter three conditions are associated with radiation of pain to the lower back.
  2. **Extra-abdominal** causes include the following:
     a. Acute myocardial infarction: do ECG for all patients presenting with upper abdominal pain/dyspepsia (refer to Chapter 36, *Coronary Syndromes, Acute*).
     b. Pneumonia (refer to Chapter 46, *Pneumonia*).
     c. Pulmonary embolism (refer to Chapter 41, *Pulmonary Embolism*).
     d. Diabetic ketoacidosis: abdominal pain may well be the first presentation for DKA. Screen hypocount (refer to Chapter 60, *Diabetic Ketoacidosis*).
- Establish peripheral intravenous lines.
- Administer crystalloids at the maintenance rate.
- Labs: bedside blood sugar; FBC; serum amylase; urea/electrolytes/creatinine; cardiac enzymes if suspicious.
- Do ECG.

- Do erect CXR and KUB.
- Give adequate analgesia.
- Keep the patient nil by mouth.
- **Disposition**: the patient can be discharged to follow-up in General Surgery if pain settles, abdomen remains benign, and investigations are normal; otherwise admit to General Surgery.

DIFFERENTIAL DIAGNOSIS OF COLICKY CENTRAL ABDOMINAL PAIN

- The colicky nature of a pain generally indicates obstruction or irritation of a hollow viscus. Consider the following:
  1. Acute gastroenteritis (refer to Chapter 6, *Diarrhoea and Vomiting*).
  2. Intestinal obstruction in large or small bowel (refer to Chapter 52, *Intestinal Obstruction*).
  3. **Mesenteric ischaemia**: associated with high mortality and prompt diagnosis is crucial albeit often difficult. Sudden severe pain associated with minimal abdominal signs and forceful bowel evacuation in a patient with risk factors should greatly heighten suspicion for the diagnosis. Risk factors include advanced age, atherosclerosis, low cardiac output states, cardiac arrhythmias, especially atrial fibrillation, severe cardiac valvular disease, recent myocardial infarction, and intra-abdominal malignancy. (Refer to Chapter 53, *Ischaemic Bowel*.)

NOTE: **Adhesion colic** as a diagnosis probably does not exist since uncomplicated adhesions are not thought to cause pain. However, in the setting of a postoperative patient, an incomplete or subacute bowel obstruction due to adhesions can produce a typical colicky pain.

References/Further Reading

1. Davis MA. Abdominal pain. *J Emerg Med Acute Pri Care*. 2001; 5325(20): 5991–6247.
2. Kamin RA, Nowicki TA, Courtney DS, Powers RD. Pearls and pitfalls in the emergency department evaluation of abdominal pain. *Emerg Med Clin North Am*. 2003; 21: 61–72.
3. Hendrickson M, Naparst TR. Abdominal surgical emergencies in the elderly. *Emerg Med Clin North Am*. 2003; 21: 937–969.
4. Gallagher EJ, Esses D, Lee C, et al. Randomized clinical trial of morphine in acute abdominal pain. *Ann Emerg Med*. 2006; 48: 150–160.
5. Ranji SR, Goldman LE, Simel DL, Shojania KG. Do opiates affect the clinical evaluation of patients with acute abdominal pain? *JAMA*. 2006; 296: 1764–1774.
6. Pineg JM, Everett WM. *Evidence-based Emergency Care. Diagnostic Testing and Clinical Decision Rules*. Oxford: BMJ Books; 2008: 189–193.

14   Pain, Chest, Acute

Shirley Ooi

CAVEATS

- A **good history** remains the cornerstone of the **diagnosis** of life-threatening causes of chest pain (Table 1).
- After excluding the 6 life-threatening causes, the important but not life-threatening causes shown in Table 2 should then be excluded.

TABLE 1   Life-threatening causes of chest pain

Causes	Key clinical features
Acute myocardial infarction (AMI)	Refer to Chapter 36, *Coronary Syndromes, Acute*
Unstable angina (as it carries a similar short-term prognosis as AMI)	Refer to Chapter 36, *Coronary Syndromes, Acute*
Aortic dissection	Refer to Chapter 34, *Aortic Emergencies*
Pulmonary embolism (PE)	Refer to Chapter 41, *Pulmonary Embolism*
Tension pneumothorax	Refer to Chapter 94, *Trauma, Chest*
Oesophageal rupture (Boerhaave's syndrome)	Chest pain following violent vomiting and CXR showing pneumomediastinum

Note: AMI and unstable angina are also known as **acute coronary syndromes (ACS)**.

TABLE 2   Important but not life-threatening causes of chest pain

Cardiac	• Stable angina • Prinzmetal angina • Pericarditis/myocarditis
Respiratory	• Simple pneumothorax • Pneumonia with pleurisy
Gastrointestinal	• Reflux oesophagitis • Oesophageal spasm (this is often a diagnosis by exclusion as it mimics ischaemic chest pain very closely)
Referred pain	• Gastritis/peptic ulcer disease • Biliary disease • Subphrenic abscess/inflammation

- Note that **benign causes**, e.g. musculoskeletal pain, costochondritis, psychogenic chest pain, and early herpes zoster neuralgia, should be **diagnoses by exclusion**.

- Although a consensus exists about what represents a **typical ischaemic chest pain** (in 1768, Heberden described it as a painful sensation in the breast accompanied by a strangling sensation, anxiety, and occasional radiation of pain to the left arm, associated with exertion and relieved by rest), the equivalent definition of atypical chest pain is less clear.

- Panju et al. synthesized data on the clinical features of patients with symptoms suggestive of ACS from 14 studies representing >30,000 patients. Patients with pain radiating to the left arm, right shoulder, or both arms and diaphoresis were more likely to have an AMI. In fact, radiation to both the right and left arms had a likelihood ratio (LR) of 7.1 (95% CI, 3.6–14.2) compared to the left arm with an LR of 2.3 (95% CI, 1.7–3.1) and the right shoulder with an LR of 2.9 (95% CI 1.4–6.0). Patients with pain described as pleuritic, sharp or stabbing, positional, or reproduced with palpating had a decreased likelihood of having an AMI (LR of 0.2–0.3). However, because these data were extracted from large cohorts of patients that included those who were clinically unstable and those with diagnostic ECGs on presentation, the clinical utility is marginal in some patients.[6]

- A more problematic group of patients are those with an **intermediate likelihood** of ACS. Goodacre et al. studied 893 patients with intermediate probability of ACS. They excluded high-risk patients with ECG changes consistent with ischaemia or new left bundle branch block (LBBB), those with comorbidities such as heart failure or arrhythmia or a serious alternative pathology, and those with definite unstable angina. They also excluded those with minimal risk of coronary artery disease (CAD), such as those <25 years old or whose pain was related to recent trauma. Goodacre et al. showed that the **duration of pain and associated symptoms (nausea, vomiting, or diaphoresis) had no value** in the diagnosis of ACS. A **burning or indigestion type of pain was associated with an odds ratio (OR) of 4.0 for ACS**, while crushing pain was associated with an OR of 0.9 in these intermediate-risk patients. The presence of chest wall tenderness was associated with a reduced risk for AMI (OR of 0.2).[7]

- In the Multicenter Chest Pain Study (MCPS), chest discomfort that is similar to a prior MI or worse than the patient's usual angina remains the strongest independent risk factors for MI and the likelihood of acute coronary ischaemia.

- Note that **radiation of pain to both arms** is highly suggestive of AMI/ACS.

- Chest pain indicative of ACS is typically described as having a **crescendo pattern**, reaching maximal intensity after several minutes. In contrast, pain from aortic dissection is **maximal** and abrupt in onset.

- **Pain lasting for >30 minutes** is indicative of AMI or non-ischaemic pain.

- **Recurrent pain** that lasts for many hours or days with each episode is unlikely to be cardiac. Pain that lasts only seconds is rarely indicative of ischaemic chest pain.

- **Rest** characteristically relieves the pain associated with stable angina within 1–5 minutes. If pain continues for longer than 10 minutes after rest, the patient is experiencing unstable angina, an AMI, or non-cardiac chest pain.

- The following are risk factors for **painless AMI**:
  1. Prior heart failure.
  2. Prior stroke.
  3. Age >75 years.
  4. Diabetes mellitus.
  5. Non-white.
  6. Women.
- Chest pain is **pleuritic** or **exacerbated by movement** in 5–8% of patients with AMI.
- 5% of known cases of AMI have **concomitant chest wall tenderness**.
- The following 3 features together make **chest pain very unlikely** to be due to **cardiac ischaemia**:
  1. Chest pain is sharp or stabbing.
  2. No history of angina or MI.
  3. Pain is reproducible by palpating chest wall or has a positional or pleuritic component.
- The **associated symptoms**, i.e. diaphoresis, dyspnoea, and syncope, are seen in AMI, PE, and aortic dissection and so may not help differentiate among these diagnoses, but they are important clues that a serious illness is present. There is **no association** between AMI and relief of chest pain with **nitroglycerin**.
- A **GI cocktail** cannot be used to differentiate between cardiac and oesophageal pain.
- The **single best historical predictor** of ACS is a known history of **AMI** or known **CAD**. The risk of a coronary event is 5 times more likely in persons with established CAD.
- **Traditional risk factors** from the Framingham study (e.g. age, male gender, smoking, hypertension, diabetes mellitus, hypercholesterolaemia, family history) have been shown to be predictive of patients who will develop CAD over a 14-year period in an outpatient setting, but were never developed or intended to identify which chest pain patient in the ED suffered acute cardiac ischaemia. They have been shown to perform poorly in this setting. In fact, **no single specific risk factor** has the power to predict AMI or acute coronary ischaemia independently. Thus, the risk factor profile cannot be depended on in isolation to risk-stratify or to predict the presence of ischaemic heart disease in the ED.
- **New emerging risk factors for CAD** include systemic lupus erythematosus, rheumatoid arthritis, and HIV.
- Think of **aortic dissection** in any patient with chest pain suggestive of AMI but with **neurological** symptoms as well. (For further tips, refer to Chapter 34, *Aortic Emergencies*.)
- In chest pain, a normal ECG does not rule out ACS, but it places the patient at less risk of subsequent adverse events. Only 65–78% of ECGs of patients admitted are definite or probable in presenting MI. The key is to repeat serial ECGs.
- People **over the age of 65** are more likely to have atypical presentations with delayed or missed diagnoses.

- Do not assume that the standard CXR completely rules out **pneumothorax** as up to one third of pneumothoraces may be missed on initial CXR. In most cases, an upright inspiratory CXR is all that is required to diagnose pneumothorax. If pneumothorax is strongly suspected and a pleural line is not visualized, an expiratory CXR (although a randomized controlled trial revealed no difference between an expiratory and an inspiratory CXR for detecting pneumothoraces) or lateral decubitus CXR can be obtained.

- Antecedent retching or vomiting is absent in 21% of cases of **Boerhaave's syndrome**. Hence the diagnosis should not be excluded in the absence of this historical feature.

  NOTE: **Mackler's triad** (chest pain, vomiting and subcutaneous emphysema) occurs in only 14% of patients with Boerhaave's syndrome.

⇨ **SPECIAL TIPS FOR GPs**
- Refer all patients with the following to the ED:
  1. Typical history of AMI but a normal ECG.
  2. Atypical history but with risk factors for CAD.
- The **major risk factors for CAD** are as follows:
  1. Diabetes mellitus.
  2. Systemic hypertension.
  3. Hyperlipidaemia.
  4. Smoking.

NOTE: A patient who has stopped smoking for <2 years is considered to have smoking as a risk factor for CAD.

- Give aspirin 300 mg stat for all patients with acute coronary syndrome before sending them to the hospital.
- All cases of AMI should be sent by ambulance to the hospital.

MANAGEMENT

- Ensure vital signs are stable. If unstable, and the patient is in distress and diaphoretic, bring the patient to the resuscitation area immediately. Attend to patients with obvious acute coronary syndrome immediately.

- Put the patient on oxygen supplementation, pulse oximetry, continuous ECG monitoring, and blood pressure monitoring.

- Do an immediate 12-lead ECG. The **role of ECG** in chest pain includes diagnosis of AMI, ischaemia, and PE.

- If the ECG is normal or suspicious but non-confirmatory of acute coronary syndrome, repeat serial ECGs at close intervals.

- Set up an IV plug and take blood tests for cardiac enzymes and other biomarkers, e.g. myoglobin and troponin T.

Table 3   **Cardiac markers**

Cardiac markers	Release kinetics			Advantages
	Detected within	Peak levels	Normalized by	
Myoglobin	1–2 hours	6–9 hours	24–36 hours	1. Earliest marker to rise in AMI 2. Useful in ruling out AMI early as myoglobin is raised in nearly all AMI at 6 hours
Creatine kinase–MB (CK-MB)	4–6 hours	18–24 hours	48–72 hours	1. Serologic gold standard of AMI, used in the World Health Organization's criteria for diagnosis of AMI

Troponin T and I	4–6 hours (standard)
	2–3 hours (high sensitivity)
		12–120 hours (standard)
		Peaked much earlier for the high-sensitivity assays
			10–14 days	1. The most widely used cardio-specific marker but not necessarily due to MI.
				2. By 2–3 hours after onset of AMI, up to 80% of AMI will have troponin elevations in the high-sensitivity assays. Hence the high-sensitivity assays are useful to rule out NSTEMI.
				3. Other causes of raised troponins include:
				  a. Acute cardiopulmonary condition, e.g. pulmonary embolism (PE) (*NOTE:* The troponin elevation in PE is more modest and resolves within 40 hours), myocarditis, heart failure, and tachy- or bradydysrhythmias
				  b. Non-cardiopulmonary condition, e.g. renal failure, sepsis
				  NOTE: The 2007 joint ESC/ACCF/AHA/COHF task force recommends that an elevated value of cardiac troponin, in the absence of clinical evidence of ischaemia, should prompt a search for other causes of myocardial necrosis.

T_0 = time of presentation; T_s = serial biomarkers.

NOTE: The new high-sensitivity troponins T and I have a diagnostic accuracy of up to 92% at 3 hours! These newer, more sensitive troponin assays will allow earlier detection (or exclusion) of MI, but whether they will improve patient outcomes remains to be seen as the specificity has decreased. Undetectable hs-cTnT at presentation has 100% sensitivity for ruling out AMI.

Disadvantages	Sensitivity (%) for diagnosis of AMI (95% CI)	Specificity (%) for diagnosis of AMI (95% CI)

1. Not specific for cardiac muscle. Other conditions associated with raised myoglobin include the following:
  a. Skeletal muscle or neuromuscular disorders
  b. Renal failure
  c. Intramuscular injections
  d. Strenuous exercise
  e. Postcoronary bypass surgery
  f. Heavy use of ethanol
Hence myoglobin should not be used alone but with another more cardiac-specific marker
	T_0 49 (43–55)
	T_s 89 (80–94)
		T_0 91 (87–94)
		T_s 87 (80–92)

1. Not specific for cardiac muscle 2. May be falsely elevated in renal failure patients 3. Narrow diagnostic window 4. Failure of total CK to rise to abnormal values in all AMI. To improve the sensitivity and specificity, the **relative %** **index** defined as $$\frac{\textbf{CK–MB (ng/ml)}}{\textbf{CK (U/L)}} \times \textbf{100\%}$$ is used. ≥5% is suggestive of AMI	T_0 42 (36–48) T_s 79 (71–86)	T_0 97 (95–98) T_s 96 (95–97)
	T_0 39 (26–53) T_s 93 (85–97) (for standard troponins)	T_0 93 (90–96) T_s 85 (76–91) (for standard troponins) *NOTE:* The sensitivity in high-sensitivity troponins are much better at T_0 but the specificity is reduced.

NOTE: Do not get a false sense of security in excluding ischaemic chest pain from normal troponin T/cardiac enzymes upon presentation at the ED. See Table 3 for a proper interpretation of the various cardiac markers.

- Give pain relief depending on provisional diagnosis.
- Do chest X-ray. The **role of CXR** in chest pain includes diagnosis of the following:
  1. Complications of AMI, e.g. heart failure and pulmonary oedema.
  2. Aortic dissection.
  3. Respiratory causes, e.g. pneumothorax, pneumonia, lung malignancy, and rib fractures.
  4. Peripheral PE.
  5. Pneumomediastinum, e.g. spontaneous rupture of lung bullae and oesophageal rupture.
- Some guidelines about the **disposition** of patients with chest pain:
  1. Admit acute coronary syndromes with ECG changes or continuing pain to the **coronary care unit**.
  2. Admit unstable angina with no ECG changes, or if the pain has subsided, to the **cardiology general ward**.
  3. Admit patients with a diagnosis of atypical chest pain syndrome with risk factors for CAD to the **cardiology general ward** unless your ED has a chest pain observation unit for further work-up of the patient.
  4. Stable angina can be discharged with medications started (aspirin 300 mg stat and then cardiprin 100 mg OM, isosorbide dinitrate 5–10 mg tds, propranolol 20 mg bd), provided there are no contraindications, and referred to the cardiology specialist clinics. (However, this group of patients is probably not common as patients with CAD would not have presented to the ED if the history is that of their usual stable angina. Hence, it is advisable to admit all chest pain patients with a known history of CAD.)
  5. Admit patients with aortic dissection to the cardiothoracic ICU.

NOTE: Recent-onset angina that appears to be stable from history is considered unstable angina. Hence, all **new-onset angina** should be **admitted** to the hospital, even if the ECG is normal.

- For treatment of the first five life-threatening causes, please refer to the individual chapters in Section 2.

References/Further Reading

1. Wu AHB, ed. *Cardiac Markers*. Totowa, NJ: Humana Press; 1998: 104–107, 120–121, 205–209, 231–235, 237–239.
2. Balk EM, Joannidis JP, Salem D, et al. Accuracy of biomarkers to diagnose acute cardiac ischemia in the emergency department: A meta-analysis. *Ann Emerg Med*. 2001; 37(5): 478–494.
3. Wilkinson K, Severance H. Identification of chest pain patients appropriate for an emergency department observation unit. *Emerg Med Clin North Am*. 2001; 19(1): 37–40.

4. Lee TH, Juarez G, Cook EF, et al. Ruling out acute myocardial infarction. A prospective multicenter validation of a 12-hour strategy for patients at low risk. *N Engl J Med*. 1991; 324: 1239–1246.

5. Clifford JS, Nagurney JT. Value and limitations of chest pain history in the evaluation of patients with suspected acute coronary syndromes. *JAMA*. 2005; 294(20): 2623–2629.

6. Panju AA, Hemmelgarn BR, Guyatt GH, et al. The rational clinical examination. Is this patient having a myocardial infarction? *JAMA*. 1998; 280(14): 1256–1263.

7. Goodacre S, Locker T, Morris F, et al. How useful are clinical features in the diagnosis of acute undifferentiated chest pain? *Acad Emerg Med*. 2002; 9(3): 203–208.

8. Lee TH, Cook EF, Weisberg MC, et al. Acute chest pain in the emergency room. Identification and examination of low risk patients. *Arch Intern Med*. 1985; 145: 85–89.

9. Canto JG, Shlipak MG, Rogers WJ, et al. Prevalence, clinical characteristics, and mortality among patients with myocardial infarction presenting without chest pain. *JAMA*. 2000; 283: 3223–3229.

10. Winters ME, Katzen SM. Identifying chest pain emergencies in the primary care setting. *Prim Care Clin Office Pract*. 2006; 33: 625–642.

11. Seow A, Kazerroni EA, Pernicano PG, et al. Comparison of upright inspiratory and expiratory chest radiographs for detecting pneumothoraces. *Am J Roentgenol*. 1997; 168: 842–843.

12. Reichlin T, Hochholzer W, Bassetti S, et al. Early diagnosis of myocardial infarction with sensitive cardiac troponin assays. *N Engl J Med*. 2009; 361: 858–867.

13. Body R, Carley S, McDowell G, et al. Rapid exclusion of acute myocardial infarction in patients with undetectable troponin using a high-sensitivity assay. *J Am Coll Cardiol*. 2011; 58(13): 1333–1339.

14. Than M, Cullen L, Reid CM, et al. A 2-h diagnostic protocol to assess patients with chest pain symptoms in the Asia-Pacific region (ASPECT): A prospective observational validation study. *Lancet*. 2011; 377: 1077–1084.

15. Thygesen K, Alpert JS, White HD, Joint ESC/ACCF/AHA/WHF Task Force for the Redefinition of Myocardial Infarction. Universal definition of myocardial infarction. *Eur Heart J* 2007; 28; 2525

15   Pain, Joint, Peripheral

Keith Ho • Shirley Ooi

CAVEATS

- **Septic arthritis** is a surgical emergency that threatens life and limb. It is a feared diagnosis in monoarticular arthritis. Missing the diagnosis can result in the development of osteomyelitis, cartilage destruction and subsequent joint displacement or generalised sepsis.
- In the sexually active population, **gonococcal arthritis** must always be considered, especially in pregnant or menstruating women and/or patients with a complement deficiency.

APPROACH TO DIAGNOSIS

- Distinguish between articular and periarticular joint pain (see Table 1).
    1. **Articular pain** involves the entire joint capsule. It is associated with painful and decreased range of movement in all planes of movement. There is joint line tenderness and an effusion is usually present.
    2. **Periarticular pain** involves the structures surrounding the joint capsule. It is usually exacerbated with movement involving the affected muscles or tendons.
- Distinguish between inflammatory and non-inflammatory joint disorders:
    1. **Inflammatory joint disorders** usually present with morning stiffness for >30 minutes and relief of symptoms with exercise. The hallmark of inflammatory arthropathy is synovitis, which is appreciated clinically as a spongy swelling around the joint. Arthrocentesis will reveal a synovial fluid white blood cell count of >2000/mm^3.
    2. **Non-inflammatory joint disorders** present with limited morning stiffness, increasing pain with movement/weight-bearing, and relief with rest.

TABLE 1   Differential diagnosis of joint pain: anatomical classification

Articular		Periarticular
Monoarticular	**Polyarticular**	**Periarticular**
Osteoarthritis	Rheumatoid arthritis	Bursitis
Infection/septic arthritis	Systemic lupus erythematosus	Cellulitis
Crystal-induced gout, pseudogout	Seronegative spondyloarthropathies	Fasciitis
Neoplasm	Viral arthritis	Tendinitis
Trauma/haemarthrosis	Rheumatic fever	Ligament injury
Avascular necrosis	Lyme disease	Epicondylitis
	Drug-induced	

TABLE 2 Differential diagnosis of joint pain: inflammatory vs non-inflammatory

Inflammatory	Non-inflammatory

• Infection
  1. Septic arthritis
  2. Disseminated gonorrhoea
  3. Mycobacteria
  4. Fungal
  5. Viral
  6. Lyme arthritis
  7. Endocarditis
	• Osteoarthritis

• Crystals
  1. Monosodium urate
  2. Calcium pyrophosphate
  3. Hydroxyapatite
	• Osteonecrosis

• Autoimmune diseases
  1. Rheumatoid arthritis
  2. Juvenile chronic arthritis
  3. Systemic lupus erythematosus
  4. Sarcoidosis
  5. Scleroderma
  6. Polymyositis/dermatomyositis
  7. Ankylosing spondylitis
  8. Reiter's syndrome
  9. Psoriatic arthritis
	• Neoplasm

- The presence of trauma merits the consideration of fracture, or internal derangement, especially if the patient has osteoporosis.

INVESTIGATIONS

- **Laboratory**:

NOTE: Serum blood testing is only of modest utility in the ED workup of monoarticular arthritis.

1. **FBC**: elevated total white blood cell count with a left shift may point towards septic arthritis, but has poor sensitivity and specificity.
2. **ESR** and **C-reactive protein**: non-sensitive and non-specific acute-phase reactants that are elevated in inflammatory states, infection, and malignancy.
3. **Uric acid**: not useful as patients with acute gouty arthritis often have normal uric acid levels.
4. **Rheumatoid factor**, **antinuclear antibody**, and **HLA-B27**: useful for follow-up, but have no role in the acute ED setting.
5. **Blood cultures** are positive in up to 50% of *Staphylococcus aureus* infections.

- **Radiology**

NOTE: There is little evidence to support the utility of obtaining X-rays in acute monoarthritis in the ED.

1. X-rays are indicated if there is significant trauma, or focal bone tenderness. Look for fractures, tumours, chondrocalcinosis (pseudogout), cortical erosions (septic arthritis), and osteophytes/joint space narrowing (osteoarthritis).

- **Arthrocentesis** facilitates diagnosis and may be therapeutic.
  1. **Indications**:
     a. Synovial fluid analysis.
     b. Draining tense effusions or haemarthrosis for analgesia.
     c. Instilling analgesic, anti-inflammatory medications.
  2. **Contraindications**:
     a. Infection (cellulitis/abscess) overlying the puncture site.
     b. Bleeding diathesis.
     c. Prosthetic joint.
  3. Send off the synovial fluid for analysis, Gram staining, and culture. This will help differentiate between septic arthritis, inflammatory, and non-inflammatory processes (see Table 3).

TABLE 3   Interpretation of Arthrocentesis

	Non-inflammatory Processes	Inflammatory Processes	Septic Arthritis
Colour	Clear	Yellow/white	Cloudy
Synovial Glucose		Non-specific	
Synovial Protein		Non-specific	
Synovial WBC	<25000/mm^3		>25000/mm^3
Synovial Lactate	<5.6 mmol/L	<5.6 mmol/L	>5.6 mmol/L
Synovial LDH	<250 U/L	<250 U/L	>250 U/L
Culture	Negative	Negative	Positive

Adapted from *Emergency Medicine Practice* May 2012 Volume 14, Number 5.[3]

SEPTIC ARTHRITIS

- **Predisposing factors**:
  1. Recent joint surgery.
  2. Age >80 years.

3. Prosthetic joint.

4. Skin infection.

5. Diabetes mellitus.

6. Rheumatoid arthritis.

7. IV drug abuse.

8. Alcoholism.

9. Immunocompromised states.

10. Low socioeconomic status.

- **Microbiology**:

  1. *Staphylococcus aureus* and streptococci are commonly implicated.

  2. Gram-negative bacilli are more often present after trauma, in intravenous drug users, neonates, the elderly, and patients with major immune deficiency.

- Monoarticular arthritis occurs in around 80% of cases. The knee is involved in the majority of cases. Other common sites include the wrists, ankles, and hips.

- Oligoarticular or polyarticular arthritis occurs in 20% of infections. Predisposing factors include patients with systemic connective tissue disease (e.g. rheumatoid arthritis) and patients with overwhelming sepsis.

- **Clinical presentation**:

  1. Swollen and painful joint, usually in a large joint.

  2. Fever (sensitivity 44–97%).

  3. Chills and spiking fevers are uncommon.

NOTE: Decreased range of motion of tenderness does not have sufficient evidence prognostically.

- **Investigations**:

  1. **Synovial fluid aspiration** should be performed as the definitive diagnostic test is identification of bacteria in the synovial fluid. The gold standard for diagnosis of a septic joint is a positive culture of synovial fluid—but this takes days! In the ED, the most important tests to send are Gram stain (50%–80% yield) and aerobic and anaerobic culture of the synovial fluid.

  2. **Blood cultures** are positive in 50% of patients with septic arthritis.

  3. **X-rays** of the affected joint are usually normal. Look for associated osteomyelitis or concurrent joint disease.

- **Management**:

  1. Pain relief.

  2. Empirical IV antibiotics: IV cloxacillin 2 g q6 hours or IV cefazolin 1–2 g q8 hours.

  3. There is no benefit to intra-articular antibiotic injection as most antibiotics penetrate the joint fluid well.

  4. Drainage of the septic joint via needle aspiration, arthroscopic drainage, or arthrotomy.

DISSEMINATED GONOCOCCAL INFECTION (DGI)

- Patients may **present** with the following syndromes:
  1. A triad of tenosynovitis, dermatitis, and migratory polyarthralgias without purulent arthritis. Joints affected are usually wrist, knee or ankle.
  2. Purulent arthritis without associated skin lesions.
- **History**:
  1. A history of recent sexual activity can usually be elicited in most patients.
  2. Genitourinary symptoms are present in only 25% of cases.
- **Examination**:
  1. Dermatitis typically consists of painless lesions that often are few in number. Lesions are usually pustular or vesiculopustular.
  2. Tenosynovitis often affects multiple tendons.
- **Investigations**:
  1. Synovial fluid analysis.
  2. 2 sets of blood cultures should be obtained from all patients with suspected DGI.
  3. Consider synovial, skin, urethral, or cervical cultures, and rectal cultures with Thayer-Martin media.
- Most patients with DGI respond dramatically and quickly to antimicrobial therapy:
  1. IV/IM ceftriaxone 2 g om, **or**
  2. PO ciprofloxacin 500 mg bd, **or**
  3. PO amoxicillin 500 mg qds.
  4. Treat possible concomitant chlamydia infection with PO doxycycline 100 mg bd for 7 days. Substitute doxycycline with erythromycin if the patient is pregnant.

GOUTY ARTHRITIS

- **Risk factors for gout**
  1. Hypertension.
  2. Diabetes.
  3. Obesity.
  4. Thiazide diuretic use.
  5. Cyclosporine use.
  6. Lead or radiocontrast exposure.
  7. Alcohol, purine rich diet (e.g. meat, seafood, legumes, dairy and coffee).
  8. Illness
  9. Trauma or major surgery.

- **Clinical presentation:**
  1. The majority of cases (up to 75%) involve the first metatarso-phalangeal joint (**podagra**). Other joints involved include the knee, ankle and tarsal joints.
  2. 20% of patients will have involvement of >1 joint.
  3. Patients may present with joint pain, bursitis and tenosynovitis.
- **Diagnosis**:
  1. Serum uric acid does not aid in the diagnosis of acute gout.
  2. The diagnosis of gout is made with the finding of **intracellular negatively birefringent crystals** in the synovial fluid, in the absence of organisms.
- **Management**:
  1. **NSAIDs** or **COX-2 selective inhibitors** may be used for analgesia.
  2. **Colchicine** can be given in the classical high dose of 1.2 mg PO followed by 0.6 mg/hour for 6 hours.
  3. However, the newer low-dose regimen of colchicine 1.2 mg PO followed by 0.6 mg 1 hour later has fewer side effects.
     a. Side effects include nausea, vomiting and diarrhoea.
     b. Colchicine is contraindicated in hepatic and renal impairment and is not removed by dialysis.
  4. **Steroids** can be considered for patients with contraindications to NSAIDs or colchicines.
  5. **Allopurinol** is useful in the management of chronic gout to decrease gout flares. However, there is no data about the appropriateness of their institution from the ED in the setting of an acute flare though it is generally recommended that uric acid-lowering agents should not be discontinued if the patient is already on a prophylactic regimen.
  6. Look for potential precipitants and give appropriate advice.
  7. Rest, ice and elevation can be used in conjunction with medication for pain relief.

References/Further Reading

1. Burton JH. Acute disorders of the joints and bursae. In: Tintinalli JE, Stapczynski JS, Ma OJ, et al., eds. *Tintinalli's Emergency Medicine: A Comprehensive Study Guide*. 7th ed. New York: McGraw-Hill; 2011: 1926–1932.

2. American College of Rheumatology Subcommittee on Rheumatoid Arthritis Guidelines. Guidelines for the management of rheumatoid arthritis: 2002 update. *Arthritis Rheum.* 2002; 46(2): 328–346.

3. Genes N, Chisolm-Straker M. Monoarticular arthritis update: Current evidence for diagnosis and treatment in the emergency department. *Emerg Med Pract.* 2012 May; 14(5): 1–19; quiz 19–20.

16 Pain, Low Back

Peter Manning • Lim Er Luen

CAVEATS

- Patients with acute low back pain (LBP) who require immediate care on arrival are those with the following:
  1. Haemodynamic instability (the most critical group).
  2. Significant trauma.
  3. Incapacitating musculoskeletal pain (pain score ≥7).
- Patients with concomitant back and abdominal pain are at risk for serious intra-abdominal or retroperitoneal bleeding and require prompt evaluation and close monitoring.
- Patients in severe distress from musculoskeletal back pain with stable vital signs can be safely and appropriately given potent analgesics after preliminary evaluation.
- Patients with progressive neurologic deficits or with bladder or bowel dysfunction require prompt surgical decompression.
- The **indications for plain lumbosacral spine X-rays** in the ED are few:
  1. A history of significant trauma to the spine (or relatively minor trauma in the elderly).
  2. Presentation suggests malignancy with possible metastasis to the lumbar spine.
  3. Fever and localized tenderness suggest osteomyelitis.
- However, if metastases or infectious aetiologies are strongly considered, X-rays may still be insensitive and the imaging of choice is magnetic resonance imaging (MRI).
- **Conservative treatment** is the mainstay of back pain **management** and consists of muscle relaxation facilitated by adequate analgesia, muscle-relaxing medications, and heat or ice packs. 90% of patients respond to such treatment. Patients should be encouraged to move around as tolerated but avoid heavy lifting. Strict bed rest is not recommended.
- Outpatient management is the norm, with admission usually reserved for patients with neurologic deficits or intractable pain.

CATASTROPHIC ILLNESSES

The following can present as LBP:

- **Ruptured abdominal aortic aneurysm (AAA)**: usually a middle-aged or elderly male patient with a history of hypertension and cardiovascular disease, who presents with LBP and abdominal pain combined with a rapid pulse, syncope, and borderline or actual hypotension. <20% of patients with a rupturing aneurysm present with the triad of abdominal pain, hypotension, and a pulsatile abdominal mass. Abdominal palpation is insensitive for detecting an AAA.

- **Aortic dissection**: consider this diagnosis in a middle-aged or elderly patient, especially with risk factors such as Marfan's syndrome or absent lower limb pulses.
- **Ruptured ectopic pregnancy**: a pregnancy-capable female with a history of risk factors for ectopic pregnancy, presenting with acute onset of LBP, associated vaginal bleeding, syncope, and unilateral abdominal pain.
- **Epidural compression syndrome**: an uncommon but very serious emergency, encompassing spinal cord compression, conus medullaris syndrome, and cauda equina syndrome. Aetiologies include a herniated disc, tumour or metastasis, epidural abscess, or epidural haematoma. The patient typically presents with LBP, unilateral or bilateral radiation, perineal anaesthesia, motor weakness of the lower extremities, and sphincter dysfunction (urinary retention typically precedes urinary or bowel incontinence). MRI may be the only imaging modality to confirm the diagnosis. Classically, surgical intervention within 6 hours of onset of the symptoms is considered essential to prevent permanent paralysis and bladder dysfunction.

> ⇨ **SPECIAL TIPS FOR GPs**
> - Patients presenting with musculoskeletal pain and stable vital signs may be treated with analgesics in the first instance. Severe pain with no response to medication should be referred to the ED or an orthopaedic specialist as soon as possible.
> - Back pain with neurological signs of bowel/bladder dysfunction is a surgical emergency and must be referred to the hospital immediately.
> - Always do an abdominal examination and palpate gently for aortic aneurysm.

MANAGEMENT

Patients with haemodynamic instability and/or history of significant trauma

- The patient must be managed in the critical care area.
- Intubation and resuscitation equipment must be immediately available.
- Provide supplemental high-flow oxygen via a reservoir mask.
- Establish at least 2 large-bore IV lines.
- Administer IV Hartmann's solution 1 L stat and reassess parameters.
- Administer type-specific blood if necessary.
- Labs: GXM 4–6 units, FBC, urea/electrolytes/creatinine, and urine HCG where relevant.
- Monitoring: ECG, vital signs q 5–10 minutes, and pulse oximetry.
- Bedside ultrasound to image the aorta and look for free fluid in the abdomen. (Refer to Chapter 118, *Emergency Ultrasound*).

- **Disposition**
  1. Early consultation with Cardiothoracic Surgery (for suspected AAA), **or**
  2. General Surgery and Orthopaedics (in cases of trauma), **or**
  3. Obstetrics and Gynaecology (in case of ruptured ectopic pregnancy).

Patients with severe, incapacitating musculoskeletal pain

- Must be managed in at least the intermediate care area and evaluated promptly.
- Reassure the patient and move him/her carefully.
- Monitor vital signs q 30–60 minutes.
- Analgesia:
  1. Voltaren® (diclofenac) dosage: 50–75 mg IM.
  2. Tramal® (tramadone) dosage: 50–75 mg IM or IV.
  3. Pethidine® (meperidine) dosage: 50–100 mg IM or IV.
- Muscle relaxation: Valium® (diazepam) dosage: 5–10 mg PO or 2–5 mg IV (must be in a monitored area if given via the IV route).
- Reassess after 1 hour and attempt thorough examination with the patient in four positions: standing, supine, prone, and sitting.
- Perform the **straight leg raising test**. A straight leg raise (SLR) is positive when there is pain in the posterior lateral aspect of the leg radiating below the knee with the patient lying supine and the hip flexed 60 degrees or less.
- Ask for urinary symptoms. If urinary retention is present, catheterize the patient and obtain a postvoid residual urine measurement.
- Perform rectal examination and assess anal tone.
- Assess for perianal sensory loss.
- Consider plain X-ray of the lumbosacral spine.
- **Disposition**
  1. **Uncomplicated cases**: discharge home for bed rest on a firm surface with adequate analgesics and muscle relaxants.
  2. **Complicated and in severe pain ± mild neurological changes and no symptoms of sphincter dysfunction**: admit to Orthopaedics for traction and pain management. If a short-stay ward is available, patients may also be admitted there for continued pain management and physiotherapy.
  3. If **spinal cord compression** or **cauda equina syndrome** is suspected, then consult Neurosurgery or Orthopaedics stat.
  4. Other patients to be **admitted** include the following:
     a. Those with infections who may require IV antibiotic therapy, e.g. pyelonephritis and prostatitis.

b. Those with lumbar spine compression fractures for pain management.

c. Those with transverse process fractures for evaluation of associated injuries.

d. Those with intractable pain who are unable to walk or care for themselves.

e. Those with suspected metastases to the spine as they may require IV dexamethasone to be started early (refer to Chapter 78, *Oncology Emergencies*).

References/Further Reading

1. Winters ME. Management of patients with acute back pain in the ED. In: Mattu A, Goyal D, eds. *Emergency Medicine: Avoiding the Pitfalls and Improving the Outcomes.* Malden, MA: Blackwell Publishing; 2007: 33–38.

2. Bitterman RA. Non-traumatic low back pain: Avoiding liability for missed cord compression. *ED Legal Letter.* 2008; 19: 85–96.

17   Pain, Scrotal and Penile

Brandon Koh • Peter Manning

CAVEATS

- The aetiology of an acute scrotum can usually be ascertained by history, physical examination, and urinalysis.
- Never diagnose epididymitis in a teenage boy with scrotal pain. It is testicular torsion until proven otherwise.
- When in doubt regarding the cause of acute scrotal pain, seek a urology consultation.

⇨ **SPECIAL TIPS FOR GPs**
- Always consider **torsion of the spermatic cord** as a possible diagnosis in every patient who presents with scrotal pain, whether continuous or intermittent.
- Remember that the testis can torse and detorse spontaneously.

ACUTE SCROTAL PAIN IN NEWBORNS

Torsion

- The likeliest cause is torsion due to breech delivery.
- Involves twisting of the **whole** spermatic cord (unfixed newly descended testis).
- Presents late:
  1. Almost all are necrotic.
  2. Low salvage rate.
- Pain and tenderness **are not** prominent features.
- The scrotum is usually red and swollen, with a palpable hard testicular mass.
- Surgery is almost always required to excise the damaged testis.

Trauma

- Usually affects both sides.
- Prominent cutaneous bruising.
- Most resolve but should be followed up.
- Spontaneous idiopathic scrotal haemorrhage; look for separate bruise over superficial ring.

ACUTE SCROTAL PAIN IN TODDLERS

- The least commonly affected age group.
- **Acute epididymo-orchitis** is the commonest cause:
  1. Some cases are viral but most are caused by *Escherichia coli*.
  2. Perform urinalysis to look for pyuna.
  3. Admit for the following:
     a. **Exclusion of torsion**.
     b. Thorough investigation of the urinary tract for congenital abnormalities.
- **Idiopathic scrotal oedema**:
  1. Sudden bilateral scrotal swelling with erythema.
  2. Painless.
  3. Associated with haemolytic *Streptococcus*, Henoch–Schöenlein purpura, and, rarely, acute leukaemia.

ACUTE SCROTAL PAIN IN ADOLESCENTS/ADULTS

- This age group has the highest incidence of acute scrotal pathology.

Testicular torsion

- Remember that '**Time is testicle**'.
- No single element of the history can reliably distinguish testicular torsion.
- Peak incidence is bimodal:
  1. First peak: neonates.
  2. Second peak: in puberty, between 12 and 18 years of age.

Symptoms

- The classic symptoms are as follows:
  1. **Sudden onset** of severe testicular pain which may radiate to the groin or lower abdomen.
  2. Often associated with nausea and vomiting.
- Almost half of patients with torsion have had a previous episode of similar pain which resolved spontaneously.

Signs

- There are **no specific clinical signs to differentiate torsion from epididymitis** (both may present with enlarged, tender testes).

- Signs suggestive of testicular torsion:
  1. **Horizontal lie**.
  2. **High position** in the scrotum.
  3. Enlarged, diffusely tender testis.
  4. Thickened spermatic cord.
  5. **Absence of the cremasteric reflex**:
     a. Highly sensitive for torsion.
     b. However, the presence of this reflex does **not** always exclude torsion.
- **Prehn's sign**: elevation of the scrotum relieves the pain in epididymitis, but not in torsion. However, it is **unreliable**.
- Torsion is a **clinical diagnosis**. Urinalysis has limited value. Patients with torsion may have pyuria.

Management

- **Immediate** urology consultation if torsion is suspected or cannot be ruled out.
- Colour Doppler ultrasound (in equivocal cases) is useful if available immediately, but it **must not** delay definitive care. In torsion, decreased or absent blood flow compared with the contralateral testis confirms the diagnosis.
- Surgical exploration is mandatory if the diagnosis is in doubt.
- Testicular salvage depends on the time between the onset of symptoms and surgery (**6–10 hours** is generally the accepted time interval). Salvage rates of 80–100% are possible if the pain has lasted <6 hours. After 10 hours, the salvage rate drops to around 20%.
- Manual detorsion can be performed to buy time. Procedural sedation may be required. Untwist the testis outward, in the direction of the ipsilateral thigh (akin to 'opening a book'). Successful detorsion will result in relief of the pain. Worsening of the pain indicates that detorsion should be done in the opposite direction. Even with successful detorsion, urgent scrotal exploration is still required.

Torsion of the appendix testis

- Occurs principally in prepubertal boys.
- Pain is less acute and may appear over 2–3 days.
- Tenderness is localized to the upper part of the testis.
- Patients often have a reactive hydrocoele and examination reveals a torsed and necrotic appendix testis ('**blue dot sign**'). This sign is usually visible at the early stage only. It is eventually obscured by erythema and oedema of the overlying scrotal skin.
- Doppler ultrasonography is required for diagnosis. It will demonstrate normal or increased blood flow.

- Treatment is supportive: analgesia and scrotal support.
- Most torsed appendages will calcify or degenerate in 10–14 days.

Epididymitis

- Inflammation of the epididymis, usually due to infection (most often bacterial).
- Predominantly a disease of adult men.
- Ask about sexual history.
- In heterosexual young men, it is most commonly caused by *Chlamydia trachomatis* and *Neisseria gonorrhoeae*.
- In homosexual young men, and men >35 years old, the most common organisms are coliforms, *Pseudomonas*, and Gram-positive cocci.

Symptoms

- Pain usually develops over hours to days.
- Irritative voiding symptoms are prominent.
- Urethral discharge is common.

Signs

- Initially, tenderness is localized to the epididymis.
- As infection spreads, it involves the testis, resulting in epididymo-orchitis, and generalized testicular tenderness.
- **Normal lie**.
- The **cremasteric reflex is typically present**.
- Fever.

Investigations

- Presence of pyuria on urinalysis, but not always.
- Doppler ultrasonography: normal or increased blood flow.

Management

- For **suspected sexually transmitted disease**:
  1. Single-dose IM ceftriaxone 250 mg **and**
  2. Doxycycline 100 mg bd for 10 days.
- For **suspected coliforms (homosexuals, men >35 years old)**:
  1. Ciprofloxacin 500 mg bd for 14 days **or**
  2. Ofloxacin 400 mg bd for 14 days.

- Analgesia.
- Scrotal support.
- Arrange a follow-up at the Urology SOC or Department of STI Control (DSC).
- Admit to Urology the following:
  1. Patients who have severe sepsis as a result of the infection, or who have not responded to outpatient treatment.
  2. Patients with scrotal abscesses.

Testicular tumours

- May present as acute pain in the scrotum due to intratumoral bleeding and capsular extension with associated inflammation.
- May mimic epididymo-orchitis.
- Arrange early review in the Urology SOC.

Fournier's gangrene

- Necrotizing fasciitis of the scrotum and perineum.
- A potentially life-threatening disease.
- Typically found in debilitated or immunocompromised patients, especially in diabetics and alcoholics.
- Usually originates from a colorectal or genitourinary source.
- Typically polymicrobial. Both aerobes and anaerobes are usually present, e.g. *E. coli*, *Bacteroides*, *Streptococcus*, and *Clostridium*.
- Prominent clinical features include the following:
  1. Scrotal pain.
  2. Fever.
  3. Perineal erythema, tenderness, induration, and crepitus.
  4. Early signs of systemic toxicity.
- Resuscitate with IV fluids, and vasopressors if necessary (if there is septic shock).
- **Broad-spectrum antibiotics** (after blood cultures have been drawn), depending on institutional practice. An example of a multi-drug regimen is as follows:
  1. IV ceftazidime (Fortum®) 2 g **and**
  2. IV clindamycin 600 mg **and**
  3. IV gentamicin 3 mg/kg.

  NOTE: Antibiotics are only an adjunct to surgical debridement.

- Immediate urology consultation for the following:
  1. To arrange for **emergency surgical debridement**.
  2. Admission to Surgical HD/ICU.

Other causes of acute scrotal pain

- Incarcerated/strangulated inguinal hernia.
- Henoch–Schönlein purpura (in children).
- Appendicitis: don't forget to examine the abdomen!
- Ruptured/leaking abdominal aortic aneurysm.

PENILE EMERGENCIES

Balanoposthitis

- An inflammation of the glans penis (balanitis) and the foreskin (posthitis).
- If recurrent, consider the presence of diabetes mellitus.
- Causes include the following:
  1. Poor foreskin hygiene.
  2. Sexually transmitted disease.
  3. Trauma.
- Retraction of the foreskin reveals foul-smelling, purulent material and the glans is red, swollen, and tender to palpation.

Management

- Good hygiene.
- 0.5% hydrocortisone cream.
- Topical antifungal cream (if candidal infection is suspected).
- If secondary infection is present, give broad-spectrum antibiotics, e.g. ciprofloxacin 500 mg bd PO for 7 days. If sexually transmitted disease is suspected, doxycycline 100 mg bd PO for 14 days can be added.
- Consider referral for circumcision in recurrent cases, or where there is phimosis.
- Be aware of the possibility of child abuse.
- Referral to Urology SOC.

Phimosis

- The inability to retract the foreskin over the glans.
- Physiological in uncircumcised infants. Forcible retraction should not be attempted as it may result in pathological phimosis.

- In adults, possible causes include chronic balanitis and poor hygiene.
- Rarely an emergency unless acute retention of urine occurs.

Management

- Emergency treatment, i.e. dilatation of the stenotic foreskin with artery forceps or performing a dorsal slit procedure, is not required unless the patient has acute retention of urine or vascular compromise of the glans.
- Referral to Urology for definitive therapy (circumcision).

Paraphimosis

- The inability to pull retracted foreskin distally back over the glans, because of a tight constricting band of skin.
- Oedema and venous engorgement can lead to arterial compromise and gangrene of the glans.
- Avoid iatrogenic paraphimosis: remember to replace the foreskin after catheterizing uncircumcised patients.

Management

- Urgent reduction of the foreskin: apply continuous, firm pressure to the glans penis for 5–10 minutes to reduce the oedema and then pull the foreskin over the glans. Pain may be reduced either by use of lignocaine gel (be generous!) or penile nerve block using 5 ml of 1% plain lignocaine.
- If manual reduction is unsuccessful, perform a dorsal slit procedure.
- If in doubt, obtain a urology consultation.
- If reduction is successful, ensure that the patient is able to void before discharge.
- Arrange a follow-up at the Urology SOC. Definitive treatment is circumcision.

Priapism

- A prolonged, usually painful erection that is unrelated to sexual arousal.
- The corpora cavernosa are typically rigid and filled with blood.
- The glans and corpus spongiosum remain flaccid (in low-flow priapism).

High-flow priapism

- Uncommon
- Usually results from perineal or straddle trauma. A lacerated cavernous artery may create an arteriovenous shunt into the corporal bodies.
- Patients typically have little pain.
- The entire penis is partially rigid, and the glans is hard.

- Auscultate for a penile bruit.
- Much lower risk of permanent complications, because of continuous inflow of arterial blood.
- Usually does not require emergency treatment.

Low-flow (ischaemic) priapism

- Decreased penile venous outflow produces venous stasis.
- Subsequent arterial compromise leads to ischaemia.
- Time-sensitive: irreversible cellular damage and fibrosis occur if treatment is not administered within 24–48 hours. Erectile dysfunction may result.
- Most cases are caused by sickle cell disease.
- Other causes are as follows:
    1. Drugs:
        a. Phenothiazines.
        b. Sildenafil (Viagra®).
        c. Alcohol, cocaine, and marijuana.
        d. Intracavernosal injections for impotence.
    2. Malignancy, e.g. leukaemia.
    3. Spinal cord injury.
    4. Idiopathic.
- Typically painful.
- Examination reveals a rigid penile shaft. The glans is soft.

Management

- Refer to a urologist immediately.
- Parenteral vasodilators: subcutaneous terbutaline 0.25–0.5 mg.
- For sickle cell disease:
    1. Analgesia.
    2. Hydration.
    3. Oxygen.
    4. Occasionally, exchange transfusion.
- Corporal blood aspiration, irrigation, and injection of a vasoconstrictor.
- The urologist may need to perform a surgical shunt.

Torn frenulum

- Generally occurs during overzealous masturbation.
- On examination, oozing (rarely spurting) blood is noted from the frenulum.

Management

- Direct pressure for 5–10 minutes.
- If direct pressure is unsuccessful, infiltrate frenulum with 1% plain lignocaine (without adrenaline) and place one or two 5/0 absorbable sutures to achieve haemostasis.
- Arrange a follow-up at the Urology SOC or GP.

Fracture of the penis

- Disruption of the tunica albuginea surrounding the corpora cavernosa.
- Typically occurs during vigorous sexual intercourse.
- A popping sound is heard.
- Followed by pain and swelling of the penis, and rapid detumescence.
- Examination reveals a swollen, ecchymotic penis.
- May be associated with urethral injury:
  1. Blood at the urethral meatus.
  2. Gross haematuria.
  3. Inability to void.

Management

- Analgesia.
- Immediate urology consultation (to arrange surgical repair).

References/Further Reading

1. Freeman L. Male genitourinary emergencies: Preserving fertility and providing relief. *Emerg Med Pract*. November 2000.
2. Knight PJ, Vassy LE. The diagnosis and treatment of the acute scrotum in children and adolescents. *Ann Surg*. 1984; 200: 664–673.
3. Lee LM, Wright JE, McLoughlin MG. Testicular torsion in the adult. *J Urol*. 1983; 130(1): 93–94.
4. Rabinowitz R. The importance of the cremasteric reflex in acute scrotal swelling in children. *J Urol*. 1984; 132: 89–90.
5. Edelsberg JS, Surh YS. The acute scrotum. *Emerg Med Clin North Am*. 1988; 6(3): 521–546.
6. Rosenstein D, McAninch JW. Urologic emergencies. *Med Clin North Am*. 2004; 88: 495–518.
7. Ban KM, Easter JS. Selected urologic problems. In: Marx JA, Hockberger RS, Walls RM, et al., eds. *Rosen's Emergency Medicine: Concepts and Clinical Practice*. 7th ed. Philadelphia: Mosby Elsevier; 2010: 1297–1324.

18   Palpitations

Benjamin Leong • Shirley Ooi

CAVEATS

- The underlying causes of palpitations may range from an increased **awareness** of a normal rhythm to **life-threatening dysrhythmias**.
- Both **tachydysrhythmias** and **premature complexes** arising from either the atria or ventricles may result in a complaint of palpitations.

NOTE: Bradydysrhythmias, however, are more likely to present as breathlessness, giddiness or syncope, and not likely to present as palpitations.

- **Associated features** such as (1) altered mental status or loss of consciousness, (2) heart failure and dyspnoea, (3) chest pain, or (4) shock are significant. These are frequently attributable to a **reduced cardiac output** caused by the dysrhythmia.
    1. Cardiac output (CO) is determined by the following formula: $\mathbf{CO = HR \times SV}$ (where HR = heart rate and SV = stroke volume)
- Although CO should increase with HR, **tachydysrhythmias** may result in a **reduced SV** when the HR is so fast that the ventricles do not have enough time to fill with blood, thus reducing CO.
- The **initial assessment** should include the **haemodynamic status**, **12-lead ECG**, and identification of **serious signs and symptoms**.
- This chapter will focus on specific dysrhythmias as well as some uncommon conditions that may be encountered in emergency medicine. (See Chapter 43, *Tachydysrhythmias* and Chapter 35, *Bradydysrhythmias* for respective ACLS algorithms.)

⇨ **SPECIAL TIPS FOR GPs**

- **Do not downplay** any patient's complaints of palpitations even if they appear 'well'.
- Always assess the **haemodynamic status** and look for clinical features of **serious signs and symptoms**.
- Perform a **12-lead ECG**, as far as possible when the patient is still experiencing the palpitations, as the dysrhythmias or ECG changes may be transient. This will facilitate subsequent diagnosis and management.
- Even if a definitive ECG diagnosis cannot be made, **the immediate priority is to ensure that the patient is stable**.
- Administer **oxygen** and establish peripheral **IV access**.

- **Reassess** the patient's haemodynamic status frequently, as this may change rapidly.
- Patients who are unstable or have serious signs and symptoms should be transported to hospital by **an ambulance service with continuous ECG monitoring capabilities**.
- Dysrhythmias such as VT and frequent PVCs, especially PVCs with R-on-T phenomena (Figure 10), may predispose to VF. Have a **manual** or **automatic external defibrillator** (AED) ready in case the patient collapses suddenly. Many out-of-hospital cardiac arrest (OHCA) cases occur in residential areas, and the GP is frequently the closest medical practitioner to victims.

GENERAL APPROACH

- Determine the **heart rate**.
- Determine if there are **additional (ectopic) beats** or **missing ("dropped") beats**.
- Determine if the abnormal rhythm or ectopic complexes are **broad** or **narrow**.
  1. *Narrow complexes* originate from the AV junction or above.
  2. *Broad complexes* may be due to a bundle branch block, originate from the ventricles, or due to conduction via an accessory pathway.
- Determine if the morphology of the complexes are **uniform or multiform**.
  1. Multiform complexes suggest that there may be more than one origin of the complexes.
- Look for **p-waves** and determine their relationship with QRS complexes.
  1. *P-waves are all related to QRS complexes.*
     a. The origin of the dysrhythmia is above the AV junction.
     b. Likely due to increased automaticity (sinus or atrial tachycardia).
  2. *P-waves more than QRS complexes.*
     a. Suggests some form of conduction block at the AV junction regardless of tachycardia.
  3. *P-waves less than QRS complexes.*
     a. The rhythm is originating from below the AV junction (fascicular or ventricular tachycardias).
  4. *P-waves absent (or masked).*
     a. Possibilities include atrial fibrillation, supraventricular and ventricular tachycardias.
- Look for **ectopic beats**.
  1. **Narrow QRS complex ectopic beats.**
     a. If no preceding p-wave, originate from the junction. These are termed **junctional ectopics**.
     b. If preceded by a p-wave, originate from the atria. These p-waves usually appear different from sinus p-waves and are termed **atrial ectopics**.

TABLE 1   ECG classification of tachydysrhythmias

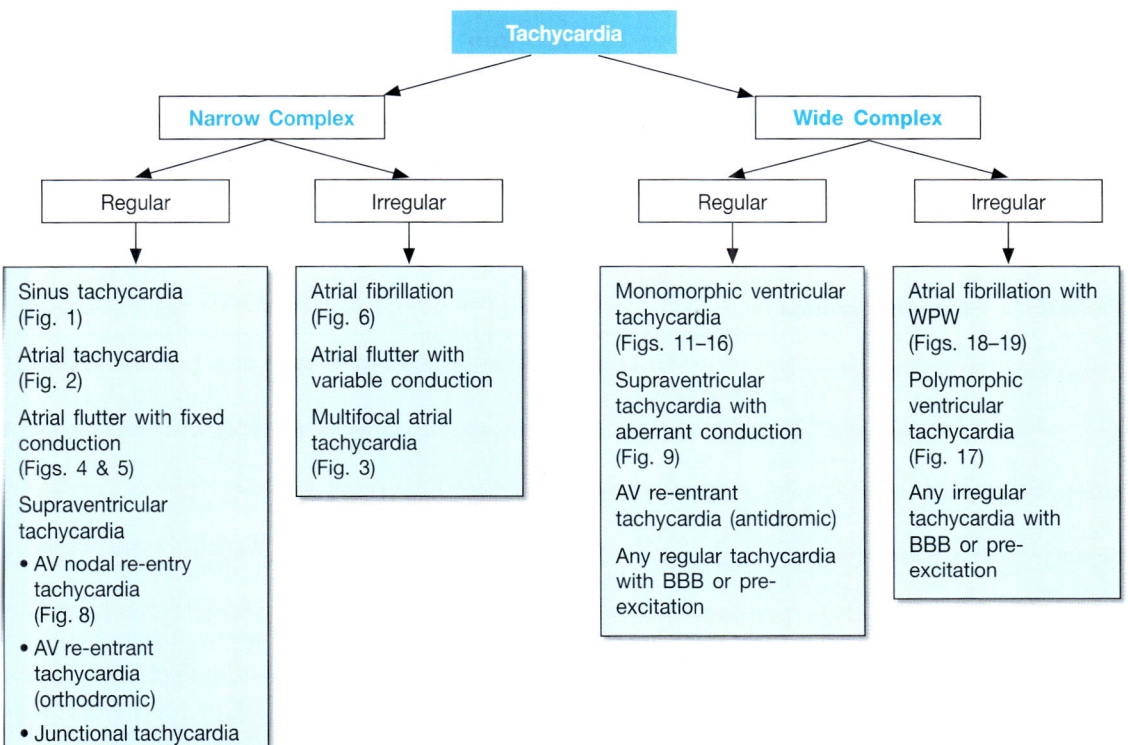

2. **Wide QRS complex ectopic beats.**
   a. Usually originate from the ventricles and are termed **ventricular ectopics**.
   b. They may also arise from the bundles of His.
   c. Less commonly, they may also be produced by an atrial ectopic with aberrant conduction, such as when the ectopic p-wave occurs during the refractory period of the right bundle, producing an RBBB pattern.

NARROW COMPLEX TACHYCARDIAS

Sinus tachycardia

- Typically defined as a heart rate >**100bpm**.
- Not by itself a dysrhythmia, but rather a physiological response to disease.
- **Causes are myriad** and include pain, anxiety, shock, sepsis, hyperthyroidism, phaeochromocytoma, pharmacological and toxicological causes.

NOTE:

   (i) **Do not assume** that sinus tachycardia is only due to **fever**. Remember that generally, the heart rate increases by only about **10 beats/min for every rise of 1°C** in temperature. *Disproportionate increases* in HR should prompt a search for other causes.

   (ii) In unexplained sinus tachycardia, consider the possibility of **myocarditis**. Checking the troponin levels may be worthwhile.

- Treatment should be directed at the underlying causes.

FIGURE 1   **Sinus tachycardia**

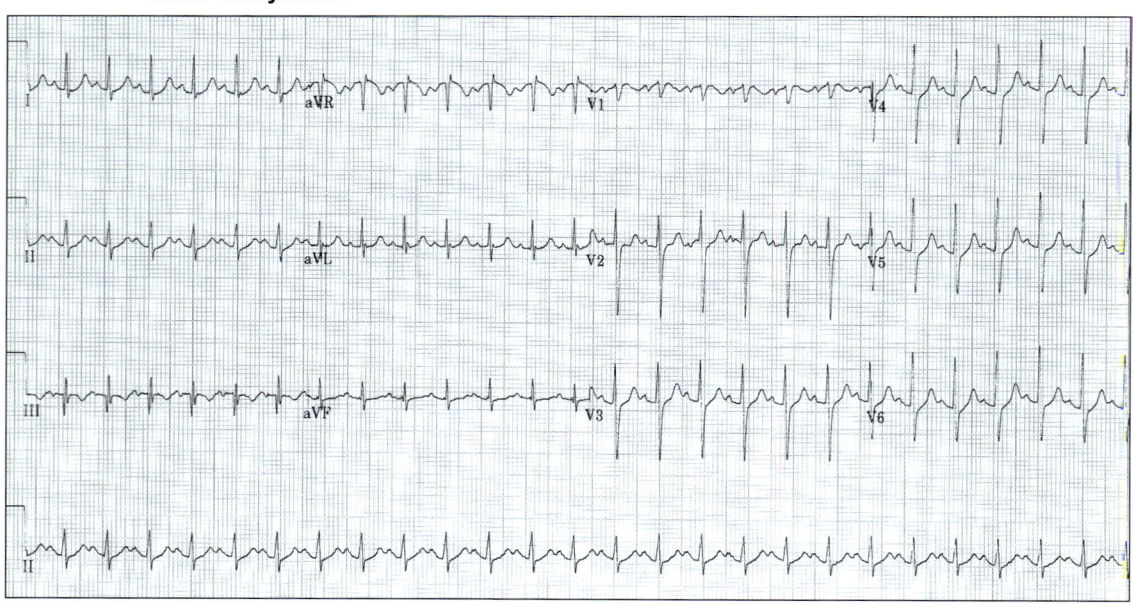

Note: (1) Regular narrow complex tachycardia. (2) All p-waves are conducted.

Atrial tachycardia

- This is due to a focus of **increased automaticity** in the atria outside of the sinus node.
- The **p-wave morphology is different** from the normal p-wave of the patient.
- *It can be impossible to differentiate from sinus tachycardia* on the ECG, if there is no previous ECG for comparison.
- If there are multiple differently sized p-waves, it is then termed Multifocal Atrial Tachycardia (MAT).
- *See Multifocal Atrial Tachycardia (next section).*

FIGURE 2 **Atrial tachycardia**

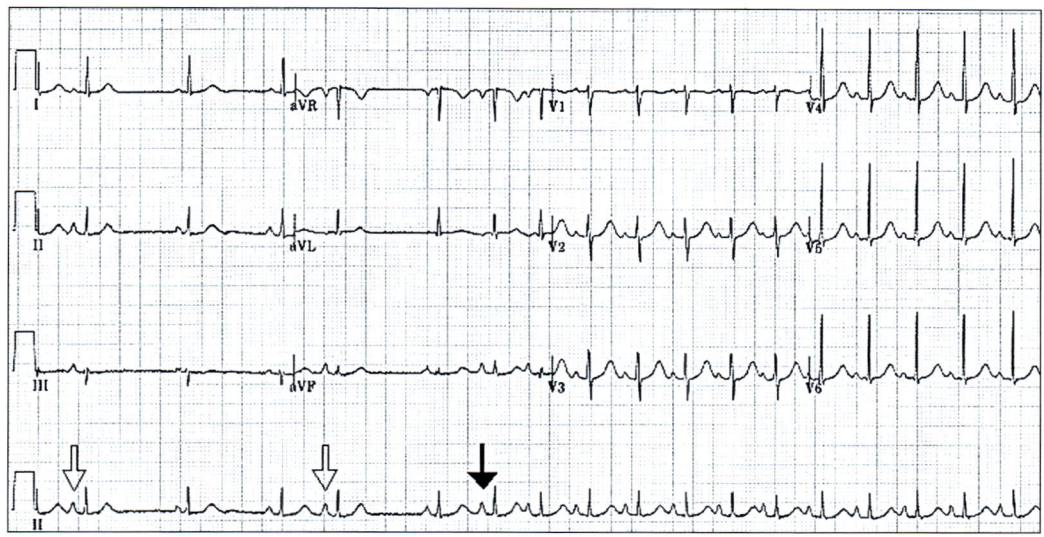

Note: (1) Normal sinus beats with normal p-waves. (2) Atrial ectopics with p-waves of a different morphology, indicated by light arrows. (3) The dark arrow indicates the start of the atrial tachycardia.

Multifocal Atrial Tachycardia

- An irregularly irregular rhythm characterised by p-waves of variable morphologies (by definition, three or more), with corresponding variations in PR intervals.
- This rhythm is most commonly encountered in patients with COPD.

FIGURE 3 **Multifocal atrial tachycardia**

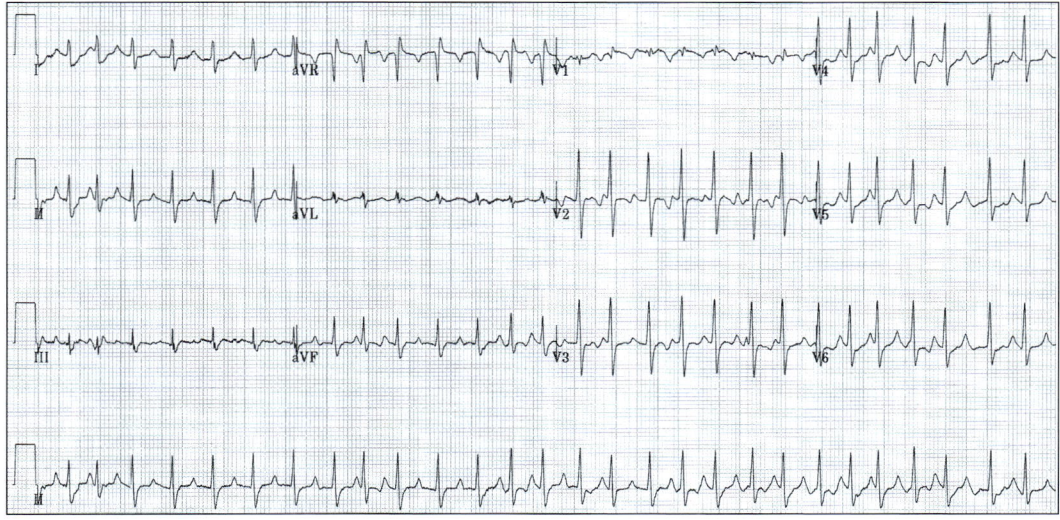

Note: Irregularly irregular tachycardia. P-waves of >3 different morphologies with varying PR intervals are seen. The QRS complexes are narrow.

Atrial Flutter

- A circus rhythm caused by cyclical depolarization of the atria at a rate of 300bpm, resulting in a **saw-toothed baseline** pattern on the ECG.
- The saw-tooth waves are also called flutter or "F" waves.
- Due to the AV nodal refractory period, conduction to the ventricles typically occurs at a **2:1** or **3:1** ratio, resulting in a ventricular rate of 150 or 100 bpm.

FIGURE 4 **Atrial flutter with 2:1 AV conduction**

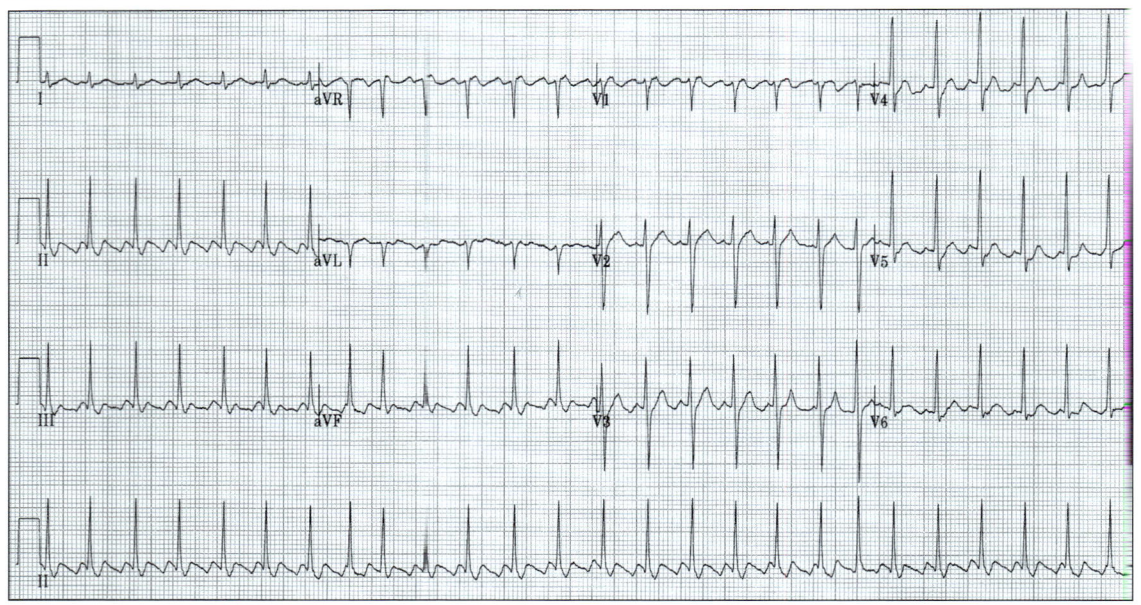

Note: (1) Regular narrow complex tachycardia of 158bpm. (2) Saw-tooth pattern is appreciable on the rhythm strip, indicating atrial flutter.

FIGURE 5 **Atrial flutter following administration of adenosine**

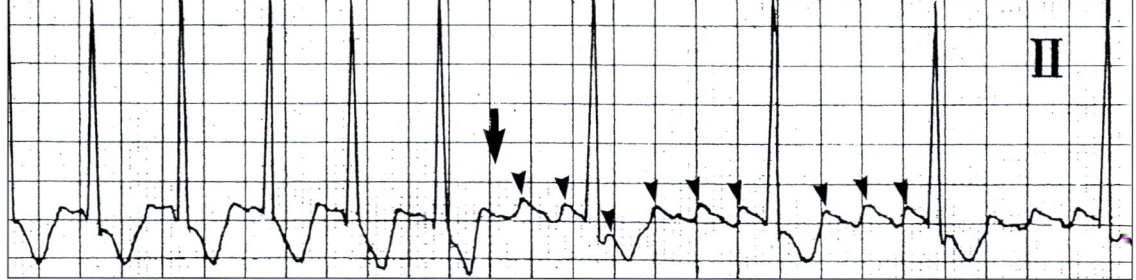

Note: During 2:1 AV conduction, the flutter ('F') waves are hidden as they are buried within the QRS complexes and the ST/T wave segments. They are evident only when the AV conductions ratio is increased to 5:1 conduction resulting in a slower ventricular rate (arrow). Arrowheads indicate flutter ('F') waves.
Image taken from *Clinical Electrocardiography* 3rd Edition, BL Chia, ©1998 World Scientific. Reproduced with permission.

Atrial Fibrillation

- A chaotic irregular rhythm of the atria resulting in an irregularly irregular ventricular rate.

FIGURE 6   Atrial fibrillation

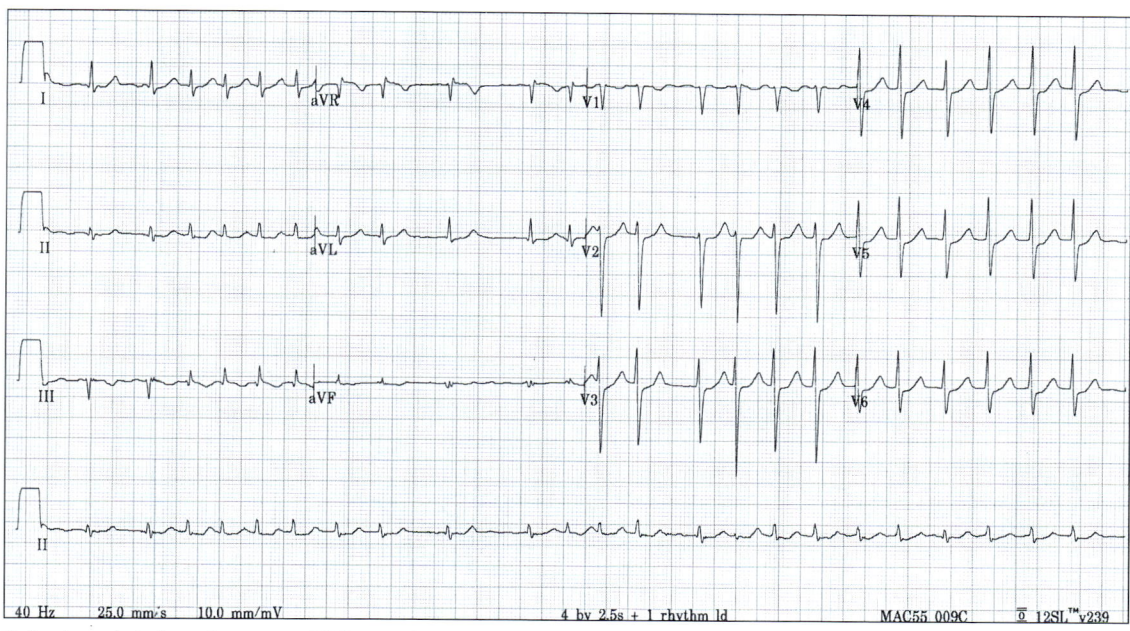

Note: Irregularly irregular narrow QRS complex tachycardia without P waves seen.

Re-entry supraventricular tachycardia (SVT)

- **AV nodal re-entrant tachycardia** (AVNRT) or **orthodromic AV re-entrant tachycardia** (AVRT) cause *narrow complex tachycardias.*
- **AVNRT** is the commonest cause of SVT in structurally normal hearts.
- It occurs due to a re-entrant circuit being formed between the slow and fast fibres of the AV node.
- **AVRT** occurs due to a re-entrant circuit being formed between the normal conduction system and an accessory bundle called the Bundle of Kent. (See Figure 7).
- **Orthodromic AVRT** is when the conduction is antegrade down the His-Purkinje bundles, and retains the normal narrow QRS complexes.
- **Antidromic AVRT** causes a wide complex tachycardia, due to the initial antegrade conduction down the accessory pathway producing a deflection before the retrograde conduction up the bundles. *Can be indistinguishable from VT on the ECG.*

FIGURE 7   (a) Orthodromic and (b) antidromic AV reentrant tachycardia

(a)   (b)

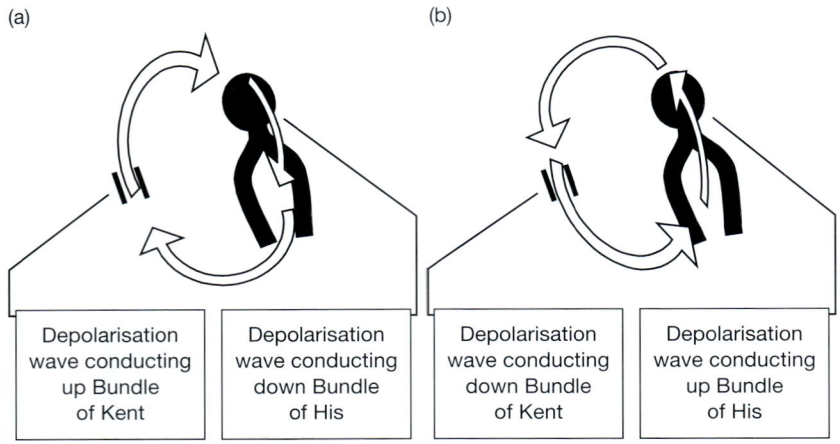

| Depolarisation wave conducting up Bundle of Kent | Depolarisation wave conducting down Bundle of His | Depolarisation wave conducting down Bundle of Kent | Depolarisation wave conducting up Bundle of His |

FIGURE 8   Supraventricular tachycardia

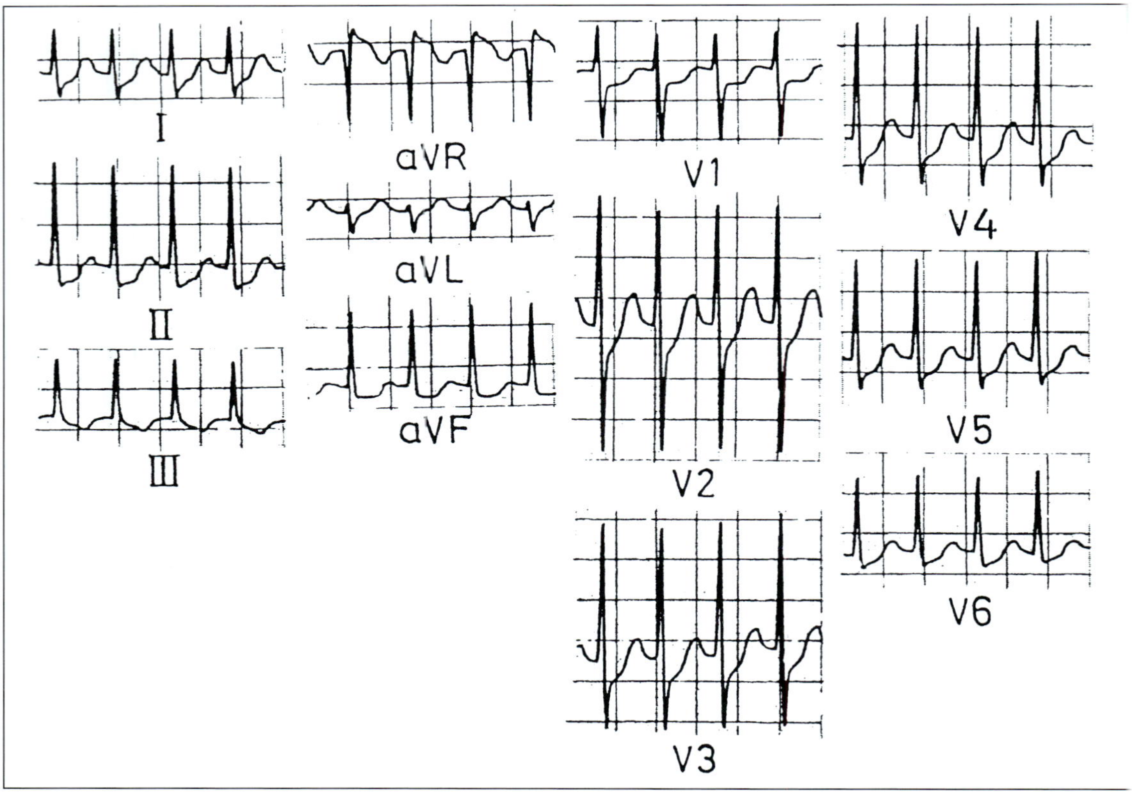

I

II

III

aVR

aVL

aVF

V1

V2

V3

V4

V5

V6

Note: (1) Regular, narrow QRS tachycardia of 157/min. (2) No p-waves are visible.
Image taken from *Clinical Electrocardiography* 3rd Edition, BL Chia, ©1998 World Scientific. Reproduced with permission.

SVT with Aberrant Conduction or Bundle Branch Block

- SVTs may appear as a *wide complex tachycardia* when associated with a *rate-related* conduction block in the bundles of His during the SVT (termed **aberrant conduction** or **aberrancy**), or when there is an existing fixed bundle branch block.
- *This may then be difficult to distinguish from VT.*
- When in doubt, treat as for VT. *See section on VT below.*

FIGURE 9   **Supraventricular tachycardia with aberrant ventricular conduction**

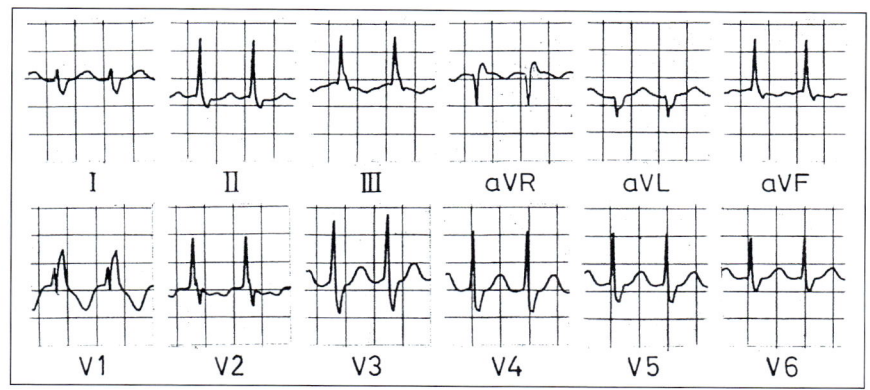

Note: (1) Rapid heart rate of 150/min. (2) Regular and wide QRS complexes (0.12s) with a typical right bundle branch block configuration (triphasic rSR' pattern in V1). (3) No clearly visible p-waves.
Image taken from *Clinical Electrocardiography* 3rd Edition, BL Chia, ©1998 World Scientific. Reproduced with permission.

Junctional tachycardia

- This is an uncommon but **distinct entity** and often easily mistaken for AVNRT or AVRT.
- The problem is one of *increased automaticity* at the AV node, as opposed to *re-entry* in PSVT.
- The result is a *narrow complex tachycardia.* The p-waves may be absent due to retrograde conduction from the AV node back into the atria.
- Causes include AMI, myocarditis, digoxin and catecholamine toxicity.

BROAD COMPLEX TACHYCARDIAS

Ventricular Arrhythmias (VA)

- A **premature ventricular contraction** (PVC) is an additional broad complex beat not preceded by a p-wave that arises from the ventricles.
- PVCs are commonly graded according to **Lown's classification**.

0	No PVCs
1	Infrequent PVCs (<30/hour)

2	Frequent PVCs (≥30/hour)
3	Multiform PVCs
4A	2 consecutive PVCs (couplets)
4B	≥3 consecutive PVCs (salvos)
5	R-on-T

- Lown's classification describes an increasing risk of morbidity and mortality, although there are overlaps between the groups.
- **Nonsustained ventricular tachycardia** is when there is a run of PVCs lasting for <30s.
- When it lasts ≥30s, it is termed **sustained VT**.

FIGURE 10   'R on T' ventricular ectopic beats and ventricular fibrillation in a patient with acute inferior infarction

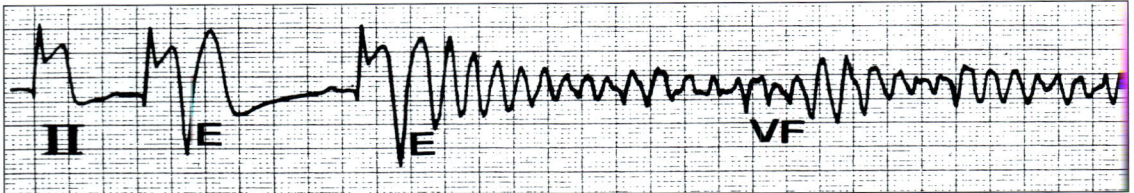

Note: (1) 'Hyperacute' changes of transmural inferior infarction as reflected by raised ST segment in II. (2) 'R on T' ventricular ectopic beats (E) initiating ventricular fibrillation (VF).
Image taken from *Clinical Electrocardiography* 3rd Edition, BL Chia, ©1998 World Scientific. Reproduced with permission (p. 94, fig 6.6).

Ventricular Tachycardia

- A regular broad complex tachycardia that is sustained for ≥30s or more.
  1. QRS complexes >120ms wide
  2. Rate >120bpm

NOTE: Wide complex tachycardias of <120bpm are unlikely to be VT. Consider differentials of hyperkalaemia, TCA overdose or accelerated idioventricular rhythm (AIVR).

- The majority of ventricular dysrhythmias occur in the presence of **structural heart disease** such as IHD, LVH and HOCM.
- An estimated 10% of VTs occurs in structurally normal hearts, when it is termed **"idiopathic VT"**.
  1. These include outflow tract VTs and fascicular VT.
  2. The classification is complex and out of the scope of this book.
- VT can be difficult to distinguish from SVT with aberrancy or BBB. Clinical and ECG features that differentiate the two are listed in **Table 2**.

TABLE 2 How to differentiate VT from SVT with aberrancy

	VT	SVT
History • Older age • Underlying IHD/CCF/cardiomyopathy • Multiple cardiovascular risk factors • Symptoms of ACS or CCF, such as chest pain, diaphoresis or breathlessness	These features support VT more than SVT	Absence of these features does not establish a diagnosis of SVT
Physical examination		
Pulse volume	Variable	Regular
Intensity of first heart sound	Variable	Regular
JVP	Cannon 'a' waves	Normal a-c-v waves
Signs of ACS or CCF	May be present	Unlikely to be present
ECG features		
(1) AV dissociation	Visible p-waves not related to ventricular rhythm Capture beats Fusion beats	Retrograde p-waves related to all QRS
(2) Praecordial lead morphology	Concordance of praecordial leads Absence of any RS complexes in **all** praecordial leads	
(3) RS interval (onset of R to nadir of S)	>100ms in **any** praecordial lead	
(4) Morphology criteria in *both* V1-2 and V6 In RBBB-like ECG (predominantly +ve QRS in V1)	*Leads V1-2* Smooth monophasic R .... qR .... Notched downslope in R (RSr' pattern. Aka 'taller left rabbit ear') .... *Lead V6* QS complex (completely negative complex) ..... R/S ratio <1	*Leads V1-2* Prominent late R wave 'Right rabbit ear'. Triphasic .... Monophasic .... *Lead V6* Triphasic qRs ....
In LBBB-like ECG (predominantly –ve QRS in V1)	*Leads V1-2* Initial R wave > 30ms duration .... R to nadir of S > 60ms duration .... Notched or slurred downslope of S wave ...... *Lead V6* (any Q wave favours VT) QS complex (completely negative complex) ..... qR complex	Absence of Q in V6 favours SVT

FIGURE 11   **Ventricular tachycardia**

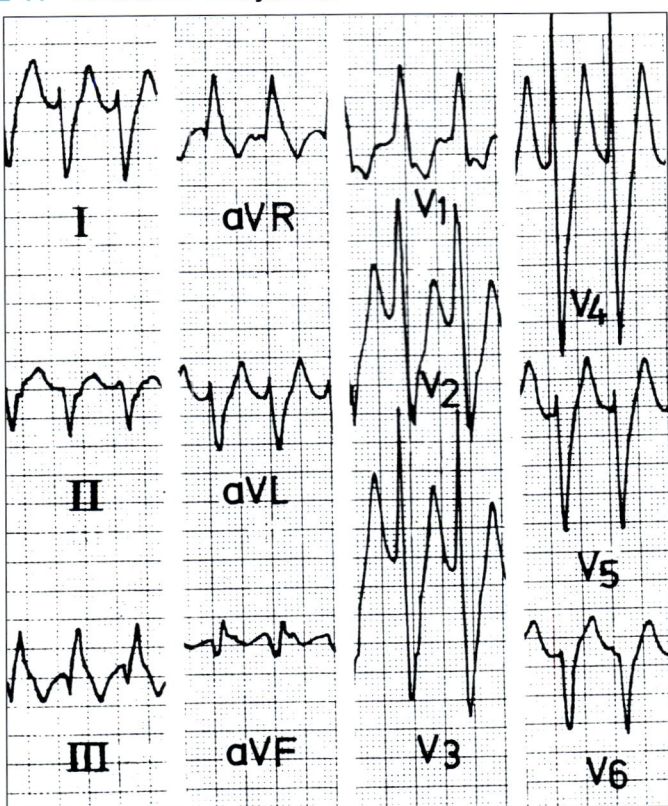

Note: (1) Rapid ventricular rate of 158/min. (2) Regular and wide (0.16s) QRS complexes. (3) Monophasic R wave in V1. (4) rS complex in V_5 and V_6. (5) Indeterminate axis of appropriately −170°.
Image taken from *Clinical Electrocardiography* 3rd Edition, BL Chia, ©1998 World Scientific. Reproduced with permission.

FIGURE 12   Ventricular tachycardia in a patient with acute myocardial infarction

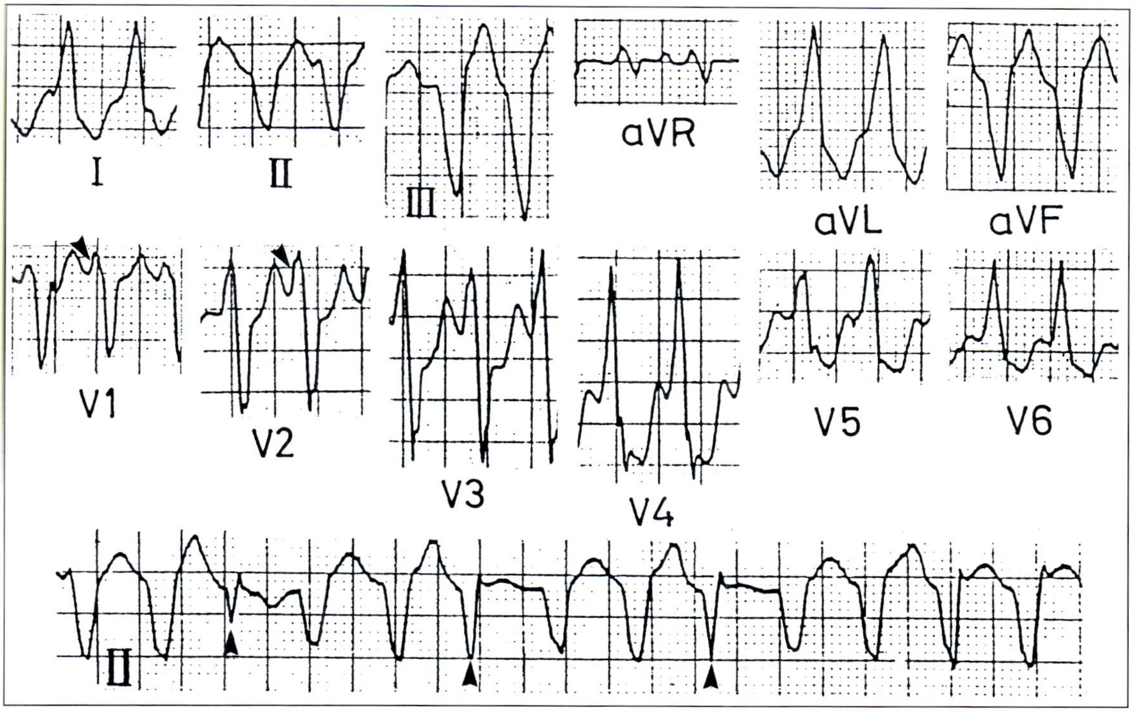

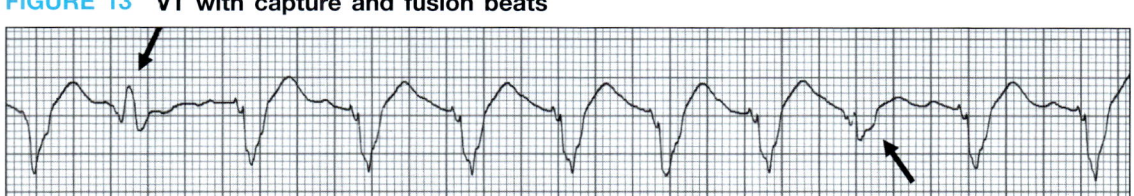

Note: (1) Regular wide QRS tachycardia of around 166/min. (2) The QRS morphology superficially resembles a left bundle branch pattern, except that the **r waves in V1 and V2** (arrowheads) are broad, thus favouring ventricular ectopy. (3) The rhythm strip in the lower part of the ECG shows **fusion beats** (arrowheads) which are of different morphologies. There is also a suggestion of **AV dissociation**, because some corresponding parts of the ST/T wave segments of consecutive ventricular complexes have slightly different morphologies and appeared deformed, most likely due to the superimposition of p-waves occurring at a rate which is different from that of the QRS complexes.

Image taken from *Clinical Electrocardiography* 3rd Edition, BL Chia, ©1998 World Scientific. Reproduced with permission (p. 98, fig 6.11).

FIGURE 13   VT with capture and fusion beats

Note: (1) Capture beat in the second QRS complex. (2) Fusion beat in the ninth QRS complex.

FIGURE 14 **Ventricular tachycardia with concordance pattern**

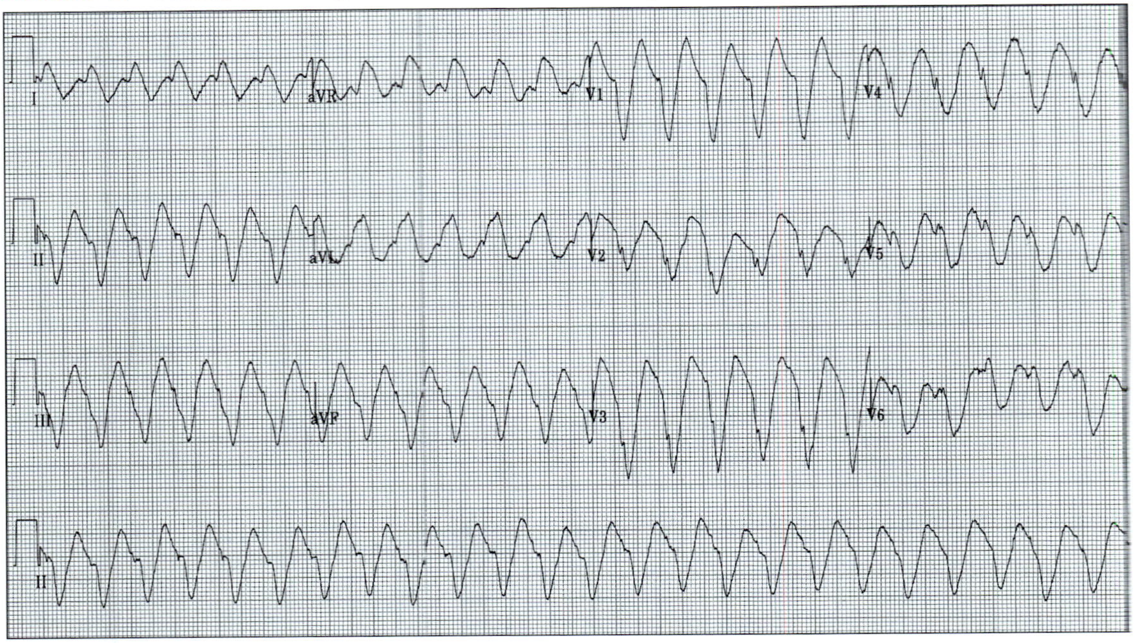

Note: (1) Regular, wide QRS tachycardia of 149bpm. (2) Negative concordance – all QRS complexes in the praecordial leads are negative in polarity.

Fascicular VT/Idiopathic Left Ventricular Tachycardia (ILVT)

- A form of **idiopathic VT**.
- Typically has an RBBB morphology with a left axis deviation.
- Has relatively narrow QRS complexes of about 120ms, hence *easily mistaken for SVT*.
- More common among young males with structurally normal hearts.
- Not responsive to Adenosine, but may respond to Verapamil. However, in general, **Verapamil is dangerous** if given to classical VT. *If in doubt, one should treat as for VT*.
- If unstable, should be treated with synchronised cardioversion.

FIGURE 15   Fascicular VT

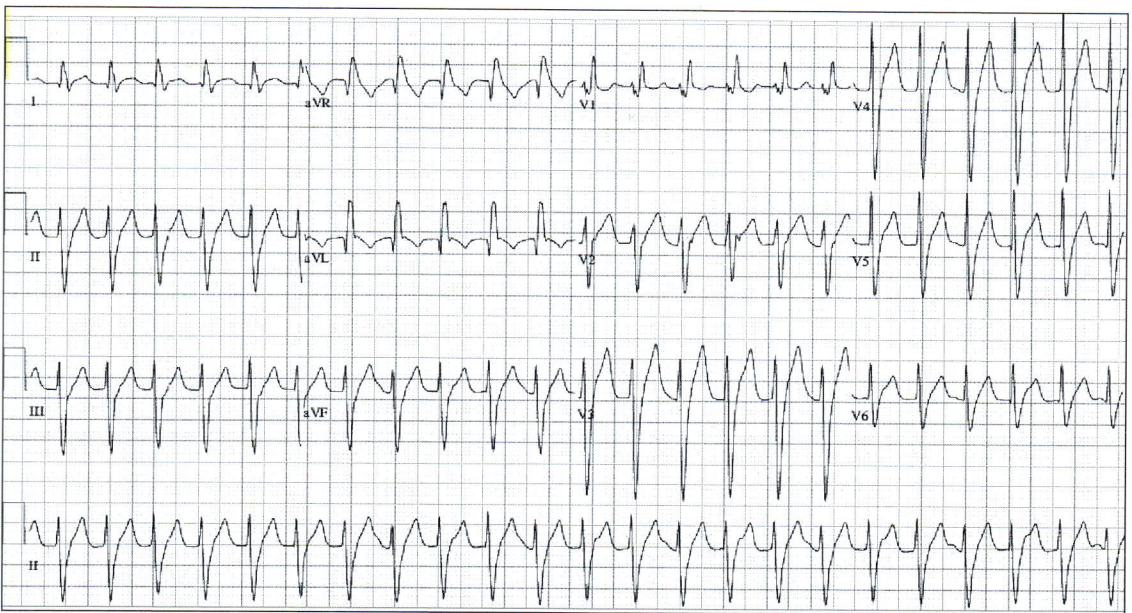

Note: (1) Relatively narrow-looking QRS complexes. (2) Left axis deviation. (3) RBBB type morphology in V1. (4) However, in V6, the R/S ratio is <1, suggesting VT rather than SVT.

FIGURE 16   Fascicular VT, post cardioversion with IV verapamil

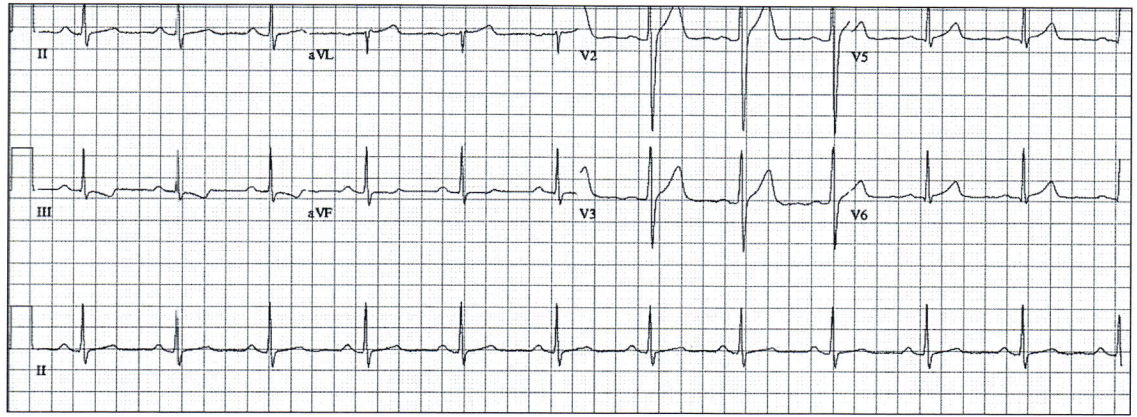

Note: The rhythm is now sinus, with narrow complexes and no more bundle branch block pattern.

Torsades de Pointes

- A form of polymorphic VT.
- See Table 3 for risk factors.
- Signs for impending Torsades de Pointes (TdP):
  a. QT or QTc >500ms
  b. QT or QTc prolonged by >60ms from baseline after commencement of pro-arrhythmic medication
  c. Polymorphic PVCs
  d. T wave alternans
  e. Non-sustained torsades de pointes

TABLE 3   Risk factors for torsades de pointes

- Women
- Elderly
- Heart disease
- Acute neurological events
- Bradydysrhythmias with long pauses
- Electrolyte disturbances
- Hypomagnesaemia
- Hypokalaemia
- Malnutrition
- Polypharmacy
- Genetics
- Long QT syndrome
- Familial history of sudden cardiac death
- Renal/hepatic dysfunction

FIGURE 17   Torsades de Pointes

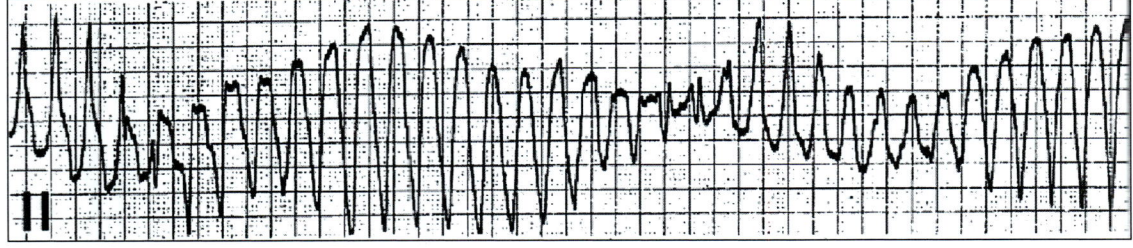

Image taken from *Clinical Electrocardiography* 3rd Edition, BL Chia, ©1998 World Scientific. Reproduced with permission. (p. 104, fig 6.19).

WPW with AF

- About 10–30% of patients with Wolff-Parkinson-White syndrome may develop atrial fibrillation.
- Also called **pre-excited AF**.
- Irregularly irregular rhythm with very fast heart rates.
- QRS complexes are variably widened, due to variable conduction down both the accessory pathway and the AV junction.
- Drugs of choice for the termination of the AF are **procainamide**, flecainide, propafenone and dofetilide.
- **AV node blocking agents**, such as adenosine, betablockers, calcium channel blockers and digoxin (aka 'ABCD' drugs) are **absolutely contraindicated**.
- Although some authors have suggested the use of amiodarone for WPW with AF, there have been reports of worsening tachycardia or even conversion to VF with its use in this setting. **Amiodarone should thus be avoided.**

FIGURE 18 **Atrial fibrillation in a patient with underlying WPW syndrome**

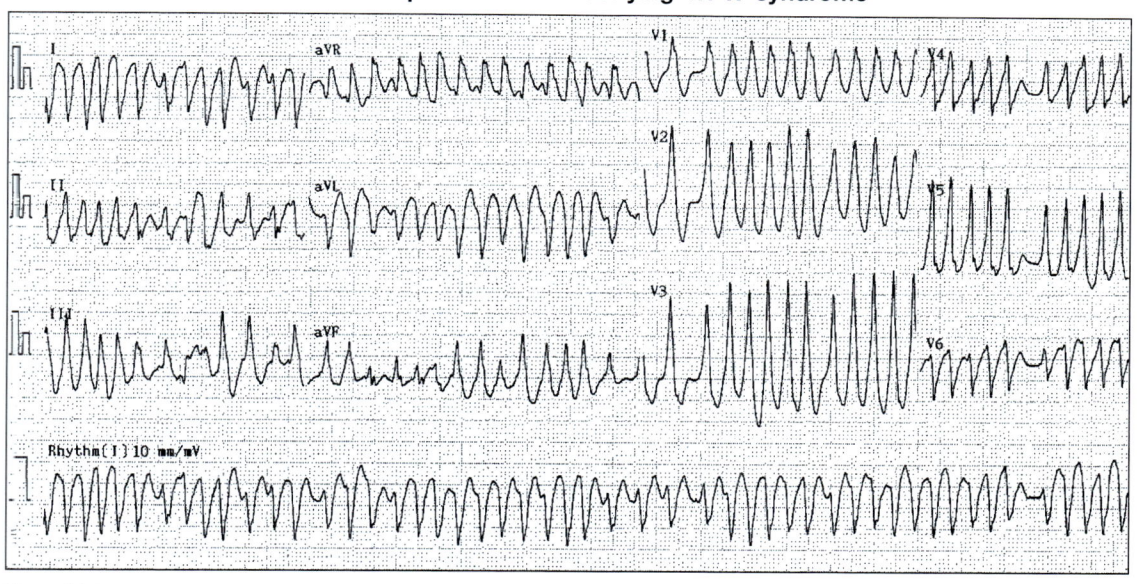

Note: (1) Irregular rhythm and very rapid ventricular rate. Some complexes approach 300bpm, a rate not seen in AF without an accessory pathway. (2) The QRS complexes are variably widened.

FIGURE 19 **Patient with WPW syndrome and AF after cardioversion to sinus with IV procainamide**

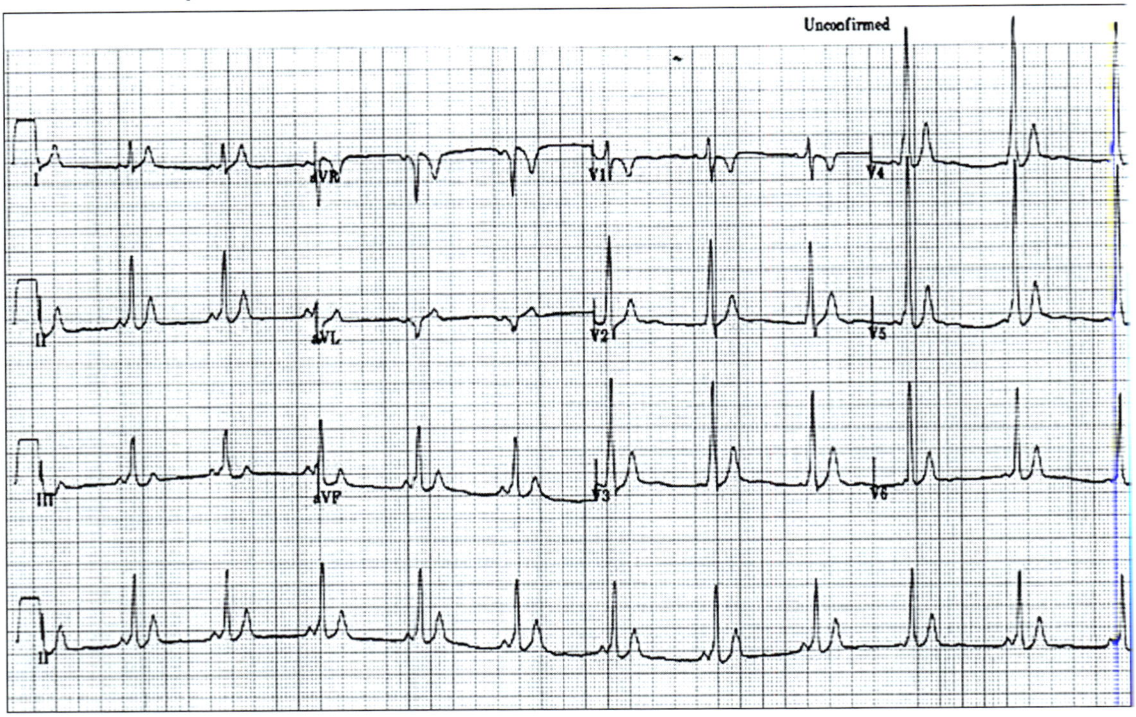

Note: (1) The rhythm is now sinus. (2) Normal QRS complexes with delta waves and shortened PR intervals are now visible.

CONDITIONS THAT PREDISPOSE TO DYSRHYTHMIAS

Brugada syndrome

- Associated with characteristic ST-T segment ECG changes with high incidence of sudden death in structurally normal hearts.
- Now believed to be the same entity responsible for Sudden Unexplained Nocturnal Death Syndrome (SUNDS) in South East Asia.
- ECG changes are often dynamic.
- May be unmasked by sodium channel blockers, fever, vagotonic agents, alpha-agonists, beta-blockers, cyclic antidepressants, combination of glucose, insulin, hyperkalaemia, hypokalaemia, hypercalcaemia and alcohol and cocaine toxicity.
- **Brugada ECG patterns** (to be differentiated from Brugada Syndrome – 3 types of ECG repolarisation patterns are recognized.

1. **Type 1** (diagnostic for Brugada syndrome) (Figure 20)
   a. J-point elevation >2mm (0.2 mV).
   b. Negative T wave in >1 right praecordial lead (V1–V3).
   c. Coved ST-T configuration.
   d. Gradually descending ST segment.
2. **Type 2** (non-diagnostic for Brugada syndrome) (Figure 21)
   a. Saddleback appearance with high take-off ST segment elevation >2mm (0.2 mV) followed by a trough displaying >1mm ST elevation.
   b. Either positive or biphasic T waves.

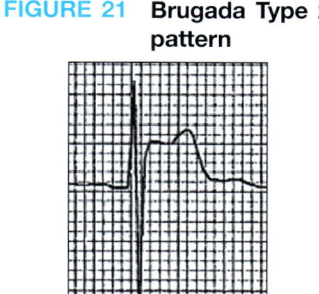

FIGURE 20 **Brugada Type 1 pattern**   FIGURE 21 **Brugada Type 2 pattern**

3. **Type 3** (non-diagnostic for Brugada syndrome)
   a. Either saddleback or coved appearance with ST segment elevation <1mm (0.1 mV).
- Brugada-like ECG patterns may occasionally be recorded in the first few hours following DC cardioversion. The significance is unclear.
- **Brugada syndrome diagnostic criteria.**
  1. Type 1 ECG pattern in >2 right praecordial leads (V1–V3), in conjunction with one of the following:
     a. Documented VF
     b. Polymorphic VT
     c. Family history of sudden cardiac death at <45 years old
     d. Coved-type ECG in family members
     e. Inducibility of VT with programmed electrical stimulation
     f. Syncope
     g. Nocturnal agonal respiration
  2. Conversion of Type 2 or Type 3 baseline ECG to Type 1 after sodium blocker administration, in conjunction with above clinical features.
- Patients with palpitations or syncope whose ECGs demonstrate Brugada ECG patterns should be referred to a cardiologist for early assessment and a view to the insertion of an **automated implantable cardiac defibrillator**.

FIGURE 22 Brugada Syndrome

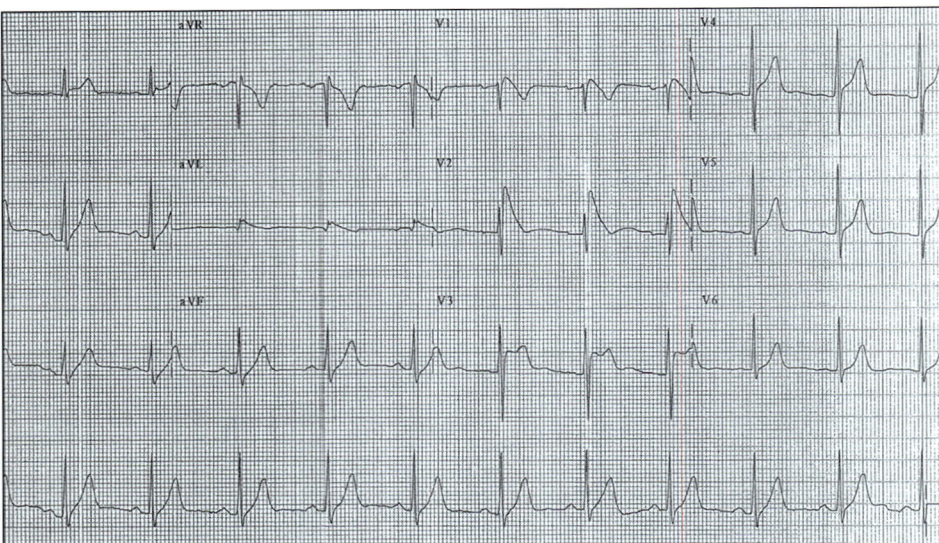

Note: (1) Coving J-point elevation >2 mm with downsloping ST segment and negative T wave in V1 and V2. (2) Brugada Type II pattern is also seen in V3.

Long QT syndromes (LQTS)

- Associated with sudden cardiac death, VF, polymorphic VT, torsades de pointes, syncope.
- $QTc = QT/\sqrt{[\text{R-R interval}]}$. (Bazett's correction for heart rate.)
- Causes of LQTS:
  1. **Congenital**
     a. Channelopathy linked to gene mutations. Twelve types known to date (LQT1—LQT12).
     b. Most well-known being **Romano-Ward Syndrome** (AD inheritance) and **Jervell-Lange-Nielsen Syndrome** (AR inheritance with congenital deafness)
  2. **Acquired**
     a. Electrolytes (Hypocalcaemia, -magnesaemia, -kalaemia)
     b. Drugs
        i. Class I or III antidysrhythmics, e.g. quinidine, procainamide, disopyramide, sotalol, amiodarone
        ii. Psychotropic drugs, e.g. phenothiazines, TCAs, haloperidol
        iii. Erythromycin
     c. Severe bradycardia with long pauses
     d. Renal dysfunction
     e. Hepatic dysfunction
     f. Heart disease

FIGURE 23 **Prolonged QT interval in an 80-year-old male with ischaemic heart disease**

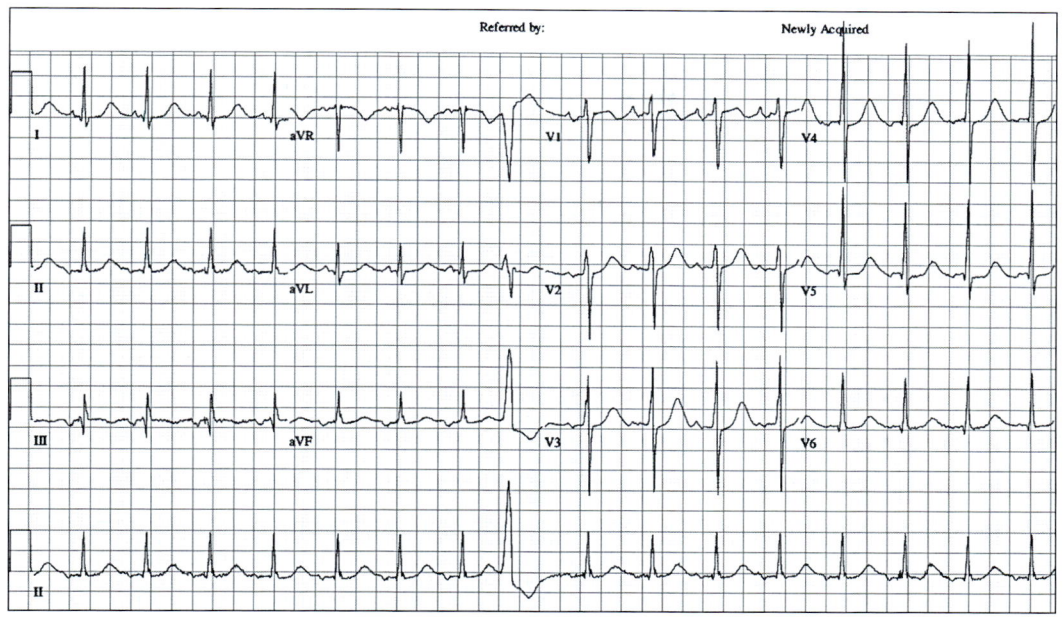

Note: (1) The ventricular rate is 97bpm. (2) QTc is 546ms. (3) QT interval is >1/2 of RR interval. (4) There is a PVC with R-on-T.

Short QT syndromes (SQTS)

• Associated with sudden death, VF, syncope, palpitations, dizziness, paroxysmal AF.

• Channelopathy linked to gene mutations. Five types known to date (SQT1–SQT5).

• QT durations do not increase despite slow heart rates, hence Bazett's correction should not be used. QT intervals should be measured at heart rates <100min.

• Very rare, only recently reported, all reported cases had QT durations <300ms.

• QT intervals below 320ms proposed as cutoff to suspect this entity.

MANAGEMENT

Refer to Chapter 43, *Tachydysrhythmias*, for a summary of details of management according to ACLS.

• Patients should be managed in the critical care area, where constant ECG monitoring can be performed, and where resuscitation equipment, e.g. defibrillator, is immediately available.

• Administer supplemental oxygen if SpO2 is decreased.

• Monitoring: ECG, vital signs q 15min, pulse oximetry.

• Establish peripheral IV line.

- **Level of consciousness:** is the patient alert, orientated and responding appropriately to questions? Decreased mentation may indicate the need for immediate synchronised electrical cardioversion (see later comments).
- **General appearance:** including presence of diaphoresis, cyanosis and tolerance of symptoms.
- Evidence does not support the use of lignocaine to discriminate between perfusing ventricular tachycardia (VT) and wide complex tachycardia of uncertain origin.
- Evidence does not support the use of adenosine to discriminate between perfusing VT and supraventricular (SVT) with aberrant ventricular conduction (SVT which is conducted to only one ventricle because of transient bundle branch block).
- **Amiodarone** is now the drug of choice in the management of stable tachydysrhythmias (except WPW with AF) due to a broad antidysrhythmic spectrum and less negative inotropic effect compared with most other agents.

References/Further Reading

1. Chia BL. *Clinical Electrocardiography*, 3rd ed. Singapore: World Scientific Publishing Co; 1998: 77, 81, 88, 94, 98–101, 104.

2. Wagner GS. *Marriot's practical electrocardiography*, 11th ed., Philadelphia: Lippincott Williams & Wilkins; 2003: 348–369.

3. Latif S, Dixit S, Callans DJ. Ventricular arrhythmias in normal hearts. *Cardiol Clin*. 2008; 26: 367–80, vi.

4. Nogami A. Idiopathic left ventricular tachycardia: assessment and treatment. *Card Electrophysiol Rev*. 2002; 6: 448–457.

5. Arya A, Piorkowski C, Sommer P, Gerds-Li JH, Kottkamp H, Hindricks G. Idiopathic outflow tract tachycardias: current perspectives. *Herz*. 2007; 32: 218–225.

6. Simonian SM, Lotfipour S, Wall C, et al. Challenging the superiority of amiodarone for rate control in Wolff-Parkinson-White and atrial fibrillation. *Intern Emerg Med*. 2010 Oct; 5(5): 421–6. Epub 2010 May 1.

7. Antzelevitch C, Brugada P, Borggrefe M, et al. Brugada syndrome: report of the second consensus conference: endorsed by the Heart Rhythm Society and the European Heart Rhythm Association. *Circulation*. 2005; 111: 659–670.

8. Zareba W, Cygankiewicz I. Long QT syndrome and short QT syndrome. *Prog Cardiovasc Dis*. 2008; 51: 264–278.

9. Pickham D, Drew BJ. QT/QTc interval monitoring in the emergency department. *J Emerg Nurs*. 2008; 34: 428–434.

19   Poisoning
General Principles
Shirley Ooi • Amila Punyadasa

CAVEATS

- The history is often unreliable in drug overdose (DO). Hence, one should have a **high index of suspicion** and assume the possibility of a **mixed overdose including alcohol intake**. See Annex for common sources of poisoning in Singapore.
- Pay special attention to the **physical examination** to get clues about the types of DOs.
- A patient with **altered mental state** and a suspicion of DO should have an **electrocardiogram** (ECG) done to exclude the possibility of cyclic anti-depressant poisoning and a **stat capillary glucose** test performed to exclude or confirm hypoglycaemia. Consider also the other various differentials of altered mental state (refer to Chapter 1, *Altered Mental State*).
- Remember that prudent management of DO includes paying attention to the emotional/psychiatric state of the patient besides managing the clinical effects of the DO.
- **Gastric lavage** should not be performed routinely for every case of DO (refer to the section *Gastric Decontamination* for details).
- **A drug screen** should not be ordered for all poisonings. History and clinical findings again are the mainstays of medical diagnosis. Seizures, coma, high anion gap metabolic acidosis and hypoventilation are conditions that may require a comprehensive toxicology screen. However, there is no replacement for good clinical judgement.

HISTORY

- Definite DO or questionable DO? Be aware that patients may not provide a completely accurate history due to personal uncertainty, subterfuge or altered mental status.
- Always consider chemicals or toxins available to the patient in question. For example, it may be necessary to screen through computer databases or call relatives, primary physicians and psychiatrists to find out the patient's recent prescriptions.
- Always obtain a corroborative history from all available sources such as family, friends or paramedics in order to aid both in the diagnosis and the management of the poisoned patient.
- Ask 'what, when, how much, how, where, why'. Any symptoms from exposure?
- Any suicidal risk? Moderate to high risk behaviour necessitates urgent psychiatric consult in the ED.
- Psychiatric and past medical history (including medications).
- Any previous suicide attempts?

PHYSICAL EXAMINATION

Vital signs

See Table 1 for details.

TABLE 1   Differential diagnoses of various vital signs in drug overdose

Temperature	Pulse rate/rhythm
HYPOTHERMIA ('COOLS')	**BRADYCARDIA ('PACED')**
C Carbon monoxide	P Propranolol (beta blocker)
O Opiates	A Anticholinesterase drugs
O Oral hypoglycaemics, insulin	C Clonidine, calcium channel
L Liquor	E Ethanol/alcohols
S Sedative hypnotics	D Digoxin
HYPERTHERMIA ('NASA')	**TACHYCARDIA ('FAST')**
N Neuroleptic malignant syndrome, nicotine	F Free base (cocaine)
A Antihistamines	A Anticholinergics, antihistamines, amphetamines
S Salicylates, sympathomimetics	S Sympathomimetics (cocaine, phencyclidine)
A Anticholinergics, antidepressants	T Theophylline
	DYSRHYTHMIAS
	Digoxin
	Cyclic antidepressants
	Sympathomimetics
	Phenothiazines
	Chloral hydrate
	Anticonvulsants

Blood pressure	Respiratory
HYPOTENSION ('CRASH')	**HYPOVENTILATION**
C Clonidine (or any antihypertensive drug)	Opioids
R Reserpine	Benzodiazepines
A Antidepressants	
S Sedative hypnotics	
H Heroin (opiates)	
HYPERTENSION ('CT SCAN')	**HYPERVENTILATION**
C Cocaine	Salicylates
T Theophylline	Central nervous system stimulant drugs
S Sympathomimetics	Cyanide
C Caffeine	
A Anticholinergics, amphetamines	
N Nicotine	

Odours

- Obvious odours: Kerosene/bleaching agents/insecticides.
- Other odours are listed in Table 2.

TABLE 2   Odours of poisons

Odours	Probable poisons
Fruity	Ethanol
Mothballs	Camphor/naphthalene
Bitter almonds	Cyanide
Silver polish	Cyanide
Stove gas	Carbon monoxide
Rotten eggs	Hydrogen sulphide
Garlic	Arsenic/parathion
Wintergreen	Methylsalicylate

Note: Carbon monoxide is odourless. Stove gas smells because of a stenching agent called mercaptans.

Neurological examination

- **Level of consciousness:** See the list below of selected drugs and toxins that cause coma or stupor.

General CNS depressants
  Anticholinergics
  Antihistamines
  Barbiturates
  Cyclic antidepressants
  Ethanol and other alcohols
  Phenothiazines
  Sedative-hypnotic agents

Cellular Hypoxia
  Carbon monoxide
  Cyanide
  Hydrogen sulfide
  Methaemoglobinaemia

Sympatholytic agents
  Clonidine
  Methyldopa
  Opiates

Other or unknown mechanisms
  Bromide
  Hypoglycaemic agents
  Lithium
  Phencyclidine
  Salicylates

- **Pupils:** Selected drugs and toxins and their effects on the pupils are listed below:

MIOSIS ('COPS')
  C Cholinergics, clonidine
  O Opiates, organophosphates
  P Phenothiazines, pilocarpine, pontine bleed
  S Sedative-hypnotics

MYDRIASIS ('AAAS')
  A Antihistamines
  A Antidepressants
  A Anticholinergics, atropine
  S Sympathomimetics (cocaine, amphetamines)

- **Fits** are caused by the substances ('**OTIS CAMPBELL**') listed below:

  O Organophosphates
  T Cyclic anti-depressants
  I Insulin, isoniazid
  S Sympathomimetics

  C Camphor, cocaine
  A Amphetamines
  M Methylxanthines
  P Phencyclidine (PCP)
  B Beta blockers
  E Ethanol
  L Lithium
  L Lead

- **Focal signs:** Look for other aetiologies, especially trauma.

Skin

- **Diaphoretic skin ('SOAP') and hypoglycaemia:**
  S Sympathomimetics
  O Organophosphates
  A ASA (salicylates)
  P PCP and hypoglycaemia

- **Dry:** Anticholinergic

- **Blistering:**
  1. Carbon monoxide
  2. Barbiturates
  3. Poison ivy
  4. Sulphur mustard
  5. Lewisite

- **Colour:**

  Red: Anticholinergic
  　　　Cyanide
  　　　Carbon monoxide

  Blue: Methaemoglobinaemia

- **Needle tracks:** Opioids

Toxidromes

Origin and definition

Toxidrome is a term that combines two Greek roots: *Toxikon* ('bow' – as arrows shot from a bow commonly have poison on their tips) and *dromos* ('race course'). Thus, toxidrome is the course that a specific poison runs or in toxicological terms, *'a syndrome that results from a specific toxin'*.

- **Opioids**
  1. Coma
  2. Respiratory depression
  3. Pinpoint pupils
  4. Hypotension
  5. Bradycardia

- **Cholinergics ('SLUDGE'):** For example, organophosphate and carbamate
  - **S** Salivation
  - **L** Lacrimation
  - **U** Urination
  - **D** Defaecation
  - **G** Gastric emptying
  - **E** Emesis

  1. 'Drowning in their own secretions'
     a. bronchorrhoea
     b. bronchospasm
     c. pulmonary oedema
  2. Altered mental state
  3. Muscle weakness and paralysis
  4. Odour of garlic
- **Anticholinergics:** For example, antihistamines, cyclic antidepressants, homatropine and scopolamine
  1. 'Hot as a hare' (hyperthermia)
  2. 'Red as a beet' (cutaneous vasodilatation)
  3. 'Dry as a bone' (decreased salivation)
  4. 'Blind as a bat' (cycloplegia and mydriasis)
  5. 'Mad as a hatter' (delirium and hallucinations)
  6. Other signs
     a. Tachycardia
     b. Urinary retention
     c. Decreased gastrointestinal motility/absent bowel sounds
- **Salicylates**
  1. Fever
  2. Tachypnoea
  3. Vomiting
  4. Lethargy (rarely coma)
  5. Tinnitus
- **Sympathomimetics:** For example, cocaine and amphetamines
  1. Hypertension
  2. Tachycardia
  3. Hyperpyrexia
  4. Mydriasis
  5. Anxiety or delirium
- **Sedative-hypnotics:** For example, barbiturates and benzodiazepines
  1. Unpredictable pupillary changes
  2. Confusion or coma
  3. Respiratory depression
  4. Hypothermia
  5. Vesicle or bullae ('barb burns')

- **Extrapyramidal:** A 'Parkinsonian' picture ('**TROD**')
  1. **T**remor
  2. **R**igidity
  3. **O**pisthotonous, oculogyric crisis
  4. **D**ysphonia, dysphagia
  This category of drugs includes the '**zines**'
  5. Chlorpromazine (Largactil®/Thorazine®)
  6. Prochlorperazine (Stemetil®/Compazine®)
  7. Haloperidol (Haldol®)
  8. Metochlopramide (Maxolon③/Reglan®)
- **Haemoglobinopathies**
  1. Carboxyhaemoglobinaemia
     a. Headache
     b. Nausea and vomiting, flu-like illness
     c. Syncope, tachypnoea, tachycardia
     d. Coma, convulsions
     e. Cardiovascular collapse, respiratory failure
  2. Methaemoglobinaemia
     a. Prominent clinical feature is cyanosis ('chocolate blood')
     b. Asymptomatic (<30% methaemoglobin level)
     c. Fatigue, weakness, dizziness, headache (30–50% methaemoglobin level)
     d. Lethargy, stupor, respiratory depression (>55% methaemoglobin level)

DIAGNOSTIC AIDS

Laboratory

- **Full blood count:** Elevated total white blood cell count = Infection/iron/theophylline/hydrocarbons
- **Serum electrolytes**
  1. 'Anion gap' = $[Na^+ + K^+] - [HCO_3^- + Cl^-]$
  2. Normal anion gap = 8–16 mEq/L
- **Metabolic acidosis/elevated anion gap**

C Carbon monoxide, cyanide	**M** Methanol
A Alcoholic ketoacidosis	**U** Uraemia
T Toluene	**D** Diabetic ketoacidosis
	P Paraldehyde
	I Iron, isoniazid
	L Lactic acidosis
	E Ethylene glycol
	S Salicylates, solvent

- **Serum urea and creatinine:** To identify any pre-existing renal dysfunction
- **Toxicology screens:** Drug levels are useful in
  1. Paracetamol
  2. Salicylates
  3. Cholinesterases
  4. Iron
  5. Lithium
  6. Theophylline
  7. Carbon monoxide

X-rays

- **Chest**
  1. Pulmonary toxic agents, e.g. hydrocarbons/toxic gases/paraquat
  2. Non-cardiogenic pulmonary oedema, e.g. opiates/phenobarbitone/salicylates/carbon monoxide
- **Abdominal: Toxins are radiopaque on X-rays (refer to mnemonic 'CHIPES')**
  - **C** Chloral hydrate
  - **H** Heavy metals
  - **I** Iron
  - **P** Phenothiazines
  - **E** Enteric-coated preps (salicylates)
  - **S** Sustained-release products (theophylline)

ECG

- Cyclic antidepressants affecting cardiac conducting system, e.g. prolonged PR, QTc and QRS intervals.
- Bradycardias and heart blocks, e.g. calcium channel blockers or beta blockers.

⇨ **SPECIAL TIPS FOR GPs**

- Do **NOT induce emesis** in a patient with DO using syrup ipecac. This is because ipecac may delay the administration or reduce the effectiveness of activated charcoal, oral antidotes and whole bowel irritation.
- It is generally safer to **refer all** patients with DOs to the emergency department by ambulance. An obvious **exception** is the child who has swallowed **oral contraceptive pills** by mistake. Reassurance can be given and the child can be discharged.
- Consider the possibility of **non-accidental injury** in a paediatric patient with a history of poisoning.
- Attend to the ABCs of the DO patient first before sending the patient to the emergency department.

MANAGEMENT

Patients with altered mental state or haemodynamic instability must be managed in the critical care area. Otherwise most DO cases can be managed in the intermediate care area.

Critical care area cases

- The first priority is always the airway.
- Airway management equipment must be immediately available.

NOTE: A patient with adequate oxygenation who has an impaired gag reflex and who needs gastric lavage will require prophylactic orotracheal intubation.

- Supportive treatment to manage the airway, breathing and circulation (ABCs) is paramount.
- Resuscitation drugs must be immediately available.
- Supplemental oxygen to maintain oxygen saturation level of at least 95%.
- Monitoring: ECG, vital signs q5–15 minutes and pulse oximetry.
- Establish a peripheral intravenous line.
- Labs (refer to *Diagnostic Aids: Laboratory*).
- Consider placement of a urinary catheter (case dependent).
- Manage seizures or dysrhythmias: Standard approach acceptable except in cases of toxicity by cyclic antidepressants, where cardiac and central nervous system complications can be prevented by alkalinization of the blood to pH of 7.5. This can be accomplished by either hyperventilation or administration of intravenous sodium bicarbonate, or both.

Ipecac

There is no evidence from clinical studies that ipecac improves the outcome of poisoned patients and its routine administration in the emergency department should be abandoned.

Concept of the 'coma cocktail'

- **Dextrose 50%:** Give only for confirmed hypoglycaemia as it may actually worsen neurologic recovery.
- **Naloxone (Narcan):**
  1. *Mechanism of action* Reverses the effects of opioids including respiratory depression, sedation and hypotension.

     Clinical effect Onset is within 2 minutes.

     Dosage Not a function of age or size (except in neonates); rather it depends on central nervous system receptor number; 2 mg for both adults and children and the same dose can be repeated up to 10 mg at intervals of 2–3 minutes. If no effect is seen with 10 mg of naloxone, the presumptive diagnosis of opioid agonist overdose must be reconsidered.

     Route of administration Intravenous, endotracheal or intralingual.

     Indications Safe but may add little to the patient's diagnostic evaluations as clinical parameters are found to be 92% sensitive in predicting responders to naloxone.

Caution There is a potential for precipitation of withdrawal symptoms when given to opioid addicts. The half-life of naloxone (60 minutes) is sometimes shorter than that of some opiates. Hence, there is a need for continued monitoring and repeat doses of naloxone.

- **Predicting opioid overdose:** See Table 3.
- **Predicting response to naloxone:** See Table 4.

TABLE 3 Predicting opioid overdose

Clinical parameter	Sensitivity (%)	Specificity (%)
Respiratory rate <12/min	79	94
Pinpoint pupils	75	85
Circumstantial evidence	67	95
Any of the above	92	76

TABLE 4 Predicting response to naloxone

Clinical parameter	N	Sensitivity (%)
Respiratory rate <12/min	20	80
Pinpoint pupils	22	88
Circumstantial evidence	15	60
Any of the above	24	96

- **Flumazenil (Anexate®):**

    Mechanism of action A benzodiazepine (BZD) is structurally related to midazolam. Flumazenil competes with other benzodiazepines at omega 1 receptor sites in the central nervous system.

    Clinical effect Onset in 1–2 minutes with peak effect in 3–5 minutes.

    Duration of effect 1–4 hours.

    Low dose reverses hypnosis, sedation of BZDs.

    High dose reverses anti-convulsant effect of BZDs.

    Indications Reverses accidental overdose of BZDs in procedural sedation, improving the patient's ventilatory status. Improves level of consciousness in known or suspected BZD overdose to avoid intubation or invasive procedures.

    Dosage Initial 0.2 mg IV; wait 30 seconds, then repeat at 0.3 mg IV; if needed, can give another 0.5 mg/min to a total dose of 3–5 mg.

    Adverse effects BZD withdrawal.

    Fits, especially in cyclic anti-depressant or BZD-dependent patients.

    Flush.

    Nausea and/or vomiting.

    Anxiety, palpitations and fear.

    Contraindications Patients taking BDZs for long-term control of fits. Anticipated use of BDZs in the near future, e.g. sedation, muscle relaxation, anticonvulsant, concomitant cyclic antidepressant toxicity and severe head trauma.

- **Thiamine:** Generally safe; indicated in all known alcoholics or the elderly, dishevelled, malnourished patient. Dosage: 100 mg IV bolus over 1–2 minutes.

Decontamination

Depending on the agent involved, proper protective gear must be worn. At the minimum level, staff should undertake full universal precautions.

- **Decontamination procedure:**
  1. Remove the patient from the contaminated area.
  2. Remove all the contaminated clothing.
  3. Brush off all powder contaminants from the patient's skin to avoid an exothermic reaction which may occur upon contact with water used for decontamination.
  4. Wash all affected skin areas with water and/or soap solution (and use shampoo for the hair). Use soft scrubs if available.
  5. Areas to concentrate on are the head, axillae, groin and back.
  6. Brush under the nails.
  7. Irrigate the eyes if specifically contaminated.
  8. Additionally decontaminate all open wounds with water.
- **End point of decontamination:**
  1. Until there is pain reduction, if primary dermal exposure is present.
  2. For eye contamination, until pain symptoms abate and/or there is a change in the colour of litmus or pH paper according to the nature of the agent involved.
  3. Uncomplicated full decontamination should take 5 to 8 minutes.

Gastric decontamination

- **Dilution:** Water or milk.
- **Gastric lavage should not be employed routinely** in the management of poisoned patients. In experimental studies, the amount of marker removed by gastric lavage was highly variable and diminished with time. There is no certain evidence that its use improves clinical outcome (Pond et al., 1995) and it may cause significant morbidity.

  Indications Should not be considered unless a patient has ingested a potentially life-threatening amount of poison and presents **within an hour of ingestion**. Even then, the clinical benefit of its use has not been confirmed in controlled studies.

  Contraindications
  Ingestion of corrosives.
  Ingestion of petroleum distillates.
  Existence of ongoing fits.
  Non-toxic ingestion.

Ingestion of sharp materials.

Significant haemorrhagic diathesis.

Procedure

Use the largest bore tube possible.

Protect the airway.

Place the patient in the left lateral and mild Trendelenburg position.

Establish correct placement of the tube.

Aspirate the stomach contents and retain specimen to be sent to the ward with the patient.

Instil lavage fluid.

Agitate stomach.

Withdraw fluid.

Repeat the procedure until the lavage fluid returns clear.

Potential complications

Aspiration

Laryngospasm

Oesophageal injury

- **Activated charcoal:**
  1. **Single dose:** Should not be administered routinely in the management of poisoned patients. Based on volunteer studies, the effectiveness of activated charcoal decreases with time; the greatest benefit is **within an hour of ingestion**.
  2. **Indications:** May be considered if a patient has ingested a potentially toxic amount of poison (which is known to be adsorbed by charcoal) within an hour; there is insufficient data to support or exclude its use after an hour of ingestion. There is no evidence that the administration of activated charcoal improves clinical outcome.
  3. **Multiple dose:** Repeated administration (>2 doses) of oral activated charcoal with the intent of enhancing drug elimination. Multiple-dose activated charcoal is thought to produce its beneficial effect by:
     a. Binding any drug which diffuses from the circulation into the gut lumen. After adsorption, a drug will re-enter the gut by passive diffusion provided that the concentration there is lower than in the blood. The rate of passive diffusion depends on the concentration gradient and blood flow. Under these 'sink' conditions, a concentration gradient is maintained and the drug passes continuously into the gut lumen where it is adsorbed by charcoal. This process has been termed '**gastrointestinal dialysis**'.
     b. Interrupting the enterohepatic and enterogastric circulation of drugs.
  4. **Indications:** Multiple-dose activated charcoal should be considered only if a patient has ingested a life-threatening amount of carbamazepine, dapsone, phenobarbitone, quinine or theophylline.

5. **Drugs adsorbed by charcoal:**

Acetaminophen	Digoxin	Meprobamate	Phenylpropanolamin
Amphetamines	Ethchlorvynol	Mercuric chloride	Phenytoin
Arsenic	Glutethamide	Methylsalicylate	Propoxyphene
Aspirin	Imipramine	Morphine	Quinidine
Chlorpheniramine	Iodine	Nortriptyline	Quinine
Chlorpromazine	Ipecac	Paraquat	Salicylates
Cocaine	Isoniazid	Phenobarbitone	Secobarbitone

6. **Substances not adsorbed by activated charcoal:**

   a. Heavy metals: Iron, lithium and cyanide

   b. Acids and alkalis

   c. Simple alcohols: Methanol and ethanol

   d. Hydrocarbons

- **Cathartics:**

   The administration of a cathartic **alone** has no role in the management of the poisoned patient and is **not recommended** as a method of gut decontamination.

   Based on available data, the routine use of cathartic **in combination** with activated charcoal is not endorsed. If a cathartic is used, it should be limited to a single dose in order to minimize adverse effects.

   Mechanism of action Decreases gastrointestinal transit time (although the data are controversial). Neutralizes the constipating effect of activated charcoal. Theoretically, they speed up gastrointestinal transit time, thus allowing activated charcoal to catch up with the pills and thus exert its effect. Cathartics may also be used for whole bowel irrigation.

   However, cathartics have **not** been proven to either

   a. reduce drug absorption or

   b. Improve outcome

   Side effects
   Vomiting
   Abdominal pain
   Electrolyte abnormalities

   Contraindications
   Pre-existing diarrhoea
   Bowel obstruction/ileus
   Volume depleted states
   Infants
   Renal failure contraindicates use of magnesium containing cathartics
   Abdominal trauma

TABLE 5 **Specific antidotes for toxins**

Toxin	Antidote	Dosage
Acetaminophen, Paracetamol	N-acetylcysteine (Parvolex®) (each ml contains 200 mg Parvolex®)	IV 150 mg/kg in 200 ml $D_5W \times 15$ min, then IV 50 mg/kg in 500 ml $D_5W \times 4$ h, then IV 100 mg/kg in 1000 ml $D_5W \times 16$ h
Arsenic, mercury, lead	BAL (dimercaprol)	5 mg/kg body weight IM
Atropine	Physostigmine	0.5–2 mg IV
Benzodiazepines	Flumazenil (Anexate®)	See section on 'coma cocktail'
Carbon monoxide	Oxygen	100% O_2 (hyperbaric for moderate-severe exposures and exposure in pregnant women) Refer to Chapter 84, Poisoning, Carbon Monoxide
Cyanide	Amyl nitrite pearls Sodium nitrite (3% sol)	Inhalation of contents of 1–2 pearls Adults: IV 300 mg (10 ml) over 2–5 min; Children: IV 0.2–0.33 ml/kg (6–10 mg)
	Sodium thiosulphate (25% sol)	Adults: 50 ml IV (12.5 g) over 10 min; can repeat half dose × 1 prn; children: 1.65 ml/kg IV over 10 min
Ethylene glycol, methanol	Ethanol (10%) mixed in D_5W	Loading dose: 800 mg/kg Maintenance: 1–1.5 ml/kg/h
Iron	Desferoxamine	15 mg/kg/h IV
Lead	EDTA: calcium disodium edetate	1000–1500 mg /m²/day IV continuous infusion
Nitrites	Methylene blue (1% solution)	1–2 mg/kg IV × 5 min
Organophosphates	Atropine	2–4 mg IV q 5–10 min prn (adult); 0.5 mg/kg IV q 5 min prn (child)
	Pralidoxime (2–PAM)	25–50 mg/kg IV (up to 1 g)
Opioids	Naloxone	See section on 'Coma cocktail'
Phenothiazines	Benztropine (Cogentin®) Diphenhydramine	2 mg IV/IM 50 mg IV/IM/PO
Isoniazid (INH)	Pyridoxine	5 g IV (can repeat if fits persist)
Digoxin, digitoxin, oleander	Digitalis Fab fragments (Digibind®)	Digoxin level unknown: 5–10 vials IV (40 µg Fab/vial): can repeat Digoxin level known: # vials Digibind $$= \frac{\frac{(serum\ digoxin) \times 5.6\ litre/kg \times wt\ in\ kg}{1000}}{0.6}$$

- **Whole bowel irrigation (WBI)**

  Prepare the bowel with an agent such as *Go-Lytely* (not absorbed) and flush drugs through the gastrointestinal tract rapidly.

  WBI is most useful when radiopaque tablets or chemicals have been ingested (providing the ability to monitor the patient's gastrointestinal tract radiographically).

  WBI should be considered for patients who have ingested substantial amounts of iron as the morbidity is high and there is a lack of other options for gastrointestinal decontamination.

  Consider in cases where activated charcoal is not useful, such as

  1. Body packing: Heroin or cocaine
  2. Overdose of sustained-release products

  Contraindications
  Bowel obstruction, bowel perforation and ileus in patients with haemodynamic instability or compromised unprotected airways.

Enhancement of elimination

- **Forced alkaline diuresis:**

  Alkalinization Alkalinizing the urine to enhance elimination of weak acids has a limited role for salicylates, phenobarbitone and herbicide 2, 4 (dichlorophenoxyacetic acid [2, 4-D]).

  Regimen A cycle of 1.5 L fluid/three hours:
  500 ml 5% dextrose + 8.4% $NaHCO_3$ at 1–2 ml/kg body weight
  500 ml 5% dextrose + 30 ml of 7.45% potassium chloride
  500 ml normal saline
  IV frusemide 20 mg at the end of each cycle
  Monitor serum pH and electrolytes: Urinary pH should be maintained at pH 8.

  Caution
  Elderly
  Cardiac patients
  Renal disease patients
  Ingestion of poisons which are cardio- and nephro-toxic.

- **Haemoperfusion:** Indications are severe intoxications with theophylline and barbiturates.

- **Haemodialysis:** Indications are
  1. Ethylene glycol
  2. Methanol
  3. Lithium (with significant central nervous system alterations)
  4. Salicylates (with fits, altered mental state, severe metabolic acidosis and serum level >100 mg/dl)

- **Specific antidotes:** See Table 5 for details.
- **Disposition:** Admission must be to General Medicine in anticipation of later transfer to Psychiatry. Non-life-threatening drug overdose without convincing suicidal intent may be discharged **after** psychiatric consultation.

ANNEX

Common sources of poisoning in Singapore

Paracetamol
Benzodiazepines
Bleaching agents
Household detergents
Antidepressants
Salicylates
Organophosphates

References/Further Reading

1. Hoffman JR. The empirical use of naloxone in patients with altered mental status: A reappraisal. *Ann Emerg Med*. 1991; 20: 246–252.

2. Chyka PA, Seger D (1997); revised by Krenzelok EP and Vale JA (2004). Position statement: Single-dose activated charcoal. The American Academy of Clinical Toxicology, European Association of Poison Centres and Clinical Toxicologists. *J Toxicol Clin Toxicol*. 1997; 35(7): 721–741.

3. Vale JA. Position statement: Gastric lavage. The American Academy of Clinical Toxicology, European Association of Poison Centres and Clinical Toxicologists. *J Toxicol Clin Toxicol*. 2004; 42(7): 933–943.

4. Barceloux D, McGuigan M, Hartigan-Go K (1997); revised by Bateman DN (2004). Position statement: Cathartics. The American Academy of Clinical Toxicology, European Association of Poison Centres and Clinical Toxicologists. *J Toxicol Clin Toxicol*. 2004; 42(3): 243–253.

5. Krenzelok EP, McGuigan M, Lheur P (1997); revised by Manoguerra AS (2005). Position statement: Ipecac syrup. The American Academy of Clinical Toxicology, European Association of Poison Centres and Clinical Toxicologists. *J Toxicol Clin Toxicol*. 2005; 42(2): 133–143.

6. Hoffman RS, Goldfrank LR. The poisoned patient with unconsciousness: Controversies in the use of a coma cocktail. *JAMA*. 1995; 274: 562–569.

7. Goldfrank LR, Flomenbaum NA, Lewin NA, et al. Principles of managing the poisoned or overdosed patient: An overview. *Goldfrank's Toxicological Emergencies*. 8th ed. New York: McGraw-Hill/Appleton & Lange; 2006: 42–50.

8. Milton T (1997); revised by Phillipe L (2004). Position statement: Whole bowel irrigation. The American Academy of Clinical Toxicology, European Association of Poison Centres and Clinical Toxicologists. *J Toxicol Clin Toxicol*. 2004; 42(6): 843–854.

9. Pond SM, et al. Gastric emptying in acute overdose: A prospective randomized controlled trial. *Med J Aust*. 1995; 163(7): 345–349.

20   Red Eye

Toh Hong Chuen • Peter Manning

CAVEATS

- The major role of the emergency department (ED) physician is to perform an appropriate eye examination and recognize potential vision-threatening disorders.
- Always perform a visual acuity on any patient with an eye problem. It defines in a simple way whether the function of this critical organ is impaired.
- Beware the combination of red eye, vomiting, frontal headache and visual loss: This is typical of **acute angle-closure glaucoma** and demands immediate attention as it is potentially vision-threatening.
- Infections and penetrating eye injuries should not be patched (photophobia can be minimized by the use of sunglasses or eye shields).
- Steroid-containing drops or ointment should not be prescribed without prior eye consultation.

⇨ **SPECIAL TIPS FOR GPs**

Refer for **immediate** ophthalmology consultation if the patient exhibits any of the following:

- Decreased visual acuity.
- Deep, rather than superficial, pain.
- Pain unrelieved by topical anaesthetics.
- Corneal oedema.
- Flare or cells in the anterior chamber.
- Ciliary flush.
- Pain in the contralateral eye on direct exposure of the unaffected eye.
- Corneal or conjunctival foreign body which cannot be removed after one attempt in the office.
- In the case or a corrosive burn, implement saline irrigation immediately prior to the patient being transported to hospital. Irrigate until the effluent is pH neutral or mildly acidic as shown by the use of blue and pink litmus paper.

MANAGEMENT

Patients are to be triaged as intermediate acuity cases or as critical care cases if there is any hint of visual impairment, e.g. acute glaucoma (with redness of eyes, vomiting, frontal headache and visual loss). They should be managed in a well-equipped eye examination room in the ED.

Examination of the eye

- There are 6 steps in an eye examination.

    1. **Visual acuity**

        The vital sign of the eye. It should be done with a standard Snellen chart, with the patient wearing glasses or contact lens if any. The patient must be able to read at least 50% of the letters on a line to be said to have that acuity. A refractive error is usually corrected with a pinhole occluder. If the patient is still unable to see, proceed with counting of fingers, movement of fingers and perception of light in this order. Topical anaesthesia may overcome reflex blepharospasm and facilitate examination. Check corneal sensation before giving topical anaesthetics.

    2. **Visual field**

        Test each eye separately. By using the normal visual field of the examiner as baseline, test the visual field with the confrontational method. This is especially important when elucidating neuro-opthalmologic visual loss.

    3. **Pupils**

        Assess the pupils for size, shape, reactivity and presence of relative afferent papillary reflex (indicating a prechiasmal defect). Pain in the contralateral eye on direct light exposure is an early sign of iritis. An irregular pupil with synechiae is seen in iritis. In **acute angle closure** glaucoma, the pupil is **mid-dilated** and very poorly responsive to light. In **iritis**, the pupil may be large or small; reactive or non-reactive depending on the extent of inflammation and posterior synechiae.

    4. **Extraocular eye movement**

        Assess the 6 cardinal positions of gaze, as well as the presence of nystagmus.

    5. **Eye lids and anterior segment**

        Conduct a careful examination of the eyelids, conjunctiva, sclera, cornea, iris, lens and anterior chamber with a pen torch. Look in particular for the following features: **Proptosis** (which may indicate retro-orbital pathology such as abscess); **ciliary flush** (which indicates anterior chamber pathology); **iridodonesis** (a shimmering movement of the iris may represent traumatic subluxation of the lens) and **corneal opacities** (e.g. keratitis or corneal ulcer). **Evert the lids** to search for a foreign body. Perform the **oblique flashlight test**[1] if acute glaucoma is suspected (with a specificity of 69%). Use the slit-lamp as an adjunct. In **iritis**, the **redness** is primarily noted at the limbus (junction between the cornea and sclera).

    6. **Posterior segment**

        Using the direct ophthalmoscope, begin with visualization of the red reflex, followed by the posterior segment of the eye including the optic cup, optic disc (and cup-to-disc ratio), retinal vessels and retina itself.

Examination adjuncts

- **The slit-lamp examination**, optimally, is used on all patients. Examine for flare and cells, posterior keratitic precipitates, and/or hyphema in the anterior chamber, indicative of an inflammatory process.
- **Tonometry** is performed after topical anaesthesia to measure intraocular pressure. An **abnormal pressure** is **>20 mmHg**. Avoid this procedure if the eye is infected or if there is the possibility of a global rupture.

  1. **Fluorescein staining** is used to elucidate corneal pathology. The stain is taken up by the hydrophilic deep layers of the cornea when the hydrophobic superficial layers are gone, as in abrasion or infection.

  2. **Imaging**: A plain film of globe soft tissue may identify a radiopaque foreign body.

  3. **Topical anaesthesia** is often useful to differentiate keratitis from iritis.

     a. Pain from conjunctivitis, a superficial foreign body, or corneal abrasion and keratitis, is relieved by a topical anaesthetic.

     b. Pain from deeper inflammation, e.g. iritis, is unrelieved by this therapy.

  4. **Homatropine**: Use of this agent, a mydriatic/cycloplegic drug, should decrease eye pain in deep inflammation of the anterior pole structures, e.g. iritis by the reduction of ciliary and iris muscle spasm.

- Refer to Table 1 for differential diagnosis of red eye.
- Refer to Table 2 for common causes of conjuncticitis.

TABLE 1   Differential diagnosis of red eye

Painful red eye	Painless red eye
Acute angle-closure glaucoma	Conjunctivitis
Scleritis	Subconjunctival haemorrhage
Uveitis	Episcleritis
Keratitis (infectious/non-infectious)	
Corneal abrasion/corneal ulcer	
Trauma/chemical injury	

TABLE 2 **Common causes of conjunctivitis**

Pathophysiology/ causative agent		Clinical presentation	Treatment
Allergic	IgE-mediated; associated with atopy	Almost always associated with itch; usually bilateral. Discharge, if any is watery and clear or mucoid	Avoid trigger. Oral anti-histamine
Viral	Adenovirus	Associated with upper respiratory tract infection; preauricular lymph nodes. Eye irritation, may spread from one eye to the other. Global conjunctivitis with follicular reaction in the inferior tarsal conjunctiva.	Symptomatic. Cold compress. Topical antibiotic. Eye and hand hygiene for two weeks
	Herpes simplex	Similar to adenovirus infection, except that there is usually significant pain, burning and a foreign body sensation. On slit-lamp examination with fluorescein: Typical dendritic pattern with bulb end, as opposed to herpes zoster dendrites with tapered ends	Topical anti-viral agents. Eye consultation
Bacteria	Gram +ve (staph/ strep) in children; Gram –ve in adult (H. influenza)	Acute onset; spread to the other eye in 48 hours. Morning crusting and difficulty opening the eyelids. If hyperacute onset occurs in sexually active population, consider *Neisseria gonorrhoea*	Topical antibiotics. Urgent referral for *Neisseria gonorrhoea* conjunctivitis as it is sight-threatening

Disposition

- Refer for **immediate** ophthalmology consultation if the patient exhibits any of the points listed in Special Tips for GPs.
- **Most patients** can be discharged home with follow-up in an eye specialist outpatient clinic within 24–48 hours.

References/Further Reading

1. Butler KH, et al. The red eye: A systematic approach to differential diagnosis and therapy. In: *Em Med Reports*. 7 Mar 1994.
2. Ahmed RM, Aneesh TN. Diagnosis and management of the acute red eye. *Emerg Med Clin N Am*. 2008; 26: 35–55.

21 Seizure

Lim Er Luen • Sim Tiong Beng • Shirley Ooi

CAVEATS

- See Table 1 for the most common causes of seizures in patients presenting to the emergency department.
- A history from a witness is vital to the diagnosis. Rule out mimickers, e.g. vasovagal syncope, hysteria/panic attacks, hypoglycaemia, transient ischemic attacks or transient cardiac arrhythmia. Presence of oral-facial injuries makes seizure more likely.
- Prolonged seizures may cause fever and vice versa.
- Ask about compliance to medication in a known epileptic with breakthrough seizure.

⇨ **SPECIAL TIPS FOR GPs**
- Check the pulse to rule out ventricular fibrillation/cardiac arrhythmia first.
- Consider meningitis in the presence of fever with or without purpuric rash and adopt universal precautions.
- Exclude hypoglycaemia and transient ischaemic attacks.

MANAGEMENT

Breakthrough seizure

- Identify any precipitants.
- Routine lab tests are not useful as they tend to have a low yield.
- Anti-epileptic drug (AED) levels are rarely indicated unless suspected drug toxicity, status epilepticus or compliance is in doubt.
  1. Encourage compliance and maintain the same dose if the patient is non-compliant. Enquire about the side effects of AEDs if any.
  2. If the patient is truly compliant with medication, check the AED level and if the level is low, increase the dose if the maximum dose has not been reached.
  3. If the maximum dose has been reached, consult the neurologist for AED options.
- **Disposition:** Admit to the observation unit and consider loading phenytoin orally 300 mg at 3-hourly intervals for 3 doses if the patient is non-compliant, elderly or the AED level is low. Discharge the patient if there is no further seizures. Educate the patient and carer that non-compliance, alcohol abuse, sleep deprivation and concurrent illness are associated with increased incidence of breakthrough seizures. Refer to the primary care physician for follow-up.

TABLE 1 Approach to seizure and its common etiologies

First seizure in a patient not known to be an epileptic

- **Well first seizure**

  1. Defined as young 'healthy' patients presenting with first seizure with return of normal mental status and neurological examination.

  2. Stat capillary blood sugar, electrocardiogram (ECG), urine HCG, serum sodium and calcium level as guided by clinical suspicion.

  3. **Disposition:** Admit to the observation unit for early electroencephalography (EEG). The earlier the EEG is performed, the more likely a helpful result will emerge from it. Magnetic resonance imaging (MRI) is the modality of choice and may be arranged as an outpatient procedure. AEDs are generally not indicated for well first seizure. Seizure first-aid advice

and counselling on home or workplace safety should be provided while the patient is in the observation unit.

- **Unwell first seizure with or without fever:** Exclude structural and metabolic causes.
  1. Stat capillary blood sugar.
  2. Labs: Full blood count, urea/electrolytes/creatinine, ionized calcium, magnesium or blood culture as guided by clinical suspicion.
  3. **ECG** in older patients to look for signs of ischaemia or dysrhythmias.
  4. Emergency head computed tomography (CT) scan is indicated for patients with head trauma, focal deficits, malignancy, shunts, human immunodeficiency virus or HIV, old cerebral vascular accidents, who are >40 years old and have a history of alcoholism and anti-coagulant use.
  5. **Disposition:**
     a. Admit the patient if he has (1) abnormal head CT; (2) persistent neurological deficits; and (3) is unreliable about follow-up.
     b. Start IV ceftriaxone 2 g if meningitis is suspected.

Status epilepticus

This is defined traditionally as ≥2 seizures without full recovery of consciousness between attacks or continuous seizure activity lasting ≥30 minutes. The emergingconsensus is any convulsive seizure >5–10 minutes to any attack that persists at the time of evaluation should be considered status epilepticus.

- **Supportive measures**
  1. Airway measures: Place patient in the recovery position.
  2. Open and maintain airway.
  3. Suction any vomitus with a Yankauer catheter.

  NOTE: If the patient is still convulsing, **do not** attempt to insert an oral airway, clear oral secretions or intubate the patient.

  4. Administer supplemental high-flow oxygen via a reservoir mask.
  5. Prepare intubation equipment in case you are unable to maintain airway and adequate oxygenation.
  6. Monitoring: Vital signs, ECG and pulse oximetry.
  7. Intravenous (IV) access.
  8. Labs:
     a. **Stat capillary blood sugar**.
     b. Full blood count, urea/electrolytes/creatinine, ionized calcium, magnesium, phosphate or arterial blood gas.

    c. Consider liver function tests, anti-convulsant levels and serum toxicology screen including ethanol.

    d. Perform a chest X-ray and urinalysis.

    e. Insert a urinary catheter.

- **Drug therapy**

1. **Benzodiazepines**

   Either IV *diazepam* or *lorazepam* are effective first-line therapies for prolonged seizures.

   Dosage: For adults, IV **diazepam** 5 mg slow bolus to be given at a rate not to exceed 2 mg/min; can be repeated at q 5 minutes (to a total of 20 mg). For infants and children, IV **diazepam** 0.02 mg/kg at a rate ≤2 mg/min; can be repeated q five minutes (to a total of 10 mg). Rectal **diazepam** 5 mg suppository is to be administered if IV access is delayed.

   IV **lorazepam** 4 mg or 0.1 mg/kg may be given over 1–2 minutes and repeated at q 5 minutes with a maximum dose of 12 mg. *Advantages* of *lorazepam* over diazepam include faster onset of action, extended duration of action and possible less cardiorespiratory depression.

   Respiratory or circulatory effects should be monitored and usually occur with doses of >20 mg of diazepam.

2. **Phenytoin**

   Dosage: IV phenytoin infusion neat at 18 mg/kg body weight at a rate ≤50 mg/min with cardiac monitoring, regardless of whether the patient is on phenytoin therapy. The infusion should not exceed 60 minutes since precipitation tends to occur after that. Loading with phenytoin at standard doses as per protocol has not been shown to result in complications even in substantial pre-infusion levels. The traditional practice of giving a half loading dose may cause a 'too slow and too low' phenomenon and complicate management.

3. IV **propofol** infusion at 50–200 mg/hr

4. Consider IV **valproate** infusion at 25–45 mg/kg at 3 mg/kg/min. In some protocols, it has been recommended as a third-line agent as it has less haemodynamic effects and has been shown in some studies to terminate seizures that have been refractory up to that stage.

5. Consider **long-acting barbiturates**: Phenobarbitone

   Dosage: IV phenobarbitone 10 mg/kg slow bolus at a rate of 100 mg/min, followed by, if necessary, IV phenobarbitone 10 mg/kg slow bolus at a rate of 50 mg/min.

6. Consider **rapid sequence intubation**: Refer to Chapter 28, *Airway Management/Rapid Sequence Intubation*.

- **Disposition:** Admit to Neurology high dependancy/medical intensive care unit after appropriate consultation.

References/Further Reading

1. ACEP Clinical Policies Committee, Clinical Policies Subcommittee on Seizures. Clinical policy: Critical issues in the evaluation and management of adult patients presenting to the emergency department with seizures. *Ann Emerg Med.* May 2004; 43(5): 605–625.

2. Duvivier EH, Pollack C. Seizures. In: Marx JA, Hockberger RS, Walls RM, eds. *Rosen's Emergency Medicine: Concepts and Clinical Practice.* 7th ed. Philadelphia, PA: Mosby-Elsevier; 2010: 1346–1355.

3. Practice parameter: Neuroimaging in the emergency patient presenting with seizure (summary statement). American College of Emergency Physicians, American Academy of Neurology, American Association of Neurological Surgeons, American Society of Neuroradiology. *Ann Emerg Med.* July 1996; 28(1): 114–118.

4. Reuber M, Hattingh L, Goulding PJ. Epileptological emergencies in accident and emergency: A survey at St. James's University Hospital, Leeds. *Seizure.* 2000; 9(9): 216–220.

5. Archibald-Taylor SK, Mills TJ. Seizures. In: Frank LR, Jobe KA, eds. *Admission and Discharge Decisions in Emergency Medicine.* Philadelphia, PA: Hanley & Belfus; 2002: 165–170.

6. Kim LG, Johnson TL, Marson AG, Chadwick DW, MRC MESS Study group. Prediction of risk of seizure recurrence after a single seizure and early epilepsy: Further results from the MESS trial. *Lancet Neurol.* Apr 2006; 5(4): 317–322.

7. Shih T. Epilepsy and seizures. In: Brust JCH. *Current Diagnosis and Treatment Neurology.* New York: McGraw-Hill Medical; 2012: 47–62.

22   Shock/Hypoperfusion States

Benjamin Leong • Shirley Ooi

DEFINITIONS

- **Shock** may be defined as a state of impaired perfusion leading to inadequate delivery of oxygen and nutrients and clearance of metabolites with consequent reversible and eventual irreversible cellular injury.
- **Shock** may be classified according to the underlying pathophysiology causing it (Table 1).
- **Hypotension** is simply a state of low blood pressure. Although often used to imply shock, a hypotensive individual may not be in shock and a normotensive individual may be in shock.

CAVEATS

Basic pathophysiology

Oxygen transport

- The principle problem in all shock states is a reduced **delivery of oxygen (DO$_2$)** to the tissues.
- As DO$_2$ falls, compensatory mechanisms result in a proportionally increased **oxygen extraction ratio (O$_2$ER)** from the blood by the tissues. The **mixed venous O$_2$ saturation** then falls, indicating that there is now less oxygen left in the venous haemoglobin.
- The tissues are thus able to maintain steady **oxygen consumption (VO$_2$)** for metabolic needs. At this stage VO$_2$ is **independent** of DO$_2$.
- Below a critical level of DO$_2$ (**DO$_2$crit**), the rate of increase in oxygen extraction cannot keep up with the falling delivery of oxygen (Figure 1).
- From this point the amount of oxygen the tissues are able to consume becomes directly **dependent** on oxygen delivery—the lower the DO$_2$, the lower the VO$_2$. This is termed **supply-dependent oxygen consumption**.
- In **pathological states**, the compensatory mechanisms that increase O$_2$ER may be impaired, thus DO$_2$crit may be higher and supply-dependent oxygen consumption begins earlier.

In **sepsis**, the situation is more complex. Maldistribution of blood flow, disruption of microvascular endothelium and impaired oxidative phosphorylation in mitochondria occur, impairing VO$_2$. Supply-dependent oxygen consumption begins earlier and therefore DO$_2$crit is also higher. The circulatory state may be hypodynamic, or more commonly hyperdynamic. In the former, the tissues are only able to consume as much oxygen as the limited delivery. In the latter, there is an improved O$_2$ delivery, but because of the microvascular and cellular derangements, the improvement may only be partial.

TABLE 1   **Types of shock**

Type	Mechanism	Examples
Hypovolaemic	Decreased preload	Reduced fluid intake, e.g. dehydration Cutaneous fluid loss, e.g. burns Gastrointestinal fluid loss, e.g. severe vomiting or diarrhoea Renal loss, e.g. diabetes mellitus and insipidus, adrenal insufficiency Third-space loss, e.g. acute pancreatitis
Haemorrhagic	Decreased preload	Trauma Gastrointestinal haemorrhage Ruptured aortic aneurysm Ruptured ectopic pregnancy
Cardiogenic	Pump impairment	Myocardial ischaemia/infarction Myocarditis Myocardial contusion Cardiomyopathy Dysrhythmias (tachy or brady) Acute valvular insufficiency Acute papillary/septal rupture
Obstructive	Pump impairment	Cardiac tamponade Tension pneumothorax Pulmonary embolism
Septic	Decreased afterload	Pneumonia Meningitis Peritonitis Cholangitis Urinary tract infections Necrotizing fasciitis
Anaphylactic	Decreased afterload	Drug allergies Insect or animal bites/stings Toxin exposures Food allergies (e.g. peanuts)
Neurogenic	Decreased afterload	Spinal cord injury
Pharmacologic	Mixed	Anti-hypertensives Sedatives Narcotics Anti-depressants Nitrates Phosphodiesterase inhibitors Toxic exposures

FIGURE 1   Relationship between oxygen delivery (DO$_2$) and oxygen consumption (VO$_2$)

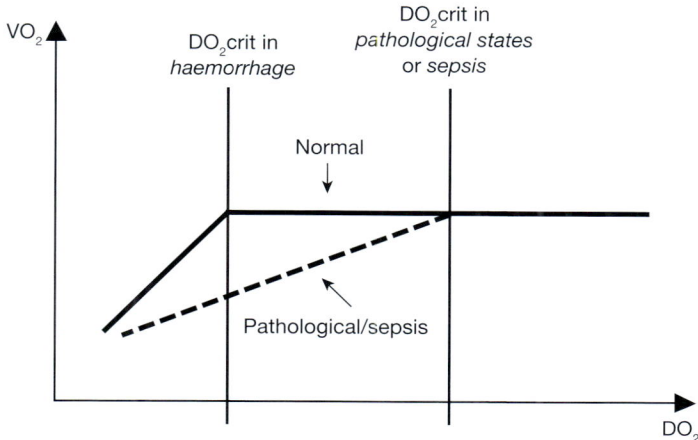

- The cells now turn to **anaerobic respiration** to make up for the shortfall in adenosine triphosphate (ATP) production (albeit very inefficiently). Lactate levels increase both due to increased production and reduced clearance.

- Therefore, at this time, the body may be described to be in **oxygen deficit**, as there is inadequate oxygen to 'spend' for its oxygen needs.

- With time, this deficit will accumulate as **oxygen debt**, which is the amount of oxygen needed to 'repay' what the body's metabolism is being owed for anaerobic respiration.

- The aim in managing shock and hypoperfusion states is therefore to **restore the delivery of oxygen** to the tissues, and the end point of resuscitation should ideally be the **complete repayment of oxygen debt**.

Acid-base physiology

- At the same time that oxygen delivery is impaired due to the low perfusion, **clearance of CO$_2$ and metabolites** from the tissue is similarly affected.

- **When perfusion is adequate**, the gaps between arterial and mixed venous pCO$_2$ and pH are small.

- However, **in severe circulatory deficit** with continued respiration (spontaneous or mechanical), two things happen:

  1. The reduced rate of blood flow to the tissues exposes the blood to the increased tissue pCO$_2$ and metabolites for a longer time. **There may then be an apparent respiratory acidosis in the venous blood, in addition to the metabolic acidosis.**

2. The rate of blood flow to the lungs is also reduced, yet because the same amount of ventilation continues for that reduced amount of pulmonary blood flow, **there may be an apparent respiratory alkalosis in the arterial blood** due to the ventilation/perfusion mismatch.

- There is thus a **widening gap** between arterial and venous pCO_2 and pH during severe shock states. This gap widens further with time, as the tissue metabolites continue to build up in the same way oxygen debt builds up.
- However, in untreated **cardiorespiratory arrest**, because there is now no ventilation, the arteriovenous gap does not widen.
- Thus, it becomes important to monitor **both** arterial and venous blood gases in severe shock states.

CLINICAL ASSESSMENT

- The initial assessment should be directed at **recognizing** a patient in shock, and identifying the **type** and **cause** of shock (refer to Table 2).
- Generally, **hypotension with classical signs of a hypoperfused** state like pallor, cool skin, tachycardia, diaphoresis or altered mental status suggests shock.
- Patients on beta blockers, athletes and patients with neurogenic shock may not exhibit tachycardia.
- Patients who have **septic shock** commonly have a hyperdynamic circulation with warm peripheries and bounding pulses. Be aware that the absence of warm peripheries does not exclude sepsis, as the patient may be in a hypodynamic circulatory state instead.
- Patients with **anaphylactic shock** may not exhibit classical clinical features of histamine release and this possibility needs to be considered.
- The **physical examination** should be directed by the presenting history.
- Even if all the commonly used clinical indicators of shock are normal, **shock** on a **cellular**, **tissue** or **organ basis** may still be present.

⇨ **SPECIAL TIPS FOR GPs**
- All patients in shock should be referred to a hospital immediately for further evaluation.
- Beware of subtle signs in geriatric and paediatric patients who may present with subtle non-specific signs of septic shock. A high index of suspicion is needed.

TABLE 2   General features of different kinds of shock

Diagnostic information	Hypovolaemic	Cardiogenic	Obstructive	Septic	Anaphylactic	Neurogenic
General features (Not all may be present, refer to the specific subgroup)			Hypotension Tachycardia Thready pulses Tachypnoea Peripheral vasoconstriction Diaphoresis Lethargy Altered mental status Reduced urine output			
Signs and symptoms	History of excessive fluid loss or reduced intake, bleeding or trauma Loss of skin turgor Dry mucosae Sunken eyes Injury patterns associated with trauma	Chest pain Dyspnoea Orthopnoea Pulmonary crackles or rhonchi Pulmonary effusion S3 gallop	Chest pain Dyspnoea Orthopnoea Signs of specific aetiology, e.g. muffled heart sounds, unilateral hyperresonant lung fields	Fever or hypothermia Bounding pulses Clinical features of respective infective aetiology	History of exposure to causative agent may or may not be available Angioedema Urticaria Stridor or rhonchi	History of spine injury Hypotension with bradycardia Peripheral vasodilation Paralysis Lax anal tone Priapism Loss of bulbocavernosus reflex
Peripheries	Cold, clammy	Cold, clammy	Cold, clammy	Hyperdynamic – warm Hypodynamic – cold	Warm and flushed or normal	Warm, dry
Heart rate	High	High or low	High	High	High	Low
Central venous pressure	Low	High	High	Low	Low	Low
Systemic vascular resistance	High	High	High	Hyperdynamic – low Hypodynamic – high	Low	Low
Mixed venous C2Sat (Normal = 70–75%)	Low	Low	Low	Hyperdynamic – high Hypodynamic – low/high	Low	Low
Cardiac output	Low	Low	Low	Hyperdynamic – high Hypodynamic – low/high	Low	Low

INITIAL MANAGEMENT OF THE PATIENT SUSPECTED OF HAVING SHOCK

- All patients exhibiting the general features of shock should be urgently transferred to a **monitored**, **critical care area** for **assessment** and **stabilization**.
- Prompt recognition and initiation of treatment is paramount to reduce morbidity and mortality.
- The patient should be put on continuous cardiac, blood pressure, heart rate and pulse oximetry monitoring. Check for orthostatic hypotension if possible.
- The airway should be maintained and oxygen given via a non-rebreather reservoir mask should be administered as far as possible. Be prepared to intubate the patient as necessary (see Chapter 28, *Airway Management/Rapid Sequence Intubation*).
- Obtain intravenous (IV) access. Place two large bore IV lines (14/16G) preferably in the antecubital veins if possible, drawing blood for lab tests concurrently.
- Begin fluid resuscitation if the patient is not suspected to be in cardiogenic shock.
- For trauma patients in shock, see Chapter 25, *Trauma Multiple, Initial Management*.

BASIC INVESTIGATIONS

- **Full blood count (FBC)**
  1. Haemoglobin (Hb) and haematocrit (HCT) are measures of concentration and unreliable in early blood loss prior to haemodilution. Pre-existing dehydration can be observed, for example, in an alcohol-dependent patient, who may have an unexpectedly elevated HCT. A very high HCT may suggest dehydration in the patient with hypovolaemic shock though rarely, may be in a patient with polycythaemia.
  2. The neutrophil count is unreliable to diagnose sepsis, as it may be high, normal or low. However, in a patient with known sepsis, a low neutrophil count carries a poor prognosis. Check if the patient is on chemotherapy. A very high neutrophil count may suggest leukaemia.

- **Urea/electrolytes/creatinine**
  1. Examine the urea and creatinine levels to identify renal impairment secondary to shock. Compare to previous results for patients with known renal disease.
  2. Elevated urea may suggest upper gastrointestinal bleeding.
  3. Na concentrations are unreliable in dehydration as they may be high, normal or low.
  4. Hyperkalaemia, hyponatraemia and hypoglycaemia may suggest acute adrenal insufficiency.
  5. Low total CO_2 (or bicarbonate) or negative base excess suggests acidosis.

- **Blood gas analysis** to identify acid-base and respiratory abnormalities.
  1. In severe shock states, a widening gap between arterial and venous pH and pCO_2 occurs, and evaluating both arterial and venous blood gases may help to identify this state. (See earlier section in this chapter, and Chapter 57, *Acid Base Emergencies*.)

2. Mixed venous O_2 saturations, if available, yield very useful information (see *Lactate* notes below).

- **Lactate** is a marker of anaerobic respiration and is a very useful measure of the state of a shock.

  1. Levels depend on the balance between production and hepatic clearance.

  2. Be aware that lactate levels rise only when compensatory mechanisms fail at the tissue level and DO_2 falls below DO_2crit. If a mixed venous O_2 saturation level or central venous ($ScvO_2$) is available, a falling level indicates increasing extraction of O_2 from the blood, and thus, implies that the DO_2 value is already falling, even prior to lactate levels rising.

- **Troponin T** and **cardiac enzymes** (see Chapter 14, *Chest Pain*).

- **Electrocardiogram** (see Chapter 14, *Chest Pain*, Chapter 43 *Tachydysrhythmias* and Chapter 35, *Bradydysrhythmias*).

- **Chest X-ray** for diagnosis of pulmonary oedema, pneumonia, clinically missed pneumothorax.

- **Coagulation profile** with a disseminated intravascular coagulation **(DIVC) screen** as coagulopathy often accompanies many shock states.

- **GXM** for patients with haemorrhagic shock and early goal-directed therapy in septic shock (see Chapter 33, *Sepsis/Septic Shock*).

- **Capillary blood glucose**

  1. Diabetic emergencies (see Chapter 60, *Hyperglycaemia*).

  2. Hypoglycaemia may occur in paediatric patients with sepsis due to a lower reserve.

- **Urine pregnancy test** Always consider the possibility of a ruptured ectopic pregnancy in females of child-bearing age with unexplained shock.

- **Blood cultures** to be drawn as needed for septic patients.

FURTHER INVESTIGATIONS

- **2D echocardiography**

  1. Ejection fraction

  2. Wall motion abnormalities

  3. Cardiac tamponade

  4. Other structural causes of cardiogenic shock

- **Abdominal ultrasound**

  1. Perform a Focused Assessment with Sonography for Trauma (FAST) examination for trauma patients.

  2. Identify aortic aneurysms.

  3. The ultrasound 'sniff test' has been described as a non-invasive method of estimating a high or low central venous pressure.

- Perform **computed tomography (CT)** scans of the chest and abdomen as needed in trauma patients, or **helical CT** if pulmonary embolism is suspected.

MANAGEMENT

This section will focus on the resuscitation of various shock states; for definitive management of the various conditions, refer to the respective chapters.

- Resuscitation strategies for shock generally target 3 mechanisms to **restore oxygen delivery** and **repay the oxygen debt** in the tissues:
  1. Intravascular volume (preload and afterload)
  2. Cardiac output (pump)
  3. Oxygen carrying capacity and delivery (Hb content)

Hypovolaemic shock

- The main problem is clearly one of **inadequate volume**.
- **Hypovolaemic shock** is the **most common** type of **shock** encountered in the emergency department.
- Unless cardiogenic shock is suspected, aggressive fluid resuscitation with **1 to 2 L of crystalloids** should be started while assessing for response, and repeated if necessary. Further resuscitation with colloids, packed red blood cells or whole blood may be appropriate.
- **In paediatric patients**, give fluid challenge with boluses of 20 ml/kg body weight of D/S(M), or Hartman's solution if the former is unavailable.
- Ensure that adequate fluid resuscitation has taken place before starting **vasopressor support**.
  1. Give IV dopamine 5–20 µg/kg/min.
  2. Add IV noradrenaline 0.5–30 µg/min if necessary.
- Placement of a central venous pressure line may be necessary for guiding fluid therapy.

Haemorrhagic shock

- The problem here is both **inadequate volume** and **oxygen carrying capacity**.
- Remember that **fluid resuscitation does not stop the haemorrhage**. If the haemorrhage does not stop spontaneously, it has to be stopped surgically.
- **Control all external haemorrhage** and obtain **urgent review** *early* by the appropriate surgical disciplines.
- **Low versus high volume** resuscitation strategies for trauma patients have been debated.
  1. In general, **prior** to definitive surgical haemorrhage control, avoid excessive fluid resuscitation **if the patient's blood pressure is normal** or near normal, as this may dislodge the blood clots that are spontaneously limiting the haemorrhage.
  2. If the patient is significantly **hypotensive with ongoing blood loss**, obtain 6 units of GXM and **transfuse early** with whole blood, or combined packed red blood cells, fresh frozen plasma and platelets. **There is *no need* to wait** until after the administration of the traditional 2 litres of crystalloids before ordering blood. Contact the surgeon urgently.
- There is little place for the use of inotropes or vasopressors in the management of haemorrhagic shock, unless the haemorrhage has definitively been controlled.

Cardiogenic shock

- The problem here is one of the **pump**.
- **Acute myocardial infarction with left ventricular failure** is the most common cause of cardiogenic shock.
- If the systolic blood pressure is <70 mmHg, start **IV dopamine 5–20 μg/kg/min** for inotropic support.
- If the systolic blood pressure is 70–100 mmHg, start **IV dobutamine 0.2–20 μg/kg/min** to reduce systemic vascular resistance and improve stroke volume.
- **Avoid excessive fluid resuscitation** as this may worsen pulmonary oedema, although controlled fluid resuscitation may be given if the patient is not in overt heart failure.
- The insertion of an **intra-aortic balloon pump** by the cardiologist may be performed to provide further haemodynamic augmentation.
- **Cardiogenic shock with right ventricular failure** may respond better to fluid resuscitation. Give IV 500 ml boluses with frequent review.
- Add dopamine, dobutamine or noradrenaline if fluid boluses are not effective.
- Futher definitive management will depend on the underlying pathology. This includes percutaneous coronary intervention for **ST-elevation myocardial infarctions**, positive pressure ventilation for **pulmonary oedema**, **rhythm control** and surgical management for structural conditions such as **critical aortic stenosis** or **valve insufficiency**.
- See Chapter 31, *Cardiogenic Shock*.

Obstructive shock

- The problem here is one of the **pump**.
- **Tension pneumothorax** should be suspected and diagnosed clinically in the initial examination. Immediate relief by needle thoracotomy followed by definitive tube thoracostomy should be performed.
- For suspected **cardiac tamponade**, perform a FAST examination, obtain an urgent cardiothoracic consult and prepare for pericardioentesis.
- For massive **pulmonary embolism** with circulatory compromise, consider noradrenaline, adrenaline or dopamine.

Septic shock

- Sepsis can affect the **capacitance**, **pump** and end-organ delivery of **oxygen**.
- **Early goal-directed therapy** has revolutionized the way septic shock is managed, with the following principles.
  1. Intravascular volume resuscitation targeting central venous pressure (CVP).
  2. Haemodynamic optimization targeting mean arterial pressure (MAP).
  3. Oxygen transport optimization targeting $ScvO_2$.
- See Chapter 33, *Sepsis/Septic Shock*.

Anaphylactic shock

- The problems are the abnormally increased **capacitance** and depressed **cardiac contractility**.
- Aggressive **fluid resuscitation** is necessary to restore preload due to the vasodilation. Give **IV 1–2 L of crystalloids**, reassess and repeat as necessary.
- **Adrenaline** is the vasoactive agent of choice, as it reverses many of the other effects of anaphylaxis.
  1. Give IM or SC adrenaline 0.3 mg. Repeat every 3 to 5 minutes according to response.
  2. If in refractory hypotension, start IV adrenaline infusion 5–15 µg/kg/min.
- See Chapter 29, *Allergic Reactions/Anaphylaxis*.

Neurogenic shock

- The problem is loss of sympathetic vascular tone leading to **vasodilation**, as well as loss of sympathetic input to the heart, resulting in **bradycardia** from unopposed parasympathetic input.
- Aggressive **fluid resuscitation** is necessary to restore preload due to the vasodilation. Give **1–2 L of IV crystalloids**, reassess and repeat to target an MAP of about 90 mmHg.
- **Vasopressors** are important to counter the vasodilation.
  1. IV dopamine 5–20 µg/kg/min.
  2. Add IV noradrenaline 0.5–30 µg/min if necessary.
- Urgent orthopaedic consult is necessary. Refer to the chapters on Chapter 102, *Trauma, Spinal Cord* and Chapter 32, *Neurogenic Shock*.

Pharmacological causes of shock

- The mechanism of shock will depend on the agent.
- Continue supportive therapy with fluid resuscitation and ventilatory support as needed.
- Carry out drug-specific management as appropriate.

End points of resuscitation and monitoring

- The volume, pump and oxygen carrying capacity of the blood are the mechanisms targetted in management to optimize *delivery* of oxygen, whereas the end point is whether these measures have worked to improve actual consumption of oxygen and repayment of oxygen debt.
- The ideal target would be complete **repayment of oxygen debt**, which is unfortunately not readily measured.
- **Clinical end points** are highly variable and difficult to generalize and unreliable.
- **Haemodynamic end points** such as blood pressure per se may reflect the general direction of illness progression or recovery, but by themselves are inadequate.
- **Metabolic end points** include pH, base excess, bicarbonate and lactate.

- **Lactate levels** returning to normal indicate that anaerobic respiration has ceased or has reduced. This is a useful guide of therapy efficacy, but will not reflect the state at which the body is still compensating by increasing oxygen extraction. A single measurement is not as useful as the trend.

- **pH, base excess and bicarbonate levels** are measures of metabolic acidosis, and in the shock state, lactic acidosis is a major contributor. However, these are indirect measurements and may be confounded by other acid-base disorders (see Chapter 57, *Acid Base Emergencies*). Nevertheless, these are very helpful surrogates without a lactate level.

- During resuscitation of the severe shock state, as tissue perfusion improves, there may be a transient rise in **pCO2** and fall in **pH** in the arterial blood, due to wash-out of accumulated tissue metabolites. With continued treatment, this will be resolved together with the widened arteriovenous pH and pCO_2 gaps.

- Other measures that have been utilized include buccal/sublingual or gastric tonometry, near infra-red spectroscopy (NIRS) and orthogonal polarization spectral imaging (OPSI).

- There is currently no one marker that has demonstrated clear prediction of survival, though repeated measures of these markers will be very useful in guiding therapy.

Disposition

- All patients in shock should be admitted to the high dependency ward or to the intensive care unit of the appropriate discipline after proper prior consultation.

- If there is associated multisystem trauma, the trauma team should be activated. Refer to Chapter 25, *Trauma, Multiple*.

References/Further Reading

1. Pennington DG. Emergency management of cardiogenic shock. *Circulation*. 1989; (suppl 1): 6.

2. Perkins RM, Levin DL. Shock in the paediatric patient. *J Paediatr*. 1982; 101: 163.

3. Lucke WC, Thomas H Jr. Anaphylaxis: Pathophysiology, clinical presentations and treatment. *J Emerg Med*. 1983; 1(1): 83–95.

4. Rivers E, Nguyen B, Havstad S, et al. Early goal-directed therapy in the treatment of severe sepsis and septic shock. *N Engl J Med*. 8 Nov 2001; 345(19): 1368–1377.

5. Rivers EP, Coba V, Visbal A, et al. Management of sepsis: Early resuscitation. *Clin Chest Med*. 2008; 29: 689–704, ix–x.

6. Ellender TJ, Skinner JC. The use of vasopressors and inotropes in the emergency medical treatment of shock. *Emerg Med Clin North Am*. 2008; 26: 759–786, ix.

7. Cocchi MN, Kimlin E, Walsh M, Donnino MW. Identification and resuscitation of the trauma patient in shock. *Emerg Med Clin North Am*. 2007; 25: 623–642, vii.

8. Tobin MJ. *Principles and Practice of Intensive Care Monitoring*. New York: McGraw-Hill; 1998.

9. Dabrowski GP, Steinberg SM, Ferrara JJ, Flint LM. A critical assessment of endpoints of shock resuscitation. *Surg Clin North Am*. June 2000; 80(3): 825–844.

10. Englehart MS, Schreiber MA. Measurement of acid-base resuscitation endpoints: Lactate, base deficit, bicarbonate or what? *Curr Opin Crit Care*. 2006; 12: 569–574.

11. Bilkovski RN, Rivers EP, Horst HM. Targeted resuscitation strategies after injury. *Curr Opin Crit Care*. 2004; 10: 529–538.

23 Stridor

Kuan Win Sen • Peng Li Lee

CAVEATS

- If the patient has an airway that is patent and maintained, **do not** disturb or manipulate the airway.
- Permit the patient to assume a position of comfort, e.g., a child will probably want to sit on his mother's lap.
- **Do NOT** allow the patient to be unattended or to leave the department e.g., to obtain X-ray.

⇨ **SPECIAL TIPS FOR GPs**
- **Do not** stimulate the oropharynx in a futile attempt to make a definitive diagnosis.
- Permit the patient to assume a position of comfort e.g., a child will probably want to sit on mother's lap
- Organize transfer of patient to hospital by ambulance rather than private car.

MANAGEMENT

- Refer to Table 1 for features that differentiate croup/acute laryngo-tracheo-bronchitis (ALTB) from epiglottitis.

Supportive care

- The moderate to severe cases should be managed in the critical care area. Only the milde cases of croup can stay in the intermediate acuity area (Table 2).
- See Table 3 for the do's and don'ts for the child with stridor.
- Airway management equipment, including a cricothyrotomy set, must be immediately available.
- Assemble immediately a team comprising senior members in Anaesthesia and ENT surgery.
- Resuscitation drugs must be immediately available.
- Administer supplemental high-flow oxygen to maintain $SpO_2 > 95\%$.
- Monitoring: ECG, vital signs q 5–15 min, pulse oximetry.
- Establish peripheral IV line.
- **Labs:** optional
  1. FBC, urea/electrolytes/creatinine preoperative
  2. ABGs, COHb in smoke inhalation
  3. Blood cultures in suspected epiglottitis
- Lateral soft tissue X-ray of the neck and CXR if time and patient's condition permit.

TABLE 1   Differentiating croup/ALTB from epiglottitis in paediatrics

	Croup/ALTB	Epiglottitis
Age	3½–5 years	2–7 years
Organism	Usually viral: *Parainfluenza*	Bacterial: *H. influenza*
Onset	Days	Hours
Prodrome	Yes	Absent
Appearance	Non-toxic	Toxic
Fever	+/–	++
Cough	Barking	Nil
Voice	Hoarse	Muffled
Drooling	Nil	Yes
Severity	Variable	Usually severe
X-ray	Steeple sign on CXR	Thumb sign on lateral soft tissue neck firm

TABLE 2   Suggested management for croup based on clinical assessment of severity

Severity	Clinical appearance	Treatment
Mild	No retractions, normal mentation and colour	Treat with cool mist only; follow up as outpatient next day
Mild to moderate	Mild retractions, normal colour, restless if disturbed	Treat as outpatient only if patient improves after mist in emergency department, is older than 6 months and has a reliable family
Moderate	Mild stridor at rest, cyanotic and lethargic	Admit and use adrenaline nebulizers
Severe	Cyanotic with severe retractions, severe stridor at rest	Treat with adrenaline nebulizers and admit to ICU

TABLE 3   Dos and don'ts for child with stridor

Do	Don't
Be gentle	Look into the throat
Allow child to assume most confortable position	Force child to lie down
Give humidified oxygen	Perform venepuncture before airway assessment by anaestheist
Assemble airway team; inform anaesthetist and ENT	Insist on lateral neck X-ray
Arrange for ICU bed if necessary	

Drug therapy

- **In angioedema**:
  1. **Adrenaline** 1:10,000 solution 5 μg/kg (0.05 ml/kg) IV slowly or via ETT. To give the first half as a bolus and titrate the second half according to clinical response, or
  2. **Adrenaline** 1:1000 solution 10 μg/kg (0.01 ml/kg) deep IM, to a maximum of 0.3 ml in children and 0.5 ml in adults.

3. **Diphenhydramine** 2 mg/kg IV in infants/children and 12.5–25 mg IV in adults.

4. IV **hydrocortisone** 5 mg/kg IV.

- **In suspected epiglottitis: ceftriaxone** (Rocephin®) 2 g IV for adults, **or** 100 mg/kg IV stat dose for children.

- **In croup** (mild/moderate)**:** 5 ml of normal saline as cool mist nebulizer q 15 min.

- **In croup** (severe): **adrenaline** nebulization – 5 ml of 1:1000 adrenaline in 2.5 ml sterile water **once only**.

- **Disposition**: Moderate to severe cases should be admitted to ICU or OT setting following consultation. Croup that clears with one saline neb can be discharged but follow up within 24 hours must be arranged.

- **Admission criteria for croup** include:

  1. A toxic appearance.

  2. Dehydration or inability to retain oral fluids.

  3. Worsening stridor or retractions at rest.

  4. Unreliable parents.

  5. No improvement with adrenaline nebulization, or worsening at 2–3 hours following adrenaline administration.

SPECIFIC ENTITIES PRESENTING WITH STRIDOR

Epiglottitis

- Traditionally thought of as a childhood illness, but nowadays occurs more commonly in adult due to routine infant vaccination with HIB conjugate vaccines.

- Common causative organisms are *H. influenzae, S. pneumoniae* and beta-haemolytic *streptococcus*

- **Clinical features**

  1. Abrupt onset and rapid progression especially in children.

  2. Severe sore throat associated with odynophagia (painful swallowing).

  3. High fever

  4. Muffled voice 'hot potato voice'

  5. Drooling

  6. Shortness of breath

  7. Stridor

  8. Patient tends to sit erect and bend forward to reduce obstructive symptoms secondary to supra-glottic swelling.

- If a film of **neck lateral soft tissue** is obtained, look for the following:

  1. An enlarged epiglottis: '**thumb sign**' (Figure 1)

  2. Enlarged aryepiglottic folds

- Imaging is seldom necessary from a diagnostic perspective, except in subacute cases with diagnostic uncertainty.
- Provide humidified supplemental oxygen.
- 2 key principles for management of epiglottitis are maintenance of the airway and administration of appropriate antibiotics.
  1. In patients with signs of near-total airway obstruction, control of the airway should always be performed before further diagnostic evaluation.
  2. Administer IV **ceftriaxone** 2 g and **clindamycin** 600 mg

NOTE: Direct evidence of the benefit from the use of glucocorticoids in epiglottitis is lacking.

Retropharyngeal/peritonsillar abscess

- Should be considered in children presenting with fever, neck stiffness, dysphagia and cervical adenopathy.
- Adults usually present subacutely with fever, nuchal rigidity, drooling and posterior pharyngeal oedema.
- X-rays are optional and may waste valuable time. If a lateral soft tissue of neck film is obtained, look for the following:
  1. Soft-tissue swelling anterior to the vertebral bodies (**normal** is up to 1/3 width of vertebral body) (Figure 2)
  2. Air-fluid levels in retropharyngeal space (uncommon)
- If immediate airway intervention is required, consider positioning the head in a downward and hyperextended position to avoid aspiration should the abscess rupture.
- Administer IV antibiotics effective against oral pathogens including anaerobes. Drug of choice is **penicillin** with **clindamycin** as an acceptable alternative.
- Specialist team should arrange immediate transfer to the OT.

Tracheobronchial foreign body aspiration

- Tends to occur at the extremes of age with adults presenting more acutely with cardiopulmonary arrest; the FB is generally found during airway interventions.

FIGURE 1 Epiglottitis showing 'thumb sign' as shown by arrow

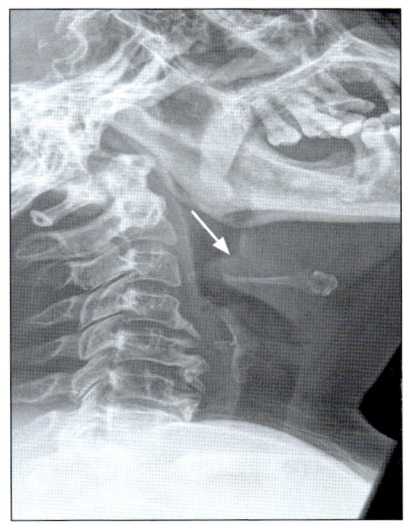

FIGURE 2 Prevertebral soft tissue swelling in retropharyngeal abscess as indicated by arrow

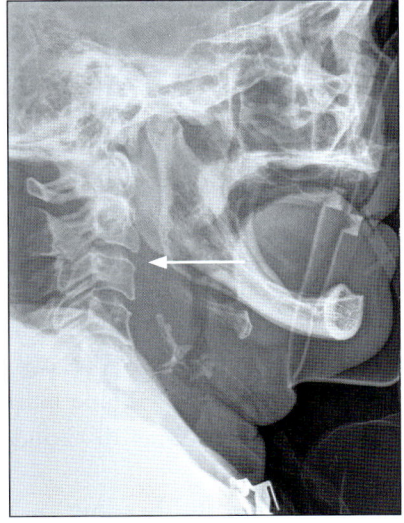

- In children, the pertinent facts are:
  1. 80% of cases occur in those <3 years of age (earlier age if a child is in environment with older children)
  2. The majority of FBs are lodged in the bronchi (>85%)
  3. The majority of aspirated FBs are radio-opaque (>90%)
  4. 24% of children with aspirated FBs have previously been misdiagnosed as chest infections
  5. Oesophageal FBs can also cause airway compromise through tracheal compression
- Immediate treatment of patients with upper airway FB and respiratory failure consists of a series of 5 back blows and 5 chest thrusts in those <1 year of age, and the Heimlich manoeuvre in those >1 year, including adults. Directly inspect the oropharynx between thrusts and **do not perform blind finger sweeps**.
  1. If the above is unsuccessful, directly inspect the hypopharynx via laryngoscope. Remove the FB with Magill forceps if it is accessible.
  2. If the above is unsuccessful, consider endotracheal intubation or a surgical airway under controlled conditions.
  3. The specialist team should arrange for laryngoscopy or bronchoscopy.

Angioedema/anaphylaxis

- Airway patency and protection is the first priority in management.
- Administer supplemental oxygen taking care not to increase agitation and precipitate respiratory arrest.
- Establish peripheral IV access for fluid challenge with crystalloid solutions.
- **Drug therapy:** see main text on *Stridor*.

Smoke inhalation

- Injury is managed initially with cool mist oxygen therapy.
- An artificial airway may be needed, as secretions may be copious.
- **Indications** for **endotracheal intubation**:
  1. Hypoxaemia unresponsive to supplemental oxygen
  2. Elevated pCO_2
  3. Worsening airway obstruction
- Draw arterial blood gas specimen (includes COHb). Refer to Chapter 84, *Poisoning, Carbon Monoxide*.
- Perform ECG to exclude ischaemia.
- Perform chest X-ray to exclude barotraumas.

References/Further Reading

1. Doherty GM, Way LW. *Current Surgical Diagnosis & Treatment*. McGraw-Hill Professional, 2005.
2. Sobol SE, Zapata S. Epiglottitis and croup. *Otolaryngol Clin North Am*. 2008 Jun; 41(3): 551–66.
3. Baren JM, Rothrock SG, Brennan JA, Lance Brown. *Pediatric Emergency Medicine*. Elsevier – Health Sciences Division, 2007.
4. Bailey BJ, Johnson JT, Newlands SD. *Head & Neck Surgery – Otolaryngology*. Lippincott Williams & Wilkins, 2006.

24 Syncope

Sim Tiong Beng • Shirley Ooi

DEFINITION

Syncope is a sudden, **brief** loss of consciousness due to transient impairment of cerebral circulation (whatever the cause), with spontaneous return to baseline neurologic function requiring no resuscitative efforts, usually occurring in the absence of organic or cerebrovascular disease.

CAVEATS

- There are many possible **causes** of syncope but the commonest, based on published evidence, are as follows:
  1. Cardiac (4–25%)
  2. Vasodepressor vasovagal (8–37%)
  3. Orthostatic hypotension (4–10%)
  4. Micturition syncope (1–2%)
  5. Hypoglycaemia (2%)
  6. Unknown aetiology (13–41%)

  Refer to Figure 1 for the causes of syncope.

NOTE: Vasovagal Syncope, although the commonest, should be a diagnosis by exclusion as it is usually benign.

- Most vasovagal syncope occurs when patient is in an upright position. Thus, when syncope occurs when patient is in a supine or sitting position, consider more serious aetiology. Similarly, exertional/effort syncope is always significant.
- Blood loss is a life-threatening cause of syncope. The possibility of gastrointestinal bleeding must be sought in all patients. For female patients who are pregnancy capable, ectopic pregnancy must be considered.
- Other life-threatening causes of syncope include: haemorrhage (e.g. gastrointestinal, abdominal aortic aneurysm rupture/aortic dissection, and trauma), cardiac syncope from arrhythmia/acute coronary syndrome/structural abnormalities, subarachnoid haemorrhage, and pulmonary embolism.
- Risk of adverse outcomes after syncope gradually increases with age and should be considered in the context of other risk factors, particularly heart disease.
- Orthostatic syncope caused by volume depletion, medication effect, and autonomic dysfunction is common among elderly patients. However, clinicians should remain cautious because orthostasis can also occur with cardiac syncope.
- The search for the cause of syncope should not necessarily end once postural hypotension is discovered.

FIGURE 1   Causes of syncope

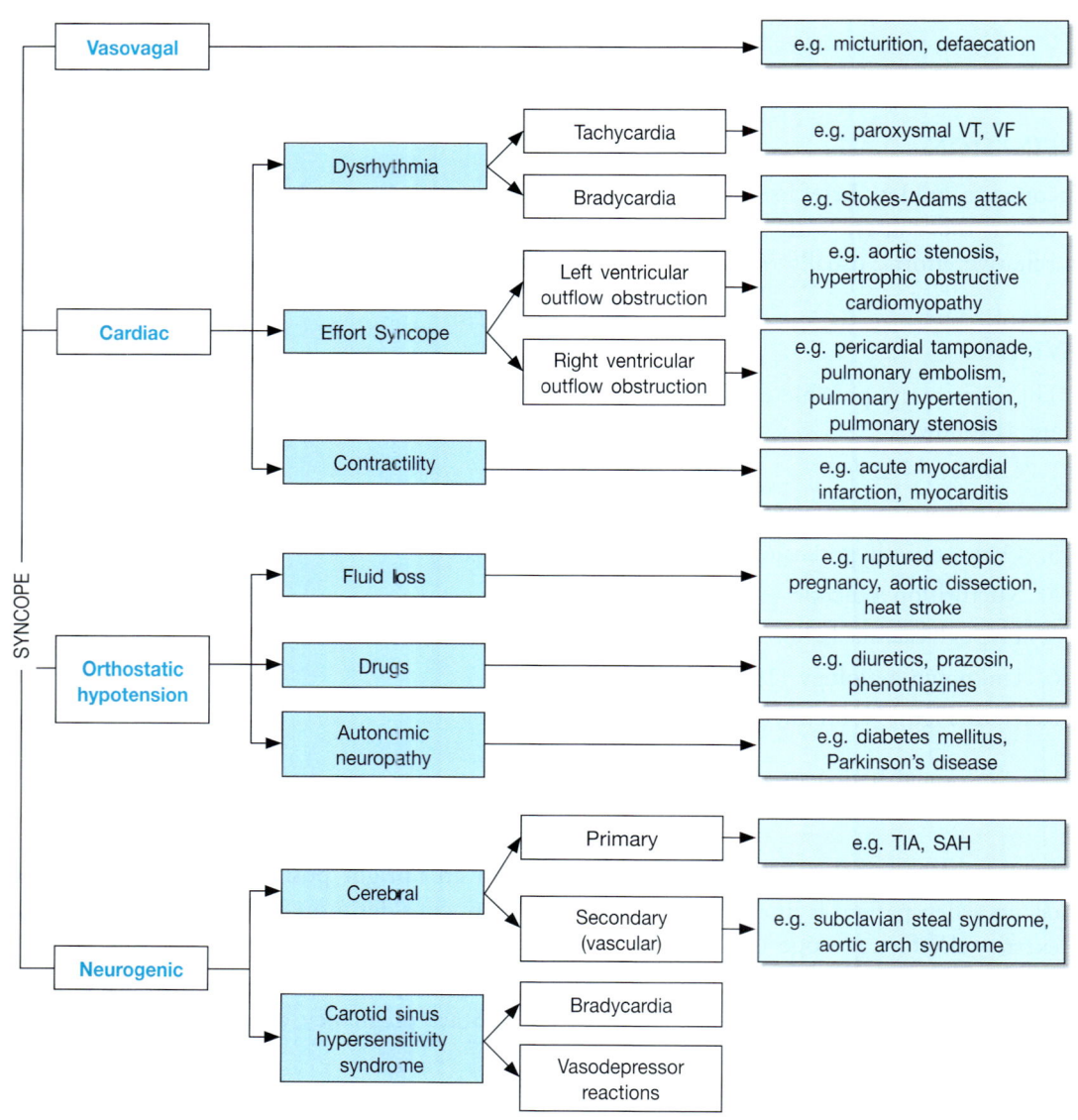

⇨ **SPECIAL TIP FOR GPs**

- Although vasovagal mechanism is the most benign cause, it should be a diagnosis by exclusion. Consider other serious causes first, such as cardiac-related illnesses, haemorrhage, and ectopic pregnancy.

INITIAL MANAGEMENT OF PATIENTS WITH SYNCOPE

- In the hospital setting, such cases are usually brought to the attention of the triage nurse early. The patient should be transferred to the critical care area if his parameters are found to be unstable. Those who are stable should be rested in the intermediate care area.
- The patient should be placed on pulse, blood pressure, and cardiac rhythm monitoring.
- The patient's airway, breathing and circulation must be quickly assessed and low-flow oxygen via nasal prongs should be provided.
- Intravenous line should be considered, especially if the initial parameters of the patient are not normal or if there is a high suspicion that the cause is due to a cardiac problem or volume loss (e.g. haemorrhage).

PATIENT ASSESSMENT

- History: Is this a true syncope? Are there clear life-threatening causes? If not, are there high-risk features? See this chapter, *Risk Stratification*.
- A thorough history is difficult to obtain because very often, the patient cannot remember the details surrounding the event. It is also difficult at times to differentiate a syncopal event from a seizure (Table 1). Other conditions, such as seizure, stroke, hypoglycaemia and head injury, do not meet the technical definition of syncope but should be considered during the initial assessment.
- **Physical findings** important in the evaluation of syncope include these:
  1. Signs of blood loss: Pallor; tachycardia; and erect and supine blood pressure.
  2. Conscious state of patient: If drowsy, think of post-ictal state, subarachnoid haemorrhage or hypoglycaemia.
  3. Cardiovascular examination for abnormal heart rhythm, murmurs and signs of heart failure.
  4. Carotid bruit may suggest transient ischemic attack as a cause.
  5. Evidence of neurological deficit, indicating an ischaemic event.
  6. Rectal examination for blood.
  7. Associated secondary injuries from the syncope, e.g. head injury, subdural/haematoma fractures.
- **Blood pressure** monitoring must be performed in all patients. It should be carried out in the following manner (2 persons are needed to prevent the patient from falling):
  1. Take supine blood pressure and pulse after 10 minutes of supine positioning.
  2. Stand the patient up for 2 minutes.
  3. Take standing blood pressure and pulse.
  4. If the patient is not tolerant, take sitting parameters instead, with legs hanging down the side of the trolley.
  5. Definition of postural hypotension: Decrease in systolic blood pressure (SBP) of >20 mmHg or increase in pulse rate of >20 beats per minute.

TABLE 1 Differential diagnosis of syncope

	Seizure	Syncope
Position of patient	Any position	Rarely in recumbent position except in Stokes-Adams attack
Colour of patient	May not change, although there may be cyanosis	Pallor
Onset	With aura. Injury from frequent falling	Without aura and more deliberate. Hence, injury from falling is rare. However, more likely to have sweating or nausea prior to event
Tonic-clonic movements with upturning of the eyes, tongue biting	Common	Absent although brief clonic seizure-like activity can accompany fainting episodes
Period of unconsciousness	Longer	Shorter
Urinary incontinence	Frequent	Seldom
Return of consciousness	Slow	Prompt
Sequelae	Mental confusion, headache, drowsiness and aching muscles are common	Physical weakness with a clear sensorium
Repeated spells of unconsciousness in a young person	May be present	Usually absent

INVESTIGATIONS

- **Electrocardiogram (ECG)** should be performed in all patients:
  1. Normal ECG makes cardiac ischaemia less likely as the cause but does not exclude dysrhythmia.
  2. Abnormal ECG indicates the risk of association between the syncopal event and cardiovascular disease. Look for conditions which predispose to dysrhythmias, e.g. Wolff-Parkinson-White syndrome (refer to Chapter 18 Figure 19), prolonged QT syndrome (refer to Chapter 18 Figure 23) or Brugada syndrome (refer to Chapter 18 Figures 20, 21 and 22) as well as hypertrophic cardiomyopathy (HOCM).
- **Optional investigations** depending on index of suspicion include:
  1. Capillary blood sugar for hypoglycaemia.
  2. Urine HCG (human chorionic gonadotropin) for suspected ectopic pregnancy.
  3. A computed tomography (CT) scan of the head if a central nervous system pathology is suspected.
  4. Electrolyte and full blood count tests have low yield and should not be performed routinely.

RISK STRATIFICATION

- During emergency department evaluation, however, the cause of syncope often remains unclear and management must focus on risk stratification to differentiate among patients safe for discharge and those who require emergent investigation and in-hospital management.

- The **San Francisco Syncope Rule (SFSR)** predicts adverse outcomes at 7 and 30 days. Significant predictors of adverse events (primarily arrhythmia) include a history of congestive heart failure, a complaint of shortness of breath, an abnormal ECG (non-sinus rhythm or new changes), a haematocrit of <30%, and a systolic blood pressure of <90 mmHg at triage. It has a **sensitivity** of 98% (89–100%, 95% confidence interval) and a **specificity** of 56% (52–60%, 95% confidence interval) at 30 days. Among several subsequent, independent validation studies, 3 found comparable sensitivity for the detection of adverse events and one did not. Cases that could be missed by SFSR include acute bleeding GIT, small sentinel SAH bleed and pulmonary embolism. Further study is needed to determine whether the SFSR can be applied to all emergency department patient populations. It should only be used as an aid in clinical decision making.

- The American College of Emergency Physicians (ACEP) has published evidence-based guidelines on the management and disposition of patients with syncope. This policy statement is based primarily on the risk stratification data presented above. (Refer to Table 2.)

- Using clinical judgement augmented by risk stratification may reduce hospital admissions and cost. However, clinicians must be careful to apply risk stratification tools to appropriate patients. Patients who have significant pathology (e.g. suspected acute coronary syndrome with normal ECG and no high-risk criteria but obviously require admission) and patients who do not reflect the population in which the stratification tool was studied are not appropriate subjects, e.g. length of coma from head injury, illicit drug/alcohol abuse should be excluded from SFSR.

TABLE 2 **High-risk features for adverse outcomes**

1 History of cardiac disease, e.g. *congestive cardiac failure*

2 Shortness of breath/chest pain/exertional syncope with event or during evaluation

3 Persistently low blood pressure (*SBP <90 mmHg*)

4 *Haematocrit <30%*

5 *Abnormal ECG* (bifascicular block, second-degree atrioventricular block, complete heart block, sinus block/pause >3 seconds, sinus bradycardia <50/min, prolonged QT, Brugada syndrome, negative T waves in the right precordial leads suggestive of arrhythmogenic right ventricular dysplasia, Q waves suggestive of myocardial infarction, small voltages suggestive of pericaridial effusion, pre-excitation, e.g. Wolff-Parkinson-White syndrome)

6 Family history of *sudden cardiac death*

7 *Older age* and associated comorbidities, e.g. ischaemic heart disease

8 Abnormal findings on cardiorespiratory or neurologic examination

Source: Adapted from Decker, Quinn, Perron, et al. (2007).

- **Low-risk patients** with obvious neurocardiogenic syncope who have returned to baseline and are asymptomatic without injury should be discharged. **High-risk** patients with obvious cardiac or neurologic causes, as with those with concerning symptoms or signs, warrant further **inpatient** evaluation. **Intermediate-risk patients** may be managed in the **observation unit**.

High-risk category

- Acute myocardial infarction, myocarditis, dysrhythmias, second and third heart block, pacemaker dysfunction, ventricular tachycardia, prolonged QT syndrome, Brugada syndrome, arrhythmogenic ventricular dysplasia (negative T waves in right precordial leads), ectopic pregnancy, antepartum haemorrhage, severe gastrointestinal bleeding, pulmonary embolism, heat stroke, and subarachnoid haemorrhage.

- Actions:
  1. Transfer the patient to the critical care area if this has not been done.
  2. Administer immediate resuscitation.
  3. Consider admission to intensive care.
  4. Contact the relevant in-house discipline stat.

Moderate-risk category

- Clinical evidence of left ventricular outflow obstruction, e.g. aortic stenosis, hypertrophic obstructive cardiomyopathy (exertional syncope), suspected mild cerebral vascular accident or transient ischaemic attack, blood loss from mild to moderate gastrointestinal bleeding/menorrhagia, orthostatic syncope from autonomic dysfunction or volume loss, e.g. dehydration from severe gastric emptying (GE) or heat exhaustion, hypoglycaemia, patients with ischaemic heart disease, mild to moderate congestive cardiac failure or supraventricular tachycardia and drug-induced syncope (e.g. anti-hypertensives, diuretics/anti-arrhythmics) and carotid sinus hypersensitivity.

- Actions:
  1. Stabilize the patient.
  2. Consider admitting the patient to the observation unit.

Low-risk category

- Vasovagal/neurocardiogenic syncope (micturition/defaecation syncope, postprandial, tussive) psychogenic syncope, anxiety and panic disorder, hyperventilation, supine hypotension in pregnant women at or near term (after obstetrics and gynaecology review) and unexplained syncope (otherwise normal).

- The emergency clinician should look for a history consistent with neurocardiogenic syncope, as these patients are low risk. A prodrome generally precedes neurocardiogenic syncope, and often includes a sense of warmth, nausea and vomiting, diaphoresis and pallor, either just prior to or shortly after the event. Inquiring about potential triggers is also helpful. Triggers commonly associated with neurocardiogenic syncope include strong physical or emotional stress, micturition, defaecation, coughing, swallowing and prolonged standing in a warm environment.

- Actions:

    1. Exclude all high-risk and moderate-risk conditions.
    2. Observe for a period of ≥2 hours.
    3. Discharge if the patient is alert and attentive and parameters are stable.
    4. For patients with recurrent vasovagal syncope, consider referral to the cardiology unit for a tilt table test.

References/Further Reading

1. Meyer M, Handler J. Evaluation of the patient with syncope: An evidence based approach. In: Masellis M, SWA Gunn, eds. *Emergency Clinics of North America*. Philadelphia, PA: WB Saunders; 1999: 17(1): 189–201.

2. Soteriades ES, Evans JC, Larson MG, et al. Incidence and prognosis of syncope. *N Engl J Med*. 2002; 347: 878.

3. Sarasin FP, Louis-Simonet M, Carballo D, et al. Prevalence of orthostatic hypotension among patients presenting with syncope in the ED. *Am J Emerg Med*. 2002; 20: 497.

4. Quinn JV, Stiell IG, McDermott DA, et al. Derivation of the San Francisco Syncope Rule to predict patients with short-term serious outcomes. *Ann Emerg Med*. 2004; 43: 224.

5. Quinn J, McDermott D, Stiell I, et al. Prospective validation of the San Francisco Syncope Rule to predict patients with serious outcomes. *Ann Emerg Med*. 2006; 7: 448.

6. Quinn J, McDermott D, Kramer N, et al. Death after emergency department visits for syncope: How common and can it be predicted? *Ann Emerg Med*. 2008; 51: 585.

7. Sun BC, Mangione CM, Merchant G, et al. External validation of the San Francisco Syncope Rule. *Ann Emerg Med*. 2007; 49: 420.

8. Birnbaum A, Esses D, Bijur P, et al. Failure to validate the San Francisco Syncope Rule in an independent emergency department population. *Ann Emerg Med*. 2008; 52: 151.

9. Huff JS, Decker WW, Quinn JV, et al. Clinical policy: Critical issues in the evaluation and management of adult patients presenting to the emergency department with syncope. *Ann Emerg Med*. 2007; 49: 431.

10. Shen WK, Decker WW, Smars PA, et al. Syncope Evaluation in the Emergency Department Study (SEEDS): A multidisciplinary approach to syncope management. *Circulation*. 2004; 110: 3636–3645.

11. Decker WW, Quinn JV, Perron AD, et al. Clinical policy: critical Issues in the evaluation and management of adult patients presenting to the emergency department with syncope. *Ann Emerg Med*. 2007; 49(4): 431–444.

12. Tan C, Sim TB, Thng SY. Validation of the San Francisco Syncope Rule in two hospital emergency departments in an Asian publication. *Acad Emerg Med*. 2013; 20: 487–49.

25   Trauma, Multiple

Initial management

Shirley Ooi • Victor Ong

INTRODUCTION

The treatment of the seriously injured patient requires rapid assessment of the injuries and initiation of life-preserving therapy. This is called **initial assessment** and includes:

- Preparation
- Triage
- Primary survey (which follows the ABCDE sequence)
- Resuscitation of vital functions
- '**AMPLE**' history of event (**A**llergies, **M**edications, **P**ast medical history, **L**ast meal eaten, **E**vents leading to the injury)
- Secondary survey (head-to-toe evaluation)
- Continued post-resuscitation monitoring
- Reevaluation
- Definitive care

NOTE:

- Primary and targeted secondary surveys should be repeated frequently to ascertain any deterioration.
- This sequence is presented as a longitudinal sequence of events. This is to facilitate an organized stepwise management of a trauma patient in a single doctor scenario. In the actual clinical situation, many of these activities occur concurrently as more than one medical and nursing staff will be attending to this patient.
- Prehospital traumatic cardiac arrest is uniformly fatal if it persists for >5 minutes or is due to problems that cannot be rapidly corrected.

IN-HOSPITAL PREPARATION

Advanced planning for the trauma patient's hospital arrival is essential. Each hospital should have a trauma activation protocol. The emergency department should have its own protocols for managing major trauma patients.

TRIAGE

This is normally a prehospital phenomenon, but *could* be instituted in the emergency department occasionally:

- When facilities are not over-extended: The sickest patients will be seen first.
- When facilities are over-extended: The most salvageable patients will be seen first.

Arrival of the trauma patient at the emergency department

The major trauma patient should be assumed to have injured the spine as a result of the trauma. Hence, transfer of the patient should be done with a view of preventing further spinal injuries. Thus, a team approach with a team leader controlling the cervical spine and coordinating the transfer, together with at least two persons on each side of the patient, is needed to safely transfer the patient from one platform to another. The use of the patient scoop, capable of being dismantled in half, is appropriate in this situation.

PRIMARY SURVEY (ABCDE) AND RESUSCITATION

During the **primary survey**, **life-threatening conditions** are identified and management is begun simultaneously. Remember that logical sequential treatment priorities must be established based on overall patient assessment.

NOTE: Priorities for the care of paediatric patients are basically the same as for adults, although quantities of blood, fluids, and medications may differ (refer to Chapter 137, *Trauma, Paediatric*).

Airway assessment with cervical spine control

- **Assessment: Ascertain patency and inspect for:**
  1. Foreign bodies in the oral cavity.
  2. Facial/mandibular fractures.
  3. Laryngeal/tracheal fractures (neck swelling and bruises).
- **Rapidly assess for suggestions of airway injury with potential obstruction**
  1. Inspiratory stridor.
  2. Blood/mucus/foreign bodies in the oral cavity.
  3. Voice change.
  4. Subcutaneous crepitus over the neck/face.
  5. Swelling/bruises over the neck.
- **Management: Establish a patent airway**
  1. Perform a jaw thrust manoeuvre.
  2. Clear the airway of foreign bodies. (Use a Yankauer suction catheter attached to suction equipment where possible.)
  3. Insert an appropriately-sized oropharyngeal or nasopharyngeal airway.
  4. Establish a definitive airway:
     a. Orotracheal or nasotracheal intubation.
     b. Needle cricothyrotomy with jet insufflation of the airway.
     c. Surgical cricothyrotomy.

- **Caveats**

  1. Assume the presence of a cervical spine injury in a multisystem trauma, especially with loss of consciousness or a blunt injury above the clavicle.

  2. The absence of neurological deficit does not exclude injury to the cervical spine.

  3. Assess for the presence of a difficult airway before paralyzing the patient (refer to Chapter 28, *Airway Management/Rapid Sequence Intubation*).

  4. When intubating a trauma patient, place the largest tube possible as smaller tubes limit instrumentation of the endotracheal tube for cultures and bronchoscopy and are more prone to muropurulent plugging from airway secretions.

  5. Causes of cardiopulmonary arrest during or just after endotracheal intubation are as follows:

     a. Excessive ventilatory pressures causing a tension pneumothorax.

     b. Inadequate oxygenation of the patient before intubation.

     c. Oesophageal intubation.

     d. Excessive ventilatory pressures retarding venous return.

     e. Air embolism.

     f. Vasovagal response.

     g. Excessive respiratory alkalosis.

Breathing and ventilation (airway patency does not ensure adequate ventilation and oxygenation)

- **Assessment**

  1. Expose the neck and chest: Ensure immobilization of the head and neck.

  2. Determine the rate and depth of respiration.

  3. Inspect and palpate the neck and chest for tracheal deviation, chest wall movements, use of accessory muscles, and any signs of deformity/wounds or crepitus.

  4. Auscultate the chest bilaterally, from the bases to the apices.

  5. If breath sounds are not equal, percuss the chest for presence of dullness or hyperresonance to determine haemothorax or pneumothorax, respectively.

  6. The following may acutely impair ventilation and oxygenation:

     a. Tension pneumothorax.

     b. Flail chest with pulmonary contusion.

     c. Open pneumothorax.

     d. Massive haemothorax.

- **Management**

  1. Attach the patient to a pulse oximeter.

  2. Administer high concentration of oxygen. The use of a non-rebreather mask with a reservoir achieves a fraction of inspired oxygen (FiO_2) of 0.7.

3. Consider the need to ventilate with a bag-valve-mask if saturation of peripheral oxygen (SpO_2) is <92% despite the non-rebreather mask application.

4. Attach an end-tidal carbon dioxide (CO_2) monitoring device (if available) to monitor for adequacy of ventilation.

5. Alleviate **tension pneumothorax** by rapidly inserting a large bore needle into the second intercostal space in the mid-clavicular line of the affected haemithorax, followed by chest tube insertion into the fifth intercostal space, anterior to the mid-axillary line (slightly posterior to the mid-axillary line in women to avoid the posterior margin of the breast).

6. Seal the **open pneumothorax** with sterile occlusive dressing, large enough to overlap the wound's edges, and tape securely on 3 sides to create a flutter-valve effect. Then insert a chest tube away from the wound site.

7. **Haemothoraces** should be managed with tube thoracostomy. The tube size should be the largest available (usually at least 28–32F) and directed posteriorly and downwards towards the spine and diaphragm.

8. In situations where **haemopneumothoraces** may be present, choose a large size chest tube for drainage.

- **Caveats**
  1. It is often difficult to differentiate ventilation from airway problems, e.g. if a ventilation problem is produced by a pneumothorax or tension pneumothorax but is mistaken for an airway problem and the patient is intubated, the patient could deteriorate further.

  2. Intubation and ventilation could produce a pneumothorax; hence, chest X-rays should be performed soon after intubation and ventilation as is practical.

  3. Do not force all trauma patients to lie flat on a trolley especially when they obviously breathe better sitting up.

Circulation with haemorrhage control

- Hypotension following injury must be considered to be hypovolaemic in origin until proven otherwise. Identify the source of external, exsanguinating haemorrhage.

- Rapid and accurate assessment of the patient's haemodynamic status is essential. **4** rapid clinical observations will yield key information within seconds:
  1. **Level of consciousness**: Reduced cerebral perfusion pressure, hence a reduced Glasgow Coma Scale (GCS) score, can result from hypovolaemia.

  2. **Skin colour**: Pinkness is helpful since it rarely goes with significant hypovolaemia. Ashen and grey skin of the face and white skin of the extremities are ominous signs of hypovolaemia; they usually indicate a blood volume loss of ≥30%.

  3. **Pulse**: This is often the earliest sign of hypovolaemic shock.
     a. Presence of rapid, weak, thready, or absent pulses.
     b. If radial pulse is present, the blood pressure (BP) is >80 mmHg.

    c. If only carotid pulse is present, the BP is >60 mmHg.

    d. An irregular pulse suggests the possibility of cardiac impairment.

4. **Blood pressure**: This may be low only after a significant amount of circulating blood volume (usually at least 2 litres) is lost, corresponding to class III/ IV shock.

- **Management**
  1. Apply direct pressure to the external bleeding site.
  2. Insert 2 large-calibre intravenous (IV) catheters, i.e. 14G or 16G into large veins (preferably antecubital/femoral or jugular veins).
  3. Obtain 4 to 6 units of blood for group and cross match (GXM), full blood count, urea/ electrolytes/creatinine, coagulation profile, and arterial blood gas (ABG).

NOTE: If no O negative blood is available, use type specific blood.

  4. Base excess (BE) on ABG of <–2 is indicative of perfusion deficit due to hypovolaemia.
  5. Initiate vigorous IV fluid therapy with warmed crystalloids (normal saline or Hartmann's). Consider blood replacement with whole blood or packed red blood cells with platelets and fresh frozen plasma in a ratio of 1:1:1 if there is ongoing blood loss or after 2 litres of crystalloids where there is little or no haemodynamic response.

NOTE: Do not resuscitate shock with glucose-containing solutions as the fluids will leak into the extravascular space.

  6. Apply **electrocardiogram (ECG) monitoring**:
     a. Dysrhythmia → Consider cardiac tamponade.
     b. Pulseless electrical activity → Consider cardiac tamponade, tension pneumothorax, and profound hypovolaemia.
     c. Bradycardia, aberrant conduction, ventricular ectopics → hypoxia and hypoperfusion.
  7. Insert urinary and nasogastric catheters unless contraindicated.

NOTE: Urinary output is a sensitive indicator of the volume status of the patient. **Urinary catheterization** is **contraindicated** when urethral injury is suspected, i.e. if:

    a. There is blood at the urethral meatus.

    b. There is a scrotal haematoma.

    c. The prostate is high-riding or cannot be palpated.

  8. A **gastric tube** is indicated to reduce stomach distention and decrease risk of aspiration. **Blood in the gastric aspirate** may represent the following:
     a. Oropharyngeal (swallowed) blood.
     b. Traumatic insertion.
     c. Actual injury to the upper gastrointestinal tract.

If there is epistaxis or cerebrospinal fluid rhinorrhoea suggestive of a cribriform plate fracture, insert the gastric tube orally instead of nasally.

9. Use a Bair Hugger or space blanket to prevent hypothermia.

- **Caveats**

   1. Persistent hypotension in trauma patients is usually due to hypovolaemia from continued bleeding.

   2. The elderly, children, athletes, and others with chronic medical conditions do not respond to volume loss in a similar manner. For example, elderly patients may not show a normal tachycardia response to blood loss, thus obscuring one of the earliest signs of volume depletion. This is worse if these patients are on beta blockers. Children have abundant physiologic reserve and often demonstrate few signs even of severe hypovolaemia.

   3. The following sites for **venous access** can be attempted but with certain provisos:

      a. **Jugular/neck**: If there is no evidence of anterior neck swelling/bruises or injuries.

      b. **Subclavian**: Preferably not used if chest injury is present.

      c. **Femoral**: If there is no evidence to suggest abdominal or pelvic injuries.

      d. If **central lines** are used for resuscitation they should be of large calibre (>8F).

   NOTE: The **femoral access** is logistically the easiest because it is remote from any airway and thoracic evaluation and resuscitative efforts as well as unhindered by the c-collar. However, it carries a significantly higher rate of venous thrombosis (up to 25%) and infection (4.4%) when compared with a subclavian line thrombosis (1.5–12.5%) and sepsis (1.5%).

   4. Elderly patients may not show tachycardia in the face of shock due to medications and underlying physiology.

Disability (neurological evaluation)

Establish the patient's level of consciousness, pupillary size, and reaction to light.

Glasgow Coma Scale (GCS) is a universally accepted standard for assessing trauma patients' level of consciousness. It is based on three parameters:

1. E (best eye movement) 1–4

2. V (best verbal response) 1–5

3. M (best motor response) 1–6

GCS is the total of the three scores, i.e. E + V + M. Scores range from 3 to 15.

Generally speaking, GCS 13–14 represent mild head injury, 9–12 represent moderate head injury and 3–8 represent severe head injury.

Assess the pupils for size, equality, and reaction to light. Unequal pupils can indicate raised intracranial pressure due to intracranial haemorrhage in trauma.

- **Caveats**

   1. Do not assume that **altered mental state** in a trauma patient is due to head injury only.

Consider the other causes such as:

a. Hypoxia.

b. Shock.

c. Alcohol/drug intoxication.

d. Hypoglycaemia.

2. Conversely, do not assume that altered mental state is due to alcohol or drug intoxication. Brain injury needs to be excluded.

Exposure/environmental control

Completely undress the patient by cutting off the clothing as appropriate. This is to help identify external injuries and bleeding. However, prevent hypothermia by covering him with blankets or a Bair Hugger. Use of warmed fluids and blood is strongly encouraged.

Adjuncts to primary survey

- Continue **monitoring** the pulse rate, blood pressure, pulse oximetry, ECG, and urinary output.
- **Perform essential X-rays for all multiple trauma patients**:
  1. Cervical spine: Anterior-posterior/lateral and open mouth view.
  2. Anteroposterior chest.
  3. Anteroposterior pelvis.

Do remember that in primary survey, one should ensure that each step of the ABCDE approach is addressed and corrective resuscitative measures are taken before moving to the next step, though with an emergency department team set up, very often the steps can be managed concurrently.

- **FAST (Focused Assessment with Sonography in Trauma)** could be performed at this stage to help investigate the possible source of bleeding in a patient with hypotensive shock.
- The 4 sites for FAST evaluation include the right hypochondrium (Morrison's pouch), left hypochondrium (splenorenal angle), hypogastrium (pouch of Douglas in females and rectovesical area in males) and subxiphoid/epigastrium region (a four-chamber view of the heart and pericardium). (Refer to Chapter 118, *Emergency Ultrasound*, for further discussion.)

NOTE: Pregnant patients should not have indicated radiographs withheld. Used judiciously, the radiation dose is not significant. Optimizing the mother's treatment will affect the best outcomes for both the mother and her unborn baby.

- **An arterial blood gas test** to obtain base excess at this stage will aid in evaluating the extent of hypovolaemic shock and as an assessment tool for response to fluid and blood resuscitation.

SECONDARY SURVEY

- This is a head-to-toe evaluation of the trauma patient, including a reassessment of vital signs. Blood pressure, pulse, respirations, temperature, and GCS.

- It does not begin until the primary survey is completed, resuscitation is initiated and the patient's ABCs are stabilized.
- It may be summarized as '**tubes and fingers in every orifice**'.
  1. It starts with '**AMPLE** history':
     Allergies
     Medications currently taken
     Past illnesses
     Last meal
     Events/environment related to the injury

Head and face

- **Assessment**
  1. Inspect for lacerations, contusions, and thermal injury.
  2. Palpate for fractures.
  3. Test the cranial nerve functions.
  4. Reevaluate the pupils for equality and reaction to light and consensual movement.
  5. Take a close look at the eyes to check for haemorrhage, corneal haziness, penetrating injury, visual acuity, lens dislocation, and presence of contact lenses.
  6. Inspect the ears and nose for cerebrospinal fluid leakage and haemotympanum.
  7. If intubated, ensure that the endotracheal tube is in the correct position and well anchored with correct connections to the ventilator.
  8. Examine the oral cavity for foreign bodies and bleeding.
- **Management**
  1. Ensure continual airway patency.
  2. Control haemorrhage by compression.
  3. Prevent secondary brain injury (refer to Chapter 95, *Trauma, Head*).
  4. Remove any contact lenses.

Neck

- **Assessment**
  1. Inspection: Blunt and penetrating injury and use of accessory breathing muscles.
  2. Palpation: Tenderness, deformity, swelling, subcutaneous emphysema, and tracheal deviation.
  3. Auscultation: Carotid arteries for bruits.
  4. If the patient is GCS 15, has no cervical spine tenderness and is able to move his neck without any pain, one can clinically clear the cervical spine.
- **Management**
  1. Maintain adequate in-line immobilization (cervical collar and head blocks) of the cervical spine in all cases where the spine cannot be clinically cleared.
  2. Order anterior-posterior/lateral/open mouth X-ray views of the cervical spine if they have not been done.

Chest

- **Assessment**
    1. Inspection: Blunt and penetrating injury, use of accessory breathing muscles and bilateral respiratory excursions.
    2. Palpation: Blunt and penetrating injury, subcutaneous emphysema, tenderness, and crepitus.
    3. Percussion: Dull or resonant.
    4. Auscultation: Breath and heart sounds.
- **Management**
    1. Carry out a chest tube insertion for non-tension haemopneumothorax if present.
    2. Ensure the chest tube is oscillating well.
    3. Perform a chest X-ray if this has not been done.

    Look out for pericardial effusion/tamponade during the FAST examination.

NOTE: **Emergency room thoracotomy** is preferred in patients with evidence of cardiac tamponade. Salvage rates are low but best in patients with penetrating chest or abdominal wounds, and recent witnessed cardiac arrest. Salvage rates are dismal in patients who have sustained blunt trauma. Therefore, this procedure is generally not indicated in blunt trauma.

Abdomen/Pelvis

- **Assessment**
    1. Inspection: Blunt and penetrating injury and evisceration.
    2. Palpation: Distension, tenderness, and guarding.
    3. Percussion: Rebound tenderness.
    4. Auscultation: Bowel sounds.
    5. X-ray of the pelvis.
- **Management**
    1. In a multiple-injured trauma patient, a clinical exam is frequently not sufficient to rule out an intra-abdominal injury. Therefore, further adjuncts such as a FAST exam, abdominal CT scan or peritoneal lavage are indicated (refer to Chapter 93, *Trauma, Abdominal*).
    2. Transfer the patient to the operating theatre when indicated (refer to Chapter 93, *Trauma, Abdominal*).

Perineal and rectal exam (commonly done when the patient is log-rolled to assess the back)

- **Evaluation**
    1. Blood at the urethral meatus.
    2. Scrotal bruising and haematoma.
    3. Perineal bruising and haematoma.
    4. Perineal wounds and tears.

- **Perineal assessment**
  1. Contusions, haematomas.
  2. Lacerations.
- **Vaginal assessment**
  1. Presence of bleeding in vaginal vault.
  2. Vaginal lacerations.
- **Rectal assessment**
  1. Anal sphincter tone.
  2. Perianal sensation.
  3. Bowel wall integrity.
  4. Bony fragments from the pelvis.
  5. Prostate position (a high-riding prostate can be a sign of a pelvic fracture in males).
  6. Rectal bleeding.

Back

- **Log-roll the patient to evaluate for the following:**
  1. Bony tenderness and deformity along the entire length of the spine and the sacroiliac joints of the pelvis.
  2. Evidence of penetrating or blunt trauma over the back.
- **Caveats**
  1. The patient should be removed from the backboard as soon as possible because:
     a. The backboard does not adequately stabilize the spine nor maintain it in the appropriate position any better than when the patient is lying on a gurney.
     b. Log-rolling minimizes excessive movement in the patient's spine.
     c. Even in healthy patients, increased duration of time on a backboard leads to increased discomfort and poor tissue oxygenation.
  2. With newer CT scanners spinal CTs can be reformatted from abdominal CTs. Due to its superior sensitivity, patients in whom there is a high suspicion for spinal injury should have a spinal CT scan done.

Extremities

- **Assessment**
  1. Inspection: Deformity and expanding haematoma.
  2. Palpation: Tenderness, crepitation, and abnormal movement.
  3. Assessment of neurovascular status: Pulses, power, and sensation.
- **Management**
  1. Select a splint appropriate to the severity of the fractures.
  2. Provide pain relief with splinting and analgesia.

3. Photograph the injured sites.

4. Cover the wounds and apply a pressure bandage over the bleeding regions.

5. Immunize against tetanus.

6. Treat open wounds and fractures with antibiotics.

Neurologic

- **Assessment: Reevaluate the pupils and level of consciousness**
  1. GCS score.
  2. Pupillary size, equality, and reaction to light.
  3. Eye movements and presence of nystagmus.
  4. Cranial nerves.
  5. Lateralizing signs.
  6. Sensory deficits.
- **Management**
  1. Ensure appropriate padding to pressure areas and protection to paralyzed limbs.

DEFINITIVE CARE/TRANSFER

- If the patient's injuries exceed the institution's immediate treatment capabilities, the process of transferring the patient is initiated as soon as the need is identified.

References/Further Reading

1. *Advanced Trauma Life Support Student Course Manual*. 7th ed. Chicago, IL: American College of Surgeons; 2012.

2. Wilson RF, Walt AJ, eds. *Management of Trauma: Pitfalls and Practice*. Baltimore, MD: Williams & Wilkins; 1996: 10–11, 24–27, 46–47, 346.

3. Kirkpatrick AW, et al. Acute resuscitation of the unstable trauma patient: Bedside diagnosis and therapy. *Canadian Surg*. 2008; 51(1): 57–69.

4. D'Amours SK, Sugrue M, Deane SA. Initial management of the polytrauma patient: A practical approach in an Australian Major Trauma Service. *Scand J Surg*. 2002; 91: 23–33.

5. Malone DL, Hess JP, Fingerhut A. Massive transfusion practice around the globe and a suggestion for a common massive transfusion protocol. *J Trauma*. 2006; 60: S91–6.

6. Paledino L, Sinert R, Wallace D, et al. The utility of base deficit and arterial lactate in differentiating major from minor injury in trauma patients with normal vital signs. *Resuscitation*. 2008; 77: 363–368.

7. Moylan M, Newgard CD, Ma OJ, et al. Association between a positive ED FAST and therapeutic laparotomy in normotensive blunt trauma patients. *J Emerg Med*. 2007; 33(3): 265–271.

8. Hauswald M, Hus M, Stockoff C. Maximizing comfort and minimizing ischaemia: A comparison of focus methods of spinal immobilization. *Prehosp Emerg Care*. 2000; 4(3): 250–252.

9. Mauthey DE, Nicks BA. Trauma management in the ED. In: Mattu A, Goyal D, eds. *Emergency Medicine. Avoiding the Pitfalls and Improving the Outcomes*. Reading, MA: Blackwell Publishing; 2007: 55–62.

26 Urinary Retention, Acute

Brandon Koh • Peter Manning • Shirley Ooi

Acute urinary retention is defined as the sudden inability to void despite the presence of a distended, full bladder.

- It is usually secondary to some form of bladder outlet obstruction.

> ⇨ **SPECIAL TIPS FOR GPs**
> - A history of urinary obstruction and fever is a urological emergency and must be referred to the nearest hospital/emergency department immediately. Always assess the vital signs in such cases.
> - In cases of chronic retention of urine (painless), do not place a urinary catheter without setting up an intravenous line line first as the resulting diuresis may precipitate hypovolaemia and shock.

CAUSES

Obstructive

- Benign prostatic hyperplasia (most common).
- Prostate cancer.
- Urethral stricture.
- Faecal impaction.
- Phimosis and paraphimosis.
- Bladder stones.
- Bladder tumours.
- Blood clot retention.
- Urethral foreign bodies.

Infectious

- Acute prostatitis.
- Urethral herpes.
- Periurethral abscess.
- Vulvovaginitis.

Pharmacologic

- Drugs with anticholinergic effects (most common):
  1. Antihistamines.
  2. Alpha-adrenergic (α-adrenergic) agonists in decongestants (e.g. pseudoephedrine).
  3. Phenothiazine anti-psychotics.
  4. Hyoscine butylbromide (Buscopan®).

- Tricyclic anti-depressants.
- Non-steroidal anti-inflammatory drugs.[4]

Neurologic

- Cerebrovascular accident.
- Spinal cord trauma.
- Spinal cord compression (secondary to metastatic cancer).
- Lumbar disc herniation.
- Peripheral neuropathy in diabetes mellitus.

Others

- Postoperative complications.
- Trauma
  1. Urethral and bladder injuries.

NOTE: In women, consider pregnancy/pelvic masses as possible causes of urinary retention!

MANAGEMENT

- Relevant history, especially
  1. Recent drug use.
  2. Recent surgery.
  3. Constipation.
  4. Lower urinary tract symptoms.
- Relevant examination.
  1. Abdomen.
     a. Look for masses.
  2. Digital rectal examination.
     a. Evaluate the prostate gland.
     b. Rule out faecal impaction.
  3. Genitalia.
  4. Neurological system.
- Immediate and complete decompression of the bladder through catheterization.
  1. When catheterizing men who are likely to have **benign prostatic hypertrophy**, start with a size 14F Foley catheter.
     a. If passage past the bladder neck cannot be achieved, repeat the process with a **larger**, not smaller, catheter, i.e. 16F.
     b. The larger-sized catheters have more rigidity and this additional rigidity often permits easy passage.

2. Patients with **recurrent urethral strictures** should be approached with a small catheter.

3. Patients with **prostatitis** (fever, chills, and an exquisitely tender prostate gland on digital rectal examination) are better served by a suprapubic catheter initially.

4. Never force the passage of a urinary catheter.

   a. If attempts at urethral catheterization are unsuccessful, obtain a urology consultation, or consider inserting a suprapubic catheter (this procedure is best left to the experienced practitioner).

5. Traditionally, gradual rather than rapid decompression of the bladder is recommended.

   a. To prevent complications such as haematuria, hypotension, and postobstructive diuresis.

6. There is, however, **no** evidence that gradual decompression reduces the risk of these complications.[6]

7. Hence, rapid and **complete** emptying of the bladder is recommended.

8. Record residual urine volume (RU) in the notes for the benefit of the reviewing urologist.

9. **Urinary obstruction plus fever** is a **urological emergency** and mandates admission of the patient.

   a. In this situation, urinalysis may be unreliable and 'miss' pyuria.

DISPOSITION

- Uncomplicated cases of acute retention of urine can be discharged with an indwelling urinary catheter and an early follow-up appointment at the urology specialist outpatient clinic.

   1. Home catheter care must be taught before discharge.

- Consider admission to Urology if there is gross haematuria or signs of severe infection.

References/Further Reading

1. Lawson DM. Urologic emergencies. *J Emerg Med Acute Pri Care*. 2001; 5325(20): 5991–6247.

2. Curtis L, Dolan TS, Cespedes RD. Acute urinary retention and urinary incontinence. *Emerg Clin North Am*. 2001; 19: 591–619.

3. Rosenstein D, McAninch JW. Urologic emergencies. *Med Clin N Am*. 2004: 88: 495–518.

4. Verhamme KM, Dieleman JP, Van Wijk MA, et al. Nonsteroidal anti-inflammatory drugs and increased risk of acute urinary retention. *Arch Intern Med*. 2005; 165(13): 1547–1551.

5. Selius BA, Subedi Rajesh. Urinary retention in adults: Diagnosis and initial mangement. *Am Fam Physician*. 2008; 77(5): 643–650.

6. Nyman MA, Schwenk NM, Silverstein MD. Management of urinary retention: Rapid versus gradual decompression and risk of complications. *Mayo Clin Proc*. 1997; 72(10): 951–956.

7. Bau KM, Easter JS. Selected urologic problems. In: Marx JA, Walls R, Hockberger R, eds. *Rosen's Emergency Medicine: Concepts and Clinical Practice*. 7th ed. Philadelphia, PA: Mosby-Elsevier; 2010: 1319–1322.

27   Violent and Psychotic Patients

Peter Manning

Violent patients make their presence obvious and require immediate attention.

CAVEATS

- The principal role of the emergency physician is to delineate, if possible, organic from inorganic causes of psychosis. Agitation should be presumed to be organic, i.e. delirium, until proven otherwise.
- A potentially life-threatening aetiology must be sought and addressed.
- Never leave a violent patient alone: Enlist the assistance of at least 5 uniformed security staff to stand in the background as a *show of force* if necessary. If the patient is female, at least one female staff member must be present at all times.

⇨ **SPECIAL TIPS FOR GPs**

- If you are evaluating such a patient in your office, do not allow yourself to become trapped by him to come between you and the door; you must have immediate access to the door.
- Notify uniformed services according to local practice at the first hint of aggression; you may need their assistance sooner than you think.
- Your patient may cooperate with **oral** doses of the drugs mentioned below should you have them available in your office. They can be given in larger doses than the parenteral route (e.g. 20 mg PO of either diazepam or haloperidol) and are less threatening to the patient than injections.

MANAGEMENT

- **Supportive care**
    1. The patient should be managed in either the intermediate or critical care area of the emergency department depending on the patient's general condition. Continual observation of the patient is maximized this way.
    2. Pay attention to the ABCs (airway, breathing, and circulation): Hypoxaemia, hypercarbia, or hypoperfusion of the brain may be the cause of disruptive behaviour.
    3. Assess for any classic toxidrome, e.g. opioid, anticholinergic, sympathomimetic or cholinergic.
    4. Take a full set of vital signs if the patient permits: Abnormalities may suggest an underlying organic, infectious, or toxicological cause of the behaviour.

5. Monitor the electrocardiogram (ECG), vital signs q30–60 minutes, and pulse oximetry, if the patient permits.

6. Stat capillary blood sugar and serum electrolytes, if the patient permits.

7. Urgent and standard approaches to ingestions or traumatic presentations must be undertaken.

8. Consider the use of **restraints**: Physical restraints to prevent self-harm or other harm should be a recurrent thought process for the physician in charge.

9. Attempt to **build rapport** with the patient: Patient privacy (the pulling of curtains partially around the cubicle), patient comfort and an empathetic non-judgemental approach may elicit cooperation and enhance the ability of the team to gain accurate information, evaluate, and effect appropriate interventions.

10. After the initial assessment and interventions, the physical examination is focused on the detection of lateralizing or focal neurological findings that will direct one to perform computed tomography (CT) imaging of the brain (non-contrast). CT imaging should also be considered in those cases where no obvious reversible aetiology is evident.

Delirium is an organic mental syndrome and is common among medically compromised patients; the elderly are also highly vulnerable.

The clinician's most important and difficult task is to differentiate delirium from dementia using the **Confusion Assessment Method (CAM)** algorithm.

CAM algorithm
1. Acute onset and fluctuating course
2. Inattention, distractibility
3. Disorganized thinking, illogical, or unclear ideas
4. Alteration in consciousness
Diagnosis of delirium needs 1 and 2, plus 3 or 4.

• **Pharmacological therapy:** If the patient is violent, consider the use of anti-psychotic or tranquilizing agents, either singly, or better, in combination.

• **Monotherapy rather than polytherapy is preferred especially in the medically ill and elderly, in whom the underlying disease process and impaired metabolisms may affect pharmacokinetics, leading to significant side effects.**

• The intravenous (IV) route is preferred for psychotic patients requiring rapid tranquilization. However, depending on the level of agitation this may not be possible or even safe, hence the intramuscular (IM) route is a good alternative.

Drug WD/ intoxication	Aggressively violent/rapid sedation needed	Agitation with undifferentiated aetiology	Elderly
Lorazepam IM or IV—begin with 1 mg and titrate upwards	*Midazolam* IM or IV 2–5 mg as needed, **OR** *Haloperidol* 2–5 mg and *Lorazepam* 1–2 mg IM or IV titrated one at a time as needed	*Haloperidol* IM/IV 2–5 mg, **OR** *Lorazepam* IM/IV 1–2 mg, **OR** *Midazolam* IM/IV 2–5 mg, **OR** *Haloperidol* 2–5 mg and *Lorazepam* 1–2 mg IM or IV titrated one at a time as needed	*Haloperidol* IM or IV 1–2 mg, **OR** *Midazolam* IM or IV 1–2 mg, **OR** *Lorazepam* IM or IV 0.5 mg

- A useful medication administration alternative in a small number of psychotic patients is oral administration since they may feel less threatened, and hence less aggressive, than when confronted with a needle.

  Dosage: Haloperidol (Haldol®) 20 mg PO (concentrate form)

  Diazepam (Valium®) 20 mg PO

- **Disposition:** Make early psychiatry consultation, preferably prior to sedation, though this may not always be possible due to the nature of the patient's presentation.

Reference/Further Reading

1. ED Management of Delirium and Agitation. *Emergency Medicine Practice*. Jan 2007.

PART 2
SPECIFIC CONDITIONS

28   Airway Management/Rapid Sequence Intubation

Shirley Ooi • Peter Manning • Gene Chan

DEFINITION

Rapid sequence intubation (RSI) is the administration, after preoxygenation, of a potent induction agent followed immediately by a rapidly acting neuromuscular blocking agent (NMBA) to induce unconsciousness and motor paralysis for tracheal intubation.

Assumptions for RSI:

- Patient **unfasted** before intubation and is therefore at **risk for aspiration**
- **A predicted difficult airway is no longer considered a contraindication to RSI.**
- Administration of the drugs is preceded by a **preoxygenation phase** (refer to second 'P' of RSI for further details) to permit a period of apnoea to occur safely between the administration of the drugs and intubation of trachea **without interposed assisted ventilation.**
- Use of **cricoid pressure or Sellick's manoeuvre** was previously recommended to prevent aspiration of gastric contents, but has been shown to impair glottic visualization in some cases, and evidence supporting its use is dubious, at best. It is **no longer recommended during emergency intubation.**

INDICATIONS

The decision to intubate is based on 3 fundamental clinical assessments:

1. **Failure of airway maintenance or protection?**

NOTE: Adequacy of airway is confirmed by having the patient speak. Possible inadequate airway includes the inability to phonate properly, stridor and altered mental state precluding response to questions. A gag reflex is neither sensitive nor specific as an indicator of loss of airway protective reflexes. The presence of pooled secretions produced by the patient's inability to swallow is a much more sensitive indicator for need of airway protection.

NOTE: A low GCS is not, in and of itself, an indication for orotracheal intubation

2. **Failure of ventilation** (e.g. status asthmaticus) **or oxygenation** (e.g. severe pulmonary oedema)?

3. **Anticipated deterioration in clinical course?**

Currently acceptable anatomy and physiology may be predicted to deteriorate or patient's work of breathing will be overwhelming in the face of multiple major injuries.

MAIN EMERGENCY AIRWAY ALGORITHM

The main emergency airway algorithm is illustrated in Figure 1. It begins once the decision to intubate is made and it ends when the airway is finally secured with a cuffed endotracheal tube.

FIGURE 1   **Main Airway Algorithm**

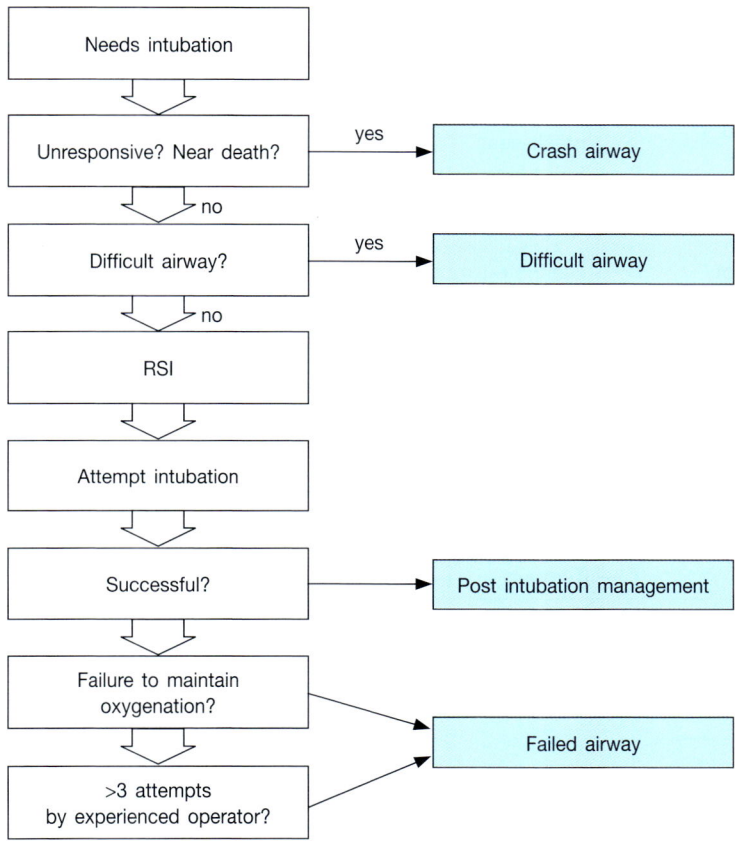

Source: Wall, et al. (2012).[1]

Once it has been decided that the patient requires intubation based on the above mentioned three indications, there is a set of questions to be answered – going down the main emergency airway algorithm.

- **Question 1: Is this a crash airway?** If the patient presents in cardiorespiratory arrest or *in extremis* with agonal efforts, the airway needs to be secured immediately. RSI is not required. Once a crash airway is identified, exit this main algorithm and manage as per crash airway.

- **Question 2: Is this a difficult airway?** Every patient who requires intubation but is not identified as a crash airway needs to be evaluated for a difficult airway. We assess for difficult laryngoscopy and intubation (LEMON), difficult Bag-Valve-Mask ventilation (MOANS), difficult extraglottic device (EGD) placement (RODS), and difficult cricothyrotomy (SMART) – See Figure 2. If a difficult airway is identified, exit this main airway algorithm and manage according to the difficult airway algorithm illustrated in Figure 3.

- **Proceed with RSI**

FIGURE 2   Predictors of a difficult airway

Difficult Bag-Valve-Mask ventilation	**M** — **M**ask seal (beard, blood or disruption that could affect mask seal)
	O — **O**besity/**O**bstruction
	A — **A**ge (the elderly are more difficult to bag)
	N — **N**o teeth (Leave the dentures in or place gauze dressings to improve the mask seal)
	S — **S**tiff lungs/**S**noring (e.g. COPD/asthma)
Difficult Laryngoscopy	**LEMON** — explained in detail below.
Difficult placement of Extraglottic Device	**R** — **R**estricted mouth opening
	O — **O**besity/**O**bstruction
	D — **D**istorted anatomy (e.g. penetrating neck injury, expanding haematoma, pharyngeal/laryngeal distortion)
	S — **S**tiff lungs (COPD/asthma)
Difficult cricothyrotomy	**S** — **S**urgery (scarring may affect sthe normal anatomy)
	M — **M**ass (e.g. haematoma, abscess, soft tissue)
	A — **A**ccess/**A**natomy
	R — **R**adiation (causing deformity and scarring)
	T — **T**umour

FIGURE 3   Difficult Airway Algorithm

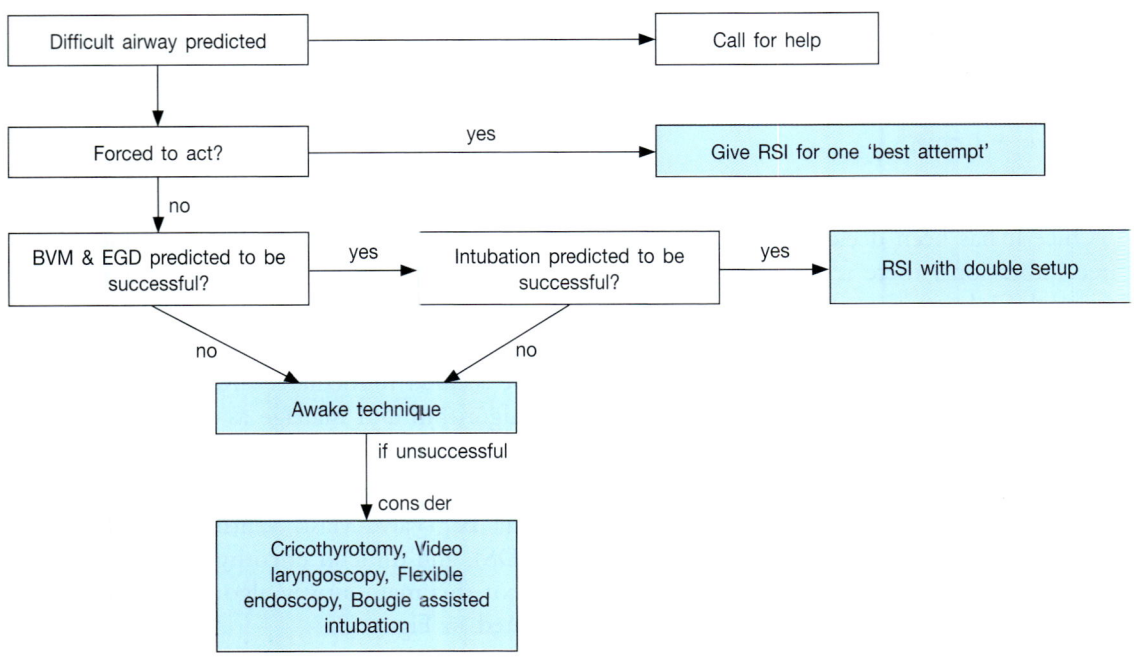

Source: Wall, et al. (2012).[1]

- **Question 3: Was intubation successful and oxygenation maintained?** Once intubation has been successfully performed and position confirmed, proceed with post intubation management. If intubation was unsuccessful, attempts at second laryngoscopy may be reasonable if oxygen saturations remain >90%. If oxygen saturations fall to <90%, Bag-Valve-Mask ventilation needs to be performed to improve oxygen saturation

- **Question 4: Is it a failed airway?** A failed airway is defined as: a) 3 failed attempts at intubation by an experienced operator; and b) 'Can't intubate, can't oxygenate'. In the event of a failed airway, an extraglottic device should be inserted or a cricothyrotomy performed.

If laryngoscopy is unsuccessful, consider the following:

1. **Is the position of the patient optimal?** Correct **alignment** of the **3 axes** of the oral cavity, pharynx and trachea (See Figure 4) is necessary to facilitate smooth and atraumatic orotracheal intubation. Consider using the concept of the **tragal line** (See Figure 5) to determine appropriate position of the patient's head on the neck [see following diagrams]. Another way of looking at the airway axes is to consider that the tragus needs to be anterior to a line drawn across the shoulders or level with the anterior chest wall.

2. Use **straight blade** if **epiglottis is long**, **floppy** or in the way.

3. Did the person performing **Sellick's manoeuvre push** the **airway out of midline** obscuring landmarks?

4. **BURP** (**B**ackward, **U**pward, **R**ightward, **P**ressure) displacement of larynx.

FIGURE 4   Airway Axes

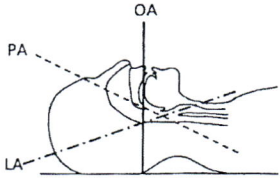

Anatomical neutral position

The oral (OA), pharyngeal (PA), and laryngeal (LA) axes are at greater than a right angle to one another.

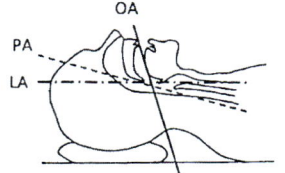

Head extended on pillow, neutral position

Flexion of the lower cervical spine aligns the pharyngeal (PA) and laryngeal (LA) axes.

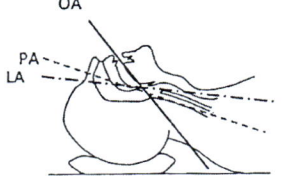

Head extended on cervical spine

The oral axis (OA) is aligned with the pharyngeal (PA) and laryngeal (LA) axes, creating the optimum 'sniffer's position'.

FIGURE 5   **Tragal Line**

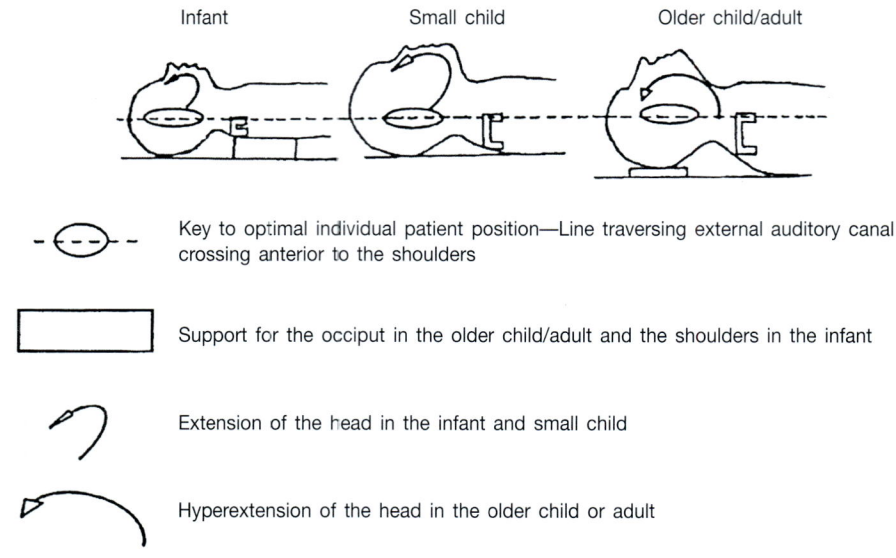

Infant   Small child   Older child/adult

Key to optimal individual patient position—Line traversing external auditory canal crossing anterior to the shoulders

Support for the occiput in the older child/adult and the shoulders in the infant

Extension of the head in the infant and small child

Hyperextension of the head in the older child or adult

⇨ **SPECIAL TIPS FOR GPs**

- **If the initial or standard bag-valve-mask fails**, ask yourself the following 4 questions:
  1. Do I have the patient in the **optimum sniffing position**? Proceed with caution in the trauma patient.
  2. Have I utilized all of my **upper airway adjuncts**?
  3. Do I have an **optimum mask seal**? For example,
     a. Applying KY jelly to a beard,
     b. Filling out hollowed cheeks with gauze placed between teeth and cheek mucosa,
     c. Reinserting patient's dentures.
  4. Have I **recruited another person** to help optimize BVM technique?

GUIDELINES ON WHEN NOT TO INTUBATE

- If you are uncomfortable with intubation techniques required and ventilation is adequate
- If the patient's condition improves during intubation attempts
- If the respiratory arrest is reversible with a drug (naloxone, flumazenil)
- If the patient has a deformity of the airway or neck (and is stable)
- If the patient has a **do not resuscitate** order

MANAGEMENT

Remember the **seven Ps of RSI**.

- **Preparation**
  1. Patient must be managed in a resuscitation area.
  2. Monitoring: ECG, pulse oximetry, vital signs q 5 min.
  3. Have sedating agents and paralyzing drugs immediately available (see below).
  4. Prepare airway equipment including stylets, different size blades, oropharyngeal airways or cricothyroidotomy tray immediately available.
  5. Have an alternative plan should you fail to intubate.
  6. Have a skilled assistant.
  7. Establish at least 2 peripheral IVs: Hartmann's or NS
  8. Always **anticipate vomiting** in all injured patients. Should a patient vomit, there are 3 manoeuvres to deal with it:
     a. Immediate suction with a large bore Yankauer sucker
     b. Rotate the patient to the lateral position or the 'recovery position'
     c. Put the patient in a Trendelenburg position (if possible)
  9. The **assessment of the difficult airway** should be done. Use the '**LEMON Law'** (mnemonic taken from Ref. 1 but details are modified) **or** 4D approach:

     L **Look externally** (e.g. maxillofacial trauma, penetrating neck trauma, blunt neck trauma, and identify difficult ventilation scenarios such as a bearded patient, morbid obesity, extreme cachexia, edentulous mouth with sunken cheeks, abnormal facies)

     E **Evaluate** the '**3-3-2 Rule**', i.e.

     First 3: 3 fingers for mouth opening-interincisor distance or Patil's test (indicates adequate **MOUTH** opening),

     Second 3: 3 fingers should fit the space between **the mentum to the hyoid bone (UNDER CHIN)**

     2: 2 fingers should fit upper border of the thyroid cartilage and the inner border of mentum, i.e., the **thyromental distance** (indicates that the floor of the mouth is adequate in size to accommodate the tongue)

     NOTE: For 3-3-2 rule, patient's own fingers are used.

     M **Mallampati score** (Figure 6) **and grade of laryngeal view** (Figure 7) for prediction of airway difficulty. Mallampati score (oropharyngeal visualization) correlates with laryngeal visualization.

  Some emergency physicians consider Mallampati and the 3-3-2 assessment to be inadequate for the emergency setting and more appropriate for an Anaesthesia elective case 'night before' assessment. Most emergency department patients are supine, which makes Mallampati difficult to assess, and the 3-3-2 assessment requires use of the patient's own fingers (not practical with large IVs placed in forearms or antecubital fossae).

FIGURE 6   Diagrams of the Mallampati Score

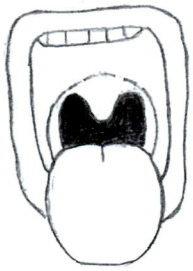 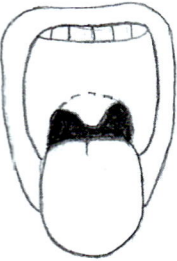 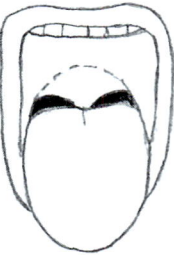 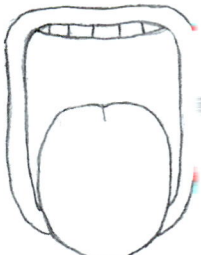

Class I:
Soft palate, uvula,
fauces, pillars visible
No difficulty

Class II:
Soft palate, uvula,
fauces visible
No difficulty

Class III:
Soft palate, base
of uvula visible
Moderate difficulty

Class IV:
Hard palate only
visible
Severe difficulty

FIGURE 7   Grade of laryngeal view: Cormack-Lehane laryngoscopic grading system

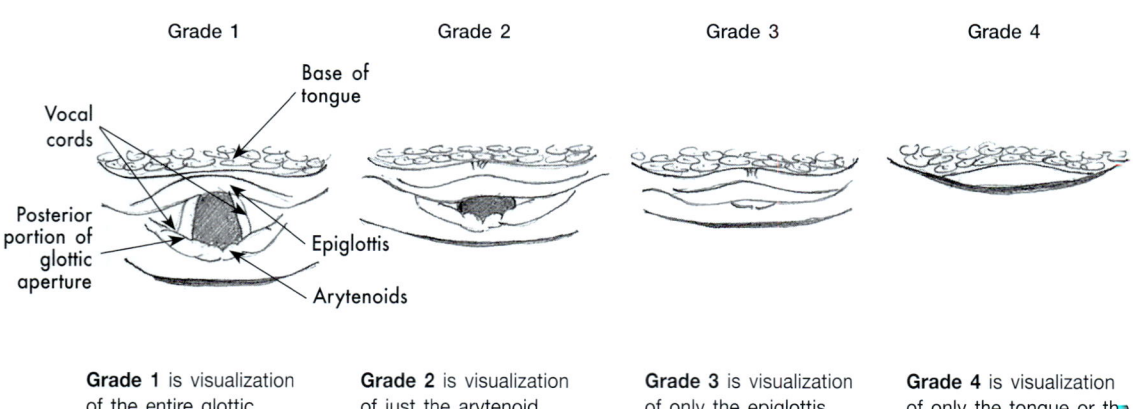

Grade 1 is visualization of the entire glottic aperture.

Grade 2 is visualization of just the arytenoid cartilaces or the posterior portion of the glottic aperture.

Grade 3 is visualization of only the epiglottis.

Grade 4 is visualization of only the tongue or the tongue and soft palate.

Instead, one might use the **4D approach**:

Dentition – large or loose teeth, dentures

Distortion – presence of vomitus, secretions, blood, bone fragments obscuring airway

Disproportion – receding chin with large tongue; buck teeth

Dysmotility – TMJ and neck mobility

Classes I and II Mallampati views are associated with superior laryngeal exposure (laryngeal grades 1 and 2) at the time of intubation and low intubation failures. In contrast, Mallampati views classes III and IV are associated with poor laryngeal visualization (laryngeal grades 3 and 4) and with higher intubation failure rates. In the ED, the formal assessment of Mallampati score sitting up is often not possible although examination of the supine patient with a tongue blade may be useful.

O Obstruction (e.g. presence of foreign body in airway, disruption of integrity of airway)

N Neck mobility: for successful ventilation, patient's neck should be positioned in the '**sniffing morning air position**', i.e. flexion at cervical spine and extension at atlanto-occipital joint. There is decreased neck mobility in the immobilized trauma patient and those with systemic arthritis.

- **Preoxygenation**

1. This is the establishment of an oxygen reservoir within the lungs and body tissue to permit several minutes of apnoea to occur without arterial oxygen desaturation. This is essential to the 'no bagging' principle of RSI.

2. Administration of **100% oxygen** with **non-rebreathing** mask for **5 min** replaces the nitrogen of room air in the Functional Residual Capacity (FRC) in the lungs with oxygen, allowing several minutes of apnoea time (in a healthy 70 kg adult, up to 8 min of apnoea time) before SpO_2 < 90%. If the patient is unable to attain an SpO_2 of ≥95%, then **CPAP** via NIV can be initiated [set at 5–15 cm H_2O].

3. If patient is **unable to be preoxygenated for 5 min** before paralytic drug is administered, get patient to take **3 to 5 vital capacity breaths** in rapid sequence from a 100% oxygen source.

4. If the discomfort and delirium of hypoxia and hypercapnia prevents patient tolerance of conventional preoxygenation, **delayed sequence intubation (DSI)** can be considered. DSI consists of the administration of specific sedative agents which do not blunt spontaneous ventilations or airway reflexes, followed by a period of preoxygenation before the administration of a paralytic agent. Another way to think about DSI is as a procedural sedation, the procedure in this case being effective preoxygenation. After the completion of this procedure, the patient can be paralyzed and intubated. An ideal agent to use in DSI which will not blunt patient's respiration or airway reflexes and provide a dissociative state, allowing the application of a NRM, or preferably NIV, is **ketamine** 1–1.5 mg/kg by slow intravenous push. This will produce a calmed patient within ~45 s.

5. The patient should receive preoxygenation in a **head-elevated position** [approximately 20°] whenever possible. For those immobilized for spinal precautions, use the reverse Trendelenburg position. The obese or heavily pregnant woman can both be preoxygenated in the upright position with mild reverse Trendelenburg positioning.

6. *Apnoeic Oxygenation* can extend the duration of safe apnoea during efforts of intubation. This technique uses a nasal cannula set at 15L/min, left in situ throughout the process of securing a tube. It has been shown that oxygen continues to diffuse into the alveoli during

periods of apnoea due to differences in pressure gradient. This permits maintenance of oxygenation without spontaneous or administered ventilations. Please note however, that carbon dioxide levels will continue to rise during periods of apnoea.

- **Pre-Treatment**
  1. This is the administration of drugs (Table 1) to mitigate the adverse effects associated with intubation.
  2. It is given 3 min prior to intubation.

TABLE 1   Pretreatment drugs for RSI

Lignocaine (1.0–1.5 mg/kg)	For reactive airway disease ('**tight lungs**') or high intracranial pressure (ICP) or '**tight brains**'#
Fentanyl (2 µg/kg given over 30–60 sec)	When **sympathetic responses** should be blunted (high ICP, aortic dissection, ruptured aortic or berry aneurysm, ischaemic heart disease)*

Notes:
There appears to be little high quality evidence available to show that IV lignocaine suppresses the rises in ICP associated with RSI in HI patients
* There was no significant difference in the haemodynamic responses to orotracheal intubation by laryngoscopy with or without pretreatment with IV fentanyl.

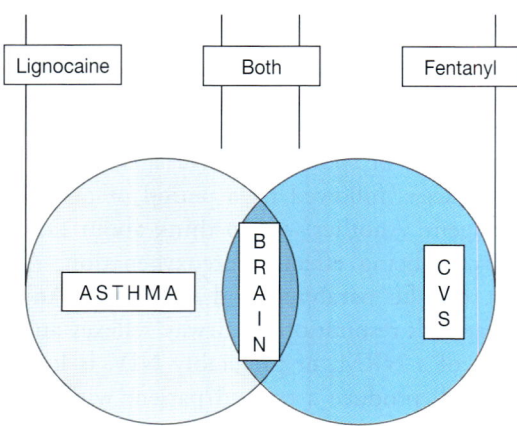

- **Paralysis with Induction** (See Table 2 for Summary of Induction Agents)
  1. This is the most vital step of the sequence.
  2. Induction agent is given as a rapid push followed immediately by a rapid push of succinylcholine.

TABLE 2 Summary of induction agents

Induction agent (Dosage)	Onset	Full recovery	Advantages	Disadvantages	Side effects/caution	Special uses
Midazolam 0.2–0.3 mg/kg	120–180 sec	0.5–2 h	Amnestic Sedative	Hypotention Suppresses respiration	Terrible induction agent as the dose required for induction is massive	
Etomidate 0.3 mg/kg (large vein)	15–30 sec	15–30 min	Cerebroprotective Haemodynamic stability		Nausea Vomiting Pain on injection Myoclonic movements Hiccups Adrenal suppression	Although considered a haemodynamically stable induction agent, it can lower BP Head injury Hypotensive patient Avoid using it in septic patients
Ketamine 2 mg/kg	15–30 sec	15–30 min	Releases catecholamines Analgesic Amnestic	Raises ICP	Raises ICP	Bronchospastic patients Hypotensive patients without head injury (HI) HI patients with normal or low BP Haemodynamic instability due to cardiac tamponade or myocardial disease Septic shock patients

- **Protection and Positioning**
  1. Sellick's manoeuvre or application of cricoid pressure is now considered optional. If it is performed, it should be initiated immediately upon the observation that patient is losing consciousness. Current opinion is that Sellick's is mandatory during positive pressure ventilation with an Ambu bag device.
  2. Patient is then positioned for laryngoscopy
- **Placement and Proof**
  1. Tube placement within the trachea should be confirmed using end-tidal CO_2 monitoring and aspiration techniques such as the oesophageal detection device.
  2. Cricoid pressure is released after confirmation of correct tube placement and endotracheal tube has been secured.
- **Postintubation Management**
  1. Secure endotracheal tube
  2. Initiate mechanical ventilation
  3. Do chest x-ray to ensure main stem intubation has not occurred. However, a more rapid way is to ensure that the proximal end of the cuff is placed 2–3 cm distal to the vocal cords or where the black marking of the ETT is located.
  4. Check BP. See Table 3 for hypotension in the post intubation period.
  5. Current philosophy is 'analgesia always, sedation often, paralysis sometimes'. Post-intubation pain and awareness MUST be avoided. Fentanyl infusion +/− propofol infusion will achieve good postintubation conditions.

     NOTE: Fentanyl is more haemodynamically neutral than propofol. This is a consideration in the borderline patient where use of propofol might cause significant hypotension.

TABLE 3   Hypotension in the Postintubation period

Cause	Detection	Action
Tension pneumothorax	Increased peak inspiratory pressure (PIP), difficulty bagging, decreased breath sounds	Immediate thoracostomy
Decreased venous return	Usually seen in patients with high PIPs secondary to high intrathoracic pressure	Fluid bolus, treatment of airway resistance (bronchodilators) Increase expiratory time. Try lowering tidal volume
Induction agents	Other causes excluded	Fluid bolus, expectant
Cardiogenic	Usually in compromised patient. ECG. Exclude other causes	Fluid bolus (caution), pressors

Source: Table reproduced with permission[1], Pg 13, Box 2.3.

PRECAUTIONS WHEN DIFFICULT AIRWAY PREDICTED

- Do not immediately do a RSI. Consider doing an **awake oral intubation**.
  1. Sedate patient with IV midazolam 1–2 mg.
  2. Spray the pharynx and larynx with a liberal amount of lignocaine, or initiate nebulization with 2% lignocaine 4 ml.
  3. Do laryngoscopy and attempt to visualize larynx/vocal cords.
  4. Spray liberally on the vocal cords.
  5. Intubate if there is fear that patient will deteriorate.
  6. If not, get ready for RSI.
  7. Further sedation may be needed, followed by IV succinylcholine 1.5 mg/kg in an adult.

ALTERNATIVE TECHNIQUES IF INTUBATION FAILS

This can be divided into 2 groups of techniques based on the ability for BVM to maintain SpO_2 >90%.

- If **BVM is able to maintain SpO$_2$ >90%**, consider the following airway techniques:
  1. intubating laryngeal mask airway
  2. lighted stylets
  3. retrograde intubation
  4. cricothyrotomy
- If **BVM is unable to maintain SpO$_2$ >90%**, cricothyrotomy is the procedure of choice

DRUG THERAPY

Induction agents

Essential for patients who are awake when RSI is being performed to significantly blunt the psychological effects of the procedure and their memory of it. (See Table 2 for summary of induction agents.)

Different Intubation Scenarios

- **Hypovolaemia** (with low BP): etomidate or ketamine. No drugs if shock is severe. **Avoid** thiopentone and midazolam
- **Isolated closed head injury** with high ICP, normal or high BP (the desired action is lower cerebral oxygen consumption, and cerebral blood flow leading to lower ICP): either thiopentone, etomidate or midazolam. **Avoid** ketamine [though current evidence suggests that ketamine helps in patients with increased ICP by maintaining cerebral perfusion], the jury is still out on this topic. Ketamine might be the victim of medical dogma dating back 40 years on the basis of 3 scientific 'papers' none of which dealt with patients suffering from traumatic head injuries!]

- **Closed head injury** (high ICP) and **Hypovolaemia** (with low BP: unresponsive to fluid): etomidate or ketamine. **Avoid** midazolam.
- **Asthma**: either ketamine, etomidate or midazolam.

Paralyzing agents

The optimum drug has a rapid onset of action and short duration. Depolarizing agents are superior to non-depolarizing agents for RSI.

The current philosophy is that it is better to mildly overdose with a neuromuscular blocking agent rather than underdosing, since one wants to obtain as ideal intubation conditions as possible.

- **Succinylcholine**: the primary agent used in emergency paralysis for airway control. Significant **side effects** include:

  1. bradycardia (especially in children and those with preexistent bradycardia)
  2. increased intracranial/intraocular pressures (contraindicated in penetrating globe trauma)
  3. increased intragastric pressure (may precipitate emesis)
  4. hyperkalaemia (especially in patients with **chronic** muscle paralysis, e.g. cerebrovascular accidents and spinal cord injuries or chronic neuromuscular disease, e.g. GBS, Myasthenia Gravis. Avoid after 5 days from acute insult until 6 months post CVA/Spinal injury.

  NOTE: Increase in plasma potassium after succinylcholine administration is modest (generally <0.5 mmol/l)

  5. hyperkalaemia in chronic renal failure patients before serum potassium known

  NOTE: There is recent evidence that succinylcholine is generally safe in hyperkalaemia, although the risk undoubtedly rises with increasing potassium levels. The best approach is to avoid succinylcholine use in patients with known, significant hyperkalaemia with serum K^+ >6 mmol/l; rocuronium is a good alternative in such cases. If the K^+ level is not known and morphology on ECG is normal, using succinylcholine is reasonable, even in patients with ESRF. In addition to its consistent, rapid attainment of excellent intubating conditions and its short duration of action, succinylcholine is eliminated independently or renal excretion, a desirable property in ESRF.

  6. fasciculation: aggravated additional musculoskeletal trauma
  7. rarely, malignant hyperthermia

  Dosage of succinycholine: administer 1.0–1.5 mg/kg ACTUAL body weight IV (2 mg/kg in children)

NOTE: Rocuronium is considered an alternative to succinylcholine due to its rapid onset of action at 1 min. However, it has a prolonged duration of action unlike succinylcholine.

- **Rocuronium**: a non-depolarizing agent used as an alternative to succinylcholine providing more prolonged paralysis during procedures, e.g. CT scans

  Dosage: administer 1.0–1.2 mg/kg IDEAL body weight IV bolus. Effective duration of action is 20–45 minutes

- **Atracurium (Tracium®)**: a non-depolarizing agent

Dosage: 0.3–0.6 mg/kg IV bolus. A disadvantage of this drug is substantial histamine release; beware in known asthmatics.

SEQUENCE OF EVENTS USING COUNT DOWN MODE

Time (minutes):

-5.00: **Preparation**
-5.00: **Preoxygenation**
-3.00: **Pretreatment (Consider lignocaine and fentanyl)**
 0.00: **Paralysis with induction**
+0.30: **Protection**
+0.45: **Placement and proof**
+1.00: **Postintubation management**
+10.00: **CXR to check depth of ETT placement**

DISPOSITION

Patients undergoing RSI are candidates for an ICU setting or go straight to the OT following appropriate consultation.

Acknowledgements

The authors would like to thank Dr Chong Chew Lan for drawing Figures 4 and 5 and Ms Sandra Han for Figures 6 and 7.

References/Further Reading

1. Wall RM, Luten RC, Murphy MF, et al. *Manual of Emergency Airway Management*. 4th ed. Philadelphia: Lippincott William & Wilkins; 2012.

2. Scott D. Weingart, MD, Richard M. Levitan, MD. Preoxygenation and prevention of desaturation during emergency airway management. *Ann Emerg Med 2012*; 59(3): 165–175

3. Hals G, Sayre M. The difficult airway: Access, intervention, and stabilization. Part I: Step-by-step techniques for advanced clinical management. *Emerg Med Rep*. 1996; 17: 23–34.

4. Hals G, Sayre M. The difficult airway: Targeting clinical applications. Part II: Indications and contraindications for intubation and invasive management. *Emerg Med Rep*. 1996; 17: 35–42

5. Schow AJ, Lubarsky DA, Olson RP, et al. Can succinylcholine be used safely in hyperkalemic patients? *Anesth Analg*. 2002; 95: 119–122.

6. Walls RM. Is succinylcholine safe in patients with hyperkalemia? *J Watch Emerg Med* 2002; 828: 3.

7. Butler J. Lignocaine premedication before RSI in head injuries. *Best BETS*.

8. Adachi YU, Satomoto M, Higuchi H, et al. Fentanyl attenuates the hemodynamic response to endotracheal intubation more than the response to laryngoscopy. *Anesth Analg*. 2002; 95: 233–237

9. Weingart SD. Preoxygenation, reoxygenation, and intubation in the ED: Delayed sequence intubation. *J Emerg Med*. 2011; 40(6): 661–7

Peter Manning • Keith Ho • Irwani Ibrahim

DEFINITIONS

- **Urticaria**: Oedematous and pruritic plaques with a pale centre and raised borders. Caused by blood vessel dilatation and oedema developing at the dermis.
- **Angiooedema**: Well-defined, non-pitting, non-pruritic swelling caused by oedema of the deeper layers of the skin (deeper layers have fewer mast cells and sensory nerve endings) but may cause burning, numbness, or pain.
- **Anaphylaxis**: A severe, potentially fatal, systemic allergic reaction to an antigen that is precipitated by the abrupt release of chemical mediators in a previously sensitized patient. The following scenarios constitute anaphylaxis:
  1. The acute onset of a reaction (minutes to hours) with involvement of the skin, mucosal tissue or both (e.g. generalized urticaria, pruritus or flushing, swollen lips-tongue-uvula) and at least one of the following: (a) Respiratory compromise (e.g. dyspnoea, wheeze, stridor, hypoxaemia) or (b) reduced blood pressure or symptoms of end-organ dysfunction (e.g. hypotonia [collapse], syncope, incontinence).
  2. ≥2 of the following occur rapidly after exposure to a likely allergen for that patient: (a) Involvement of the skin/mucosal tissue, (b) respiratory compromise, (c) reduced blood pressure or associated symptoms, (d) persistent gastrointestinal symptoms (e.g. crampy abodominal pain, vomiting).
  3. Reduced blood pressure after exposure to a known allergen.
- **Anaphylactoid reactions** resemble anaphylactic reactions but do not require prior exposure because they are not immunologically mediated. Rather, they are due to direct histamine release from mast cells and macrophages.

CAVEATS

- These states represent a spectrum of hypersensitivity reactions ranging from the mild urticaria to life-threatening anaphylaxis; progression from a milder form to full-blown anaphylaxis may occur.
- **Frequency (approximate ratios)**

Urticaria	Angiooedema	Anaphylaxis
200 cases	20 cases	1 case

- These reactions are immunoglobulin E (IgE) or immunoglobulin G4 (IgG_4)-mediated and are responsible for the majority of anaphylactic reactions that occur, e.g. drug-induced reactions (penicillin and non-steroidal anti-inflammatory drugs are the most common causes). Other common causes of anaphylactic reactions include the following:
  1. Foods (e.g. shellfish, egg white, and peanuts)
  2. Hymenoptera venoms (e.g. bees, wasps, and hornets)
  3. Environmental reactions (e.g. dust and pollens)

ANAPHYLAXIS

Shock/stridor/bronchospasm: A deadly but often preventable emergency.

Clinical evolution of symptoms
- **Early signs of impending anaphylaxis**
  1. Nasal itching or stuffiness.
  2. A lump in the throat (laryngeal or uvular oedema) or hoarseness.
  3. Lightheadedness and syncope.
  4. Chest pain, shortness of breath, and tachypnoea.
  5. Skin complaints: Warmth and tingling of the face (especially the mouth), upper chest, palms, or soles are usually the first clinical manifestations of anaphylaxis.
  6. Gastrointestinal complaints: Nausea, vomiting, diarrhoea with tenesmus, or crampy abdominal pain.
- **Full-blown anaphylaxis**
  1. The syndrome includes angiooedema of the tongue, soft palate, and larynx that can lead quickly to acute upper airway obstruction with stridor.
  2. Other symptoms are hypotension, tachycardia (or other dysrhythmias), altered mental state, dizziness, wheezing, and cyanosis that can lead quickly to cardiopulmonary arrest.

  NOTE: Coughing is an ominous sign that often portends the onset of pulmonary oedema.

  3. The skin may or may not show the classic wheal-and-flare reaction. If the patient has poor skin perfusion, or is dark-skinned, a skin reaction may be difficult to see.

⇨ **SPECIAL TIPS FOR GPs**

- It is safer to refer all patients with various presentations of allergic reactions to the emergency department, except for those with a mild and isolated urticarial rash.
- Always ask the patient regarding 'a lump in the throat' and treat with **subcutaneous** (SQ) **adrenaline** (assuming there are no contraindications such as ischaemic heart disease), **before** sending the patient to the emergency department by ambulance, as this is an early sign of laryngeal or uvular oedema.
- Adrenaline is the mainstay of treatment in anaphylaxis. In normotensive patients, administer SQ or intramuscular (IM) adrenaline 1:1000 0.01 ml/kg (up to 0.3 ml). In hypotensive patients, administer intravenously 0.1 ml/kg (up to 5 ml) of a 1:10,000 solution over 5 minutes, or by deep IM injection if intravenous (IV) access is unavailable.
- Set up a peripheral IV line and give crystalloid infusions and antihistamines before sending an anaphylactic patient to the emergency department by ambulance.

Management

- **Supportive measures**

  1. The patient must be managed in a resuscitation area.
  2. Provide supplemental high flow oxygen.
  3. Monitoring: Electrocardiogram (ECG), pulse oximetry, and vital signs q5 minutes.
  4. Be prepared for intubation or cricothyroidotomy.

  NOTE: Extreme caution is indicated in the consideration of sedation and paralysis prior to intubation. Consider using 'awake oral intubation'; refer to Chapter 28, *Airway Management Rapid Sequence Intubation* for details. Sedation and paralysis are contraindicated because a distorted airway may preclude intubation after paralysis.

  5. Obtain immediate anaesthesia/ear, nose, and throat consultations for assistance in airway management.
  6. Circulatory support: Establish large bore IV × 1 (14/16G). Give 2l Hartmann's or normal saline as bolus.
  7. Consider vasopressors (e.g. IV dopamine 2–20 µg /kg/min) to keep the systolic blood pressure greater than 90 mmHg.
  8. If relevant, stop administration of the suspected agent such as blood transfusion.
  9. If relevant, flick out the insect stinger with a tongue blade. **Do not squeeze the stinger**, as this may result in further envenomation by the originally partially discharged sac.
  10. If an allergen was ingested, consider gastric lavage and activated charcoal.
  11. If there is no pulse, commence external cardiac massage.
  12. Labs: None immediately necessary.

- Drug therapy

  1. **Adrenaline**: This is the drug of choice. The following doses are advised:

     a. Normotensive patient: 0.01 ml/kg (up to 0.5 ml) of a **1:1000 solution** given by **deep IM injection**.

     b. Hypotensive patient: 0.1 mg of a **1:10,000** solution given slowly **intravenously** over 5 minutes. Consider IV infusion 1–4 µg/min (administer via deep IM injection if IV access is unavailable).

     c. In either case half the calculated dose may be infiltrated around a causative sting.

  2. **Glucagon**: Consider its use when adrenaline is relatively contraindicated, e.g. in patients with ischaemic heart disease, severe hypertension, pregnancy, patients on beta blockers or if there is no response to adrenaline. Dosage: 1–5 mg IV over 5 minutes, followed by an infusion of 5–15 µg/min titrated to clinical response.

  3. Choose one of the following H_1 **antihistamines** listed in Table 1.

NOTE: Promethazine is a vesicant which is highly caustic to the intima of blood vessels and surrounding tissues. Formulated with phenol, it has a pH between 4 and 5.5. Where possible, intravenous administration should be avoided.

TABLE 1 Types of antihistamines and dosage

Types of antihistamines	Dosage
Diphenhydramine	Adult: 25 mg IM/IV Paediatrics 1 mg/kg IM/IV
Chlorpheniramine (Piriton®, a H_1-blocker)	10 mg IM/IV
Promethazine (Phenergan®)	Adult:　　　　25 mg IM Child >6 years: 12.5 mg IM Child <6 years: 6.25–12.5 mg IM

  4. H_2-blockers **cimetidine** (Tagamet®) 200–400 mg IV bolus or ranitidine 25–50 mg diluted in 20 ml D5% IV infusion over 5 minutes for persistent symptoms unresponsive to the above treatment.

  5. **Nebulized bronchodilators** for persistent bronchospasm. Administer salbutamol (Ventolin®) 2:2 via nebulizer q 20–30 minutes.

  6. **Corticosteroids** to potentiate the effects of adrenaline and decrease capillary permeability: Effects are not immediate. Dosage: Hydrocortisone 200–300 mg IV bolus; can be repeated q6 hours.

- Disposition

  Patients should be admitted to the intensive or high dependency unit, following appropriate consultation, for observation and repeated doses of antihistamines and steroids.

ANGIOOEDEMA

Drug-induced angiooedema

Angiotensin-converting enzyme (ACE) inhibitors are a common cause; other causes are those of urticaria (see below).

- **Clinical presentation**: Body areas that are typically affected include the face and neck (with a predeliction for the lips, soft palate, and laryngeal structures); foreskin and scrotum; and hands and feet.

- **Management** is symptomatic but one must be ready to establish a definitive airway since deterioration to anaphylaxis can occur at any time.

- **Supportive measures**
  1. The patient should be managed in at least the intermediate care area.
  2. Monitoring: Vital signs q15 minutes, pulse oximetry, and ECG.
  3. Establish peripheral IV plug as a precaution.
  4. Provide supplemental oxygen to maintain SpO_2 greater than 94%.
  5. Be prepared for intubation or cricothyroidotomy: See cautionary note above regarding sedation and paralysis. Consider using 'awake oral intubation'; refer to Chapter 28, *Airway Management/Rapid Sequence Intubation* for details.

- Drug therapy
  1. **Adrenaline**
     a. IM 0.3–0.5 ml 1:1000 solution in adults of >45 kg body weight
     b. IM 0.01 ml/kg (up to 0.3 ml) 1:1000 solution in children and adults of <45 kg body weight
  2. **Antihistamine**: Refer to the dosages in Table 1.
     a. Diphenhydramine
     b. Chlorpheniramine
     c. Promethazine
  3. **Prednisolone**
     a. Dosage: 40–60 mg PO (by mouth) in adults
     b. 2 mg/kg body weight PO in children

- Disposition: Admit for 12–24 hours of observation since a rebound may occur 6–12 hours after the initial onset and apparently successful treatment. If eyelid swelling is the sole symptom/sign, then the patient may be discharged following resolution.

Hereditary angiooedema (HAE)

Caused by a deficiency of C_1-esterase inhibitor and is precipitated in most cases by trauma or stress.

- **Clinical presentation**
  1. Marked facial oedema, swelling of lips and tongue, soft palate and laryngeal structures.
  2. Abdominal pain with nausea, vomiting, and diarrhoea are common.

- **Management**
  1. Treat with fresh frozen plasma (contains C_1 inhibitor).
  2. Adrenaline doses as stated above may also be effective.

  NOTE: Cases of HAE often do not respond to corticosteroids, antihistamines, or standard doses of adrenaline, and a definitive airway may be needed.

- **Disposition**: Admit all such cases to a high dependency unit for 12–24 hours given the tendency for resistance to treatment.

URTICARIA

Table 2 identifies the common causes of urticaria.

- **Management**: This is symptomatic in most cases but be aware that progression to anaphylaxis has been known.
- **Supportive measures**: The patient should preferably be managed in the intermediate care area of the emergency department. Management in the low acuity area is feasible but frequent reevaluations are necessary to detect deterioration early.

TABLE 2   Common causes of urticaria

Drug reaction	Beta-lactams (penicillin/cephalosporins)
	Aspirin
	Sulphonamides
	Non-steroidal anti-inflammatory drugs
	Traditional Chinese Medicines
	Local anaesthetic agents
Infection	Infectious mononucleosis
	Hepatitis B
	Coxsackie virus
	Parasitic infestations
Others	Food: Peanuts, food dyes, and flavourings
	Exposure to sun, heat, and cold
	Malignancies
	Pregnancy
	Autoimmune

- **Drug therapy**
  1. **Antihistamines**: Refer to Table 1 for the recommended dosages.
     a. Diphenhydramine
     b. Chlorpeniramine
     c. Promethazine
  2. **Prednisolone**: Dosage: 40–60 mg PO in adults if lesions are extensive, or this is a recurrent episode, or patient has had angiooedema before. Prescribe a five-day home course and no tapering of dose is required.
- **Disposition**
  1. The patient can be discharged if the response to treatment is prompt and there is no angiooedema.
  2. Discharge with at least a 3-day course of antihistamines.
  3. Consider admission if the patient has a past history of admission for urticaria.

ANAPHYLACTOID REACTIONS

Anaphylactoid reactions resemble anaphylactic reactions but do not require prior exposure because they are not immunologically mediated. They are due to direct histamine release from mast cells and macrophages.

Management

- **Commonly implicated agents include** radiographic contrast media, aspirin, non-steroidal anti-inflammatory drugs, and opiates.
- **Treatment**: The same as that for anaphylaxis.

References/Further Reading

1. Joint Task Force on Practice Parameters for the American Academy of Allergy, Asthma and Immunology; the American College of Allergy, Asthma and Immunology; and the Joint Council of Allergy, Asthma and Immunology. The diagnosis and management of anaphylaxis: An updated practice parameter. *J Allergy Clin Immunol.* 2005; 115(3): S483–S523.

2. American Heart Association guidelines for cardiopulmonary resuscitation and emergency cardiovascular care. Part 10.6: Anaphylaxis. *Circulation.* 2005; 112 (Suppl I): IV–143–IV–145.

3. Walls RM. Airway. In: Marx JA, Hockberger RS, Walls RM et al, eds. Rosen's *Emergency Medicine: Concepts and Clinical Practice.* 7th ed. Philadelphia, PA: Mosby-Elsevier; 2010.

4. Sampson HA, Munoz-Furlong A, Campbell RL, et al. Second symposium on the definition and management of anaphylaxis: Summary report—Second National Institute of Allergy and Infectious Disease/Food Allergy and Anaphylaxis Network symposium. *J Allergy Clin Immunol.* 2006; 117(2): 391–397.

5. Oswalt ML, Kemp SF. Anaphylaxis: Office management and prevention. *Immunol Allergy Clin North Am.* 2007; 27: 177.

30   Cardiac Arrest Algorithms

Benjamin Leong

CAVEATS

- **Cardiac arrest** may be defined as the 'cessation of cardiac mechanical activity as confirmed by the absence of signs of circulation'.
- Cardiac arrest is often classified as **witnessed** vs **unwitnessed** and **out-of-hospital cardiac arrest** (OHCA) vs **in-hospital cardiac arrest** (IHCA).
- The '**Chain of Survival**' concept is central to the management of cardiac arrests and illustrates the importance of an integrated approach consisting of:
  1. Early Access
  2. Early CPR
  3. Early Defibrillation
  4. Early Advanced care and Post resuscitation management
- The **3-phase time-sensitive model** of cardiac arrest describes the following:
  1. **Electrical Phase**. This is within the first 4 minutes following onset of cardiac arrest. Management of VF in this phase is immediate defibrillation.
  2. **Circulatory Phase**. This is approximately 4 to 10 minutes following the onset of cardiac arrest. A period of chest compressions to perfuse the myocardium prior to defibrillation increases successful conversion.
  3. **Metabolic Phase**. This is approximately after 10 minutes following the onset of cardiac arrest. Metabolic management such as therapeutic hypothermia may be beneficial.
- International resuscitation guidelines are reviewed and revised every 5 years, by the **International Liaison Committee On Resuscitation** (ILCOR).
- In Singapore, the **National Resuscitation Council** (NRC) reviews and issues our Resuscitation Guidelines in the light of these revisions.
- At the time of writing, the last ILCOR guideline revision was in **2010**, followed by our NRC guidelines in **2011**.
- The 2011 NRC guidelines continues the previous emphasis on **good quality CPR.**
  1. **Coronary perfusion pressure (CPP)** is defined as the difference between **aortic** and **right atrial pressures** in **diastole**.
     a. **Hard and fast chest compressions** increase the aortic pressures.
     b. Aortic pressures take time to build up during chest compressions due to fluid inertia, but **fall rapidly when chest compressions are interrupted** for various interventions such as airway control, ventilations, delivery of multiple shocks, rhythm and pulse checks. Delays in commencing and frequent interruptions during chest compressions are thus detrimental.

   c. Complete chest recoil is paramount in allowing the **right atrial pressure to fall to their lowest point** during relaxation. Failure to completely release the pressure on the chest wall during relaxation prevents that, and narrows the difference between aortic and right atrial pressures, resulting in lower CPP.

Major points and changes in the 2011 Singapore NRC guidelines

- **Basic Cardiac Life Support (BCLS) and defibrillation**

  The initial A-B-C sequence of assessment has been retained, but with the following changes:

  1. **Omission of initial 2 rescue breaths** after look-listen-feel. This is to minimize delays in initiating chest compressions.
  2. **Laypersons do not need to perform a pulse check**, whilst **healthcare providers should still perform it**.
  3. After **10s**, if there is no breathing or pulse, commence CPR immediately.
  4. Compression rate should be at least **100 bpm**.
  5. Compression depth has been increased to **at least 5 cm**, from 4–5 cm previously.
  6. **Complete chest wall recoil** is important to allow return of blood and improve CPP.
  7. Tidal volumes of **400–600 mls** per breath to avoid unnecessary increases in intra-thoracic pressures.
  8. Compression-Ventilation ratio for CPR remains as **30:2.**
  9. Laypersons untrained in CPR should at least perform **compression-only CPR**. This may be guided by telephone instructions from the 995 dispatch centre.
  10. **Immediate defibrillation** upon recognition of VF/pulseless VT (or a shockable rhythm as analysed by an AED). The previous distinction between witnessed and unwitnessed arrest has been removed.
  11. Resumption of CPR immediately after delivery of shocks without rhythm or pulse checks to minimise interruptions in CPR.

- **Advanced Cardiac Life Support (ACLS)**

  Airway & Breathing

  1. The insertion of **advanced airway devices** should not delay or interrupt chest compressions unnecessarily.
  2. The routine use of **cricoid pressure** for intubation is no longer recommended, as it may distort the airway, and impede intubation and ventilation. If performed (such as for the patient who is actively regurgitating), it may need to be **adjusted, relaxed or released** during airway insertion.
  3. **Confirmation of tube placement** should be performed by the following methods with respective caveats:
     a. **5-point auscultation**: for symmetry of breath sounds and absence of gastric insufflation. May be unreliable.

b. **Bilateral chest expansion**: for effective ventilation. May be asymmetrical in pneumothorax.

c. **Tube misting and de-misting**. May be unreliable.

d. **ETCO$_2$** (quantitative or semi-quantitative).

e. The presence of expired CO_2 returning from the endotracheal tube is indicative of successful tracheal incubation.

f. The gastric bubble may contain small amounts of CO_2. After the patient has been bagged 6 breaths, if the ETCO$_2$ detector continues to show a colour change, then it is unlikely to be due to gastric CO_2.

g. Cardiac arrest patients generally already have very low ETCO$_2$ levels (<10 mmHg), due to the absence of circulation returning tissue CO_2 to the lungs.

h. Good quality CPR should increase ETCO$_2$ levels, by generating forward flow of blood to the tissues and back.

i. A sudden sustained recovery of ETCO$_2$ up to normal levels is indicative of ROSC.

4. **CXR**. Not practical during resuscitation. Only reliable for assessing tube depth, such as right main bronchus intubation. The oesophagus is a midline structure like the trachea, and a tube in the midline on an anteroposterior CXR may not be in the trachea. A clue is if the tube outline is outside the tracheal outline, it is likely to be outside the trachea.

Circulation

1. Alternative vascular access to intravenous routes are **intra-osseous** (IO) and **central venous lines**.

2. **Endotracheal administration of drugs** is no longer recommended, as the doses needed have been found to be far in excess of previous recommendations.

Drugs

1. The following **drugs** have been removed from routine use due to lack of evidence for efficacy:

2. **Atropine** removed from asystole/PEA algorithm (but retained in symptomatic bradycardia management).

3. **Sodium bicarbonate** removed from routine prolonged resuscitation (only use in conditions such as hyperkalaemia, tricyclic acid overdose).

• **Post Resuscitation bundle**:

Airway and Ventilatory goals

1. Insert definitive airway if not yet done.

2. Maintain **SpO$_2$ 94–98%**.

a. Hyperoxaemia should be avoided, as that may worsen reperfusion injury. FiO$_2$ should be titrated down to achieve this.

3. Maintain **normocapnia ($PaCO_2$ 35–45 mmHg)**.

   a. Hypocapnia causes cerebral vasoconstriction and is deleterious.

4. Maintain $ETCO_2$ 35–40 mmHg.

5. Target **low tidal volumes (6–8ml/kg body weight)** to avoid increased intra-thoracic pressures

Circulatory goals

1. Maintain **MAP >65mmHg**. Fluid resuscitation and inotropic support as appropriate.

2. Target **$ScvO_2$ >70%**.

Metabolic goals

1. **Glucose control** to **6–10 mmol/L**, as hyperglycaemia has been shown to be detrimental.

Neurological goals

1. **Therapeutic hypothermia** has been shown to improve neurological outcomes in comatose survivors of cardiac arrest, in particular OHCA with initial VF and is promising for n Hospital Cardiac Arrest (IHCA) as well.

2. The target temperature is **32–34°C** within 4 hours and maintained for 24 hours, followed by gradual rewarming over 12 hours.

3. Conscious level and seizure monitoring should be performed and seizures controlled.

4. Neurological prognostication is unreliable before 72 hours and should only be performed after that.

⇨ **SPECIAL TIPS FOR GPs**

- GPs can play a critical role in the **first 3 rings of the 'Chain of Survival'**, and should thus be competent in BCLS and use of Automated External Defibrillators (AED).
  1. They are often in the community.
  2. They can provide early good quality CPR.
  3. They can provide early defibrillation with an AED.
  4. They may also deliver rhythm specific drugs if available.
- GPs can play a vital role in educating their patients on the following:
  1. Early recognition of pre-arrest and cardiac arrest states.
  2. Promotion of CPR training in the community.
  3. Advice to seek medical attention early.
  4. Planning on end-of-life issues.
- GPs may be integrated into the pre-hospital response for cardiac arrests.

Management Algorithms

Based on Singapore National Resuscitation Council 2011 Guidelines and ILCOR 2010 Resuscitation Guidelines. Where there are differences, the NRC guidelines are given precedence here.

- Note that the following section describes the ACLS cardiac arrest algorithms as delivered by a single healthcare provider.

- In an Emergency Department where teams are organised to attend to a patient in cardiac arrest, many of the activities should be performed concurrently, but the sequences described here should be a guide for the priority of actions to be undertaken.

- Non cardiac arrest rhythm algorithms are covered in separate sections (see Chapter 18, *Palpitations*, Chapter 43, *Tachydysrhythmias* and Chapter 35, *Bradydysrhythmias*)

- With the continuing emergence of new evidence, these algorithms will be updated and revised.

- Successful completion of an ACLS provider course will also equip the provider with practical skills not covered in this section.

UNIVERSAL ALGORITHM (see Figure 1)

The algorithmic approach to ACLS has been retained, but is now presented in a cyclical rather than linear form.

- The initial response to a suspected victim of cardiac arrest begins with the **universal algorithm**.

- **Assess responsiveness**

  1. **Shake and shout** loudly "Hello, are you ok?" to elicit for response.

- If there is **no response**,

  1. Call for **help** (activate crash team or equivalent in hospital, or call emergency medical services 995 if out of hospital)

  2. Call for **defibrillator** or **Automated External Defibrillator** (AED)

  3. In the Emergency Department, have the patient brought to the **resuscitation area** immediately.

PRIMARY ABCD SURVEY

Focus on good quality CPR and early defibrillation

A – Airway

- **Clear the airway**

  1. Perform the **head-tilt, chin-lift manoeuvre**.

     a. If **cervical trauma** cannot be excluded, use the **jaw thrust** or **tongue-jaw lift** manoeuvres instead, with concurrent **in-line cervical immobilisation**.

  2. **Inspect** the airway for foreign bodies.

FIGURE 1 ACLS Universal Algorithm

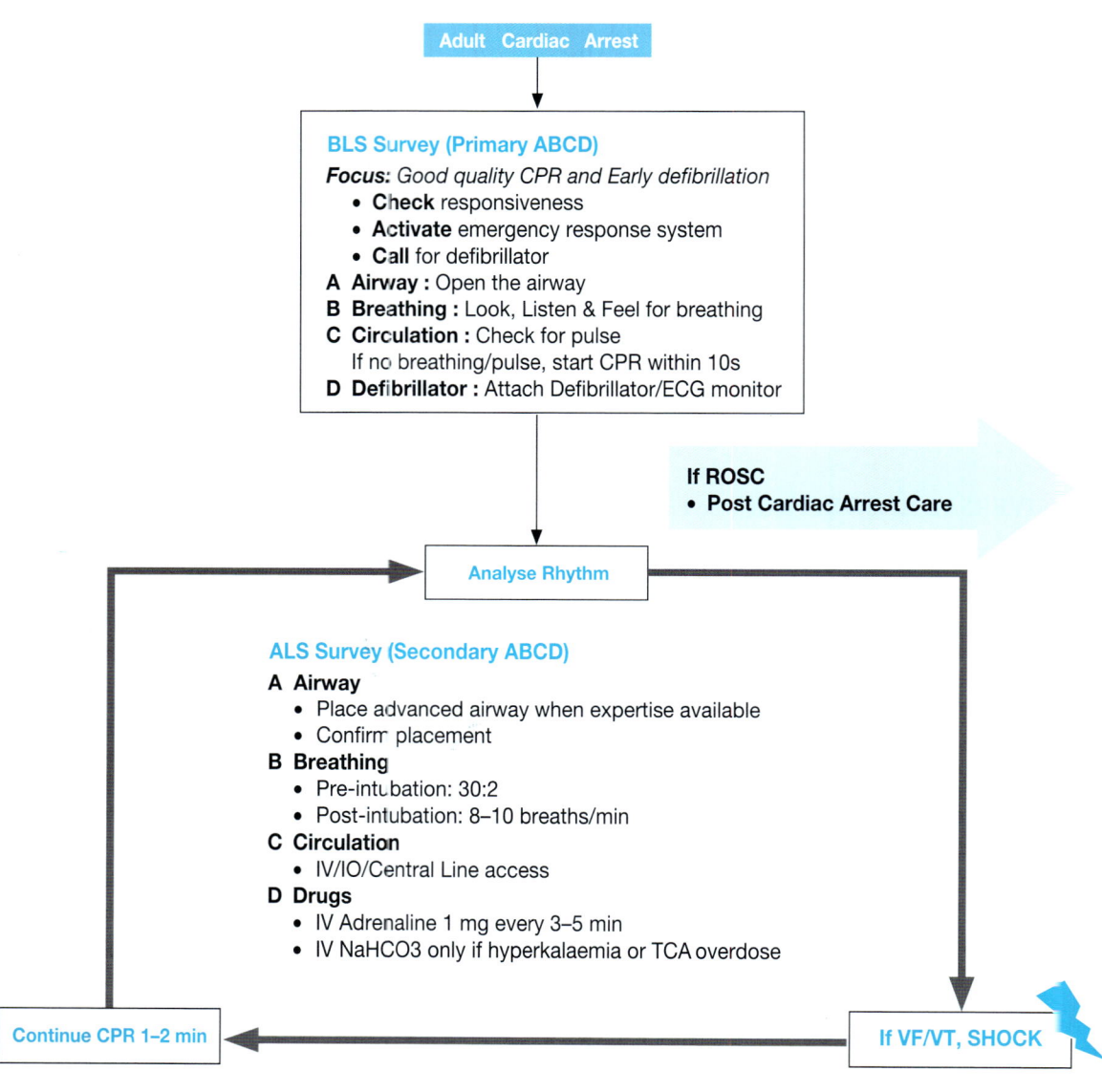

3. Use a **suction device** to remove oral secretions and vomitus.

4. Larger foreign bodies may be removed by performing a **finger sweep**.

NOTE: **Finger sweeps** should be performed only if solid material is visible in the oropharynx. If performed incorrectly, finger sweeps may exacerbate airway obstruction by pushing any non-visualised foreign material deeper in.

5. Foreign bodies that are lodged in the airway may be expelled by performing **chest compressions** or **abdominal thrusts**.

6. Airway adjuncts such as **oro-** or **nasopharyngeal airways** may be used to support the airway.

B – Breathing

- **Look, Listen and Feel** for breathing.
  1. Lean forward with the cheek near the patient's nose. Look with the **eyes** at the chest, listen with the **ears** and feel with the **cheek** for breathing.
  2. Note that **gasping** (agonal) respirations should NOT be mistaken for normal breathing.

NOTE: Omit the 2 rescue breaths under previous guidelines

C – Circulation

- **Check for a pulse** by palpating the carotid artery concurrently whilst checking for breathing.
- Do not take **>10 seconds for both** *Look-Listen-and-Feel* and *Pulse-check*.
- If there is no breathing, no pulse, the patient is unresponsive and does not exhibit any other signs of life, the patient is in **cardiac arrest**.
  1. Begin **CPR** immediately.

CPR standards

- The new guidelines emphasise **good quality of CPR**.
  1. **Chest compressions** should be delivered:
     a. at a **rate of at least 100/min**
     b. to a **depth of ≥5 cm**
     c. ensuring **complete chest recoil** between compressions
     d. with **minimal interruptions** to the chest compressions
  2. **Ventilations** should be delivered:
     a. 400–600mls per breath
     b. at **1 second** per breath
     c. enough for visible **chest rise**

3. **Compressions and ventilations** should be **synchronized** at a ratio of 30 compressions to 2 ventilations (**30:2**) until a definitive airway has been secured (See Secondary ABCD survey).

    a. Synchronization of compressions and ventilations reduces gastric insufflation that may occur when ventilations are delivered at the same time the chest is compressed.

4. NRC guidelines allow for **compression only CPR** during dispatcher-guided CPR (when a caller calls 995), or if the rescuer is unable or unwilling to perform ventilations during CPR.

D – Defibrillator

- Once a **defibrillator** is available, **analyse the rhythm** for **shockable or non-shockable rhythms**.

1. *Shockable rhythms* are **ventricular fibrillation (VF)** as **pulseless ventricular tachycardia (VT)**.

2. *Non-shockable rhythms* are **asystole** and **pulseless electrical activitiy (PEA)**.

3. **Automated External Defibrillators** (AED) detect **shockable rhythms** automatically, but may prompt the operator to check for a pulse.

NOTE: VT *with a pulse* is managed differently (see Chapter 43, **Tachydysrhythmias**).

4. If a shockable rhythm is present (VF/pulseless VT), perform defibrillation immediately (see Box 1 under section on **VF/pulseless VT**), then continued on to Secondary ABCD survey.

5. If no shockable rhythm is present (see section on **PEA/Asystole**), proceed to Secondary ABCD survey.

SECONDARY ABCD SURVEY

Focus on advanced airway, ventilatory support and rhythm specific drugs

A – Airway

- Placement of an **advanced airway device** with one of the following.

1. Endotracheal intubation

2. Laryngeal mask airway (LMA)

NOTE: Only endotracheal intubation with a cuffed endotracheal tube is considered a definitive airway. The rest are advanced supraglottic airways.

- **Confirm placement** of the airway device (See Chapter 28, *Airway Management/Rapid Sequence Intubation*).

NOTE: The need for insertion of an advanced airway must be balanced against interruptions to chest compression.

1. Rule of thumb: attempts should be ≤**30s,** or the time the doctor performing the intubation can **hold his own breath**.

2. If it is possible to perform the intubation without interrupting the chest compression at all, then chest compressions should be continued.

3. If repeated attempts are unsuccessful (rule of thumb: 3 attempts), **do not interrupt chest compressions further**, but continue with bag-mask ventilation.

- **Secure** airway device with tape or commercial airway holder.

B – Breathing

- Once an advanced airway device is **confirmed to be in place**, there is **no longer a need to synchronise compressions with ventilation**.

1. Compressions should now be **continuous without pause** at **100 bpm**.

2. Ventilations should be delivered continuously at **8 to 10 per minute**.

3. This is termed **asynchronous compression and ventilation**.

4. **Avoid hyperventilating the patient** – it is very easy and common for a healthcare provider to inadvertently bag the patient too fast or too deeply per breath in the excitement of attending to a cardiac arrest.

   a. Use only 1 hand to bag about 1/3 of the bag, as most bags are about 1.5–1.8L in size.

- **Confirm** effective oxygenation and ventilation.

C – Circulation

- Obtain **IV access**.

1. Large proximal veins such as the antecubital veins or external jugular veins are preferred for **intravenous** (IV) access.

2. If peripheral vascular access is not possible, alternative routes are the placement of an **intra-osseus needle** or insertion of a **central venous catheter**.

3. *Endotracheal administration of drugs is no longer recommended.*

- Attach **monitors** once available.

D – Drugs (see respective sections)

- Give IV **adrenaline** 1mg every 3–5 mins for all cardiac arrest cases
- IV **amiodarone** 300 mg is indicated for persistent VF. It may be repeated once at 150 mg at the physician's discretion.

1. IV lignocaine 1.0–1.5 mg/kg is an alternative, and can be repeated once.

NOTE: Use only amiodarone or lignocaine, but not both, as the use of multiple agents may be pro-arrhythmic.

2. IV **magnesium sulphate** 1–2 gm may be given if torsades de pointes is suspected.

3. IV NaHCO3 may be given if hyperkalaemia or TCA overdose is suspected.

4. The routine use of atropine for PEA and asystole has been removed from the guidelines.

5. It takes continuous CPR of 30 to 60s after drug administration for drug to circulate to heart.

D – Differentials

- Consider potentially reversible causes ("**5H's** **and 5T's**").

  Hypoxia   **T**ablets (Drug OD)
  Hypovolaemia   **T**amponade, cardiac
  Hydrogen ion – acidosis   **T**ension pneumothorax
  Hyper-/hypokalaemia, metabolic   **T**hrombosis, coronary (ACS)
  Hypothermia   **T**hrombosis, pulmonary (embolism)

Repeat cycle

- **Reassess patient and rhythm** after 1–2 mins of CPR.

  1. Briefly pause CPR to assess rhythm

     a. If the rhythm has returned to **sinus**, assess ABCs in reverse order.

        i. **Check pulse.** If there is a pulse, **Return of Spontaneous Circulation (ROSC)** has occurred. (see section on **Post Resuscitation Care**).

        ii. **Check for breathing.** If no spontaneous breathing, support ventilation.

        iii. **Reassess airway.** If not secured, prepare for intubation.

     b. If the rhythm is **VF/pulseless VT** or **PEA/asystole**, go to respective sections and repeat cycle.

     c. Ensure CPR is not interrupted or delayed unnecessarily.

VF / PULSELESS VT (see Figure 2)

- **VF or pulseless VT** is identified during the rhythm analysis.
- **Prepare to defibrillate** the patient (see Box 1).

NOTE: Do not confuse the terms *Defibrillation* and *Cardioversion*

1. **Defibrillation** is the process of stopping ventricular fibrillation by the delivery of a controlled electric shock to the heart.

   a. **Defibrillation is NOT synchronized to the cardiac rhythm,** as ventricular fibrillation is completely disorganized, making synchronization irrelevant and impossible.

2. **Cardioversion** refers to the conversion of a perfusing but unstable rhythm to sinus rhythm, and may be *electrical, pharmacological*, or *non-pharmacological*.

   a. **Electrical cardioversion MUST be synchronized**, as the rhythm is organized, and has a vulnerable period when an electric shock may trigger ventricular fibrillation instead. The shock is thus electronically timed to discharge immediately after the large R- or S-wave, avoiding the vulnerable repolarization period near the apex of the T-wave.

FIGURE 2   VF/Pulseless VT Algorithm

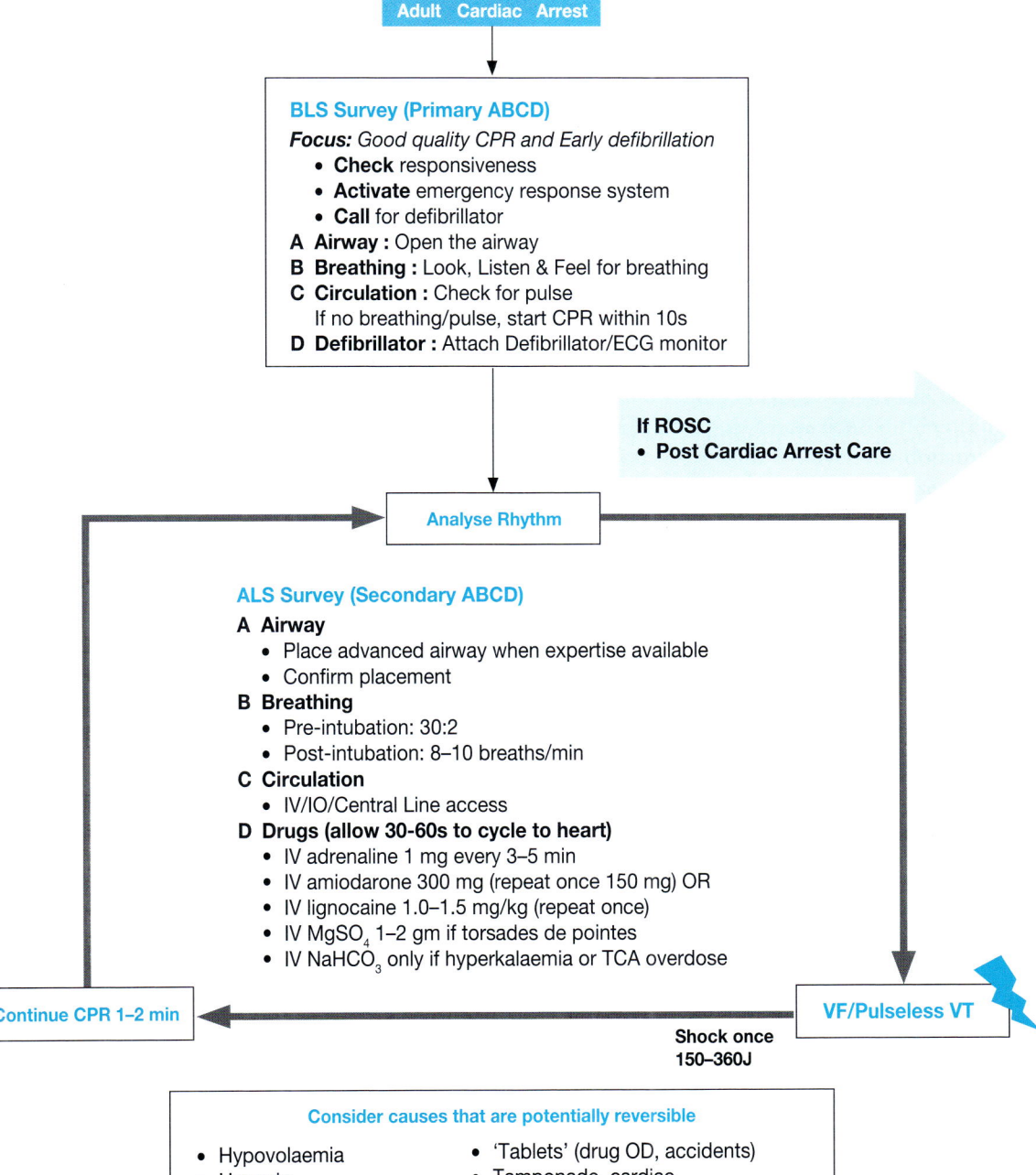

BOX 1 **Procedure for Defibrillation**

1. Apply **gel pads** or **self-adhesive defibrillator pads** to patient.
2. Ensure **synchronizer** ('sync') is OFF.
   a. If the 'sync' is on during VF, there may be no markers as the rhythm is too irregular for the defibrillator to detect any R waves.
   b. The defibrillator will then not discharge when the triggers are pulled.
3. Select energy level and charge defibrillator.
   a. **Biphasic defibrillator**
      i. 150J–360J *(AHA: 120J–360J)*
      ii. Recommended energy levels are device specific
   b. **Monophasic defibrillator**
      i. 360J *(Escalating energy levels are no longer recommended)*
   c. **Continue CPR whilst charging** the defibrillator.
4. Ensure all personnel are '**clear**', checking all the way to the foot of the bed.
5. **Re-confirm** rhythm.
6. **Deliver 1 shock** *(Stacks of 3 shocks are no longer recommended)*.
   a. If using **defibrillator paddles**, hold on to the triggers and maintain pressure on the paddles until the shock is delivered.
   b. If using **self-adhesive defibrillation pads** press the appropriate button on the defibrillator to deliver shock.
7. After the shock, **do not pause to check the rhythm or a pulse**.
8. **Resume CPR immediately for 1 to 2 mins** *(AHA: 5 cycles of 30:2 or 2 mins)* before reassessing the patient.

- Perform **Secondary ABCD Survey** if not already done.

NOTE: Ensure that **chest compressions are not interrupted** throughout this process

- Administer **drugs** appropriate for rhythm.
  1. **Adrenaline** 1 mg IV/IO every 3 to 5 minutes.
  2. If persistent VF, give **amiodarone** 300mg IV/IO or **lignocaine** 1.0–1.5mg/kg IV/IO and continue CPR for 30 to 60s.
  3. Prepare to shock within 1 min (see Box 1.)
  4. IV **magnesium sulphate** 1–2gm may be given if torsades de pointes is suspected.
- Repeat cycle, continue CPR, rhythm/pulse checks.
  1. If the rhythm is **VF/pulseless VT** or **asystole**, go to respective sections.
  2. If ROSC occurs, go to section on **post resuscitation care**.

PULSELESS ELECTRICAL ACTIVITY/ASYSTOLE (see Figure 3)

- There is **no shockable rhythm** identified after rhythm analysis.
  1. *Any* rhythm or electrical activity (ie other than VF or pulseless VT) that fails to generate a palpable pulse is considered to be **pulseless electrical activity (PEA)**.
     a. The definition of PEA includes a **spectrum** ranging from broad to narrow complex brady- to tachydysrhythmias, and thus the management is highly dependent on the underlying cause.
  2. **Asystole** is the *absence* of rhythm, and appears as a 'flatline'. Differentials include **disconnected leads**, an organized rhythm in a plane 90 degrees **perpendicular** to the selected rhythm leads, **fine VF**, and **true asystole**.
     a. Perform the 'flatline' checks to exclude other causes of flatline
        i. **Check connections** of ECG cables and leads.
        ii. **Select different leads** on the monitor to identify presence of organized rhythms in other planes.
        iii. **Increase gain** on defibrillator monitor to identify fine VF.
- Perform **Secondary ABCD Survey** if not already done.

NOTE: Ensure that **chest compressions are not interrupted** throughout this process.

- Administer **drugs** appropriate for rhythm
  1. **Adrenaline** 1 mg IV/IO every 3 to 5 minutes.
  2. IV **NaHCO$_3$** may be given if hyperkalaemia or TCA overdose is suspected.
- Repeat cycle, continue CPR, rhythm/pulse checks.
  1. If the rhythm is **VF/pulseless VT** or **asystole**, go to respective sections.
  2. If ROSC occurs, go to section on **post resuscitation care**.

MONITORING DURING CARDIAC ARREST

- Conventionally, monitoring of the patient's status during cardiac arrest management is based on continuous **ECG rhythm monitor** and **palpation of pulses**, and this is reflected in the algorithms above. Other modalities are also described below.
  1. **ECG monitor**
     a. Look for the restoration of an organized rhythm.
     b. However this only shows the electrical status of the heart but does not represent actual flow.
  2. **Palpation of pulses**
     a. Although universally used in assessment of the circulatory status of the cardiac arrest victim, this may be unreliable, as the strength of pulsations generated during CPR does not equate to forward flow.

FIGURE 3   **PEA/Asystole Algorithm**

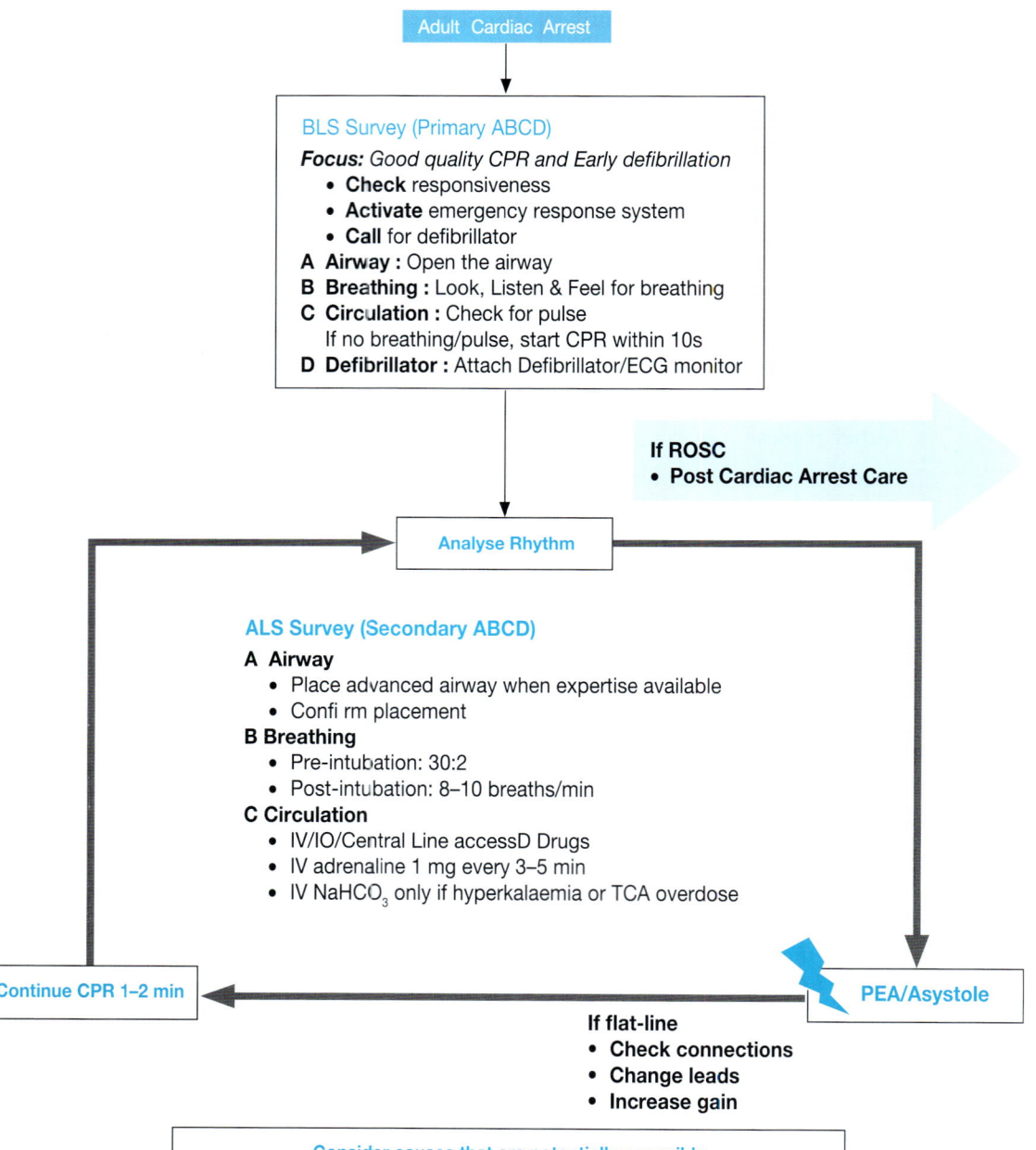

3. **Blood pressure monitoring**
   a. Non-invasive blood pressure monitoring may be difficult and unreliable.
   b. Intra-arterial monitoring may detect small deflections, but do not represent actual tissue perfusion

4. **Pulse oximetry**
   a. This is unreliable in cardiac arrest situations

5. **Metabolic monitoring**
   a. Measurement of blood gases and lactate may be unreliable and difficult to interpret in cardiac arrest situations, but will be helpful for post resuscitation therapeutic monitoring.

6. **End tidal CO_2** ($PetCO_2$) reflects tissue production of CO_2 and cardiac output carrying that CO_2 to the lungs.
   a. The normal value of $PetCO_2$ is usually about 38 mmHg.
   b. A $PetCO_2$ of <10 mmHg is associated with cardiac arrest.
   c. An increase in $PetCO_2$ from such low levels is seen during effective, good quality CPR.
   d. $PetCO_2$ may thus be used as a real-time feedback to guide quality of CPR.
   e. A study has found that if $PetCO_2$ does not rise above 10 mmHg after 20 mins of CPR, mortality is 100%.
   f. ROSC is associated with significant increase in $PetCO_2$.

POST RESUSCITATION CARE

- There is a new emphasis on post resuscitation care in the latest NRC guidelines.
- **Return Of Spontaneous Circulation (ROSC)**
  1. Signs of ROSC include a **palpable pulse**, spontaneous **breathing** (more than an occasional gasp), **coughing**, **movement**, a measurable **blood pressure** or **arterial waveform**, sudden sharp rise in end-tidal CO_2.
  2. This has been defined as the restoration of a spontaneous perfusing rhythm that provides evidence of more than an occasional gasp, fleeting palpable pulse, or arterial waveform for approximately >30 seconds.
- **Sustained ROSC**
  1. This is deemed to have occurred when signs of circulation persist without need for chest compressions for a period of **>20 mins**.

Post resuscitation investigations and monitoring:

- **Investigations**
  1. 12 lead ECG
  2. CXR

3. FBC

4. Urea/electrolytes/creatinine/glucose

5. Cardiac enzymes/troponins

6. ABG, lactate

7. Echocardiography

8. CT/MRI

- **Monitoring** (depending on Emergency Department and ICU setup, some of these measures may be initiated in the ICU)

  1. Continuous ECG monitor

  2. Blood pressure

  3. Pulse oximetry

  4. Capnography

  5. Temperature

  6. Urine output

  7. CVP or Swan-Ganz Catheter

  8. $ScvO_2$

  9. EEG monitoring

The management targets for post cardiac arrest care are:

- **Early Haemodynamic Optimization**

  1. MAP 65–100 mmHg

  2. CVP 8–12 mmHg

  3. $ScvO_2$ >70%

  4. Urine output >1 ml/kg/hour

  5. These targets reflect the aim to maximize tissue perfusion and repay oxygen debt

- **Oxygenation**

  1. SaO_2 94–98%

  2. Post ROSC ventilation with 100% O_2 in the first hour was associated with worse neurological outcome compared to immediate adjustment of FiO_2 to targeted SaO_2 levels, possibly due to generation of excess oxygen free radicals.

  3. Oxygen therapy should thus be limited to avoid unnecessary hyperoxia.

- **Ventilation**

  1. $PaCO_2$ 40 mmHg (normocarbia).

  2. Hyperventilation may result in cerebral vasoconstriction and hypoventilation in hypoxia and hypercarbia.

  3. If therapeutic hypothermia (see below) is employed, note that the reduced metabolism may result in reduced ventilatory needs.

- **Circulatory Support**
  1. Volume expansion
  2. Vasopressors
  3. Intra-aortic balloon pump (IABP)
  4. Extracorporeal membrane oxygenation (ECMO)
- **Management of ACS**
  1. If post resuscitation ECG shows STEMI, immediate coronary angiography with PCI is indicated.
  2. If PCI is unavailable, thrombolytic therapy is an accepted alternative.
  3. If ACS is suspected, coronary angiography may still be considered.
- **Therapeutic hypothermia**
  1. Mild hypothermia is the only therapy applied in the post cardiac arrest setting shown to improve survival rates.
  2. Initial evidence supports the use of post resuscitation hypothermia for VF patients, though some benefit has been noted in patients with non-VF rhythms.
  3. Additionally whilst initial recommendations were for induction of hypothermia after ROSC, there is increasing promise that initiating therapeutic hypothermia before ROSC may be beneficial.
  4. Target temperature should be 32 to 34°C for 12 to 24 hours.
  5. Methods for cooling the patient include non-invasive (e.g. cooling pads) and invasive (e.g. cooling catheters).
  6. IV saline 2L at 4°C may be used to initiate cooling.
  7. Pyrexia is common in the first 48 hours after cardiac arrest and should be prevented or treated with antipyretics or active cooling.
- **Sedation and Neuromuscular Blockade**
  1. This should be considered for mechanical ventilation and therapeutic hypothermia.
  2. Continuous EEG monitoring may be needed to monitor for seizure activity.
- **Seizure control and Prevention**
  1. Treat seizures if they occur, but there is no evidence for routine prophylactic anticonvulsant use as yet.
  2. Sedated patients and patients on neuromuscular blockade would benefit from EEG monitoring.
- **Glucose Control**
  1. Close monitoring of glucose should be performed to avoid hypo- or hyperglycaemia.
  2. Recommended targets are 4.4 mmol/L to 6.1 mmol/L or 8 mmol/L.
- **Other measures include**
  1. Neuroprotective pharmacology
  2. Adrenal dysfunction

3. Renal failure

4. Infection

5. Placement of AICDs

- **Post Cardiac Arrest Prognostication**

  1. Post resuscitation neurological prognostication should be performed only after 72 hours.

  2. Factors that may affect outcomes include pre-, intra-, and post-cardiac arrest factors.

  3. Tests for prognosis include neurophysiological tests, neuroimaging and biochemical markers.

References/Further Reading

1. Anantharaman V, Gunasegaran K. Advanced Cardiac Life Support guidelines 2011. *Singapore Med J.* 2011 Aug; 52(8): 548–55

2. Deakin CD, Morrison LJ, Morley PT, et al; Advanced Life Support Chapter Collaborators. Part 8: Advanced life support. 2010 International Consensus on Cardiopulmonary Resuscitation and Emergency Cardiovascular Care Science with Treatment Recommendations. *Resuscitation.* 2010 Oct; 81 Suppl 1: e93–e174.

3. Deakin CD, Nolan JP, Soar J, et al. European Resuscitation Council Guidelines for Resuscitation 2010 Section 4. Adult advanced life support. *Resuscitation.* 2010 Oct; 81(10): 1305–52.

4. Jacobs I, Nadkarni V, Bahr J, et al. Cardiac arrest and cardiopulmonary resuscitation outcome reports: update and simplification of the Utstein templates for resuscitation registries: a statement for healthcare professionals from a task force of the International Liaison Committee on Resuscitation (American Heart Association, European Resuscitation Council, Australian Resuscitation Council, New Zealand Resuscitation Council, Heart and Stroke Foundation of Canada, InterAmerican Heart Foundation, Resuscitation Councils of Southern Africa). *Circulation.* 2004; 110: 3385–3397.

5. Weisfeldt ML, Becker LB. Resuscitation after cardiac arrest: a 3-phase time-sensitive model. *JAMA.* 2002; 288: 3035–3038.

6. Ward KR, Barbee RW, Ivatury RR. Monitoring techniques during resuscitation. In: Ornato JP, Peberdy MA, Eds. *Cardiopulmonary Resuscitation.* Humana Press, Totowa New Jersey, 2005.

7. Neumar RW, Nolan JP, Adrie C, et al. Post-cardiac arrest syndrome. epidemiology, pathophysiology, treatment, and prognostication a consensus statement from the International Liaison Committee on resuscitation (American Heart Association, Australian and New Zealand Council on Resuscitation, European Resuscitation Council, Heart and Stroke Foundation of Canada, InterAmerican Heart Foundation, Resuscitation Council of Asia, and the Resuscitation Council of Southern Africa); the American Heart Association Emergency Cardiovascular Care Committee; the Council on Cardiovascular Surgery and Anesthesia; the Council on Cardiopulmonary, Perioperative, and Critical Care; the Council on Clinical Cardiology; and the Stroke Council. *Circulation.* 2008; 118: 2452–2483.

31 Cardiogenic Shock

Kuan Win Sen • Shirley Ooi

CAVEATS

- Cardiogenic shock is a result of *decreased myocardial contractility* and *inadequate systemic vasoconstriction* from a systemic inflammatory response to extensive myocardial damage.
- It is primarily diagnosed based on clinical findings supported by haemodynamic measurements (e.g. cardiac index is less than 2.2 L/min/m^2 and pulmonary artery wedge pressure is more than 18 mmHg). Clinical signs of hypoperfusion include altered mental state, cold, clammy skin, and oliguria.
- Examples of non-cardiac conditions mimicking cardiogenic shock include pulmonary embolism and aortic dissection.
- Cardiogenic shock has a very high mortality rate.

TABLE 1 Causes of cardiogenic shock

Myopathic	Mechanical
Acute myocardial infarction	Acute mitral regurgitation
Myocarditis	Ventricular septal/free wall/aneurysm rupture
Dilated cardiomyopathy	Left ventricular inflow/outflow tract obstruction
Right ventricular failure	

CLINICAL PRESENTATION

- Laboured breathing with audible coarse crackles or wheezing.
- Impaired circulation: Tachycardia (may be absent if patients are on beta blockers), delayed capillary refill, hypotension, diaphoresis, and poor peripheral pulses.
- End-organ dysfunction (e.g. decreased mental function and urinary output).
- Jugular venous distension as evidence of right ventricular failure.
- Pulmonary oedema from left ventricular dysfunction.
- Loud murmurs may indicate valvular dysfunction.
- Beck's triad (diagnostic features are jugular venous distension, pulsus paradoxus and muffled heart sounds) may be present to suggest tamponade.
- Gallop (especially the S3 heart sound which is pathognomonic of congestive heart failure).

The presence of pulmonary oedema in the setting of hypotension increases the likelihood of cardiogenic shock.

⇨ **SPECIAL TIPS FOR GPs**

- Not all patients with cardiogenic shock present with all the 'classic' signs of severe systemic hypotension, systemic hypoperfusion, and respiratory distress.
- Cardiogenic shock is more commonly seen with *anterior* myocardial infarctions due to a larger area of myocardium involvement.
- The severity of hypotension defining cardiogenic shock varies. Hypotension alone should not be the basis for diagnosis in the absence of signs of peripheral hypoperfusion.

MANAGEMENT

- **Aims in the emergency department**
  1. Make diagnosis.
  2. Prevent ischaemia.
  3. Treat the underlying cause (e.g. coronary artery perfusion in acute myocardial infarction).
- Airway, breathing and circulation (ABCs)
  1. Endotracheal intubation and mechanical ventilation for patients with excessive work of breathing.
  2. High flow oxygen given via a mask to maintain SpO_2 at >90%.
  3. Intravenous fluids to maintain adequate preload (consider central venous pressure monitoring, pulmonary capillary wedge pressure monitoring, and sonographic assessment of inferior vena cava filling).
- Intravenous opioids (e.g. morphine 2–4 mg) to relieve pain, induce sedation, block adrenergic discharge, and lessen cardiac stress.
- Intravenous vasopressors provide inotropic support to increase perfusion.
  1. To be used with **caution** to avoid extreme heart rates which may increase myocardial oxygen consumption, increase infarct size, and impair cardiac pump ability.
  2. **Dobutamine** is the **drug of choice to improve cardiac contractility**.
     a. β_1-adrenergic agonist with minimum chronotropic and peripheral vasoconstrictive effects.
     b. Does not cause the release of norepinephrine.
     c. Relatively mild α_1-adrenergic (vasoconstrictor) receptor effect countered by more potent β effect.
     d. Minimal effects on myocardial oxygen demand.
     e. Does not increase infarct size or elicit dysrhythmias.
     f. May be infused up to doses of 40 μg/kg/min without significantly increasing the heart rate.

3. **Dopamine**

   a. **Low doses** ('**renal doses**') (2–5 µg/kg/min) increase coronary perfusion, renal perfusion, cerebral blood flow, and splanchnic flow. However, 'renal dose' of dopamine is not evidence-based; rather attempt to attain a mean arterial pressure of more than 60 mmHg).

   b. **Moderate doses** (**5–10 µg/kg/min**) have direct β-**adrenergic** receptor effects, which increase cardiac contractility without significant effects on blood pressure.

   c. **Higher doses** elevate systemic vascular resistance by stimulating α-**adrenergic** receptors, cause tachycardia, and vasoconstriction of renal and splanchnic beds.

   d. Use with caution in patients with cardiogenic shock (moderate and high doses) as it may adversely influence the balance of myocardial oxygen delivery and consumption.

4. **Digoxin**

   a. Modest inotropic effects. Useful for treatment in patients with atrial fibrillation with rapid ventricular response.

- **Intra-aortic balloon pump**

  1. Consult with the cardiologist early if cardiogenic shock is not readily reversed with pharmacological therapy.

  2. This therapy is recommended as a stabilizing measure and combined with thrombolytic therapy if angiography and revascularization are not readily available.

  3. Counter-pulsation reduces left ventricular afterload and improves coronary artery blood flow.

- Early cardiology consult.

References/Further Reading

1. Bongard FS, Sue DY. *Current Critical Care Diagnosis and Treatment.* 2nd ed. New York: McGraw-Hill; 2002: 262–266.

2. Hollenberg SM, Bates ER. *Cardiogenic Shock.* Armonk. New York: Futura Publishing Company, Inc.; 2002.

3. Hasdai D, Berger PB, Battler A, Holmes DR. Cardiogenic Shock: *Diagnosis and Treatment.* Totowa, NJ: The Humana Press; 2002.

32 Neurogenic Shock
Rakhee Yash Pal

DEFINITION

- Neurogenic shock is a form of distributive shock, the other two being septic shock and anaphylactic shock.
- Neurogenic shock is the rarest form of shock.
- It is caused by a sudden loss of sympathetic tone to regions distal to the level of injury, resulting in vasodilatation as well as restricting both the reflex tachycardia, and vasoconstriction responses to hypovolaemia.
- The decreased peripheral resistance and hypotension can lead to pulmonary oedema.

CAVEATS

- In trauma patients with hypotension in the absence of tachycardia, haemorrhagic shock must still be considered as the patient may not be able to mount the tachycardic response, e.g. a patient on beta blocker therapy.
- Also, the most common cause of shock in the trauma patient is loss of circulating blood volume from haemorrhage, though it may coexist with neurogenic shock. Thus, patients should be treated as for haemorrhagic shock, until specific etiologies can be ruled out.
- Haemorrhagic shock can reduce spinal blood flow, causing further neurological injury.

CAUSES

- Injury to cervical and upper thoracic spinal cord.
- Severe brain stem injury at the medulla level.
- Regional anaesthesia and drugs.

CLINICAL FEATURES

- Hypotension with bradycardia.
- Warm, flushed skin.
- Accompanying neurological deficits.

MANAGEMENT

- **Intravenous fluids**: Large volumes may be needed to restore normal haemodynamics but care should be taken not to overload as it may precipitate pulmonary oedema. Monitor the urinary output with an indwelling urinary catheter.

- **Inotropic support**: Dopamine is often used.
- **Atropine**: Increase heart rate and improve cardiac output.
- **Vasopressors**: If hypotension remains refractory to treatment.
- Urgent orthopaedic and/or neurosurgical consult.

References/Further Reading

1. American College of Surgeons Committee on Trauma. Spine and spinal cord trauma. *Advanced Trauma Life Support for Doctors Manual*. 8th ed. Chicago, IL: American College of Surgeons; 2008.

2. Kirk RM, Ribbans WJ. *Clinical Surgery in General: RCS Course Manual*. 4th ed. New York: Elsevier Health Sciences; 2004.

3. Delamarter RB, Coyle J. Acute management of spinal cord injury. *J Am Acad Orthop Surg*. 1999; 7: 166–175.

33 Sepsis/Septic Shock

Irwani Ibrahim • Kuan Win Sen

DEFINITIONS

- **Infection**: A microbial phenomenon characterized by an inflammatory response to the presence of microorganisms or the invasion of normally sterile host tissues by those organisms.

- **Bacteraemia**: The presence of viable bacteria in the blood without mention of the host response.

- **Systemic inflammatory response syndrome (SIRS)**: The systemic inflammatory response to a variety of severe clinical insults which may or may not be infective in nature. The response is manifested by at least two of the following conditions:

  1. Temperature >38°C or <36°C.

  2. Heart rate of >90 beats per minute.

  3. Respiratory rate of >20 breaths per minute or carbon dioxide partial pressure ($PaCO_2$) of <32 mmHg.

  4. White blood cell count of >12,000/mm^3, <4000/mm^3, or >10% immature (band) forms.

- **Sepsis**: The systemic response to *infection*. The response is identical to SIRS.

- **Severe sepsis**: Sepsis complicated by organ dysfunction, perfusion abnormalities, or hypotension. Perfusion abnormalities may include (but are not limited to) lactic acidosis, oliguria, or an acute alteration in mental state. Hypotension is defined as a systolic blood pressure of <90 mmHg, mean arterial pressure of <65 mmHg or a reduction of >40 mmHg from baseline in the absence of another known cause for hypotension.

- **Septic shock**: Sepsis with hypotension (as defined above) despite adequate fluid resuscitation, along with the presence of perfusion abnormalities (as defined above). Patients who are receiving inotropic support or vasopressor agents may not be hypotensive at the time perfusion abnormalities are measured, yet may still be considered to be in septic shock.

- **Cryptic shock**: Global tissue hypoxia, evidenced by elevated blood lactate of ≥4 mmol/L in the setting of normotension. Severe sepsis with cryptic shock carries a mortality rate similar to overt septic shock.

- **Multiple organ dysfunction syndrome (MODS)**: Presence of altered organ function in an acutely ill patient such that homeostasis cannot be maintained without intervention.

CAVEATS

- In the elderly, the very young or immuno-compromised, the clinical presentation may be atypical and non-specific with no fever or localizable source of infection (refer to Chapter 81, *Geriatric Emergencies*).

- Symptoms of sepsis include fever, chills, and constitutional symptoms of fatigue, malaise, anxiety, or confusion. These symptoms are not pathognomonic for infection and may be seen in a variety of non-infectious inflammatory conditions. They may be absent in serious infections especially in the elderly, who commonly present with only tachypnoea and altered mental state (delirium).

- Abnormal vital signs such as tachypnoea, tachycardia, and increased pulse pressure may suggest sepsis even if fever is absent.

NOTE: In the early stages of sepsis, cardiac output is well maintained or increased, resulting in warm skin and extremities. As sepsis progresses, the patient will start to show signs of poor distal perfusion, e.g. cool skin and extremities. Hence, late septic shock without fever is indistinguishable from other types of shock and a high index of suspicion is required. It is often a diagnosis of exclusion.

- The most frequent sites of infection are the lungs, abdomen, urinary tract, and skin (Table 1). Among patients older than 65 years of age, urinary tract is the most common source of infection.

TABLE 1   Predisposing factors for Gram-negative and Gram-positive bacteraemia

Gram-negative bacteraemia	Gram-positive bacteraemia
Diabetes mellitus	Vascular catheters
Lymphoproliferative disease	Indwelling mechanical device
Cirrhosis of the liver	Burns
Burns	Intravenous (IV) drug injections
Chemotherapy	

⇨ **SPECIAL TIPS FOR GPs**
- If delay to the nearest hospital is anticipated, start intravenous fluid resuscitation immediately.
- In patients with signs of meningococcaemia, start intravenous crystalline penicillin 4 mega units immediately as patients can deteriorate rapidly within a few hours.

MANAGEMENT

Principles

- Early recognition.
- Source control.

- Early and adequate antibiotic therapy.
- Ventilatory support.
- Early haemodynamic resuscitation and support.
- The patient must be managed in the resuscitation area.
- Monitoring: Electrocardiogram (ECG), vitals signs q5 minutes and pulse oximetry.
- **Labs**:
  1. Capillary blood sugar.
  2. Full blood count.
  3. Blood cultures (draw from two different sites).
  4. Disseminated intravascular coagulopathy screen.
  5. Urea/electrolytes/creatinine.
  6. Arterial blood gas.
  7. Urine culture.
- **Chest X-ray** to look for consolidation and signs of ARDS (adult respiratory distress syndrome).
- Consider **ECG**.
- Insert a **urinary catheter** to monitor the urine output.
- Maintain **airway**, give supplemental high flow oxygen. Endotracheal intubation should be considered if the airway is not secured or ventilation and oxygenation are inadequate. The induction agent, etomidate, should be used with caution as it causes adrenal suppression. Ketamine is an alternative agent for induction.
- **Haemodynamic stabilization**:
  1. Establish two large bore IV lines and aggressively correct the hypotension with fluid resuscitation (i.e. rapid fluid administration of at least 1–2 L crystalloid or 20–40 ml/kg). Consider inserting a central venous catheter, especially if a potent vasopressor is required.
  2. Vasoactive agent support may be needed if there is no response to fluid challenge. **Noradrenaline** is the agent of choice in septic shock, starting at 1 µg/kg/min. Alternatively, **dopamine** can be used (dosage at 5–20 µg/kg/min).
  3. Successful fluid resuscitation is indicated by stabilization of mentation, blood pressure, respiration, pulse rate, skin perfusion, and good urine output.

NOTE: In selected centres, **early goal-directed therapy (EGDT)** for severe sepsis and septic shock can be instituted. This technique involves aggressive treatment to achieve specific resuscitation goals originally central venous pressure (CVP), mean arterial pressure (MAP), and central venous oxygen saturation ($ScvO_2$) within 6 hours of presentation. Patients receive intensive monitoring which includes the $ScvO_2$ (central venous oxygen saturation) via a catheter.

$ScvO_2$ is a **global index of perfusion** and reflects the balance between oxygen delivery and consumption. The **normal** $ScvO_2$ is **70–75%**. A decreased $ScvO_2$ indicates insufficient oxygen delivery, reflecting exhausted compensation and indicates a poor outcome. An increased ScvO$_2$ signifies adequate cardiac function, but may indicate poor oxygen consumption and extraction. This situation may reflect impending cellular death, since oxygen is not being consumed by the affected tissue. It too carries a poor prognosis.

Current evidence suggests **dynamic haemodynamic parameters** (e.g. change in stroke volume index, passive leg raising, and pulse pressure variation) to be more accurate than static measures (e.g. CVP) in predicting **fluid responsiveness** of the patient. **Lactate clearance** has been evaluated as an important index to independently predict survival in patients with severe sepsis or septic shock.

- **Infection control**:
  1. It is paramount that the **right** antimicrobial therapy is started as soon as possible.
  2. The three principal considerations are host immune response (immuno-competent or compromised), organism (community or hospital acquired) and severity of illness (severe or non-severe sepsis).

NOTE: Table 2 is only a guide. The spectrum of bacteria and their sensitivities vary in different hospitals.

TABLE 2 **Suggested antibiotics**

Suspected infection	Suggested antibiotics
Immuno-competent without an obvious source	Third-generation cephalosporin (e.g. IV ceftriaxone) or for penicillin allergy, quinolones (e.g. IV ciprofloxacin 200 mg)
Immuno-compromised without an obvious source	Anti-pseudomonal antibiotic (e.g. IV ceftazidime 1 g) or for penicillin allergy, quinolones plus aminoglycosides (e.g. gentamicin 80 mg)
Severe community-acquired pneumonia (CAP)	IV augmentin 2.4 g plus IV ceftazidime 2 g plus IV azithromycin 500 mg for severe CAP or see Chapter 46, *Pneumonia, Community Acquired*
Skin and soft tissue infection	IV cefazolin 2 g. Consider IV vancomycin 1 g if there is a history of penicillin allergy or there is a history of IV drug abuse or indwelling catheter. For necrotizing fasciitis, IV clindamycin 600 mg plus IV penicillin G 2–4 MU
Acute meningitis	Third-generation cephalosporin (IV ceftriaxone 2 g)
Urinary tract	Third-generation cephalosporin (IV ceftriaxone 2 g)
Intra-abdominal infection	Third-generation cephalosporin (IV ceftriaxone 2 g) and IV metronidazole 500 mg
Biliary tract infection e.g. acute cholangitis and acute cholecystitis	Third-generation cephalosporin (IV ceftriaxone 2 g)

3. Source control measures such as abscess and empyema drainage, tissue debridement (e.g. for necrotizing fasciitis) and removal of infected prostheses should be discussed with the attending surgeons.

- The use of **corticosteroids** in septic shock is still controversial. However, it plays a primary role if adrenal insufficiency is suspected or documented.
- Consult the Intensive Care team for transfer to their care.

References/Further Reading

1. Levy MM, Fink MP, Marshall JC, et al. 2001 SCCM/ESICM/ACCP/ATS/SIS International Sepsis Definitions Conference. *Intensive Care Med*. Apr 2003: 29(4): 530–538.

2. Rivers E, Nguyen B, Havstad S, et al. Early goal-directed therapy in the treatment of severe sepsis and septic shock. *N Engl J Med*. Nov 2001: 8: 345(19): 1368–1377.

3. Catenacci MH, King K. Severe sepsis and septic shock: Improving outcomes in the emergency department. *Emerg Med Clin North Am*. Aug 2008; 26(3): 603–623.

4. Jansen TC, van Bommel J, Schoonderbeek FJ, et al. LACTATE study group. Early lactate-guided therapy in intensive care unit patients: A multicenter, open-label, randomized controlled trial. *Am J Respir Crit Care Med*. Sep 2010: 15: 182(6): 752–761.

5. Arnold RC, Shapiro NI, Jones AE, et al. Emergency Medicine Shock Research Network (EMShockNet) Investigators. Multicenter study of early lactate clearance as a determinant of survival in patients with presumed sepsis. *Shock* July 2009; 32(1): 35–39.

34 Aortic Emergencies
Shirley Ooi • Gene Chan

AORTIC DISSECTION

DEFINITIONS

- Aortic dissection occurs due to an aortic intimal tear, intramural haematoma, or separation of the tunica media creating a false lumen. Propagation of the dissection from the initial tear accounts for the varied clinical manifestations.
- **Predisposing factors** include patients with hypertension, smoking, atherosclerosis, pregnant patients, or patients with disorders of collagen, or vasculitis (giant cell arteritis or Marfan's syndrome).
- Two primary types of classifications are in use: the DeBakey and Stanford classifications.
- The **DeBakey system** is divided into 3 types:
  1. Type I involves the ascending aorta, aortic arch, and the descending aorta.
  2. Type II involves the ascending aorta, but does not extend beyond the left subclavian artery.
  3. Type III involves only the descending aorta, starting at, or distal to, the left subclavian artery.
- The **Stanford system** is divided into two groups:
  1. Type A involves the ascending aorta (with or without involvement of the descending aorta).
  2. Type B involves only the descending aorta.

  The Stanford classification is simpler and it helps to delineate treatment (see below).

CAVEATS

- Consider the **diagnosis of aortic dissection** in any patient with the following:
  1. Sudden, severe, tearing chest pain/upper abdominal pain radiating to the back, maximal at the outset.
  2. Migratory pain from the chest to the abdomen to the lower limbs (**ILEAD**, i.e. **I**schaemia of the **L**ower **E**xtremities due to **A**ortic **D**issection). As a rule, the pain of acute myocardial infarction (MI) is *not* migratory, and when the two occur together, the dissection typically begins first and leads to the MI.
  3. Chest pain with associated neurological symptoms, syncope, transient ischaemic attack, stroke, or paraplegia.
  4. Chest pain with increased risk of aortic dissection, e.g. hypertension, Marfan's syndrome, Ehlers–Danlos syndrome, and pregnancy.
  5. Pulse deficits or difference in systolic blood pressure in both arms (>20 mmHg) or blood pressure in the upper limbs is greater than in the lower limbs.

6. Chest pain with new onset aortic regurgitation murmur.

7. Chest pain with widened mediastinum of >8 cm on the posteroanterior chest X-ray.

8. Myocardial infarction is usually due to inferior MI because of the lesions in the right coronary artery affecting the coronary ostia (1–7%).

NOTE: The absence of pulse deficit or widened mediastinum does not exclude the diagnosis of aortic dissection.[5]

- **Diagnoses** that may be **confused** with **thoracic aortic dissection** include the following:
  1. Myocardial infarction or unstable angina.
  2. Abdominal disease.
  3. Stroke.
  4. Lower extremity ischaemic thrombosis.
  5. Pneumonia.
  6. Pericardial disease.

NOTE: Aortic dissection can occur together with any of the above diagnoses.

- When a patient is **initially evaluated for aortic dissection** and the entity is not found, **remember** the following points:
  1. In some cases, multiple tests (e.g. transoesophageal echocardiography followed by computed tomography (CT) aortogram, etc.) are needed to detect the disease.
  2. The next most likely cause of the patient's complaints may be another type of serious cardiac disease.
  3. If a patient needs to be evaluated for aortic dissection, it is usually done with admission as the ultimate disposition, regardless of the diagnostic test results.
  4. Patients with a negative evaluation for aortic dissection have a high rate (23%) of acute myocardial infarction or unstable angina, both of which should not be overlooked even if dissection is excluded.

⇨ **SPECIAL TIPS FOR GPs**

- Aortic dissection is a serious condition that is very easily missed unless one specially looks for it. It should be considered very seriously if the electrocardiogram (ECG) done for a suspected acute myocardial infarction is normal or in chest pain patients with concomitant neurological deficits. Remember that it is one of the six life-threatening causes of chest pain!
- Once the diagnosis is suspected, do not send the patient to the emergency department in his own transport. Call the ambulance. Meanwhile, if possible, set up one or two intravenous (IV) lines, control the patient's blood pressure and alleviate pain.
- If aortic dissection is suspected, remember that anti-platelet agents and thrombolytic therapy are contraindicated.

- Remember that acute aortic dissection is 2 to 3 times more common than ruptured abdominal aneurysm, and the misdiagnosis rate is as high as 90%. Furthermore, the mortality of untreated type A dissection is 1% per hour in the first 48 hours.

MANAGEMENT

NOTE: The **goal of treatment** is to prevent death and irreversible end-organ damage. The **aim of medical therapy** is to lower the rate of rise of blood pressure (dP/dT) and to lower the mean blood pressure and heart rate.

- Monitor the vital signs (including cardiac activity) in the critical care area.
- Give high flow supplemental oxygen.
- Set up 2 large bore IV lines. Send **blood** for the following:
  1. Full blood count.
  2. Urea/electrolytes/creatinine.
  3. Coagulation profile.
  4. GXM 4 to 6 units packed cells; if hypotensive, two units rapid match blood as well.
  5. Cardiac enzymes.
- Do a 12-lead **ECG** to exclude concomitant acute myocardial infarction.
- Order **chest X-ray**. See Table 1 for features suggestive of aortic dissection.

NOTE: The screening upright chest X-ray will be abnormal in 80–90% of cases of aortic dissection. However, a normal chest X-ray does *not* exclude the diagnosis.

- Bedside **2-Dechocardiography** can be done to look for widened aortic root of >3cm in proximal aortic dissection.
- Bedside **transoesophageal echocardiography (TEE)** is the definitive diagnostic study of choice in aortic dissection in an unstable patient.
- Arrange for **CT aortogram** once diagnosis is suspected.
- Give **pain relief** with IV morphine 2.5–5.0 mg titrated to clinical need.
- Insert a **urinary catheter** to monitor the urine output and to exclude anuria/oliguria suggesting possible involvement of both renal arteries.

NOTE: Most patients with acute aortic dissection present with significant hypertension. A small percentage will present with hypotension from aortic rupture into the pleural space or into the pericardium with subsequent tamponade.

- Put the patient on the circulation and neurological observation chart.
- Start **hypotensive therapy** if the patient is hypertensive. Aim to **reduce systolic blood pressure to 100–120 mmHg**, provided the urine output remains at more than 30 ml/hr.

TABLE 1   Chest X-ray findings in aortic dissection

1. Widened superior mediastinum (>3 cm on a posteroanterior film; most common, i.e. 75% of chest X-rays).
2. Extension of aortic shadow more than 5 mm beyond its calcified wall ('eggshell' or 'calcium' sign; this is due to the acute dissection separating the adventitia and the calcified intima; the most specific physical sign of aortic dissection although not common).
3. Obliteration of the aortic knob or localized bulge.
4. Aortic enlargement.
5. Double density of the aorta (false lumen less radiopaque).
6. Loss of space between the aorta and the pulmonary artery.
7. Widening of the paravertebral stripe.
8. New pleural effusion (free haemothorax).
9. Apical pleural cap (localized apical haemothorax).
10. Depression of the left main stem bronchus to more than 140°.
11. Shift and elevation of the right main stem bronchus.
12. Deviation of the trachea/endotracheal/nasogastric tube to the right (away from the developing haematoma).

Give:

1. IV **labetalol**: Initial treatment with IV beta blocker helps reduce the heart rate to below 60 beats per minute. The fall in both blood pressure and rate of rise of systolic pressure will minimize aortic wall stress.

    a. IV **labetalol** may be more readily accessible and is a good alternative as it produces both alpha-adrenergic (α-adrenergic) and beta-adrenergic (β-adrenergic) blocks. Make up a solution of 1 mg/ml by diluting 50 mg (10 ml) to 40 ml normal saline or 5% dextrose solution. Start infusion at 2 mg/min titrated up to 8 mg/min every 15 minutes as necessary. Alternatively, for more rapid control of blood pressure, give IV labetalol 20 mg bolus over 2 minutes initially followed by repeat or double doses every 10 minutes until the target heart rate is reached or a maximum of 150 mg has been given, then start continuous infusion at 2 mg/min titrated up to 8 mg/min.

    NOTE: Although labetalol is a combined alpha and beta blocker, it is actually 7× more of a beta blocker for all intents and purposes, and the provider should always be prepared to add nitroprusside because labetalol is usually insufficient when used as a single agent

    b. IV **propranolol** can also be used.

    c. IV **esmolol** may be preferable in the acute setting due to its short half-life and ability to be titrated to effect. However, cost and availability is an issue.

2. IV **nitroprusside infusion plus IV propranolol**

    Make a solution of 100 μg/ml nitroprusside by adding 50 mg to 500 ml 5% dextrose. Start infusion at 6 ml/hr (10 μg/min) and increase it by steps of 10 μg/min every 5 minutes as necessary, and give IV propranolol 1 mg every 5 minutes until a **target**

heart rate of 60–80 beats per minute is achieved (give **before** or **simultaneously** with nitroprusside as nitroprusside may produce reflex tachycardia).

- If hypotensive, start IV fluid resuscitation. Treatment for cardiac tamponade not responding to fluid resuscitation is immediate pericardiocentesis. Inotropic agents should be avoided since they will increase aortic shear stress and worsen the dissection.

NOTE: All patients receive medical therapy initially, regardless of dissection type. Medical therapy will lower the blood pressure and decrease the velocity of left ventricular contraction. This decreases aortic shear stress and minimizes the tendency for propagation of the dissection.

- Patients with documented aortic dissection who are **normotensive** or have no pain should still be treated with a medical regimen. Further decreases of their blood pressure and heart rate to the aforementioned ranges are unlikely to cause harm and will help stop progression of the dissection in the same manner as in hypertensive patients.
- Contact the cardiothoracic surgeon as soon as diagnosis is suspected and while medical therapy is being instituted.
- The **indications for surgical repair** of aortic dissection include:
  1. All Stanford type A dissections.
  2. Type B dissections with complications (rupture, severe distal ischaemia, intractable pain, progression, and uncontrolled hypertension). Otherwise, type B dissections can be managed medically.
  3. Uncontrolled hypertension.
  4. Progression of dissection.

References/Further Reading

1. Hals G. Acute thoracic aortic dissection: Current evaluation and management. Part I: Pathophysiology, risk factors, and clinical presentation. *Emerg Med Rep*. 2000; 21(1): 1–10.
2. Hals G. Acute thoracic aortic dissection: Current evaluation and management. Part II: Definitive diagnosis, patient evaluation, and outcome optimizing management in the emergency department. *Emerg Med Rep*. 2000; 21(2): 11–22.
3. UptoDate—Clinical manifestations and diagnosis of aortic dissection. Updated 31 July 2008.
4. UptoDate—Management of aortic dissection. Updated 14 Sept 2007.
5. Chua M, Ibrahim I, Neo X, et al. Acute aortic dissection in the ED: risk factors and predictors for missed diagnosis. *Am J Emerg Med* 2012 Oct; 30(8): 1622–1626.

ABDOMINAL AORTIC ANEURYSM (AAA)

DEFINITIONS

- A localized dilatation of an artery of >50% of the normal diameter. A dilatation of <50% of the normal arterial diameter is termed *ectasia*.

CAVEATS

- Occurs in 5–7% people over 60 years old.
- In Singapore, the male:female ratio approximates 2:1, with an apparent lower incidence in Indians.
- May **present** as:
  1. Catastrophic intraperitoneal rupture causing collapse, shock and death. Most have a sentinel bleed into retroperitoneum, which then ruptures intraperitoneally.
  2. Abdominal, flank or back pain (sometimes mimicking ureteric colic).

  NOTE: The back pain could be either due to the expansion of the AAA with erosion of the spinal vertebrae or it could represent rupture of the aneurysm, which is a surgical emergency.

  3. Abdominal mass, often pulsatile, but occasionally not.
  4. Syncope with postural hypotension.
  5. Embolization causing acute ischaemic limb or mottling of the lower trunk and extremities. Peripheral embolization could cause **blue toe syndrome**.
  6. Aortoenteric fistula presenting as melaena.
  7. Compression of the bowel, stomach or oesophagus may lead to dysphagia, early satiety, nausea and/or vomiting.

  NOTE: The majority (75%) are asymptomatic.

- Diffuse and non-specific nature of a symptomatic AAA may lead to errors in diagnosis. Any elderly patient presenting with hypotension, shock and back pain must have a ruptured AAA excluded. Most diagnostic **errors** are due to the **failure to palpate pulsatile mass**.
- Look for **expansile versus transmitted pulsation** by placing fingers alongside pulsation; deviation of the fingers laterally is due to aneurysm.
- All patients with a pulsatile mass >3 cm should have an ultrasound evaluation.
- Mortality rate from emergency surgery is 75–90%, whereas it is only 3–5% in an elective repair.

PATHOPHYSIOLOGY

- Most aortic aneurysms are associated with atherosclerosis, while other common aetiologies include cystic medial necrosis, Ehlers-Danlos syndrome, and dissection.

RISK FACTORS

- Hypertension: seen in at least 40% of AAAs.
- Smoking: 8 times greater likelihood of having AAA compared with non-smokers.
- Hyperlipidaemia and hyperhomocysteinaemia.

RISK OF RUPTURE

- Aortic aneurysms have an exponential expansion rate and the risk of rupture is proportional to the diameter of the aneurysm:
  1. Aneurysms 4–5.5 cm diameter have 5% risk of rupture
  2. Aneurysms 6–7 cm have 33% risk of rupture
  3. Aneurysms >7 cm have 95% risk of rupture
- Some studies suggest hypertension and COLD are strong predictors of rupture in small aneurysms.
- Recent trials such as the UK Small Aneurysm trial and ADAM trial have shown no long-term survival benefit for surgery in aneurysms <4 cm diameter.

⇨ **SPECIAL TIPS FOR GPs**
- Aortic aneurysm may present as abdominal pain, back pain, colic or ischaemic leg pain.
- Diagnosis is often made by a physical examination of the abdomen.
- Diagnosis may be confirmed by B-Mode ultrasound.
- Elective surgical intervention is indicated for most patients with AAA >5 cm diameter to prevent rupture/death.
- Smaller aneurysms should be monitored by regular ultrasound measurements.

MANAGEMENT OF RUPTURED AORTIC ANEURYSM

General measures

- Manage patient in the critical care area.
- Intubation and resuscitation equipment must be immediately available.
- Inform appropriate surgical team stat according to local protocols.
- ABC primary survey, ensure patent airway and perform resuscitative measures as needed.
- Monitor ECG, vital signs, pulse oximetry.
- Establish at least 2 large-bore IV lines with normal saline as infusate but **do not** over-resuscitate patient. Permit hypotension of 90–100 mm Hg systolic.
- **Labs:** GXM 6 units whole blood, FBC, urea/electrolytes/creatinine, coagulation profile, ABG. Order group-specific blood as necessary if delay in full cross-match.
- Portable CXR (look for dissection/mediastinal widening).
- **Plain abdominal films** will show calcification in approximately 50% of cases, but needs to be seen in both lateral and AP films to diagnose an AAA. If the classical 'egg-shell' appearance is present, the degree of confidence in diagnosis is high. A negative plain x-ray does **not** exclude the diagnosis of AAA and limits the value of this study.
- Place urinary catheter.

Specific measures

- Do not allow repeated abdominal palpation once diagnosed.
- **Bedside ultrasound** is useful in the ED to diagnose the presence of an aneurysm but is operator-dependent. It may not detect a contained rupture. An aortic diameter of >3cm suggests the possibility of AAA.
- Ruptured AAA is a surgical emergency and the patient must be prepared for operation as soon as possible. There is no place for routine abdominal or CT films.
- However, if patient is **stable**, then **CT scan** has become the investigation of choice with regard to the diagnosis of AAA, but **must not delay definitive treatment** of a ruptured or leaking AAA.

Disposition

- Admit to Cardiothoracic Surgery or General Surgery according to local practice protocols

References/Further Reading

1. Hals G. The clinical challenges of abdominal aortic aneurysm: Rapid, systematic detection and outcome-effective management. *Emerg Med Rep*. 2000; 21(11): 121–140.

2. UK small aneurysm trial. *Lancet*. 1998; 352: 1649–1655.

3. Noel AA, Cherry KJ. Ruptured abdominal aortic aneurysms. *J Vasc Surg*. 2001; 34(1): 41–46.

4. Powell JT, Brown LC. The natural history of abdominal aortic aneurysms and their risk of rupture. *Acta Chir Belg*. 2001; 101(1): 11–16.

5. Hsiang YN, Turnbull RG. Predicting death from ruptured abdominal aortic aneurysms. *Am Surg*. 2001; 181 1): 30–35.

35 Bradydysrhythmias

Benjamin Leong • Shirley Ooi

CAVEATS

- The peri-arrest arrhythmias in **Advanced Cardiac Life Support** (ACLS) are divided into the tachycardias and bradycardias.
- This section covers the **bradycardias** and the algorithmic approach to their management.
- International resuscitation guidelines are reviewed and revised every five years, by the **International Liaison Committee on Resuscitation** (ILCOR).
- In Singapore, the **National Resuscitation Council** (NRC) reviews and issues the Resuscitation Guidelines in the light of these revisions.
- At the time of writing, the last ILCOR guideline revision was in **2010**, followed by the NRC guideline revision in **2011**.

> ⇨ **SPECIAL TIPS FOR GPs**
>
> Serious signs and symptoms of bradydysrhythmias include altered mental status, giddiness, hypotension, and syncope (**Stokes–Adams attack**).
> - Patients with such presentations should have an **electrocardiogram** (**ECG**) done.
> - In general, in the absence of haemodynamic instability or serious signs and symptoms, the low heart rate may be left untreated.
> - However, if the ECG shows potentially lethal rhythms such as a type II second-degree or third-degree heart block, these patients should be transferred to the emergency department for admission to hospital, even if they appear stable.
> - Refer all unstable patients to the emergency department immediately via ambulance.

Sinus bradycardia

- Any heart rate that is <60 beats per minute.
- Every P wave is associated with a QRS complex.
- Causes include high vagal tone, acute myocardial infarction, hypothyroidism, sick sinus syndrome, electrolyte disorders, toxic exposures, and beta blocker use.

First-degree heart block

- PR interval is >0.20 seconds.
- PR interval is constant.
- Every P wave is associated with a QRS complex.

NOTE: **Hyperkalaemia** may present with first-degree heart block.

FIGURE 1   **Approach to bradydysrhythmias**

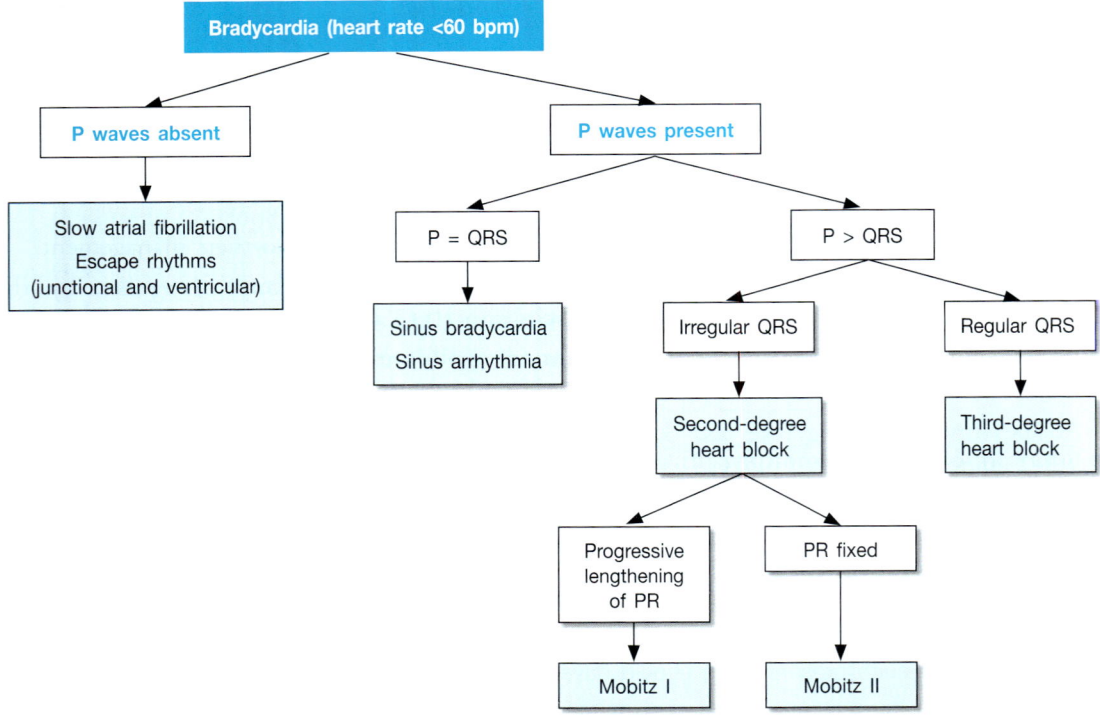

FIGURE 2   **First-degree heart block**

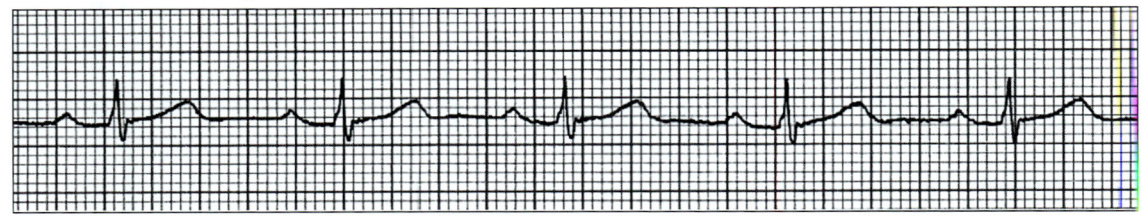

Notes:
1. Prolonged PR interval of 222 milliseconds.
2. Every P wave is conducted.

Mobitz type I second-degree heart block

- Also called **Wenckebach phenomenon**.
- **Progressive lengthening of the PR interval** followed by a **P wave** that is **not conducted**.
- The R-R interval shortens until the blocked beat.
- The cycle then restarts with resetting of the PR interval.
- This results in '**clusters**' of beats.
- Typically due to a **high vagal tone**.

- Usually **narrow QRS complexes**, unless bundle branch block coexists.
- Traditionally considered benign, but recent evidence suggests the benefit of pacemakers in these patients too.

FIGURE 3   **Mobitz type I second-degree heart block**

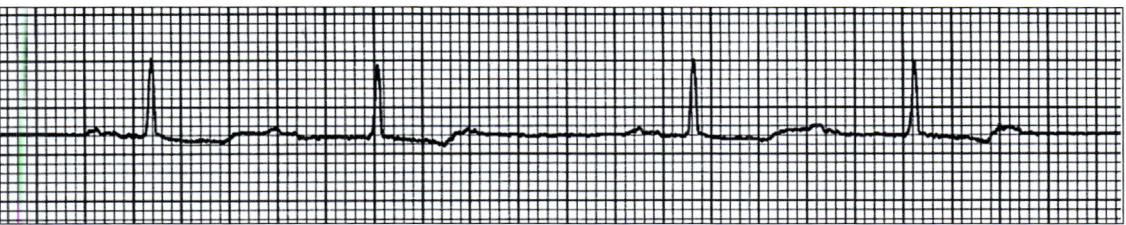

Notes:
1. Increasing P-R intervals followed by a non-conducted P wave.
2. Clustering of beats.

Mobitz type II second-degree heart block

- **Fixed PR interval**.
- Unpredictable **non-conduction of P wave**.
- No clustering of beats.
- More likely to be infranodal in origin and hence associated with **widened QRS complexes**, though it may be narrow also.
- Risk of deteriorating into complete heart block.
- If two or more P waves are not conducted, it is a **high-grade AV block**.

FIGURE 4   **Mobitz type II second-degree heart block**

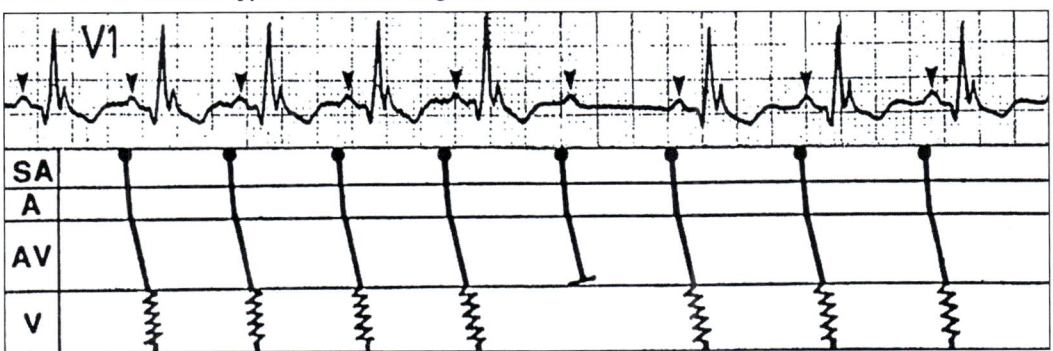

Notes:
1. PR interval is constant at 0.16 seconds.
2. The sixth beat is not conducted.
3. The QRS complexes are broad.
Image taken from *Clinical Electrocardiography* 3rd Edition, BL Chia, ©1998 World Scientific. Reproduced with permission.

2:1 second-degree heart block

- This can be easily mistaken for complete heart block, as the QRS intervals are constant.
- The difference is that the P-R intervals for the conducted P waves are constant, as opposed to being non-constant in complete heart block.
- The level of the block may be supra- or infra-Hisian but it is often clinically difficult to distinguish between the two.

FIGURE 5   2:1 second-degree heart block

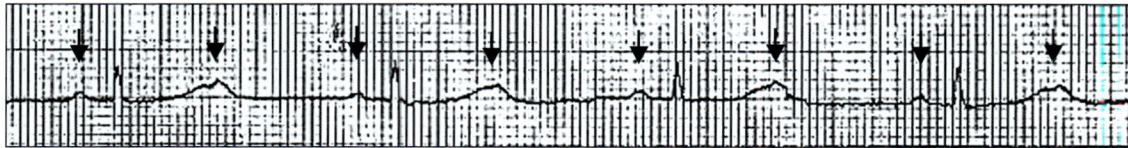

Notes:
1. P waves (arrowed) are present for every alternate QRS complex.
2. The P-R intervals for the conducted P waves are constant.
3. The non-conducted P waves are superimposed over the T waves. This is not complete heart block.

Third-degree heart block (also called complete heart block)

- This is a potentially unstable rhythm.
- There is **complete dissociation** of P waves from QRS complexes.
- QRS complexes are regular escape rhythms, as opposed to type II heart blocks, when they are irregular due to dropped beats.
- **Narrow QRS complexes** suggest a block at the level of the atrioventricular (AV) node. The heart rate is typically between 40–60 beats per minute, and is responsive to atropine.
- **Broad QRS complexes** suggest an infranodal block, and the heart rate is typically 40 beats per minute or below.
- Infranodal blocks are unlikely to respond to atropine.

FIGURE 6   Third-degree heart block

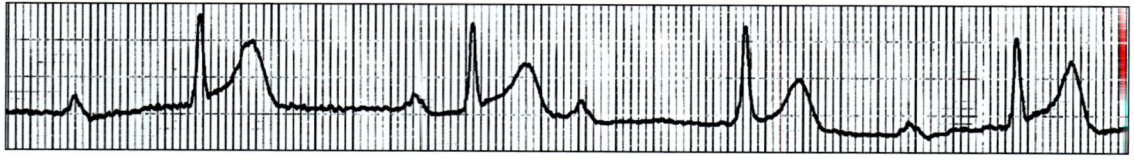

Notes:
1. During AV dissociation, P waves and QRS complexes demonstrate independent rhythms.
2. There is no clustering of beats.
3. The ventricular rhythm is regular.

Management algorithms

NOTE: Based on the Singapore National Resuscitation Council 2011 Guidelines and ILCOR 2010 Resuscitation Guidelines. Where there are differences, the NRC guidelines are given precedence here.

Universal algorithm

- The initial response to a patient with tachycardia begins with the **universal algorithm** (Figure 7).
- If the patient is unresponsive, call the Cardiac Arrest team (see Chapter 30, *Cardiac Arrest Algorithms*).

FIGURE 7 **Initial assessment and management of bradydysrhythmias**

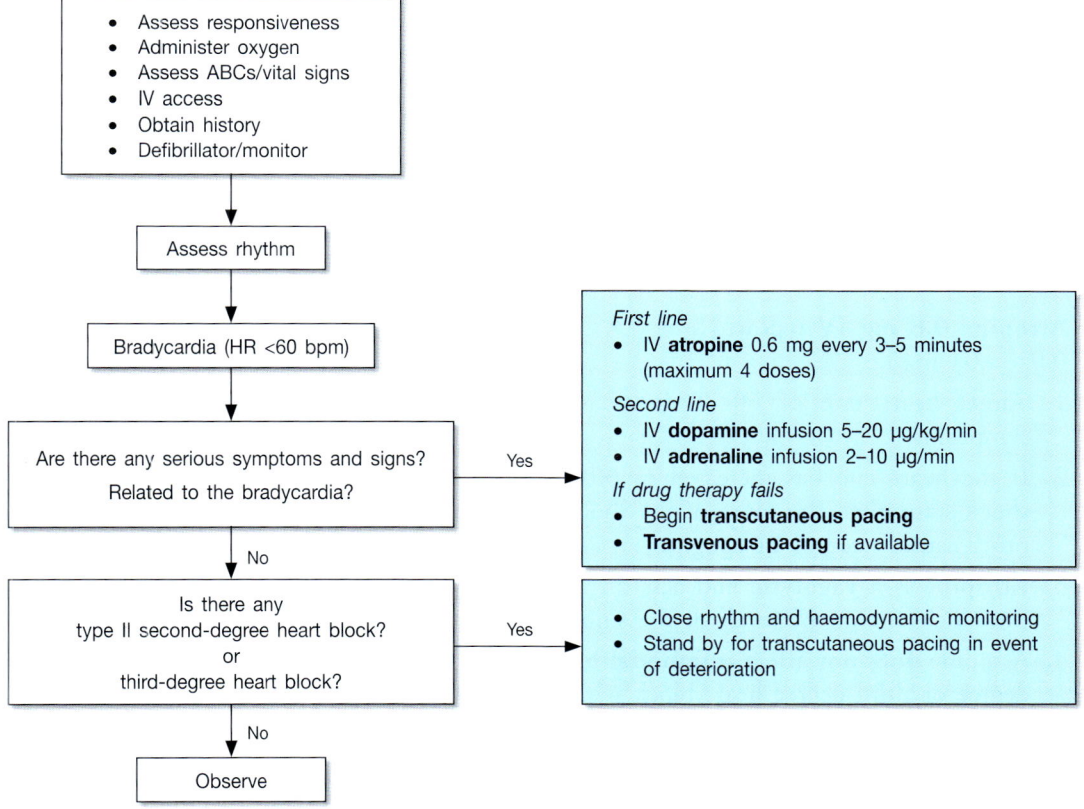

ABCD survey

- Assess, clear, and support the **airway, breathing and circulation**.
- Give **supplemental oxygen**.

- Establish **intravenous access**.
- Attach **defibrillator/ECG monitor** once available and **assess rhythm**.
  1. Absolute bradycardia is defined as any heart rate below 60 beats per minute.
- Assess **vital signs**, brief targeted **history**, and **physical examination** findings.
- Obtain a **12-lead ECG** when available.
- Look for **serious symptoms or signs** that are *associated with bradycardia*:
  1. **Breathlessness**
  2. **Altered mental status**
  3. Systolic blood pressure of **<90 mmHg** and clinical features of **shock**
  4. Clinical features of **heart failure**
- If **serious signs and symptoms are present** and attributable to bradydysrhythmia, proceed to **intervention sequence for bradydysrhythmias**.
- If there are no serious signs and symptoms, is there any **type II second-degree AV block or third-degree AV block**?
  1. If present, these patients need to be **closely monitored** with **preparations for pacing**, as they may deteriorate.
  2. If not, the patients may be observed.

INTERVENTION SEQUENCE FOR BRADYDYSRHYTHMIAS

- **Atropine 0.6 mg IV** repeated every 3 to 5 minutes, up to a maximum dose of 2.4 mg or 0.03–0.04 mg/kg.
  1. Target heart rate of 60–70 beats per minute, with resolution of serious signs and symptoms.
  2. If the heart rate has increased to 60–70 beats per minute without improvement in the shock state, then the cause of the shock is unlikely to be due to the heart rate *per se*, and other causes need to be sought.
  3. **Atropine** is a **vagolytic** and acts on bradydysrhythmias that are vagally mediated, where the blocks are at the levels of the sinoatrial (SA) or AV nodes.
  4. Atropine **does not affect infranodal blocks**, and thus is *unlikely* to work in type II second-degree or third-degree heart block with **broad QRS complexes**.
  5. Administration of atropine doses <0.6 mg may induce paradoxical bradycardia.
  6. Avoid atropine with transplanted hearts as it may induce paradoxical bradycardia or asystole.
  7. Patients with transplanted hearts will respond better to intravenous catecholamines or theophylline.
- **Second-line drugs**
  1. **Dopamine** 5–20 µg/kg/min IV infusion
  2. **Adrenaline** 2–10 µg/min IV infusion

- If drugs fail to resolve the bradycardia, and the patient remains symptomatic, prepare for **transcutaneous pacing** (see Box 1).
- **Other drugs and modalities**
  1. IV **theophylline** may be considered for the denervated heart (transplanted heart) or denervated muscles in patients with spinal cord injury.
  2. IV **glucagon** and **calcium gluconate** may be used for β-blocker or calcium channel blocker overdose.
  3. Percussion (fist) pacing may be considered in haemodynamically unstable patients as a temporizing measure while preparing for electrical pacing.
- Admit all **patients with symptomatic bradydysrhythmias**.
- **Lab tests** should include full blood count, urea/electrolytes/creatinine, and cardiac biomarkers.

NOTE: Severe hyperkalaemia can cause bradydysrhythmias, and may not respond to typical ACLS interventions. Maintain a high index of suspicion in patients with end-stage renal failure, severe metabolic acidosis, etc. Look for tall T waves (see Chapter 63, *Renal Emergencies*).

- All patients on **pacing** should be admitted to the **coronary care unit**.

BOX 1 Transcutaneous pacing (see Figures 8a to 8d)

- **Explain the procedure** to the patient.
- **Administer IV sedation** and **analgesia**, **preoxygenate** the patient.
- Apply **self-adhesive pacing pads** to the patient.
  1. Place one pad inferior to the right clavicle and the other over the apex
  or
  2. Place one pad anterior to the apex and the other behind the thorax, just medial to the scapula.
- Set the **pacing mode**.
  1. FIXED mode will deliver a fixed number of beats regardless of the patient's intrinsic heart rate.
  2. DEMAND mode (preferred) will only deliver beats when the patient's heart rate falls below the set rate.
- Set the **heart rate** to about 60–70 beats per minute (higher rates are unnecessary).
- Set starting **current output level** to the minimal setting.
  1. **Note** that in pacing, the setting is **current** (mA), not **energy** (J).
  2. The amount of energy delivered in each pacing impulse is less than 1/1000 of a defibrillation shock, and is safe for healthcare providers.
- Turn pacer ON.
  1. Note the presence of **pacing spikes** (Figure 8b) on the ECG monitor, indicating that pacing impulses are being delivered.
  2. Increase the current slowly. The usual range is 0 to 200 mA.

3. Watch for **electrical capture**; this is when pacing spikes are followed by a **broad QRS complex** with **T wave** (Figure 8c).

   a. If no T waves are associated with the broad QRS complex, that is likely to be an artifact and not a true cardiac depolarization.

4. Once electrical capture has occurred, check for **mechanical capture** by feeling for palpable pulses associated with the broad QRS complexes.

5. The minimum current at which capture occurs is the **threshold**. Set the **current output level** at about just above the threshold (approximately 10%) (Figure 8d).

- If **capture** has taken place, recheck the patient's vital signs, 12-lead ECG labs and arrange for transfer.

- If there is no capture, consider alternative placement of adhesive pads, consult the cardiologist for transvenous pacing and start second-line drugs.

FIGURE 8a   Unstable bradycardia

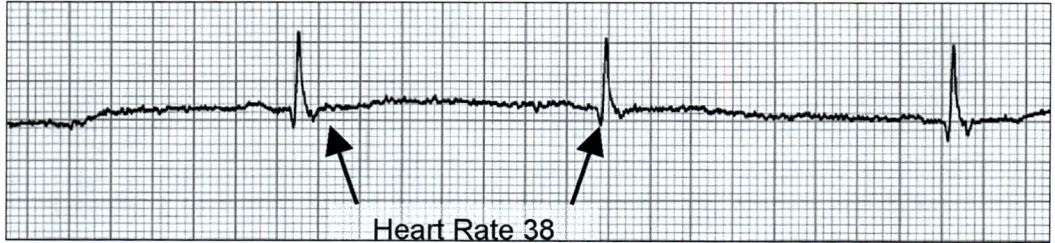

Heart Rate 38

FIGURE 8b   Pacing, no capture

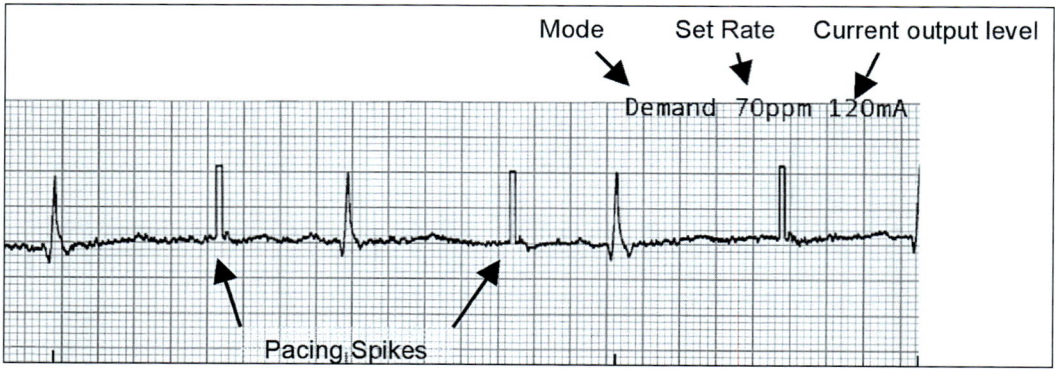

Mode   Set Rate   Current output level

Demand 70ppm 120mA

Pacing Spikes

FIGURE 8c **Capture threshold**

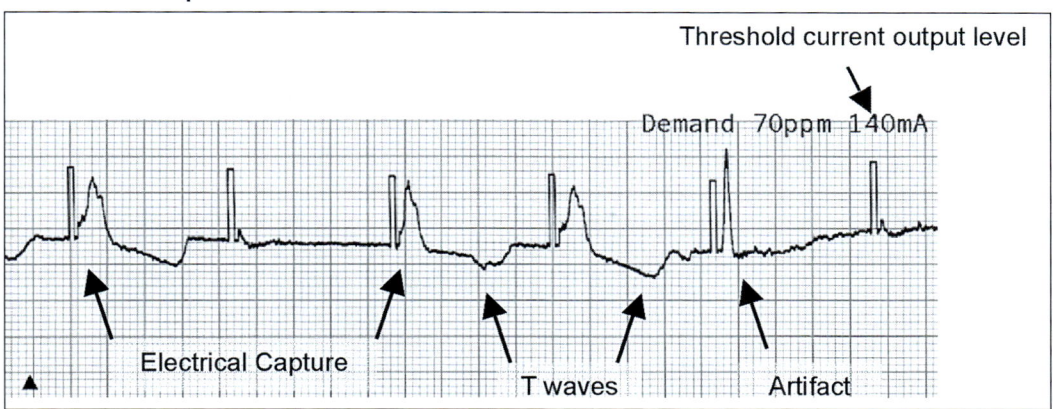

FIGURE 8d **Capture**

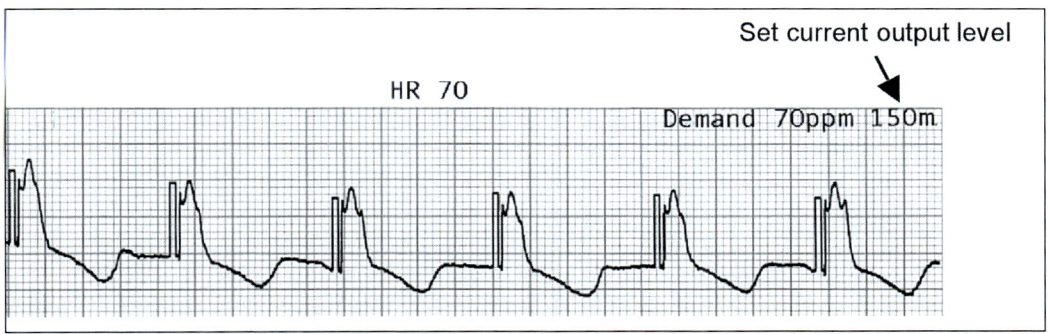

DISPOSITION

* Unstable patients should be admitted to the coronary care unit or high dependency ward.
* Patients who are stable but who may have potentially serious arrhythmias should be admitted to a ward with cardiac monitoring capabilities (see Table 1 for indications for telemetry admission).

TABLE 1   Indications for telemetry admission

Good evidence for cardiac monitoring

- Automatic implantable cardiac defibrillator fired
- AV block
- Prolonged QT with associated ventricular arrhythmias
- Acute heart failure/pulmonary oedema
- Admitted acute cerebrovascular disease
- Acute coronary syndrome
- Patients requiring massive blood transfusions

Cardiac monitoring may be beneficial

- Patients evaluated for syncope
- Patients with gastrointestinal haemorrhage after endoscopy
- Patients with atrial arrhythmias receiving therapy for rate control
- Patients with electrolyte imbalance
- Patients with subacute congestive heart failure

No evidence for telemetry

- Patients requiring blood transfusions
- Patients evaluated for chest pain
- Patients with exacerbations of chronic obstructive pulmonary disease
- Stable patients with pulmonary embolism receiving anti-coagulation

Adapted from Chen and Hollander (2007).

References/Further Reading

1. Chia BL. *Clinical Electrocardiography*. 3rd ed. Singapore: World Scientific; 1998: 115.

2. Anantharaman V, Gunasegaran K. Advanced Cardiac Life Support guidelines 2011. *Singapore Med J*. Aug 2011; 52(8): 548–555.

3. Deakin CD, Morrison LJ, Morley PT, et al. Advanced Life Support Chapter Collaborators. Part 8: Advanced life support. 2010 International Consensus on Cardiopulmonary Resuscitation and Emergency Cardiovascular Care Science with Treatment Recommendations. *Resuscitation*. Oct 2010; 81(Suppl 1): e93–e174.

4. Deakin CD, Nolan JP, Soar J, et al. European Resuscitation Council Guidelines for Resuscitation 2010. Section 4: Adult advanced life support. *Resuscitation*. Oct 2010; 81(10): 1305–1352.

5. Bessman ES. Emergency cardiac pacing. In: Roberts JR, Hedges JR, eds. *Clinical Procedures in Emergency Medicine*. 4th ed. Philadelphia, PA: WB Saunders; 2004.

6. Syverud SA, Dalsey WC, Hedges JR. Transcutaneous cardiac pacing. *Ann Emerg Med*. 1984; 13: 982.

7. Shaw DB, Gowers JI, Kekwick CA, et al. Is Mobitz type I atrioventricular block benign in adults? *Heart*. 2004; 90: 169–174.

8. Chen EH, Hollander JE. When do patients need admission to a telemetry bed? *J Emerg Med*. 2007; 33: 53–60

36   Coronary Syndromes, Acute

Kuan Win Sen • Shirley Ooi

DEFINITION

Acute coronary syndromes (ACS) include conditions that share the same pathophysiology of myocardial ischaemic states, i.e. unstable angina (**UA**), non-ST elevation myocardial infarction (**NSTEMI**) and ST-segment elevation myocardial infarction (**STEMI**).

Since an elevation of cardiac enzymes or troponin may not be detectable for hours after initial presentation, **UA** and **NSTEMI** are frequently indistinguishable at first evaluation. The differentiation can only be made over time where those with UA have no elevated cardiac biomarkers in circulation and have usually transient, if any, electrocardiogram (ECG) changes of ischaemia compared to those with NSTEMI who will have elevated biomarkers and/or ECG repolarization abnormalities. The management of UA and NSTEMI are somewhat similar. Unstable angina develops at rest or with minimal exertion and should be differentiated from *stable angina*.

STEMI occurs when there is complete occlusion of a coronary artery with transmural (full thickness) myocardial wall infarction. The ECG will show ST-segment elevations in the area of the heart fed by the affected blood vessel. The criteria for the diagnosis of STEMI (based on the 2007 Joint ESC/ACCF/AHA/WHF Task Force and modified by the 2009 Expert Panel of the AHA/ACC/HRS) are as follows:

- **Men 40 years of age and older**: J-point elevation of at least **2 mm** in leads **V2** and **V3** and at least **1 mm** in **all other leads**.
- **Men younger than 40 years**: J-point elevation of at least **2.5 mm** in leads **V2** and **V3**.
- **Women:** J-point elevation of at least **1.5 mm** in leads **V2** and **V3** and at least **1 mm** in **all other leads**.
- **Men and women**: J-point elevation of at least 0.5 mm in leads V3R and V4R (≥1 mm in males <30 years).
- **Men and women**: J-point elevation of at least 0.5 mm in leads V7 through V9.
- **Men and women**: J-point depression of at least 0.5 mm in V2 and V3 and at least 1 mm in **all other leads**.

NOTE: The J-point is the point marking the end of the QRS complex and the beginning of the following part that merges into the T-wave in an ECG.

CAVEATS

- Patients with UA usually present with one of the following patterns of symptoms:
  1. New onset (<2 months) of severe angina.
  2. Abrupt worsening of previous angina, with symptoms becoming more frequent, more severe, or more prolonged and less responsive to glyceryl trinitrate (GTN).
  3. Prolonged (>15 minutes) angina occurring at rest.

- About 2–4% of all cases of myocardial infarction (MI) are inappropriately discharged home. The majority of these cases involve young patients with unsuspected acute myocardial infarction (AMI) and elderly patients with atypical presentations (refer to Chapter 81, *Geriatric Emergencies*). Hence, AMI should be excluded in *older patients* as well as *diabetic* patients presenting with unexplained cardiac, respiratory, and neurologic symptoms.

- The criteria for diagnosis of AMI were revised in 2000 and again in 2007 by several international cardiovascular societies. The essentials for diagnosis include a *high level of suspicion*, *serial ECGs*, and *troponin* levels.

- Factors leading to the **missed diagnosis of MI** cited in successful litigation include the following:

  1. Failure to order study (ECG or serum marker).
  2. Failure to consider diagnosis.
  3. Inappropriate discharge from the emergency department.
  4. Incorrect interpretation of tests (ECG or serum marker).
  5. Over-reliance of negative studies (both ECG and a *single* negative serum marker).

- The following are characteristics of the **atypical AMI presentation**:

  1. Personality traits such as masculinity, calmness, independence, and low anxiety.
  2. Behaviour pattern (low rates of physician presentation for past medical issues, the stoic patient, and the patient in denial).
  3. Higher pain thresholds (both non-cardiac and cardiac pain issues).
  4. Major depression or psychosis.
  5. Demented patient or other factors reducing effective communication.
  6. Physician and patient misinterpretation of symptoms and signs resulting from AMI.
  7. Sensory, motor, and autonomic neuropathy.
  8. Impaired central nervous system recognition of the ischaemia.

- The following are **anginal equivalent complaints, syndromes, and presentations**:

  1. **Anginal equivalent complaints**: Dyspnoea, nausea/vomiting, diaphoresis, weakness/dizziness, cough, and syncope.
  2. **Anginal equivalent syndromes**: Delirium, confusion, and cerebrovascular accident.
  3. **Anginal equivalent presentations and findings**: Cardiac arrest, new onset arrhythmia, new onset congestive cardiac failure, unexplained bronchospasm, unexplained tachycardia, and peripheral oedema.

- The following are **risk management tips** for patients with possible MI:

  1. Age and gender (although women are at lower risk of MI than men) should not rule out the diagnosis of ischaemia or infarction.
  2. History of heart disease is a critical factor. For the patient with a known history of angina or MI who presents with a potentially new ischaemic event, risk factors have limited diagnostic significance since the presence of cardiovascular disease is a known fact.

3. The following are risk factors relevant in patients with chest pain: Family history, diabetes mellitus, hypertension, hyperlipidaemia, smoking, and a history of cocaine use.

4. Consider implementing a policy of old ECG retrieval as a normal departmental routine in any patient with a potential cardiac-related presentation.

5. Chest pain in the presence of a new left bundle branch block should be considered an AMI. All new left BBB with consistent chest pain should be considered for reperfusion therapy.

6. Resting chest pain in a patient with known heart disease should be considered an ominous finding.

- Diagnosis of **UA** is made on clinical grounds, based on the fact that there are no ECG changes or non-specific ECG changes present and that the patient is already free of chest pain.

- **NSTEMI** should be diagnosed in any patient whose cardiac enzymes are raised without evidence of ST elevation MI. An NSTEMI does not need to have ECG changes present.

The **ECG** may show the following:

1. ST-segment depression

2. Transient ST-segment elevation that resolves spontaneously or after glyceryl trinitrate treatment

3. T-wave inversion

4. Evidence of previous myocardial infarction

5. Left bundle branch block

6. Minor non-specific changes

The ECG can also be normal. It should **not** show persistent acute ST-segment elevation.

- **Cardiac enzymes** (CK-MB, troponin, and myoglobin) may be normal or elevated. Elevated **troponin T** or **I** concentration is highly specific for myocardial damage and identify patients at high risk for complications.

- The higher the troponin concentration the greater the risk of death within 30 days of presentation. Normal or previously undetectable troponin concentrations >12 hours after the onset of symptoms identify patients at low risk of early complication.

- Meta-analysis comparing troponin T and I indicates that the two markers are equally sensitive and specific, have similar prognostic significance and support their role in risk stratification.

- **TIMI** (Thrombolysis In Myocardial Infarction) investigators have developed a 7-variable risk stratification tool (TIMI risk score) that predicts the risk of death, reinfarction, or urgent revascularization at 14 days after presentation:

1. ≥65 years of age.

2. Presence of ≥3 cardiac risk factors.

3. ST-segment deviations of ≥0.5 mm on ECG at presentation.

4. ≥2 anginal events in the preceding 24 hours.

5. Increased cardiac biomarkers.

6. Aspirin use in the preceding seven days.

7. Prior coronary artery stenosis of 50% or more.

NOTE: TIMI score is intended to be used ONLY for patients in whom the decision has already been made to admit; TIMI is not intended to be used for undifferentiated chest pain patients and therefore even the lowest TIMI should never be used to decide to send a patient home.

- Patients are considered to be **high risk** if their TIMI risk score is ≥**5** and low risk if the score is ≤**2**. High risk patients have a greater benefit from early percutaneous intervention and use of glycoprotein IIb/IIIa inhibitor and low molecular weight heparin than lower risk patients.

- **Low risk categories**: A normal cardiac troponin at 12 hours after the onset of symptoms can identify a group of people at low risk of immediate cardiac events; furthermore, these patients who also have a normal ECG and normal cardiac enzymes (CK-MB) do not need admission to the coronary care or high dependency unit.

- **Treatment** aims consist of control of symptoms and prevention of MI and death. This can be achieved by instituting **anti-ischaemic** and **anti-thrombotic therapy** in the first instance, and if this is not successful, follow up with mechanical revascularization.

- It is important to manage **hypertension and heart failure** in the acute phase of ACS, as treatment can diminish wall stress and myocardial ischaemia and can help to stabilize the patient.

- **Thrombolytic treatment** has **not** been shown to be of benefit in patients with ACS without ECG ST-segment elevation (except for those with suspected acute MI and left bundle branch block).

⇨ **SPECIAL TIPS FOR GPs**
- Patients with AMI may present atypically clinically and from ECGs.
- Beware of the atypical presentation of AMI in the elderly, diabetic, and the young with risk factors.
- Refer all cases of acute coronary syndrome to the emergency department.
- Once AMI is diagnosed **do not** send the patient to the emergency department using his own transport! Call for the ambulance.
- Give **aspirin** 300 mg stat before sending the patient to hospital.

MANAGEMENT

The goals of management are as follows:

1. To confirm diagnosis by ECG and serum biomarker.
2. To estimate risk of death, reinfarction or urgent revascularization (using e.g. the TIMI risk score).
3. To relieve ischaemic pain.
4. To correct the abnormal haemodynamic state.
5. To reduce myocardial oxygen consumption.
6. To initiate anti-platelets, anti-coagulants and reperfusion therapy if required.

- Monitor the patient's vital signs in the critical care area.
- Give oxygen via mask.
- Start dual anti-platelet therapy with aspirin and either ticagrelor or clopidogrel.
- Treat with **aspirin 300 mg** orally.

NOTE: Aspirin achieves platelet inhibition within an hour. Avoid enteric-coated aspirin because its onset of action is delayed for 3 to 4 hours. Aspirin reduces the risk of cardiac death and non-fatal myocardial infarction by about 50% at 3 months.

- For **high risk** patients with non-ST elevation ACS with dynamic ST changes or positive cardiac markers, give oral **ticagrelor** 180 mg (See Figure 1) and admit for early cardiac catheterisation.
- For **low risk** non-ST elevation ACS with no dynamic ST or negative markers, give oral **clopidogrel** (Plavix®) 600 mg (See Figure 1).

FIGURE 1 NUH ACS algorithm

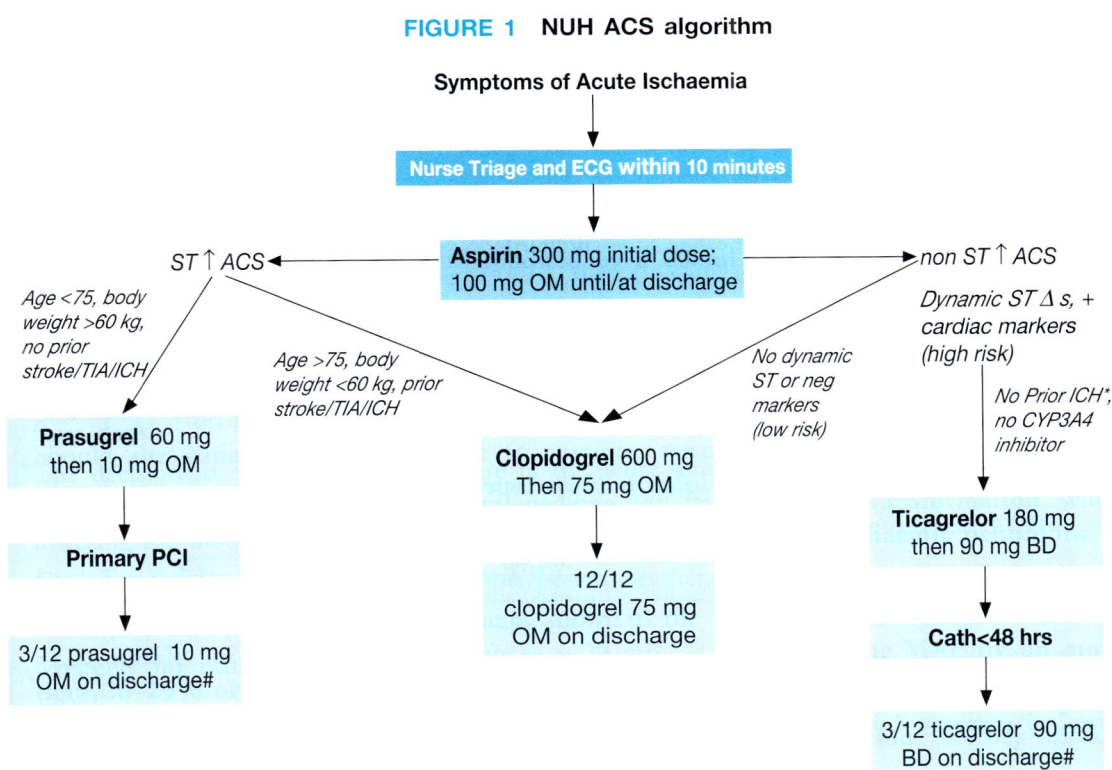

* ICH = intracranial haemorrhage; please consult cardiology registrar on-call re antiplatelet therapy
\# remaining 9/12 prescription will be as outpatient. Follow-up within 3/12 of discharge

- Conduct **IV plug** and **blood tests**, i.e. full blood count, urea/electrolytes/creatinine, cardiac enzymes, cardiac troponin T or I, coagulation profile, type and screen for packed cells.
- Give sublingual **glyceryl trinitrate (GTN)** in patients with ischaemic type chest pain. If a patient has persistent pain after two sublingual GTNs, proceed with IV GTN 20–200 µg/min at 5- to 10-minute intervals until the chest pain resolves or mean arterial pressure decreases by 10%. Discontinue if hypotensive.

NOTE: IV GTN is especially useful in patients with ACS and hypertension/heart failure. There is no evidence that administration by IV infusion is more efficacious than equipotent doses of long-acting nitrates given by other routes, but titration of dose may be quicker and easier to manage with IV administration. GTN is **contraindicated** in right ventricular infarction and patients with a history of phosphodiesterase inhibitor intake for erectile dysfunction in the prior 24 hours.

- Give IV **morphine** in titratable doses for pain relief if chest pain and anxiety persist despite IV GTN.
- Give **beta blockers** to reduce the risk of infarction if there are no contraindications, e.g. heart failure, respiratory failure, more than or equal to second-degree heart block, and hypotension (systolic blood pressure <90 mmHg).

  Cardioselective intravenous atenolol/metoprolol is useful in patients with severe hypertension. Otherwise, oral beta blockers can be started later if a patient is haemodynamically compromised with gradual titration upwards once more stable.

NOTE: IV beta blockers should ONLY be used in the setting of severe hypertension, but in others IV beta blockers are considered harmful. In fact in the new guidelines, beta blockers should really be given only orally, and there is no risk; they can be given orally at some point within the first 24 hours, and avoided entirely if there is a contraindication.

- **Heparin**, when used intravenously, reduces the incidence of recurrent ischaemia and progression to Q-wave MI.

  Use of IV heparin requires careful monitoring of the level of anti-coagulation. Heparin is associated with a rebound in unstable angina when discontinued which can be blunted with the use of aspirin.

  The use of low molecular weight heparins has advantages of a lower incidence of heparin-induced thrombocytopaenia (HIT), ease of administration without a need for monitoring, a more predictable action due to their almost complete bioavailability and lower degree of platelet aggregation.

NOTE: The following have been shown to reduce the risk of complications in patients with unstable angina and non-STEMI:

1. Unfractionated heparin without aspirin is more effective than placebo.
2. Unfractionated heparin combined with aspirin may be more effective than aspirin alone.
3. Low molecular weight heparin combined with aspirin is more effective than aspirin alone.

- High risk cases should be treated with an **intravenous small molecule platelet glycoprotein IIb/IIIa inhibitor** for up to 96 hours. It should also be given to those with elevated troponin T who are scheduled to undergo percutaneous coronary intervention using unfractionated heparin. This should commence before intervention. Examples include eptifibatide and tirofiban. Abciximab has not been shown to be beneficial in patients with NSTEMI in the GUSTO IV trial.

- **Detection and correction of an obvious precipitating factor**, e.g. anaemia, fever, thyrotoxicosis, hypoxia, tachydysrhythmias, aortic stenosis, or sympathomimetic drugs, avoids potential complications.

- Do a chest X-ray to exclude other causes of chest pain and to look for complications of ACS.

Specific management for STEMI

- Consider **reperfusion therapy (method of choice for STEMI)**, i.e. percutaneous coronary intervention (PCI) versus thrombolysis. PCI is the **preferred** strategy when available as multiple randomized controlled trials have shown enhanced survival compared to fibrinolysis with a lower rate of intracranial haemorrhage and recurrent MI.

Table 1 **Advantages and disadvantages of thrombolysis versus PCI**

	Thrombolysis	Percutaneous coronary intervention
Advantages	• Rapid administration • Widely available • Convenient	• Better clinical efficacy, i.e. superior vessel patency, TIMI grade 3 flow rates and reduced occlusion rates • Less haemorrhage • Early definition of coronary anatomy allows tailored therapy and more efficient risk stratification
Disadvantages	• Patency ceiling, i.e. infarct-related artery is restored in only 60–85% of patients, with a normal TIMI grade 3 epicardial coronary flow in only 45–60% of patients • Less clinical efficacy, i.e. optimal reperfusion is not achieved in more than 50% of patients, and re-occlusion of infarct vessel occurs in 5–15% of patients at week 1 and 20–30% within 3 months • Risk of haemorrhage	• Delay limits efficacy • Less widely available • Requires expertise

Consider whether the patient is a candidate for **thrombolytic therapy** by reviewing the criteria for thrombolysis, which are as follows:

1. Typical chest pain of AMI.
2. ST-segment elevation fulfilling the criteria stated in *Definition* above.
3. Chest pain <12 hours from onset.
4. Patients <75 years of age.

If patients satisfy the criteria for consideration of **thrombolysis**, review the following list of **contraindications**:

- **Absolute**
  1. History of intracranial haemorrhage.
  2. History of ischaemic stroke in the past 3 months (except acute ischaemic stroke within 3 hours).
  3. Presence of cerebral vascular malformation or intracranial malignancy.
  4. Suspected aortic dissection.
  5. Bleeding diathesis or active bleeding (except menses).
  6. Significant head trauma or facial trauma in the past 3 months.

- **Relative**
  1. Severe hypertension (blood pressure >180/110 mmHg).
  2. History of ischaemic stroke >3 months.
  3. The presence of dementia.
  4. Known intracranial disease that is not an absolute contraindication.
  5. Traumatic or prolonged cardiopulmonary resuscitation (CPR) that lasted more than 10 minutes.
  6. Major surgery within 3 weeks.
  7. The presence of active peptic ulcer.
  8. Internal bleeding within the last 2 to 4 weeks.
  9. Non-compressible vascular punctures.
  10. Pregnancy.
  11. On warfarin therapy.
  12. For streptokinase, prior exposure (more than 5 days ago) or history of allergic reaction.

If the answer to **any** of the above is 'yes', **do not** administer thrombolytics. Discuss the case with the cardiologist-on-call first.

If there are no contraindications, consider the **choice of thrombolytics**, i.e. streptokinase (SK) versus recombinant tissue plasminogen activator (rtPA):

SK	rtPA
1. The most commonly used and cost-effective choice.	1. Can be used in either gender.
2. The better choice when the risk for intracranial haemorrhage is the highest (e.g. in the elderly) because the use of rtPA results in increased likelihood of intracranial haemorrhage.	2. Patients are <50 years of age.
	3. Patients have an anterior AMI.
	4. Chest pain of <12 hours.

Obtain consent (verbal or written) from patients and their relatives. Inform them of the benefits, risks, and alternatives of thrombolytic therapy.

- The risk of intracranial bleeding (1%) is higher in the following situations:
  1. The patient is >65 years of age.
  2. The patient has a body weight of <70 kg.
  3. The patient has hypertension on presentation.
  4. The drug rtPA is used (compared to SK).

- **SK allergy** occurs in approximately 5% of patients treated for the first time, especially those with a recent streptococcus infection. About 0.2% of patients experience a serious anaphylactic reaction.

- **Hypotension** occurs during IV SK infusion (15%), but this type of low blood pressure responds to decreasing the rate of infusion and volume expansion.

Dosage of thrombolytic therapy

SK	rtPA
1. IV SK 1.5 mega units in 100 ml normal saline over 1 hour.	1. 100 mg rtPA is dissolved in 100 ml sterile water.
	2. Administer 15 mg IV bolus.
	3. Administer IV infusion of 0.75 mg/kg over 30 minutes (not to exceed 50 mg).
	4. Followed by IV infusion of 0.5 mg/kg over 60 minutes (not to exceed 35 mg).

- If the patient is in **shock**, always look for precipitating causes:
  1. Do a gentle rectal examination to look for **gastrointestinal bleeding**.
  2. Is the patient **bradycardic**? Treat according to ACLS guidelines.
  3. Is the patient **tachycardic**? Treat according to ACLS guidelines.
  4. Is the patient having a **right ventricular infarct**?
     a. Do right-sided leads in the presence of ST elevation in II and III and aVF as in inferior AMI (Figure 1a). Look for at least 1 mm ST elevation in V4R, V5R, and V6R (Figure 1b).
     b. If so, give fluid challenge of 100–200 ml normal saline over 5 to 10 minutes and assess response.
     c. This can be repeated if the patient does not become breathless and there are no clinical signs of pulmonary oedema.
     d. Start inotropes (IV dobutamine/dopamine 5–20 μg/kg/min) if the blood pressure remains low despite IV fluid administration of 500 ml.

FIGURE 1a   **Inferoposterior STEMI**

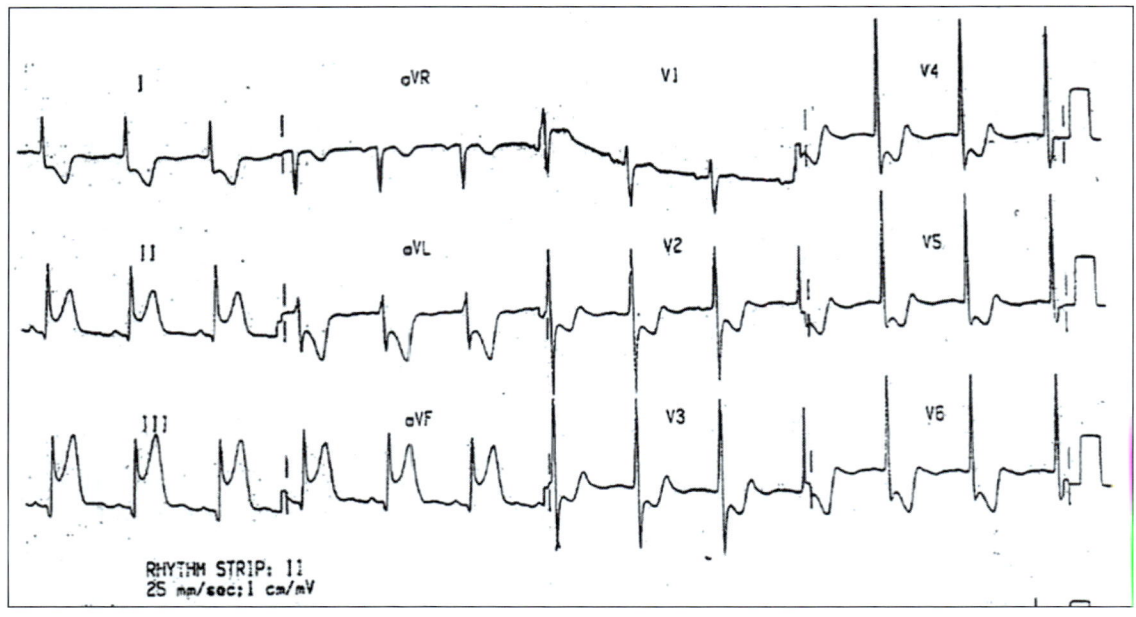

ECG shows ST elevation in the inferior leads (II, III and aVF) with reciprocal ST depression in I and aVL. ST depression in V2 and V4 indicate presence of posterior infarction.

FIGURE 1b   **Inferoposterior and right ventricular STEMI**

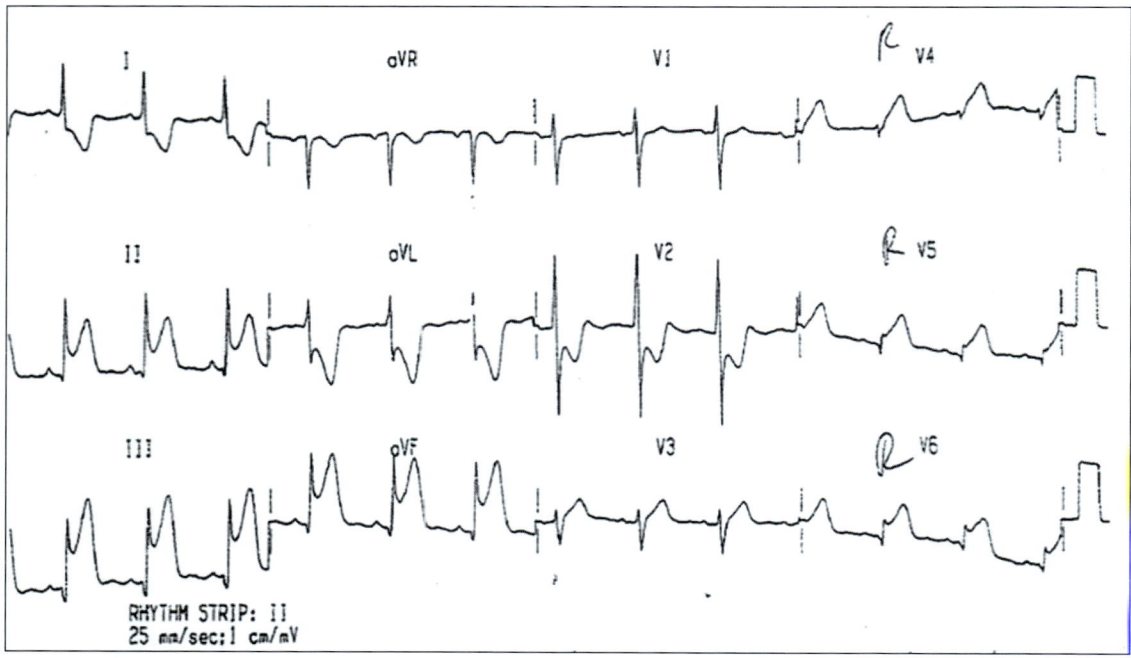

Right ventricular infarction is seen as ST elevation in the right-sided leads in V4R, V5R and V6R.

5. Is the patient in **cardiogenic shock** because of **mechanical complications**, e.g. papillary muscle dysfunction or rupture, septal rupture or cardiac tamponade from free wall rupture?

    a. Call the cardiologist and cardiothoracic surgeon.

    b. Meanwhile, start inotropic support, e.g. IV dobutamine/dopamine 5–20 μg/kg/min.

- Catheterize the patient to measure the urine output.
- Admit to coronary care unit.

References/Further Reading

1. Gibler WB, Cannon CP, Blomkalns AL, et al. Practical implementation of the guidelines for unstable angina/non-ST-segment elevation myocardial infarction in the emergency department. *Ann Emerg Med*. 2005; 46: 185.

2. ACC/AHA 2007 guidelines for the management of patients with unstable angina/non-ST-elevation myocardial infarction: A report of the American College of Cardiology/American Heart Association Task Force on Practice Guidelines (Writing Committee to Revise the 2002 Guidelines for the Management of Patients with Unstable Angina/Non-ST-Elevation Myocardial Infarction) developed in collaboration with the American College of Emergency Physicians, the Society for Cardiovascular Angiography and Interventions, and the Society of Thoracic Surgeons endorsed by the American Association of Cardiovascular and Pulmonary Rehabilitation and the Society for Academic Emergency Medicine. *J Am Coll Cardiol*. Aug 2007: 14: 50(7): e1-e157. [Erratum in: *J Am Coll Cardiol*. Mar 2008: 4; 51(9): 974.]

3. Grech ED, Ramsdale DR. Acute coronary syndrome: Unstable angina and non-ST segment elevation myocardial infarction. *BMJ*. 7 June 2003; 326(7401): 1259–1261.

4. Pope JH, Selker HP. Acute coronary syndromes in the emergency department: Diagnostic characteristics, tests, and challenges. *Cardiol Clin*. Nov 2005; 23(4): 423–451.

5. Wagner GS, Macfarlane P, Wellens H, et al. AHA/ACCF/HRS recommendations for the standardization and interpretation of the electrocardiogram. Part VI: Acute ischemia/infarction: A scientific statement from the American Heart Association Electrocardiography and Arrhythmias Committee, Council on Clinical Cardiology; the American College of Cardiology Foundation; and the Heart Rhythm Society. Endorsed by the International Society for Computerized Electrocardiology. *J Am Coll Cardiol*. 2009; 53: 1003.

6. Thygesen K, Alpert JS, White HD; Joint ESC/ACCF/AHA/WHF Task Force for the Redefinition of Myocardial Infarction. Universal definition of myocardial infarction. *J Am Coll Cardiol*. 27 Nov 2007; 50(22): 2173–2195.

7. Bates ER. Fibrinolytic reperfusion. *Reperfusion Therapy for Acute Myocardial Infarction*. *Informa Healthcare*. 2008: 42–58.

37 Other Heart Conditions
(Pericarditis, Myocarditis, Infective Endocarditis, and Cardiomyopathy)
Ong Pei Yuin

⇨ **SPECIAL TIPS FOR GPs**

- The diagnosis of **myocarditis** requires a **high index of suspicion** due to its non-specific and variable presentation. Symptoms of fever, vomiting, or respiratory distress are often mistakenly diagnosed as gastritis or a viral illness. Acute myocarditis should be suspected whenever a patient, especially a young male, presents with otherwise unexplained, new onset cardiac abnormalities such as heart failure, myocardial infarction, cardiac dysrhythmias (including unexplained sinus tachycardia), or conduction disturbances. A history of recent upper respiratory infection or enteritis may also be elicited in a majority of cases of viral myocarditis.

- Always consider a **cardiac aetiology** for **sudden unexplained syncope**, even in a young, fit person. Ask about previous episodes of syncope, palpitations, family history of sudden death, and perform an electrocardiogram (ECG) for all presentations of syncope.

- Signs of **intravenous drug abuse** include needle track marks on antecubital and femoral veins and a cachexic appearance. In such patients with unexplained high fever, consider **infective endocarditis** as a source.

PERICARDITIS

- Pericarditis: An inflammation, infection, or infiltration of the pericardial sac, with or without pericardial effusion. Acute pericarditis is rapid in onset and may lead to cardiac tamponade. Chronic constrictive pericarditis results from chronic inflammation leading to thickening of the pericardium.

- **Multiple aetiologies** can result in pericarditis:

  1. Infective: Viral (e.g. adenovirus, varicella, and cytomegalovirus), bacterial (e.g. staphylococcus, streptococcus, haemophilus, and tuberculosis), fungal, and protozoa.

  2. Neoplastic infiltration (especially lung, breast, lymphoma, and leukaemia malignancies).

  3. Uraemia.

  4. Myxoedema.

  5. Pancreatitis.

  6. Amyloidosis.

  7. Postmyocardial infarction (Dressler's syndrome).

  8. Autoimmune disorders such as systemic lupus erythematosus, rheumatoid arthritis, and scleroderma.

  9. Post-irradiation.

Symptoms and signs/diagnostic considerations

- **Symptoms** include these:
  1. Chest pain that is commonly sharp, pleuritic, fairly sudden in onset. May be relieved by sitting up and leaning forward.
  2. Fever.
  3. Dyspnoea and cough.
  4. Nausea and anorexia.
- **Signs** include the following:
  1. Tachypnoea and tachycardia.
  2. Pericardial friction rub best heard along the lower left sternal edge.
  3. Signs of cardiac tamponade that include muffled heart sounds, distended neck veins, and hypotension (**Beck's triad** – an uncommon finding). One is more likely to encounter two out of the three features.
  4. Signs of biventricular heart failure in constrictive pericarditis including lung crepitations, jugular venous pressure elevation, peripheral oedema, hepatomegaly, and ascites.

Investigations

- **Lab tests**:
  1. Full blood count shows an increase in the number of white blood cells.
  2. Erythrocyte sedimentation rate and C-reactive protein are elevated.
  3. Cardiac enzyme levels are raised.
- The **ECG** in pericarditis evolves through four stages:
  1. Stage 1 (hours to days): Diffuse ST elevation with reciprocal ST depression in leads aVR and V1. There is also an elevation of the PR segment in lead aVR and depression of the PR segment in other limb leads (see Figure 1).

  NOTE: ST elevation is maximum in lead II in pericarditis in contrast to lead III in inferior myocardial infarction. T-waves in pericarditis are not tall.

  2. Stage 2: Normalization of the ST and PR segments.
  3. Stage 3: Development of diffuse T-wave inversions.
  4. Stage 4: Normalization of ECG or persistence of T-wave inversions.
- The chest X-ray may be normal or show cardiomegaly.
- Echocardiography is used to detect pericardial effusion.
- Thoracic computed tomography can delineate the extent of the pericardium thickening and pericardial fluid.

FIGURE 1   An ECG showing pericarditis

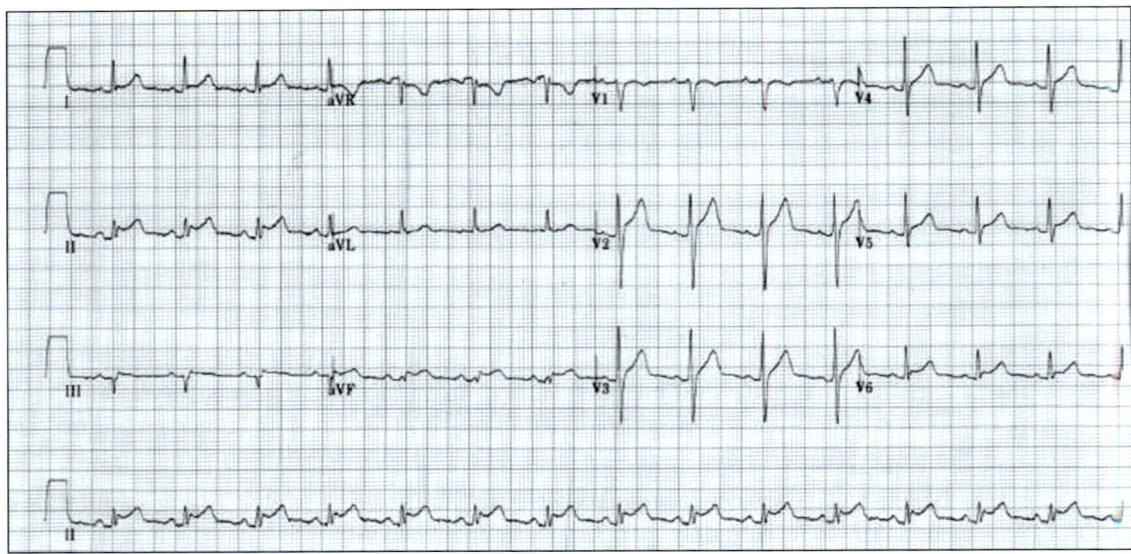

Note widespread ST elevation which does not follow an anatomic distribution with PR depression in the same leads; ST depression and PR elevation in aVR. Note also ST elevation is maximal in lead II rather than lead III.

Management

- Airway, breathing and circulation (ABCs), supplemental oxygen, cardiac monitoring, pulse oximetry, and intravenous access.
- Full blood count, urea/creatinine, troponin, and creatine kinase, erythrocyte sedimentation rate, PT/PTT, and GXM.
- Refer to the cardiologist for echocardiography. This should be arranged urgently if tamponade is suspected.
- Perform ultrasound-guided pericardiocentesis if there are any signs of haemodynamic compromise.
- **Drugs**:
    1. **Non-steroidal anti-inflammatory drugs** (NSAIDS): Ibuprofen 400–800 mg orally q6 to 8 hours is preferred due to rare side effects and good impact on coronary blood flow. Alternatively, aspirin 800 mg q6 to 8 hours for a week, followed by gradual tapering, can be given, and this is preferred if the pericarditis is associated with an acute myocardial infarction.
    2. **Colchicine**: 0.5–1 mg/day in addition to NSAIDS is efficacious in preventing the recurrence of viral and idiopathic pericarditis.
    3. **Glucocorticoids**: For example, prednisolone 1 mg/kg/day should be considered only for patients refractory to NSAIDS and colchicines, and should only be used for acute pericarditis due to connective tissue disease, immune-mediated pericarditis or uraemic pericarditis.
- Specific treatment is dependent on the underlying aetiology (e.g. anti-tuberculous medications).

Disposition

- Admit to a general ward or intensive care unit depending on the severity of the patient's clinical condition.

MYOCARDITIS

- Myocarditis: An inflammation of the heart that is characterised by myocyte necrosis, often resulting in cardiac dysfunction and heart failure. Half of patients will report an antecedent viral illness.
- **Aetiologies**:
  1. **Infective**: Viral (e.g. adenovirus, varicella-zoster virus, influenza, and enterovirus), bacterial (e.g. tuberculosis, diphtheria, and group A streptococcus), protozoa (e.g. leishmaniasis, malaria and toxoplasmosis), spirochetes (e.g. syphilis) and fungal.
  2. **Drugs** (e.g. ampicillin, acetaminophen, penicillin, hydrochlorothiazide, chemotherapy agents, etc.).
  3. **Autoimmune** disorders such as systemic lupus erythematosus, Kawasaki disease, Wegener's granulomatosis, sarcoidosis, and giant cell arteritis.
  4. **Environmental toxins** from scorpion and snake bites.
  5. Myocarditis can also occur as a complication of **other cardiomyopathies** such as cardiac amyloidosis, hypertrophic cardiomyopathy, and arrhythmogenic right ventricular cardiomyopathy.

Symptoms and signs

- The clinical presentation of myocarditis is variable, depending on the location of the inflammation and the severity of the disease. Myocardial inflammation may be focal or diffuse, and may involve any of the cardiac chambers. Subtle cardiac symptoms are often overshadowed by the more prominent viremic symptoms of fever and myalgia.
- **Symptoms** are often non-specific and they include the following:
  1. Fever.
  2. Malaise and fatigue.
  3. Chest pain that is commonly pleuritic, sharp, often associated with pericarditis.
  4. Dyspnoea on exertion, reduced exercise tolerance.
  5. Palpitations.
  6. Syncope (a risk factor for sudden death).
- **Signs** include these:
  1. Fever and tachypnoea.
  2. Unexplained tachycardia disproportionate to fever.
  3. Cyanosis.
  4. Pericardial rub may be heard.

5. Signs of heart failure including lung crepitations, jugular venous pressure elevation, peripheral oedema, **hepatomegaly**, and ascites.

6. Patients with rapidly evolving myocarditis can present with cardiogenic shock or sudden cardiac death due to acute pump failure or ventricular fibrillation.

Investigations

- **Lab tests:**
    1. Full blood count (elevated white blood cell counts in 25% of patients).
    2. Erythrocyte sedimentation rate (elevated in 60% of patients).
    3. Cardiac enzymes are elevated in only a minority of patients. Normal cardiac enzymes do not exclude myocarditis.
- The **ECG** may be normal or abnormal in myocarditis. Abnormalities are usually non-specific unless there is associated pericarditis. Sinus tachycardia is the most frequent finding. There may be transient, non-specific ST- and T-wave changes, dysrhythmias, and heart blocks. ECG findings may mimic acute myocardial infarction.
- The **chest X-ray** may be normal or show cardiomegaly or features of heart failure.
- **Echocardiography** may show impaired left ventricular function, segmental wall motion abnormalities, decreased ejection fraction, pericardial effusion, and ventricular thrombus (in 15% of patients).
- Cardiovascular **magnetic resonance imaging** can detect myocardial oedema and myocyte injury.
- Endomyocardial biopsy and **polymerase chain reaction** identification of **viral infection** from **pericardial** or other **body fluids** can help to confirm the specific aetiology of the myocarditis.

Management

- ABCs, supplemental oxygen, cardiac monitoring, pulse oximetry, and intravenous access.
- Full blood count, urea/creatinine, troponin, and creatine kinase, erythrocyte sedimentation rate, PT/PTT, and GXM.
- Manage patients as for acute heart failure.
- Treat dysrhythmias if present.
- High-grade heart blocks may require cardiac pacing.
- Refer to the cardiologist for urgent echocardiography.
- **Medications**:
    1. Angiotensin-converting enzyme (ACE) inhibitors: **Captopril** 6.25 mg orally (PO) 3 times a day (tds), titrate to a maximum of 50 mg tds.
    2. **Digoxin** 0.125–0.375 mg PO/day.
    3. **Frusemide** PO or IV 20–80 mg two times a day (bd) to tds; titrate for fluid overload.

4. Intravenous **immunoglobulin** (IVIG) 2g/kg IV may be of benefit in viral aetiologies.

5. **Immuno-suppressive therapy** is of unproven medical benefit.

- Avoid NSAIDS, sympathomimetics, and beta blocker drugs as they increase myocardial necrosis.

Disposition

- Admit the patient to a monitored area (telemetry or high dependency bed) as appropriate to his clinical condition.

INFECTIVE ENDOCARDITIS

- A microbial infection of the endothelial surface of the heart, characterized by vegetations.
- **Risk factors** include structural heart disease (especially mitral and aortic regurgitation), IV drug abusers (IVDAs), prosthetic heart valves, congenital heart disease, long-term indwelling catheters, and poor dental hygiene.
- **Organisms**:
  1. Bacterial agents: *Streptococcus viridans*, *Staphyloccus aureus* (especially IVDAs), β-haemolytic streptococci, enterococci, haemophilus, and Gram-negative bacteria.
  2. Candida and aspergillus (found in particular in IVDAs, patients with prosthetic valves, and immuno-compromised patients).
  3. Non-bacterial thrombotic endocarditis: Malignancy, uraemia, burns, and systemic lupus erythematosus.
- **Symptoms** and **signs** include these:
  1. Fever, the most common symptom, usually moderate, remitting.
  2. Fatigue, chills, diaphoresis, nausea, night sweats, arthralgias, myalgias, and weight loss.
  3. Cardiac signs such as new or changing murmurs (especially mitral and aortic regurgitation) in 80% of patients, unexplained heart failure and pericarditis (secondary to local invasion).
  4. Splenomegaly (up to 50% of patients).
  5. Anaemia.
  6. Cutaneous signs: **Splinter haemorrhages**, **Osler's nodes** (painful indurations on the palms and soles), **Janeway lesions** (non-tender erythematous macules on the palms and soles), **Roth spots** (red retinal haemorrhages), '**blue-toe syndrome**' (tender cyanotic digits or toes), and clubbing.
  7. Chronic subacute bacterial endocarditis can present as a chronic wasting disease, similar to human immunodeficiency virus (HIV) or malignancies.

A patient has to satisfy the Duke criteria on presentation to establish a diagnosis of infective endocarditis. Established in 1994, the Duke criteria are a collection of major and minor diagnostic parameters. The following conditions must be fulfilled to establish a definite diagnosis: Two major or one major + three minor or five minor criteria, without a clear alternative diagnosis.

- **Major criteria**:
  1. Positive blood cultures (≥2) with typical infective endocarditis microbes.
  2. New murmur or positive echocardiogram for cardiac oscillating mass, abscess or prosthetic valve dehiscence.
- **Minor criteria**:
  1. Predisposing cardiac condition or intravenous drug use.
  2. Fever of ≥38.0°C.
  3. Vascular phenomena.
  4. Immunologic phenomena.
  5. Echocardiogram consistent with endocarditis but not meeting major criteria.
  6. Positive blood culture, but not meeting major criteria, or positive serology or molecular test for compatible microbe.

Complications of infective endocarditis

- Cardiac: Heart failure, valve abscess, pericarditis, and fistula formation.
- Neurologic: Embolic stroke, brain abscess, and brain haemorrhage.
- **Embolization**: Septic pulmonary emboli, especially tricuspid valve infections in IVDAs, appear as fluffy infiltrates on chest X-rays and present with fever, and dyspnoea. Emboli to limbs and other organs cause ischaemic extremities and organ failures.
- Renal failure from infarction, nephritis, and abscess formation.
- Mycotic aneurysms.
- Metastatic abscesses.

Prognosis

Overall mortality for infective endocarditis is 20–25%. Aggressive organisms such as *Staphylococcus aureus* are more lethal than *Streptococcus viridans*. Increased duration of infection, embolic phenomena causing major organ damage and more extensive heart valve damage with increasing likelihood of heart failure and heart surgery, also increase mortality.

Investigations

- **Lab tests**:
  1. Full blood count shows haemolytic anaemia and leucocytosis.
  2. Blood cultures.
  3. Erythrocyte sedimentation rate and C-reactive protein are elevated.
  4. Urinalysis may show microscopic haematuria.
- The **ECG** may show tachycardia, dysrhythmias, or heart blocks.

- The **chest X-ray** may show features of heart failure or septic pulmonary emboli (fluffy infiltrates) in right-sided endocarditis.
- **Echocardiography** detects acute valvular lesions, abscesses, and vegetations.

Management

- ABCs, supplemental oxygen, cardiac monitoring, pulse oximetry, and intravenous access.
- Send blood for full blood count, urea and electrolytes, troponin and creatine kinase, erythrocyte sedimentation rate, C-reactive protein, PT/PTT, and GXM.
- Take at least 2 sets of blood cultures from different sites.
- **IV antibiotic therapy**:
  1. Native valve or congenital abnormality: IV penicillin G 4 MU + IV cloxacillin 2 g + IV gentamicin 1 mg/kg (if allergic to penicillin, give IV vancomycin 15 mg/kg in place of penicillin and cloxacillin).
  2. Prosthetic valve or IVDA: IV vancomycin 15mg/kg + IV gentamicin 1 mg/kg + PO rifampicin 600 mg.
- Refer to the cardiologist for urgent echocardiography.

Disposition

- Admit unstable patients to the cardiac intensive care unit. Stable patients require at least a monitored bed.

CARDIOMYOPATHY

- Cardiomyopathies are a heterogeneous group of diseases of the myocardium associated with mechanical and/or electrical dysfunction of the heart.
- They are classified into the following types, each of which has multiple different causes: Dilated cardiomyopathy, hypertrophic obstructive cardiomyopathy (HOCM), restrictive cardiomyopathy, dysrhythmogenic right ventricular cardiomyopathy (DRVC), and others due to specific systemic diseases, e.g. alcoholic cardiomyopathy or peripartum cardiomyopathy (or those that do not have a specific identifiable cause).
- Genetic causes account for 20–30% of cases.
- Cardiomyopathies can be divided into those with systolic dysfunction and diastolic dysfunction.
  1. **Systolic dysfunction** is characterized by a decrease in myocardial contractility. Left ventricular enlargement occurs in order to maintain cardiac output. However, eventually compensatory mechanisms are overwhelmed and cardiac output decreases. This is characteristic of dilated cardiomyopathy.
  2. **Diastolic dysfunction** is characterized by abnormal left ventricular relaxation and filling and results in elevated filling pressures. This is characteristic of hypertrophic and restrictive cardiomyopathy, and sometimes also seen in dilated cardiomyopathy.

- **Causes** of cardiomyopathies include the following:
  1. **Dilated cardiomyopathies**: There are multiple causes such as ischaemia, valvular causes, viral infections, and genetic abnormalities.
  2. **HOCM:** The majority of HOCM cases are caused by mutations in the sarcomeric contractile protein genes (autosomal dominant), others by genetic causes, e.g. Noonan syndrome, metabolic diseases, mitochondrial diseases, and recessive glycolipid storage diseases.
  3. **Restrictive cardiomyopathies** are secondary to infiltrative diseases, e.g. amyloidosis, sarcoidosis, storage diseases, or endomyocardial diseases (e.g. secondary to radiation, chemotherapy, or toxic agents).
  4. **DRVC** is associated with genetic cellular mutations leading to replacement of the right ventricle with fibrous or fatty tissue.

Symptoms and signs/diagnostic considerations

- History of an antecedent viral illness, HIV, chemotherapy or underlying systemic condition (e.g. sarcoidosis), pregnancy, and depositional disorders (haemochromatosis).
- Family history of sudden death.
- Episodes of syncope or dyspnoea.
- **Symptoms and signs**:
  1. **Dilated cardiomyopathy** causes fatigue, dyspnoea, orthopnoea, and chest pain. Clinical signs of heart failure may be present: S4 gallop, jugular venous pressure elevation, and liver enlargement.
  2. **HOCM** causes exertional syncope or near-syncope, dyspnoea, and heart failure. Arrhythmias include paroxysmal atrial fibrillation, supraventricular tachycardia, non-sustained ventricular tachycardia, and ventricular fibrillation which can lead to sudden death. Examination may be normal or show features of outflow tract obstruction: Mid-systolic murmur at the left sternal edge radiating to the aortic and mitral areas. Mitral regurgitation murmur may also be present.
  3. **Restrictive cardiomyopathies** cause decreased effort tolerance, fatigue, and dyspnoea. Examination findings include mitral regurgitation murmurs and jugular venous pressure (JVP) elevation with Kussmaul sign (rise in JVP with inspiration), ascites, and peripheral oedema.
  4. **DRVC** causes giddiness, syncopal/near-syncopal episodes, palpitations, dysrhythmias, heart failure, and sudden death.

Investigations

- **Lab tests**: Full blood count, renal panel, and cardiac enzymes.
- **Chest X-ray**:
  1. **Dilated cardiomyopathy**: Cardiomegaly, pulmonary congestion, and pleural effusions.
  2. **HOCM**: May be normal or show a bulge along the left heart border due to left ventricular hypertrophy (LVH).
  3. **Restrictive cardiomyopathy**: Normal cardiac silhouette with pulmonary congestion.

- **ECG**:
    1. **Dilated cardiomyopathy**: Atrial fibrillation, heart blocks and conduction abnormalities, and Q waves may be seen in anterior and inferior leads.
    2. **HOCM**: Normal in 15% of patients. Abnormal ECGs show ST and T abnormalities, LVH with strain, QRS complexes tallest in mid-chest leads, and deep Q waves in inferio-lateral leads. (See Figure 2)
    3. Various dysrhythmias such as new onset AF and VT may also be seen.

- **Echocardiography** shows depressed ejection fraction and excludes pericardial tamponade. Systolic outflow obstructions and abnormal diastolic filling are also seen.

FIGURE 2   ECG showing HOCM

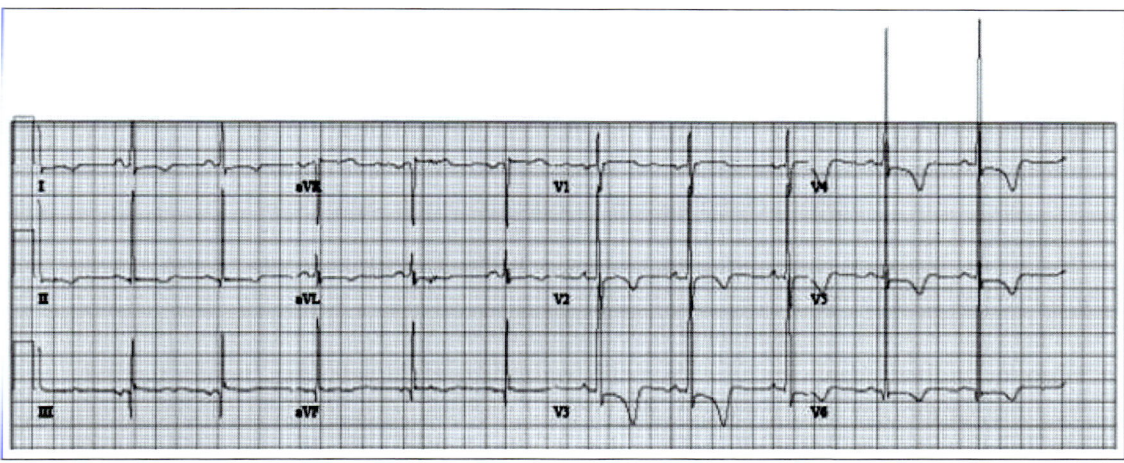

ECG shows tall QRS complexes in leads V2-6. Narrow deep Q waves are seen in III and aVF.

Management

- ABCs, supplemental oxygen, cardiac monitoring, pulse oximetry, and intravenous access.
- Send blood for full blood count, renal panel, and cardiac enzymes. Do an arterial blood gas test if patients are breathless.
- **For left ventricular heart failure**: Give oxygen, start IV GTN 5–50 μg/min titrated to blood pressure response, IV frusemide 40–120 mg, and IV morphine 2–5 mg titrated to the severity of the condition. Perform a bladder catheterization to monitor the urinary output. For patients in severe respiratory distress, intubation for positive pressure ventilation, or continuous positive airway pressure (CPAP) may be needed.
- For **HOCM**, treatment depends on the presentation such as dysrhythmia, heart failure, or ischaemia. Place patients in the supine position. Control heart rate with beta blockers or β-blockers (IV propranolol 1–3 mg slow bolus) and reduce obstruction with calcium channel blockers (IV verapamil 2.5–10 mg over 2 minutes). IV amiodarone 150 mg over 10 minutes

followed by 60 mg per hour for 6 hours can be given for dysrhythmias. **Avoid vasodilatory drugs** in HOCM as this may further impair cardiac filling and cause cardiovascular collapse. If this occurs, give fluid bolus.

- **Electrical cardioversion** may be needed for unstable dysrhythmias.
- Consider **anti-coagulation** for dilated cardiomyopathy as per atrial fibrillation management to reduce the risk of systemic embolization.

Disposition

Admit patients with suspected cardiomyopathy, unexplained syncope with possible cardiac aetiologies, or significant heart failure. Admit to telemetry beds for patients with arrhythmias or history of sudden syncope. Unstable patients or intubated patients should be admitted to the coronary care unit.

References/Further Reading

1. Schaider JJ, Hayden SR, Wolfe RE, et al., eds. *Rosen & Barkin's 5-Minute Emergency Medicine Consult*. Philadelphia, PA: Lippincott Williams & Wilkins; 2007.

2. Crawford MH, Durack DT. Clinical presentation of infective endocarditis. *Cardiol Clin*. 2003; 21: 159–166.

3. Troughton RW, Asher CR, Klein AL. Pericarditis. *Lancet*. 2004; 363: 717.

4. Spodick DH. Acute pericarditis: Current concepts and practice. *JAMA*. 2003; 289: 1150.

5. Imazio M, Bobbio M, Cecchi E, et al. Colchicine in addition to conventional therapy for acute pericarditis: Results of the COlchicine for acute PEricarditis (COPE) trial. *Circulation*. 2005; 112: 2012.

6. Imazio M, Demichelis B, Parrini I, et al. Day-hospital treatment of acute pericarditis: A management program for outpatient therapy. *J Am Coll Cardiol*. 2004; 43: 1042.

7. Maisch B, Seferovic PM, Ristic AD, et al. Guidelines on the diagnosis and management of pericardial diseases executive summary; The task force on the diagnosis and management of pericardial diseases of the European Society of Cardiology. *Eur Heart J*. 2004; 25: 587.

8. Olinde KD, O'Connell JB. Inflammatory heart disease: Pathogenesis, clinical manifestations, and treatment of myocarditis. *Annu Rev Med*. 1994; 45: 481.

9. Dec G, Waldman H, Southern J, et al. Viral myocarditis mimicking acute myocardial infarction. *J Am Coll Cardiol*. 1992; 20: 85.

10. Theleman KP, Kuiper JJ, Roberts WC. Acute myocarditis (predominantly lymphocytic) causing sudden death without heart failure. *Am J Cardiol*. 2001; 88: 1078.

38 Heart Failure, Acute

Zulkarnain Ab Hamid • Shirley Ooi

INTRODUCTION

Acute heart failure (AHF) is a clinical syndrome that may result from any structural or functional cardiac disorder that impairs the ability of the heart to fill with or eject blood, resulting in congestion and failure of the heart to maintain circulation that is adequate for organ and peripheral perfusion.

Regardless of the aetiology, AHF manifests as a consequence of **increased preload**, **increased afterload**, **reduced cardiac output** or a combination of the above.

FIGURE 1 **Pathophysiology of Acute Decompensated Heart Failure**

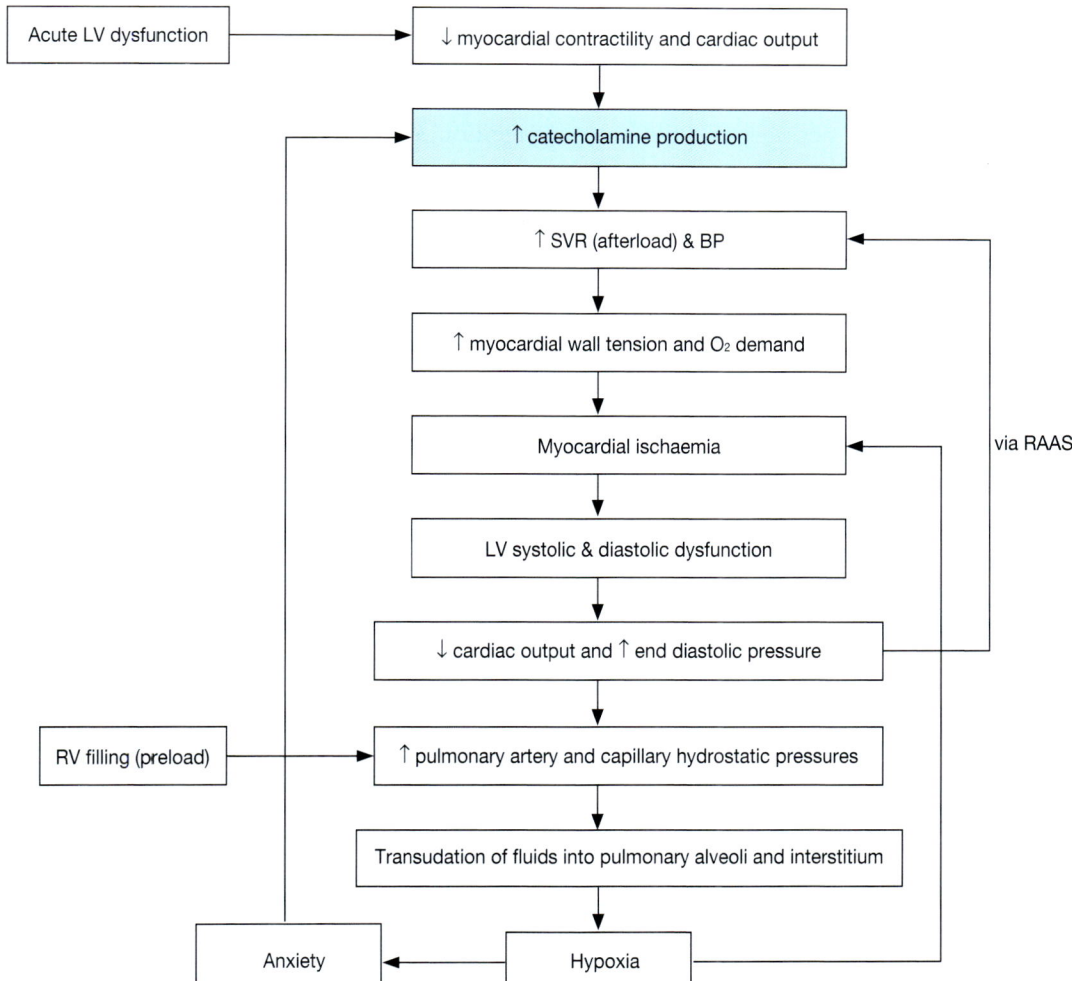

Note: LV – left ventricular, O_2 – oxygen, RAAS – Renin-Angiotensin-Aldosterone system, SVR – systemic vascular resistance

CAVEATS

- A patient with AHF can present in any of 7 clinical categories[1,2]:

  1. **Acute decompensation of chronic left heart failure (ADHF)**. This conventionally refers to an acute presentation by someone with pre-existing chronic heart failure (CHF). They typically present with signs of congestion and fluid retention such as orthopnoea, pedal oedema, weight gain and progressive exertional dyspnoea.

  2. **Acute cardiogenic pulmonary oedema**. This is usually the result of an acute left heart failure in someone who does not have pre-existing CHF, primarily affecting the lungs, and is not usually accompanied by other signs of congestion and fluid retention as mentioned above.

  3. **Cardiogenic shock** (refer to Chapter 31, *Cardiogenic Shock*).

  4. **Acute coronary syndrome (ACS)-related heart failure**. Patients present with the clinical picture (history and electrocardiogram) and biomarker evidence (troponins) of an ACS. AHF occurs in 15% of patients with ACS, and are frequently associated with or precipitated by episodes of dysrhythmias.

  5. **Hypertensive acute heart failure**. Patients present with symptoms and signs of heart failure accompanied by high blood pressure but relatively preserved left ventricular function.

  6. **High output failure**. This is characterized by high cardiac output, manifesting with high heart rate, warm peripheries, pulmonary congestion and sometimes with hypotension.

  7. **Isolated right heart failure**. This is characterized by low output syndrome, jugular venous distension, congestive hepatomegaly and hypotension.

NOTE: The focus of this chapter is on presentation 1 and 2 above, the management of which is basically the same.

- Cardiogenic pulmonary oedema does not equate to systemic volume overload. Inappropriate and overaggressive diuresis risks hypotension and deterioration of renal function. In fact, 50% of cardiogenic pulmonary oedema is euvolaemic. Thus, the aim of treatment is **redistribution**

- Exclude **renal failure** as a cause of fluid overload before diagnosis of heart failure.

- Heart failure may present as **non-specific complaints**:
  1. Weakness
  2. Lightheadedness
  3. Abdominal pain
  4. Malaise
  5. Wheezing
  6. Nausea

- History and physical examination, supplemented with appropriate diagnostic investigations remain the cornerstone in the diagnosis of heart failure. Clinical elements that increase the likelihood that a presentation is ADHF include:

  1. *History*: previous heart failure positive likelihood ratio (LR+) of ADHF: 5.8; myocardial infarction, LR+ 3.1; coronary artery disease, LR+ 1.8.

  2. *Symptoms*: paroxysmal nocturnal dyspnoea, LR+ 2.8; orthopnoea, LR+ 2.2; oedema, LR+ 2.1.

  3. *Signs*: S3 heart sound, LR+ 11; hepatojugular reflux, LR+ 6.4; jugular venous distension, LR+ 5.1; rales/crackles, LR+ 2.8; peripheral oedema, LR+ 2.3; wheezing, LR+ 0.52.

4. ***Diagnostic findings***: pulmonary venous congestion (on CXR), LR+ 12; interstitial oedema on CXR, LR+ 12; alveolar oedema on CXR, LR+ 6; atrial fibrillation, LR+ 3.8; cardiomegaly on CXR, LR+ 3.3; new T-wave changes, LR+ 3.0.

- Where the diagnosis is uncertain, **BNP or NT-proBNP** is useful in distinguishing between cardiac and non-cardiac causes of dyspnoea. The significant value is dependent on age. In general, **BNP >500 pg/ml or NT-proBNP >1000 pg/ml** is diagnostic for ADHF.

NOTE: **Causes of raised BNP or NT-proBNP** include:

- Cor pulmonale
- Acute pulmonary embolism
- Renal failure
- Primary pulmonary hypertension
- Liver cirrhosis
- Advancing age
- Gender (women have higher levels than men)

- Always look for **precipitating causes** of heart failure (**Table 1**), so that the management of these may be incorporated into the treatment strategy. Ischaemia is the most common precipitant of new-onset AHF.
- The cardiac conditions combined with asthma or symptoms of chronic obstructive airway disease are difficult clinical challenges and will require a multidisciplinary approach. The presence of these co-morbid conditions confounds the diagnostic process. Furthermore, these conditions may present concomitantly, thus presenting the clinician with a management challenge.

Patients with coexisting insulin-dependent diabetes mellitus have a significantly increased mortality rate.

TABLE 1 Precipitating causes of heart failure

Cardiac	Non-Cardiac
• Myocardial ischaemia or infarction	• Pulmonary embolism
• Dysrhythmias	• Superimposed systemic infection, especially pneumonia
• Valvular heart disease	
• Acute myopathies (e.g. post-partum cardiomyopathy, acute myocarditis)	• Systemic illness, e.g. severe hypertension, severe anaemia, thyrotoxicosis, heavy alcohol consumption
• Non-compliance with therapeutic regimen including failure to restrict fluid intake	• Drugs: cocaine, amphetamines, excess use of bronchodilators, 1st-generation calcium antagonist, beta-blockers, NSAIDS
• Bacterial endocarditis	• Pregnancy

⇨ **SPECIAL TIPS FOR GPs**

- Always look for a cause of heart failure in patients especially if they have been stable and on medication for a long time. Coronary events or renal impairment must be identified.
- Patient in severe heart failure may present with wheezing. This is **cardiac asthma** and will require aggressive management in the ED before it deteriorates to pulmonary oedema. Ventolin nebulization will not make the patient improve symptomatically. Nitrates have been shown to be safely instituted as an empirical first line therapy in the prehospital setting.
- Elderly patients have altered autonomic regulation and are sensitive to the side effects of the drugs used in the therapy for heart failure. Special precaution is necessary to tailor the therapy.

MANAGEMENT

- Manage patient in a monitored area: vital signs, pulse oximeter and continuous ECG monitoring.
- Maintain airway. Patient with ADHF, unless having altered mental state or severe respiratory distress, need not be intubated at the onset, but may be treated first, as the symptoms improve rapidly with appropriate treatment.
- Administer supplemental oxygen 100% via non-rebreather face mask.
- Obtain IV access and obtain bloods for FBC, urea/electrolytes/creatinine and cardiac markers (troponins).
- Do **ECG** to diagnose cardiac ischaemia or dysrhythmia, prior MI, or LVH (from chronic hypertension or other causes)
- Order **CXR**. Aside from features of heart failure (see above), the CXR can be used to look for other causes of respiratory distress or hypotension, including pneumonia, pneumothorax, widened mediastinum of aortic dissection and pericardial effusion.

NOTE: The classic radiographic findings (Figure 2) are not always found at the time of initial 2-hour presentation. As much as a 12-hour delay may occur between the onset of symptoms and the development of significant radiographic abnormalities when the onset of ADHF is abrupt.

- The **aims of pharmacological management** of ADHF are:
  1. To decrease right-sided filling (preload) (e.g. GTN, frusemide, morphine)
  2. To increase left-sided emptying by
     a. decreasing systemic vascular resistance (afterload) (e.g. nitrates, angiotensin-converting enzyme inhibitor, hydralazine and nitroprusside).
     b. improving left ventricular contractility (using inotropic support); sometimes necessary.
- **1ˢᵗ line drug: Nitrates**.
  1. Give sublingual GTN first for rapid initiation of treatment. This can be followed by topical GTN patch for mild to moderate ADHF and IV GTN for severe ADHF.
     NOTE: GTN reduces both preload and afterload.

FIGURE 2 Chest radiograph showing classic radiographic findings of ADHF: cardiomegaly, upper lobe diversion, hilar pulmonary congestion and alveolar oedema. Bilateral infiltrates in a 'bat wing' pattern and Kerley B lines are not so obvious on this x-ray

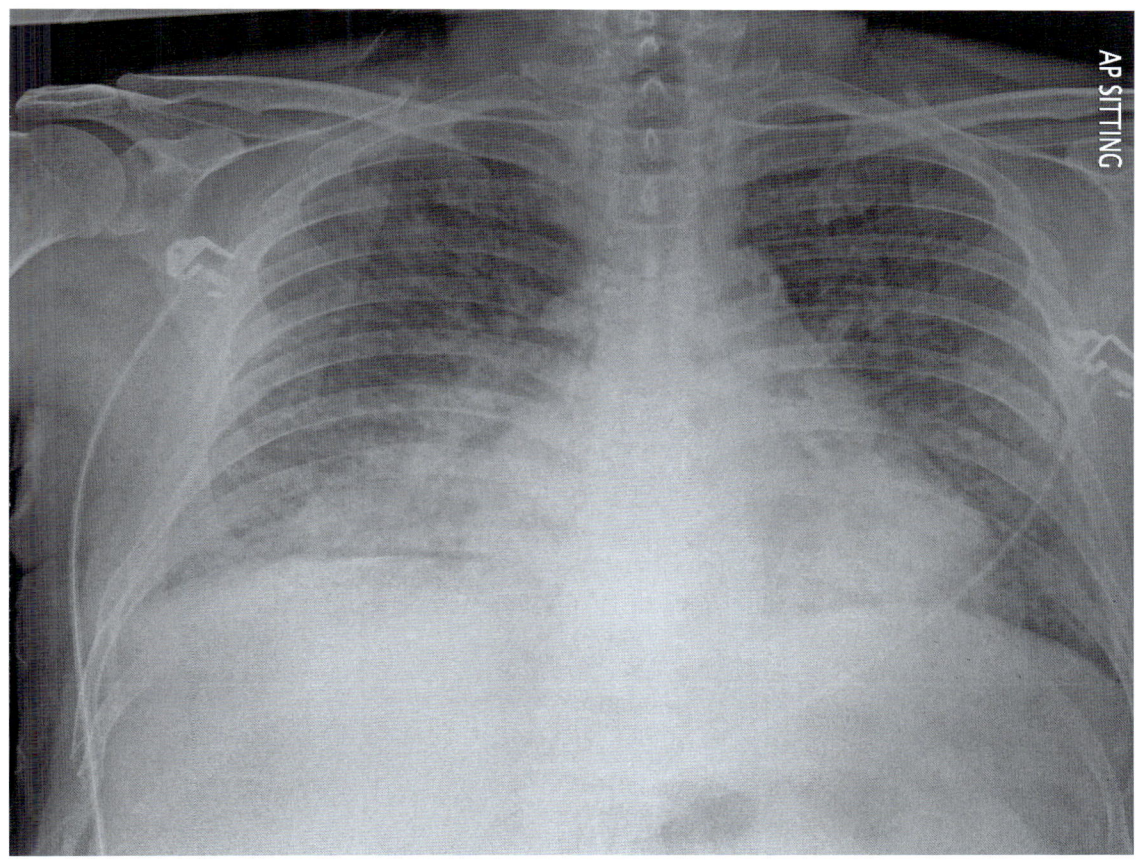

AP SITTING

2. Reasons for nitrates being a 1st line drug:

   a. Rapid (effect seen within 5 mins with S/L GTN), reliable preload reduction

   b. Moderate/high doses reduces afterload and maintains or improves stroke volume and cardiac output.

   c. Its short half-life means that even if there is a pre-hospital misdiagnosis, the effects are easily reversed.

NOTE: The key is to start with IV GTN of 20–50 µg/min titrating upwards rapidly to >100 µg/min. Tail down the dose of IV GTN if patient goes hypotensive. BP returns to normal value within 5–10 mins of discontinuing the IV GTN.

Caution:

1. Hypotension
2. Right ventricular infarct
3. Acute mitral regurgitation
4. Aortic stenosis (dependence of preload to maintain BP)
5. Pulmonary hypertension (dependence of preload to maintain BP)
6. Patients taking medications for erectile dysfunction e.g. sildenafil (Viagra®) – will cause precipitous drop in BP.

- **2ⁿᵈ line drug: ACE-inhibitor (ACE-I).**

1. For mild to moderate ADHF, give SL **captopril** 12.5 mg if SBP <110 mmHg and 25 mg if SBP >110 mmHg.

NOTE: SL captopril can be prepared by dipping regular captopril tablet in water before administering sublingually.

2. For moderate to severe ADHF, IV captopril or **enalapril** can be administered.
3. Captopril, like GTN, reduces both preload and afterload. Effect can be seen in 6–12 minutes!
4. Effect of combined ACE-I and nitrates exceeds each drug alone.
5. ACE-I is an acceptable alternative to IV GTN as 1ˢᵗ line drug in those with contraindications to GTN.

- **3ʳᵈ line drug: Diuretics**

NOTE: IV frusemide (Lasix®) should not be a first line but rather a 3ʳᵈ line drug for APO. The reasons are as follows:

1. Initial adverse haemodynamic effects of increased afterload, decreased stroke volume and decreased cardiac output.
2. No direct preload reducing effect
3. The decrease in preload through diuresis is a delayed effect taking 45–120 minutes to produce effective diuresis because ADHF patients have elevated afterload resulting in markedly diminished renal perfusion. Hence, diuretics may ultimately worsen renal function further; this effect is more pronounced in the elderly.

NOTE: These adverse effects may be blunted by administration of preload-reducing (GTN or ACE-I) and afterload-reducing medications (high dose GTN or ACE-I) *before* frusemide.

- Do **NOT give morphine** as there is no evidence of its venodilatory effect but can potentially worsen symptoms. Histamine-related side effects may increase catecholamines. Morphine may also cause respiratory and myocardial suppression. If it is for anxiolysis, benzodiazepines will be better although not necessary in the management.

- For moderate to severe ADHF with evidence of pulmonary oedema, and with intact mental state and no evidence of ST-elevation MI, prepare for **non-invasive ventilation (NIV)**. The benefit of NIV is seen only if **used early**, and its use, when strongly indicated, supercedes the use of pharmacological agents. Check response to treatment, including subjective improvement as reported by patient, oxygenation (with SpO_2 monitoring and half-hourly arterial blood gas) and blood pressure.

NOTE: NIV has been shown to **decrease mortality** besides reducing the need for intubation.

- Monitor urine output to assess response to therapy.
- Patients who develop worsening respiratory distress or altered mental state should be **intubated** for the purpose of protecting the airway and improve breathing and ventilation. During rapid sequence induction, pretreatment with IV fentanyl is recommended to reduce catecholamine release.
- Patients who are hypotensive at the onset (and for which none of the above treatments can be initiated) should be administered **inotropes** to increase cardiac output. There is no difference in mortality in use of the different types of inotropes. One can start with intravenous dopamine or dobutamine started at 20 μg/kg/min and titrated downwards according to response.

DISPOSITION

There are 3 options for disposition for patients with ADHF:

1. Admission to cardiac ward
2. Admission to short-stay or observational ward
3. Discharge.

Admission to cardiac ward

The vast majority of the patients with ADHF are admitted. Discharging a patient without adequate treatment may be associated with reattendances and increased short-term morbidity and mortality. Table 2 shows instances where admission is recommended or strongly advised.

Admission to Observation Units

- There has been growing interest in the assignment of patients with ADHF to ED observation units. However, there are as yet, no randomised studies performed to date to substantiate its use. Admission to such admission units should be protocolised to reduce the possibility of inappropriate admissions. As such, both inclusion and exclusion criteria should be laid down, in consultation with cardiologists to determine appropriate patient selection.

TABLE 2   Recommendations for admission to cardiac ward

Heart Failure Society of America Recommendations for Admission of ED patients with Heart Failure (modified)	
Admission is recommended	Severe ADHF • Hypotension • Worsening renal function • Altered mental status or syncope Dyspnoea at rest Arrhythmia with haemodynamic compromise, including new-onset atrial fibrillation Acute coronary syndrome
Admission should be required	Worsening congestion (pulmonary or systemic) Significant electrolyte disturbance Associated comorbidities: • Pneumonia • Pulmonary embolism • Diabetic ketoacidosis • Transient ischaemic attack New-onset (de novo) heart failure

- Examples of **inclusion criteria**:
  1. Patients presenting to the ED with mild to moderate ADHF.
  2. Anticipated length of stay not more than 24–48h (depending on departmental policy).
  3. Adequate follow-up and social support anticipated at time of discharge.

- Examples of **exclusion criteria**:
  1. No previous history of CAD (i.e. de novo AHF)
  2. Diagnostic uncertainty, e.g. possible COPD, PE, etc.
  3. Severe haemodynamic instability that would warrant admission:
     a. Heart rate >130 or <50/min
     b. Hypotensive (systolic BP <90 mmHg or requiring inotropic support)
     c. BP > 220/110 mm Hg.
  4. Temperature >38°C
  5. Raised cardiac markers (troponins or CKMB/CK)
  6. New ischaemic changes on ECG
  7. Severe electrolyte imbalances
  8. Patients on dialysis or with significant renal impairment
  9. Syncope
  10. Multiple severe comorbidities which are likely to complicate disposition and management.

Discharge

- The patient may be discharged if he:
  1. Has no chest pain or concomitant illness
  2. Responds to diuretics given at the ED (comfortable at rest on room air, SpO_2 on room air ≥95%).
  3. Shows no radiographic evidence of chronic heart failure.
- Discharge with the following and refer patient for follow-up at the cardiology outpatient clinics:
  1. SL GTN 500 µg PRN, to be used as first line, when there is an acute exacerbation while in outpatient setting. There should be an appropriate care plan for the patient to inform when there is a need for emergent treatment at the emergency department.
  2. Loop diuretics, e.g. Lasix® 40 mg OM, and potassium supplements, e.g. span K 1.2 mg OM if patient is not dehydrated, not on diuretics before and urea/electrolytes/creatinine are normal.
  3. Increase dose of loop diuretics if patient is already on diuretics.
  4. If patient has **concurrent hypertension**, besides loop diuretics, angiotensin converting enzyme inhibitor, eg captopril 6.25–12.5 mg tds or hydralazine 25 mg tds may be given.
  5. Dietary advice to decrease salt intake and fluid restriction.

References/Further Reading

1. European Society of Cardiology. ESC guidelines for the diagnosis and treatment of acute and chronic heart failure 2008. *Eur Heart J* 2008: 29; 2388–2442.

2. Gardner RS, McDonagh TA, Walker NL. *Oxford Specialist Handbook in Cardiology: Heart Failure*. Oxford: Oxford University Press; 2007: 343–368.

3. ACEP subcommittee on acute heart failure syndromes. Clinical Policy: Critical issues in the evaluation and management of adult patients presenting to the emergency department with acute heart failure syndromes. *Ann. Emerg. Med*. 2007; 49: 627–669.

4. Ooi S, Niemann JT. Congestive heart failure and cor pulmonale. In: Wolfson, AB ed. *Harwood-Nuss' Clinical Practice of Emergency Medicine*. Philadelphia: Lippincott Williams & Wilkins; 2010: 469–474.

5. Adams JG, ed. *Emergency Medicine*. Philadelphia: Saunders Elsevier; 2008: 523–536.

6. Mushlin SB, Greene HL. *Decision Making in Medicine, An Algorithmic Approach, 3rd Ed*. Philadelphia: Mosby Elsevier; 2010: 82–91, 96–97.

7. Simel DL, Rennie D, Keitz SA, eds. *The Rational Clinical Examination, Evidence-Based Clinical Diagnosis*. McGraw-Hill; 2009: 183–214.

8. Brashers VL. *Clinical Applications of Pathophysiology, An Evidence-Based Approach, 3rd Ed*. Missouri: Mosby Elevier; 2006: 53–63.

9. Fauci AS, Braunwald E, et al. *Harrison's Principles of Internal Medicine, 17th Ed*. McGraw-Hill; 2008: 1452–1453.

10. Mattu A, Martinez JP, Kelly BS. Modern management of cardiogenic pulmonary edema. *Emerg Med Clin N Am* 2005; 23: 1105–1125.

39   Hypertensive Crises

Benjamin Leong • Peter Manning

DEFINITIONS

- **Hypertension** is defined as blood pressure levels of ≥140/90 mmHg, though it should be recognised that blood pressure levels are a continuous variable.

    The Eighth Report (JNC 8) does not address the definitions of hypertension and prehypertension but thresholds of pharmacologic treatment were defined.

- **Hypertensive crises** are a heterogeneous group of clinical situations associated with markedly elevated blood pressures. They are classically categorized into *hypertensive emergencies* and *hypertensive urgencies*. As this categorization is somewhat arbitrary, specific definitions often differ from author to author, and can be very confusing.

    1. **Hypertensive emergencies**: It is the target organ dysfunction rather than the absolute blood pressure level *per se* that defines a hypertensive emergency. Perhaps the best definition for hypertensive emergencies is from the Sixth Report of the JNC: 'Situations that require immediate blood pressure reduction (not necessarily to the normal range) to prevent or limit target organ damage'.

    2. **Hypertensive urgencies**: For the purposes of this chapter, hypertensive urgencies are defined as '**clinical scenarios with markedly elevated blood pressures (>180/120 mmHg) without obvious end-organ dysfunction**'.

CAVEATS

General

- Hypertensive crises occur mostly in patients known to have hypertension, though some can present *de novo*, with no previous history.
- **Do not simply treat a number**; treatment of hypertensive crises should be guided by the overall clinical status of the patient.
- **Do not 'treat the physician'**: A dilemma often faced by the physician is whether or not to treat his family members or himself. This is akin to the decision of whether or not to lower blood pressure, which can be very difficult and should be carefully weighed against causing unintended tissue hypoperfusion.
- In the vast majority of severely hypertensive patients, blood pressure may be reduced with **oral medications**, and long-term control of blood pressure is probably the most important factor in influencing prognosis.
- The **follow-up care** of a patient presenting with a hypertensive crisis is just as important as the emergent care, to ensure proper chronic blood pressure control and prevent future episodes.
- The terms '**accelerated hypertension**', '**malignant hypertension**', and '**accelerated-malignant hypertension**' describe severe hypertension with associated retinal changes according to the

Keith–Wagener–Barker grading. While it was previously found that grades 3 and 4 were associated with poorer outcomes, recent authors have found no difference based simply on these fundoscopic findings.

Basic pathophysiology

- **Blood pressure = CO × TPR** (CO = Cardiac output; TPR = Total peripheral resistance).
- **CO = HR × SV** (HR = Heart rate; SV = Stroke volume).
- Therefore, **blood pressure is affected by changes in TPR, HR, and SV**.
- The **regulation** of blood pressure is now understood to depend on interactions in the following mechanisms:
  1. **Renin-angiotensin-aldosterone** (RAA) system. Renal hypoperfusion triggers renin release from the juxtaglomerular complex, converting angiotensinogen to angiotensin I, which is then further converted to angiotensin II by angiotensin-converting enzyme in the lungs. Angiotensin II is a very potent vasoconstrictor and also stimulates aldosterone release, leading to sodium and water retention.
  2. **Endothelial function** Vasoactive substances secreted by the endothelium include nitric oxide, prostacyclin, and endothelin.
  3. **Sympathetic nervous system** Acute pain, emotional stress, or exercise affects the blood pressure through this mechanism, leading to arterial vasoconstriction and increased cardiac output. Vascular bed autoregulation then results in arteriolar vasoconstriction to protect the distal tissue bed from the elevated blood pressures.
  4. **Humoral system** Bradykinin is a potent vasodilator that is inhibited by angiotensin II, and atrial natriuretic peptides promote renal sodium and water excretion.
  5. In both chronic hypertension and hypertensive crises, pathological conditions affecting **TPR, HR,** and **SV** will lead to changes in **blood pressure** (see Table 1).
  6. In **hypertensive crises**, although not completely understood, an abrupt elevation in vascular resistance appears to be the initiating step that triggers vicious cycles leading to marked increases in blood pressure.
  7. **Vascular endothelial damage** then occurs when compensatory mechanisms are overwhelmed, leading to **excessive fluid shear stress**, **increased vascular permeability**, **fibrin deposition**, and activation of the **coagulation cascade** resulting in **fibrinoid necrosis** of arterioles, and **end-organ hypoperfusion**.
  8. Activation/amplification of the **renin-angiotensin system** is another major driver of hypertensive crises. Angiotensin II induces further **vasoconstriction**, as well as the release of **pro-inflammatory cytokines**, further adding to vascular damage and leading to a **vicious cycle**. However, not all hypertensive emergencies are associated with high renin states; e.g. in pre-eclampsia, the renin level actually falls.
  9. **Pressure natriuresis** may also occur, where salt and water reabsorption in the proximal tubules decreases. This then results in volume depletion and further activation of the renin-angiotensin system.

TABLE 1   Causes of hypertensive emergencies

Essential hypertension

Renal parenchymal disease
Acute glomerulonephritis
Vasculitis
Haemolytic uraemic syndrome
Thrombotic thrombocytopaenic purpura

Renovascular disease
Renal artery stenosis (atheromatous or fibromuscular dysplasia)

Pregnancy
Eclampsia

Endocrine
Phaeochromocytoma
Cushing's syndrome
Renin-secreting tumours
Mineralocorticoid hypertension (rarely causes hypertensive emergencies)

Drugs
Cocaine, sympathomimetics, erythropoietin, cyclosporin and antihypertensive withdrawal
Interactions with monoamine-oxidase inhibitors (tyramine), amphetamines, and lead intoxication

Autonomic hyper-reactivity
Guillain-Barré syndrome and acute intermittent porphyria

Central nervous system disorders
Head injury, cerebral infarction/haemorrhage, and brain tumour

Source: Vaughan CJ, Delanty N. Hypertensive emergencies. *Lancet.* 2000; 356: 411–417.

10. **The rate of rise of the blood pressure** is more important than the absolute level of the blood pressure itself. In patients with chronic hypertension, adaptive changes in the vasculature provide some protection, and end-organ dysfunction may only occur at much higher blood pressures, while in contrast, a previously normotensive patient will suffer complications at lower blood pressures. The presence of those same adaptive vascular changes in chronic hypertensive patients also means that **over-zealous correction** of the blood pressure in these patients may be **hazardous** leading to **strokes or acute myocardial infarction**.

11. Regardless of the initial cause of the hypertension, when **end organs** are affected requiring rapid lowering of blood pressures, these constitute **hypertensive emergencies**.

12. The presentation and specific management of hypertensive emergencies will depend on the **underlying causes** and the **end-organ systems** affected by the blood pressure (see Table 2). The management of these will be discussed below.

TABLE 2 Presentations of hypertensive emergencies

1. Hypertensive encephalopathy
2. Acute ischaemic stroke
3. Intracranial haemorrhage/subarachnoid haemorrhage
4. Acute left ventricular failure (acute pulmonary oedema)
5. Aortic dissection
6. Acute myocardial infarction/acute coronary syndrome (ACS)
7. Acute renal failure
8. Pre-eclampsia/eclampsia
9. Sympathetic crises

CLINICAL ASSESSMENT

Is the blood pressure reading correct?

- If the blood pressure measured by a monitoring device is too high (or too low), repeat using a *manual* sphygmomanometer.
- Is the cuff the correct size, and, is the arrow located correctly, i.e. over the brachial artery?
- Check the other arm.
- Recheck about 1 hour later if the patient is otherwise asymptomatic.

Is it a hypertensive emergency?

- Look for evidence of **end-organ damage**.
- **A clinical examination should include the following**:
  1. Fundoscopy for haemorrhages, exudates, and papilloedema.
  2. Neurological examination for altered mental states and focal deficits.
  3. Cardiovascular examination for left ventricular failure, new aortic regurgitation murmurs, and evidence of dissection.
- **Bedside investigations should include the following**:
  1. ECG.
  2. Urine dipstick for haematuria and proteinuria.
  3. Urine pregnancy test in females of child-bearing age with new hypertension.
- **Lab investigations should include the following**:
  1. Full blood count.
  2. Creatinine, urea, and electrolytes.
  3. Liver function tests if the patient is pregnant to identify **HELLP** (**H**aemolysis, **E**levated **L**iver enzymes, and a **Low Platelet** count) syndrome.
  4. Cardiac enzyme screen and troponin T test.

- **Radiology should include the following**:
  1. Chest X-ray for left ventricular failure and widened mediastinum.
  2. Computed tomography of the brain for patients with altered mental state.

⇨ **SPECIAL TIPS FOR GPs**

- Do not treat the patient based on a single blood pressure reading alone. Recheck the blood pressure when the patient is comfortable, using an appropriately-sized blood pressure cuff.
- The use of commercially available home blood pressure machines by patients at home can provide very good insight into their blood control, especially for patients with reactive ('white coat') hypertension. The home readings should be compared with manual blood pressure readings at the GP clinic to verify accuracy.
- Good blood pressure control of patients with hypertension reduces the number of cases presenting with hypertensive emergencies or urgencies.
- In the patient with a suspected hypertensive crisis presenting to the GP clinic, rest the patient in a quiet and comfortable environment and arrange for transfer to hospital.
- For the patient who has defaulted on his medication, an oral dose of the patient's regular medication (if the patient is able to swallow and protect the airway) is reasonable while awaiting transfer.
- The use of sublingual nifedipine, though popular in the past, lowers blood pressures imprecisely and has been found to be associated with serious adverse events. Its use is now an unacceptable practice.

MANAGEMENT

- All patients with **hypertensive emergencies** must be managed in a closely monitored area as the clinical state may change rapidly.
- Monitor **ECG** and **pulse oximetry** and check **vital signs** every 5 to 10 minutes.
- Give supplemental low flow **oxygen** and obtain **intravenous access. Invasive arterial blood pressure monitoring**, if available, is preferred.
- The general aim is to control the blood pressure without compromising circulation to the end organs.
- Patients with severely elevated blood pressures without evidence of end-organ dysfunction (**hypertensive urgencies**) may be managed in an intermediate care area (see below).

SPECIFIC CONDITIONS

Hypertensive encephalopathy

- Hypertensive encephalopathy is often considered an organic brain syndrome associated with marked hypertension.

- New understanding links this to an entity presently called **posterior reversible encephalopathy syndrome** (PRES). PRES is associated with vasogenic oedema predominantly in the posterior brain seen on brain imaging. It has been documented in a variety of clinical syndromes including hypertensive encephalopathy, eclampsia/pre-eclampsia, sepsis, cancer chemotherapy, autoimmune disease, and transplantation.

- The exact **mechanism** is uncertain with two conflicting theories – hypertension with failed autoregulation and hyperperfusion versus vasoconstriction with hypoperfusion and ischaemia.

- The **clinical features** include headache, nausea/vomiting, visual disturbances or loss, weakness and lethargy, seizures, confusion, and papilloedema. Focal signs have also been documented, making the distinction between altered mental status due to a stroke and PRES difficult in the emergency department.

- Hypertensive encephalopathy/PRES is **generally reversible** with treatment of the blood pressure, though some cases have been documented to have irreversible sequelae.

- The **treatment goal** is to **lower the mean arterial pressure (MAP) within an hour to 20–25% below presenting level, or diastolic blood pressure (DBP) to no less than 100–110 mmHg,** then further towards **160/100 mmHg over the next 2 to 6 hours**. If the neurological status deteriorates during treatment, stop or lower the dose of medication. If the patient remains stable and is tolerating the lowered blood pressure, a further gradual reduction towards normal blood pressure may be implemented over the next 8–24 hours.

- **Labetalol, fenoldopam, nicardipine**, and **enalapril** are generally effective.

- **Nitroprusside** is frequently recommended by many authors, but should be reserved as a therapy of last resort today.

Acute ischaemic stroke

- Acute ischaemic stroke (AIS) is frequently associated with hypertension, and is likely to reflect a **compensatory mechanism** to restore cerebral perfusion pressure (CPP) to the ischaemic brain. The elevated blood pressure frequently returns to pre-stroke levels within **four days**.

- The decision to treat the blood pressure in the acute setting is very difficult; leaving it high exposes the patient to a risk of **cerebral oedema** and **haemorrhagic transformation**, while lowering the blood pressure may compromise the circulation to the **ischaemic penumbra**.

- **Current recommendations** are that antihypertensive therapy is not routinely indicated.

- Initiate blood pressure lowering therapy only if the systolic blood pressure (SBP) is >220 mmHg, or diastolic blood pressure is >120 mmHg, and **lower the MAP by no more than 20–25% or DBP to no less than 100–110 mmHg**.

- If the patient is a candidate for **thrombolytic therapy**, the **target blood pressure is lower than 180/110 mmHg**.

- Therapeutic options include **labetalol, fenoldopam, nicardipine**, and **enalapril**.

- **Nitroprusside** is frequently recommended by many authors, but should be reserved as a therapy of last resort today.

Intracerebral haemorrhage (ICH) and subarachnoid haemorrhage (SAH)

- **Cerebral perfusion pressure** (CPP) is the difference between **MAP** and **intracranial pressure** (ICP).
- CPP = MAP – ICP.
- **Cerebral autoregulation** maintains a constant blood flow to the brain over a wide range of MAP from **50** to **150 mmHg**.
- This ability is **lost** in ICH, and an elevated systemic blood pressure will directly result in excessive blood flow to the haemorrhaging area.
- On the other hand, the expanding haematoma also leads to increased ICP.
- Thus, the **blood pressure goal** in reducing the MAP to limit haemorrhage must be balanced against reductions in CPP.
- **Labetalol** is the agent of choice for acute blood pressure control.
- Specifically in SAH, **nimodipine** is specially indicated as it reduces cerebral arterial vasospasm due to irritation by blood. Nimodipine may cause **transient hypotension** and blood pressure medications need to be adjusted accordingly. It should, however, not be used as the sole treatment for SAH.

Aortic dissection

- This must always be considered when a patient presents with **hypertension** and **acute chest pain** or **acute myocardial infarction** (when the dissection affects the coronary arteries, most commonly the right coronary artery) or a **new aortic regurgitation murmur** is detected. The classical history of tearing pain radiating to the back may **not** be present (see Chapter 34, *Aortic Emergencies*).
- Once recognized, the **therapeutic goal** in this setting is to rapidly lower the **SBP to about 100–120 mmHg** within 5 to 10 minutes.
- The preferred drug in this case is **labetalol**, as it effectively lowers the dP/dt (see below). Alternatively, a **β-blocker** administered concurrently with **nitroprusside** or α-**blocker** is appropriate.
- **Avoid** drugs that increase **reflex tachycardia** (e.g. GTN, nitroprusside, calcium channel blockers, hydralazine, or ACE inhibitors) unless paired with a β-**blocker**.
- Urgent cardiothoracic consult is indicated.

Acute left ventricular failure

- Commonly labelled as acute pulmonary oedema, this occurs when the severe hypertension results in acute left ventricular failure from excessive afterload, causing decompensation (see Chapter 38, *Heart Failure, Acute*).
- Clinically the patient is typically sitting up, in respiratory distress, with cold and clammy peripheries, diaphoresis and frank pulmonary rales, or rhonchi.
- The **therapeutic goal** is to control the blood pressure until **alleviation of the signs of heart failure**.

- **GTN** IV is the drug of choice in this setting to reduce the preload and afterload of the heart.
- IV **diuretics** is only a 3rd line drug.

Acute myocardial infarction/acute coronary syndrome

- This occurs when the severe hypertension leads to increased ventricular wall tension and myocardial oxygen demands, or it could be due to pain, anxiety, and increased sympathetic tone.
- A blood pressure of more than 180/110 mmHg is a contraindication to thrombolysis.
- The therapeutic options include **GTN**, **β-blockers**, and **ACE inhibitors**.
- **Avoid** pure vasodilators such as nitroprusside that increase **reflex tachycardia** as this condition increases myocardial oxygen demands.

Acute renal failure

- This is both a **cause** and **consequence** of markedly raised blood pressure.
- This should be considered in a patient with severe hypertension and **new onset renal failure** or **rapidly worsening renal function** in a patient with known renal impairment.
- The goal is to reduce the blood pressure while maintaining renal blood flow.
- **Fenoldopam** has the advantage of increasing renal blood flow.
- Other therapeutic options include **calcium channel blockers**, **α-blockers**, **β-blockers**, **hydralazine**, and **nitroprusside**.
- **Avoid** ACE inhibitors.

Pre-eclampsia/eclampsia (see Chapter 108)

- This must be considered in all hypertensive (blood pressure >140/90 mmHg) pregnant women after **20 weeks of amenorrhoea**.
- Without a clear history, it may be hard to distinguish from pre-existing hypertension.
- Pre-eclampsia is associated with increased 24-hour urinary protein (>300 mg/dL), but a urine dipstick test at any point in time may be negative, as the proteinuria fluctuates throughout the day. Oedema was a classical sign of pre-eclampsia, but that is now not used to diagnose pre-eclampsia since oedema is also a classical sign of pregnancy.
- The **HELLP syndrome** (**H**aemolysis, **E**levated **L**iver enzymes, and a **L**ow **P**latelet count) is a severe manifestation of pre-eclampsia.
- **Eclampsia** occurs when a patient with pre-eclampsia develops a **seizure**. However, other causes of seizures need to be ruled out, including epilepsy and intracranial haemorrhage.
- Recent evidence links it to **posterior reversible encephalopathy syndrome** (PRES) (see the section on *Hypertensive Encephalopathy* above).
- The definitive treatment of eclampsia and pre-eclampsia is delivery of the baby, the timing of which needs to be planned by the obstetrician.

- Treatment with **magnesium sulphate** ($MgSO_4$) is essential to prevent evolution into eclampsia. $MgSO_4$ should be given until deep tendon reflexes are lost.
- **Blood pressure control** in pre-clampsia is essentially a balance of preventing maternal complications and maintaining placental blood flow.
- The **therapeutic goal** is to maintain the blood pressure **<160/105 mmHg**, but not to lower the DBP <90 mmHg, as placental perfusion is reduced in these patients.
- **Methyldopa** is commonly used to treat hypertension in pregnancy due to its safety profile.
- For *acute* blood pressure control of pregnancy-induced hypertension, **hydralazine** has been the mainstay for years, but its drawback is the induction of reflex tachycardia. **Labetalol** does not have that disadvantage and its use is increasing.
- **ACE inhibitors** are contraindicated in pregnancy and **nitroprusside** should be avoided as it may cause profound reflex bradycardia and hypotension and also accumulate in the placenta.

Catecholamine crises

- Also called **sympathetic crises**, these may be caused by **catecholamines** from **endogenous** (phaeochromocytoma) or **exogenous** sources (sympathomimetic drugs of abuse such as cocaine or amphetamines), **rebound phenomena** from clonidine withdrawal, and may also occur in patients with **autonomic dysfunction** such as Guillain-Barré syndrome.
- Clinical features include severe hypertension, tachycardia, diaphoresis, and pyrexia.
- **Isolated β-blockade** in this group of patients leads to **unopposed α-adrenergic activity** and further increased blood pressure.
- **Labetalol** is traditionally the drug of choice in this situation, but it has been found not to relieve the coronary vasospasm of cocaine.
- Therapeutic options include **nicardipine**, **fenoldopam**, **verapamil** with **diazepam**, or **phentolamine**.

DRUG THERAPY IN HYPERTENSIVE EMERGENCIES (Refer to Table 3)

Sodium nitroprusside

- This powerful arterial and venous dilator acts directly on smooth muscles of resistance and capacitance vessels.
- It is able to lower blood pressure for all forms of hypertensive emergencies regardless of pathophysiology.
- However, its use stimulates reflex tachycardia and reactive renin secretion, which may be pathophysiologically unfavourable.
- Due to its extreme potent efficacy, rapid onset and short half-life, its safe use should only be by constant infusion with concurrent intra-arterial blood pressure monitoring.

- It is degraded in light and needs to be administered in opaque containers and tubing.
- It is **not** suitable for use in **pregnancy** (e.g. for those women with eclampsia) due to placental accumulation.
- Cyanide toxicity also limits its use, due to accumulation of its toxic metabolites, thiocyanate and cyanide after prolonged administration (24–48 hours), especially in patients with renal or hepatic dysfunction.
- Although many authorities still recommend its use as a first-line agent in hypertensive crises, with various newer and pathophysiologically more appropriate drugs being available, it should be probably reserved as an agent of last resort – when the blood pressure remains dangerously high despite all other attempts at lowering it.
- Intravenous infusion starts at 0.25 µg/kg/min; titrate to response. The average effective dose is 3 µg/kg/min, with a range of 0.25–10 µg/kg/min (do not use the maximum dose for more than 10 minutes).

Labetalol hydrochloride

- A selective α_1-receptor and non-selective β-receptor blocker.
- Effectively reduces peripheral vascular resistance without reflex tachycardia.
- Useful for patients with ischaemic heart disease in reducing myocardial oxygen demand and tachycardia.
- Very effective in aortic dissection by reducing the force of systolic ejection, thus reducing aortic dP/dt (rate of change of blood pressure over time) and endothelial shear stress.
- Contraindicated in patients with asthma, chronic obstructive lung disease (COLD), congestive cardiac failure, bradycardia, and atrioventricular block.
- While useful for phaeochromocytoma, low doses may result in paradoxical hypertension because the β-blocking effect is stronger than the α-blocking effect.
- Does not reverse the coronary vasospasm caused by cocaine, though it does reduce the blood pressure.
- Give IV 20 mg bolus, followed by 20–80 mg every 10 minutes, or start at an infusion rate of 0.5–2.0 mg/min. The maximum dose is 300 mg per day.

Propranolol

- Non-selective β-blocker.
- May be used in conjunction with nitroprusside for aortic dissection and with phentolamine for catecholamine crises.
- Contraindicated in patients with asthma, COLD, congestive cardiac failure, bradycardia, and atrioventricular block.
- Give IV 1 mg bolus and titrate.

TABLE 4   Drug Therapy in Hypertensive Emergencies

Drug	Mechanism of action	Special indications	Adverse effects	Contraindications/ conditions to avoid	Dosage	Onset/ duration
Nitroprusside	Arterial and venous vasodilation		Reflex tachycardia Nausea/vomiting Flushing Headache Muscle spasm Thiocyanate and cyanide toxicity	Pregnancy	0.25–10 μg/kg/min infusion	Instantaneous/ 1–2 min
Nitroglycerin	Venodilation	Acute pulmonary oedema	Reflex tachycardia Flushing Headache Vomiting Methaemoglobinaemia Tachyphylaxis		5–100 μg/min infusion	1–5 min/ 3–5 min
Nicardipine	Calcium channel blocker Vasodilation		Reflex tachycardia Flushing Headache Nausea Oedema	Heart failure	5–15 mg/hr IV	5–10 min/ 1–4 hr
Hydralazine	Vasodilation	Pre-eclampsia/ eclampsia	Reflex tachycardia	Aortic dissection	5–10 mg IV	5–15 min/ 3–8 hr
Enalapril	Angiotensin II production inhibition Vasodilation		Hyperkalaemia Renal impairment Hypotension in high renin states	Pregnancy Renal artery stenosis	1.25–5 mg PO every 6 hours	30 min/ 6 hr
Enalaprilat	Angiotensin II production inhibition Vasodilation		Hyperkalaemia, Renal impairment Potential hypotension in high renin states Headache Dizziness	Pregnancy	1.25–5 mg IV	15 min/ 4–6 hr

Drug	Action	Indications	Adverse effects	Contraindications	Dose	Onset/Duration
Fenoldopam	Dopamine-1 receptor agonist, Vasodilation, Renal arterial dilation and natriuresis		Reflex tachycardia, Nausea, Headache, Flushing, Increased intra-ocular pressure		0.1–0.6 µg/kg/min	5 min/ 10–15 min
Esmolol	Cardioselective β-blocker, Reduced heart rate, Reduced cardiac contractility	Aortic dissection (used in combination with an α-blocker), Postoperative hypertension	Heart failure, Heart block, Bronchospasm, Flushing, Nausea, Infusion site pain	Heart failure, Asthma/chronic obstructive pulmonary disease	200–500 µg/kg/min IV infusion for 4 minutes, then 150–300 µg/kg/min; 500 µg/kg loading dose over 1 minute, followed by infusion at 25–50 µg/kg/min, increase by 25 µg/kg/min every 10–20 minutes to a maximum of 300 µg/kg/min	1–2 min/ 10–20 min
Phantolamine	α_1-blocker, Vasodilation		Reflex tachycardia, Flushing, Headache, Nausea		5–15 mg IV, Maximum dose 15 mg	1–2 min/ 3–10 min
Labetalol	α_1, β-blocker, Vasodilation, Reduced heart rate, Reduced cardiac contractility	Aortic dissection	Heart failure, Heart block, Bronchospasm, Nausea, Dizziness, Paraesthesias	Heart failure, Asthma/chronic obstructive pulmonary disease	20–80 mg IV every 10 minutes, 0.5–2 mg/min IV infusion	5–10 min/ 3–6 hr
Clonidine	Central α_2-agonist		Sedation, Dry mouth, Bradycardia		0.1–0.2 mg PO hourly, to a maximum 0.8 mg in 24 hours	30–60 min/ 6–12 hr

Esmolol

- An ultra-short-acting cardioselective β-blocker with no vasodilatory effects.
- May be used in conjunction with nitroprusside for aortic dissection and with phentolamine for catecholamine crises.
- Contraindicated in patients with asthma, COLD, congestive cardiac failure, bradycardia, and atrioventricular block.
- Give IV 250–500 µg/kg/min boluses, then 50–100 µg/kg/min infusion; may repeat IV bolus after 5 minutes or increase infusion up to a maximum of 300 µg/kg/min.

Phentolamine

- A potent α_1-blocker.
- Generally used for catecholamine crises in conjunction with β-blockers.
- May cause tachycardia and orthostatic hypotension.
- Give IV 5–15 mg boluses.

Nitroglycerin

- A direct venodilator. It also causes some arterial vasodilation at high doses.
- Useful in **acute myocardial infarction/acute coronary syndrome** and **acute left ventricular failure**.
- Causes **reflex tachycardia** and increases **fluid shear stress**, and should be **avoided** in the treatment of aortic dissection, unless given concurrently with β-**blockers**.
- Other side effects include headache and vomiting. Thus, it may be of limited value in patients with hypertensive encephalopathy.
- IV infusion at 5–100 µg/min. Titrate to response.

Hydralazine

- A direct arteriolar vasodilator.
- Useful for acute blood pressure control in pre-eclampsia and eclampsia.
- Causes **reflex tachycardia**, and in some patients a lupus-like syndrome.
- Give IV 5–10 mg boluses q 15 minutes and titrate.

Nicardipine

- A second-generation dihydropyridine calcium channel blocker.
- Has strong cerebral and coronary vasodilatory effect, reduces afterload and increases cardiac output, and has been found to reduce myocardial and cerebral ischaemia.
- Contraindicated in heart failure.
- May cause reflex tachycardia and headache.

- Give IV 5–15 mg/hr infusion. Infusion rate may be increased by 2.5 mg/hr every 5 minutes to a maximum of 15 mg/hr, until desired blood pressure reduction is achieved, following which the infusion rate should be decreased by 3 mg/hr.

Fenoldopam

- A peripheral dopamine-1 receptor agonist, causing vasodilation, activating dopamine receptors in the kidney and increasing renal blood flow.
- May cause increased intra-ocular pressure.
- Lowers diastolic blood pressure.
- Give IV 0.1–0.6 µg/kg/min infusion.

Enalaprilat

- This is an intravenous ACE inhibitor.
- Avoid administration in patients with renal artery stenosis.
- May cause renal failure.
- Give IV 1.25–5 mg every 6 hours.

HYPERTENSIVE URGENCY

- The most common situation is a known hypertensive patient who has been non-compliant with his regular medications.
- There may be some non-specific symptoms such as headache and nausea, though one must be very careful not to miss a hypertensive emergency such as hypertensive encephalopathy in this situation.
- These symptoms are expected to resolve with treatment.
- Over-aggressive lowering of blood pressure in this group of patients may do more harm than good.
- The goal is to lower blood pressure gradually over a period of 24–48 hours to a target DBP of 100–110 mmHg.
- Oral medications are preferred over intravenous forms.
- The patient's own medications may be given if compliance is poor.

DRUG THERAPY FOR HYPERTENSIVE URGENCY

Many options are available, some of which are listed below:

- **Felodipine**: 2.5 mg orally, PO (age >65 years) or 5 mg PO (age <65 years)
- **Amlodipine**: 5–10 mg PO
- **Extended release nifedipine**: 30 mg PO

- **Captopril**: 12.5–25 mg PO
- **Labetalol**: 100–200 mg PO
- **Prazosin**: 1–2 mg PO
- **Clonidine** 0.1–0.2 mg PO (previous practice of clonidine loading has fallen out of favour)

Disposition

- *Hypertensive emergency*: Patients should be admitted to an intensive care unit in consultation with General Medicine and the respective subspecialities involved.
- *Hypertensive urgency*: Patients can be discharged **if** response is prompt and the blood pressure is acceptable after 4 hours of monitoring; however, follow-up must be arranged within 48 hours. In patients with newly diagnosed hypertension where the cause is uncertain, admit to General Medicine for evaluation and exclusion of secondary causes of hypertension.

References/Further Reading

1. Sixth Report of the Joint National Committee on Prevention, Detection, Evaluation, and Treatment of High Blood Pressure. *Arch Intern Med*. 1997; 157: 2413–2446.
2. Chobanian AV, Bakris GL, Black HR, et al. Seventh Report of the Joint National Committee on Prevention, Detection, Evaluation, and Treatment of High Blood Pressure. *JAMA*. 2003; 289: 2560–2572.
3. Chobanian AV, Bakris GL, Black HR, et al. Seventh Report of the Joint National Committee on Prevention, Detection, Evaluation, and Treatment of High Blood Pressure. (Complete Report). *Hypertension*. 2003; 42: 1206–1252.
4. Alderman MH. JNC 7: Brief summary and critique. *Clin Exp Hypertens*. 2004; 26: 753–761.
5. Varon J. The diagnosis and treatment of hypertensive crises. *Postgrad Med*. 2009; 121: 5–13.
6. Hebert CJ, Vidt DG. Hypertensive crises. *Prim Care*. 2008; 35: 475–487, vi.
7. Marik PE, Varon J. Hypertensive crises: Challenges and management. *Chest*. 2007; 131: 1949–1962.
8. Aggarwal M, Khan IA. Hypertensive crisis: Hypertensive emergencies and urgencies. *Cardiol Clin*. 2006; 24: 135–146.
9. Gilmore RM, Miller SJ, Stead LG. Severe hypertension in the emergency department patient. *Emerg Med Clin North Am*. 2005; 23: 1141–1158.
10. Blumenfeld JD, Laragh JH. Management of hypertensive crises: The scientific basis for treatment decisions *Am J Hypertens*. 2001; 14: 1154–1167.
11. Vaughan CJ, Delanty N. Hypertensive emergencies. *Lancet*. 2000; 356: 411–417.
12. Hypertensive crisis. How to tell if it's an emergency or an urgency. *Postgrad Medicine*. 1 May 1999; 105(5) 119–26, 130.
13. Gray RO. Hypertension. In: Marx J, Hockberger R, Walls R, eds. Rosen's *Emergency Medicine: Concepts and Clinical Practice*. 7th ed. Philadelphia, PA: Mosby-Elsevier; 2010: 1076–1087.
14. Wyatt JP, Illingworth RN, Graham CA, et al. *Oxford Handbook of Emergency Medicine*. 3rd ed. Oxford, UK: Oxford University Press; 2006: 92–93.
15. Pula JH, Eggenberger E. Posterior reversible encephalopathy syndrome. *Curr Opin Ophthalmol*. 2008; 19 479–484.

16 Bartynski WS. Posterior reversible encephalopathy syndrome. Part 1: Fundamental imaging and clinical features. *AJNR Am J Neuroradiol*. 2008; 29: 1036–1042.

17 Bartynski WS. Posterior reversible encephalopathy syndrome. Part 2: Controversies surrounding pathophysiology of vasogenic edema. *AJNR Am J Neuroradiol*. 2008; 29: 1043–1049.

18 Boehrer JD, Moliterno DJ, Willard JE, et al. Influence of labetalol on cocaine-induced coronary vasoconstriction in humans. *Am J Med*. 1993; 94: 608–610.

19 Guyton AC, Coleman TG, Cowley AV, et al. Arterial pressure regulation. Overriding dominance of the kidneys in long-term regulation and in hypertension. *Am J Med*. 1972; 52: 584–594.

20 James PA, Oparil S, Carter BL. 2014 evidence-based guideline in the management of high blood pressure in adults. Report from panel members appointed to the 8th Joint National Committee (JNC8). *JANA* 2014; 311(5): 507–520.

40 Acute Limb Ischaemia

Kuan Win Sen

CAVEAT

- Acute limb ischaemia is defined as a sudden decrease in limb perfusion that causes a potential threat to limb viability in patients who present within two weeks of the acute event.

AETIOLOGY

TABLE 1 Causes of acute arterial occlusion

Thrombosis	Embolus	Trauma
Vascular grafts	Cardiac source (atrial fibrillation, acute myocardial infarction, endocarditis, and prosthetic valves)	Blunt
Thrombosis of aneurysm	Arterial source (aneurysm)	Penetrating
Hypercoagulable state		
Low flow state		

- 80% of **emboli** are from a cardiac source. Emboli are typically lodged in an acute narrowing of the artery, e.g. atherosclerotic plaques and at the bifurcation points of blood vessels.
- Ischaemia from arterial **thrombosis** in underlying atherosclerosis is usually less severe than that following acute embolus. This is due to collateral circulation that has developed over time.
- Arterial **trauma** can be from iatrogenic causes (vascular/cardiac diagnostic and interventional procedures). Intimal flaps and dissection are frequently the cause of occlusion.

CLINICAL PRESENTATION

- The **6 Ps** of acute limb ischaemia are as follows:
  1. **Pain**: Sudden dramatic development consistent with embolus. Gradual increase in the symptoms consistent with chronic ischaemia.
  2. **Pallor**: The level of arterial obstruction is usually one joint above the line of demarcation between the normal and ischaemic tissue.
  3. **Poikilothermia**
  4. **Pulselessness**: Presence of pulse deficit in the asymptomatic *contralateral* extremity indicative of underlying chronic arterial occlusive disease. Conversely, the presence of a strong pulse in the asymptomatic contralateral extremity indicates that the underlying occlusion is acute.

5. **Paraesthesia**: Subjective sensory deficits suggest early nerve dysfunction. The anterior compartment of the lower leg is most sensitive to ischaemia. Sensory deficits over the dorsum of the foot are often the earliest neurologic sign of vascular insufficiency.

6. **Paralysis**

- In addition, the '**blue-toe syndrome**' can occur from small vessel occlusion.

   1. Appearance of a cool, painful, cyanotic toe, or forefoot in the presence of strong pedal pulses and a warm foot.

- Perform a focused **physical examination** to look for:

   1. Atrial fibrillation.

   2. Signs of **chronic peripheral vascular disease** (suggestive of thrombotic aetiology).

      a. Shiny hyperpigmentation of the skin

      b. Hair loss

      c. Muscle atrophy

      d. Skin ulceration

   3. Sensation and motor control.

   4. All peripheral pulses (use Doppler ultrasound if the patient does not have a palpable pulse).

- Clinical categories of acute limb ischaemia:

   1. **Viable**: No sensory loss or muscle weakness.

   2. **Marginally threatened** (salvageable if treated promptly): Minimal sensory loss (more distally), no muscle weakness, and arterial Doppler inaudible.

   3. **Immediately threatened** (salvageable with immediate revascularization): Sensory loss more proximal, rest pain, mild to moderate muscle weakness and arterial Doppler inaudible.

   4. **Irreversible**: Sensory loss and muscle weakness profound, possible rigour, arterial, and venous Doppler signals inaudible. Require amputation.

⇨ **SPECIAL TIPS FOR GPs**

- **Time** is **limb** and **life**.
- There is a window of approximately **6 hours** before **irreversible** neuromuscular damage to a limb occurs.
- The amputation rate is 6–20% whereas the mortality rate is 6–12%.
- Always consider limb ischaemia as a cause of limb pain or neurological deficit.

MANAGEMENT

- Manage the patient in a monitored care area.
- Emergency management:

   1. Aspirin.

2. Unfractionated heparin.

3. Dependent positioning.

4. Avoidance of extremes of temperature.

5. Analgesia.

- Provide oxygen.
- Perform ECG to look for atrial fibrillation.
- Order full blood count, renal panel, coagulation panel and type, and screen tests.
- Refer to the vascular surgeon promptly.
- Imaging: Use digital subtraction **angiography** as the gold standard for acute limb ischaemia (benefit of concurrently diagnosing and treating occlusion).
- Alternative:

  1. Use **duplex ultrasonography** if the patient is allergic to contrast agents or at high risk of contrast-induced nephropathy.

  2. Perform **computed tomography/magnetic resonance angiography** if an equivocal examination and no immediate intervention are needed.

- Treatment recommendation by the Seventh American College of Chest Physicians (ACCP) Consensus Conference on Antithrombotic Therapy and the 2007 TASC II Consensus:

  1. IV **heparin** followed by continuous infusion of heparin.

- Patients with threatened extremities should receive emergent surgical revascularization:

  1. **Endovascular intervention**: Intra-arterial thrombolysis and percutaneous thrombectomy

  2. **Surgery**: Open thrombectomy and bypass grafting

- Patients with non-viable extremities should undergo prompt amputation without imaging to reduce risk of infection, myoglobinuria, acute renal failure, hyperkalaemia, multi-organ failure, and cardiovascular collapse.

References/Further Reading

1. Norgren L, Hiatt WR, Dormandy JA, Nehler MR, Harris KA, Fowkes FG; TASC II Working Group. Inter-society consensus for the management of peripheral arterial disease (TASC II). *J Vasc Surg*. Jan 2007; 45(Suppl S): S5–67.

2. Lin M. Acute limb ischemia: What are the newest diagnostic treatment options? *American College of Emergency Physicians Scientific Assembly 2007*.

3. Hirsch AT, Haskal ZJ, Hertzer NR, et al. ACC/AHA 2005 Practice guidelines for the management of patients with peripheral arterial disease (lower extremity, renal, mesenteric, and abdominal aortic): A collaborative report from the American Association for Vascular Surgery/Society for Vascular Surgery, Society for Cardiovascular Angiography and Interventions, Society for Vascular Medicine and Biology, Society of Interventional Radiology, and the ACC/AHA Task Force on Practice Guidelines (Writing Committee to Develop Guidelines for the Management of Patients with Peripheral Arterial Disease): Endorsed by the American Association of Cardiovascular and Pulmonary Rehabilitation; National Heart, Lung, and Blood Institute; Society for Vascular Nursing; TransAtlantic Inter-Society Consensus; and Vascular Disease Foundation. *Circulation*. 2006; 113: e463.

41   Pulmonary Embolism

Shirley Ooi • Gene Chan

CAVEATS

- Thrombotic pulmonary embolism (PE) is not an isolated disease of the chest but a complication of venous thrombosis. Deep venous thrombosis (DVT) and PE are therefore part of the same process, venous thromboembolism.

- Leg DVT is found in 70% of patients with PE. Conversely, PE occurs in 50% of patients with proximal DVT of the legs (involving popliteal and/or more proximal veins), and is less likely when the thrombus is confined to the calf veins.

- As PE is preceded by DVT, the **factors predisposing** to the two conditions are the same and broadly fit Virchow's triad of venous stases, injury to the vein wall, and enhanced coagulability of the blood (Table 1).

NOTE: In **surgical series**, the risk of venous thromboembolism rises rapidly with age, length of anaesthesia and the presence of previous venous thromboembolism, or cancer. The incidence is highest in those undergoing emergency surgery (e.g. for hip fractures) following trauma and pelvic surgery. In **medical series**, venous thromboembolism is frequent in patients with cardiorespiratory disorders (e.g. congestive heart failure and irreversible airways disease), leg immobility (caused by stroke and other neurological disease), and cancer.

TABLE 1   Some common risk factors for venous thromboembolic disease

Flow stasis	Prolonged immobilization due to long journeys, a stroke, etc.
	Major trauma or surgery within 4 weeks
	Congestive heart failure
	Obesity
	Advanced age
	Spinal cord injuries
	Shock syndromes
Endothelial damage	Local trauma
	Surgery of legs and pelvis
	Vasculitis
	Burns
	Electric shock
	Infection
	Previous history of thromboembolism
Coagulation abnormalities	Polycythaemia
	Platelet abnormalities
	Oral contraceptive drugs with high estrogen content
	Malignant neoplasia
	Deficiency of antithrombin III, protein C or S

NOTE: The identification of risk factors not only aids in the clinical diagnosis of venous thromboembolism, but also guides decisions about prophylactic measures and repeat testing in borderline cases.

- **Case fatality rate** is <5% in treated patients who are haemodynamically stable at presentation but approximately 20% in those with persistent hypotension.
- **PE** can be **classified** into 3 main types as shown in Table 2.

TABLE 2   Clinical forms of pulmonary embolism

Pulmonary embolism	History	Vascular obstruction	Presentation
Acute minor	Short, sudden onset	<50%	Dyspnoea with or without pleuritic pain and haemoptysis
Acute massive	Short, sudden onset	>50%	Right heart strain with or without haemodynamic instability and syncope
Subacute massive	Several weeks	>50%	Dyspnoea with right heart strain

Notes:
1. Massive PE without hypoxaemia is so rare that if the arterial oxygen tension (PaO_2) is normal, an alternative diagnosis should be considered.
2. Although PE impairs the elimination of carbon dioxide, hypercapnia is rare.
3. A patient with massive PE is obviously dyspnoeic but **not orthopnoeic**.
4. The third and least common presentation, i.e. subacute massive PE, mimics heart failure or indolent pneumonia, especially in the elderly.
Source: Table adapted with permission from Riedel (2001), Table 3.

- Nearly all patients with PE will have **one or more** of the following **clinical features**:
  1. Dyspnoea of sudden onset
  2. Tachypnoea (>20 breaths/minute)
  3. Chest pain (pleuritic or substernal)

NOTE: If the clinician remembers these 3 features, the possibility of PE will rarely be overlooked. When these clinical features are associated with electrocardiogram (ECG) signs of right ventricular strain and/or radiologic signs of plump hilum, pulmonary infarction or oligaemia, the likelihood of PE is high. It is further strengthened in the presence of risk factors for venous thromboembolism and arterial hypoxaemia with hypocapnia. On the contrary, the absence of all these three clinical features virtually excludes the diagnosis of PE.

- Table 3 shows the estimation of the pretest clinical likelihood of PE.

NOTE: In patients with low pretest probability for PE, if the D-dimer ELISA (enzyme-linked immunosorbent assay) test is found to be negative, PE can be confidently excluded. In contrast, if D-dimer is found to be positive in patients with low pretest probability for PE, the patient should be reevaluated. A negative D-dimer test cannot be used confidently to exclude a PE in intermediate or high risk patients.

TABLE 3 Estimation of the (pretest) clinical likelihood of pulmonary embolism

High (>85% likely)	Otherwise unexplained sudden onset of dyspnoea, tachypnoea or chest pain and at least two of the following:
	Significant risk factor present (immobility, leg fracture, and major surgery)
	Fainting with new signs of right ventricular overload in ECG
	Signs of possible leg DVT (unilateral pain, tenderness, erythema, warmth, or swelling)
	Radiographic signs of infarction, plump hilum, or oligaemia
Intermediate (15–85% likely)	Neither high nor low clinical likelihood
Low (<15% likely)	Absence of sudden onset of dyspnoea, tachypnoea, and chest pain
	Dyspnoea, tachypnoea, or chest pain present but explainable by another condition
	Risk factors absent
	Radiographic abnormality explainable by another condition
	Adequate anticoagulation control (international normalized ratio >2 or activated partial thromboplastin time >1.5 times) during the previous week

Source: Table reproduced with permission from Riedel (2001), Table 4.

⇨ **SPECIAL TIPS FOR GPs**

- Remember that PE is one of the 6 life-threatening causes of chest pain!
- Clinical features of PE are deceivingly non-specific, but PE is highly unlikely in the absence of all of the following: dyspnoea, tachypnoea, and chest pain.
- Do not rely on the clinical triad of pleuritic chest pain, dyspnoea, and haemoptysis as they are rarely found.
- When an ECG is done for chest pain and T-wave inversion is seen in lead III, look for the presence of S1Q3T3 and the other associated ECG features of PE.

MANAGEMENT

In cases of massive PE with signs of haemodynamic instability:

- Monitor the patient's vital signs in the critical care area.
- Give **oxygen** via a non-rebreather mask or intubate if unable to maintain oxygenation.

NOTE: Intubation may cause the haemodynamic situation to deteriorate further by impeding venous return.

- Set up 2 **large bore intravenous (IV) lines** and send blood for investigation. Start fluid resuscitation.

NOTE: When thrombolytic treatment is considered, the antecubital route should be preferred and insertion of arterial lines avoided.

- If blood pressure is still low despite fluid resuscitations, start **inotropes**.

NOTE: Inotropes may do no more than precipitate dysrhythmias when the cardiac output is reduced, the dilated right ventricle is hypoxic and already near maximal stimulation from the high concentration of endogenous catecholamines. The judicious use of IV noradrenaline titrated against a moderate increase in blood pressure may be beneficial.

- Give **pain relief**.

NOTE: Opiates should be used with caution in the hypotensive patient.

- Contact the cardiothoracic registrar-on-call for admission to the cardiothoracic intensive care unit.

General emergency investigations
- **ECG** findings in PE:
  1. ECG changes are usually non-specific.
  2. The commonest ECG change is **T-wave inversion** in the anteroseptal and inferior leads found in 68% of patients with PE. The number of inverted T-waves in the anterior and inferior distribution increase with severity of right heart strain, cor pulmonale, and resulting subepicardial ischaemia, and predicts early complication from PE. Reversal of T-wave before the 6th day is associated with a more favourable outcome.
  3. In minor PE, there is no haemodynamic stress and, thus, the only finding is sinus tachycardia.
  4. In acute or subacute massive PE, evidence of **right heart strain** may be seen:
     a. Rightward shift of the QRS axis.
     b. Transient right bundle branch block.
     c. T-wave inversion in leads V_{1-3}.
     d. P pulmonale
     e. Classical $S_1Q_3T_3$ (only present in 12% of massive PE)
  5. Normal ECG in 6% of massive PE.
  6. The main value of ECG is in excluding other potential diagnoses, such as myocardial infarction or pericarditis. Refer to Figure 1 for the ECG in PE.

- **Arterial blood gas**: The characteristic changes are a **reduced PaO_2 and a $PaCO_2$ that is normal or reduced** because of hyperventilation. The PaO_2 is almost never normal in massive PE but can be normal in minor PE, mainly due to hyperventilation. In such cases, the widening of the alveolo-arterial PO_2 gradient ($AaPO_2$ >20 mmHg) may be more sensitive than PaO_2 alone. (For further details, refer to Chapter 57, *Acid Base Emergencies* and Chapter 143, *Useful Formulae*). Both hypoxaemia and a wide $AaPO_2$ may obviously be due to many other causes. Blood gases, therefore, may heighten the suspicion of PE, but are of insufficient discriminant value to permit proof or exclusion of PE. Note the patient's fraction of inspired oxygen (FiO_2) at the time of blood sampling.

- Full blood count.

- Urea/electrolytes/creatinine.

- The **D-dimer** ELISA test has a sensitivity of 85–94% for diagnosing pulmonary embolism. However, its specificity is only 67–68%. A normal D-dimer ELISA test result is useful in excluding PE in patients with a low pretest probability of PE or a non-diagnostic lung scan. However, an abnormal result (however high) does not imply significantly increased probability of PE.

- GXM 4 to 6 units of packed red blood cells.

- **Chest X-ray** findings in PE:

  1. In general, the chest X-ray (CXR) is not specific or diagnostic in PE, but comparison with previous films may be helpful.

  NOTE: The main benefit of CXR is to rule out other conditions mimicking PE (e.g. pneumothorax, pneumonia, left heart failure, tumour, rib fracture, massive pleural effusion, and lobar collapse), but PE may coexist with other cardiopulmonary processes.

  2. The **findings** may show the following:
     a. Normal CXR (~40%).

NOTE: A normal film is compatible with all types of acute PE. In fact, a normal film in a patient with severe acute dyspnoea without wheezing is very suspicious of PE.

     b. **Fleischner sign** (distended central pulmonary artery due to the presence of a large clot)
     c. Evidence of pulmonary infarction: Peripheral opacities, sometimes wedge-shaped with the apex pointing towards the hilum or semicircular, with its base against the pleural surface (**Hampton's hump**).
     d. Focal pulmonary oligaemia in the parts of the lung affected by emboli (**Westermark sign**) but this is difficult to diagnose on the type of film usually available in the acute situation.
     e. Long bands of focal atelectasis seen in pulmonary infarction (**Fleischner lines**).
     f. Small pleural effusions.
     g. Raised hemidiaphragm.

FIGURE 1   ECG of a 71-year-old man who presented with right-sided chest discomfort, dyspnoea, and coughing

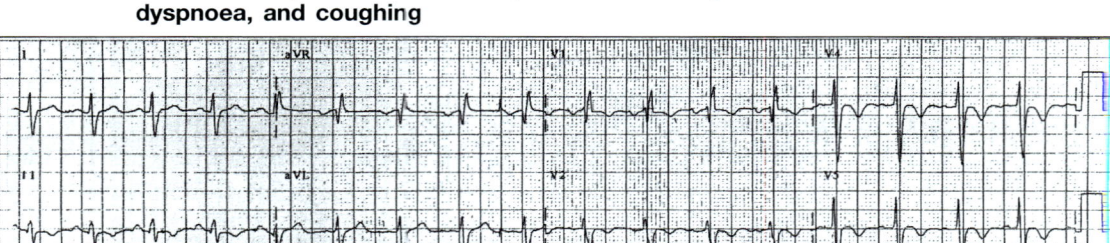

Figure 1 shows the ECG of a 71-year-old man who presented with right sided chest discomfort, dyspnoea and coughing. A spiral computed tomography scan confirmed pulmonary embolism. Note the following ECG changes: Sinus tachycardia, $S_1Q_3T_3$, right axis deviation, right bundle branch block (RBBB), T inversion in V_{1-5} and P pulmonale.

NOTE: Aletectas, small pleural effusions and raised diaphragm have low specificity for PE.

    h. Localized infiltrate.

    i. Consolidation.

Venous Compression Ultrasonography (CUS)

- CUS of the lower extremities is another diagnostic tool utilized to increase or decrease suspicion for PE in certain situations.
- Single CUS had a sensitivity of only 54%, a specificity of 97. A **single CUS should not be used to rule out PE**, particularly when the test results are discordant with the clinical assessment of risk. For these reasons, follow-up CUS examinations are obtained approximately 5 to 7 days later to assess for clot progression.

Bedside Cardiac Echocardiography

- With the increase in emergency physician-performed bedside ultrasonography, focused bedside cardiac echocardiography is becoming an important tool in the assessment of the patient with possible PE.
- The role of ultrasound in patients with suspected pulmonary embolus is to prioritize further testing, assess the differential diagnosis, and assist with treatment decisions for haemodynamically significant emboli in the severely compromised patient.

- In an acute massive (haemodynamically significant) or submassive (haemodynamically stable with enlargement of the right ventricle) pulmonary embolus, the **right ventricle can be dilated** and have reduced function or contractility.

- In patients with haemodynamically significant pulmonary embolus, the left ventricle can be underfilled and hyperdynamic.

- The presence of right ventricular enlargement and dysfunction in patients with pulmonary embolus is prognostically important and associated with significantly higher inhospital mortality. It is also one of the best predictors of poor early outcome.

Definitive investigations

- **Computed Tomographic Pulmonary Angiography (CTPA)**

  1. CTPA has become the primary radiologic study ordered for evaluation of PE.

  2. Although CTPA alone does detect the majority of PE, it is not sensitive enough to detect all subsegmental PE. However, subsegmental PE does not confer the same risk to the patient as larger clots.

  3. The main **advantage** of PE is that the imaging of lung parenchyma and great vessels is possible (e.g. pulmonary mass, pneumonia, emphysema, pleural effusion, and mediastinal adenopathy) and diagnosis can be made if PE is absent. Hence, CTPA can help in diagnosing alternative causes of dyspnoea. CTPA can also detect right ventricular dilatation, thus indicating severe, potentially fatal PE.

  4. Main disadvantages of CTPA.

     a. Exposure to radiation of 15 mSv (equivalent to approximately 150 2-view CXRS)

     b. Adverse reactions to iodinated intravenous contrast media.

        i. development of anaphylaxis or other systemic allergic reaction.

        ii. contrast-induced nephropathy

- **Lung scintigraphy**

  1. A normal perfusion scan essentially excludes the diagnosis of a clinically relevant recent PE because occlusive PE of all types produces a defect of perfusion.

  2. However, many conditions other than PE, such as tumours, consolidation, left heart failure, bullous lesions, lung fibrosis, and obstructive airway disease, can also produce perfusion defects.

  3. PE usually produces a defect of perfusion but not ventilation ('mismatch') while most of the other conditions produce a ventilation defect in the same area as the perfusion defect (matched defects).

  4. The probability that perfusion defects are caused by PE can be assessed as high, intermediate, or low depending on the type of scan abnormality (Table 4).

TABLE 4 **Probability of underlying pulmonary embolism according to the criteria of the PIOPED* study**

Clinical likelihood	Scan probability (%)			
	Normal/very low	Non-diagnostic		
		Low	Intermediate	High
Low	2	4	16	56
Intermediate	6	16	28	88
High	0	40	66	96

Note: *Prospective Investigation of Pulmonary Embolism Diagnosis study.
Table reproduced with permission from Riedel (2001), Table 5.

Suspected PE

- Start IV heparin 5000 U bolus or SC fraxiparine 0.4 ml for patients weighing less than 50 kg, 0.5 ml for those weighing between 50 and 60 kg, and 0.6 ml for those heavier than 65 kg.
- Investigate.
- Contact the general medical or respiratory medical registrar.
- Admit the patient to Respiratory Medicine.

References/Further Reading

1. Riedel M. Acute pulmonary embolism 1: Pathophysiology, clinical presentation, and diagnosis. *Heart.* 2001; 85: 229–240.

2. Riedel M. Acute pulmonary embolism 2: Treatment. *Heart.* 2001; 85: 351–360.

3. Kline JA, Israel EG. Diagnostic accuracy of a bedside D-dimer assay and alveolar dead-space measurement for rapid exclusion of pulmonary embolism: A multi-center study. *JAMA.* 2001; 14: 285: 761–768.

4. Ginsberg JS, Wells PS, Kearon C, et al. Sensitivity and specificity of a rapid whole-blood assay for D-dimer in the diagnosis of pulmonary embolism. *Ann Intern Med.* 1998; 129: 1006–1011.

5. Lim TK. Non-invasive tests for acute pulmonary embolism: What are the real advances? *Singapore Med J.* 2001; 42(10): 446–449.

6. Brown MD, Rowe BH, Reeves M. The accuracy of the enzyme-linked immunosorbent assay D-dimer test in the diagnosis of pulmonary embolism: A meta-analysis. *Ann Emerg Med.* 2002; 40(2): 133–144.

7. Church A, Tichauer M. The emergency medicine approach to the evaluation and treatment of pulmonary embolism, *Emergency Medicine Practice*, Dec 2012; vol 14, no. 12.

42   Venous Emergencies

Kuan Win Sen

CAVEATS

- Venous conditions warranting assessment in the emergency department include infection, inflammation, and/or thrombosis of the vein, both deep and superficial.
- The concept of **Virchow's triad** is important in understanding the pathogenesis of venous thromboembolism:
    1. Venous stasis
    2. Vascular endothelial injury
    3. Hypercoagulable state (inherited or acquired)
- Life-threatening conditions like pulmonary embolism may be preceded by deep vein thrombosis of the lower limbs. Other venous emergencies include superior vena cava syndrome and superficial phlebitis/thrombophlebitis.

> ⇨ **SPECIAL TIPS FOR GPs**
> - In up to 60% of patients, **superior vena cava (SVC) obstruction** may be the first presentation of an underlying **malignancy**.
> - Superficial thrombophlebitis of the lower extremity may progress to deep vein or deep venous thrombosis (DVT) and subsequently pulmonary embolism if left untreated especially in deep proximal lower limb veins.
> - There may not necessarily be a correlation between the location of symptoms and the site of thrombosis in patients with DVT, therefore a high index of suspicion is required especially in patients with risk factors for developing DVT.
> - Suspect **IV drug abuse** in thrombophlebitis affecting unusual sites especially in the presence of multiple hyperpigmented sites over the limbs.

Deep Venous Thrombosis

- **Clinical features**
    1. Oedema, principally **unilateral**.
    2. Leg pain occurs in 50% of patients, but this is entirely non-specific.
    3. Tenderness occurs in 75% of patients but is also found in 50% of patients without objectively confirmed DVT.
    4. Fullness of the lower limb that increases with standing or walking.
    5. Pain in the lower extremities on coughing or sneezing which is different from the electric-type pain with cough or sneeze associated with sciatica.

6. The affected limb is often warmer than the normal side.

7. Palpable 'cords' which are very specific, although insensitive for thrombosis.

- Risk factors for DVT include age, obesity, inactivity, history of thrombosis and medical conditions such as heart failure and cancer (refer to Chapter 41, *Pulmonary Embolism*).

- DVT is usually unilateral unless vena cava occludes, a rare and catastrophic event.

    1. *Phlegmasia cerulea dolens* is an uncommon form of massive proximal venous thrombosis of the lower extremities and carries a high morbidity often leading to circulatory collapse and shock.

- DVT usually occurs over several days. A sudden, severe pain is more likely due to muscle strain/tear or a **popliteal (Baker's) cyst rupture**.

- A combination of clinical signs and symptoms that include tenderness, swelling, redness, and the assessment of **Homan's sign** (pain in the posterior calf or knee on forced dorsiflexion of the foot) cannot adequately differentiate patients with or without DVT as more than 50% of patients without DVT may exhibit a positive Homan's sign.

- DVT is **unlikely** to be the cause if body temperature **is >39°C**.

- A lack of discrepancy in calf size does not rule out DVT. However, **asymmetric calf swelling of >3 cm** is almost always a significant finding in DVT.

- A meta-analysis in 2005 concluded the following:

    1. Only a difference in calf diameters is of potential value for ruling in DVT (likelihood ratio [LR] 1.8; 95% confidence interval [CI] 1.5–2.2).

    2. Only the absence of calf swelling (LR 0.67; 95% CI 0.58–0.78) and absence of difference in calf diameters (LR 0.57; 95% CI 0.44–0.72) are of potential value for ruling out DVT.

TABLE 1   Modified Wells score*

Clinical characteristic	Score
Active cancer (receiving treatment ≤6 months or currently on palliative treatment)	1
Paralysis, paresis or recent plaster immobilization of lower extremities	1
Recently bedridden for at least 3 days or have had major surgery within 12 weeks (GA/RA**)	1
Localized tenderness along distribution of deep venous system	1
Entire leg swollen	1
Calf swelling at least 3 cm larger than asymptomatic side (measured 10 cm below tibial tuberosity)	1
Pitting oedema confined to symptomatic leg	1
Collateral superficial veins (non-varicose)	1
Previously documented DVT	1
Alternative diagnosis at least as likely as DVT	–2

Notes: *A score of ≥2 indicates likely probability of DVT.
         **GA: General anaesthesia; RA: Regional anaesthesia.

TABLE 2   Hamilton score*

Clinical characteristics	Score
Plaster immobilization of the lower limb	2
Active malignancy (≤6 months or current)	2
Strong clinical suspicion of DVT by emergency department physicians with no other diagnostic possibilities	2
Bed rest (>3 days) or recent surgery (<4 weeks)	1
Male sex	1
Difference in calf circumference >3 cm on the affected side (10 cm below tibial tuberosity)	1
Erythema	1

Note: *A score of 3 or more indicates likely probability of DVT.

- **Clinical prediction rules for DVT**: Modified Wells and Hamilton scores have similar performance characteristics.
- **Compression ultrasonography** is the non-invasive approach of choice for diagnosis of symptomatic patients with a first episode of suspected DVT.
- A **D-dimer** test can be used to rule out DVT (the D-dimer has a sensitivity of ~98.5% for proximal DVTs).
  1. A negative D-dimer in conjunction with a low **pretest** clinical probability by the modified Wells or Hamilton scores may be useful in excluding DVT without the need for ultrasound testing.
  2. A negative result does exclude the possibility of a distal DVT.
  3. The test may not be suitable for the exclusion of DVT or PE when the patient has been presenting symptoms for more than seven days.
  4. False negative results may occasionally arise, and the level of clinical suspicion must be taken into account when evaluating the test result.
  5. A drawback of all D-dimer methods is low specificity for the diagnosis of venous thromboembolism.
  6. Causes of **false positive results** include **infection**, **malignancy**, recent **surgery**, and **trauma**. Thus, while a **negative result** is **useful in ruling out venous thromboembolism**, a positive result is not useful for confirming the diagnosis.
- **Treatment:** Anti-coagulant therapy is indicated for patients with symptomatic proximal DVT as pulmonary embolism will occur in about 50% of untreated patients within days or weeks of the event.
  1. IV **heparin** 80 U/kg bolus followed by 18 U/kg/hr maintenance infusion
  2. **Lower molecular weight heparin** (e.g. SC enoxaparin 0.1 mg/kg bd)
  3. SC fondaparinux (inhibits factor Xa)

- **Other treatment modalities**
  1. Consultation with the interventional radiologist for catheter-directed intrathrombus thrombolysis in patients with ileofemoral DVT.
  2. Thrombectomy is reserved for patients with massive ileofemoral vein thrombosis with vascular compromise when thrombolysis is contraindicated.

Pulmonary Embolism

This is the sudden blockage of one or more arteries in the lung. For more details, refer to Chapter 41, *Pulmonary Embolism*.

Superior Vena Cava Syndrome

- This is the obstruction of blood flow in the superior vena cava (SVC) either from invasion or external compression of the SVC.
- **Causes**
  1. Malignancy (lung cancer and lymphoma account for 95% of the cases) is the most common cause of SVC syndrome.
  2. Thoracic aortic aneurysms.
  3. Iatrogenic causes (indwelling central venous devices, dialysis access, and pacemaker leads may cause thrombosis).

Clinical presentation

- **Symptoms**
  1. Dyspnoea.
  2. Headache and giddiness.
  3. Facial swelling, especially when bending forward or lying down.
  4. Upper limb swelling.
  5. Chest pain.
  6. Dysphagia.
- **Signs**
  1. Facial oedema/plethora.
  2. Venous distension of the neck, chest wall, and upper limbs, especially when the patient raises the upper limbs.
     a. **Pemberton's manoeuvre** (patient raises both arms above the head vertically for 60 seconds, which exacerbates obstructive symptoms by decreasing the thoracic inlet area).
  3. Cyanosis.
  4. Horner's syndrome, paralysis of the vocal cords, and paralysis of the phrenic nerve are rare.

- **Investigations**
  1. A **CXR** will provide clues as to the cause of the obstruction if it is from an external compression. Up to 84% of CXRs are abnormal in one series. The most common findings are **mediastinal widening** and **pleural effusion**.
  2. Thoracic computed tomography, venography, or magnetic resonance imaging may also be used.
- **Treatment goals**: Treat the underlying condition and palliate the symptoms:
  1. Manage the patient in the **resuscitation** area.
  2. Give high flow **oxygen** and with the patient in an **upright** position.
  3. Administer IV **dexamethasone** 4 to 8 mg stat.
  4. Only consider diuretics in the presence of cerebral or airway oedema as their routine use in the emergency department has not shown consistent benefit.
  5. Endotracheal intubation and mechanical ventilation may be necessary if the patient develops signs of impending airway compromise.
  6. In malignant causes, the primary aim is to treat the malignant process.
  7. **Emergency radiotherapy** is no longer recommended except when the patient presents with **stridor** due to central airway obstruction or severe laryngeal oedema.
  8. Consider consultation with the vascular surgeon for iatrogenic causes of SVC syndrome for stenting.

Superficial Phlebitis

- This is due to inflammation, infection, and/or thrombosis in a superficial vein.
- The **superficial femoral vein** is a **deep vein** and evidence of thrombophlebitis in it will require treatment for DVT.

Clinical presentation

- Tenderness, pain and erythema along a superficial vein.
- Palpable **cord** with warmth and surrounding erythema.
- Suspicion of a thrombus arises when the palpable cord persists after lifting the limb against gravity.
- Low grade **fever** may accompany an uncomplicated superficial phlebitis but a high fever and the presence of **purulent** discharge suggest a **septic thrombophlebitis**.
- A cord may be palpable for weeks to months after an episode of superficial phlebitis.

Predisposing conditions

- Disruption in Virchow's triad.
- Infection (bacterial pathogens: *Staphylococcus aureus, Staphylococcus epidermidis, Enterobacteriaceae, Pseudomonas aeruginosa, and Enterococci*).

- IV cannulation (patient with burns or are immuno-compromised).
- IV drug abuse (especially intravenous buprenorphine and midazolam locally).
- Use of oral contraceptives or hormone replacement therapy.
- IV medications (**potassium chloride**, **calcium chloride/gluconate**, and hypertonic solutions, e.g. **dextrose 50%**).

Association with DVT

- Superficial venous thrombosis may occur together with DVT due to direct extension of the thrombus.
- The risk of progression to DVT is greater if the superficial thrombosis is present in the proximal greater saphenous vein or the saphenous-femoral junction.
- Upper extremity superficial thrombophlebitis is unlikely to lead to DVT.

Imaging

- **Compression ultrasound** is the modality of choice for confirmation of the diagnosis of DVT especially in occult cases.

Treatment

- Remove the IV cannula if thrombophlebitis occurs in the setting of an IV catheter.
- Treat uncomplicated superficial phlebitis with heat, elevation, and non-steroidal anti-inflammatory drugs. Compression stockings are also useful.
- The use of low molecular weight heparin has been advocated by some for lower extremity superficial thrombophlebitis.
- Administer IV antibiotics (from another IV site) if there are signs of cellulitis.
- Administer IV antibiotics and perform surgical drainage in the presence of suppurative thrombophlebitis.

References/Further Reading

1. Goodacre S, Sutton AJ, Sampson FC. Meta-analysis: The value of clinical assessment in the diagnosis of deep venous thrombosis. *Ann Intern Med.* 2005; 143: 129.

2. Subramaniam RM, Snyder B, Heath R, et al. Diagnosis of lower limb deep venous thrombosis in emergency department patients: Performance of Hamilton and modified Wells scores. *Ann Emerg Med.* Dec 2006; 48(6): 678–685.

3. Wilson LD, Detterbeck FC, Yahalom J. Clinical practice. Superior vena cava syndrome with malignant causes. *N Engl J Med.* 2007; 356: 1862.

4. Rice TW, Rodriguez RM, Light RW. The superior vena cava syndrome: Clinical characteristics and evolving etiology. *Medicine (Baltimore).* 2006; 85: 37.

5. Di Nisio M, Wichers I, Middledorp S. Treatment for superficial thrombophlebitis of the leg. *Cochrane Database Syst Rev.* 2007: CD004982.

Benjamin Leong • Shirley Ooi

CAVEATS

- The peri-arrest arrhythmias in **Advanced Cardiac Life Support** (ACLS) are divided into the tachycardias and bradycardias.
- This section covers the **tachycardias** and the algorithmic approach to their management.
- For the diagnostic approach, refer to Chapter 18, *Palpitations* for more details.
- International resuscitation guidelines are reviewed and revised every 5 years by the **International Liaison Committee on Resuscitation** (ILCOR).
- In Singapore, the **National Resuscitation Council** (NRC) reviews and issues the Resuscitation Guidelines in the light of these revisions.
- At the time of writing, the last ILCOR guideline revision was in **2010**, followed by the NRC guidelines in **2011**.

> ⇨ **SPECIAL TIPS FOR GPs**
> - Patients with palpitations should be assessed carefully for serious signs and symptoms of instability and by a 12-lead ECG.
> - Refer all unstable patients to the emergency department immediately via ambulance.

Management Algorithms

NOTE: Based on the Singapore National Resuscitation Council 2011 Guidelines and ILCOR 2010 Resuscitation Guidelines. Where there are differences, the NRC guidelines are given precedence here.

- Note that the following section describes the ACLS tachycardia algorithms as delivered by a single healthcare provider.
- In an emergency department where teams are organized to attend to critically ill patients, many of the activities should be performed concurrently, but the sequences described here should be a guide for the priority of actions to be undertaken.
- With the continuing emergence of new evidence, these algorithms will be updated and revised.
- Successful completion of an ACLS provider course will also equip the provider with practical skills not covered in this section.
- **There have been no major changes** in the 2011 guidelines for the management of tachydysrhythmias.

Universal algorithm

- The initial response to a patient with tachycardia begins with the **universal algorithm** (Figure 1).
- **Assess responsiveness:** If the patient is unresponsive, (see Chapter 30 *Cardiac Arrest Algorithms*).

FIGURE 1   **Management approach to tachydysrhythmias**

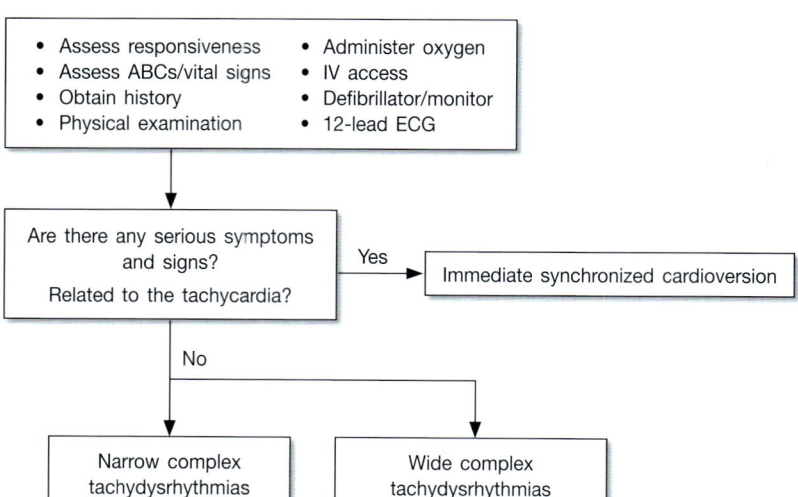

ABCD survey

- Assess, clear, and support the **airway, breathing, and circulation (ABCs)**.
- Give **supplemental oxygen**.
- Establish **intravenous access**.
- Attach **defibrillator/ECG monitor** once available and **assess rhythm**.
- Tachycardia is defined as any heart rate >100 beats per minute.
- Wide complex: QRS complex is >120 ms in duration.
- Narrow complex: QRS complex is <120 ms in duration.
- Assess **vital signs**, brief targeted **history**, and **physical examination**.
- Obtain a **12-lead ECG** when available.
- Look for **serious signs or symptoms** that are *associated with tachydysrhythmias*:
  1. **Chest pain**
  2. **Breathlessness**
  3. **Altered mental status**
  4. Systolic blood pressure of **<90 mmHg** and clinical features of **shock**
  5. Clinical features of **heart failure**

     NOTE: Tachydysrhythmias with rates of **<150 beats per minute** are unlikely to cause serious signs and symptoms in the *healthy heart*, though patients with significant myocardial dysfunction or comorbidities may be symptomatic at lower heart rates.
- If **serious signs and symptoms are present** and attributable to the tachydysrhythmia, prepare for **synchronized cardioversion** (Box 1).

NOTE: Sinus tachycardia **should not** be cardioverted.

- If there are no **serious signs and symptoms** it is recommended that further treatment options await expert consultation because treatment has the potential for harm (see the *Narrow* and *Wide Complex Tachydysrhythmias* sections in this chapter).

BOX 1   Procedure for synchronized cardioversion

NOTE: Tachydysrhythmias with rates of <150 beats/min rarely need cardioversion.

1. **Explain the procedure** to the patient.
2. **Administer IV sedation** and **analgesia, preoxygenate** the patient.
3. Apply **gel pads** or **self-adhesive defibrillator pads** to the patient.
4. Ensure **synchronizer** ('sync') is ON.
   a. This will time the delivery of the shock to the R wave of the QRS complex, so as to avoid shock delivery during the 'vulnerable period' when ventricular fibrillation may be triggered.
   b. **Check for 'sync' markers** above the R wave. If the 'sync' is on but there are no markers, the rhythm is too irregular for the defibrillator to synchronize the shock.

   NOTE: If cardioversion is necessary but it is impossible to synchronize the shock due to an irregular rhythm, use high energy (defibrillation dose) *unsynchronized* shocks.

      i. Low energy unsynchronized shocks are more likely to induce ventricular fibrillation.
5. Select the appropriate energy level and charge the defibrillator.
   a. **Wide complex tachydysrhythmia**
      i. 100 J, 150 J, 200 J, 300 J, and 360 J
   b. **Narrow complex tachydysrhythmia** (supraventricular tachycardia or atrial fibrillation)
      i. 50 J, 100 J, 150 J, 200 J, 300 J, and 360 J
6. Ensure all personnel are '**clear**' of the patient.
7. **Re-confirm** rhythm.
8. **Deliver shock.**
   a. Note that there is a brief moment before the synchronized shock is delivered.
   b. If using **defibrillator paddles**, hold on to the triggers and maintain pressure on the paddles until the shock is delivered.
   c. If using **self-adhesive defibrillation pads** and pressing a button on the defibrillator to shock, note that some models may require the operator to press and hold until the synchronized shock is delivered.
9. **Reassess the patient and rhythm.**
   a. If the rhythm has converted to sinus, reassess the airway, breathing and circulation, and obtain a 12-lead ECG.
   b. If the rhythm has not converted, escalate the energy levels and repeat shock.
   c. If the patient has become pulseless, commence cardiopulmonary resuscitation (CPR) immediately, and proceed according to the cardiac arrest universal algorithm (Chapter 30, *Cardiac Arrest Algorithms*).
   d. If rhythm has become VF, perform immediate defibrillation, and proceed according to VF protocol (see Chapter 30, *Cardiac Arrest Algorithms*)

NARROW COMPLEX TACHYDYSRHYTHMIAS

- **Narrow complex tachydysrhythmias** (QRS <120 ms) may be divided into **regular** or **irregular** (Figure 2).
- Causes of **regular narrow complex tachydysrhythmias**:
  1. Sinus tachycardia
  2. Paroxysmal supraventricular tachycardia (PSVT)
     a. AV nodal re-entrant tachycardia (AVNRT), the most common type of re-entrant supraventricular tachycardia
     b. AV re-entrant tachycardia (AVRT), which is associated with Wolff-Parkinson-White (WPW) syndrome
  3. Atrial flutter with regular atrioventricular conduction (e.g. 2:1)

FIGURE 2   **Narrow complex tachydysrhythmias (with a pulse)**

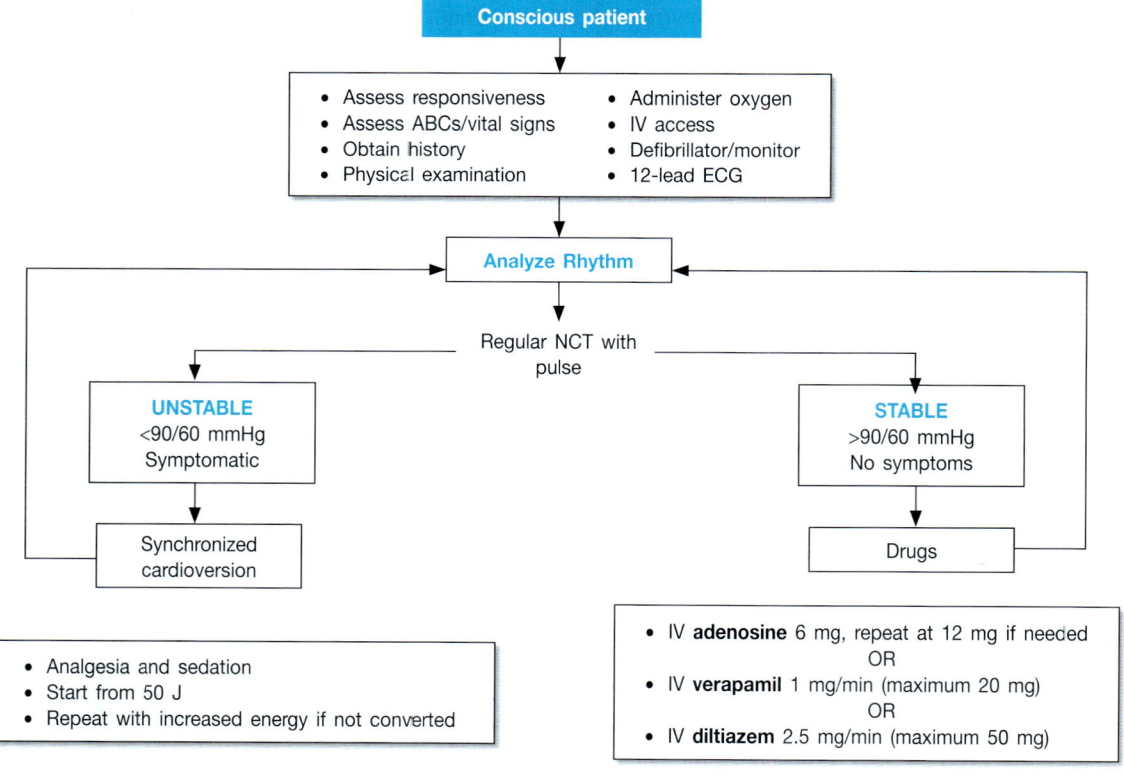

- Causes of **irregular narrow complex tachydysrhythmias**:
  1. Atrial fibrillation (AF) is the most common
  2. Atrial flutter with variable block
  3. Multifocal atrial tachycardia (MAT)

Paroxysmal supraventricular tachycardia (PSVT)

- **Non-pharmacological methods (vagal manoeuvres)** should be the first line of treatment for stable PSVT, and properly performed, should convert 20–25% of cases.
- The 2 most common techniques are the **Valsalva manoeuvre** (Box 2A) and **carotid sinus massage** (Box 2B).
- If vagal manoeuvres are unsuccessful, proceed to **chemical cardioversion**.
- The main drug options are **adenosine, verapamil**, and **diltiazem**.
- Before attempting chemical cardioversion with any of these drugs, beware of a suspected **atrial fibrillation with Wolff-Parkinson-White (WPW) syndrome** (see **Note** under Atrial Fibrillation).
- In these cases the heart rate may be so rapid as to *appear* regular. However, the QRS complexes will exhibit varying morphologies (narrow and/or wide), whereas in PSVT, the QRS complexes should be monomorphic.
- Depending on availability and experience, either of these drugs may be used as a first line, and if conversion is unsuccessful, the other one is to be used next.
- **Adenosine** is given as a rapid bolus followed by a 20 ml saline flush in a proximal vein (Box 3).
- **Verapamil** is given as a constant infusion at 1 mg/min IV, up to a maximum of 20 mg. **Diltiazem** is given at 2.5 mg/min up to 50 mg. Stop the infusion when the rhythm converts to sinus.
- Should the patient become **unstable** at anytime, **synchronized electrical cardioversion** (Box 1 and Figure 3) should be performed without delay.
- **Once conversion has taken place**, recheck the **vital signs** and record a 12-lead **ECG**.
- Look for a **delta wave** on the ECG in WPW.
- **ST depressions** may also occur in what is known as the 'post-tachycardia syndrome'.
- There is no utility for *routine* cardiac biomarkers in the management of most cases of PSVT.
- Most patients may be discharged after a **2-hour monitoring period**, if they remain haemodynamically stable and exhibit no ECG changes.
- **Most patients do not require anti-arrhythmic medications** on discharge until reviewed by Cardiology, though patients with frequent episodes despite being already on anti-arrhythmic medications should be reviewed by a cardiologist early for more definitive treatment such as electrophysiological studies with radio frequency ablation.

BOX 2A   Vagal manoeuvre – Valsalva manoeuvre

1. **Explain the procedure** to the patient.
2. The **supine position** is preferred.
3. Possible **techniques** include these:
   a. Having the patient blow into a tube leading to a **manometer** and maintaining a pressure of **40 mmHg** at least.
   b. Having the patient blow into a **20 ml syringe** to push the plunger out.
   c. Having the patient blow against a **closed glottis** like straining to have a bowel movement.
4. Have the patient **maintain** the Valsalva manoeuvre for about **30 seconds**.
   a. The **heart rate** will **increase** above the supraventricular tachycardia rate during this period, as a compensatory response to the reduced venous return due to the increased intra-thoracic pressure.
   b. Allow the patient to **release the strain** after about 30 seconds.
   c. Immediately after the release of the intra-thoracic pressure, due to the **sudden return of blood** to the heart (which is still beating fast at this point), there will be an **overshoot response** of blood pressure.
   d. The sudden increase in blood pressure will trigger a **reflex bradycardia. Conversion**, if successful, will take place at this time.
5. The effectiveness of the Valsalva manoeuvre is affected by patients with autonomic dysfunction.

BOX 2B   Vagal manoeuvre – Carotid sinus massage

1. Do not perform in the elderly due to possible underlying **atherosclerotic disease** and **risk of stroke**.
2. **Auscultate for carotid bruits** – do not proceed if present.
3. **Explain the procedure** to the patient.
4. **Record ECG lead** during the procedure.
5. Position the patient in the **Trendelenburg position** to distend carotid sinuses, with the head turned to one side.
   a. Some references describe carotid sinus massage (CSM) in the **sitting position**.
   b. It has also been found that performing CSM with concurrent Valsalva may improve success rates.
6. **Palpate for carotid pulse** in the groove between the sternocleidomastoid and trachea.
7. Position the index and middle fingers over the **superior-most** point of a palpable carotid pulse, behind the angle of the jaw.
8. Apply digital pressure **backwards and medially**, compressing the carotid sinus against the cervical vertebrae, but take care **not** to occlude it.
9. Perform **massaging motions** (circular or longitudinal) with the fingertips on the carotid sinus for **no more than 5 to 10 seconds**, to stimulate the carotid baroreceptors and increase atrioventricular junctional refractoriness and reduce conductivity.
10. **Stop** if the patient experiences giddiness or unilateral weakness.
11. Watch the ECG monitor for **conversion to sinus rhythm**.
12. If unsuccessful, you may repeat once after 1 minute, then retry on the opposite side.
13. Do not perform multiple attempts if both sides are unsuccessful.

BOX 3 Technique for delivering intravenous adenosine

1. **Explain the procedure** to the patient, warning of transient chest discomfort, flushing, and nausea.
2. **Record ECG lead** during the procedure.
3. Obtain IV access in a **large proximal vein** such as an antecubital vein with a three-way tap connected to the cannula.
4. Raise the arm and rapidly deliver **adenosine 6 mg IV push** followed by a **20 ml saline flush** through the three-way tap.
   a. Conduction through the atrioventricular node will be slowed or even completely blocked, resulting in a brief period of asystole, followed by conversion to sinus rhythm in most cases.
   b. If unsuccessful, repeat **up to 2 more times** with **12 mg** after 1 to 2 minutes between attempts.
5. The most common cause of failure is injecting too slowly, as the half-life of adenosine is less than 10 seconds.
6. In cases of tachycardia of indeterminate origin, the ventricular rate may be slowed down transiently enough for diagnosis to be made.
7. Adenosine may cause **ventricular fibrillation**. Thus, this should be performed in a **monitored area** with a **defibrillator** and other resuscitation equipment immediately available.

FIGURE 3 Synchronized cardioversion

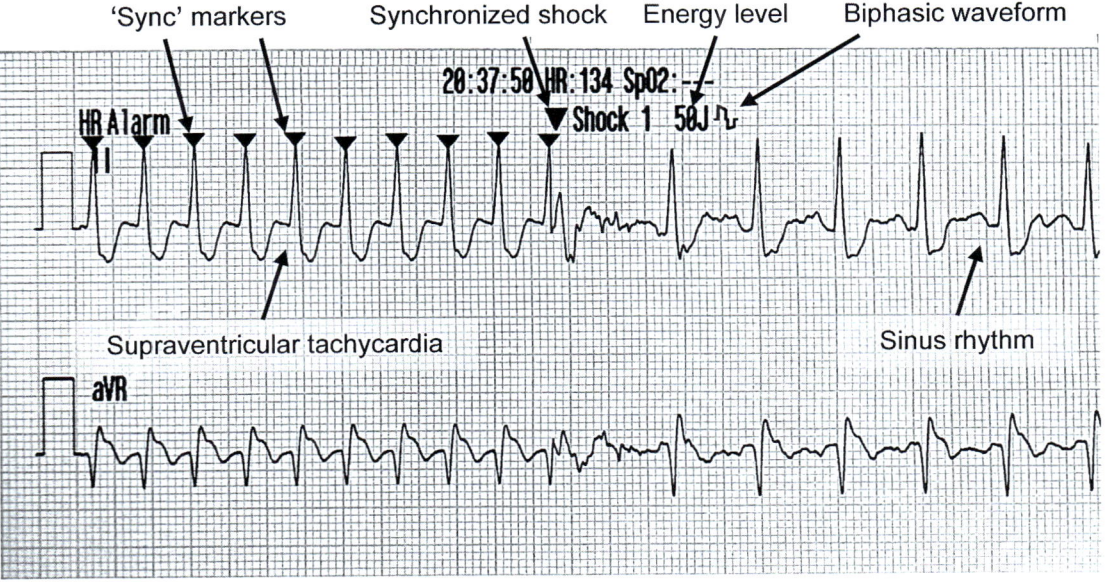

- All discharged patients should be given **advice on vagal manoeuvres** if they are able to understand and perform them.
- **The following patients should be admitted**:
  1. Those who have failed chemical cardioversion.
  2. Those who present with recurrent PSVT after conversion.
  3. Those with haemodynamic instability.
  4. Those who show ECG changes
  5. All patients who have electrical cardioversion.

Atrial fibrillation or flutter

- The initial aim of management of acute atrial fibrillation (AF) is **ventricular rate control**. Clearly defined target heart rates are not available, though a reasonable level would be about 100–110 beats per minute or less.
- The following drugs may be used:

If no heart failure

- **Nondihydropyridine calcium channel blockers**
  1. **Diltiazem** 2.5 mg IV every 3 minutes up to a maximum of 50 mg
  2. **Verapamil** 1 mg/min IV up to a maximum of 20 mg

NOTE: Diltiazem is preferred over verapamil as it has less negative inotropic effects.

  3. **Avoid** in
     a. Hypotension.
     b. Heart failure.
     c. AF with WPW (see **Note** below).
     d. Patients on concurrent β-blockers.
- **β-blockers**
  1. β-blockers are the drugs of choice in AF due to thyrotoxicosis.
  2. **Esmolol** 500 µg/kg IV over 1 minute, followed by infusion at 50–200 µg/kg/min.
  3. **Metoprolol** 2–5 mg IV every 5 minutes up to 15 mg.
  4. **Propanolol** 100 µg/kg IV in 3 divided doses at 2- to 3-minute intervals.
  5. **Avoid** in
     a. Hypotension.
     b. Heart failure.
     c. WPW with AF (see **Note** below).
     d. Patients on concurrent calcium channel blockers.

If there is heart failure

- **Digoxin**
  1. Digoxin 0.5 mg IV.
  2. Indicated in AF with heart failure.
  3. Avoid in
      a. WPW with AF (see **Note** below).

- **Amiodarone**
  1. Amiodarone 150 to 300 mg IV over 30 minutes followed by 900 mg over 24 hours. Maximum dose is 2.2 g/day.
  2. Indicated in AF with heart failure.
  3. May cause hypotension due to its solvent. Reduce infusion rate.
  4. Avoid in
      a. WPW with AF (see **Note** below). Although some references describe the use of amiodarone in this setting, the atrioventricular nodal blocking effect of amiodarone may occur preferentially.

NOTE: In **WPW with AF**, AVOID all agents that selectively block the atrioventricular node (adenosine, beta blockers, calcium channel blockers, and digoxin aka 'ABCD' drugs), as this will promote conduction of fibrillatory waves across the accessory bundle without the protective refractory period of the atrioventricular node.

- **Procainamide**
  1. Procainamide 20 mg/min IV until arrhythmia suppression, hypotension, QRS widened by >50% or maximum dose of 17 mg/kg.
  2. Indicated in **AF with pre-excitation (WPW)**, as it blocks both the AV node and the accessory bundle.
  3. **Avoid** in
      a. Patients on concurrent drugs that prolong QT interval.
      b. Pro-arrhythmic in hypokalaemia, hypomagnesaemia, or acute myocardial infarction.
- **Rhythm control** in AF aims to return the patient to sinus rhythm.
- In **stable** patients, this should not be necessary in the emergency department and is best performed under the care of a specialist.
- The main concern is whether an **atrial thrombus** has formed due to the fibrillation.
- This is likely to have occurred if the AF has been present for **>48 hours**.
- Conversion of the rhythm to sinus would restore organized atrial contractions capable of dislodging and creating an **embolization** of the clot.
- **Transoesophageal echocardiography** may be employed to identify the presence of one.

- If a clot is present, or there is any doubt, the patient should be fully **anti-coagulated** prior to any attempts at converting the rhythm to sinus, unless the patient is **unstable**, in which case **electrical cardioversion** should be attempted immediately, followed by anti-coagulation without delay.
- **Chemical cardioversion** may be performed with the following drugs:
  1. Amiodarone.
  2. Flecainide.
  3. Ibutilide.
  4. Propafenone.
- **Electrical cardioversion** (See Box 1 above) is employed when the patient is unstable, but may be used as an elective procedure if chemical cardioversion is contraindicated.
- For thromboprophylactic therapy, the **CHA$_2$DS$_2$-VASc** score is now used instead of the **CHADS$_2$** score for risk stratification in patients with AF (Box 4).

NOTE: Options for primary stroke prevention include aspirin, dual antiplatelet therapy, vitamin K antagonists (VKA) such as warfarin, and new oral anticoagulants such as dabigatran, apixaban, rivaroxaban. Risk and benefits must be discussed with the patient.

BOX 4   CHADS$_2$ vs CHA$_2$DS$_2$-VASc scores

Risk Factors	Points	
	CHADS$_2$	CHA$_2$DS$_2$-VASc
Congestive heart failure	1	1
Hypertension	1	1
Age		
>75	1	
>/= 75		2
Diabetes Mellitus	1	1
Stroke / TIA	2	2
Vascular Disease		1
Age 65–74		1
Sex **c**ategory (female)		1
Total possible	0–6	0–9

European Society for Cardiology Guidelines (2010)

CHA$_2$DS$_2$-VASc = 0: No therapy or aspirin (preferred: no therapy)
CHA$_2$DS$_2$-VASc = 1: Oral anticoagulant or aspirin (preferred: oral anticoagulant)
CHA$_2$DS$_2$-VASc >/= 2: Oral anticoagulant

WIDE COMPLEX TACHYDYSRHYTHMIAS

- **Wide complex tachydysrhythmias** (QRS >120 ms) may be **regular** or **irregular** (Figure 4).
- Causes of **regular wide complex tachydysrhythmias**:
  1. Ventricular tachycardia (VT).
  2. SVT with abberant conduction.
- Causes of **irregular wide complex tachydysrhythmias**:
  1. Polymorphic VT and torsades de pointes.
  2. AF with abberancy.
  3. AF with WPW.

FIGURE 4   Wide complex tachydysrhythmias (with a pulse)

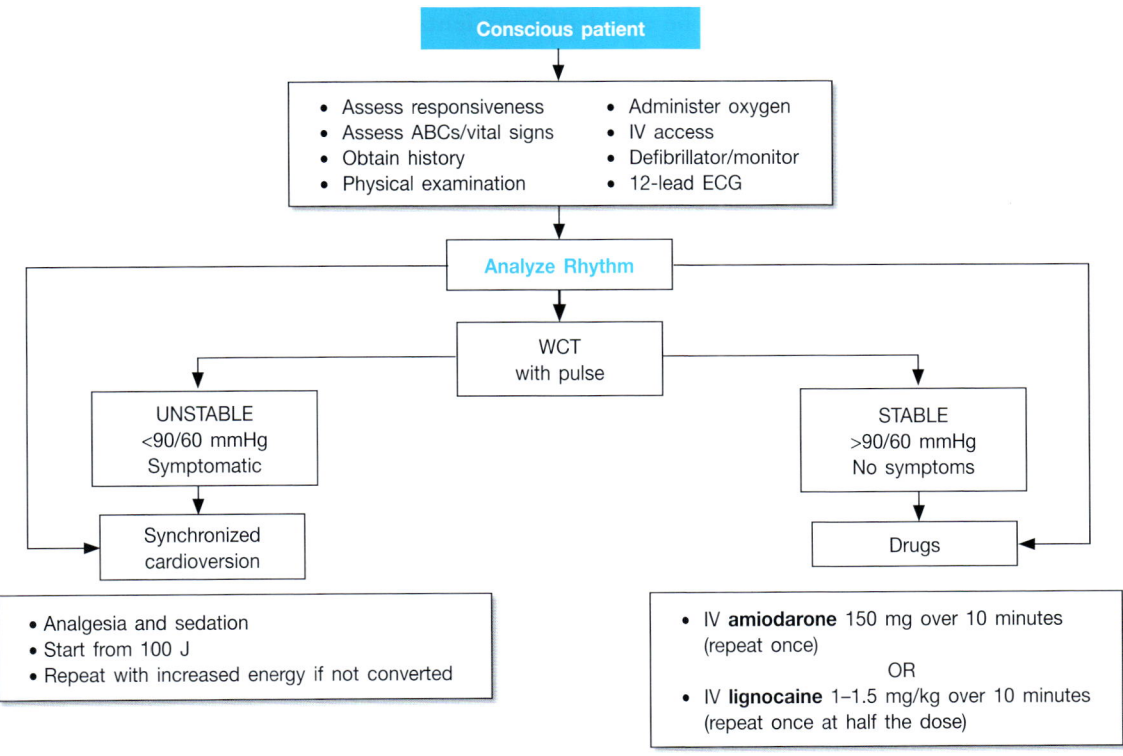

Ventricular tachycardia

- Based on the current Singapore NRC guidelines, the two main drug options are **amiodarone** and **lignocaine**.
- **Amiodarone** is given as 150 mg over 10 minutes, and repeated once if necessary, followed by an infusion of 1 mg/min for 6 hours then 0.5 mg/min. The maximum daily dose is 2.2 g.
- **Lignocaine** is given as 1–1.5 mg/kg IV push, repeated once at half the dose, if necessary, after about 5 to 10 minutes, up to a maximum of 3 mg/kg.
- **AHA: Procainamide** and **sotalol** are additional options that have been found to be superior to lignocaine.
- **Procainamide** is given at a rate of 20–50 mg/min or 100 mg every 5 minutes, until arrhythmia is suppressed, hypotension ensues or the QRS complex is prolonged by 50%, up to a maximum of 17 mg/kg.
- **Sotalol** may be given at a rate of 100 mg or 1.5 mg/kg over 5 minutes.
- Procainamide and sotalol should be **avoided in patients with prolonged QT intervals and heart failure**.
- **Do not give more than one** anti-arrhythmic agent at any one time.
- If either drug fails, the next step should be **elective synchronized cardioversion**.
- If the patient is **stable**, then he should be admitted for the procedure to be performed by the cardiologist.
- If the patient becomes **unstable**, then perform synchronized cardioversion in the emergency department without delay (Box 1).
- As VT may degenerate into VF, the patient should be managed in a **monitored area** and a **defibrillator** and other resuscitation equipment should be immediately available.

SVT with aberrancy

- If **SVT with aberrancy** is strongly suspected, a **trial of adenosine** may be given (see Box 3)
- When in doubt or if adenosine is unsuccessful, the patient should be treated as for VT.

Polymorphic VT and torsades de pointes

- **Polymorphic VT** may be classified based on whether the underlying QT interval (during sinus rhythm) is prolonged or not.
- Where the **underlying QT is prolonged**, this is **torsades de pointes**.
- Correct **electrolyte abnormalities** giving rise to the prolonged QT (hypoMg and hypoK).
- Give **IV magnesium sulphate** 1–2 g over 60–90 seconds, followed by an infusion of 1–2 g/hr.
- Consider **overdrive pacing** under the care of a cardiologist.
- **Drugs that prolong the QT interval**, such as class I (quinidine, disopyramide, and procainamide) and class III (amiodarone, and sotatol) anti-dysrhythmics, phenothiazines, tricyclic antidepressants, and macrolides should be avoided.

- Where the **underlying QT is not prolonged**, this is polymorphic VT.
- **Amiodarone** may be effective for chemical cardioversion.
- Magnesium and lignocaine **are not** likely to be effective.
- If the patient is **unstable**, use **defibrillation energy doses** and **unsynchronized** direct current shock (Box 1).
- As polymorphic VT and torsades may degenerate into VF, the patient should be managed in a **monitored area** and a **defibrillator** and other resuscitation equipment should be immediately available.
- **If conversion has taken place**, recheck the **vital signs**, and record a 12-lead **ECG**.
- Look for evidence of **ischaemia** as ventricular tachydysrhythmias are most commonly associated with ischaemia.
- Perform **lab investigations** including full blood count, urea/electrolytes/creatinine, and cardiac biomarkers.
- All patients should be **admitted** for monitoring in a telemetry or coronary care unit, unless the diagnosis of SVT with aberrancy is certain, in which case the patient may be managed as for SVT.

References/Further Reading

1. Anantharaman V, Gunasegaran K. Advanced Cardiac Life Support guidelines 2011. *Singapore Med J*. Aug 2011; 52(8): 548–555.

2. Deakin CD, Morrison LJ, Morley PT, et al. Advanced Life Support Chapter Collaborators. Part 8: Advanced life support. 2010 International Consensus on Cardiopulmonary Resuscitation and Emergency Cardiovascular Care Science with Treatment Recommendations. *Resuscitation*. Oct 2010; 81(suppl 1): e93–e174.

3. Deakin CD, Nolan JP, Soar J, et al. European Resuscitation Council Guidelines for Resuscitation 2010. Section 4: Adult advanced life support. *Resuscitation*. Oct 2010; 81(10): 1305–1352.

4. Waxman MB, Wald RW, Sharma AD, et al. Vagal techniques for termination of paroxysmal supraventricular tachycardia. *Am J Cardiol*. 1980; 46: 655–664.

5. Porth CJ, Bamrah VS, Tristani FE, et al. The Valsalva maneuver: Mechanisms and clinical implications. *Heart Lung*. 1984; 13: 507–518.

6. Pomeroy PR. Augmented carotid massage. *Ann Emerg Med*. 1992; 21: 1169–1170.

7. Lim SH, Anantharaman V, Teo WS, et al. Comparison of treatment of supraventricular tachycardia by Valsalva maneuver and carotid sinus massage. *Ann Emerg Med*. 1998; 31: 30–35.

8. Lim SH, Anantharaman V, Teo WS. Slow-infusion of calcium channel blockers in the emergency management of supraventricular tachycardia. *Resuscitation*. 2002; 52: 167–174.

9. Gage BF, Waterman AD, Shannon W, et al. Validation of clinical classification schemes for predicting stroke: Results from the National Registry of Atrial Fibrillation. *JAMA*. 13 June 2001; 285(22): 2864–2870.

10. Camm AJ, Kirchhof P, Lip GYH, et al. Guidelines for the management of atrial fibrillation: the Task Force for the Management of Atrial Fibrillation of the European Society of Cardiology (ESC). Eur Heart J 2010; 31(19): 2369–429.

11. Odum LE, Cochran KA, Aistrope DS, et al. The CHADS2 versus the new CHA2DS2-VASc scoring systems for guiding antithrombotic treatment of patients with atrial fibrillation: review of the literature and recommendations for use. Pharmacotherapy. 2012 Mar; 32(3): 285–96.

44   Asthma
Goh Ee Ling • Malcolm Mahadevan

DEFINITION

- Asthma is a chronic inflammatory disorder characterized by variable airway obstruction with recurrent or chronic wheeze and/or cough.
- Because the underlying pathophysiology is that of bronchial hyper-reactivity due to airway inflammation, the cornerstone of therapy is **steroids**.

CAVEATS

- **'All that wheezes is not asthma'**. Differentials to consider include the following:
  1. Congestive cardiac failure.
  2. Upper airway obstruction.
  3. Bronchogenic carcinoma with obstruction.
  4. Bronchiectasis.
  5. Metastatic carcinoma with lymphangitic metastasis.
  6. Gastroesophageal reflux (GERD).
  7. Chronic obstructive pulmonary disease (COPD).
- Physical signs may be absent at the time of examination as symptoms are often transient but this does not exclude the diagnosis of asthma.
- Absence of rhonchi on auscultation may indicate a silent chest in severe, life-threatening asthma.

CLINICAL ASSESSMENT

- The **aims** of **clinical assessment** are as follows:
  1. Determine the severity of acute asthmatic attack and treat accordingly (see Table 1).
  2. Identify patients who are at high risk of dying from asthma (see Table 2).
  3. Establish the patient's current treatment and level of asthma control (see Table 3).
- **History**
  1. Presenting symptoms: Triad of asthma symptoms are dyspnoea, wheezing and cough.
  2. Precipitating factors, e.g. dust and upper respiratory tract infection.
  3. High risk features (see Table 2).
  4. Current medications including compliance.
- **Physical examination**
  1. General appearance: Mental state (agitated or drowsy), signs of respiratory distress and cyanosis.
  2. Vitals signs: Especially oxygen saturation levels (SaO_2).
  3. Respiratory: Prolonged expiratory phase, rhonchi, crepitations, and air entry.

TABLE 1   Classifying severity of asthma exacerbations

	Mild	Moderate	Severe	Respiratory arrest imminent
Symptoms				
Breathlessness	While walking Can lie down	While talking Prefer to sit	While at rest Sit upright	Exhausted Feeble respiratory effort
Speech	Speak in sentences	Speak in short phrases	Speak only a few words	Hardly able to talk
Mental state	May be agitated	Usually agitated	Usually agitated	Drowsy or confused
Signs				
Respiratory rate	Increased	Increased	Often >30/min	Decreased
Use of accessory muscles	Usually not	Commonly	Usually	Paradoxical thoracoabdominal movement
Wheeze	Moderate, often only end expiratory	Loud, throughout exhalation	Usually loud; throughout inhalation and exhalation	No wheeze ('silent chest')
Pulse/minute	<100	100–120	>120	Bradycardia
SaO$_2$% (room air)	>95%	91–95%	<91%	Clinically cyanosed
Peak expiratory flow (PEF) after initial bronchodilator OR % predicted or % personal best	>80%	60–80%	<60% or response lasts <2 hours	

TABLE 2   Risk factors for death from asthma

Past history of sudden severe exacerbations

Prior intubation and mechanical ventilation for asthma

Prior admission for asthma to an intensive care unit

Two or more hospitalizations for asthma in the past year

Three or more emergency care visits for asthma in the past year

Hospitalization or an emergency care visit for asthma within the past month

Use of more than two canisters per month of inhaled short-acting β$_2$-agonist

Current use of systemic corticosteroids or recent withdrawal from systemic corticosteroids

Difficulty perceiving airflow obstruction or its severity

Comorbidity, as from cardiovascular diseases or chronic obstructive pulmonary disease

Serious psychiatric disease or psychosocial problems

Low socioeconomic status and urban residence

Illicit drug use

Not currently using inhaled corticosteroids

TABLE 3   Levels of asthma control

Characteristic	Controlled	Partly controlled	Uncontrolled
Daytime symptoms	None (≤2x/week)	>2x/week	>3 features or partly controlled asthma present
Limitations of activities	None	Any	
Nocturnal symptoms/awakening	None	Any	
Need for reliever/rescue treatment	None (≤2x/week)	>2x/week	
Lung function (PEF rate or forced expiratory volume in 1 second (FEV1))	Normal	<80% predicted or personal best	
Exacerbations	None	≥1/year	One in any week

- **Investigations**

  Not indicated in most cases and guided by clinical assessment.

  1. **Chest X-ray**: Indicated in patients not responding to initial therapy. Look for pneumothorax, pneumonia, or congestive cardiac failure.

  2. **Arterial blood gas**: Usual in severe asthmatic exacerbations to look for hypercarbia (an ominous sign) and hypoxia.

  3. **Others**: Full blood count and renal panel (especially for hypokalaemia due to nebulized salbutamol).

⇨ **SPECIAL TIPS FOR GPs**

- During an acute asthma attack, the early use of an **oral corticosteroid** will reduce the risk of asthma death. Thus, nearly all patients who need nebulized treatment for acute severe asthma in the clinic need a course of oral prednisolone approximately 0.5 mg/kg/day for 7 to 10 days without the need to tail down.

- Patients who need frequent (more than once in 6 to 12 months) nebulizations for acute asthma are at high risk of dying from it.

- Daily use of a **low dose inhaled corticosteroid** will reduce the risk of severe exacerbations and thus reduce asthma deaths in high risk patients very cost effectively.

MANAGEMENT

- The **aims of emergency department therapy** for asthma are as follows:

  1. Ensure adequate oxygenation.

  2. Reverse airflow obstruction.

  3. Relieve inflammation.

- See Figure 1 for the asthma management flowchart.

- **Supportive measures**
  1. The patient should be placed in at least a monitored area. In the presence of severe asthmatic attack, the patient should be managed in the critical care area.
  2. Monitoring: Electrocardiogram, pulse oximetry, and vital signs.
  3. Support airway, breathing and circulation:
     a. Secure airway in patients with severe asthma or imminent respiratory arrest.
     b. Administer supplemental oxygen.
     c. Obtain intravenous access (not necessary in mild attacks).
- **Drug therapy**
  1. **Bronchodilators**

     Continuous inhaled short-acting beta-agonist salbutamol in combination with ipratropium via nebulization every 20 minutes for 1 hour.

     Addition of ipratropium has been shown to produce additional bronchodilation with minimal side effects.
  2. **Steroids**

     It reduces inflammation and also has an acute bronchodilator effect.

     Give oral prednisolone 0.5–1 mg/kg or intravenous hydrocortisone 200–400 mg.

     Steroids administered via the oral route are as rapid in onset and effective as that given via the intravenous route.
  3. **Magnesium sulphate**

     Indicated in poor responders to bronchodilator therapy with moderate to severe asthma.

Its mechanism of action is likely to inhibit smooth muscle contraction, decrease histamine release from mast cells, and inhibit acetylcholine release.

Give 1–2 g as an infusion over 30 minutes.

NOTE: Watch for hypotension.

- **Disposition**
  1. Patients who are intubated and require mechanical ventilation will be admitted to a medical intensive care unit.

  NOTE: Use **low tidal volumes** with slow respiratory rate of 6–8/min for patients that get intubated, keep plateau pressure <35 mmHg, as with COPD; about 35 mmHg is when risk for barotrauma increases significantly.

  2. Admit the following patients to a general ward under Respiratory Medicine or an observation unit if available in the emergency department.
     a. Patients who respond partially and whose PEFR is <50% of predicted within 60 minutes.

FIGURE 1 Flowchart showing the management of asthma

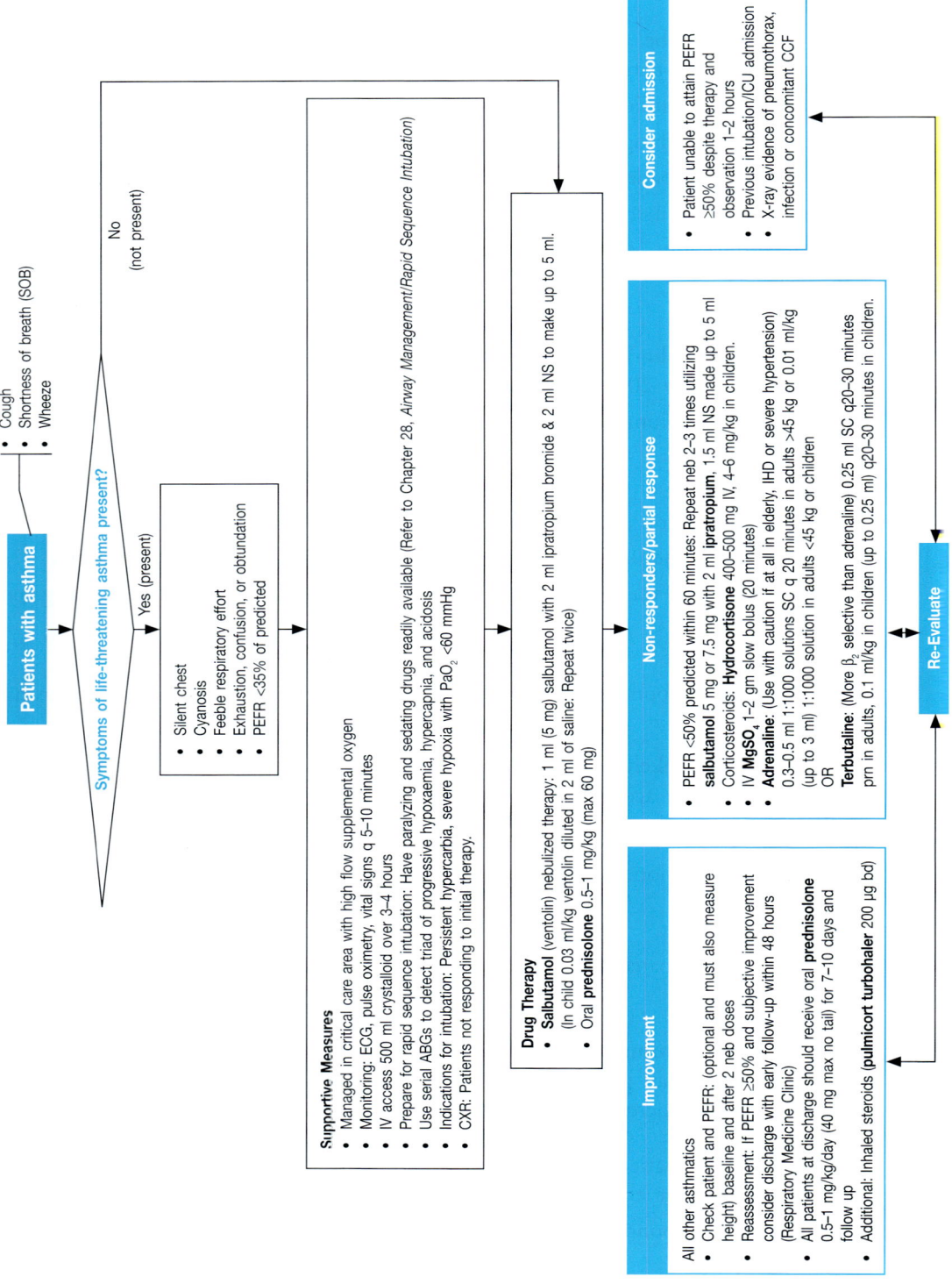

Patients with asthma
- Cough
- Shortness of breath (SOB)
- Wheeze

Symptoms of life-threatening asthma present?

Yes (present)
- Silent chest
- Cyanosis
- Feeble respiratory effort
- Exhaustion, confusion, or obtundation
- PEFR <35% of predicted

No (not present)

Supportive Measures
- Managed in critical care area with high flow supplemental oxygen
- Monitoring: ECG, pulse oximetry, vital signs q 5–10 minutes
- IV access 500 ml crystalloid over 3–4 hours
- Prepare for rapid sequence intubation: Have paralyzing and sedating drugs readily available (Refer to Chapter 28, *Airway Management/Rapid Sequence Intubation*)
- Use serial ABGs to detect triad of progressive hypoxaemia, hypercapnia, and acidosis
- Indications for intubation: Persistent hypercarbia, severe hypoxia with PaO₂ <60 mmHg
- CXR: Patients not responding to initial therapy.

Drug Therapy
- **Salbutamol** (ventolin) nebulized therapy: 1 ml (5 mg) salbutamol with 2 ml ipratropium bromide & 2 ml NS to make up to 5 ml.
  (In child 0.03 ml/kg ventolin diluted in 2 ml of saline: Repeat twice)
- Oral **prednisolone** 0.5–1 mg/kg (max 60 mg)

Non-responders/partial response
- PEFR <50% predicted within 60 minutes: Repeat neb 2–3 times utilizing **salbutamol** 5 mg or 7.5 mg with 2 ml **ipratropium**, 1.5 ml NS made up to 5 ml
- Corticosteroids: **Hydrocortisone** 400–500 mg IV, 4–6 mg/kg in children.
- IV **MgSO₄** 1–2 gm slow bolus (20 minutes)
- **Adrenaline:** (Use with caution if at all in elderly, IHD or severe hypertension) 0.3–0.5 ml 1:1000 solutions SC q 20 minutes in adults >45 kg or 0.01 ml/kg (up to 3 ml) 1:1000 solution in adults <45 kg or children
  OR
  Terbutaline: (More β₂ selective than adrenaline) 0.25 ml SC q20–30 minutes prn in adults, 0.1 ml/kg in children (up to 0.25 ml) q20–30 minutes in children.

Consider admission
- Patient unable to attain PEFR ≥50% despite therapy and observation 1–2 hours
- Previous intubation/ICU admission
- X-ray evidence of pneumothorax, infection or concomitant CCF

Improvement

All other asthmatics
- Check patient and PEFR: (optional and must also measure height) baseline and after 2 neb doses
- Reassessment: If PEFR ≥50% and subjective improvement consider discharge with early follow-up within 48 hours (Respiratory Medicine Clinic)
- All patients at discharge should receive oral **prednisolone** 0.5–1 mg/kg/day (40 mg max no tail) for 7–10 days and follow up
- Additional: Inhaled steroids (**pulmicort turbohaler** 200 µg bd)

Re-Evaluate

   b. Patients who require second-line therapy with magnesium sulphate.

   c. Patients who respond to treatment but have high risk features.

   d. Patients who improve symptomatically and whose PEFR is 50% or greater.

3. Check inhaler technique.

4. Assess control of asthma using **asthma control test (ACT)**, a 5-item self-administered questionnaire used to objectively monitor control, and guide therapy for both doctors and patients.

5. Advise patients to avoid precipitating factors, e.g. dust and fumes.

6. Emphasize the importance of compliance with regard to follow-up and taking medications.

   a. Arrange for early follow-up with a respiratory specialist outpatient clinic.

References/Further Reading

1. Emerman CL, Cydulka RK, McFadden ER. Comparison of 2.5 mg vs 7.5 mg inhaled albuterol in the treatment of acute asthma. *Chest*. 1999; 115(1): 92–96.

2. Brenner B, Kohn MS. The acute asthmatic patient in the ED: To admit or discharge. *Am J Emerg Med*. 1998; 16(1): 69–75.

3. McFadden ER, Casale TB, Edwards TB, et al. Administration of budesonide once daily by means of turbuhaler to subjects with stable asthma. *J. Allergy Clinical Immunol*. 1999; 104(1): 46–52.

4. Quadrel M, Lavery RF, Jaker M, et al. Prospective randomized trial of epinephrine, metaproterenol and both in the prehospital treatment of asthma in the adult patient. *Ann Emerg Med*. 1995; 26(4): 469–473.

5. Lin RY, Rehman A. Clinical characteristics of adult asthmatics requiring intubation. *J Med*. 1995; 26(5–6): 261–277.

6. National Asthma Education and Prevention Program Expert Panel Report 2. Guidelines for the diagnosis and management of asthma. NIH. Publication No. 97-4051 July 1997. Available at: www.nhlbi.nib.gov/guidlines/asthma/asthgdln.pdf.

7. Global Initiative for Asthma. Global Strategy for Asthma Management and Prevention. Revised 2006. Available at: www.ginasthma.org.

8. Nathan RA, Sorkness CA, Kosinski M, et al. Development of the asthma control test: A survey for assessing asthma control. *J Allergy Clin Immunol*. 2004; 113(1): 59–65.

9. Silverman RA, Osborn H, Runge J, et al. IV magnesium sulfate in the treatment of acute severe asthma. *Chest*. 2002; 122: 489–497.

10. MOH Clinical Practice Guidelines 1/2008. Management of Asthma.

45   Chronic Obstructive Pulmonary Disease (COPD)

Goh Ee Ling • Quek Lit Sin • Malcolm Mahadevan

DEFINITION

- Chronic obstructive pulmonary disease (COPD) is characterized by airflow limitation which is progressive, worsening, and is not fully reversible.
- It is associated with the exposure of the lungs to noxious particles or gases.
- **Key features** to make a **diagnosis** of COPD:
  1. Chronic cough
  2. Chronic sputum production
  3. Dyspnoea: Progressive and worsening with time. Worse with exercise and during respiratory infections.
  4. History of exposure to risk factors, e.g. smoke, occupational dusts, etc.
- See Table 1 for the classification of the severity of COPD.

TABLE 1   **Classification of COPD by severity according to the Global Initiative for Chronic Obstructive Lung Disease (GOLD)**

0: At risk	Normal spirometry Chronic symptoms (cough and sputum production)
I: Mild	FEV_1/FVC <70% FEV_1 ≥80% of predicted With or without chronic symptoms (cough and sputum production)
II: Moderate	$FEV1_1/FVC$ <70% 50% ≤FEV_1 <80% of predicted With or without chronic symptoms (cough and sputum production)
III: Severe	FEV_1/FVC <70% 30% ≤FEV_1 <50% of predicted With or without chronic symptoms (cough and sputum production)
IV: Very severe	FEV_1/FVC <70% FEV_1 <30% of predicted or FEV_1 <50% of predicted plus chronic respiratory failure*

Note: *Respiratory failure = Arterial partial pressure of oxygen (PaO_2) <8.0 kPA (60 mmHg) with or without arterial partial pressure of CO_2 ($PaCO_2$) >6.7 kPa (50 mmHg).

CAVEATS

- About 10% of patients with COPD have no smoking history.
- About 10% of patients with COPD have clinical features of asthma and hence should be treated as for asthma cases.
- There are 2 features that point to the diagnosis of asthma rather than COPD:
  1. Complete bronchoreversibility to bronchodilators.
  2. Diurnal variation in peak flow of >20%.

CLINICAL ASSESSMENT

- An acute exacerbation of COPD is defined as an acute event with worsening of the patient's usual symptoms.
- **History**
  1. Presenting symptoms: Worsening dyspnoea, increased cough with increased sputum production, and/or purulence and fever.
  2. Past medical history including frequency of exacerbations/admissions, previous admissions needing non-invasive ventilation (NIV), or intubation.
  3. Current medications including compliance.
  4. Severity of COPD including end-of-life or do-not-intubate issues have been discussed.
- **Physical examination**
  1. General appearance: Drowsy (may indicate hypercarbia) and signs of respiratory distress.
  2. Vital signs: In particular oxygen saturation level (SpO_2) and respiratory rate and fever (indicating infection).
  3. Respiratory conditions: Barrel chest, rhonchi, prolonged expiratory phase, signs of pneumonia/pneumothorax, and air entry.
- **Investigations**

  Much guided by clinical assessment and response to therapy.
  1. **Chest X-ray**: Should be considered in all patients. Will show hyperinflated lung fields with flattened diaphragms. Look for pneumothorax and pneumonia.
  2. **Arterial blood gas**: Should be performed after at least two nebulizations in order to determine the need for NIV (refer to Chapter 48, *Respiratory Failure, Acute*).
  3. **Others**: ECG (usually sinus tachycardia. P pulmonale may be present in patients with cor pulmonale), full blood count, urea/electrolytes.

⇨ **SPECIAL TIPS FOR GPs**
- Advise all patients with COPD to quit smoking as this is the most important intervention.
- Flu vaccination should also be considered for patients aged 65 years and older as it has been shown to reduce hospitalizations and mortality risk.

MANAGEMENT

- The **aims** of management are these:
  1. Treatment of acute exacerbations via reversal of bronchospasm, relief of inflammation, and relief of precipitating factors.
  2. Early non-invasive ventilation for suitable patients with type 2 respiratory failure.
  3. Appropriate disposition and follow-up.

- **Supportive measures**
  1. The patient should be placed in a monitored area. Those with severe respiratory distress or failure should be in the critical care area.
  2. Monitoring: ECG, pulse oximetry, and vital signs.
  3. Obtain intravenous access (not necessary in all patients).
  4. Support airway, breathing and circulation (ABCs).
     a. Secure airway for patients who are in imminent respiratory arrest or in type 2 respiratory failure with contraindications to NIV.

     NOTE: **Ventilatory settings** should be **low rates**, **low tidal volumes**, **and prolonged expiratory phase**.

     b. Supplemental low flow controlled oxygen for all patients with respiratory distress or SpO_2 less than 90% aiming for SpO_2 of 92–95% via nasal prongs or ventimask.
     c. **Non-invasive ventilation** should be initiated as early as possible for suitable patients. It reduces mortality, the need for intubation, complications and length of stay when compared with standard medical treatment (refer to Chapter 48, *Respiratory Failure, Acute*).
     d. **Fluid administration**. Should be judicious unless patients are in shock as these patients are usually elderly and may have diminished cardiac function such as cor pulmonale.

- **Drug therapy**
  1. **Bronchodilators**

     Continuous inhaled short-acting beta-agonist salbutamol administration in combination with ipratropium via nebulization every 20 minutes for one hour.

     Addition of ipratropium has been shown to produce additional bronchodilation and with minimal side effects.

  2. **Steroids**

     It reduces inflammation and also has an acute bronchodilator effect.

     Give oral prednisolone 0.5–1 mg/kg or intravenous hydrocortisone 200–400 mg.

     Steroids given via the oral route **are as rapid and effective** as that administered via the intravenous route

  3. **Antibiotics**

     Should be started when there is a history of purulent sputum/increased shortness of breath/increased sputum purulence, clinical signs of pneumonia, or consolidation on the chest X-ray. Common colonizers of respiratory tract include *Strep pneumonia, Haemophilus influenzae, Moxarella catarrhalis, Klebsiella, Mycoplasma, Pseudomonas,* and *Streptococcus.*

     The choice of antibiotics can be any of the following for a duration of 5 days to a week.

     a. Beta-lactam-lactamase inhibitor combination, e.g. amoxicillin–clavulanate.
     b. Second-generation macrolide, e.g. azithromycin and clarithromycin.

    c. Second-generation cephalosporin, e.g. cefuroxime.

    d. Quinolones, e.g. levofloxacin.

4. Others

    a. Methylxanthines (aminophylline) have **not** been shown to improve forced expiratory volume in one second (FEV_1) or affect hospital admission.

    b. Magnesium sulphate has not been found to be useful for **chronic obstructive pulmonary disease** (COPD).

- **Disposition**
- Patients who can be discharged must satisfy the following criteria:

1. Inhaled β_2-agonist therapy required no more frequently than every 4 hours.

2. The patient who is previously ambulant is able to walk comfortably.

3. The patient has been clinically stable for 12–24 hours.

4. Arterial blood gases (ABGs) have been stable for 12–24 hours.

5. The patient or caregiver fully understands how to administer the correct medications.

6. Follow-up and home care arrangements have been completed.

7. The patient, his family, and physician are confident that the patient can manage successfully.

- Check inhaler technique.
- Advise to stop smoking.
- Refer to the COPD nurse before discharge and early outpatient review at Respiratory Medicine.
- Discharge with a 7–10 days supply of steroids and antibiotics (if need be).
- Those who respond partially and do not satisfy the discharge criteria should be admitted to a general ward or observation unit in the emergency medicine department (if available).
- Those who are intubated or require NIV should be admitted to the high dependency or intensive care unit.

References/Further Reading

1. Barnes PJ. New therapies for COPD: *Thorax*. 1998; 53(2): 137–147.

2. Barnes PJ. Mechanism in COPD: Differences from asthma: *Chest*. 2000; 117: 2(supp l):10s–14s.

3. Friedman M. Combined bronchodilator therapy in the management of chronic obstructive pulmonary disease. *Respirology*. 1997; 2(suppl 1): S19–S23. Review.

4. Campbell S. For COPD a combination of ipratropium bromide and albuterol sulfate is more effective than albuterol base. *Arch Intern Med*. 1999; 159(2): 156–160.

5. Gross N, Tashkin D, Miller R, et al. Inhalation by nebulization of albuterol-ipratropium combination (Dey combination) is superior to either agent alone in the treatment of chronic obstructive pulmonary disease. Dey Combination Solution Study Group. *Respiration*. 1998; 65(5): 354–362.

6. Routine nebulized ipratropium and albuterol together are better than either alone in COPD. The COMBIVENT Inhalation Solution Study Group. *Chest*. 1997; 112(6): 1514–1521.

7. Wood-Baker R, Walters EH, Gibson P. Oral corticosteroids for acute exacerbations of chronic obstructive pulmonary disease. *Cochrane Database Syst Rev.* 2001; (2): CD001288.

8. Barr RG, Rowe BH, Camargo CA Jr. Methylxanthines for exacerbations of chronic obstructive pulmonary disease. *Cochrane Database Syst Rev.* 2001; (1): CD002168.

9. Kramer N, Meyer TJ, Meharg J, et al. Randomized, prospective trial of non-invasive positive pressure ventilation in acute respiratory failure. *Am J Respir Crit Care Med.* 1995; 151(6): 1799–1806.

10. Bott J, Carroll MP, Conway JH, et al. Randomised controlled atrial of nasal ventilation in acute ventilatory failure due to chronic obstructive airway disease. *Lancet.* 1993; 341(8860): 1555–1557.

11. Mehta S, Hill NS. Noninvasive ventilation. *Am J Respir Crit Care Med.* 2001; 163(2): 540–577.

12. MOH Clinical Practice Guidelines 4/2006. Chronic Obstructive Pulmonary Disease.

13. Executive Summary: Global Strategy for the Diagnosis, Management and Prevention of COPD. Revised 2007.

46   Pneumonia, Community Acquired (CAP)

Goh Ee Ling • Malcolm Mahadevan • Shirley Ooi

DEFINITION

Pneumonia is defined as an acute infection of the pulmonary parenchyma. Community-acquired pneumonia (CAP) is diagnosed if there are:

- **Infiltrates on the chest X-ray which are consistent with pneumonia**.
- **Altered breath sounds and/or localized crepitations**.

Patients must not be hospitalized patients or residents of a long-term facility 14 days before symptom onset.

CAVEATS

- Pneumonia can only be diagnosed reliably on chest X-rays as physical examination alone has poor sensitivity and specificity.
- Pneumonia is the most common cause of death from an infective cause in Singapore. Hence, prompt diagnosis and treatment are essential.

MICROBIOLOGY

- The most **common bacterial pathogens** include these:
  1. *Streptococcus pneumoniae* (65%).
  2. *Haemophilus influenzae* (10%).
  3. Atypicals: *Mycoplasma* and *Legionella* (10%).
  4. *Staph aureus* (2%).
  5. Rare Gram-negatives (1%).
  6. Multiple infections (5–10%).
- There is a dramatic increase in the incidence of penicillin-resistant (40%) and multiple drug-resistant *Streptococcus pneumoniae*. Hence, this affects the choice of empirical antibiotics used in patients with severe CAP.
- There is a higher incidence and virulence of Gram-negative CAP in Singapore. *Burkholderia pseudomallei* and *Klebsiella pneumoniae* account for approximately 25% of severe CAP and are associated with a mortality of >50%.
- Tuberculosis accounts for 15–20% of CAP in Singapore and should be considered in all patients, especially the elderly.
- Patients with human immunodeficiency virus (HIV) usually present with *Pneumocystis carinii* pneumonia **(disproportionate hypoxaemia with mild CXR abnormalities) or pulmonary tuberculosis (extensive)**.

CLINICAL ASSESSMENT

- The aims of clinical assessment are:
  1. Confirm the diagnosis of CAP.
  2. Define the appropriate risk stratification.
  3. Choose the right antibiotic treatment.
  4. Identify the appropriate disposition.
- **History**
  1. **Presenting symptoms**
     a. Lower respiratory tract infection (≥2 symptoms may be present): Fever/hypothermia, rigours, sweats, new cough with/without sputum, chest pain, and dyspnoea
     b. Non-specific: Fatigue, myalgia, abdominal pain, anorexia, and headache.
  2. **Past medical history, in particular for risk factors for mortality including the following**
     a. Old age.
     b. Alcoholism.
     c. Active malignancy.
     d. Neurological disease.
     e. Heart failure.
     f. Diabetes mellitus.
     g. Previous pneumonia, pneumonia due to Gram-negatives and aspiration pneumonia.
  3. **Prior treatment for current illness, e.g. prior antibiotics**.

PHYSICAL EXAMINATION

- General appearance: Altered mental state, signs of respiratory distress, dehydration, and signs of toxicity.
- Vital signs: Tachypnoea, fever, and signs of shock (tachycardia and hypotension).
- Respiratory: Crepitations, pleural effusion, and rhonchi.

INVESTIGATIONS

- **CXR**: Extent of consolidation, parapneumonic effusion, and cavitation
- **Bloods**:
  1. Full blood count and renal panel.
  2. Blood cultures in moderate to severe CAP only.
  3. Arterial blood gas (if necessary).
  4. Lactate for prognostication in severe CAP.
- **Others** (determined by clinical assessment): Electrocardiogram (ECG), capillary blood sugar, and urine culture.

MANAGEMENT

- **Risk stratification**: This provides the basis for clinical decision making on the site of treatment (inpatient versus outpatient), intensity of diagnostic evaluation, and initial choice of antibiotics. Risk stratification tools should be used in conjunction with clinical assessment and not employed to replace the physician's judgement.
  1. **Fine pneumonia severity index**
     a. This is a prediction rule that stratifies patients into five classes for risk of death from all causes within 30 days of presentation (see Figure 1). It determines the initial site of care based on the risk class that correlates with mortality rates.
     b. It has been validated in a large number of patients in the US.

FIGURE 1 **Identifying patients in risk class I in the derivation of the prediction rule**

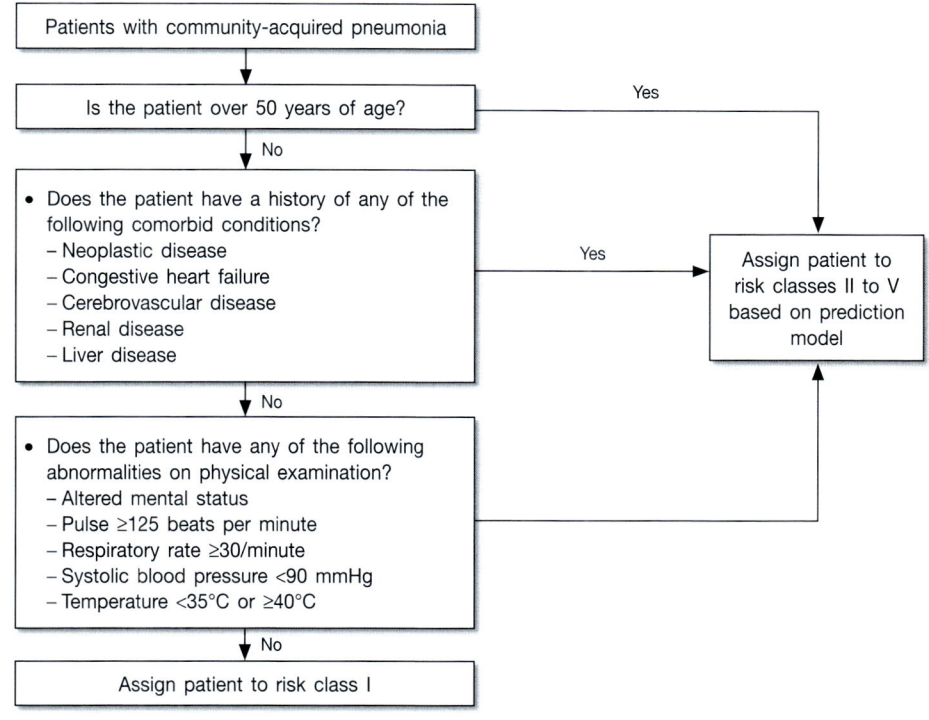

Source: Fine, et al. (1997), Figure 1, p. 246.[2]

c. A risk score (total point score) for a given patient is obtained by summing patient age in years (age − 10 for females) and the points for each applicable patient characteristic (Tables 1 and 2).

d. Oxygen saturation of <90% is considered abnormal.

2. **CURB-65**.

- A simpler clinical prediction rule that is based on the following 5 factors with each being given 1 point, validated for predicting mortality in CAP:

1. Confusion.

2. Urea ≥7 mmol/L.

3. Respiratory rate of >30 breaths per minute.

4. Blood pressure (systolic <90 mmHg or diastolic ≤60 mmHg).

5. Age ≥65 years.

- See Table 4 for the application of CURB-65.

TABLE 1   Scoring system for identification of patient risk for persons with community-acquired pneumonia

Patient characteristic	Points assigned[1]
Demographic factors	
• Age: Males	Age (in years)
Females	Age (in years) −10
• Nursing home resident	+10
*Comorbid illnesses**	
• Neoplastic disease	+30
• Liver disease	+20
• Congestive heart failure	+10
• Cerebrovascular disease	+10
• Renal disease	+10
*Physical examination findings**	
• Altered mental state	+20
• Respiratory rate ≥30/min	+20
• Systolic blood pressure <90 mmHg	+20
• Temperature <35°C or ≥40°C	+15
• Pulse ≥125/min	+10
Laboratory findings	
• pH <7.35	+30
• BUN ≥10.7 mmol/L	+20
• Sodium <130 mEq/L	+20
• Glucose ≥13.9 mmol/L	+10
• Haematocrit <30%	+10
• pO_2 <60 mmHg or oxygen saturation <90%	+10
• Pleural effusion	+10

Source: Fine, et al. (1997), Table 2, p. 247.[2]

TABLE 2 Stratification of risk score

Risk	Risk class	Based on
	I	Absence of features marked with asterisks in Table 1 and age ≤50 years
Low	II	≤70 total points
	III	71–90 total points
Moderate	IV	91–130 total points
High	V	>130 total points

Source: Fine, et al. (1997), Table 3, p. 248.[2]

TABLE 3 Risk class mortality for CAP patients

Risk class	No. of points	Mortality (%)	Recommendations for site of care
I	0	0.1	Outpatient
II	≤70	0.6	
III	71–90	2.8	Inpatient
IV	91–130	8.2	
V	>130	29.2	

Source: Fine, et al. (1997), Table 3, p. 248.

Table 4 Application of CURB-65

Factors	30-day mortality (%)	Risk level	Site of care
0	0.7	Low	Outpatient
1	2.1	Low	
2	9.2	Moderate	Inpatient (ED observation unit) or closely supervised outpatient
3	14.5	Moderate high	Inpatient; consider intensive care unit (ICU) admission
4 or 5	40	High	ICU

Note: Pneumonia Severity Index (PSI) has a higher discriminatory power for short-term mortality, and thus is more accurate for low risk patients than the CURB-65. However PSI is more complicated and requires arterial blood gas sampling and other tests; thus CURB-65 score is more easily used in primary care settings.
Source: Lim WS et al. (2003).[5]

- **Supportive measures**
    1. The patient should be placed in isolation in at least a monitored area or critical area if he is in septic shock or respiratory failure.
    2. Monitoring: ECG, vital signs, and pulse oximetry.
    3. Obtain intravenous access.
    4. Support airway, breathing and circulation (ABCs).
        a. Secure airway in the presence of refractory shock or respiratory failure.
        b. Give supplemental oxygen.
        c. Administer fluid resuscitation for patients in shock (refer to Chapter 33, *Sepsis/Septic Shock*). Consider inotropes for patients who respond poorly to fluid resuscitation.
- **Antimicrobial therapy**
    1. The initial choice of antibiotics should be based on risk category and the relative prevalence of common pathogens.
    2. Use of quinolones should be reserved for severe CAP in category III and above only as this may promote drug resistance as well as delay diagnosis and treatment of pulmonary tuberculosis.
    3. Patients with severe CAP needing intensive care unit admission will require broad spectrum antibiotics that will cover penicillin-resistant *Streptococcus pneumoniae*, *Burkholderia pseudomallei*, *Klebsiella pneumoniae*, *Staphylococcus aureus*, and atypical pathogens.
    4. See Table 5 for the choice of antibiotics.
    5. See Table 6 for likely types of microorganisms in pneumonia found in different clinical settings.

TABLE 5 **Empiric antibiotic therapy for community-acquired infections in hospitalized adults**
(*Please obtain cultures before antibiotic administration and tailor therapy according to microbiological results*)

Infection	Suggested antibiotics	Alternative(s) if penicillin allergy/Comment(s)
Community-acquired Pneumonia		
Hospitalized, not in ICU	Ceftriaxone IV 1g q12h + Clarithromycin PO 500 mg q12h[1]	Levofloxacin PO 750 mg q24h[1]
Suspect aspiration	Amoxicillin-clavulanic acid IV 1.2g q8h[2]	Ceftriaxone IV 1g q12h + Metronidazole PO 400 mg q8h/IV 500 mg q8h
Severe pneumonia	Amoxicillin-clavulanic acid IV 1.2g q6h + Azithromycin PO/IV 500 mg om + Ceftazidime IV 2g q8h	Ceftazidime IV 2g q8h + Levofloxacin IV 750 mg q24h

Source: National University Hospital, Singapore antibiotic guidelines.

TABLE 6   Likely types of microorganisms in pneumonia in different clinical settings

Fenicillin and multi-drug resistant pneumococci	• Age >65 years • Beta-lactam therapy within the past 3 months • Alcoholism • Immune suppressive illness • Exposure to a child in day care centres
Enteric Gram-negatives	• Resident in a nursing home • Underlying cardiopulmonary disease • Multiple comorbidities • Recent antibiotic therapy
Pseudomonas aeruginosa	• Bronchiectasis • Corticosteroid therapy • Broad spectrum antibiotic therapy • Malnutrition

• **Disposition**

Patients who are to be managed as an inpatient should be admitted in isolation to Respiratory Medicine. Those who are discharged should be followed up at respiratory specialist outpatient clinics within a week for review.

References/Further Reading

1. Lim TK. Emerging pathogens for pneumonia in Singapore. *Ann Acad Med S'pore*. 1997; 26: 651–658.

2. Fine MJ, Auble TE, Yearly DM, et al. A prediction rule to identify low risk patients with community acquired pneumonia. *N Eng J Med*. 1997; 336: 243–250.

3. Koh TH, Lui RVTP. Increasing antimicrobial resistance in clinical isolates of Strep pneumoniae. *Ann Acad Med S'pore*. 1997; 26: 604–608.

4. Lee KH, Hui KP, Lim TK. Severe community acquired pneumonia in Singapore. *S'pore Med J*. 1996; 37: 374–377.

5. Lim WS, van der Eerden MM, Laing R, et al. Defining community acquired pneumonia severity on presentation to hospital: An international derivation and validation study. *Thorax*. 2003; 58(5): 377–382.

6. Bauer TT, Ewig S, Marre R, et al. CRB-65 predicts death from community acquired pneumonia. *J Intern Med*. 2006; 260: 93.

7. Mandell LA, Wunderink RG, Anzueto A, et al. IDSA/ATS guidelines for CAP in adults. *Clinical Infectious Disease* 2007; 44: S27–72.

8. Lim WS, Baudouin SV, George RC, et al. British Thoracic Society guidelines for the management of community acquired pneumonia in adults: update 2009. *Thorax* 2009; 64: iii1–iii53.

47　Pneumothorax

Amila Punyadasa • Shirley Ooi

CAVEATS

- The management of pneumothorax is dependent on the size, clinical state of the patient, and whether the lung is diseased or normal.
- **Tension pneumothorax** is a medical emergency that requires a clinical diagnosis and treatment before chest X-ray (CXR) screening. Tracheal displacement is a **late** development in tension pneumothorax.
- It is important to give appropriate advice to all patients discharged from a health facility.

CLASSIFICATION OF SPONTANEOUS PNEUMOTHORAX

- Spontaneous pneumothorax has no antecedent traumatic or iatrogenic cause.
- It can be divided into two types:
  1. **Primary:** Where there is no underlying lung abnormality or underlying disease that predisposes to pneumothorax.
  2. **Secondary:** Where the underlying lung is diseased (e.g. COPD and pneumonia).

⇨ **SPECIAL TIPS FOR GPs**
- Pneumothorax must be considered in all patients presenting with acute shortness of breath or a young Marfanoid patient with a sudden onset of unilateral chest pain.
- Suspect a **tension pneumothorax** in patients with severe dyspnoea, tachycardia, signs of impaired peripheral perfusion, diminished breath sounds in one hemithorax, and raised jugular veins. Do **immediate needle decompression** by inserting a 14G IV venula into the second intercostal space in the mid-clavicular line and remove the metal stylet before sending the patient by ambulance to hospital. If not, the patient will die! (For further details, refer to Chapter 94, *Trauma, Chest*.)

INITIAL MANAGEMENT

- A patient with suspected pneumothorax and unstable vital signs must be managed in a resuscitation area. Other patients with pneumothorax can be managed in the intermediate care area.
- Measure vital signs and monitor the patient for electrocardiogram (ECG), vital signs and pulse oximetry.
- Administer 100% oxygen.
  1. The **rate of reabsorption** of the pneumothorax, assuming no persistent air leak, is between **1.25% and 2.2%** of the volume of **hemithorax per day**.

2. The addition of **high flow oxygen therapy** (10 L/min) increases this reabsorption rate four-fold **(6% per day)**, during that period of supplementation.

Investigation

- The main investigation is the chest X-ray although it tends to underestimate the size of the pneumothorax.
- The **size of the pneumothorax** may be determined by the following although the size does not correlate well with the clinical manifestations, the symptoms being more severe in secondary than primary pneumothoraces:
    1. The **distance from the lung apex to the ipsilateral cupola** (apex of the lung) at the parietal surface:
        a. Small pneumothorax (<3 cm) and large pneumothorax (≥3 cm) [**ACCP guidelines**].
    2. **The interpleural distance**:
        a. Small pneumothorax (<2 cm) and large pneumothorax (>2 cm) (**British Thoracic Society, BTS, guidelines**). This is the protocol that we adopt in Singapore.

FIGURE 1   **Quantification of the size of a pneumothorax**

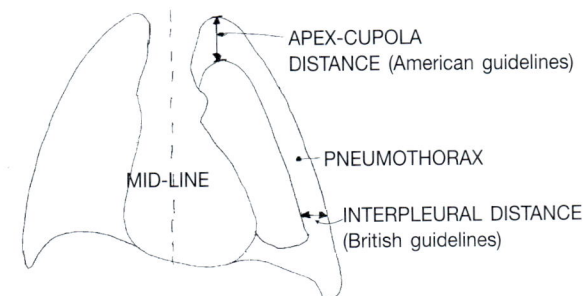

MANAGEMENT

- Management depends on the following factors:
    1. Stability of the patient.
    2. Size of the pneumothorax.
    3. Type of pneumothorax.
    4. Refer to Figure 2.

FIGURE 2 The National University Hospital of Singapore's (NUH) Emergency Medicine Department's pneumothorax protocol and clinical pathway

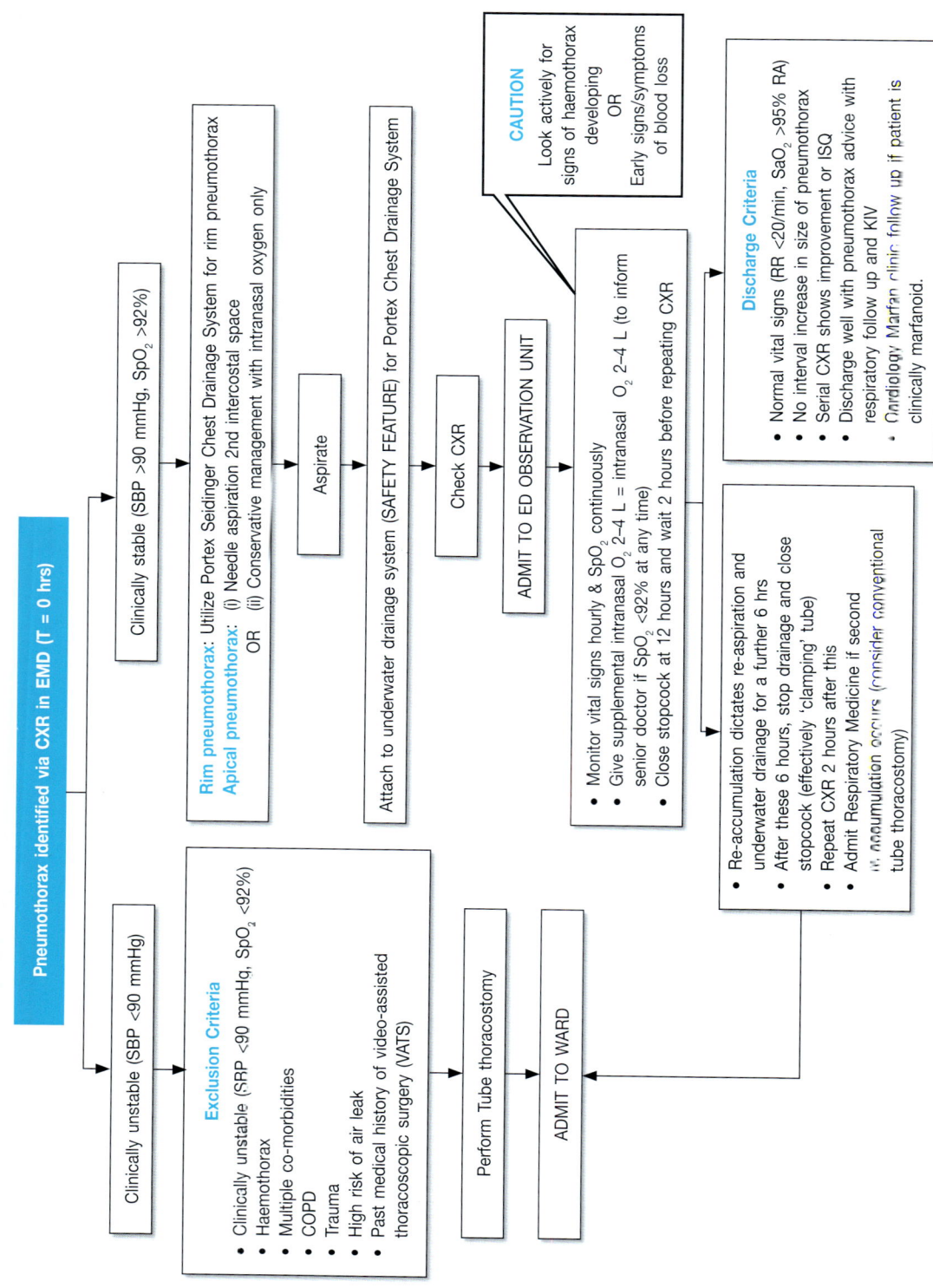

Small primary pneumothorax (stable patient) – <2 cm rim

- Observe the patient in the emergency department for 3 to 6 hours.
- Thereafter the patient may be discharged if:
  1. The patient is clinically stable.
  2. A repeat CXR does not show enlargement of the pneumothorax.
- Give comprehensive pneumothorax advice (see below).
- Schedule a follow-up appointment with a respiratory specialist for symptom and CXR surveillance (timing not specified by the BTS guidelines but, assuming symptom resolution, an interval review at one week should suffice).

Large primary pneumothorax (stable patient)

- Drain the pneumothorax with an aspiration technique. At the National University Hospital of Singapore a Portex® Seldinger Chest Drainage Kit with capabilities for both manual aspiration and conventional underwater drainage is used.
- Admit the patient for observation to either the observation unit or respiratory medicine general ward.

Unstable patient with large pneumothorax

- If the patient has tachypnoea and/or tachycardia only, the pneumothorax should be drained expediently with a 24–28 French chest tube or other equivalent.
- If the patient is hypotensive,
  1. The patient should be considered to have tension pneumothorax.
  2. Needle thoracostomy using a 14G IV venula should be performed stat in the second intercostal space in the mid-clavicular line.
  3. Thereafter, a 24–28 French chest tube should be inserted.
- The patient must be admitted.

Patient with secondary pneumothorax

- All patients should be admitted for at least 24 hours and receive supplemental oxygen as the air leak is less likely to settle spontaneously, so most patients will require active intervention.
- Aspiration is less likely to be successful.
- Most patients require the insertion of a small-bore chest drain.

PNEUMOTHORAX ADVICE

- Pneumothorax advice should be given to all patients discharged from the emergency department, regardless of whether the lungs have expanded or not.

- **Absolute contraindications**, even after complete resolution of the pneumothorax include these activities:
  1. Mountain climbing.
  2. Deep sea diving.
- **Relative contraindications**, until complete resolution of the pneumothorax (demonstrated clinically and on X-rays) include:
  1. Air travel (BTS Air Travel Working Party) for 6 weeks.
  2. Strenuous activity (e.g. pushing and pulling heavy weights) for 4 weeks.

References/Further Reading

1. Management of spontaneous pneumothorax. An American College of Chest Physicians Delphi Consensus Statement. *Chest*. 2001; 199: 590–602.

2. Mackenzie SJ, Gray A. Primary spontaneous pneumothorax: Why all the confusion over first line treatment? *J R Coll Physicians Edinb*. 2007; 37: 335–338.

3. Baumann MH. Management of spontaneous pneumothorax. *Clin Chest Med*. (2006); 27: 369–381.

4. MacDuff A, Arnold A, Harvey J. Management of spontaneous pneumothorax: British Thoracic Society pleural disease guideline 2010. Thorax 2010, 65(Suppl 2): ii18–ii31.

5. Noppen M, Alexander P. Manual aspiration versus chest tube drainage in first episodes of primary spontaneous pneumothorax. *American Journal of Respiratory and Critical Care Medicine*. 2002; 165: 1240–1244.

6. Faruqi S, Gupta D, et al. Role of simple aspiration in the management of pneumothorax. *Indian Journal of Chest Disease and Allied Science*. 2004; 46: 183–190.

7. Ayed AK, Chandrasekaran C, Sukumar M. Aspiration versus tube drainage in primary spontaneous pneumothorax: A randomized study. *European Respiratory Journal*. 2006; 27: 477–482.

48   Respiratory Failure, Acute

Goh Ee Ling • Malcolm Mahadevan

DEFINITIONS

Acute respiratory failure (RF) refers to failure of the lungs to oxygenate and/or remove carbon dioxide adequately.

- **Type I respiratory failure**: Where the arterial partial pressure of oxygen (PaO_2) is <60 mmHg.
- **Type II respiratory failure**: Where the arterial partial pressure of carbon dioxide ($PaCO_2$) is >55 mmHg with or without poor oxygenation.
- See Table 1 for causes of respiratory failure.

TABLE 1   Causes of respiratory failure

Hypoxia	Hypercapnia
Pulmonary embolism	**Decreased central respiratory drive**
Pneumonia	Drugs
Pneumothorax	Head injury
Asthma	Central nervous system lesions
Severe anaemia	Metabolic alkalosis
High altitude	Loss of hypoxic drive in chronic type 2 RF treated with oxygen
Carbon monoxide poisoning	**Airway obstruction**
	Asthma
	Chronic obstructive pulmonary disease
	Thoracic cage abnormalities
	Morbid obesity
	Chest trauma
	Kyphoscoliosis
	Neurological/neuromuscular abnormalities
	Myasthenia gravis
	Guillain-Barré syndrome
	Cervical/high thoracic injury

CAVEATS

- Patients with **type II failure alone** may look **deceptively 'comfortable'**, i.e. they are often not tachypnoeic.
- A hypercarbic patient is drowsy while a hypoxic patient is often agitated and sometimes violent.
- Pulse oximetry measures arterial oxygen saturation of haemoglobin (SaO_2) but not adequacy of ventilation (which includes the partial pressure of oxygen and carbon dioxide in the blood, i.e. pO_2, and pCO_2, respectively) which must be evaluated by arterial blood gas. See Table 3 for an interpretation of arterial blood gas.

- SaO_2 of 91% corresponds to PaO_2 of 60 mmHg in general but this is affected by pH, temperature, and 2,3-DPG level which lead to the shift of the oxyhaemoglobin dissociation curve.
- A PaO_2 level of 100 mmHg in a patient on supplemental oxygen may not be normal. Always calculate the alveolar–arterial oxygen gradient (A–a gradient, for short).
- **Do not treat the high $PaCO_2$** level in patients with chronic compensated type II respiratory failure, i.e. they have **normal pH**.
- **Do not give sodium bicarbonate to patients with low pH due to carbon dioxide (CO_2) retention!** This will exacerbate the respiratory acidosis.
- Always give as much oxygen as is necessary to correct hypoxia (keep SaO_2 at 90–92%) in chronic obstructive pulmonary disease (COPD) patients without fear of removing hypoxic drive as hypoxia kills before hypercapnia.
- **Oxygen therapy**: See Table 2.

⇨ **SPECIAL TIP FOR GPs**
- Give supplemental oxygen to all patients who are dyspnoeic until the arrival of the ambulance even if they do not look cyanosed.

MANAGEMENT

The aims of management are as follows:
- Confirm diagnosis of respiratory failure and determine the cause.
- Provide supportive measures to treat respiratory failure.
- Treat the underlying cause of respiratory failure.

Supportive measures

- Place the patient in the resuscitation room.
- Monitoring: Electrocardiogram (ECG), vital signs and pulse oximetry.
- Secure airway for airway protection and/or ventilation (refer to Chapter 28, *Airway Management/ Rapid Sequence Intubation*).
- Give supplemental oxygen. FiO_2 is determined by the patient's condition and SpO_2 level (see Box 1 for details on oxygen therapy).
- Perform an early arterial blood gas test to determine the type and severity of respiratory failure.

TABLE 2 Devices used for oxygen delivery

Device	Features	Advantages	Disadvantages	Indications
Nasal prongs	• Low flow (1–6 L/min) • FiO_2* 0.24–0.40 (approximately 3–4%/L) • FiO_2 delivered is variable	• Simple to use • Does not interfere with talking or eating • Better compliance	• Imprecise FiO_2 • Maximum FiO_2 <40%	• Mildly hypoxic patients • Patients with history of retaining CO_2
Simple mask	• Low flow (5–10 L/min) • FiO_2 0.35–0.50 (approximately 3–4%/L)	• Provides higher FiO_2 than nasal prongs	• Less comfortable, hot and confining • Interferes with talking and eating • May cause CO_2 rebreathing if flow is set too low • Variable delivered FiO_2	• Moderately hypoxic patients not known to have chronic obstructive pulmonary disease (COPD)
Venturi mask	• Provides high flow of up to 60 L/min • FiO_2 0.24–0.50	• More precise FiO_2 • Maximum FiO_2 50%	• Needs two settings and higher risk of errors in application** • Poorer compliance • CO_2 rebreathing possible if flow rate inadequate • Difficult to talk and eat	• Controlled oxygen therapy, e.g. for type II failure from COPD
Non-rebreather mask	• Low flow (6–15 L/min) • FiO_2 0.50–0.80	• Maximum FiO_2 80%	• Poorer compliance • Obstructs access to mouth • Claustrophobic	• High FiO_2 necessary to correct hypoxia

Notes: *FiO_2: Fraction of inspired oxygen.
**Correct application for Venturi masks (two diluters):
• Decide on the FiO_2 desired (use green diluter for 24–30% and white diluter for 35–50%).
• Set oxygen to the appropriate flow rate for the desired FiO_2.
• Set the size of the Venturi aperture on the face mask to the desired FiO_2.

BOX 1   **Interpreting arterial blood gas**

- **Oxygen delivery and oxygenation**
  1. It is important to document the amount of supplemental oxygen given to the patient in order to interpret the results properly.
  2. The FiO_2 delivered may be estimated by the following:
     a. Nasal prongs (2–4 L/min): 21% + 4% for every litre per minute
     b. Standard mask (6–8 L/min): FiO_2 50–60%
     c. Reservoir mask (non-rebreather mask): 80–85%
  3. Oxygen delivered by low flow systems such as intra-nasal cannulae is significantly affected by the entrainment of atmospheric air and hence the FiO_2 delivered may be inconsistent and inaccurate.
  4. Ideally, supplemental oxygen should be delivered by a fixed system such as a Venturi mask, which allows accurate FiO_2 settings.
- The **alveolar–arterial oxygen gradient (A–a gradient)** is a useful tool in evaluating how well a patient is oxygenating.
- If there is no capture, consider alternative placement of adhesive pads, consult the cardiologist for transvenous pacing and start second-line drugs.
  1. $P(A–a)O_2 = PAO_2 – PaO_2$ (mmHg)

     $$= [(760 – 47) \times FiO_2 – PaCO_2/0.8] – PaO_2$$

     where the FiO_2 is expressed as a decimal.
  2. Normal gradient = 10 to 20 mmHg. Levels of >50 mmHg suggest severe pulmonary dysfunction.
  3. The A–a gradient is known to rise with a patient's age and the FiO_2.
     a. Add 3.5 mmHg for every decade of life, or use this formula: Normal = Age/4 + 4.
     b. Add 5 to 7 mmHg for every 0.1 increase in FiO_2.
     c. Note that there is no correction for smokers.
  4. Causes of an elevated A–a gradient include V/Q mismatch (i.e. ventilation and perfusion of the lungs are not evenly matched), right to left shunt and diffusion abnormalities.
  5. However, the literature is unclear about the interpretation of a normal A–a gradient in a patient with suspected pulmonary embolism.
  6. Another tool for quick estimation of oxygenation is the PaO_2/FiO_2 ratio, sometimes called the **carrico index**.
     a. Normal = 500–600 mmHg.
     b. Levels of <200 mmHg suggest adult respiratory distress syndrome (ARDS) in patients with alveolar infiltrates in 3 of 4 pulmonary quadrants and normal pulmonary capillary wedge pressure.

Ventilatory support

- Invasive ventilation (for intubated patients): Via endotracheal tube or tracheostomy.

NOTE: Details of modes of invasive ventilation are beyond the scope of this chapter.

- **Non-invasive ventilation**
  1. Definition: The application of positive pressure ventilation to a patient in the absence of a definitive airway such as the endotracheal tube or tracheostomy.
  2. Modes of ventilation: CPAP (continuous positive airway pressure) or BiPAP (bilevel positive airway pressure).
  3. Indications: See Table 3.
  4. **Contraindications**
     a. Cardiac or respiratory arrest.
     b. Inability to use a mask because of trauma or surgery.
     c. Excessive secretions.
     d. Haemodynamic instability or life-threatening arrhythmias.
     e. High risk of aspiration.
     f. Impaired mental status or drowsiness.
     g. Uncooperative or agitated patient.
     h. Life-threatening refractory hypoxaemia.

TABLE 3   Indications of Non-Invasive Ventilation

Blood Gas Findings
Partial pressure of carbon dioxide in arterial gas ($PaCO_2$) >45 mmHg
Arterial pH <7.35 but >7.10
Ratio of partial pressure of arterial oxygen (PaO_2) to fraction of inspired oxygen ($PaCO_2/FiO_2$) <200

Clinical Inclusion Criteria
Signs or symptoms of acute respiratory distress
Moderate to severe dyspnoea
Respiratory rate greater than 24 breaths per minute
Accessory muscle use
Abdominal paradox

Diagnosis
COPD exacerbation
Acute pulmonary oedema
Pneumonia

COPD = Chronic obstructive pulmonary disease, mmHg = Millimetres of mercury.
Table used with permission from S. Sharma (2006).[3]

5. **Complications**

   a. Patient–ventilator dyssynchrony.

   b. Pneumothorax.

   c. Leakages that may compromise ventilation.

   d. Hypotension due to positive end expiratory pressure (PEEP) causing decreased venous return.

   e. Mask discomfort.

   f. Facial abrasions/skin breakdown.

Treatment of the underlying cause of respiratory failure

Disposition

The patient will be admitted to the appropriate discipline and right site of care depending upon the diagnosis and clinical status.

References/Further Reading

1. Goh SK. Respiratory failure. In: Tai DYH, Lew TWK, Loo S, eds. *Bedside ICU Handbook*. 2nd ed. Singapore: Armour Publishing; 2007: 389–391.

2. Leong A. Non-invasive mechanical ventilation. In: Tai DYH, Lew TWK, Loo S, eds. *Bedside ICU Handbook*. 2nd ed. Singapore: Armour Publishing; 2007: 391–393.

3. Sharma S. Non-invasive ventilation. In: *Business Briefing: US Respiratory Care*; 2006: 104–106.

49 Appendicitis, Acute

Sim Tiong Beng • Malcolm Mahadevan

CAVEATS

- The **classical presentation** of pain beginning periumbilically and moving to the right lower quadrant (RLQ) associated with vomiting, anorexia, rebound, and fever are reported in only 50–60% of patients.

- Vomiting following the onset of abdominal pain is more consistent with appendicitis than other diagnosis. See Table 1 for the differential diagnosis of appendicitis.

- All patients with RLQ tenderness should be diagnosed as having appendicitis until proven otherwise. Special groups of patients to be particularly vigilant include children, the elderly, women, pregnant women and the immuno-compromised.

- **Atypical/early presentations** are actually more common. Early pain may be vaguely localized to the epigastrium which makes diagnosis difficult. Retrocaecal appendix, due to its 'hidden' position, is thought to result in delayed diagnosis of acute appendicitis and increased rate of perforation.

- Healthy adult males are the only group of patients considered to be at low risk for misdiagnosis and the only patient who is safe from appendicitis is the patient who has already had his appendix removed!

- **Right lower quadrant pain** (80%) and **pain before vomiting** (100%) are more consistent for appendicitis compared with fever (67%) and nausea (58%).

- Rectal tenderness on rectal examination has only a sensitivity of 41% and a specificity of 77%. Although it used to be taught that appendicitis is very unlikely in the absence of **anorexia,** anorexia is present only in 68% of patients with appendicitis.

TABLE 1 Differential diagnosis of appendicitis

Differential diagnosis of appendicitis	
• GE	• Pancreatitis
• Non-specific abdominal pain	• Biliary tract disease
• Intestinal obstruction	• Endometriosis
• Inflammatory bowel disease	• Ovarian cyst
• Diverticulitis	• Pelvic inflammatory disease
• Meckel's diverticulitis	• Mid-cycle pain
• Adenitis	
• Henoch–Schonlein purpura	• Renal colic
	• UTI
	• Torsion testis

- Body temperatures >39°C are uncommon in the first 24 hours of illness but not uncommon after the rupture of the appendix. Think of other diagnosis (e.g. acute pyelonephritis, PID) in a patient with a high fever (>39°C) early in the onset of abdominal pain.
- **No** laboratory test can establish the diagnosis of acute appendicitis with 100% accuracy. Serial clinical examination is the key to diagnosis.
- Leucocytosis with 'left shift' is seen in 75–80% of patients with acute appendicitis. Both of these values alone have been shown not to be useful in ruling out appendicitis because of its low sensitivity (Sn), specificity (Sp), and lack of discriminative powers.
- Urinalysis should also be interpreted with caution in view of the close proximity of the appendix to the ureter; appendiceal inflammation may result in changes in urine sediment resulting in the false diagnosis of urinary tract infection.
- The only finding specific for appendicitis on abdominal X-ray is the faecolith but this is rarely seen on plain films (2% incidence) and does not justify the cost of obtaining the study.

⇨ **SPECIAL TIPS FOR GPs**
- Appendicitis is most commonly seen in 10- to 30-year-olds, although it can also be seen in patients of any age. Although rare, it has been reported in infants.
- Recurrent and chronic appendicitis is a recognized clinical entity and does occur, albeit not frequently.
- It should be included in the differential of *any* patient seen with abdominal pain. See Table 1 for the differential diagnosis of appendicitis.

MANAGEMENT

High clinical probability of acute appendicitis.

- The diagnosis begins with a history and physical examination (including pelvic and rectal).
- Withhold foods and fluids from the patient, i.e. nil by mouth.
- Set up intravenous (IV) lines and send blood for full blood count, urea/electrolytes, creatinine.
- Perform a urinalysis.
- Conduct a urine pregnancy test, if applicable.
- Give titrated IV analgesia, e.g. opiates together with an anti-emetic can be safely administered as they improve symptoms but do not mask the signs of peritonism.[8,9,10,11,12]
- Obtain surgical consultation.
- Give IV **ceftriaxone** 1 g and IV **metronidazole** 500 mg if there are signs of appendiceal perforation.
- Admit to General Surgery for appendectomy.

Borderline cases of appendicitis

- History and physical examination (including pelvic and rectal).
- Full blood count.
- Urinalysis.
- Urine pregnancy test, if applicable.
- Send the patient to the **observation** unit for serial clinical examination and **Alvarado scoring**.

  1. As appendicitis is an evolving illness, the clinical picture will become clearer during observation. With additional time, the observation unit allows the physician to evaluate patients with undifferentiated abdominal pain better.

  2. The **Alvarado score** is based on three symptoms, three signs, and two laboratory findings, as shown in Table 2. A score of 5 or 6 is compatible with the diagnosis of acute appendicitis. A score of 7 or 8 indicates a probable appendicitis, and a score of 9 or 10 indicates a very probable acute appendicitis (see Table 3). A popular mnemonic used to remember the Alvarado score factors is **MANTRELS**.

     M Migration to the right iliac fossa

     A Anorexia

     N Nausea/vomiting

     T Tenderness in the right iliac fossa

     R Rebound pain

     E Elevated temperature (fever)

     L Leucocytosis

     S Shift of leucocytes to the left

TABLE 2   Alvarado scoring system

Features	Score
Symptoms	
Migratory right iliac fossa pain	1
Nausea/vomiting	1
Anorexia	1
Signs	
Right iliac fossa tenderness	2
Fever >37.3 °C	1
Rebound pain in right iliac fossa	1
Laboratory test	
Leucocytosis (>10 × 109/L)	2
Neutrophilic shift to the left >75%	1
Total score	10

TABLE 3 **Probability of appendicitis by the Alvarado score and management strategies**

Alvarado score	Probability	Suggested management
≤4	Low	Discharge from the emergency department with abdominal pain advice and follow-up outpatient appointment
5–6	Moderate	Observation unit
≥7	High	Inpatient admission

3. The positive and negative predictive values of the Alvarado score are 77.6 and 52.4%, respectively. It is more effective in men and children, with a predictive value of 84 and 92.8%, respectively. Discriminant analysis reveals a cut-off value that is ≥6 rather than the original value that is ≥7. The sensitivity of the Alvarado score increases from 69.2% to 92% with the new cut-off value of ≥6. The Alvarado scoring system can be used in the emergency department to guide in the evaluation of patients presenting with right iliac fossa (RIF) pain. In women, additional investigations (e.g. pelvic scan to rule out gynaecological causes) may be required to confirm the diagnosis.

RESULTS

- **Ultrasonography** has been used successfully in diagnosing acute appendicitis, although the greatest experience has been in children. In adults, sensitivity and specificity are approximately 86 and 81%, respectively and is frequently insufficient or non-diagnostic.

- Reported sensitivity (Sn), specificity (Sp), positive likelihood (+ve LR), and negative likelihood ratios (–ve LR) for **computed tomography (CT)** are 94%, 95%, 13.3, and 0.09, respectively. The results show that CT is far superior to ultrasound, 86% (Sn), 81% (Sp), 5.8 (+ve LR), and 0.19 (–ve LR). CT may be particularly useful in females to reduce negative appendectomy rate. It is also useful in patients with atypical presentation, e.g. RIF pain with fever and diarrhoea (colitis) and elderly patients with malignancy.

- The benefit of **diagnostic laparoscopy** has been most evident in fertile women, in whom it is associated with an 80% reduction in the rate of negative appendectomies.

References/Further Reading

1. Prystowsky JB, Pugh CM, Nagle AP. Current problems in surgery. Appendicitis. *Curr Probl Surg*. Oct 2005; 42(10): 688–742.

2. Hals G. Acute appendicitis: Meeting the challenge of diagnosis in the ED. *Emerg Med Rep*. 1999; 20(8): 71–86. Coleman C, Thompson JE, Bennion RS, et al. WBC count is a poor predictor of severity of disease in the diagnosis of appendicitis. *Am Surg*. 1998; 64: 983–985.

3. Dueholm S, Bagi P, Bud M. Laboratory aid in the diagnosis of acute appendicitis: A blinded, prospective trial concerning the diagnostic value of leukocyte count, neutrophil differential count, and C-reactive protein. *Dis Colon Rectum*. 1989; 32: 855–859.

4. Cardall T, Glasser J, Guss DA. Clinical value of the total white blood cell count and temperature in the evaluation

of patients with suspected appendicitis. *Acad Emerg Med*. Oct 2004; 11(10): 1021–1027.

5. Malone AJ, Shetty MR. Diagnosis of appendicitis. *Lancet*. 1997; 14: 349.

6. Hoffman J, Rasmussen AB. Aids in the diagnosis of acute appendicitis. *Br J Surg*. 1989; 76: 774–779.

7. Does this patient have appendicitis? *JAMA*. 1996; 276: 1589.

8. Zollie N, Cust MP. Analgesia in the acute abdomen. *Ann Royal Coll of Surg Edin*. 1986; 68: 209–210.

9. Attard AR, Corlett MJ. Safety of early pain relief for acute abdominal pain. *BMJ*. 1992; 305: 554–556.

10. Lovechio F, Oster N. The use of analgesics in patients with acute abdominal pain. *J Emerg Med*. 1997; 15; 6: 775–779.

11. Pace S, Burke TF. Intravenous morphine for early pain relief in patients with acute abdominal pain. *Acad Emerg Med*. 1996; 3: 1086–1092.

12. Mahadevan M, Graff L. Prospective randomized study of analgesic use for ED patients with right lower quadrant abdominal pain. *Am J Emerg Med*. 2000; 18: 753–756.

13. DeKoning EP. Acute appendicitis. In: Tintinalli JE, Stapczynski JS, Ma OJ, et al, eds. *Tintinalli's Emergency Medicine: A Comprehensive Study Guide*. 7th ed. New York: McGraw-Hill; 2011: 574–578.

14. Hostetler B, Leikin JB, Timmons JA, Hanashiro PK, Kissane K. Patterns of use of an emergency department-based observation unit. *Am J Ther*. Nov–Dec 2002; 9(6): 499–502.

15. Garcia Pena BM, Mandl KD, Kraus SJ, et al. Ultrasonography and limited computed tomography in the diagnosis and management of appendicitis in children. *JAMA*. 1999; 282: 1041.

16. Carrico CW, Fenton LZ, Taylor GA, et al. Impact of sonography on the diagnosis and treatment of acute lower abdominal pain in children and young adults. *AJR Am J Roentgenol*. 1999; 172: 513.

17. Terasawa T, Blackmore CC, Bent S, Kohlwes RJ. Systematic review: Computed tomography and ultrasonography to detect acute appendicitis in adults and adolescents. *Ann Intern Med*. 5 Oct 2004; 141(7): 537–546.

18. Wagner PL, Eachempati SR, Soe K, et al. Defining the current negative appendectomy rate: For whom is preoperative computed tomography making an impact? *Surgery*. 2008; 144: 276.

19. Sauerland S, Lefering R, Neugebauer EA. Laparoscopic versus open surgery for suspected appendicitis (Cochrane Review). *Cochrane Database Syst Rev*. 2002; CD001546.

20. Shrivastava UK, Gupta A, Sharma D. Evaluation of the Alvarado score in the diagnosis of acute appendicitis. *Trop Gastroenterol*. Oct–Dec 2004; 25(4): 184–186.

21. Chan MYP, Tan C, Chiu MT, Ng YY. Alvarado score: An admission criterion in patients with right iliac fossa pain. *Surg J R Coll Surg Edinb Irel*. 2003; 1(1): 39–41.

50   Hepatic Encephalopathy, Acute

Malcolm Mahadevan • Lee Yin Mei • Lim Seng Gee

DEFINITION

Hepatic encephalopathy is defined as a syndrome of altered mental state and reversible neuropsychiatric state complicating liver disease.

CLASSIFICATION

There are two classifications each with widely differing aetiologies, clinical presentations, physical findings, and management principles:

- Encephalopathy associated with acute liver failure.
- Encephalopathy associated with liver cirrhosis and portal hypertension.

⇨ **SPECIAL TIPS FOR GPs**
- Avoid narcotics, tranquillizers, and sedatives that are metabolized in the liver.
- Be aware that not all hepatic encephalopathies arise in patients with chronic liver cirrhosis. Acute hepatic failure can arise from ingestion of toxins, recreational drug use, and hepatitis A, B, and E.

Encephalopathy associated with acute liver failure

- A medical emergency that requires prompt recognition and treatment as the patient may deteriorate into a coma and require a liver transplant.
- Typically the patient is previously well with **no history of liver disease**.
- Symptoms are vague and non-specific, i.e. malaise and fatigue with nausea, followed by jaundice and encephalopathy that may progress rapidly to coma.
- **History**: Care should be taken in the history to exclude the following:
  1. Overdose of paracetamol.
  2. Ingestion of toxins such as fenfluramin.
  3. Use of the recreational drugs cocaine and Ecstasy.
  4. Intravenous (IV) drug use.
  5. A recent travel history in an attempt to exclude hepatitis A and E.
  6. A history of recent sexual exposure significant for possible hepatitis B.

- **The physical examination** should show no signs of chronic liver disease, focal neurology or a high fever. Such findings should prompt the search for an alternative cause for encephalopathy.
- **Grades of encephalopathy**:
  1. **I** Trivial lack of awareness, anxiety, euphoria, or short attention span.
  2. **II** Lethargy or apathy with minimal disorientation for time or place. The patient may show subtle personality change or inappropriate behaviour.
  3. **III** Stupor and confusion.
  4. **IV** Coma.
- **Management**:
  1. The patient should be managed in the critical care area of the emergency department.
  2. Airway maintenance and oxygenation: If the patient is comatose or has airway compromise, perform endotracheal intubation.
  3. Monitoring: Electrocardiogram (ECG), vital signs q5 to 15 minutes and pulse oximetry.
  4. Establish peripheral IV line.
  5. Administer IV fluids: Normal saline infusion at a rate sufficient to maintain peripheral perfusion is best performed with haemodynamic monitoring.
- **Drug therapy**: Give IV mannitol 20%: 1 g/kg body weight.
- **Investigations**:
  1. Stat capillary blood sugar.
  2. Full blood count, urea/electrolytes/creatinine, coagulation profile, and liver function tests.
  3. Serum toxicology (where relevant).
  4. Hepatitis A, B, C, D, and E (anti-HAV IgM, HbsAg, anti-HBS, anti-HCV, anti-delta, and anti-HBE) screening.
  5. Urgent head computed tomography scan to detect cerebral oedema.
- **Disposition**: Consult Gastroenterology and admit to intensive care unit.

Encephalopathy associated with liver cirrhosis and portal hypertension

- The patient **has established liver disease** and has a disturbance of consciousness that develops over a short period of time and fluctuates in severity, or may be a more chronic phenomenon.
- The current classification consists of 3 categories: Episodic, persistent, or minimal. Encephalopathy in cirrhosis is caused by portosystemic shunting and altered amino acid metabolism with ammonia playing a strong role as well as other neuro-transmitters.
- **History**: The recognition of a history of established cirrhosis or liver disease is important.

- **Precipitating events** that tip patients with chronic liver disease into hepatic encephalopathy include the following:
  1. **H** Haemorrhage from the gastrointestinal tract, e.g. from varices or erosions.
  2. **E** Electrolyte imbalance (hypokalaemia, alkalosis as seen in diuretic use, and vomiting and diarrhoea) and hypoglycaemia.
  3. **P** Protein intake (excessive).
  4. **A** Azotaemia (from volume contraction) and diuretics.
  5. **T** Tranquillizers and other sedatives.
  6. **I** Infections, e.g. spontaneous bacterial peritonitis, urinary tract infection or pneumonia, and also infections arising in surgical wounds.
  7. **C** Constipation.
- The **physical examination**:
  1. May show signs of chronic liver disease, e.g. spider naevi, gynaecomastia, liver palms, leuchonychia, and a hepatic flap.
  2. May show enlargement of the liver or spleen as well as ascites.
  3. Should include a rectal examination for melaena (black tar-like stool).
- **Management**:
  1. Manage the patient in the critical care area of the emergency department.
  2. Airway maintenance and oxygenation: If the patient is comatose or has airway compromise, perform endotracheal intubation.
  3. Monitoring: Electrocardiogram (ECG), vital signs q 5 to 15 minutes, and pulse oximetry.
  4. Establish peripheral IV line.
  5. Administer IV fluids: Normal saline infusion at a rate sufficient to maintain peripheral perfusion is best performed with haemodynamic monitoring.
- **Investigations**: These are targeted to confirm the **diagnosis** of **encephalopathy** complicating cirrhosis as well as to look for the **precipitating cause**:
  1. Stat capillary blood sugar.
  2. Full blood count, urea/electrolytes/creatinine, ammonia, coagulation profile, and liver function tests.
  3. Blood cultures and urinalysis as indicated.
  4. Chest X-ray.
- **Drug therapy**:
  1. IV dextrose 50% 40 ml for hypoglycaemia and IV thiamine 100 mg if the patient has alcoholic cirrhosis.
  2. IV naloxone 2 mg if the patient has significant obtundation.
  3. IV flumazenil 0.5 mg repeated after 5 minutes (shown in small controlled trials to improve the grade of encephalopathy).

- **Reversal of encephalopathy**:

  1. **Lactulose** 30 ml given orally (PO) or a lactulose enema: Produces an osmotic diarrhoea, thus altering intestinal flora that decreases ammonia production.

  2. **Oral antibiotics:** Randomized controlled trials show no clinical benefits.

  3. **Protection of gastrointestinal mucosa:** Give **omeprazole** 20–40 mg IV slowly over 5 minutes.

- **Disposition:** Consult Gastroenterology with a view to admit to a high dependency unit (or intensive care unit if intubated).

References/Further Reading

1. Sherlock S, Dooley J. *Diseases of the Liver and Biliary system*. 10th ed. Oxford, UK: Blackwell Science; 1997.

2. Ferenci P, Lockwood A, Mullen K, et al. Hepatic encephalopathy: Definition, nomenclature, diagnosis and qualification. Final report at the 11th World Congress of Gastroenterology, Vienna, 1998.

51   Hepatobiliary Emergencies

Brandon Koh

The acute problems originating from the hepatobiliary system that present to the emergency physician are usually complications of biliary stone disease. The various forms are described below.

BILIARY COLIC

- Approximately 20% of people who have gallstones have biliary colic.
- It describes the constellation of symptoms experienced by a patient when the gallbladder contracts against an outlet obstruction.
  1. Occurs when a gallstone is lodged in the neck of the gallbladder or in Hartmann's pouch.
- Most often seen in obese women between the ages of 30 and 50 years.
- It is a **clinical diagnosis**.

Clinical features

- Sharp, cramping pain.
- Localized to the right hypochondrium or epigastrium.
- Often radiating to the right scapula or interscapular area.
- Symptoms commonly occur following large or fat-rich meals.
- The pain often occurs at night, affecting sleep.
- Associated with nausea, malaise, bloating, and belching.
- Symptoms tend to be recurrent.
- Usually resolves spontaneously or with analgesia.

Management

- Give analgesia.
- Avoid heavy meals.
- Stick to a low fat diet.
- If the symptoms resolve with treatment, discharge with an outpatient USS HBS (ultrasound scan of the hepatobiliary system) appointment, and subsequent follow-up at the general surgery specialist outpatient clinic.
- Patients who do not respond to trials of analgesia may require admission.

CAVEATS

- Always look for symptoms and signs of **obstructive jaundice** as this suggests the presence of **biliary ductal stones** rather than biliary colic *per se*.
- The presence of pain and fever, suggests that **acute cholecystitis** has occurred.
- The presence of pain, fever, and obstructive jaundice suggests the presence of **acute cholangitis**.

ACUTE CHOLECYSTITIS

- Gallstones are present in over 90% of the cases.
- Prolonged gallbladder outlet obstruction leads to acute cholecystitis.[4]
- The female to male ratio is approximately 3:1.

Clinical features

- Colicky pain in the epigastrium or right hypochondrium.
- This pain persists or escalates over 12–24 hours. Its prolonged duration distinguishes it from biliary colic.
- There is often a history of milder episodes of biliary colic, which worsen progressively.
- Associated with fever, chills, nausea, vomiting, and anorexia.
- On examination, there may be tenderness in the right hypochondrium.
- Up to 25% of patients have a palpable distended gallbladder.
- **Murphy's sign** is positive when the patient complains of increased pain and catches his breath when palpation is performed over the right hypochondrium during inspiration.
  1. This is due to the inflamed gallbladder coming into contact with the tips of the examiner's fingers during inspiration.
  2. A positive Murphy's sign is **highly sensitive (97%)** and predictive (positive predictive value 93%) of acute cholecystitis.[5]

NOTE: These physical signs may be absent in the elderly.

Investigations

- Full blood count
  1. Look for elevated white blood cells with left shift.
- Renal panel
- **Liver function tests**
  1. Bilirubin, alkaline phosphatase (ALP), aspartate aminotransferase (AST), and transaminase (ALT) may be mildly elevated.
  2. A significantly elevated bilirubin should raise the possibility of choledocholithiasis.
- **Amylase**
  1. May be mildly elevated.
  2. Look for significant elevation that may suggest concomitant pancreatitis.
- **Plain abdominal X-ray**
  1. Minimal value.
- **USS HBS** is the imaging modality of choice
  1. The following features on the USS are supportive of acute cholecystitis:
     a. Gallstones (See Chapter 118, *Emergency Ultrasound* Fig. 12)
     b. Sludge
     c. Wall thickening (>4 mm)
     d. Pericholecystic fluid (See Chapter 118, *Emergency Ultrasound* Fig. 14)
     e. Positive sonographic Murphy's sign

Management

- Keep the patient nil by mouth.
- Commence IV fluids (regime depending on the patient's hydration and haemodynamic status).
- Give analgesia.
- Administer IV antibiotics (**ceftriaxone** 1 g and **metronidazole** 500 mg).
- Admit to General Surgery.

Caveats

- In the elderly and in patients with diabetes, acute cholecystitis may present with severe sepsis or septic shock.
- Potential **complications** of acute cholecystitis include gallbladder gangrene, perforation, and empyema.
  1. These require an urgent General Surgery consult.

ACUTE CHOLANGITIS

- This occurs as a result of bacterial infection superimposed on biliary tree obstruction.
- The most common cause of obstruction is stones in the common bile duct.
- Biliary obstruction after biliary intervention carries a very high risk of cholangitis.
- Most commonly cultured organisms are *E. coli*, *Klebsiella*, *Enterococcus*, and *Enterobacter*.

Clinical features

- **Charcot's triad** is classically described.
  1. Fever (most common symptom).
  2. Pain in the right hypochondrium.
  3. Jaundice.
- More severe cholangitis presents with **Reynold's pentad**.
  1. Charcot's triad **plus**
     a. Altered mental status.
     b. Hypotension.
- Tenderness in the epigastrium/right hypochondrium.
- Patients are usually ill and show signs of toxicity.
  1. **Septic shock** may be present.

Management

- Monitor in P1.
- Check vital signs q 5 minutes.
- Give supplementary oxygen.
- Resuscitate with IV fluids.
- Administer analgesia.
- Perform laboratory tests:
  1. Full blood count (elevated white blood cells)
  2. Renal panel
     a. Correct electrolyte abnormalities if present.
  3. **Liver function tests**
     a. Significantly elevated bilirubin.
     b. Elevation in alkaline phosphatase greater than any elevation in AST/ALT.
  4. **Amylase**
     a. May be elevated, but not to a similar extent as in pancreatitis.
  5. **Coagulation profile**
     a. Disseminated intravascular coagulation (DIVC) may be present due to severe sepsis.

6. Group and cross match
7. Arterial blood gases
   a. Metabolic acidosis
8. Lactate
9. Blood cultures
- Insert a urinary catheter to monitor the urine output.
- Give IV antibiotics (**ceftriaxone** 1 g and **metronidazole** 500 mg).
  1. In patients with allergy to penicillin, ciprofloxacin is a good alternative to the cephalosporin.
- Start vasopressors if the patient is still hypotensive despite adequate restoration of circulatory volume with IV fluids.
  1. Insert a central venous line to guide fluid resuscitation.
- Admit to Gastroenterology.
  1. Definitive therapy is endoscopic retrograde cholangiopancreatography (ERCP) with intervention (bile duct clearance or drainage).
- Consider referring the patient for admission to the medical high dependency or intensive care unit for haemodynamic monitoring and further management.

Differential diagnosis

Do not forget other possible diseases presenting in a similar fashion, such as the following:
- Acute coronary syndrome.
- Peptic ulcer disease.
- Pancreatitis.
- Ureteric colic.
- Hepatitis/liver abscess.
- Basal pneumonia.

LIVER ABSCESS

Pyogenic liver abscess

Aetiology
- Intra-abdominal infections
  1. E.g. Appendicitis, diverticulitis
- Biliary obstruction (benign/malignant), stenting or instrumentation
- Haematogenous spread
  1. E.g. Bacterial endocarditis, IV drug abuse
- Hepatic trauma

- Cryptogenic (no cause found)

Diabetic/immunocompromised patients are especially susceptible.

Clinical presentation:
- Early symtoms are usually insidious and nonspecific
  1. Malaise, loss of appetite
- Late symptoms
  1. Fever, chills
  2. Abdominal pain (may not be localized to the right upper quadrant)
- Septic shock
  1. In delayed presentation or in the setting of biliary obstruction

Investigations:
- FBC
  1. Leucocytosis with left shift
- Deranged liver function test
- Blood cultures
  1. *Klebsiella pneumoniae* (more common in the Asian population)
  2. *Escherichia coli*, other Gram negative organisms
  3. Gram positive (*Strep*, *Staph aureus*)
- CXR/AXR
  1. Usually nonspecific, may show
     a. Pleural effusion/collapse of lung
     b. Elevation of diaphragm
- Ultrasound
  1. Sensitivity 75–95%
- CT scan
  1. Sensitivity 95%
  2. More accurate than ultrasound, especially with contrast enhancement

Treatment:
- Parenteral antibiotics
  1. IV ceftriaxone 1 g
  2. IV metronidazole 500 mg
- Drainage of pus
  1. Percutaneous/open

Disposition:

- Admission to Gastroenterology if patient is well (and abscess can be drained percutaneously) and to General Surgery if patient is ill (e.g. patient in septic shock, having ruptured liver abscess, peritonitis from perforated diverticulitis, gallbladder abscess, etc.)
- Consider HD/ICU care if the patient has septic shock or severe metabolic acidosis.

References/Further Reading

1. Elwood David R. Cholecystitis. *Surg Clin North America*. 2008; 88; 1241–1252.

2. Riviello RJ, Bradley WJ. Presentation and management of acute biliary tract disorders in the emergency department: Optimizing assessment and treatment of cholelithiasis and cholecystitis. *Emerg Med Rep*. 2002; 23(17): 203–210.

3. Russell RCG, et al. *Bailey & Love's Short Practice of Surgery*. 24th ed. London: Arnold; 2004.

4. Indar A, Beckingham I. Acute cholecystitis. *BMJ*. 2002; 325: 639–643.

5. Singer AJ, McCracken G, Henry MC. Thode HC Jr, Cabahug CJ. Correlation among clinical, laboratory, and hepatobiliary scanning findings in patients with suspected acute cholecystitis. *Ann Emerg Med*. 1996; 28: 267–272.

6. Yusoff Ian F, et al. Diagnosis and management of cholecystitis and cholangitis. *Gastroenterol Clin North Am*. 2003; 32: 1145–1168.

7. Attasaranya Siriboon, et al. Choledocholithiasis, ascending cholangitis, and gallstone pancreatitis. *Med Clin North Am*. 2008; 92: 925–960.

8. Kaye M. Reid-Lombardo et al., Hepatic Cysts and Liver Abscess, *Surg Clin of North Am* 2010; 90: 679–697.

52   Intestinal Obstruction

Brandon Koh • Irwani Ibrahim

CAVEATS

- The classical quartet of symptoms are:
  1. Abdominal pain, distension, vomiting, and constipation.
  2. However, vomiting may be delayed in low bowel obstruction and distension may be minimal in high bowel obstruction.
- Always examine the hernial orifices and perform a rectal examination. Impacted faeces would indicate a pseudoobstruction instead.

BACKGROUND

- Intestinal obstruction can be divided into **mechanical** (Box 1) and **non-mechanical obstructions** (Box 2).

BOX 1   Causes of mechanical obstruction

Intraluminal
Impaction
Foreign bodies
Bezoar
Gallstones

Intramural
Stricture
Malignancy

Extramural
Adhesions from previous surgery
Hernia
Volvulus
Intussusception

BOX 2   Causes of non-mechanical obstruction

- Paralytic ileus
  1. Postoperative
  2. Intra-abdominal sepsis
  3. Metabolic (uraemia, hypokalaemia)
- Mesenteric vascular occlusion
- Pseudo-obstruction

CLINICAL FEATURES

- **Pain**
    1. Sudden onset
    2. Usually severe
    3. Colicky in nature
- **Vomiting**
    1. The more distal the obstruction, the longer the interval between the onset of symptoms and the appearance of nausea and vomiting.
- **Distension**
    1. The more distal the obstruction, the greater the degree of distension.
- **Constipation**
    1. Absolute
        a. Neither faeces nor flatus is passed.
    2. Relative
        a. Only flatus is passed.
    3. Absolute constipation is a cardinal feature of complete intestinal obstruction.
- **Dehydration**
    1. Dry mucous membranes.
    2. Oliguria.
- **Bowel sounds**
    1. Initially hyperactive and high pitched (tinkling).
    2. Eventually absent due to bowel fatigue.

It is important to look for the features listed in Box 3 that suggest the presence of strangulation.

BOX 3   Evidence of strangulation

Constant pain (even despite decomposition)
Fever
Shock
Peritonitis

In a **strangulated external hernia,**
- The lump is tense, tender and irreducible, and has recently increased in size.
- There is no expansile cough impulse.

INVESTIGATIONS

- Full blood count

- Renal panel
  1. Look for electrolyte derangements and pre-renal azotemia.
- GXM
- Abdominal X-ray
  1. Look for dilated loops of small and large bowel, as well as air-fluid levels.
  2. Fluid levels appear later than gas shadows.
  3. The more pronounced the fluid levels, the more advanced the obstruction.

Small bowel

- Dilated to >3 cm in diameter.
- Centrally located.
- Presence of valvulae conniventes.
  1. Extend across the entire diameter of the lumen.

Large bowel

- Peripherally located.
- Presence of colonic haustral folds.
  1. Extend only partially across the lumen.

MANAGEMENT

- Maintain airway and provide supplemental oxygen if necessary.
- Administer IV fluids.
- Correct electrolyte abnormalities.
- Keep the patient nil by mouth.
- Insert a nasogastric tube and allow passive/free drainage to decompress the bowels.
  1. Drip and suck (bowel rest).
- Insert a urinary catheter to monitor the urine output in patients who are in shock.
- Give IV antibiotics if there is evidence of strangulation.
  1. **Ceftriaxone** 1 g and **metronidazole** 500 mg.
- Admit to General Surgery.
- If there is evidence of strangulation or peritonitis, the general surgery registrar should be called stat.
  1. To facilitate emergency surgery and admission to surgical high dependency or intensive care unit.

References/Further Reading

1. Russell RCG, et al. *Bailey & Love's Short Practice of Surgery*. 24th ed. London: Arnold; 2004.
2. Cappell Mitchell S, Batke Mihaela. Mechanical obstruction of the small bowel and colon. *Med Clin North Am.* 2008; 92: 575–597.

53   Ischaemic Bowel/Mesenteric Ischaemia

Brandon Koh

CAVEATS

- One should have a **high index of suspicion of ischaemic** bowel in at-risk patients who present with a sudden **onset** of abdominal pain, the **severity** of which is **out of proportion** to the **clinical signs**.
- The non-specific presentation of early bowel ischaemia and the lack of physical signs often result in a delayed diagnosis.
- Concrete physical signs occur late, when the intestinal infarction is already irreversible.
- Mortality is high, estimated at around 70%.[2]

PATHOPHYSIOLOGY

- **Risk factors** include these:
  1. Advanced age.
  2. Dysrhythmias, especially atrial fibrillation (predisposes to embolism).
  3. Valvular heart disease/endocarditis.
  4. Chronic congestive cardiac failure.
  5. Peripheral vascular disease/atherosclerosis.
  6. Recent myocardial infarction, with residual ventricular thrombus.
  7. Hypotension.
- **Aetiology**: Occlusion of the visceral vessels by either one of the following:
  1. An embolus (more common).
  2. A thrombus.
- The superior mesenteric vessels are the most commonly affected.
- The ischaemic bowel (and its mesentery) becomes swollen and oedematous.
- Blood-stained fluid exudes into the peritoneal cavity and bowel lumen.
- After occlusion of the vasculature, haemorrhagic infarction occurs.
  1. Gangrene and perforation of the bowel follow rapidly.

CLINICAL FEATURES

- Sudden onset of severe abdominal pain (in a patient with risk factors).
  1. Pain is typically central.
  2. Pain is **out of proportion** to the physical findings is the **hallmark** of mesenteric ischaemia.

- Persistent vomiting and diarrhoea occur early.
    1. One may be misled into thinking the problem is gastroenteritis!
    2. There is subsequent passage of altered blood.
- Tachycardia is often the first abnormal vital sign.
- Fever (but it may be absent).
- Tachypnoea (from pain or metabolic acidosis) and diaphoresis.
- Hypovolaemic shock (late finding).
- There is initially only mild abdominal tenderness.
    1. Peritonitis occurs **late**.
- Absent bowel sounds (**late** sign, after the development of complete infarction).

NOTE: However, ischaemic bowel can occur without these classic risk factors and even in the young patient.

It should be suspected when the pain seems out of proportion to the physical findings, and the patient appears too ill for his condition to be accounted for by a benign process.

A prominent surgeon previously commented on the lack of physical findings in acute mesenteric ischaemia: 'Perhaps the best overall finding was an uneasy feeling on the part of the examining physician that his patient looked sick, but that he could not say why or from what.'[5]

Hence, a high index of suspicion must be maintained.

INVESTIGATIONS

- There are **no specific laboratory tests** to diagnose mesenteric ischaemia.
- Useful **laboratory tests** include these:
    1. Full blood count.
        a. Look for haemoconcentration, and an elevated white blood cell count.
    2. Renal panel.
    3. Coagulation profile.
    4. GXM.
- An elevated serum **amylase** is found in almost half of patients with intestinal infarction.
    1. An incorrect diagnosis of pancreatitis may result.
- **Arterial blood gases**
    1. Approximately 50% of patients with mesenteric ischaemia have a metabolic acidosis.
- **Arterial lactate**
    1. Most patients with mesenteric ischaemia have an elevated lactate.
    2. It correlates with the degree and extent of ischaemia found at surgery.[6,7]
    3. Acute mesenteric ischaemia has a sensitivity nearing 100%.[6,7]

- **Electrocardiogram**
  1. Look for atrial fibrillation.

IMAGING STUDIES

- **Plain abdominal radiographs**
  1. Rarely diagnostic, and completely normal 25% of the time.
  2. Early features are non-specific.
     a. Small bowel distension with air-fluid levels or ileus.
  3. As the disease progresses, '**thumbprinting**' and separation of the bowel loops occur.
     a. This is a manifestation of bowel wall oedema and focal haemorrhage.
  4. **Pneumatosis intestinalis**
     a. When necrosis occurs, linear collections of air may be seen in the bowel wall.
- **Computed tomography (CT) scans**
  1. Recent advances enable the mesenteric vasculature to be visualized.
     a. Helical CT
     b. Use of IV contrast
     c. CT angiography
- **Angiography**
  1. Remains the gold standard for diagnosing acute mesenteric ischaemia.
  2. The sensitivity for detecting arterial occlusion is consistently more than 90%.[8,9]

⇨ **SPECIAL TIP FOR GPs**
- Abdominal pain should not be dismissed as a benign process, particularly in high risk patients.

MANAGEMENT

- Check vital signs q 5 minutes.
- Maintain airway and provide supplemental oxygen.
- Administer IV fluids.
- Keep the patient nil by mouth.
- Give intravenous antibiotics:
  1. **Ceftriaxone** 1 g and **metronidazole** 500 mg.
- Consider inserting a nasogastric tube to decompress the bowel.

- Insert a urinary catheter to monitor the urine output.
- Avoid vasoconstricting drugs like dopamine and noradrenaline if possible.
- Seek immediate consultation with the general surgery registrar.
- For definitive treatment and disposition, operating theatre/radiology/surgical intensive care unit.

References/Further Reading

1. Russell RCG, et al. *Bailey & Love's Short Practice of Surgery*. 24th ed. London: Arnold; 2004.

2. Brandt LJ, Boley SJ. AGA technical review on intestinal ischemia. *Gastroenterology*. 2000; 118: 954.

3. Martinez JP, Hogan GJ. Mesenteric ischemia. *Emerg Med Clin North Am*. 2004; 22: 909–928.

4. Shanley CJ, Weinberger JB. Acute abdominal vascular emergencies. *Med Clin North Am*. 2008; 92: 627–647.

5. Anane-Sefah JC, Blair E, Reckler S. Primary mesenteric venous occlusive disease. *Surg Gynecol Obstet*. 1975; 141: 740.

6. Lange H, Jackel R. Usefulness of plasma lactate concentration in the diagnosis of acute abdominal disease. *Eur J Surg*. 1994; 160: 381–384.

7. Lange H, Toivola A. Warning signs in acute abdominal disorders: Lactate is the best marker of mesenteric ischemia [Swedish]. *Lakartidningen*. 1997; 94: 1893–1896.

8. Klein HM, Lensing R, Klosterhalfen B, Tons C, Gunther RW. Diagnostic imaging of mesenteric infarction. *Radiology*. 1995; 197: 79–82.

9. Kim AY, Ha HK. Evaluation of suspected mesenteric ischemia: Efficacy of radiologic studies. *Radiol Clin North Am*. 2003; 41: 327–342.

54   Pancreatitis, Acute

Brandon Koh • Peter Manning

CAVEATS

- Classically, acute pancreatitis is associated with elevated serum amylase.
  1. The threshold value is >1000 U/L or ≥3× the upper limit of normal range.
  2. This, however, is not always present.
- Patients with acute exacerbations of chronic pancreatitis often have 'subthreshold' elevations of serum amylase due to a reduced volume of functioning pancreatic tissue.
- Elevated amylase levels may also be seen in other acute abdominal disease processes, but these do not classically reach threshold values.
- See Table 1 for the differential diagnoses of pancreatitis.

TABLE 1   Differential diagnoses of pancreatitis

Site of pathology	Examples	
Abdominal	Perforated peptic ulcer	
	Acute exacerbation of pain from peptic ulcer disease	
	Biliary colic	
	Acute cholangitis	
	Ischaemic bowel	
	Ruptured/ leaking abdominal aortic aneurysm	
	Abdominal aortic dissection	
Supradiaphragmatic	Basal pneumonia	
	Acute coronary syndrome	

KEY CONSIDERATIONS

When a diagnosis of acute pancreatitis is made, the emergency physician should consider the following key questions:

- **What is the cause of the pancreatitis?** (Table 2)
- The most common causes are gallstone disease (40%) and alcohol intake (35%).[1]
- **How severe is the pancreatitis?** (See *Clinical Predictors of the Severity of Pancreatitis* on page 371.)

TABLE 2   Causes of pancreatitis

Alcohol	**Vascular**
Hypertriglyceridaemia	Polyarteritis nodosa and other vasculitic disorders
Hypercalcaemia	Ischaemia
Drug induced	
Scorpion venom	**Infections**
	Mumps
Mechanical	Coxsackie B
Gallstones	Cytomegalovirus
Postoperative	Cryptococcus
Abdominal trauma	
Post-endoscopic retrograde cholangiopancreatography	**Others**
Pancreatic tumours	Genetic
	Autoimmune
	Idiopathic

CLINICAL FEATURES

- Abdominal pain
    1. Typically localized to the epigastrium.
        a. The abdominal pain may be in the right upper quadrant or left upper quadrant.
    2. Acute onset.
    3. Severe.
    4. Deep, penetrating pain, radiating to the back.
    5. Exacerbated by eating and drinking (especially alcohol).
    6. Patients may lean forward or curl up.
    7. Patients tend to be restless and agitated.
        a. As opposed to patients with a perforated viscus (who tend to keep still).
- Nausea and vomiting
    1. Very common (about 90% of patients).
- Severe pancreatitis can present with severe upper abdominal tenderness and guarding.
- Ileus may be present.
    1. Decreased bowel sounds.
    2. Epigastric distension.
- Hypovolaemia (dehydration)
    1. Tachycardia.
    2. Hypotension.
    3. Oliguria.

- **Grey-Turner's sign**
  1. Flank ecchymosis.
  2. Indicates retroperitoneal haemorrhage from haemorrhagic pancreatitis.
- **Cullen's sign**
  1. Periumbilical ecchymosis.
  2. Indicates intra-abdominal haemorrhage.

LABORATORY TESTS

- **Full blood count**
  1. Elevated white blood cells are common.
- **Renal panel**
  1. Look for electrolyte derangement and azotaemia.
  2. Elevated glucose is common.
- **Liver function tests**
  1. A significantly elevated transaminase (>150 IU/L) suggests gallstone pancreatitis.[2]
  2. A significantly elevated bilirubin suggests choledocholithiasis.
- **Amylase**
  1. >3× above normal: Highly specific for pancreatitis.
  2. Lacks specificity at lower levels.
  3. May be elevated to a lesser degree in other conditions.
  4. Insensitive in delayed clinical presentation.
     a. Amylase levels return to normal after several days.
  5. The degree of elevation of amylase is not a marker of disease severity.
- **Lipase**
  1. High sensitivity and specificity.[3]
  2. Not routinely used in all emergency departments.

IMAGING STUDIES

- **Plain abdominal X-ray** and **erect chest X-ray**
  1. Mainly ordered to exclude alternative causes of the patient's symptoms, e.g. pneumoperitoneum in a perforated viscus.
  2. Findings suggestive of pancreatitis:
     a. Dilated bowel loops with air-fluid levels from ileus.
     b. Sentinel loop.

    c. Dilated proximal bowel because of spasm of the distal bowel overlying the inflamed pancreas.[4]

  3. A pleural effusion (more common on the left side) may be evident on the chest X-ray.[5]

- CT abdomen

  1. Useful in diagnosis and prognostication.

CLINICAL PREDICTORS OF THE SEVERITY OF PANCREATITIS

- Determining the severity of pancreatitis is important for these reasons:

  1. Early recognition of complications.

  2. Decision making regarding the disposition of the patient (admission to the general ward, high dependency, or intensive care unit).

- Formal clinical scoring systems improve the accuracy of estimations of disease severity.

  1. **Ranson's criteria** is one of these scoring systems.[6]

    a. Limited use in the emergency department, as scoring can only be completed 48 hours after the initial diagnosis is made.

- Systemic complications suggestive of **severe pancreatitis** include these:[7]

  1. Refractory hypotension.

  2. Adult respiratory distress syndrome/hypoxaemia.

  3. Disseminated intravascular coagulation.

  4. Renal failure.

  5. Acidosis.

⇨ **SPECIAL TIPS FOR GPs**

- Beware of atypical presentations.

  1. The pain is often in the central abdomen or epigastrium, but this is not always so.

    a. When pancreatitis affects the pancreatic body and tail, the pain may be in the left hypochondrium rather than in the central abdomen.

    b. Acute pancreatitis must, therefore, always be considered a possible diagnosis in any patient presenting with upper abdominal pain.

MANAGEMENT

- Maintain the airway, provide supplemental oxygen.
- Keep the patient nil by mouth (rest the pancreas).

- Give IV fluids.
  1. Patients are generally severely dehydrated from the profound loss of intravascular fluid into the pancreas and abdomen ('third space losses').
  2. Correct electrolyte derangements, if any.
- Insert a urinary catheter to monitor the urine output (if the patient is hypotensive).
- Administer analgesia.
  1. Parenteral opioids.
- Perform a nasogastric tube insertion, only in the following situations:
  1. Ileus.
  2. Persistent vomiting.
- Give prophylactic antibiotics for severe pancreatitis.
  1. The use of prophylactic antibiotics for the treatment of severe pancreatitis, however, is a controversial issue.
  2. Not routinely recommended unless there is a specific infection.[8]
- Admit to General Surgery.
- For patients with severe pancreatitis with systemic complications:
  1. Consult the general surgery registrar for admission to surgical high dependency or intensive care unit.

References/Further Reading

1. Steinberg W, Tenner S. Acute pancreatitis. *N Engl J Med*. 1994; 330(17): 1198–1210.
2. Tenner S, Dubner H, Steinberg W. Predicting gallstone pancreatitis with laboratory parameters: A meta-analysis. *Am J Gastroenterol*. 1994; 89(10): 1863–1866.
3. Smith RC, Southwell-Keely J, Chesher D. Should serum pancreatic lipase replace serum amylase as a biomarker of acute pancreatitis? *ANZ J Surg*. 2005; 75(6): 399–404.
4. Davis S, Parbhoo SP, Gibson MJ. The plain abdominal radiograph in acute pancreatitis. *Clin Radiol*. 1980; 31(_): 87–93.
5. Raghu MG, Wig JD, Kochhar R, et al. Lung complications in acute pancreatitis. *JOP*. 2007; 8(2): 177–185.
6. Ranson JHC, Rifkind KM, Roses DF, et al. Prognostic signs and the role of operative management in acute pancreatitis. *Surg Gynaecol Obstet*. 1974; 139: 69–81.
7. Mitchell RMS, Byrne MF, Baille J. Pancreatitis. *Lancet*. 2003; 361: 1447.
8. Banks PA, Freeman ML. Practice guidelines in acute pancreatitis. *Am J Gastroenterol*. 2006; 101(10): 2379–2400.
9. Cappell Mitchell S. Acute pancreatitis: Etiology, clinical presentation, diagnosis, and therapy. *Med Clin North Am*. 2008; 92: 889–923.

55 Peptic Ulcer Disease/Dyspepsia

Andrea Rajnakova • Lim Seng Gee

CAVEATS

- Most patients with dyspepsia or abdominal pain do not have peptic ulcer disease.
- There are no discriminant symptoms for peptic ulcer disease although food-related symptoms, relief with antacids, and nocturnal symptoms are more common.
- Peptic ulcer disease may be asymptomatic, or present with anaemia or gastrointestinal bleeding.
- Endoscopy is the best method to diagnose or exclude peptic ulcer disease

SYMPTOMS

- The patient with an uncomplicated peptic ulcer disease usually presents with upper abdominal pain or discomfort. Poor appetite, nausea, and vomiting may also be present.
- Alarm features include weight loss, haematemesis or malaena, anaemia, dysphagia and palpable abdominal mass.
- It is not possible to differentiate between gastric and duodenal ulcers on the basis of history alone, although gastric ulcer patients tend to be older and are more likely to complain of weight loss.
- The pain is typically situated in the epigastrium, but may occur in the lower chest or right or left hypochondrium, and is typically diffuse.
- The pain typically occurs when the patient is hungry, 1 to 3 hours after meals, and may be nocturnal, and be relieved by food or antacids. It is also characterized by remission and exacerbations. Ulcer pain may occasionally radiate to the back. It should be noted that there are no discriminant symptoms of ulcer disease.
- The diagnosis of peptic ulcer cannot be established or excluded based on patient symptoms alone. Typical ulcer-like pains may occur in patients with non-ulcer dyspepsia. On the other hand, asymptomatic ulcers are more common in patients taking NSAIDs.
- Even asymptomatic ulcers may present with bleeding. The only presenting symptom may be tiredness and giddiness due to anaemia. If the bleeding is heavy, malaena with or without haematemesis, or coffee ground vomiting will be present.

⇨ **SPECIAL TIPS FOR GPs**

- *H. pylori* and non-steroidal anti-inflammatory drugs (NSAIDs) are the most common risk factors for peptic ulcer disease.
- People aged >40 years with **chronic dyspepsia** should be **investigated endoscopically** to rule out gastrointestinal malignancy.

- All patients with **dyspepsia** and **alarm features**, such as weight loss, anaemia, dysphagia, palpable abdominal mass or evidence of gastrointestinal bleeding (haematemesis or malaena) should be referred to a gastroenterologist for endoscopy.
- Always enquire into the **complications** of peptic ulcer disease such as bleeding (haematemesis or malaena) and vomiting (pyloric obstruction). These emergencies need urgent hospital referral.
- Surgery is rarely necessary and is only carried out if complications such as perforation, recurrent severe bleeding that cannot be controlled endoscopically, or obstruction develop.

MANAGEMENT

The aims of management of upper abdominal discomfort or pain are as follows:

- Make a provisional diagnosis (refer to Chapter 140, *Pain Management*).
- Relieve the symptoms.
- Decide on who to admit to hospital.
- Decide on who to refer for specialist consultation.

Symptoms management

- After **excluding life-threatening causes** which require immediate intervention and admission, e.g. acute myocardial infarction, aortic dissection, ruptured abdominal aortic aneurysm, and other important causes such as perforated peptic ulcer, hepatobiliary sepsis such as cholangitis, cholecystitis, liver abscess, and pancreatitis, the patient should be given symptomatic relief.
- Give mist **magnesium trisilicate (MMT)/aluminium hydroxide** 40–80 ml and an **antispasmodic**, e.g. IV or IM hyoscine-N-butylbromide (Buscopan®) 40 mg or oral proton pump inhibitors (PPIs).

NOTE: Statistically, peptic ulcer disease represents 10–15% of abdominal pain which will respond to MMT. There is **no role for IV proton pump inhibitors**. The evidence supports giving IV PPI for patients with upper gastrointestinal bleeding.

- Discharge patients with MMT or oral PPI or give motilium (domperidone) to dyspeptic patients while waiting for a definitive diagnosis to be made at the gastroenterology specialist outpatient clinic (SOC).
- For patients with acute abdominal pain/discomfort which resolves at emergency department treatment, no further treatment is indicated.
- There is no role for *H. pylori* eradication for undiagnosed peptic ulcer disease and non-ulcer dyspepsia in the emergency department.

DISPOSITION

Indications for hospital admission

- Bleeding: Haematemesis, malaena, and coffee ground vomiting. Admit to Gastroenterology or General Surgery depending on the hospital policy.

- Perforation: Admit to General Surgery.

- Narrowing and obstruction: Difficult to diagnose in the emergency department, but if the patient presents with vomiting or signs of intestinal obstruction, admit to General Surgery.

- Patients are non-responsive to treatment at the emergency department (this is only if they have severe symptoms): Admit to Gastroenterology.

- Abdominal pain with fever and jaundice: Admit to Gastroenterology.

Indications for outpatient referral to Gastroenterology

- Chronic dyspepsia or a recent onset of new symptoms in patients aged more than 40 years old.

- Presence of alarm features such as weight loss, loss of appetite, anaemia, dysphagia, and palpable abdominal mass.

- Persistence of symptoms despite a trial of empirical treatment, such as PPI therapy.

NOTE: **A single episode of abdominal pain/discomfort** (without any alarm features) **should not be referred to the SOC** since this complaint is very common and is usually self-limiting and non-specific.

Discharge advice

Always remember to discharge patients with advice to return to the emergency department immediately if there is fever, lower abdominal pain, persistent diarrhoea, or vomiting. Remember **upper abdominal pain** may be an **early symptom of acute appendicitis**.

References/Further Reading

1. Chan FKL, To KF, Wu JCY, et al. Eradication of *Helicobacter pylori* and risk of peptic ulcers in patients starting long-term treatment with non-steroidal anti-inflammatory drugs: A randomized trial. *Lancet.* 2002; 359: 9–13.

2. Ateshkadi A, Lam NP, Johnson CA, et al. *Helicobacter pylori* and peptic ulcer disease. *Clin Pharm.* 1993; 12(1): 34–48.

3. Hawkey CJ, Karrasch JA, Szczepanski L, et al. Omeprazole compared with misoprostol for ulcers associated with non-steroidal anti-inflammatory drugs. Omnium study. *NEMJ.* 1998; 338: 727–734.

4. Yeoh KG, Kang JY. Peptic ulcer disease. In: Guan R, Kang JY, Ng HS, et al, eds. *Management of Common Gastrointestinal Problems.* Singapore: Habbas MediMedia Asia Pte Ltd; 2000: 31–46.

5. Graham DY, Rakel RE, Fendrick AM, et al. Recognizing peptic ulcer disease: Keys to clinical and laboratory diagnosis. *Postgraduate Medicine.* 1999; 105(3): 113–133.

6. Lahaie RG, Gaudreau C. *Helicobacter pylori* antibiotic resistance: Trends over time. *Can J Gastroenterology.* 2000; 14(10): 895–899.

7. Manes G, Balzano A, Iaquinto G, et al. Accuracy of the stool antigen test in the diagnosis of *Helicobacter pylori* infection before treatment and in patients on omeprazole therapy. *Aliment Pharmacol Ther.* 2001; 15(1): 73–79.

56   Perianal Conditions
Charles Bih-Shiou Tsang

CAVEATS

- Bleeding from the anal canal is usually fresh and bright red. Blood mixed with stool suggests a more proximal aetiology.
- **Pain and bleeding** with bowel movements occur in **anal fissures**. Bleeding from **piles** is usually **painless**.
- Deep-seated anal abscesses can present with constant chronic anal pain and few physical signs. An endoanal ultrasound evaluation by a colorectal surgeon is required.
- Recurrent perianal abscesses in the same area suggest an underlying fistula-in-ano.

⇨ **SPECIAL TIPS FOR GPs**

- Do not attribute rectal bleeding in a middle-aged or elderly patient solely to bleeding piles. Refer to a colorectal surgeon to exclude lesions in the more proximal gastrointestinal tract.
- Never assume that rectal bleeding with bowel movements in a patient is due to piles without performing a digital rectal examination and anoscopy. If the bleeding persists despite conservative treatment, always exclude a more proximal aetiology, e.g. barium enema and colonoscopy.

HAEMORRHOIDS

- **Clinical features**
  1. Bright red rectal bleeding is common usually after the passage of stool.
  2. Bleeding can be variable in quantity but is usually self-limiting.
  3. The prolapsing mass requires digital reduction.
  4. A painful and prolapsing mass with a bluish hue represents thrombosis and is usually not reducible.
  5. **First-degree piles** do not appear at the anus after defaecation. The main symptom is bleeding after a bowel movement.
  6. **Second-degree piles** protrude through the anus on defaecation but spontaneously reduce.
  7. **Third-degree piles** remain outside the anus unless pushed back manually.
  8. **Fourth-degree piles** cannot be pushed back inside the anus.
- **Acute management**
  1. **Bleeding first- and second-degree piles**
     a. Provide reassurance.

b. Perform rectal examination and anoscopy to exclude a proximal aetiology.

c. Discharge with a 6-week course of bulking agents, e.g. one satchet of ispaghula husk twice daily (Fybogel®, Metamucil®, and Mucilin®) or micronized flavonoids (Daflon 500®) in a dose of 3 tabs twice a day (bd) for 3 days, then 2 tabs bd for 2 weeks.

2. **Bleeding third-degree piles with mild thrombosis**

a. Instruct the patient to lie prone with an ice pack placed in the buttock cleft to reduce oedema.

b. Administer parenteral analgesia, e.g. a non-steroidal anti-inflammatory drug (NSAID) or opioid agonist.

c. Attempt digital reduction with a generous amount of lubricant.

d. If successful, discharge the patient with analgesics, bulking agents, and flavonoid agents.

e. If unsuccessful, admit the patient for further management.

PERIANAL HAEMATOMA

- **Clinical features**

1. This is due to the rupture of blood vessels of the external haemorrhoidal venous complex.

2. On examination there is an exquisitely tender and bluish discrete pea-shaped lump.

3. The pain usually peaks within the first 2 days and settles by the 5th day.

- **Acute management**

1. In the first 2 days perform incision and drainage in the emergency department:

a. Prep perianal skin with betadine (ask the patient if he has any allergy first).

b. Infiltrate around the haematoma with 5 ml of 1% lignocaine using a 22G needle.

c. Make a small radial incision towards the anus and evacuate the haematoma by expressing it.

d. Apply direct pressure to stop any oozing.

e. Insert a small ribbon pack.

f. Discharge the patient with analgesics and bulking agents to prevent constipation or straining.

g. The ribbon pack can be removed the next day by the patient after a sitz bath. To prepare a sitz bath, fill a tub to hip height with warm water, and add two tablespoons of salt.

h. Refer the patient to a colorectal surgeon for outpatient follow-up review.

2. After 2 days, provide reassurance and discharge the patient with analgesics and bulking agents.

ANAL FISSURES

- **Clinical features**

  1. Presents with bright red rectal bleeding with bowel movements.
  2. Severe pain differentiates this condition from piles.
  3. The common aggravating causes are poor fluid intake and a fibre-deficient diet.
  4. The rectal examination reveals an acute linear tear posteriorly or anteriorly on gently effacing the anal verge. A digital rectal examination **may not be possible** due to severe anal pain and spasm.

- **Acute management**: If the pain is so severe as to preclude a proper rectal examination, admit the patient for examination under anaesthesia. Most acute fissures heal spontaneously with proper bowel regulation. However, if the symptoms persist beyond 8 weeks, the fissure may not heal without surgical intervention. Signs of chronicity include the appearance of a boat-shaped ulcer with white anal sphincter fibres seen at the base. There is often a skin tag (aka sentinel pile) at the distal margin of the fissure and a hypertrophic anal papilla at the apex. The mainstay of treatment is conservative management consisting of:

  1. A 6-week course of **bulking agents**, e.g. one sachet of ispaghula husk twice a day (Fybogel®, Metamucil®, and Mucilin®) and 2 L of oral fluids a day.
  2. **Topical analgesia**: Lignocaine jelly 2% applied around the anus before a bowel movement to help ease the pain; this can be followed by a sitz bath (see above for directions on how to prepare one).
  3. **Glyceryl trinitrat (GTN) paste** can be useful for 'chemical sphincterotomy'.
  4. Note that **stool softeners**, e.g. Agarol® and lactulose, are seldom necessary, and the resultant diarrhoea may aggravate the fissure.
  5. Arrange for outpatient follow-up with a colorectal surgeon.

ANORECTAL SEPSIS

- **Classification:** Park's classification categorizes anorectal sepsis in relation to the anal sphincter complex. Most abscesses arise from anal glands that are present within and around the anal sphincters and may be submucous, perianal, intersphincteric, ischiorectal, or supralevator in location.

- Persistent drainage from an abscess that has been drained previously (≥2 months) suggests the presence of a fistula.

- **Clinical features**

  1. **A classic abscess** presents as a red, warm and tender swelling, which may already be pointing or draining pus.
  2. **Differential diagnosis of a perianal abscess from an ischiorectal abscess**: Look at the relationship of the abscess to the pigmented perianal skin. An abscess within the pigmented skin means a perianal abscess, whereas an abscess lying more laterally outside the pigmented skin means an ischiorectal abscess.

3. A small deep-seated abscess may present with few external signs other than pain and tenderness on a rectal examination. Typically, this patient has received several courses of antibiotics or analgesics from his own doctor. Hence, chronic perianal pain should be referred to a colorectal surgeon for the exclusion of a deep-seated abscess.

4. A persistent discharging sinus or swelling for >2 months after drainage of an abscess suggests an **anal fistula**. A rectal examination often reveals an indurated subcutaneous cord running radially from the external opening towards the anus. This cord is the fistula track.

- **Acute management**
  1. **Acute abscess**:
     a. **Incision and drainage** in the emergency department under conscious sedation and local anaesthesia: A linear incision over the most fluctuant part of the abscess is then converted into a cruciate incision and the edges are trimmed to deroof the abscess.
     b. After expression of all pus, lightly pack with ribbon gauze for haemostasis (can be removed the next day after a sitz bath).
     c. Prescribe analgesics for 1–2 days with referral for review by a colorectal surgeon within a week. If pain or fever persists, advise the patient to return to the emergency department earlier as the abscess may have been incompletely drained.
        Criteria for admission:
        i. **Diabetics with perianal abscesses** for surgical drainage and control of blood sugar levels or
        ii. a high suspicion of **necrotizing fasciitis** (tender induration with crepitus around the abscess).
  2. **Recurrent perianal abscesses or suspected underlying anal fistula**: Admit for drainage by a colorectal surgeon.

PROLAPSED RECTUM

- **Clinical features**
  1. **'True' prolapse** is seen in infants and elderly females but is uncommon. The entire thickness of the rectal wall is intussuscepted through the anus. The 'pinch' test reveals a double layer or 'a sleeve within a sleeve'.
  2. **'Pseudo' prolapse** is a prolapsed haemorrhoid or rectal mucosal prolapse and is common. The 'pinch' test fails to reveal another layer of rectal wall beneath. The mucosal prolapse is often associated with a history of chronic straining. The resultant mucus seepage may also cause pruritis.

- **Acute management**
  1. **'True' prolapse**: Perform gentle digital reduction and bowel regulation in adults to avoid straining and make an early referral to a paediatrician (in the case of infant patients) or colorectal surgeon (adult patients). If reduction is not possible, then it is deemed to be incarcerated and is a surgical emergency.

2. **'Pseudo' prolapse of rectal mucosa**: Prescribe a course of bulking agents (see above) and advise adequate fluid intake to avoid straining during defaecation. Refer to a colorectal surgeon for definitive management (rubber band ligation).

POSTHAEMORRHOIDECTOMY BLEEDING

- **Clinical feature**

  <5% of such patients may present with secondary haemorrhage 7–10 days after surgery; this may occur after a difficult bowel movement with straining. The bleeding is usually self-limiting and minor. However, in a small percentage, it can be sufficient to cause hypovolaemic shock.

- **Acute management**

  1. If severe, resuscitate with rapid fluid replacement via a large bore intravenous cannulae; GXM if necessary.

  2. Prepare to inspect the anal canal, identify the bleeding point and secure haemostasis.

      a. Prepare proper lighting, proctoscope, suction equipment, 20 ml of adrenaline solution diluted 1:10,000 in a syringe with a 23G spinal needle.

      b. Keep the patient in the left lateral position and apply generous amounts of lignocaine jelly to the anus prior to the insertion of the proctoscope; evacuate the clots and slowly withdraw the proctoscope to visualize the anal canal, in particular the haemorrhoidectomy wound.

      c. Identify the bleeding point and inject the adrenaline solution.

      d. Insert an adrenaline pack and leave it in-situ for minor persistent oozing.

  3. Arrange an immediate colorectal consultation in the emergency department if the bleeding cannot be controlled. In the interim, a size 18F Foley catheter can be inserted into the anus and the catheter balloon filled with 30 ml of water and traction applied with the catheter taped to the thigh. The balloon creates a tamponade effect on the haemorrhoidectomy wound.

  4. In minor cases where bleeding has already stopped:

      a. Discharge the patient with a course of metronidazole 400 mg three times a day (tds) for a week and a course of micronized flavonoids, e.g. Daflon®.

      b. Arrange early follow-up with the patient's surgeon.

References/Further Reading

1. Misra MC, Parshad R. Randomized clinical trial of micronized flavonoids in the early control of bleeding from acute internal haemorrhoids. *Br J Surg*. 2000; 87(7): 868–872.

2. Ho YH, Tan M, Seow-Choen F. Micronized purified flavonidic fraction compared favorably with rubber band ligation and fiber alone in the management of bleeding hemorrhoids: Randomized controlled trial. *Dis Colon Rectum*. 2000; 43(1): 66–69.

3. Eu KW, Seow-Choen F, Goh HS. Comparison of emergency and elective haemorrhoidectomy. *Br J Surg.* 1994; 81(2): 308–310.

4. Keighley M. Haemorrhoidal disease. In: Keighley MRB, ed. *Surgery of the Anus, Rectum and Colon.* London: WB Saunders; 1993: 304–305.

5. Sorgi MB, Sardinas C. Anal fissure. In: Wexner SD, ed. *Clinical Decision Making in Colorectal Surgery.* Tokyo: Igaku-Shoin Medical Publishers, Inc; 1995: 123–126.

6. Grace, R. Anorectal sepsis. In: Dudley CH, Russell RCG, eds. *Atlas of General Surgery.* Kent, UK: Butterworth & Co; 1986: 614–621.

7. Goldberg S. Rectal prolapse and rectoanal intussusception in clinical decision making. In: Wexner SD, ed. *Clinical Decision Making in Colorectal Surgery.* Tokyo: Igaku-Shoin Medical Publishers, Inc; 1995.

8. Ho YH, Tan M, Seow-Choen F, et al. Prospective randomized controlled trial of a micronized flavonidic fraction to reduce bleeding after haemorrhoidectomy. *Br J Surg.* 1995; 82(8): 1034–1035.

57 Acid Base Emergencies

Goh Ee Ling • Benjamin Leong • Peter Manning

CAVEATS

- Symptoms and signs of acid base emergencies are often nebulous and wide ranging. Hence, a high index of suspicion should be maintained.
- Always consider acid base/electrolyte disorders in a patient with altered mental state.
- A complete evaluation of acid base disorders requires both arterial blood gas and serum electrolytes.
- Under most normal conditions, venous pH will be about 0.02 less than arterial pH, and can be used as an approximate. Venous blood gases (VBG), however, cannot be used as a replacement for arterial blood gases (ABG) in evaluating respiratory function.
- In shock and hypoperfusion states, the arterial and venous pH and partial pressure of carbon dioxide (pCO_2) gap will widen with time with the venous pH expected to fall further below the arterial pH, due to the accumulation of metabolites and carbon dioxide (CO_2) in the tissues. Also, in shock states with normal respiration, the reduced pulmonary blood flow will lead to a ventilation–perfusion mismatch where there may be an apparent respiratory alkalosis in the arterial blood (see Chapter 22, *Shock/Hypoperfusion States*).
- This chapter will focus on the interpretation of the acid base status.

⇨ **SPECIAL TIPS FOR GPs**

- Hyperventilation is a diagnosis of exclusion in tachypnoeic patients. Always consider metabolic acidosis (manifesting with Kussmaul's breathing), pulmonary embolism, and severe asthma.
- Early identification and treatment of acid base disorders offers the best chances of recovery or improvement.

DIAGNOSING ACID BASE DISORDERS

- Follow these steps to detect an acid base disorder:

  1. **Check the internal consistency** of the results using the H–H equation.

     Multiply the $\dfrac{pCO_2 \times 24}{[HCO_3^-]} = $ 'X' (the H^+ concentration)

     Correlate 'X' with the number in the right-hand column of the table on the next page and note the corresponding pH in the left-hand column. The pH and the measured pH in the ABG result should be equal or very close to equal. If they are not close to equal, concern must be raised about the validity of the data since they do not satisfy the Henderson–Hasselbach equation and the test should be repeated. Failure to do so has clinical implications since serious management decisions are made based on the measured data, e.g. whether to intubate or use non-invasive ventilation and sodium bicarbonate. This simple step takes only 15 seconds to perform and therefore should not be considered an impediment to a smooth and efficient workflow.

pH	Approximate (H$^+$) (mmol/L)
7.00	100
7.05	89
7.10	79
7.15	71
7.20	63
7.25	56
7.30	50
7.35	45
7.40	40
7.45	35
7.50	32
7.55	28
7.60	25
7.65	22

2. **Identify the primary abnormality** starting with the pH.

   a. pH <7.35 and [HCO$_3^-$] <20 mmol/L: Metabolic acidosis

   b. pH <7.35 and pCO$_2$ >45 mmHg: Respiratory acidosis

   c. pH >7.45 and [HCO$_3^-$] >24 mmol/L: Metabolic alkalosis

   d. pH >7.45 and pCO$_2$ <35 mmHg: Respiratory alkalosis

3. **Identify any secondary abnormality** by checking the adequacy of compensation.

   a. **Metabolic acidosis: Expected pCO$_2$ = (1.5 × [HCO$_3^-$] + 8 mmHg (±2).**

   b. **Metabolic alkalosis: Expected pCO$_2$ = (0.6 × [HCO$_3^-$ − 24]) + 40 mmHg.**

      i. If measured pCO$_2$ is lower than expected, concurrent respiratory alkalosis is present.

      ii. If measured pCO$_2$ is higher than expected, concurrent respiratory acidosis is present.

   c. **Respiratory acidosis or alkalosis:**

      i. **Acute**

         - **[HCO$_3^-$] changes 1–2 mmol/L for every change in pCO$_2$ by 10 mmHg.**

         - pH changes 0.08 for every change in pCO$_2$ by 10 mmHg.

      ii. **Chronic**

         - **[HCO$_3^-$] changes 4–5 mmol/L for every change in pCO$_2$ by 10 mmHg.**

         - pH changes 0.03 for every change in pCO$_2$ by 10 mmHg.

      iii. If the measured [HCO$_3^-$] is lower than expected, consider the presence of concurrent metabolic acidosis.

      iv. If the measured [HCO$_3^-$] is higher than expected, consider the presence of concurrent metabolic alkalosis.

BOX 1   Important formulae

- The Henderson–Hasselbalch (H–H) equation:

$$pH = 6.1 + \log \frac{[HCO_3^- \text{ (in mmol/L)}]}{0.03 \times PaCO_2 \text{ (in mmHg)}} \text{ (where 6.1 = p}K_A).$$

1. The measured venous total CO_2 levels given in some electrolyte panels include $[HCO_3^-]$ and dissolved CO_2.

   Total CO_2 = $[HCO_3^-]$ + dissolved CO_2

   = $[HCO_3^-]$ + 0.03 × $PaCO_2$ (in mmHg)

   = $[HCO_3^-]$ + 1.2 (if $PaCO_2$ = 40 mmHg)

2. Therefore the venous CO_2 may be used as an estimate of the serum bicarbonate level, bearing in mind that it is about 1 mmHg higher than the actual bicarbonate level.

- **Anion gap (AG): $[Na^+]$ – $[HCO_3^-]$ – $[Cl^-]$**

1. **Normal = 3–11 mmol/L.** Recent changes in electrolyte measuring techniques have resulted in a lowered normal range for the anion gap, and this has been validated in studies of normal healthy volunteers.

2. **Causes of low AG:**
   a. Hypoalbuminaemia (AG decreases by 2.5 mmol/L for every 1 g/dL decrease)
   b. Paraproteinaemia
   c. Hyponatraemia
   d. Hypermagnesaemia
   e. Spurious hyperchloraemia
   f. Lab errors

d. **Calculate the 'gaps':**
   i.   Anion gap (AG): $[Na^+]$ + $[K^+]$ – $[HCO_3^-]$ – $[Cl^-]$.
   ii. Excess anion gap (ΔAG): AG – 10 (+/– 4).
   iii. Bicarbonate gap (ΔHCO_3^-): 24 – HCO_3^-.
   iv. Delta gap (Δgap) = Difference between the change in AG and change in $[HCO_3^-]$.
   v.   Δgap = ΔAG – ΔHCO_3^-.
   vi. If the AG is high and the change in the anion gap is 0, the AG will rise by the same amount that the bicarbonate has fallen; this is a simple high anion gap metabolic acidosis (HAGMA).
   vii. If the AG is high and the change in the anion gap is >0, there are too many HCO_3^- ions, then there is a HAGMA and concurrent metabolic alkalosis.
   viii. If the AG is high and the change in the anion gap is <0, there are less HCO_3^- ions than expected, then there is a HAGMA and concurrent non-anion gap metabolic acidosis (NAGMA).

General rules

- **Rule 1**: The direction of the pH change is the primary abnormality. Compensatory mechanisms do not 'overcompensate' nor even fully compensate to normal.
- **Rule 2**: Any abnormality in any of the 3 variables of the H–H equation (pH, $[HCO_3^-]$ and pCO_2) is associated with an acid base disorder **without exception**.

    If the pH is normal, check for balanced acid base disorder:

    1. $[HCO_3^-]$ <20 pCO_2 <35:   Metabolic acidosis and respiratory alkalosis
    2. $[HCO_3^-]$ >24 pCO_2 >45:   Metabolic alkalosis and respiratory acidosis
    3. $[HCO_3^-]$, pCO_2 normal, AG >11:   HAGMA and metabolic alkalosis
    4. $[HCO_3^-]$, pCO_2 normal, AG normal: Normal (unlikely NAGMA and metabolic alkalosis)

- **Rule 3**: The presence of a very high anion gap (>20) suggests a HAGMA even in the presence of a normal pH or $[HCO_3^-]$. The body does not generate an elevated anion gap just to compensate for alkalosis.

    (Refer to Chapter 48, *Respiratory Failure, Acute* for interpretation of oxygenation of ABG.)

TYPES OF ACID BASE DISORDERS

Metabolic acidosis

- **Definition**: pH <7.35 and $[HCO_3^-]$ <20 mmol/L.
    1. **HAGMA**: $[HCO_3^-]$ <20 mmol/L and anion gap >11 mmol/L.
    2. **NAGMA (hyperchloraemic metabolic acidosis)**: $[HCO_3^-]$ <20 mmol/L and anion gap <11 mmol/L.
- **Causes:** The causes of HAGMA may be summarized by the mnemonics SULK (somewhat more reflective of pathogenic mechanisms) or CATMUDPILES, and the causes of NAGMA may be summarized by the mnemonics USEDCARP. See Table 1 for causes of HAGMA and Table 2 for causes of NAGMA.
- **Treatment of metabolic acidosis**: This is essentially targeted at the **underlying cause**, e.g.:
    1. Diabetic ketoacidosis (hydration and insulin therapy).
    2. Shock (hydration, inotropes and treatment for sepsis).
    3. Renal failure (dialysis).
    4. Methanol/ethylene glycol ingestion (ethanol).
- Bicarbonate therapy is controversial.
    1. Potential adverse effects include electrolyte disturbances (e.g. hypokalaemia and hypocalcaemia), paradoxical intra-cerebral, and intra-cellular acidosis, post-treatment alkalosis, hypernatraemia/hyperosmolality, and fluid overload. Furthermore, bicarbonate therapy has **not** been shown to improve survival.
    2. Possible benefits are improved myocardial contractility, response to catecholamines, and haemodynamic status.

TABLE 1   Causes of high anion gap metabolic acidosis (HAGMA)

S	Salicylates, exogenous toxins (e.g. metformin, methanol, toluene, ethylene glycol, iron, and paraldehyde)	**C**	Cyanide, carbon monoxide
		A	Alcoholic ketoacidosis
		T	Toluene
U	Uraemia	**M**	Methanol, methaemoglobin
L	Lactic acidosis (**type A:** Any cause of tissue hypoxia, e.g. shock, sepsis, cyanide, and carbon monoxide poisoning; **type B:** non-hypoxic causes, e.g. liver, renal disease, inborn errors of metabolism, metformin, phenformin, isoniazid, and iron)	**U**	Uraemia
		D	Diabetic ketoacidosis
		P	Paraldehyde
		I	Isoniazid/iron (via lactic acidosis)
		L	Lactic acidosis (e.g. any cause of shock, hypoxia, metformin, phenformin, and cyanide poisoning)
K	Ketoacidosis (diabetic, alcoholic, and starvation)	**E**	Ethylene glycol (**not** ethanol)
		S	Salicylates and solvent

TABLE 2   Causes of normal anion gap metabolic acidosis (NAGMA)

Hyperkalaemic type	*Renal*	**U**	Ureterosigmoidostomy
	Renal tubular acidosis (type IV)	**S**	Small bowel fistula
	Potassium sparing diuretics	**E**	Extra chloride
	Hypoaldosteronism/Addison's disease	**D**	Diarrhoea
	Early obstructive uropathy	**C**	Carbonic anhydrase inhibitor
	Early uraemic acidosis	**A**	Adrenal insufficiency
	Resolving diabetic ketoacidosis	**R**	Renal tubular acidosis
	Exogenous Cl⁻ gain	**P**	Pancreatic fistula
	Hydrochloric acid (HCl)		
	Ammonium chloride (NH_4Cl)		
	Lysine-HCl, arginine-HCl		
Hypokalaemic type	*Gastrointestinal*		
	Diarrhoea (HCO_3^- loss >Cl⁻ loss)		
	Urinary to bowel diversion (e.g. ureterosigmoidostomy)		
	Surgical fistulae and drains		
	Renal		
	Renal tubular acidosis (types I and II)		
	Acetazolamide (functional renal tubular acidosis)		
Dilution acidosis	Excessive sodium chloride (NaCl) infusion dilutes plasma HCO_3^-		

3. Pathophysiologically, bicarbonate therapy is more likely to benefit a patient with NAGMA than one with HAGMA, because in NAGMA it takes days before renal recovery of bicarbonate ions can be significant, and in HAGMA, treatment of the underlying cause promotes conversion of the excess anions to bicarbonate.

4. A patient should be able to ventilate the increased CO_2 load before bicarbonate therapy is given.

5. Current recommendations do **not** advocate **routine bicarbonate therapy unless** the **pH is <7.1** and the patient is **haemodynamically compromised**.

   a. Suggested targets include pH >7.1 and [HCO_3^-] >5 mmol/L.

   b. Titrate in aliquots of 50–100 ml of 8.4% $NaHCO_3$ (by slow infusion diluted in D5%) and check 30 minutes after the completion of the procedure.

NOTE: There is no perfect formula to calculate the amount of bicarbonate needed to correct the pH as the acid base status is constantly changing with disease progression and therapy.

   c. A suggested rough rule of thumb is:

$$HCO_3^- \text{ (mmol) needed} = 0.5 \times \text{Body weight (kg)} \times [\text{Target} - \text{Measured } HCO_3^-] \text{ (mmol).}$$

Respiratory acidosis

Definition: pH <7.35 and pCO_2 >45 mmHg.

Causes: Respiratory acidosis arises when there is reduced exhalation of CO_2. See Table 3 for the causes.

- **Treatment** of respiratory acidosis is targeted at the underlying cause:
  1. Ventilatory support may be necessary. Options include intubation or non-invasive positive pressure ventilation (NIPPV).
  2. Supplemental oxygen given to patients with known type II respiratory failure should be delivered by fixed systems to allow accurate titration and prevent suppression of hypoxic drive.

TABLE 3   Causes of respiratory acidosis

Central causes of reduced respiratory drive	Drugs (e.g. sedative and opiates)
	Head injury
	Central nervous system lesions
	Metabolic alkalosis
	Loss of hypoxic drive in chronic type II respiratory failure treated with oxygen
Airway obstruction	Asthma
	Chronic obstructive lung disease
Thoracic cage abnormalities	Kyphoscoliosis
	Morbid obesity
	Chest trauma
Neurological/ neuromuscular abnormalities	Myasthenia gravis
	Guillain-Barré syndrome
	Cervical/high thoracic spine injury

Metabolic alkalosis

- **Definition**: pH >7.45 and $[HCO_3^-]$ >25 mmol/L.
- **Causes**: The excess bicarbonate generated in metabolic alkalosis is usually rapidly removed by the kidneys. For metabolic alkalosis to persist, the acute cause must continue, or the renal compensatory mechanism must be impaired by a perpetuating mechanism (see Table 4 for the causes of metabolic alkalosis).

TABLE 4   Causes of metabolic alkalosis

Acute causes (initiating mechanisms of metabolic alkalosis)	
Increased HCO_3^- intake	Antacid abuse
	Excessive $NaHCO_3$ intake
	Massive blood transfusion (due to breakdown of citrate)
Acid loss	Upper gastrointestinal tract losses, such as severe vomiting (e.g. hyperemesis gravidarum and bulimia), nasogastric suction, and gastric outlet obstruction
	Lower gastrointestinal tract losses, such as severe diarrhoea (e.g. gastroenteritis and laxative abuse) when the HCO_3^- loss is less than the Cl^- loss, villous adenoma, rare causes such as chloride diarrhoea
	Renal losses, such as loop and distal diuretics
Acid shifts	Hypokalaemia
Perpetuating mechanisms of metabolic alkalosis	
Hypovolaemia	Contraction alkalosis (due to reduced volume of distribution for bicarbonate and paradoxical renal H^+ loss)
Hypochloraemia (saline responsive)	Causes of acute hydrochloric acid (HCl) losses (as above)
	Rare causes of Cl^- depletion, such as achlorhydria and cystic fibrosis
Hypokalaemia (saline unresponsive)	Increased mineralocorticoid activity, such as primary hyperaldosteronism, Cushing's disease, liquorice abuse, and Liddle's syndrome
	Renal potassium losses, such as diuretic use or abuse, rare congenital diseases (Bartter's and Gitelman's syndromes)

- **Treatment of metabolic alkalosis**:
  1. Provide supplemental oxygen, a readily available resource in the emergency department.
  2. Treat acute causes.
     a. Stop increased bicarbonate intake.
     b. Reduce acid loss.
        i. Stop nasogastric suction.
        ii. Give H_2 antagonists or proton pump inhibitors.
        iii. Stop loop or distal diuretics, change to potassium-sparing diuretics.
  3. Reduce the shift in acidity by correcting hypokalaemia.
     a. Chloride sensitive type (saline responsive):
        i. Chloride deficit (mmol/L) = $0.3 \times$ Body weight (kg) $\times (100 - [Cl^-])$.
        ii. 1 L of 0.9% NaCl contains 154 mmol of Na^+ and Cl^-.
        iii. Therefore, the amount required (L) = Cl^- deficit/154.
     b. Give potassium replacement as necessary.
     c. Reduce gastric acid loss with proton pump inhibitors or H_2 antagonists.

4. When a patient has chloride-resistant or saline unresponsive metabolic alkalosis:

   a. Give potassium replacement to limit renal preferential H^+ excretion.

   b. Give mineralocorticoid antagonism with spironolactone or triamterene.

5. Suggested targets of therapy include pH <7.55 and HCO_3^- <40 mmol/L.

Respiratory alkalosis

- **Definition**: pH >7.45 and pCO_2 <35 mmHg.
- **Causes:** See Table 5.

TABLE 5   Causes of respiratory alkalosis

Increased respiratory drive	Pain and anxiety (hyperventilation)
	Fever
	Primary central nervous system lesions (e.g. tumours, infection, and cerebrovascular accident)
	Drugs (e.g. salicylates)
	Pregnancy
Hypoxia	Pulmonary embolism
	Pneumonia
	Pneumothorax
	Mild asthma
	Severe anaemia
	High altitude
	Carbon monoxide poisoning

- **Treatment of respiratory alkalosis** is targeted at the underlying cause, e.g.

   1. Oxygen for hypoxic conditions.

   2. Analgesia for pain.

   3. Antibiotics for pneumonia.

   4. Chest tube for pneumothorax.

   5. Resuscitation for shock states.

   The respiratory alkalosis by itself does not usually require treatment, and should resolve with management of the underlying condition.

CLINICAL APPROACH TO ACID BASE DISORDERS

- The roles of the emergency physician are as follows:

   1. Recognize that there is an acid base disorder.

   2. Diagnose the cause whenever possible.

   3. Treat the underlying cause.

- **Clinical effects of acid base derangements**: The commonest encountered acid base derangement is metabolic acidosis; the clinical effects of acid base derangements are similar, whether the event is acidosis or alkalosis, with only minor differences in their manifestations:
  1. **Altered mental states**
     a. Lethargy and drowsiness.
     b. Irritability and confusion.
     c. Obtundation and coma.
     d. In addition, alkaloses may result in giddiness and headache from cerebral vasoconstriction due to hypocarbia. Carpopedal spasm, tetany, perioral numbness, peripheral numbness, and even seizures may result from the associated ionic hypocalcaemia.
  2. **Cardiovascular**
     a. Myocardial depression and hypotension.
     b. Impaired response to catecholamines.
     c. Electrocardiogram changes and dysrhythmias due to electrolyte abnormalities.
     d. Hypocalcaemia in alkaloses may have an additive cardiodepressive effect.
     e. Cardiovascular collapse.
  3. **Respiratory**
     a. Hyperventilation in metabolic acidosis and respiratory alkalosis.
     b. Hypoventilation in metabolic alkalosis.
     c. There may be tachypnoea and a sensation of shortness of breath associated with respiratory acidosis.
     d. There may be a fruity odour associated with the ketonaemia of diabetic ketoacidosis.
     e. Acidosis causes a right shift of the haemoglobin oxygen dissociation curve, resulting in poorer pulmonary uploading of oxygen to haemoglobin with downstream tissue hypoxaemia.
     f. Alkalosis causes a left shift of the haemoglobin oxygen dissociation curve, with decreased peripheral oxygen unloading and tissue hypoxaemia.
  4. **Electrolyte imbalances**
     a. Acidosis is associated with hyperkalaemia due to competitive preferential excretion of hydrogen ions.
     b. Alkalosis is associated with hypokalaemia due to preferential renal excretion of potassium ions. Further, alkalosis induces increased calcium binding to proteins, resulting in a decrease in the fraction of free ionic calcium.
  5. **Gastrointestinal**
     a. Nausea/vomiting.
     b. Diarrhoea.
     c. Abdominal pain in diabetic ketoacidosis.

- **Disposition**: The patient will be admitted to the appropriate discipline and right site of care depending on the diagnosis and clinical status.

References/Further Reading

1. Oh MS. Evaluation of renal function, water, electrolytes, and acid-base balance. In: McPherson RA, Pincus MR, eds. *Henry's Clinical Diagnosis and Management by Laboratory Methods*. Philadelphia, PA: Elsevier; 2006.

2. Effros RM, Wesson JA. Acid-base balance. In: Mason RJ, Broaddus VC, Murray JF, Nadel JA, eds. *Murray & Nadel's Textbook of Respiratory Medicine*. 4th ed. Philadelphia, PA: Elsevier; 2005.

3. Nicolau DD, Kelen GD. Acid base disorders. In: Tintinalli JE, Ma OJ, Stapczynski JS, et al, eds. *Tintinalli's Emergency Medicine: A Comprehensive Study Guide*. 7th ed. New York: McGraw-Hill; 2011: 102–112.

4. Kwek TK. Acid base disorders. In: Tai D, Lew T, eds. *Bedside ICU Handbook*. Singapore: Tan Tock Seng Hospital; 2000: 20–25.

5. Lolekha PH, Lolekha S, et al. Update on value of the anion gap in clinical diagnosis and laboratory evaluation. *Clin Chim Acta*. 2001; 307(1–2): 33–36.

6. Kraut JA, Madias NE. Serum anion gap: Its uses and limitations in clinical medicine. *Clin J Am Soc Nephrol*. 2007; 2: 162–174.

7. Ibrahim I, Ooi SB, Chan YH, Sethi S. Point-of-care bedside gas analyzer: Limited use of venous pCO_2 in emergency patients. *J Emerg Med*. 2011; 41(2): 117–23.

8. Umeda A, Kawasaki K, Abe T, Watanabe M, Ishizaka A, Okada Y. Hyperventilation and finger exercise increase venous-arterial pCO_2 and pH differences. *Am J Emerg Med*. 2008; 26: 975–980.

9. Malatesha G, Singh NK, Bharija A, et al. Comparison of arterial and venous pH, bicarbonate, pCO_2 and PO_2 in initial emergency department assessment. *Emerg Med J*. 2007; 24: 458–571.

10. Rang LC, Murray HE, Wells GA, Macgougan CK. Can peripheral venous blood gases replace arterial blood gases in emergency department patients? *CJEM*. 2002; 4: 7–15.

11. New A. Oxygen: Kill or cure? Prehospital hyperoxia in the COPD patient. *Emerg Med J*. 2006; 23: 144–146.

12. Murphy R, Mackway-Jones K, Sammy I, et al. Emergency oxygen therapy for the breathless patient. Guidelines prepared by North West Oxygen Group. *Emerg Med J*. 2001; 18: 421–423.

13. Belpomme V, Ricard-Hibon A, Devoir C, et al. Correlation of arterial pCO_2 and $PETCO_2$ in prehospital controlled ventilation. *Am J Emerg Med*. 2005; 23: 852–859.

14. Crosslet DJ, McGuire GP, Barrow PM, Houston PL. Influence of inspired oxygen concentration on deadspace, respiratory drive, and $paCO_2$ in intubated patients with chronic obstructive pulmonary disease. *Crit Care Med*. 1997; 25: 1522–1526.

15. Zhang H, Vincent JL. Arteriovenous differences in pCO_2 and pH are good indicators of critical hypoperfusion. *Am Rev Respir Dis*. 1993; 148: 867–871.

16. Van der Linden P, Rausin I, Deltell A, et al. Detection of tissue hypoxia by arteriovenous gradient for pCO_2 and pH in anesthetized dogs during progressive hemorrhage. *Anesth Analg*. 1995; 80: 269–275.

58   Adrenal Insufficiency, Acute

Goh Ee Ling • Malcolm Mahadevan

DEFINITION

- Acute adrenal insufficiency or 'Addisonian crisis' is a life-threatening condition that results from insufficient cortisol production.

CAVEATS

- Symptoms and signs are non-specific, hence, a high index of suspicion is needed.
- Mortality is significant if left untreated.
- Treatment should therefore be given based on clinical suspicion without laboratory confirmation that will delay therapy.
- Abdominal pain and tenderness are not uncommon in primary adrenal insufficiency and must be differentiated from surgical abdomen.
- An adrenal crisis may occur in a variety of situations.

TABLE 1   Situations in which an adrenal crisis may occur

- Following stress such as surgery or trauma in a patient with chronic adrenal insufficiency
- Sudden withdrawal of steroids in a patient on long-term steroids
- After bilateral adrenalectomy or damage to both adrenal glands post-trauma or haemorrhage
- Pituitary apoplexy

CLINICAL ASSESSMENT

- **History**
  1. Presenting symptoms
     a. Non-specific weakness (99%), fatigue, and weight loss are three cardinal features.
     b. Gastrointestinal upset: Nausea and vomiting, abdominal pain (34%), diarrhoea (20%), anorexia, altered mental state, confusion, coma, and lethargy.
  2. Precipitating factors, e.g. stress, fever, recent surgery, trauma, and acute myocardial infarction (AMI).
  3. Past medical history, e.g. diseases that require treatment with long-term steroids such as autoimmune disorders.
  4. Medications, e.g. use of steroids or traditional medicine.
- **Physical examination**
  1. General appearance: Dehydration, lethargy, altered mental state, and Cushingoid facies.

2. Vital signs: Look for persistent hypotension and orthostatic hypotension.

3. Hyperpigmentation in buccal mucosae, exposed areas, or areas subject to friction: Only in primary adrenal insufficiency.

4. Others: Evidence of sepsis or trauma.

- **Investigations**

1. Stat capillary blood sugar.

2. Bloods:

   a. Full blood count.

   b. Renal panel: Hyponatraemia, hyperkalaemia, elevated urea, hypoglycaemia, and metabolic acidosis.

   c. Arterial blood gas: Metabolic acidosis.

   d. Plasma cortisol (plain tube) and adrenocorticotropin (ACTH) (ethylenediaminetetraacetic acid, EDTA, and tube on ice). **Send to lab as urgent**.

3. Chest X-ray: May be normal but often reveals a small heart. There may be stigmata of an earlier infection or current tuberculosis or fungal infection, when this is the cause of Addison's disease.

4. Electrocardiogram (ECG): May show low voltage QRS tracing with non-specific ST-T wave changes and/or hyperkalaemic changes (reversible with glucocorticoid replacement) and changes of AMI.

5. Others (guided by clinical evaluation): Septic work-up – blood culture and urinalysis/urine culture.

⇨ **SPECIAL TIPS FOR GPs**
- Initial diagnosis and treatment is presumptive; delays will result in poor clinical outcome.
- Treat hypoglycaemia with dextrose and steroids concurrently.

MANAGEMENT

- **Supportive measures**

1. The patient must be managed in the critical care area since this is a potentially life-threatening condition.

2. Monitoring: ECG, pulse oximetry, and vital signs.

3. Obtain intravenous access with 2 large bore cannulas.

4. Support the airway, breathing and circulation:

   a. Secure the airway for protection if need be.

   b. Give supplemental oxygen.

   c. Administer fluids: Give IV 0.9% saline/D_5W by rapid infusion until hypotension is corrected (usual deficit approximates 2–3 L).

- **Drug therapy**

  1. Give IV dextrose 50% 40 ml to correct hypoglycaemia which may be refractory and require repeated boluses; feed with isocal if the patient is alert.

  2. Give glucocorticoid replacement: IV **hydrocortisone** 100 mg q 6 hours. It is physiological, more rapidly acting than dexamethasone and has mineralocorticoid activity, especially in the case of suspected primary adrenocortical insufficiency.

  NOTE: Draw blood for plasma cortisol and ACTH before treatment.

  3. Give IV sodium bicarbonate (if needed): 50 mmol over 1 to 2 hours; monitor the acid base status with serial arterial blood gases.

  4. Treat the precipitating cause, e.g. antibiotics for sepsis.

- **Disposition**

  Consult Endocrine/General Medicine regarding anticipated admission to the medical intensive care unit for close monitoring.

References/Further Reading

1. Werbel SS, Ober KP. Acute adrenal insufficiency. *Endocrinol Metab Clin North Am.* 1993; 22: 303.

2. Soon PC. Addisonian crisis. In: Tai DYH, Lew TWK, Loo S, eds. *Bedside ICU Handbook.* 2nd ed. Singapore: Armour Publishing; 2007: 151–152.

59   Fluid and Electrolyte Disorders

Kuan Win Sen

CAVEATS

- Body fluids are distributed between the intra-cellular space (ICF) and extra-cellular space (ECF) in a ratio of 2:1. The ECF comprises fluid in the interstitial/tissue spaces and blood vessels (25% of the ECF is plasma).
- Effective circulating volume is the part of the ECF that is effectively perfusing the tissues.
- **Methods of assessing effective circulating volume**:
  1. Clinical parameters: Heart rate, blood pressure, and jugular venous distension.
  2. Non-invasive measurement of the inferior vena cava diameter by ultrasonography.
  3. Invasive measurement of central venous pressure or pulmonary capillary wedge pressure can be used for more critically ill patients.
- **Normal** serum osmolality (**Se Osm**) **285–295 mOsm/kg**. Calculated and measured serum osmolality are within 10 mOsm/kg of each other. An osmolar gap greater than 10 mOsm/kg suggests the presence of unmeasured osmotically active substances, e.g. alcohol, acetone, and mannitol.
- **Calculated Se Osm** (mOsm/kg) = **2[Na$^+$ (mmol/L)] + Glucose (mmol/L) + Urea (mmol/L)**
- **Urine osmolality:** Average is about **500–800 mOsm/kg**. After an overnight fast, the urine osmolality should be at least three times the serum osmolality.
- A **serum osmolality** of **384 mOsm/kg** produces **stupor**. The patient may have **grand mal seizures** if the serum osmolality is **>400 mOsm/kg**. Values **>420 mOsm/kg** are **fatal**.

⇨ **SPECIAL TIPS FOR GPs**
- Symptoms of electrolyte disorders tend to be **non-specific** such as fatigue, irritability, lethargy, and generalized weakness especially in the elderly. A high index of suspicion is required especially if the patient is on poly-pharmacy.
- **Se Osm of 285 mOsm/kg** correlates with a **urine specific gravity** of **1.010**.
- Hyponatraemia (<130 mmol/L) is the most common electrolyte abnormality in general hospitalized patients. Suspect hyponatraemia in patients who are on thiazide diuretics.
- Be vigilant to diagnose **hypothyroidism** and **adrenal insufficiency** (especially with hyperkalaemia) in patients with hyponatraemia as they usually masquerade as cases of SIADH.

TABLE 1   Total body water (percentage of body weight)

Age (years)	Male (%)	Female (%)
18–40	60	50
41–60	50–60	40–50
>60	50	40

TABLE 2   Distribution of electrolytes in the body

Electrolyte	ECF (mmol/L)*	ICF*
Sodium (Na^+)	135–150	10–14 mmol/L
Potassium (K^+)	3.5–5.0	140–150 mmol/L
Chloride (Cl^-)	98–107	3–4 mmol/L
Bicarbonate (HCO_3^-)	21–27	7–10 mmol/L
Calcium (Ca^{2+})	2.15–2.55	7–10 mmol/L
Phosphate (PO_4^{3-})	0.85–1.45	4 mmol/kg**
Magnesium (Mg^{2+})	0.70–0.91	40 mmol/kg**

Notes: * Values may vary among laboratories.
** Values vary among various tissues and nutritional states.

TABLE 3   Causes of increased/decreased serum osmolality

Increased (hyperosmolality)	Decreased (hypoosmolality)
Renal disease	Sodium loss (diuretic use and low salt diet)
Congestive heart failure	Hyponatraemia
Dehydration	Adrenocortical insufficiency
Diabetes insipidus	Syndrome of inappropriate antidiuretic hormone secretion (SIADH)
Hyperglycaemia	Excessive water ingestion/replacement
Hypercalcaemia	
Hypernatraemia	
Alcohol ingestion	

DISORDERS OF SODIUM CONCENTRATION

Hyponatraemia

- **Clinical presentation**

  1. More common in the extremes of age as these groups are less able to express thirst and less able to regulate fluid intake autonomously.

  2. The symptoms are usually non-specific and attributable to cerebral oedema. They include anorexia, nausea and vomiting, confusion, lethargy, agitation, headache, muscle weakness, cramps and seizures.

3. Patients with [Na⁺] >125 mmol/L are usually **asymptomatic**. May have some gastrointestinal symptoms (nausea or vomiting).

4. The major symptoms occur when [Na⁺] is <125 mmol/L, especially when hyponatraemia occurs acutely.

5. Physical findings are of a neurological nature. Varying degrees of **cognitive impairment** to focal or generalized **seizures** may be encountered. Determining the patient's hydration status may help to establish the aetiology of hyponatraemia (Table 4).

TABLE 4 **Relationship between total body water (TBW) and total body sodium (Na⁺) and extra-cellular fluid volume (ECF)**

Fluid status	Status of TBW, Na+, ECF	Examples
Hypovolaemic hyponatraemia	TBW↓, Na⁺↓↓, ECF↓	Excessive sweating, burns, vomiting, diarrhoea, diuretics (thiazides)
Euvolaemic hyponatraemia	TBW↑, Na⁺↔, ECF↑ without oedema	SIADH
Hypervolaemic hyponatraemia	TBW↑↑, Na⁺↑, ECF↑↑ with oedema	Congestive cardiac failure (CCF), hypothyroidism, liver cirrhosis, nephrotic syndrome, psychogenic polydipsia
Redistributive hyponatraemia	TBW↔, Na⁺↔, water shifts from intra-cellular to extra-cellular compartment	Hyperglycaemia, mannitol
Pseudohyponatraemia	TBW↔, Na⁺↔, aqueous phase diluted by excessive proteins or lipids	Hypertriglyceridaemia, multiple myeloma

Notes: ↑↑: Markedly increased   ↑: Increased   ↔: Unchanged   ↓: Decreased   ↓↓: Markedly decreased

Management

- The main aim of management is to prevent the sequelae of uncorrected hyponatraemia. **Cerebral oedema** is the main complication which can lead to irreversible neurological damage and death.

- Patients are invariably managed as inpatients. The role of the emergency department in managing these patients is to:

1. Address acute life-threatening conditions and initiate supportive care.

   a. Establish a definitive airway in those with airway compromise.

   b. Treat seizures.

   c. Avoid hypotonic intravenous fluids which may exacerbate cerebral oedema.

- Acute (<48 hours) hyponatraemia is less common than chronic hyponatraemia. It is usually seen in patients with a history of sudden free water loading (e.g. patients with psychogenic polydipsia and iatrogenic intravenous hypotonic fluids postoperatively).

- Be wary of **redistributive hyponatraemia** where the simple treatment is aimed at correcting the **hyperglycaemia**.
  1. **Sodium (corrected) = Sodium (measured) + Glucose/4**
     (all values in mmol/L).
- More aggressive correction (i.e. with hypertonic 3% sodium chloride solution) is required for patients with [Na⁺] that is less than 110 mmol/L or those exhibiting severe confusion, seizures, coma, or signs of brain stem herniation. The aim is not to correct the level of [Na⁺] and keep it within the normal range but to arrest the progression of the symptoms by raising the level of [Na⁺] by 4–6 mmol/L.
- Treatment of patients with chronic hyponatraemia has been associated with the development of **osmotic demyelination syndrome (central pontine myelinolysis)**. Symptoms (dysarthria, dysphagia, seizures, altered mental state, quadriparesis, and hypotension) usually begin 2–6 days after correction of the serum sodium level. This condition is typically irreversible. Patients with hypokalaemia, history of alcoholism or liver transplant and female patients are more prone to this condition.
- Correction of chronic hyponatraemia is recommended not to exceed 10–12 mmol/L in the first 24 hours and not to exceed 18 mmol/L in the first 48 hours.
- Conivaptan (vaprisol), an arginine vasopressin antagonist has been indicated for the treatment of euvolaemic and hypervolaemia hyponatraemia.

HYPERNATRAEMIA

Causes

- Unreplaced water loss (requires an impairment in thirst or access to water).
  1. Insensible and sweat losses.
  2. Gastrointestinal losses.
  3. Central or nephrogenic diabetes insipidus.
  4. Osmotic diuresis.
  5. Hypothalamic lesions impairing thirst or osmoreceptor function.
     a. Primary hypodipsia.
     b. Reset osmostat in mineralocorticoid excess.
- Loss of water into cells.
  1. Severe exercise or seizures.
- Sodium overload.
  1. Intake or administration of hypertonic sodium solutions.
- [Na⁺] levels of >190 mmol/L usually indicate long-term salt ingestion.
- [Na⁺] levels of >170 mmol/L usually indicate diabetes insipidus.
- [Na⁺] levels of 150–170 mmol/L usually indicate dehydration.

Clinical presentation

- The mortality rate especially among elderly patients is high (>50% in most studies). Most deaths are due to an underlying disease process rather than hypernatraemia itself.
- Symptoms are non-specific. **Early signs** include anorexia, restlessness, nausea and vomiting. **Late signs** include altered mental state, lethargy, irritability, and eventually stupor and coma.
- Musculoskeletal signs such as twitching, hyperreflexia, ataxia and tremors have been documented as well as generally non-focal neurological symptoms.

Management

- Emergency department management involves the restoration of normal serum tonicity and diagnosis and treatment of the underlying aetiology.
- Address the airway, breathing and circulation (ABCs). **Hypovolaemic** patients with tachycardia and hypotension should receive volume resuscitation with **isotonic sodium chloride** solution (NOT hypotonic solutions as they leave the intravascular space quickly and do not help to correct the hypotension).
- When possible, provide free water orally to patients.
- Do not correct at a rate >0.5 mmol/L/hr.
- Monitor input and output.
- **Euvolaemic** patients can be treated with **hypotonic fluids** orally or intravenously (e.g. dextrose 5%, 0.45% saline).
- Patients with renal failure may require dialysis.

HYPOKALAEMIA AND HYPERKALAEMIA

Refer to Chapter 63, *Renal Emergencies*.

HYPOCALCAEMIA

Causes

- Hypoalbuminaemia: The most common cause (e.g. due to cirrhosis, nephrosis, malnutrition, burns, or sepsis).
  1. **Calcium (corrected, mmol/L)**
     = Calcium (measured, mmol/L) + [(40 − Albumin (g/L)) × 0.02]
- Hypomagnesaemia: Causes parathyroid hormone end-organ resistance.
- Hyperphosphataemia: Occurs in critically ill patients and patients on phosphate-containing enemas. Phosphate binds to calcium strongly.
- Post-parathyroid resection.
- Vitamin D deficiency/resistance.

- Others
  1. Acute pancreatitis.
  2. Rhabdomyolysis.
  3. Sepsis.
  4. Osteoblastic malignancies.
  5. Hydrofluoric acid burn/ingestion.

Clinical presentation

- Patients may complain of muscle cramping, dyspnoea due to bronchospasm, tetanic contractions, peripheral limb numbness, and tingling sensations.
- Acute hypocalcaemia may lead to syncope, angina, and congestive cardiac failure.
- Neurological manifestations include irritability, confusion, hallucinations, dementia, extra-pyramidal effects, and seizures.
- Classic peripheral neurological findings include the following:
  1. **Chvostek sign**: Twitching of the branches of the facial nerve when tapped about 2 cm anterior to the tragus of the ear.
  2. **Trousseau sign**: Carpal spasm on inflation of a blood pressure cuff above the systolic pressure (ulna and median nerve ischaemia).
- Electrocardiogram (ECG) may show **prolonged QT** interval and dysrhythmias.

Management

The role of the emergency department is in management of patients with severe hypocalcaemia with life-threatening symptoms.

- Supportive treatment includes monitoring vital signs, administering oxygen, and establishing intravenous (IV) access.
- IV calcium for symptomatic patients (tetany and seizures), prolonged QT interval and asymptomatic patients with corrected serum calcium less than 1.9 mmol/L. Oral calcium can be used for those with milder symptoms (paraesthesia).
- IV calcium (10–20 ml of calcium gluconate 10%, equivalent to 90–180 mg elemental calcium, in 50 ml of dextrose 5%) can be infused over 10–20 minutes. Although calcium chloride contains more elemental calcium (10 ml contains 272 mg elemental calcium), it is not recommended due to risk of **tissue necrosis** in the event of extravasation. (See Joint Commission International [JCI]: International Patient Safety Goal #3 – High Risk Medications.)

HYPERCALCAEMIA

Causes

TABLE 5   Causes of hypercalcaemia

Parathyroid hormone-mediated	Parathyroid hormone-independent
Primary hyperparathyroidism (adenoma(s), carcinoma)	Hypercalcaemia of malignancy (multiple myeloma, breast cancer, lung cancer)
Familial (MEN-I, MEN-IIa, familial hypercalciuric hypercalcaemia)	Vitamin D intoxication
Secondary hyperparathyroidism (chronic kidney disease, vitamin D deficiency)	Chronic granulomatous disease (sarcoidosis, tuberculosis, leprosy, histoplasmosis)
Tertiary hyperparathyroidism (excessive secretion of parathyroid hormone after long-standing secondary hyperparathyroidism following a successful renal transplantation)	Medications (thiazides, lithium, theophylline toxicity)
	Endocrine causes (hyperthyroidism, acromegaly, phaeochromocytoma, adrenal insufficiency)
	Immobilization
	Parenteral nutrition

Clinical presentation

- 'Bones, stones, abdominal groans and psychic moans': Usually caused by hyperparathyroidism.
- Musculoskeletal signs: Bone pain, muscle weakness, osteopaenia, or osteoporosis.
- Renal symptoms: Nephrolithiasis, nephrocalcinosis, polyuria, and polydipsia.
- Gastrointestinal symptoms: Nausea, vomiting, constipation, pancreatitis, and peptic ulcer disease.
- Neurological symptoms: Decreased concentration, confusion, stupor, depression, and headache.
- Cardiovascular signs: Hypertension, bradycardia, shortened QT interval, prolonged T waves and coving of ST segments, and left ventricular hypertrophy.
- Elderly patients are more likely to be symptomatic from moderate elevations of calcium levels.
- Patients with hypercalcaemia from malignancy may lack many features associated with hypercalcaemia caused by hyperparathyroidism.

Management

- Patients with asymptomatic or mildly symptomatic (e.g. constipation) hypercalcemia (<3.0 mmol/L) do not require immediate treatment.
- **A serum calcium level of 3.0–3.5 mmol/L** may be well-tolerated chronically, and may **not require immediate treatment**.

- An acute rise to these concentrations may cause marked changes in sensorium, which requires more aggressive measures. Patients with a serum calcium concentration **>3.5 mmol/L require treatment**, regardless of the symptoms.

- **Treatment goals in the emergency department**:
  1. Stabilize and reduce calcium level.
  2. Ensure adequate hydration.
  3. Increase urinary calcium excretion.
  4. Discontinue pharmacologic agents causing hypercalcaemia.

- Hydration with **isotonic saline** decreases calcium level through dilution. Expansion of extra-cellular volume increases renal calcium clearance by inhibiting proximal and loop reabsorption of sodium, thereby reducing the passive reabsorption of calcium.

- The rate of fluid administration depends on the degree of hypercalcaemia, severity of dehydration, and ability of patients to tolerate hydration (e.g. history of congestive cardiac failure and renal failure).

- As a guide, isotonic saline can be administered at an initial rate of 200–300 ml/hr that is then adjusted to maintain the urine output at 100–150 ml/hr.

- Careful monitoring is required to observe for signs and symptoms of fluid overload.

- **Loop diuretics (frusemide)** may be used in patients who are fluid overloaded at presentation or have impaired renal function. However, in patients with renal failure, dialysis may be necessary to remove excess calcium.

- Loop diuretics should **not** be used routinely due to the following reasons:
  1. Potential fluid and electrolyte complications may result from a massive saline infusion and frusemide-induced diuresis such as hypokalaemia, hypomagnesaemia and volume depletion if the diuretic-induced losses are not replaced.
  2. The availability of drugs such as the bisphosphonates and calcitonin that inhibit bone resorption, which is primarily responsible for the hypercalcaemia.

References/Further Reading

1. Porth C, Gaspard KJ, Matfin G. *Essentials of Pathophysiology: Concepts of Altered Health States*. Philadelphia, PA: Lippincott Williams & Wilkins, 2006.

2. McPhee SJ, Papadakis MA, Tierney LM. *Current Medical Diagnosis and Treatment*. New York: McGraw-Hill Professional; 2007.

3. Adrogué HJ, Madias NE. Hyponatremia. *N Engl J Med*. 25 May 2000; 342(21): 1581–1589.

4. Verbalis JG, Goldsmith SR, Greenberg A, Schrier RW, Sterns RH. Hyponatremia treatment guidelines 2007: Expert panel recommendations. *Am J Med*. Nov 2007; 120(11 suppl 1): S1–21.

5. Adrogue HJ, Madias NE. Hypernatremia. *N Engl J Med*. 18 May 2000; 342(20): 1493–1499.

6. Cooper MS, Gittoes NJ. Diagnosis and management of hypocalcaemia. *BMJ*. 2008; 336: 1298.

7. LeGrand SB, Leskuski D, Zama I. Narrative review: Furosemide for hypercalcemia: An unproven yet common practice. *Ann Intern Med*. 19 Aug 2008; 149(4): 259–263.

Diabetic Ketoacidosis (DKA) and Hyperosmolar Hyperglycaemic State (HHS)

Peter Manning • Shirley Ooi • Sim Tiong Beng

DKA

CAVEATS

- DKA is caused by a combination of absolute or relative insulin deficiency, and an increase in counterregulatory hormones, leading to increased gluconeogenesis, accelerated glycogenolysis, and impaired glucose utilization by peripheral tissues, lipolysis and unrestrained hepatic fatty acid oxidation to ketone bodies, culminating in hyperglycaemia and ketonaemia.

- **Diagnostic criteria** are:
  1. Hyperglycaemia with blood glucose ≥14 mmol/l
  2. Acidaemia with arterial pH <7.3, bicarbonate <15 mmol/l
  3. Ketonaemia or ketonuria

- High plasma glucose level leads to osmotic diuresis with sodium and water loss, hypotension, hypoperfusion and shock. Patients present with significant polyuria, polydipsia, weight loss, dehydration, weakness and clouding of sensorium.

- Younger undiagnosed diabetics frequently present with DKA developing over 1–3 days. Plasma glucose level may not be grossly raised.

- GI complaints are common presenting symptoms, especially in the young. There may be nausea, vomiting and diffuse abdominal pain. This can be severe and misdiagnosed as 'acute surgical abdomen'. Serum amylase level is often elevated in the absence of pancreatitis. Hyperglycaemic crisis also results in non specific elevation of hepatic transaminases, creatinine kinase, lactate dehydrogenase, and lipase and must therefore be interpreted with caution.

- Inflammatory markers like CRP are often elevated in DKA, but return to normal values after with resolution of DKA.

- Leucocytosis up to 15K is a rule in DKA and may not necessarily indicate infection. It is thought to be due to stress and may be correlated to elevated levels of cortisol and noradrenaline. However, TW >25K may designate infection.

- The admission serum sodium is usually low due to the osmotic influx of water from intracellular to extracellular space in the presence of hyperglycaemia. Therefore, an increased or even normal sodium indicates a rather profound dehydration

- Investigate abdominal pain if the DKA is mild or if the pain persists after resolution of ketoacidosis or in the presence of peritoneal signs.

- Hyperventilation with deep rapid breathing ('air hunger/kussmaul's breathing') and the smell of acetone on the breath is characteristic of DKA.

- A superimposed metabolic alkalosis from vomiting may mask the severity of ketoacidosis.

- 10% of DKA population presents with euglycaemia. This could be due to exogenous insulin injection en route to the hospital, antecedent food restriction, and inhibition of gluconeogenesis.
- DKA can potentially exist even when the patient is tested negative for urine ketones. This is because urine dipstick test uses the nitroprusside method which detects only acetoacetate and acetone and not beta-hydroxybutyrate (the main metabolic product in ketoacidosis) and may potentially miss a DKA predominant in beta-hydroxybutyrate.
- **Causes**:
  1. Insufficient insulin/Non compliance to insulin therapy
  2. Infection: common foci are UTI, respiratory tract, skin
  3. Infarction: myocardial, CVA, GIT, peripheral vasculature
- Signs of infection are often masked or deceptive. Temperature is rarely raised and increased total white count may only reflect ketonaemia; however, any fever, even low grade, indicates sepsis. If in doubt, it is probably safest to treat with a broad spectrum antibiotic.
- Over-rapid fluid replacement can cause cardiac failure, cerebral oedema, and ARDS, especially in patients with underlying cardiac disease or the elderly. CVP monitoring may be needed.

⇨ **SPECIAL TIPS FOR GPs**
- Have a high index of suspicion when seeing patients with complaints of nausea and vomiting, with or without abdominal pain, especially if the vital signs were abnormal or if the patient has rapid shallow kussmaul's breathing. The 'viral gastritis' may turn out to be DKA.
- Check bedside blood sugar level for all toxic-looking febrile patients.
- Check bedside blood sugar level and urine dipstick for ketones if the diagnosis is suspected.
- Put up a normal saline infusion and give IV/IM insulin stat before sending to hospital by ambulance.

MANAGEMENT

Supportive measures

- Patient must be managed in a monitored area.
- Supplemental high-flow oxygen.
- Monitoring: ECG, pulse oximetry, vital signs q 15–30 min, blood levels of glucose, ketones, potassium and acid base balance q1–2 hours.
- Labs: FBC, urea/electrolytes/creatinine/calcium/magnesium/phosphate (to include venous glucose), cardiac enzymes, DIC screen (if septic), urinalysis (for ketones and leucocytes), serum ketones (beta-hydroxybutarate), serum osmolality, and arterial blood gas.
- Consider blood culture (**at least** 7.5 ml blood per bottle).
- 12-lead ECG, CXR, urine dipstick: looking for a cause of the DKA.

- Circulatory support: IV normal saline as the basic resuscitation fluid, switching to 0.45% NS as perfusion improves and BP normalizes, then D_5W/45% NS as serum glucose level drops. Total fluid loss in DKA averages 4–6 litres.
- Urinary catheter to monitor urine output.

Specific measures

The therapeutic goal of DKA hinges on correcting underlying pathophysiologic abnormalities. The cornerstones involve fluid resuscitation, acid-base and electrolyte correction, insulin therapy, and identification of precipitating factors, and above all, frequent meticulous patient monitoring. The comatose with or without vomiting patient warrants immediate intubation to reduce aspiration risk.

- **IV volume replacement**: directed toward correction of intravascular and extravascular volume deficits and improving renal function. It also lowers blood glucose independently of insulin therapy.

  1. **If patient is in shock**: if in septic shock, administer **IV Hartmann's solution 20–30 ml/kg** over 30 mins, start IV antibiotics and admit to ICU. If patient is in cardiogenic shock, admit to ICU for vasopressors and haemodynamic monitoring

  2 **If patient has severe hypovolaemia without shock**: Administer **0.9% NaCl 1 L/hr**. If BP remains low after 2L of NaCl, consider colloids/Hartmann's solution and HD/ICU care.

  3. **If patient is neither hypotensive nor severely dehydrated**: Administer **0.9%NaCl 1 L/hr (15–20 ml/kg/h)** in the first hour. Further fluid therapy will depend on haemodynamic/ perfusion status, sodium level and urinary output.

  4. If corrected **serum sodium is low**, administer **0.9 % NaCl 250-500 ml/h** depending on hydration status. If patient is haemodynamically stable and if the **corrected sodium is normal/elevated**, infuse **0.45% NaCl** at 4–14 ml/kg/h (i.e., 250–500 mls 0.45% NaCl per hour) evenly over the 24 hours with careful monitoring of the serum glucose level.

NOTE: **Corrected serum sodium = Measured serum sodium + 0.3 (venous glucose in mmol/l – 5.5)**

  Switch to **5% dextrose** when serum **glucose level falls below 14 mmol/l**. Normal or half strength NS may be continued in conjunction with IV dextrose 5% to correct fluid/electrolyte derangements. Monitor urine output hourly, and check electrolytes and creatinine every 2–4 hours till stable.

NOTE: Fluid replacement should correct estimated deficits (4–6 litres) within the first 24 hours, but serum osmolality should not decrease by more than 3 mOsm/kg/h to avoid cerebral oedema.

- **Insulin administration**: large doses are not needed to reverse DKA. In addition, hypoglycaemia and hypokalaemia are more likely to occur with large-dose insulin therapy.

  1. Administer a bolus dose of **0.1 units/kg body weight of IV SI** in adults, followed by a low-dose continuous infusion of **0.1 units/kg body weight/hour** in both adults and children, or give a IV dose of **0.14 units/kg BW insulin** if the bolus insulin dose is

omitted. If the blood glucose does not decrease by ≥10% in the first hour, increase the insulin infusion. Adjust the infusion rate to obtain a drop serum glucose level by approx. **3–4 mmol/l per hour**. If the target glucose lowering is not achieved, then the insulin infusion may be doubled every hour for possible insulin resistance which may occur in sepsis, or occult infection. Monitor blood glucose hourly.

2. When blood glucose level decreases to ≤**14 mmol/l**, **halve** the IV SI infusion rate to **0.05–0.1 units/kg/h** and start IV D5% to aim for blood glucose level of **8–12 mmol/l for DKA and 12–16 mmol/l for HHS.** Maintain the SI infusion until acidosis clears (pH > 7.3 and HCO$_3$ > 15). SC SI q4 h can then be instituted within an overlap period of 1–2 hours. Do **not** stop IV SI simply because blood glucose has normalized.

- **Restoration of electrolyte balance**: early potassium replacement is now standard. Establish that there is urine output of 50 ml/hr first, then replace as follows:

   1. **Serum K$^+$ < 3.3 mmol/l**, withhold insulin and give 20–40 mEq KCl per hour until K > 3.3 mmol/l.

   2. **Serum K$^+$ 3.3–5.2 mmol/l**, give 20–30 mEq K$^+$ in each litre of IV fluid to keep serum K between 4–5 mmol/l. (This can be given as 2/3 KCL and 1/3 KHPO$_4$; phosphate replacement is indicated when serum phosphate < 0.3 mmol/l or if patient is anaemic or in cardiorespiratory distress.)

   3. **Serum K$^+$ > 5.2 mmol/l**, withhold potassium but check serum potassium every 2 hours.

NOTE: A low initial serum potassium concentration reflects severe total body potassium deficiency and warrants immediate replacement and even consideration to withhold insulin therapy till potassium is restored >3.3 mEq/L to prevent catastrophic respiratory failure and life-threatening cardiac dysrhythmia.

Monitor serum K$^+$ 2 hrly.

NOTE: Hyperglycaemia may give rise to pseudohyponatraemia. An elevated serum sodium level indicates profound dehydration and requires more aggressive fluid therapy.

- **Restoration of acid-base balance**: sodium bicarbonate is to be given only if severe hyperkalaemia with ECG changes or if the arterial **pH is <6.9**, since IV volume replacement and, later, insulin will improve the metabolic acidosis. If pH is < 6.9, give IV 8.4% NaHCO$_3$ 100 mls with 20 mmol of KCl over 2 hrs. Monitor ABG and serum K$^+$ every 2 hours. Repeat IV NaHCO$_3$ and KCl every 2 hrs until pH is ≥7.0.

NOTE: No beneficial but deleterious effects can occur when given at higher pH.

NOTE: Venous blood gas pH has been shown to correlate very well with the arterial blood gas pH and can therefore be used as a good substitute of arterial pH to assess response to therapy, and avoiding pain and complications from repeated arterial punctures. Initial blood gas analysis, however, should still be an arterial sample as recommended by the American Diabetes Association (ADA).

Potential complications that the clinician needs to be aware of while managing hyperglycaemic crisis

These include:

1. hypoglycaemia,
2. hypokalaemia,
3. hyperchloraemia,
4. fluid overload,
5. ARDS,
6. thromboembolism and
7. rhabdomyolysis.

Disposition

- Patients with severe DKA (pH<7.0 and bicarbonate <10), hypotension or oliguria refractory to initial rehydration, or who have mental obtundation/coma, with total serum osmolality >340 mOsm/kg, should be considered for HD or MICU admission.
- Stable cases can be admitted to general ward.

HYPEROSMOLAR HYPERGLYCAEMIC STATE (HHS) ALSO KNOWN AS HYPEROSMOLAR HYPERGLYCAEMIC NON-KETOTIC STATE

The diagnostic criteria for HHS:

1. Blood glucose >33 mmol/l
2. Arterial pH >7.3, HCO_3 >18
3. Absence of severe ketonaemia or ketonuria
4. Effective serum osmolality (2 × Na + glucose) > 320 mOsm/Kg H_2O

HHS usually has worse fluids deficit up to 10 L, and tends to occur over a few days. Mixed picture of DKA and HHS can prevail in the same patient.

⇨ **SPECIAL TIPS FOR GPs**
- Consider the diagnosis of HHS in an elderly patient with abnormalities in vital signs or mental state, or with complaints of weakness, anorexia or fatigue.
- HHS may be unexpectedly found in patients who present with concurrent medical insults such as acute CVA, severe burns, MI, infection, pancreatitis or drugs (e.g. diuretics, beta-blockers, glucocorticoids, neuroleptics, phenytoin and calcium channel blockers). Hence check the bedside glucose level in an elderly patient fairly liberally to avoid missing HHS or DKA.
- Put up a normal saline infusion before sending the patient by ambulance to hospital.

MANAGEMENT OF HHS

- Similar to DKA, except insulin bolus is not required and more fluids needed.

References/Further Reading

1. Kitabchi AE, Umpierrez GE, Murphy MB, Kreisberg RA. Hyperglycemic crises in adult patients with diabetes: a consensus statement from the American Diabetes Association. *Diabetes Care* 2009 July; 32(7): 1335–1343.

2. Cydulka RK, Maloney GE. Diabetes mellitus and disorders of glucose homeostasis. In: Marx JA, Hockberger RS, Walls RM, eds. *Rosen's Emergency Medicine: Concepts and Clinical Practice.* 7th ed. Philadelphia: Mosby, Inc; 2010: 1633–1649.

3. Kelly AM. The case for venous rather than arterial blood gases in diabetic ketoacidosis. *Emerg Med Australas* 2006 Feb; 18(1): 64–7.

4. Kreshak A, Chen EH. Arterial blood gas analysis: are its values needed for the management of diabetic ketoacidosis? *Ann Emerg Med* 2005; 45(5): 550–1.

5. Kitabchi AE, Umpierrez GE, Murphy MB, et al. Hyperglycemic crises in diabetes. *Diabetes Care* 2004 Jan; 27 Suppl 1: S94–102

6. Umpierrez G, Freire AX. Abdominal pain in patients with hyperglycemic crises. *J Crit Care* 2002 Mar; 17(1): 63–7.

7. Magee MF, Bhatt BA. Management of decompensated diabetes. Diabetic ketoacidosis and hyperglycemic hyperosmolar syndrome. *Crit Care Clin* 2001 Jan; 17(1): 75–106.

8. Vantyghem MC, Haye S, Balduyck M, et al. Changes in serum amylase, lipase and leukocyte elastase during diabetic ketoacidosis and poorly controlled diabetes. *Acta Diabetol* 1999 Jun; 36(1–2): 39–44.

9. Wyatt JP, Illingworth RN, Graham CA, et al, eds. *Oxford Handbook of Accident and Emergency Medicine.* Oxford: Oxford University Press 3rd ed; 2006: 150–151.

10. Singapore Ministry of Health Clinical Guidelines on Diabetes Mellitus 1999.

61 Hypoglycaemia

Sim Tiong Beng • Benjamin Leong

DEFINITION OF HYPOGLYCAEMIA

- Sympton of hypoglycaemia with or without verous blood glucose level that is <4.0 mmol/L in patients with diabetes mellitus on treatment, OR.
- Venous glucose levels fall <2.8 mmol/L, with or without symptoms.
- Adrenergic symptoms and signs:
  1. Hunger.
  2. Sweatiness.
  3. Palpitations.
  4. Tachycardia.
- Neuroglycopaenic symptoms and signs:
  1. Headaches, dizziness, and confusion.
  2. Drowsiness, fits, and coma.

CAVEATS

- Always check stat capillary blood sugar of any patient presenting with altered mental state, focal neurological signs, e.g. hemiplegia or seizures.
- If an **Addisonian crisis** is suspected, give intravenous **(IV) hydrocortisone** 100 mg and IV D/S in addition to correction of hypoglycaemia.
- Although easily reversible, hypoglycaemia can cause permanent brain damage and death if it is severe and prolonged.
- Bedside capillary glucose test kits generally provide fairly accurate glucose readings, except at extremes, in the presence of hypotension, hypothermia and oedema; hence, always confirm the presence of hypoglycaemia with a venous sample. Otherwise, they are acceptable and crucial in ensuring early diagnosis and prompt treatment.
- Suspect **recreational drug abuse** in a well non-diabetic patient with hypoglycaemia.
- Remember that patients with varying degrees of baseline glycaemic control will have varying presenting symptoms; a sudden drop in glucose levels in a patient with chronic hyperglycaemia might produce extensive autonomic symptoms, even if levels are in the euglycaemic range, whereas a modest drop in glucose in a tightly-controlled patient might not produce symptoms.

Causes

- Most cases are diabetic patients on treatment with insulin or sulphonylureas.
- **Causes of hypoglycaemia** in a **healthy-appearing patient:**
    1. Medications/drugs
        a. Insulin and oral hypoglycaemic agents (OHGA) especially glibenclamide (see Tables 1 and 2)
        b. Alcohol
        c. Salicylates
        d. Non-selective beta blockers (which attenuate the adrenergic response to stress)
        e. Recreation drug, e.g. Power One Walnut
    2. Intense exercise or missed meal
    3. Insulinoma (very rare!)

TABLE 1 Types of insulin

Insulin type	Onset of action	Peak effect	Duration of action
Rapid-acting (Human insulin analogues) • Lispro (humalog) • Aspart (novorapid)	5–20 minutes	1–3 hours	3–5 hours
Short-acting (Recombinant human regular insulin) • Humulin Regular ®/SI • Actrapid	30–60 minutes	2–4 hours	6–8 hours
Intermediate-acting • Neutral Protamine Hagedorn (NPH) • Lente	1–4 hours	8–12 hours	12–20 hours
Long-acting • Ultralente/ultratard/Humulin U • Glargine (lantus) • Detemir (lemevir)	3–5 hours 1–4 hours 1–4 hours	10–16 hours Peakless	18–24 hours 24 hours 18–24 hours
Premixed insulins • Mixtard 30 or Humulin 30/70 (premixed 30% regular insulin + 70% intermediate-acting insulin)	30–60 minutes	2–8 hours	24 hours
• Mixtard 50 or Humulin 50/50 (premixed 50% regular insulin + 50% intermediate-acting insulin)	30–60 minutes	2–8 hours	24 hours
• Biphasic insulin analogue 1. Novomix 30 (premixed 30% insulin aspart + 70% protaminated)	10–20 minutes	1–3 hours	24 hours
2. Humalog Mix 25/75 (premixed 25% insulin lispro + 75% protaminated insulin lispro)	10–20 minutes	1–3 hours	24 hours

TABLE 2 Oral hypoglycaemic agents

Oral hypoglycaemic agent (OHGA)	Duration of action	Mode of action	Risk of hypoglycaemia
Sulfonylureas		Stimulate pancreatic insulin secretion	Yes, especially long-acting agents
• First generation			
Chlorpropamide	24–72 hours		
Tolbutamide	6–10 hours		
Tolazamide	14–16 hours		
• Second generation			
Glipizide	6–10 hours		
Gliclazide	12–18 hours		
Glyburide	24 hours		
Glibenclamide	24 hours		
• Third generation			
Glimepiride (amaryl)	24 hours		
Meglitinides		Stimulate pancreatic insulin secretion	Yes, but less so than sulfonylureas
• Repaglinide	<4 hours		
• Nateglinide	4 hours		
Biguanide		Decrease hepatic glucose production	Minimal or none
• Metformin	6–12 hours		
Thialidinedione		Increase peripheral glucose utilization	Minimal or none
• Rosiglitazone	Weeks		
• Pioglitazone	4 weeks		
α-glucosidase inhibitors		Decrease gastrointestinal tract absorption of glucose	No
• Acarbose	3–4 hours		
• Miglitol	3–4 hours		

- **Causes of hypoglycaemia in an ill-appearing patient**:
  1. Sepsis and shock.
  2. Infection: Malaria, especially with quinine or quinidine treatment.
  3. Liver failure.
  4. Cardiac failure (diffuse liver dysfunction).
  5. Renal failure (impaired gluconeogenesis).
  6. Endocrine.
     a. Hypothalamus/pituitary or adrenal insufficiency of cortisol.
     b. Insulin antibodies.
  7. Starvation and anorexia nervosa.
  8. Non-islet cell tumour, e.g. sarcoma and mesothelioma.
  9. Congenital liver problems including defects of carbohydrate, amino acid, and fatty acid metabolism.

⇨ **SPECIAL TIPS FOR GPs**

- Educate patients and their caregivers on oral hypoglycaemic agents, insulin, and appropriate meal and snack plans.
- Educate patients about **sick day management plans**.
- **Avoid long-acting sulphonylureas, especially glibenclamide** and chlorpropamide, in patients who are elderly, or who have liver, renal, or cardiac impairment.
- Aim for tight glucose control in general (aim for HbA1C 6.5–7%), but must take into account age, renal function, and comorbidities. For the elderly, aim for less tight glucose control.
- Self-blood glucose monitoring will help to reduce the incidence of hypoglycaemia.
- Encourage **medication safety at home**.
  1. Keep drugs locked up and out of the reach of children.
  2. Discourage the practice of taking medication out of their original blister packs and filling them into recycled containers to prevent confusion.
  3. Label packages clearly.

MANAGEMENT

- **Manage the patient in a monitored area**
  1. Monitoring: Electrocardiogram (ECG), pulse oximetry, and vital signs.
  2. Administer supplemental low flow oxygen if required.
- **History and examination**
  1. Risk factors of hypoglycaemia:
     a. Food intake due to acute sepsis and meal-related issues (e.g. urinary tract infection with decreased appetite).

     PLUS

     b. Elderly, aged >65 years.
     c. Chronic renal failure with serum creatinine ≥130 mmol/L.
     d. HbA1c (glycated haemoglobin) <7%.
     e. Those who have a duration of diabetes mellitus of >10 years.
     f. Those who have ≥3 comorbidities.
     g. Polypharmacy patients taking >10 tablets a day.
     h. Use of glibenclamide or insulin, recent increment in OHGA, or insulin.
     i. No self-monitoring of blood glucose or hypoglycaemia education from diabetic nurse educator.
- **Investigation**
  1. **Venous blood glucose**, urea/electrolytes/creatinine, liver function tests, full blood count.
  2. If the patient is not diabetic, take **1 to 2 extra plain tubes of blood on ice** for serum insulin, C-peptides and cortisol especially if the patient is hypotensive with abnormal electrolytes.

- The **treatment** depends on the level of consciousness and cooperation of the patient.

  1. **Conscious and cooperative patient**

     a. **Oral therapy** is preferred.

     b. Give a **carbohydrate-rich drink** (e.g. Ensure, Isocal and Nepro). Note that a can of Ensure/Isocal has 250 calories and a can of Nepro has 500 calories, compared with a pint of D5W, which has only 100 calories.

  2. **Unconscious or uncooperative patient**

     a. **If IV access is available**, give **IV dextrose 50% 40–50 ml** and flush with normal saline to minimize phlebitis. Recovery is almost immediate.

     b. **If IV access is unavailable** or if the patient is very uncooperative, **intramuscular (IM) or subcutaneous (SC) glucagon 1 mg** may be given. Note that IM or SC glucagon takes a few minutes longer to work than IV dextrose. Glucagon is also not suitable for use in hypoglycaemia secondary to sulphonylureas or liver failure.

  3. If chronic alcoholism is suspected, give **IV thiamine 100 mg**.

  4. If the patient does **not respond to dextrose**, some **differentials** to be considered are:

     a. **Adrenal insufficiency**: Take a plain tube for serum cortisol and then give **IV hydrocortisone 100–200 mg**.

     b. Sepsis.

     c. **Insulinoma or factious insulin/recreational drug abuse**: Do proinsulin and C-peptide and maintain on IV dextrose 10% as hypoglycaemia is recurrent.

     d. **Intracranial pathology** including cerebral oedema, intra-cerebral haemorrhage, and subarachnoid haemorrhage. Obtain a head computed tomography (CT) and manage accordingly.

     e. **Drug overdose** such as tricyclic anti-depressants, salicylate, opioids, anti-malarials, e.g. quinine.

     f. **Heat stroke**.

     If there are associated injuries, give **tetanus prophylaxis**.

- **Monitoring**

  1. Check the capillary blood glucose hourly until it is >10 mmol/L on 2 consecutive readings followed by every 2 hours × 2 hours then 8 hourly if glucose control is between 8–12 mmol/L.

  2. Consider repeat doses if there is poor response to therapy, or a continuous infusion of dextrose 10%. Omit IV dextrose only if the patient is feeding well and if capillary blood glucose is >10 mmol/L on 2 consecutive readings. Consider giving Isocal/Ensure if intake is poor.

  3. If there is a **persistent altered mental state** despite normalization of blood capillary glucose, get a **brain CT scan** to rule out intracranial pathology.

- **Disposition**
  1. The disposition of the patient depends on several factors, which include the following:
     a. **Aetiology** of the hypoglycaemia, including the causal agent.
     b. **Severity** of the neurological deficit and its response to treatment.
     c. **Response** of the blood glucose levels and the need for continuous replacement.
     d. Concurrent issues, e.g. head injury.
     e. **Social/psychiatric circumstances**, such as availability of a responsible caregiver, or suicidal patients.
  2. Consider **discharge from the emergency department** if
     a. The insulin or OHGA is short acting.
     b. The patient missed a meal or had prior intense exercise.
     c. There is good response to dextrose therapy and dextrose infusion is able to maintain euglycaemia.
     d. The patient is able to tolerate feeds well.
     e. The patient and his caregiver are motivated and competent to monitor blood capillary glucose at home and have a clear management and follow-up plan.
  3. Consider **observation unit admission** (if any of the above is not met) for further monitoring and management. Refer the patient to a diabetic nurse educator and dietician. It is important to counsel the patient on medication on insulin/OHGA reduction, hypoglycaemia symptoms, and management plan. Identify precipitating factors leading to the hypoglycaemia, e.g. poor intake from mild sepsis. Stop giving glibenclamide if the patient is on it and convert to short-acting OHGA. Stop metformin if serum creatinine is >150 mmol/L to reduce lactic acidosis risk.
  4. Consider **inpatient care** if there are multiple comorbidities or medical issues, poor social support, suspected recreational drug abuse (risk of recurrent hypoglycaemia).
  5. Consider **intensive care unit admission** if massive overdose of OHGA, acute liver failure, or severe sepsis is present.
  6. If the cause of hypoglycaemia has been clearly recognized and reversed (such as a diabetic who missed a meal after injecting insulin) with good clinical recovery, the patient may be discharged home under the care of a responsible caregiver and follow up with his primary care physician.

References/Further Reading

1. Tan C. Hypoglycemic emergencies in diabetic patients. *Critical Decisions in Emergency Medicine*. June 2008; 22(10): 9–9–19.

2. Diabetes Mellitus. Clinical Practice Guidelines. *MOH Clinical Practice Guidelines 3/2006*.

3. de Galan BE, Schouwenberg BJ, Tack CJ, et al. Pathophysiology and management of recurrent hypoglycemia and hypoglycemia unawareness in diabetes. *Neth J Med*. 2006; 64(8): 269–279.

4. Mohammad Jalili. Type 2 diabetes mellitus. In: Tintinalli JE, Ma OJ, Stapczynski JS, et al., eds. *Tintinalli's Emergency Medicine: A Comprehensive Study Guide*. 7th ed. New York: McGraw-Hill, 1430–1432.

5. Cryer PE, Davis SN, Shamoon H. Hypoglycemia in diabetes. *Diabetes care*. 2003; 26(6): 1902–1912.

6. Caroll MF, Burge MR, Schade DS. Severe hypoglycemia in adults. *Rev Endocr Metab Disord*. 2003; 4(2): 149–157.

7. Miller CD, Phillips LS, Ziemer DC, et al. Hypoglycemia in patients with type 2 diabetes mellitus. *Arch Intern Med*. 2001; 161: 1653–1659.

8. Wyatt JP, Illingworth RN, Graham CA, et al., eds. *Oxford Handbook of Accident and Emergency Medicine*. Oxford, 3rd ed. UK: Oxford University Press, 2006.

9. Service JF. Classification of hypoglycemic disorders. *Endocrinol Metab Clin North Am*. 1999; 28: 501–517.

62   Thyroid Emergencies
– Thyroid Crisis and Myxoedema
Malcolm Mahadevan • Goh Ee Ling

THYROID CRISIS

CAVEATS

- A thyroid crisis is defined as a sudden severe life-threatening exacerbation of hyperthyroidism associated with multiple-organ decompensation.
- Suspect the existence of **thyroid storm** in any **known case of hyperthyroidism developing a fever**.
- Thyroid storm is fatal if untreated: Mortality rate is 20–50%.
- Avoid aspirin-based antipyretics: They release free T4 and free T3 from protein-bound sites.
- **Clinical presentation**
  1. **Fever** as an indicator of underlying sepsis or a consequence of thyroid storm.
  2. **Tachycardia out of proportion to fever** classically persists during sleep.
  3. **Accentuated thyrotoxic symptoms and signs** such as weight loss and tremors.
  4. **Multi-organ dysfunction**:
     a. Central nervous system dysfunction: Altered mental state with mental confusion, delirium, agitation, stupor, and coma.
     b. Gastrointestinal dysfunction: Abdominal pain, diarrhoea, and vomiting may simulate a surgical abdomen; jaundice may occur with liver dysfunction.
     c. Cardiovascular system dysfunction: Systolic hyper- or hypotension, heart failure, rapid atrial fibrillation, or flutter.
  5. Recent history of thyroid disease requiring treatment or a precipitating event, e.g. sepsis, recent surgery, and iodinated computed tomography (CT) contrast.
  6. Trauma patient with increasing pulse and blood pressure.
  7. Volume depletion from fever, increased metabolism, and diarrhoea.
- Beware atypical presentation especially in the elderly where a high index of suspicion is essential. They may only present with weakness, heart failure or atrial fibrillation, and goitre may not be evident.
- **Physical examination findings**
  1. Hyperpyrexia is an indicator of underlying sepsis or a consequence of thyroid storm.
  2. Systolic hyper- or hypotension, heart failure, rapid atrial fibrillation, or flutter.
  3. Tachycardia out of proportion to fever.
  4. Altered mental state (**mandatory** diagnostic criterion) delirium, agitation, stupor, and coma.

5. Volume depletion from fever, increased metabolism, and diarrhoea.

6. Stigmata of hyperthyroidism is goitre, tremors, lid lag/retraction, and myopathy.

⇨ **SPECIAL TIP FOR GPs**

- Thyroid storm must often be recognized and treated based on clinical grounds because laboratory confirmation of the disease cannot be obtained in a timely manner.

MANAGEMENT

Supportive measures

- The patient must be managed in the critical care area due to the life-threatening nature of this disease entity.
- Administer supplemental high flow oxygen by a non-rebreather reservoir mask.
- Monitoring: Electrocardiogram (ECG), vital signs q 10–15 minutes, and pulse oximetry.
- Establish large bore peripheral intravenous (IV) lines.
- Administer IV fluids: Dextrose saline by slow infusion with appropriate electrolytes and vitamins; **correct volume depletion cautiously** to avoid precipitating or worsening heart failure. However, immense fluid losses may require replacement of 3–5 L/day. Electrolyte abnormalities include mild hypercalcaemia and hyperglycaemia.
- **Investigations**:
  1. Full blood count.
  2. Urea/electrolytes/creatinine, calcium, and venous blood glucose.
  3. Liver panel.
  4. Thyroid screen to include thyroid stimulating hormone, free T4. Send the blood tube to the ward with the patient.
  5. Chest X-ray for evidence of heart failure and infection.
  6. ECG to determine presence of ischaemia, infarction, or dysrhythmia.
  7. Urinalysis by dipstick reagent and culture and sensitivity (C&S) if sepsis is suspected.
- Correct precipitating factors, e.g. sepsis and acute myocardial infarction.
- Administer paracetamol, tepid sponging, or other cooling techniques to relieve fever.

Drug therapy

A multi-drug approach with emphasis on medication sequence is vital.

- **Beta blockers**: Crucial even in the presence of high cardiac output heart failure.
  1. Give ultra-short acting IV **esmolol**; test dose 250 µg/kg followed by an infusion of 50 µg/kg/min if available, or

2. Give IV **propranolol** 1 mg q 5 minutes until severe tachycardia is controlled. If the patient is able to tolerate oral therapy, then **propranolol 60 mg PO q 4 hours** or **80 mg PO q 8 hours** can be given (takes an hour to have an effect).

NOTE: Treat other cardiovascular complications with conventional means, e.g. digoxin and diuretics.

- **PTU** (propylthiouracil) blocks iodination as well as the conversion of T4 to T3.
  Dosage: 400–600 mg stat orally or via Ryle's tube, followed by 200–300 mg q 4 hours.

NOTE: Per rectal PTU can be given if the patient is kept nil by mouth (NBM). Dissolve in a paediatric Fleet enema and give through a Nelaton catheter.

- **Iodine** solution inhibits the release of thyroid hormone; **must** give 1 to 2 hours post-PTU therapy.
  Dosage: Lugol's iodine 5 drops PO or via Ryle's tube q 8 hours.

NOTE: If the patient is kept NBM, give IV sodium iodide 1 g/500 ml saline q 12 hours.

- **Hydrocortisone** 100 mg 8 hourly; also block conversion of freeT4 to freeT3.

Disposition

- Consult with Endocrine/General Medicine regarding anticipated admission to the medical intensive care unit.

References/Further Reading

1. Smallridge RC. Metabolic and anatomic thyroid emergencies: A review. *Crit Care Med.* 1992; 20: 276–291.

2. Nayak B, Burman K. Thyrotoxicosis and thyroid storm. *Endocrino Metab Clin North Am.* 2006; 35: 663–686.

MYXOEDEMA

DEFINITION

- Myxoedema is defined as severe hypothyroidism characterized by 2 hallmark features of **decreased mental status** and **hypothermia**.
- **Clinical manifestions**
  1. **Neurological symptoms**: Confusion, lethargy, psychosis (**myxoedema madness**), and seizures.
  2. **Hypothermia**: Due to impaired thermogenesis.
  3. **Hyponatraemia**: Due to renal impairment or the syndrome of inappropriate antidiuretic hormone secretion (SIADH).
  4. **Hypoventilation** with respiratory acidosis: Due to depression of the central ventilatory drive.

5. **Hypoglycaemia**: Due to decreased gluconeogenesis or associated adrenal insufficiency.

6. **Cardiovascular**: Bradycardia, heart failure, pericardial effusion, and hypotension.

CAVEATS

● Myxoedema is an endocrine emergency which remains a clinical diagnosis.

● The mortality rate is 30–40% and is higher in elderly patients and those with cardiovascular complications.

● Treatment should therefore be given based on clinical suspicion without laboratory confirmation that will delay therapy.

CLINICAL ASSESSMENT

● **History**

1. Presenting symptoms, e.g. lethargy and altered mental state.
2. Symptoms of hypothyroidism, e.g. weight gain and voice change.
3. Precipitating factors, e.g. infection and trauma.
4. Past medical history, e.g. surgery or radio-iodine therapy.
5. Medication history, e.g. amiodarone and lithium (which can lead to hypothyroidism).

● Causes of hypothyroidism

Results from severe, long-standing hypothyroidism, or precipitated by acute events.

See Table 1 for causes of hypothyroidism.

TABLE 1 Causes of hypothyroidism

Long-standing hypothyroidism	Autoimmune thyroiditis Previous surgery or radio-iodine treatment for hyperthyroidism Medications, e.g. amiodarone and lithium
Precipitating factors	Infection Trauma Acute myocardial infarction (AMI) Cold exposure Sedative drugs, e.g. opiates and benzodiazepines Stroke

● **Physical examination**

1. General appearance: Altered mental status
2. Vital signs: Look for bradycardia, hypotension, hypothermia, and hypoventilation.
3. Cardiovascular signs: Muffled heart sounds (in pericardial effusion) and elevated jugular venous pressure/pedal oedema/S3 (in cardiac failure).

4. Neurological signs: Focal neurological deficits, tongue laceration (in seizures), and slow ankle reflexes.

5. Skin: Puffy face and carotinaemia.

6. Others: Thyroidectomy scar and evidence of sepsis.

- **Investigations**
  1. Stat capillary blood glucose
  2. Bloods:
     a. Full blood count: Anaemia, raised total white cell count or leucocytosi in sepsis
     b. Renal panel: Especially for hyponatraemia
     c. Creatine kinase: Should be >1000 iu/L
     d. Arterial blood gas: Type 2 respiratory failure
     e. Thyroid function test: Free T4 and thyroid-stimulating hormone
     f. Serum cortisol: Look for associated hypocortisolism
  3. Chest X-ray: Cardiomegaly, pleural effusion, pulmonary oedema, and pneumonia.
  4. ECG: Changes of acute myocardial infarction, bradycardia, J waves (in hypothermia), and low voltages of QRS complexes (in pericardial effusion).

⇨ **SPECIAL TIPS FOR GPs**
- Myxoedema must be treated based on clinical grounds and not delayed for laboratory confirmation which cannot be obtained in a timely manner.
- Always check capillary blood glucose levels in patients with suspected myxoedema and initiate treatment for hypoglycaemia which is a common associated finding.

MANAGEMENT

- **Supportive treatment**
  1. The patient must be managed in the critical care area.
  2. Monitoring: ECG, vital signs, and pulse oximetry.
  3. Obtain intravenous access.
  4. Support the airway, breathing and circulation.
     a. Secure the airway for protection if need be.
     b. Give supplemental oxygen.
     c. Administer fluid resuscitation for hypotension. Add on vasopressors if the patient does not respond to fluids. Avoid hypotonic fluids in hyponatraemic patients.
  5. Passively rewarm the patient with a heating blanket.
  6. Give IV **hydrocortisone** 100 mg 8 hourly (to stop later if serum cortisol is normal).

- **Thyroid hormone replacement**
  1. Can be given orally or intravenously.
  2. Either T3 (triiodothyronine) or T4 (L-thyroxine).
  3. T3 has the advantages of a rapid onset of action and greater biological activity.
  4. Dose:

     T3: 2.5 µg 8 hourly followed by double doses every 2 to 3 days to the target dose of 30–40 µg/day.

     T4: 25 µg as test dose then increase dose to 500 µg on the first day. Subsequent dosing 25–100 µg/day.

     Maintenance dose should be lower in elderly patients and those with ischaemic heart disease.

- **Treat the precipitating causes and complications**
  1. Hypoglycaemia: Correct with IV dextrose 50% followed by IV dextrose 10% drip.
  2. Hyponatraemia: Correct slowly with normal saline.
  3. Cardiac failure: Give diuretics and vasodilators.
  4. Sepsis: Give antibiotics.

- **Disposition**

  Patients with myxoedema should be admitted to the high dependency or intensive care unit for close monitoring.

References/Further Reading

1. Yamamoto T, Fukuyama J, Fujiyoshi A. Factors associated with mortality of myxedema coma: Report of eight cases and literature survey. *Thyroid*. 1999; 9: 1167.

2. Soon PC, Loh KC. Hypothyroid (myxoedema) coma. In: Tai DYH, Lew TWK, Loo S, eds. *Bedside ICU Handbook*. 2nd ed. Singapore: Armour Publishing; 2007: 154–155.

3. Cheah JS. Myxoedema coma. In: Lee KH, Wong J, Tan CC, eds. *Survival Guide to Acute Medicine*. 1st ed. Singapore: Singapore University Press; 1998: 140–141.

63 Renal Emergencies

Peter Manning • Keith Ho

HYPERKALAEMIA

Caveats

- The severity of hyperkalaemia is related to the plasma potassium level but there is considerable inter-patient and intra-patient variability. The rapidity of the development of hyperkalaemia has a significant bearing on the clinical severity. **Do not** wait for the potassium level results to come back from the lab if either clinical state or electrocardiogram (ECG) suggests hyperkalaemia; rather, treat empirically.

- Clinical manifestations can be protean. ECG changes when present are useful but may be difficult to interpret and may even be absent in some patients with severe hyperkalaemia. Metabolic acidosis and hypocalcaemia can worsen the severity of hyperkalaemia.

- In the appropriate clinical setting (e.g. chronic renal failure, diabetic with nephropathy, etc.) with ECG changes consistent with severe hyperkalaemia (see Figure 1), it is appropriate to consider empiric therapy if the serum potassium result is anticipated to be unavailable immediately.

- A serum potassium level >5.5 mmol/L is considered hyperkalaemia. Pseudohyperkalaemia is most commonly due to extravascular haemolysis. Other causes include severe thrombocytosis and leucocytosis.

- **The severity of hyperkalaemia** can be classified as follows:

  1. **Mild**: The potassium level is <6.0 mmol/L and the ECG may be normal or show only peaked T waves.

  2. **Moderate**: The potassium level is between 6.0 and 7.0 mmol/L and the ECG may show peaked T waves.

  3. **Severe**: The potassium level is between 7.0 and 8.0 mmol/L and the ECG shows flattening of the P wave and QRS with T wave (sine wave) that leads to atrioventricular (AV) dissociation, ventricular dysrhythmias, and death.

Four-step Management of Hyperkalaemia

- **Step 1: Stabilization of membrane potential**

  1. Administer **calcium gluconate** 10%: 10 to 20 ml intravenously over 3 to 10 minutes, to a maximum of 20 ml. Onset in 1 to 2 minutes. Repeat the same dose if there is no improvement. The duration of effect is 30–60 minutes.

NOTE: Intravenous (IV) calcium should be **used only** when there is ECG evidence of severe hyperkalaemia (IV calcium is not required when the ECG shows peaked T waves alone), significant neuromuscular weakness, or a serum potassium level that is >7.0 mmol/L. The drug should be

FIGURE 1   Electrocardiographic manifestations of hypokalaemia and hyperkalaemia

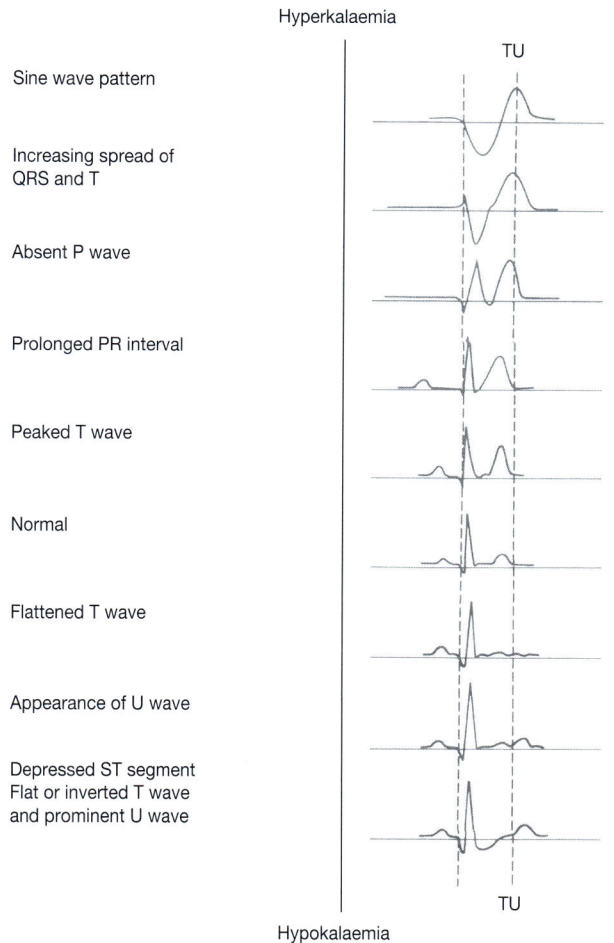

Hyperkalaemia

Sine wave pattern

Increasing spread of
QRS and T

Absent P wave

Prolonged PR interval

Peaked T wave

Normal

Flattened T wave

Appearance of U wave

Depressed ST segment
Flat or inverted T wave
and prominent U wave

Hypokalaemia

Figure reproduced with permission.[2]

used with absolute caution in patients on digoxin as it can bring about severe digitalis toxicity. Ensure the IV line is working well because extravasation of calcium chloride into the subcutaneous tissue can cause skin necrosis. That is why calcium gluconate rather than calcium choride is a safer choice.

● **Step 2: Shift the potassium in the extra-cellular fluid into the intra-cellular fluid**

1. Administer **dextrose/insulin**: 40–50 ml D50W IV over 5 to 10 minutes and 10 units of regular insulin as separate boluses. Onset in 30 minutes and duration of effects is between 4 and 6 hours. This treatment is recommended over sodium bicarbonate therapy.

2. Administer **sodium bicarbonate** 1 mEq/kg body weight IV as a bolus over 5 minutes in patients with moderate to severe metabolic acidosis; repeat in half an hour in patients with severe metabolic acidosis. Onset is 5 minutes and duration of effect is between 1 and 2 hours.

NOTE: Sodium bicarbonate therapy is most useful in the severely acidotic patient (may have no effect in the non-acidotic patient). It should be used with caution in chronic renal failure patients since it may lead to fluid overload and provoke hypocalcaemic tetany or fits due to acute alkalosis.

- Administer **salbutamol**: Add 5 mg salbutamol to 3–4 ml saline and nebulize over 10 minutes. Onset is half an hour and duration effect is 2 hours. Salbutamol should be used with caution in patients with known or suspected ischaemic heart disease.
- **Step 3: Remove potassium from the body**
  1. **Resonium A**: 15 g orally (PO) 4 to 6 hourly. Onset is between 1 and 2 hours and duration effect is 2 hours. Use with caution in patients with significant constipation or ileus.
  2. **Haemodialysis** (contact Renal Medicine first): Onset in minutes and it has a duration of 4 hours.
- **Step 4: Prevent further potassium increase**
  1. Review all medications, e.g. Span K, ACE inhibitors, and beta blockers.
  2. Review diet and give advice.

NOTE: Steps 3(1) and 4 usually suffice for stable mild to moderate hyperkalaemia. However repeat a serum potassium level to ensure there is no continued increase in potassium and an improvement in the serum potassium level.

RENAL FAILURE

Definitions

- **Acute renal failure:** An abrupt (within 48 hours) reduction in kidney function:
  1. An absolute increase in serum creatinine of ≥26.4 mol/L.
  2. A percentage increase in serum creatinine of ≥50% from the baseline level.
  3. A reduction in urine output (documented oliguria of <0.5 ml/kg per hour for >6 hours)

The above criteria include both an absolute and a percentage change in creatinine to accommodate variations related to age, gender, and body mass index, and to reduce the need for a baseline creatinine but do require ≥2 creatinine values within 48 hours. The above criteria should be used in the context of the clinical presentation and following adequate fluid resuscitation when applicable.

- **Chronic kidney disease**
  1. Structural kidney damage or decreased kidney function (decreased glomerular filtration rate, GFR) for ≥3 months.
- **End-stage renal disease (kidney failure)**
  1. The GFR is <15 ml/min per 1.73 m^2, which is accompanied in most cases by signs and symptoms of uraemia, or
  2. A need to start kidney replacement therapy (dialysis or transplantation).

Chronic Renal Failure with Fluid Overload and not on Dialysis

- Manage the patient in the critical care area.*
- Place the patient in an upright position.*
- Administer supplemental high flow oxygen.*
- Monitoring: ECG, vital signs q 5 to 10 minutes, and pulse oximetry.*
- Preserve one upper-limb vessel for future arteriovenous access (no blood taking or drip setting).
- Draw blood for full blood count, urea/electrolytes/creatinine, and arterial blood gas; also for cardiac enzyme tests if cardiac ischaemia is suspected.
- Drug therapy
  1. **GTN** 0.5 mg sublingually (SL) or nitroderm patch 5–10 mg or IV 10–200 µg/min.
  2. **Morphine** 2–5 mg IV (if there is severe pulmonary oedema).
  3. **Felodipine** 2.5 mg PO if the blood pressure is high.
  4. **Frusemide** 120–240 mg IV.
- Consider dialysis if there is severe fluid overload, hyperkalaemia, metabolic acidosis, or the patient is not responding to the above measures (contact the renal physician-on-call).

Coronary Renal Failure with Fluid Overload without Accessible Peripheral Venous Access

- See the asterisked steps in the previous section.
- Drug therapy
  1. **GTN** 0.5 mg SL or nitroderm patch 5–10 mg.
  2. **Felodipine** 2.5 mg PO if the blood pressure is high.
  3. **Frusemide** 120–240 mg PO.

SEVERE METABOLIC ACIDOSIS

Caveats

- Patients often present with non-specific symptoms. Its clinical effects are overshadowed by the signs and symptoms of the underlying disorder.
- Metabolic acidosis should be suspected in any patient with hyperventilation, altered mental state, and haemodynamic instability.

Management

- **Supportive measures**
  1. The patient should be managed in the critical care area.
  2. Ascertain airway patency and manage accordingly.
  3. Monitoring: ECG and vital signs q 5 to 10 minutes.

4. Establish peripheral IV access with normal saline at 'keep open' rate.

5. **Labs**: Full blood count, urea/electrolytes/creatinine, stat capillary blood glucose, arterial blood gas, serum osmolality, urinalysis, and ECG.

6. **X-rays:** No specific role in acid base states. However, a kidney, ureter, and bladder X-ray may be useful to identify an ingested substance, e.g. iron tablets, or a gastrointestinal problem causing or complicating the acid base imbalance, e.g. bowel obstruction or ischaemic bowel.

Decision Priorities

- Once the lab values are available, and assuming they are accurate, 3 steps are followed in the **evaluation** for an **acidotic state**. Refer to Chapter 57, *Acid Base Emergencies* and Chapter 143, *Useful Formulae* for more details.

1. Determine primary and secondary acid base abnormalities.

2. Calculate the osmolal gap to detect the presence of low molecular weight osmotically active substances (refer to Chapter 143, *Useful Formulae*).

3. Review the potassium level in relation to the abnormal pH (refer to Chapater 143, *Useful Formulae*).

Specific Therapy

- Bicarbonate therapy is reserved for severe organic acidosis or those not easily reversed. The goal is to raise the arterial pH >7.2. There is no need to correct the pH if it is ≥7.2 unless there is some life-threatening problem that needs to be addressed. No perfect formula exists but the following is useful: **Dose of NaHCO$_3$ [mEq] = (Desired [HCO$_3^-$] – Measured [HCO$_3^-$] × 50% body weight in kg**. Half this dose is given initially with the remainder depending on repeat laboratory evaluation. Do not aim to correct bicarbonate to normal levels.

- **Dosage:** Bolus therapy is recommended only for those with severe acidosis or when there is haemodynamic compromise. Patients with less life-threatening acidosis may be treated with IV bicarbonate infusion. Add 100–150 mEq NaHCO$_3^-$ (2–3 ampoules of 8.4% NaCHO$_3^-$) to 1 L of D5W and run over 1 to 2 hours with repeated arterial blood gases as a guide to therapy.

- **Potential complications of the therapy** are hypernatraemia, hyperosmolality, volume overload, hypokalaemia, and post-treatment alkalosis.

INDICATIONS FOR DIALYSIS

- Severe pulmonary oedema.

- Severe uncontrollable hypertension from severe fluid overload not responding to diuretics.

- Hyperkalaemia refractive to medical treatment.

- Severe metabolic acidosis refractive to medical treatment.

- Some poisoning, e.g. methanol, ethylene glycol, and salicylates (severe).

- Uraemia, including pericarditis and encephalopathy.

PROBLEMS ASSOCIATED WITH DIALYSIS

Haemodialysis

Vascular access-related complications

- **Bleeding**
    1. Apply digital pressure for 5 to 10 minutes but **do not** occlude/thrombose the vessel with excess pressure.
    2. Document the presence of a thrill following the procedure. Observe the patient for 1 to 2 hours thereafter.
    3. Continued bleeding mandates consultation with the Dialysis Access team and Renal Medicine.
- **Loss of thrill in shunt**: Seek immediate consultation with the Dialysis Access team and Renal Medicine. Do not forcefully manipulate vessel.
- **Infection** (2–5% of arteriovenous fistulas; 10% of functional grafts).
    1. While the classic signs are common, patient may present with fever only.
    2. Draw blood for full blood count and first blood culture; administer the first dose of antibiotics, e.g. IV ceftazidime 1–2 g.
    3. Admit to Renal Medicine; inform the renal physician-on-call if the patient is overtly septic.

Non-vascular access-related complications

- **Hypotension**
    1. Post-haemodialysis hypotension may be due to a reduction in circulating intravascular volume in a patient whose compensatory mechanisms are inadequate. The most common cause is excessive ultrafiltration from underestimation of the patient's dry weight. Check with the patient how much fluid was removed during the haemodialysis session.
    2. This may be seen in patients on peritoneal dialysis. Again, check with the patient how much negative balance was achieved with the peritoneal dialysis session.
    3. Most cases respond to observation post-dialysis, but may require IV fluid.
    4. However, consider and exclude the following:
        a. Occult haemorrhage: Do a per rectal examination to detect gastrointestinal bleeding.
        b. Acute myocardial infarction/dysrhythmias or pericardial tamponade.
        c Life-threatening hyperkalaemia: Treat empirically if there are severe changes of hyperkalaemia.
        d. Infection.
        e. Pulmonary or air embolism and acute haemolysis in haemodialysis.

- **Dyspnoea**
  1. Most commonly due to volume overload; consider sudden cardiac failure, pericardial tamponade, pleural effusion, severe acidosis, severe anaemia (from acute and chronic blood loss), and sepsis.
  2. Exclude acute myocardial infarction: Others include pulmonary or air embolism and acute haemolysis in haemodialysis.

- **Chest pain**
  1. Commonly ischaemic in origin with underlying ischaemic heart disease exacerbated by the transient hypotension and hypoxaemia associated with the dialysis process. Also consider pulmonary embolism, acute haemolysis, and air embolism in haemodialysis.
  2. Management: ECG, monitoring, and cardiac enzymes.
  3. Conduct appropriate consultations with Renal Medicine and/or Cardiology.
  4. Consider non-ischaemic causes of chest pain including pericarditis, lung/pleural disease, reflux oesophagitis, gastritis, or peptic ulcer disease.

- **Neurological dysfunction**
  1. Exclude electrolyte abnormalities, infection, and major intracranial catastrophes.
  2. Management:
     a. Draw stat capillary blood sugar, urea/electrolytes/creatinine, and arterial blood gas.
     b. Monitoring: ECG, vital signs q5–15 minutes, and pulse oximetry.
     c. Search for new focal neurological abnormalities and perform head computed tomography (CT) scan.
  3. Fits: Treat as per normal. Consult the renal physician-on-call and/or Neurology.

- **Dialysis disequilibrium**
  1. This usually occurs at the end of a dialysis treatment and the patient initially presents with headache, nausea, disorientation, restlessness, and blurred vision. This may progress to seizures, coma, and death.
  2. Treatment involves stopping dialysis and administering IV mannitol to increase serum osmolality.
  3. However, consider and exclude the following:
     a. Uraemia
     b. Intracranial events: Subdural haematoma, cerebral infarction, and intra-cerebral haemorrhage
     c. Meningitis
     d. Metabolic disturbances (hyponatraemia and hypoglycaemia)
     e. Drug-induced encephalopathy

Peritoneal dialysis

Dialysis access-related complications include these:

- **Peritonitis**
  1. Cloudy effluent, non-specific abdominal pain, malaise, fever, and chills in mild to moderate cases.
  2. Vomiting, severe pain, shock, and classic signs of peritonitis in more severe cases.
  3. Management:
     a. Draw full blood count, urea/electrolytes/creatinine, and first blood culture.
     b. Call the continuous ambulatory peritoneal dialysis (CAPD) nurse for rapid exchanges of fluid lavages.
     c. Inform the physician-on-call regarding the case.
     d. Administer intra-peritoneal (IP) antibiotics, e.g. IP vancomycin 1 g and IP gentamycin.
- **Leaking catheter**: Admit and inform renal physician-on-call of admission.
- **Hypotension**: See above.
- **Acute abdomen**
  1. This is often due to a serious intra-abdominal condition whose presentation mimics peritonitis.
  2. Obtain combined Renal Medicine and General Surgery consultations.

NOTE: CAPD patients are at risk for developing abdominal/inguinal herniae due to chronically elevated intra-abdominal pressures and intestinal obstruction secondary to adhesions.

- **Infection of tunnel/catheter exit site**
  1. Often difficult to detect clinically.
  2. Consult with Renal Medicine.

References/Further Reading

1. Sinert R, Spektor M. Emergencies in renal failure and dialysis patients. In: Tintinalli JE, Ma OJ, Stapczynski JS, et al., eds. *Tintinalli's Emergency Medicine: A Comprehensive Study Guide*. 7th ed. New York: McGraw-Hill; 2011: 624–630.
2. Zull DN. Disorders of potassium metabolism. In: Wolfson AB, ed. Endocrine and metabolic emergencies. *Emerg Med Clinics North Am*. 1989; 7(4)783.
3. Mehta RL, et al. and the Acute Kidney Injury Network. Acute Kidney Injury Network: Report of an initiative to improve outcomes in acute kidney injury. *Critical Care*. 2007: 11: R31.
4. K/DOQI clinical practice guidelines for chronic kidney disease: Evaluation, classification, and stratification. Kidney Disease Outcome Quality Initiative. *Am J Kidney Dis*. 2002; 39: S1–246.
5. Piraino B, et al. Peritoneal dialysis-related infections recommendations: 2005 update. *Perit Dial Int*. Mar–Apr 2005; 25(2): 107–131.

64   Urinary Tract Infections
Chiu Li Qi

CAVEATS

- Urine dipstix may be false negative for nitrites in UTI caused by organisms which do not convert nitrates to nitrites.
- Treatment of asymptomatic bacteriuria is not indicated except in the pregnant and before urological intervention.
- Consider infection with a fastidious organism in symptomatic patients with negative urine cultures. Such organisms include *Chlamydia, Mycoplasma, Gonococci, Trichomonas, Candida* and *Mycobacteria.*
- Pregnant patients with asymptomatic UTI should be treated and referred for follow up.
- **Upper UTI + obstruction/hydronephrosis = urological emergency!** Start intravenous antibiotics and refer to urology for decompression.

Classical presentation

- UTIs are more common in females.
- Common organisms include *E. Coli, Proteus, Klebsiella* species and *Staphylococcus saprophyticus.*
- **Lower UTI (urethritis, cystitis)**: dysuria, frequency, haematuria, suprapubic discomfort/pain, urgency, burning, cloudy urine with an offensive smell. Fever is usually absent and acute phase reactants are not elevated.
- **Upper UTI (pyelonephritis, pyelonephrosis)**: fever, loin and/or back pain, vomiting, rigors, malaise, and occasionally with signs of sepsis/septic shock.
- **Uncomplicated UTI**: Infections in otherwise healthy female with structurally normal urinary tract and voiding function.
- **Complicated UTI**: Infections of urinary tracts which are anatomically or functionally altered.

Predisposing factors

- Female gender
- Sexual intercourse
- Diaphragm contraceptive/vaginal spermicide
- Diabetes mellitus
- Immunosuppression
- Pregnancy
- Menopause
- Urinary tract obstruction
- Instrumentation
- Genitourinary malformations

High risk features

- Children
- Male (recurrent UTI)
- Pregnancy
- Renal impairment
- Immunosuppression
- Underlying genitourinary malformations
- Renal transplant
- Long-term urinary catheter treatment

Differential Diagnoses

- Appendicitis
- Drug-induced/radiation-induced cystitis
- Sexually-transmitted diseases
- Urethritis
- Urological cancer
- Vaginitis

Laboratory tests evaluation

- Full blood count, urea, creatinine and electrolytes (high risk patients or those with complicated UTIs)
- Dipstix urinalysis: may show positive for nitrites, leucocytes and/or blood
- Urine FEME
- Mid-stream urine: $>10^5$ colony-forming units per mL of urine
- Blood cultures (if signs of sepsis/shock)

⇨ **SPECIAL TIPS FOR GPs**

- Any patient presenting with symptoms of an upper UTI and obstruction should be referred to the Emergency Department
- UTI in children under 2 years old do not present classically. Do a urine dipstix or urine FEME in all febrile preverbal children without other clear source(s) of infection.
- **Prevention of UTIs:**
  1. Encourage adequate fluid intake.
  2. Void when the need is felt; do not hold it in.
  3. Girls and ladies wipe from front to back after going to the toilet.
  4. Void after sexual intercourse.

MANAGEMENT

TABLE 1 A guide to suggested antibiotics

Infection	Suggested antibiotics	Alternative(s) if penicillin allergy
Acute uncomplicated cystitis	PO amoxicillin-clavulanate 625mg q8h (3 days) *or* PO co-trimoxazole 160/800mg q12h (3 days)	PO ciprofloxacin 500mg q12h (3 days) *or* PO nitrofurantoin 50mg q6h (7 days)
Pyelonephritis/ complicated UTI	IV ceftriaxone 2g q24h	PO ciprofloxacin 500mg q12h (7days) *or* IV gentamicin 5mg/kg q24h
Cystitis (in pregnancy)	PO amoxicillin-clavulanate 625mg q8h (3 days)	
Pyelonephritis (in pregnancy)	IV ceftriaxone 2g q24h	

Disposition

- **Uncomplicated lower UTI**: oral antibiotics and discharge.

- **Uncomplicated upper UTI**: urine culture and consider oral antibiotics in well, low-risk patients with a follow up; admit unwell patients or those with high-risk features for intravenous antibiotics.

- **Complicated lower UTI**: urine culture, oral antibiotics in well, low-risk patients with a follow-up; admit patients with high-risk features for intravenous antibiotics.

- **Complicated upper UTI**: urine culture, admit all patients for intravenous antibiotics.

- **Unwell, septic patients**: consider escalation of antibiotics, early imaging and urology referral in the Emergency Department.

References/Further reading

1. Franz M, Hörl WH. Common errors in diagnosis and management of urinary tract infection. I: pathophysiology and diagnostic techniques. *Nephrol Dial Transplant* 1999; 14(11): 2746–53

2. Gupta K, Hooton TM, Naber KG, et al. International clinical practice guidelines for the treatment of acute uncomplicated cystitis and pyelonephritis in women: a 2010 update by the Infectious Diseases Society of America and the European Society for Microbiology and Infectious Diseases. *Clin Infec Dis* 2011; 52(5): e103–20

3. Grabe M, Bjerklund-Johansen TE, Botto H, et al. Guidelines on urological infections. EAU guidelines 2010 edition. *Arnhem: European Association of Urology*. 2011: 1–112.

4. Bjerklund-Johansen TE, Naber K, Wagenlehner F, Tenke P. Patient assessment in urinary tract infections: symptoms, risk factors and antibiotic treatment options. *Surgery* 2011; 29(6): 265–71

5. Hsueh PR, Hoban DJ, Carmeli Y, et al. Consensus review of the epidemiology and appropriate antimicrobial therapy of complicated urinary tract infections in Asia-Pacific region. *J Infect.* 2011; 62(2): 114–23

6. Salvatore S, Salvatore S, Cattoni E, et al. Urinary tract infections in women. *Eur J Obst & Gyne and Reprod Bio*. 2011; 156(2): 131–6.

65   Urolithiasis

Toh Hong Chuen • Shirley Ooi

CAVEATS

- A rupturing abdominal aneurysm can mimic urolithiasis (causing both ureteric colic and haematuria). Exercise caution before diagnosing ureteric colic in patients aged >50 years, especially male patients with cardiovascular risk factors and no past history of urolithiasis or nephrolithiasis.
- **Obstructive uropathy** in the presence of **urinary tract infection** is a **urological emergency**! Obtain a urologic consult at the emergency department.
- Relevant history in the assessment and management of patients with renal calculi include:
    1. Occupation/dehydration.
    2. Renal impairment/solitary kidney.
    3. Hyperparathyroidism/inflammatory bowel disease (calcium oxalate stone).
    4. Recurrent urinary tract infection (struvite stones).
    5. Gout (uric acid stones).
    6. Family history (cystinuria has an autosomal recessive inheritance).
- Irreversible renal damage may occur after 1 to 2 weeks with complete obstruction, with the presence of infection as a major contributor of progressive renal damage.
- 90% of stones are radiopaque (except uric acid stones). 75% of the stones are found in the distal third of the ureter. The rate of spontaneous passage for renal calculi is inversely proportional to the size of the calculi (with sizes <5 mm, 5–8 mm, and >8 mm at 90, 15, and 5%, respectively).

CLINICAL FEATURES

- Pain: Usually starts at night or early hours of the morning. It has an abrupt onset with 'crescendo' intensity, starts in the flank, extends into the abdomen and radiates to the groin. A stone high in the ureter may be referred to the testis/ovary; whereas one approaching the bladder may be referred to the scrotum/vulva. The character is severe and colicky (hyperperistalsis of calyces, pelvis, and ureter) in the background of dull constant ache (distention of renal capsule). The patient experiencing renal colic is usually rolling around and not keeping still as there is no comfortable position.
- Fever is absent (the presence of fever suggests infection!) and the abdomen is soft. Pay careful attention to the presence of a pulsatile mass or abdominal bruit indicating an abdominal aortic aneurysm.
- Struvite stones tend to be insidious in formation and grow into a staghorn over weeks or months. Patients present with recurrent urinary tract infection, gross haematuria, vague abdominal pain, or urosepsis rather than the typical colic seen with calcium stones.

DIFFERENTIAL DIAGNOSIS   (See Table 1)

TABLE 1   Differential diagnosis of renal/ureteric colic

Appendicitis
Salpingitis
Diverticulitis
Pyelonephritis
Ovarian torsion
Prostatitis
Bowel obstruction
Ectopic pregnancy
Leaking abdominal aortic aneurysm
Carcinoma

⇨ **SPECIAL TIPS FOR GPs**

- Most kidney stones can be treated conservatively.
- Loin to groin pain with haematuria is indicative of kidney stones.
- Men with pain in the right iliac fossa have appendicitis until proven otherwise.
- Always consider ectopic pregnancy in women and seek a menstrual history and perform a urinary human chorionic gonadotrophin (HCG) test.
- Provide adequate analgesia with non-steroidal anti-inflammatory drugs (NSAIDs).
- Obstructive uropathy with fever is a urological emergency and should be referred to hospital urgently!

MANAGEMENT

Investigations

- **Urine dipstick**: While 4.9% of patients with urolithiasis documented by intravenous (IV) urography have no microscopic haematuria, the absence of haematuria should prompt the consideration of an alternative diagnosis.[7] An elevated urine pH (>7.6) may suggest the presence of urea-splitting organism; while uric acid stones are often associated with a urine pH of <5
- **Blood investigations** such as full blood count and renal panel are not routinely required in the management. They should be done if complications (e.g. infection) are suspected, or in high risk population groups (e.g. those with chronic renal failure and a solitary kidney).
- There is no need to do a **kidney, ureter, and bladder (KUB) X-ray** at the emergency department. While most stones are radiopaque, the most common radiographic densities seen on KUB are phleboliths in the pelvic veins. These can be done at the outpatient setting (with prior bowel preparation) on the day of the urologic consultation.
- **Non-contrast computed tomography (CT) imaging** in patients with suspected kidney stones improves the diagnostic accuracy and can provide important information about other unsuspected conditions, some of which may require emergency treatment. In general, CT

imaging has a higher sensitivity and specificity than ultrasound (sensitivity 96% versus 61%; specificity both 100%) CT imaging has also a higher sensitivity and specificity compared to intravenous urography (sensitivity 94.1% versus 85.2%; specificity 94.2% versus 90.4%).

Treatment

- **Dietary modification**
  1. Increase fluid intake to maintain a urine output of 2 L per day.
  2. Keep salt intake low, around 2000–3000 mg per day (for calcium and cystine stones).
  3. Most patients do not need to modify their calcium intake. A modest calcium intake can be advocated for patients who are known to be hypercalciuric.
  4. Restriction of oxalate-rich food, such as nuts, chocolate, tea, and dark roughage is recommended. Limit vitamin C supplement to 500 mg or less per day (ascorbic acid is converted to oxalate in vivo).
- **Drug therapy**
  1. The priority in emergency department management here is **pain control**. NSAIDs are first-line agents as they reduce pain of ureteric colic by reducing ureterospasm and renal capsular pressure. Treat nausea and vomiting symptomatically (e.g. consider IM stemetil 12.5 mg).
  2. Consider **allopurinol** 300 mg per day for patients with a history of gout (uric acid stones).

Disposition

- Refer to Urology for **admission** if:
  1. Infection is present.
  2. There is persistent pain despite being treated with analgesia.
  3. Stone size is more than 8 mm on KUB (if performed).
  4. The patient has a known solitary kidney.
- Refer pregnant patients for early outpatient appointment.

References/Further Reading

1. Rosen's Emergency Medicine: Concepts and Clinical Practice. 6th ed. Philadelphia, PA: Mosby-Elsevier; 2006: Chap 98: 1586–1593.
2. Park S, et al. Pathophysiology and management of calcium stones. *Urol Clin North Am.* 2007; 34: 323–334.
3. Cameron MA, et al. Uric acid nephrolithiasis. *Urol Clin North Am.* 2007; 34: 335–346.
4. Healy KA, et al. Pathophysiology and management of infectious staghorn calculi. *Urol Clin North Am.* 2007; 34: 363–374.
5. Sheafor DH, Hertzberg BS, Freed KS, et al. Nonenhanced helical CT and US in the emergency evaluation of patients with renal colic: Prospective comparison. *Radiology.* 2000; 217: 792–797.
6. Pfister SA, Deckart A, Laschke S, et al. Unenhanced helical computed tomography vs intravenous urography in patients with acute flank pain: Accuracy and economic impact in a randomized prospective trial. *European Radiology.* 2003; 13: 2513–2520.
7. Ooi SB, Kour NW, Mahadev A. Haematuria in the diagnosis of urinary calculi. *Ann Acad Med* Singapore 1998; 27: 210–214.

66 Meningitis

Goh Ee Ling • Francis Lee • Shirley Ooi

DEFINITION

- Meningitis is an inflammatory disease of the leptomeninges.
- See Table 1 for the causes of meningitis.

TABLE 1 Causes of meningitis

Viruses	*Enteroviruses* *Human immunodeficiency virus* (HIV) infection *Herpes simplex meningitis* Mumps
Bacteria	*Haemophilus influenzae* *Streptococcus pneumoniae* *Neisseria meningitides* *Listeria monocytogenes* *Staphylococcus aureus*
Fungal	*Cryptococcus neoformans* *Coccidioides immitis*
Tuberculosis	
Others	Spirochetes, e.g. syphilis, Lyme disease Drugs, e.g. non-steroidal anti-inflammatory drugs (NSAIDs), bactrim Tick-borne disease Neoplasms

CAVEATS

- The classic triad of fever, neck rigidity, and altered mental state is only present in 44% of all cases of meningitis especially in the extremes of age who may present atypically, e.g. irritability, nausea, and vomiting. On the other hand, at least 2 of the 4 signs – fever, neck stiffness, change in mental status, and headache occur in 95% of cases; 4% have only 3 symptoms, and 1% have none.
- At least one finding of the triad should be present in patients with meningitis. This has a high sensitivity (99–100%).
- Delays in administration of antibiotics are associated with adverse outcomes. Hence, antibiotics should be started immediately after blood cultures are taken even if lumbar puncture is delayed. The algorithm is antibiotics, then computed tomography (CT), and lumbar puncture.

NOTE: The argument that antibiotics will render the cerebrospinal fluid (CSF) non-diagnostic is also unfounded. Initial antibiotic therapy does not change CSF cell counts or protein or glucose. Grain stain and culture may also remain positive despite antibiotic administrations.

CLINICAL ASSESSMENT

● **History**

1. Presenting symptoms:

   a. Classic triad: Fever, neck rigidity and altered mental state.

   b. Neurological symptoms: Seizures, photophobia, focal neurological deficits (including cranial nerve palsies), hearing loss, and headache.

   c. Non-neurological symptoms: Skin rash (purpura or petechiae and maculopapular), arthritis, vomiting, and nausea.

2. Past medical history, e.g. immuno-compromised states such as HIV infection.

3. Travel history.

4. Contact history (important to administer antibiotic prophylaxis to close contacts).

● **Physical examination**

1. General appearance: Altered mental state, signs of toxicity, and consciousness level.

2. Vital signs: Look for hypotension and tachycardia (indicating septic shock).

3. Signs of meningism:

   a. Neck rigidity.

   b. Brudzinski and Kernig signs (late features of meningitis).

   c. Jolt accentuation of headache via horizontal rotation of the head at a frequency of 2 to 3 times per second.

4. Neurological examination: Focal neurological deficits, cranial nerve palsies, and papilloedema.

5. Others: Skin rash, signs of an immuno-compromised state such as oral thrush and cachexia.

● **Risk stratification**

This is based on 3 basic clinical features (hypotension, altered mental state, and seizures) that stratify the patient into 3 risk groups (no clinical risk factors, 1 clinical risk factor, and 2 or 3 clinical risk factors).[6]

   It correlates with adverse outcomes of in-hospital mortality or a neurological deficit at discharge.

⇨ **SPECIAL TIPS FOR GPs**

- If **meningococcaemia** is suspected, **IV crystalline penicillin 4 mega units** can be given stat if there is a delay in getting the patient to the hospital by ambulance.
- Chemoprophylaxis should be considered for office staff – **ciprofloxacin 500 mg × 1 dose**.

MANAGEMENT

- **Investigations**

  1. Stat capillary blood sugar.

  2. Bloods: Full blood count, renal panel, blood cultures, lactate (in occult sepsis or septic shock), disseminated intravascular coagulation (DIVC) screen (in suspected meningococcaemia) and arterial blood gas.

  3. **CT head:** To rule out mass lesions and indicated in patients who have the following:

     a. Focal neurological deficits.

     b. New onset seizures.

     c. Depressed level of consciousness.

     d. Evidence of raised intracranial pressure such as papilloedema.

     e. Immuno-compromised states, e.g. HIV infection.

     f. Head injury.

  4. **Lumbar puncture** (usually performed inpatient): Prior administration of antibiotics will not affect CSF culture of pathogens in most patients for up to a few hours. May be done prior to CT head in the absence of the above indications.

     a. Tube 1: Cell count and cytospin for cell and differential count.

     b. Tube 2: Protein and glucose.

     c. Tube 3: Microbiology (gram stain, culture and sensitivity C&S), acid-fast bacillus smear, tuberculosis culture, Indian ink, and fungal culture).

     d. Tube 4: Crytococcal antigen, bacterial antigens, i.e. *Streptococcus pneumoniae*, *Neisseria meningitides*, *Haemophilus influenzae B* and *Group B streptococcus*.

     e. Tube 5: Virology studies if viral meningitis is suspected.

See Table 2 for the interpretation of CSF analysis.

TABLE 2   CSF picture in bacterial and viral meningitis

	Normal	Bacterial meningitis	Viral meningitis
Colour	Clear	Cloudy	Clear
Opening pressure	<18 cm H_2O	>20 cm H_2O	<18 cm H_2O
White blood cell count	0	200–10,000/mm^3	25–1000/mm^3
Glucose	>40 mg/dl	<40 mg/dl (<50% of blood glucose)	>40 mg/dl (>50% of blood glucose)
Protein	<40 mg/dl	100–500 mg/dl	50–100 mg/dl

- **Cryptococcal meningitis** shares a similar CSF picture to that of bacterial meningitis except for a lower white blood cell count. Definitive diagnosis depends on a positive Indian ink and cryptococcal antigen results.
- **Tuberculous meningitis** also produces CSF changes similar to viral meningitis. Definitive diagnosis depends on acid-fast bacilli stain and culture.
  1. **Others (guided by clinical assessment):** Urine culture, chest X-ray, and electrocardiogram (ECG).
- **Supportive measures**
  1. The patient should be placed in a monitored or critical care area under isolation.
  2. Medical staff taking care of the patient must take universal precaution.
  3. Monitoring: ECG, vital signs, and pulse oximetry.
  4. Obtain intravenous (IV) access.
  5. Support the airway, breathing and circulation (ABCs).
     a. Secure the airway for airway protection in patients with a depressed level of consciousness or refractory shock.
     b. Give supplemental oxygen.
     c. Administer fluid resuscitation for patients in septic shock. The rate and amount are determined by the patient's haemodynamic status and response (refer to Chapter 33, *Sepsis/Septic Shock*).
- Symptomatic treatment, e.g. antipyretics and anti-emetics.

Drug therapy

- **Antibiotics**
  1. Antibiotics should be initiated as soon as blood cultures are taken.

  See Table 3 for antibiotic choices.

- **Steroids**
  1. Mainly indicated in adults with known or suspected pneumoccal meningitis especially if the Glasgow Coma Scale is 8–11.
  2. As an adjuvant therapy to reduce mortality and neurological complications such as hearing loss or focal neurological deficits.
  3. Dose: IV **dexamethasone** 10 mg 6 hourly for a total of 4 days.
  4. First dose of steroid must be given 15 minutes before or concomitant with the first dose of antibiotics because the theoretical mechanism for steroid efficacy is to prevent immunological response to lysis bacterial proteins.
- **Chemoprophylaxis** for meningococcal meningitis
  1. Should be given to the following close contacts:
     a. Prolonged close contact with the case patient during the 7 days before onset of illness.
     b. Contact at child care centres.
     c. Close contact where there was exposure to the patient's secretions, e.g. during endotracheal intubation.

TABLE 3   **Empirical antibiotic regime for bacteria meningitis**

Group	Suspected organisms	Empiric therapy
Immuno-competent adults (<60 years old)	*Streptococcus pneumoniae* *Neisseria meningitidis* *Haemophilus influenza* Less common: *Listeria monocytogenes* *Group B streptococcus*	IV ceftriaxone 2 g 12 hourly OR IV cefotaxime 2 g 4–6 hourly
Immuno-competent adults(≥60 years old)	*Streptococcus pneumoniae* *Listeria monocytogenes* Less common: *Group B streptococcus* *Neisseria meningitides* *Haemophilus influenza*	As above PLUS IV ampicillin 200 mg/kg/day in 4–6 divided doses
Immuno-compromised	*Listeria monocytogenes* Gram-negative bacilli *Streptococcus pneumoniae*	IV ceftazidime 2 g 8 hourly PLUS IV ampicillin 2 g 4 hourly
Indwelling central nervous system devices (ventricular–peritoneal shunt)	Coagulase +ve *Staphylococcus aureus* *Streptococcus pneumoniae* *Neisseria meningitidis* *Haemophilus influenza* *Enterobactericae*	IV ceftriaxone 2 g 12 hourly OR IV vancomycin 1 g 12 hourly
Nosocomial (post-neurosurgical) **Penetrating central nervous system trauma**	*Staphylococcus aureus* *Streptococci* Gram-negative bacilli Coagulase-negative *Staphylococci*	IV ceftazidime 2 g 8–12 hourly
Meningococcaemia	*Neisseria meningitidis*	IV penicillin G 400,000 units 4 hourly OR IV ceftriaxone 2 g 12 hourly OR IV ampicillin 2 g 4–6 hourly

2. Choice of antibiotics
   a. **Rifampicin**
      i. Adults: 600 mg 12 hourly for 2 days.
      ii. Children (1–6 years): 10 mg/kg 12 hourly for 2 days.
      iii. Children (3–11months): 5 mg/kg 12 hourly for 2 days.
   b. **Ciprofloxacin**
      i. Adults: Single dose 500 mg.
   c. **Ceftriaxone**
      i. Adults: Intramuscular 250 mg as a single dose.
      ii. Children (<15 years): Intramuscular 125 mg as a single dose.

- **Disposition**

All patients with meningitis should be admitted under Neurology isolation for further management. Those with septic shock or require ventilatory support should be admitted to the high dependency or intensive care unit.

References/Further Reading

1. Meurer WJ. Lavoie FW. Central nervous system infections. In: Marx JA, ed. *Rosen's Emergency Medicine: Concepts and Clinical Practice*. 7th ed. Philadelphia, PA: Mosby-Elsevier; 2010: 1417–1429.
2. Van de Beek D, de Gans J, Spanjaard L, et al. Clinical features and prognostic factors in adults with bacterial meningitis. *N Engl J Med*. 2004; 351: 1849.
3. Proulx N, Frechete D, Toye B, et al. Delays in the administration of antibiotics are associated with mortality from adult acute bacterial meningitis. *QJM*. 2005; 98: 291.
4. Auburtin M, Wolff M, Charpentier J, et al. Detrimental role of delayed antibiotic administration and penicillin-nonsusceptible strains in adult intensive care unit patients with pneumococcal meningitis: The PNEUMOREA prospective multicenter study. *Crit Care Med*. 2006; 34: 2758.
5. Van De Beek D, de Gans J, Melntyre P, Prasad K. Corticosteroids for acute bacterial meningitis. *Cochrane Database Syst Rev*. 2007; CD004405.
6. *MOH Clinical Practice Guidelines* 1/2006. Use of Antibiotics in Adults.

67   Migraine and Cluster Headache

Sim Tiong Beng

CAVEATS

- Primary headaches are those not associated with an underlying pathology. They include tension-type headache, migraine with or without aura, and cluster headache.
- The ability to make a rapid and accurate diagnosis is crucial to the successful management of primary headache disorder. The clinical diagnosis of tension-type headache or migraine should be guided by the International Headache Society criteria (Tables 1 to 4).

TABLE 1   Characteristics of primary headache disorders

	Migraine	Tension-type	Cluster
Location	Unilateral	Bilateral	Strictly unilateral
Intensity	Moderate to severe	Mild to moderate	Severe
Duration	4–72 hours	30 minutes to 1 week	15–90 minutes
Quality	Throbbing	Tightening	Severe
Associated symptoms	Yes	No	Autonomic symptoms
Gender	More common in females	More common in females	More common in males

- Tension-type headache is the most common type of primary headache. Specific diagnostic criteria for primary headaches are listed in Table 2.

TABLE 2   Tension-type headache diagnostic criteria

- Tension-type headache
  1. Infrequent: 1 attack/month
  2. Frequent: 1–15 attacks/month
  3. Chronic: >15 attacks/month
- Headache lasting from 30 minutes to 7 days
- Headache has ≥2 of the following characteristics:
  1. Bilateral location.
  2. Pressing/tightening (non-pulsating) quality.
  3. Mild or moderate intensity.
  4. Not aggravated by routine physical activity such as walking or climbing stairs.
- Both of the following:
  1. No nausea or vomiting (anorexia may occur).
  2. No more than one of photophobia or phonophobia.
- Not attributed to another disorder.

TABLE 3   Migraine without aura diagnostic criteria

- ≥5 attacks lasting 4–72 hours (untreated or unsuccessfully treated)
- Headache has ≥2 of the following characteristics:
    1. Unilateral location.
    2. Pulsating quality.
    3. Moderate or severe pain intensity.
- During headache ≥1 of the following is present:
    1. Nausea and/or vomiting.
    2. Photophobia and phonophobia.
- Not attributed to another disorder.

TABLE 4   Migraine with aura diagnostic criteria

A. ≥2 attacks fulfilling ≥3 of the following:

- ≥1 *fully reversible* aura symptoms indicating focal cerebral cortical and/or brain stem functions:
    1. Visual symptoms including positive features (e.g. homonymous haemianopia, blind spots, flashes of light, and zigzag lines) and/or negative features (i.e. loss of vision).
    2. Sensory symptoms including positive features (i.e. pins and needles) and/or negative features (i.e. numbness).
    3. Dysphasic speech disturbance.
- ≥1 aura symptom develops gradually over >4 minutes, or ≥2 symptoms occur in succession.
- No aura symptom lasts >60 minutes; if ≥1 aura symptom is present, accepted duration is proportionally increased.
- Headache follows aura with free interval of ≥60 minutes (it may also simultaneously begin with the aura).

B. ≥1 of the following **aura features** establishes a diagnosis of migraine with typical aura:

- Homonymous visual symptoms.
- Unilateral paresthesias and/or numbness.
- Unilateral weakness.
- Aphasia or unclassifiable speech difficulty.
- Signs or brain stem dysfunction, such as diplopia, ataxia, or vertigo.

TABLE 5   Cluster headache diagnostic criteria

A. ≥5 attacks of severe unilateral orbital, supraorbital, and/or temporal pain lasting from 15 to 180 minutes untreated, with ≥1 of the following signs occurring on the same side as the pain:

- Conjunctival injection.
- Lacrimation.
- Nasal congestion.
- Rhinorrhoea.
- Forehead and facial sweating.
- Miosis.
- Ptosis.
- Eyelid oedema.

B. Attacks have a frequency of 1 every other day to 8 per day.

⇨ **SPECIAL TIPS FOR GPs**

- Do not diagnose migraine if the first episode of severe headache occurs after the age of 50 years old.
- A validated 3-item questionnaire (ID-Migraine) covering disability, nausea, and sensitivity to light should be used by the primary physician if screening for migraine is required.
- Use standardized self-assessed questionnaires, e.g. Migraine Disability Assessment (MIDAS) and Headache Impact Test-6 (HIT-6) to determine migraine disability (see Appendices 1 and 2).
- **Migraine 'comfort' signs** include:
  1. Positive family history of migraine.
  2. Headaches related to the menstrual cycle.
  3. Headaches preceded by typical aura.
  4. Headaches remaining periodic and stable over time.
  5. Normal physical and neurological findings.
- Advise the patient to take the analgesic early during an acute attack to abort it.
- When to refer to a specialist: Diagnostic uncertainty, treatment failure, suspicion of secondary headache syndrome, chronic daily headache, and reassurance for patient or provider.

MANAGEMENT

- **Tension-type headache**
  1. Simple analgesics and non-steroidal anti-inflammatory drugs are effective and may be used for acute treatment of tension-type headaches at the following doses. Caffeine can be used as an analgesic adjuvant for acute treatment of tension-type headache.

Drugs	Dosage	Grade and level
Aspirin	500–1000 mg	Grade A, level 1–
Paracetamol	1000 mg	Grade A, level 1–
Ibuprofen	400–800 mg 8 hourly as needed	Grade A, level 1–
Ketoprofen	25–50 mg	Grade A, level 1–
Naproxen	275–550 mg 8–12 hourly as needed (maximum: 1250 mg in 24 hours)	Grade B, level 1–
Diclofenac	50 mg 8 hourly as needed or 75 mg intramuscularly	Grade B, level 1–

  2. Medication overuse should be avoided as it increases the risk of developing chronic daily headache.
  3. **Prophylactic treatment**, e.g. **amitriptyline** 10–75 mg, should be considered when headaches are frequent. Start at low doses and titrate up to therapeutic effects to minimize the side effects. Patients must be counselled of possible side effects and continue to take the medications for 4 weeks and more to see relief.

Migraine

1. A non-oral route is preferred for patients with nausea or vomiting.

2. **Over-the-counter medications**, e.g. paracetamol and Panadol Extra, should be tried early as a **first-line** acute treatment of migraine.

3. If paracetamol is ineffective, **non-steroidal anti-inflammatory drugs (NSAIDs)** listed in the above table should be used in the treatment of acute migraine episode (grade A, level 1+).

4. **Anti-emetics** IV metoclopramide 10 mg or IM stemetil 12.5 mg may also be used in combination with NSAIDs (grade B, level 1+).

5. Migraine-specific drugs (*triptans, ergotamine*) should be tried if NSAIDs are ineffective or contraindicated:

   a. Non-specific 5-hydroxytryptamine receptor agonists, e.g. **ergotamine** 1–2 mg 1 hourly (up to a total of three doses) and caffeine (Cafergot) (grade A, level 1++).

   b. Selective 5-hydroxytryptamine receptor agonists, e.g. **Zolmig** 2.5 mg 4 hourly (maximum two doses a day) is an alternative but its use is limited by its cost (grade A, level 1++).

6. The danger of medication-overuse headache developing with excessive use of symptomatic migraine medication should be emphasized to the patient.

7. **Prophylaxis**:

   a. These patients require prophylaxis:

      i. Those who have ≥2 attacks a month.

      ii. Those who have severe attacks, failed or have intolerance to acute treatment, comorbidities, and migraines with prolonged aura.

   b. **Medication use**:

      i. Start at low dose and titrate upwards gradually until clinical effects are achieved in the absence of adverse events.

      ii. Give each treatment at least a month to see the clinical benefits and if benefit is seen, a course of medication ideally lasting at least 6 months should be given.

      iii. Long-acting medication may improve compliance.

   c. **Patient education**:

      i. Discuss the rationale for a particular treatment and possible side effects and how long it will take to achieve clinical benefits.

      ii. Keep headache diaries to address frequency, duration, severity, medication response, and side effects.

Cluster headache

1. This is a primary headache disease characterized by recurrent short-lasting attacks (15–180 minutes) of excruciating unilateral periorbital pain accompanied by ipsilateral autonomic signs (lacrimation, nasal congestion, ptosis, miosis, lid oedema, and redness of the eye). During the attacks, patients tend to be restless. Diagnosis is a clinical one.

TABLE 6 Dose and frequency of migraine prophylactic medications

Drugs	Dosage and frequency	Grade and level
• **Beta blockers**		
Atenolol	50–100 mg OM (every morning)	Grade A, level 1++
Propranolol	40–240 mg/day	Grade A, level 1++
Metoprolol	50–300 mg/day	Grade A, level 1++
Bisoprolol	5 mg/day	Grade B, level 1+
• **Calcium channel blockers**		
Flunarizine	5–10 mg ON (every night)	Grade A, level 1++
Verapamil	240 mg OM	Grade A, level 1++
• **Anti-depressants**		
Amitriptyline	10–150 mg ON	Grade A, level 1++
Fluoxetine	10–40 mg OM	Grade B, level 1+
Venlafaxine	75–150 mg/day	Grade B, level 1+
• **Anti-convulsants**		
Sodium valproate	500–1500 mg/day	Grade A, level 1++
Topiramate	50–200 mg/day	Grade A, level 1++
Gabapentin	1200 mg/day	Grade B, level 1+
• **Non-steroidal anti-inflammatory drugs**		
Naproxen sodium	550 mg bd (twice daily)	Grade A, level 1++
• **Serotonin receptor antagonist**		
Pizotifen	0.5–2 mg tds (three times daily)	Grade A, level 1++
• **Angiostensin blockers**		
Candesartan	16 mg/day	Grade B, level 1+
Lisinopril	10–20 mg/day	Grade B, level 1+
• **Others**		
Magnesium	400–600 mg/day	Grade B, level 1+
Riboflavin	200 mg bd	Grade B, level 1+
Coenzyme Q10	300 mg/day	Grade B, level 1+

2. It affects young adults, predominantly males. Prevalence is estimated at 0.5–1.0/1000.

3. Cluster headache has a circannual and circadian periodicity, attacks being clustered (hence the name) in bouts that can occur during specific months of the year. During bouts, attacks may happen at precise hours, especially during the night. The disease course over a lifetime is unpredictable. Some patients have only one period of attacks, while in others the disease evolves from episodic to chronic form.

4. Alcohol is the only dietary trigger of cluster headache; strong odours (mainly solvents and cigarette smoke), and napping may also trigger attacks.

5. Acute treatment is based on subcutaneous administration of sumatriptan and high flow oxygen. Verapamil, lithium, methysergide, prednisone, greater occipital nerve blocks, and topiramate may be used for prophylaxis.

APPENDIX 1   The Migraine Disability Assessment (MIDAS) questionnaire to assess migraine disability

1. On how many days in the last 3 months did you miss work or school because of your headaches?

2. How many days in the last 3 months was your productivity at work or school reduced by half or more because of your headaches? (Do not include days you counted in question 1 where you missed work or school.)

3. On how many days in the last 3 months did you not do household work because of your headaches?

4. How many days in the last 3 months was your productivity in household work reduced by half or more because of your headaches? (Do not include days you counted in question 3 where you did not do household work.)

5. On how many days in the last 3 months did you miss family, social, or leisure activities because of your headaches?

Total score: Add up the number of days given in response to the questions above.

Interpretation

Grade	Definition	Score
I	Minimal or infrequent disability	0–5
II	Mild or infrequent disability	6–10
III	Moderate disability	11–20
IV	Severe disability	21+

Source: Lipton RB. Clinical utility of an instrument assessing migraine disability: The Migraine Disability Assessment (MIDAS) questionnaire. Headache. Oct 2001; 41(9): 854–861.

APPENDIX 2   Headache Impact Test-6 (HIT-6) questionnaire to determine migraine disability

Rated on a five-point scale of:
- Never: 6 points
- Rarely: 8 points
- Sometimes: 10 points
- Very often: 11 points
- Always: 13 points

The score ranges from 36 to 78 points.

1. When you have headaches, how often is the pain severe?

2. How often do headaches limit your disability to do usual daily activities?

3. When you have a headache, how often do you wish you could lie down?

4. In the past 4 weeks, how often have you felt too tired to do work or daily activities because of your headaches?

5. In the past 4 weeks, how often have you felt fed up or irritated because of your headaches?

6. In the past 4 weeks, how often did headaches limit your disability to concentrate on work or daily activities?

Interpretation

Less than 50 points	Little or no headache impact
50–54 points	Some impact
55–58 points	Substantial impact
More than 59 points	Very severe impact

References/Further Reading

1. MOH Clinical Practice Guidelines 5/2007. Diagnosis and management of headache.

2. Headache Classification Subcommittee of the International Headache Society. The International classification of headache disorders. *Cephalalgia*. 2004; 24(suppl 1): 1–160.

3. Cerbo R, Barbanti P, Fabbrini G, et al. Amitriptyline is effective in chronic but not in episodic tension-type headache: Pathogentic implications. *Headache*. 1998; 38(6): 453–457.

4. Moja PL, Cusi C, Sterzi PR, Canepari C. Selective serotonin re-uptake inhibitors (SSRIs) for preventing migraines and tension type headaches. *Cochrane Database Syst Rev*. 20 July 2005; (3): CD002919.

5. Lipton RB, Dodick D, Sadovsky R, et al. A self-administered screener for migraine in primary care: The ID Migraine validation study. *Neurology*. 12 Aug 2003; 61(3): 375–382.

6. Lipton RB, Stewart WF, Sawyer J, et al. Clinical utility of an instrument assessing migraine disability: The Migraine Disability Assessment (MIDAS) questionnaire. *Headache*. Oct 2001; 41(9): 854–861.

7. Nachit-Ouinekh F, Dartigues JF, Henry P, et al. Use of the headache impact test (HIT-6) in general practice: Relationship with quality of life and severity. *Eur J Neurol*. Mar 2005; 12(3): 189–193.

8. Gladstone JP, Dodick DW. Current and emerging treatment options for migraine and other primary headache disorders. *Expert Rev Neurotherapeutics*. 2003; 3: 89–116.

9. Coppola M, Yealy DM, Leibold RA. Randomised, placebo-controlled evaluation of prochlorperazine versus metoclopramide for emergency department treatment of migraine headache. *Ann Emerg Med*. 1995; 26(5): 541–546.

10. Matchar D, et al. Evidence-based guidelines for migraine headache in the primary care setting: Pharmacological management of acute attacks. *US Headache Consortium, American Academy of Neurology*.

68 Stroke

Peng Li Lee • Lim Er Luen • Shirley Ooi

DIAGNOSIS

- Acute stroke is characterized by the sudden onset of focal neurological deficits, usually referable to a brain vascular territory. Common clinical presentations include hemiparesis, hemisensory loss, facial weakness, dysarthria, aphasia, and visual disturbance, occurring alone or in combination.
- **Strokes** are **classified** as follows (refer to Table 1):
  1. **Ischaemic** strokes (IS, 70–90%, higher incidence in Caucasians). Common aetiologies include large artery atherothrombosis, cardioembolism, and small vessel disease (lacunar strokes).
  2. **Haemorrhagic** strokes, which are **intra-cerebral haemorrhage** (ICH, 10–30%, higher incidence in non-Caucasian ethnic groups), and **subarachnoid haemorrhage** (SAH, about 2%).

NOTE: SAH patients often have no focal neurological deficits (refer to Chapter 69, *Subarachnoid Haemorrhage*).

TABLE 1 Clinical features of three types of stroke

Clinical features	Haemorrhagic	Ischaemic Thrombotic	Embolic
Onset	Sudden	Gradual	Sudden
Conscious level	Often decreased	Often normal unless large	Often normal
Headache	Usually +	+/−	Usually −
Nausea, vomiting	++	Usually −	Usually −
Past medical history	Hypertension On anti-coagulants Coagulopathies	Similar factors for coronary artery disease	Atrial fibrillation
Vital signs	Usually severe hypertension	Usually moderate or normal blood pressure	Variable blood pressure but usually no hypertension

+ = Present
− = Absent

CAVEATS

- Although the diagnosis of stroke is often straightforward, some common 'stroke mimics' should be considered (Table 2). Always perform a **capillary (fingerstix) glucose level to exclude hypoglycaemia**.
- Stroke is recognized as a time-sensitive emergency, especially with the more common use of intravenous **rt-PA (alteplase)** treatment for acute ischaemic stroke within **3 hours of symptom** onset. Patients with suspected stroke should be transported by ambulance to the nearest emergency department to expedite triage and management.
- It is important to define the time of stroke symptom onset. For patients unable to provide this information or who awaken with stroke symptoms, the time of onset is defined as when the patient was last awake and symptom-free or known to be 'normal'.
- Neurological deficits associated with headache, nausea, vomiting, a decreased conscious level and grossly elevated blood pressure are more likely to occur in **haemorrhagic strokes** (refer to Table 1).
- Treatment of hypertension in acute stoke is often controversial and should be approached cautiously (see the following discussion).

TABLE 2 Differential diagnosis of stroke

- Hypoglycaemia/hyperglycaemia
- Postepileptic (Todd's) paralysis
- Complicated migraine
- Hypertensive encephalopathy
- Head trauma (epidural/subdural haematoma)
- Brain tumour/abscess
- Meningitis/encephalit s
- Aortic dissection
- Bell's palsy
- Functional (psychiatric) conditions

⇨ **SPECIAL TIPS FOR GPs**

- Stroke patients who are **potential candidates for thrombolysis** should be transferred to the emergency department (ED) by ambulance without delay, given the narrow time window for this treatment.
- Most patients with suspected stroke should also be assessed emergently at the ED for timely management. Home visit and outpatient assessment are not advisable except for patients who present with mild non-disabling symptoms which are non-progressive and have already lasted for more than 48 hours.
- The general practitioner can play an important role in educating at-risk patients (e.g. those with hypertension, diabetes mellitus, hypercholesterolaemia, cardiac disease, smoking and a history of stroke or transient ischaemic attack (TIA)s, and their families to recognize common stroke symptoms, thus facilitating early presentation when stroke occurs.

- Always check the **capillary blood sugar level** to exclude hypoglycaemia.
- **Bell's palsy** is often confused with stroke. Bell's palsy (isolated lower motor neuron-type facial nerve palsy) usually presents with complete paralysis of the entire half of the face **without** sparing the forehead muscles.
- Patients who present with a **recent TIA** (acute neurological deficits attributed to a cerebrovascular aetiology with complete remission within 24 hours of symptom onset) are at high risk of suffering from ischaemic stroke early in the post-TIA period. They require urgent referral to a neurologist or a stroke clinic. If a same-day neurology appointment is not available, an anti-platelet agent (e.g. aspirin 150–300 mg stat, followed by 75–100 mg daily) may be commenced if not contraindicated. Patients with recurrent TIAs or crescendo TIAs should be urgently referred to the ED.

MANAGEMENT

The management of a suspected stroke patient in the ED includes:

- Maintenance of optimal physiological status, including oxygenation, hydration, and satisfactory blood glucose level. All patients should initially be put on nil by mouth, and started on maintenance IV isotonic saline. Arterial hypotension, if present, should be investigated and fluid replacement initiated. Fever should be investigated for infective sources and controlled with anti-pyretic agents. Airway protection (including intubation) may be necessary. Blood pressure management is discussed below.

- Definitive diagnosis of stroke and the stroke subtypes (IS, ICH, or SAH). This requires a head computed tomography (CT) scan that should be performed on all patients with suspected stroke within 24 hours of admission.

- Capillary blood glucose monitoring (see discussion above).

- Electrocardiogram should be done as stroke patients commonly have cardiac abnormalities.

- An **emergent head CT scan** to be performed in the ED is indicated in:

    1. IS patients who are candidates for thrombolytic or anti-coagulant therapies, e.g. present within 3 to 4.5 hours of symptom onset (see Figures 1 and 2 for CT brain findings in ischaemic stroke).

    2. Suspected ICH, e.g. grossly elevated blood pressure, headache, vomiting, possibly drowsiness, low platelet count, impaired clotting profile, anti-coagulant use or use of stimulant drugs (see Figure 3 for CT brain in ICH).

    3. Suspected SAH, e.g. worst headache of life, meningism or loss of consciousness (refer to Chapter 69, *Subarachnoid Haemorrhage*).

    4. Patients at risk of early deterioration, e.g. severe cortical stroke with hemiplegia, forced eye deviation, and aphasia or hemineglect; suspected stroke in the posterior fossa.

FIGURE 1   This image shows a hypodense lesion over the right parietal lobe consistent with a chronic infarct. There is ex-vacuo dilatation of the posterior horn of the lateral ventricle due to compensatory expansion secondary to cortical atrophy

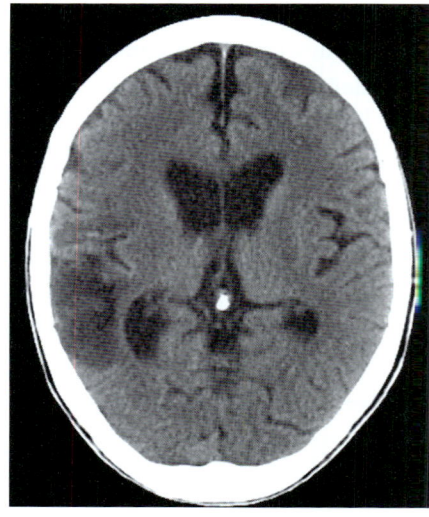

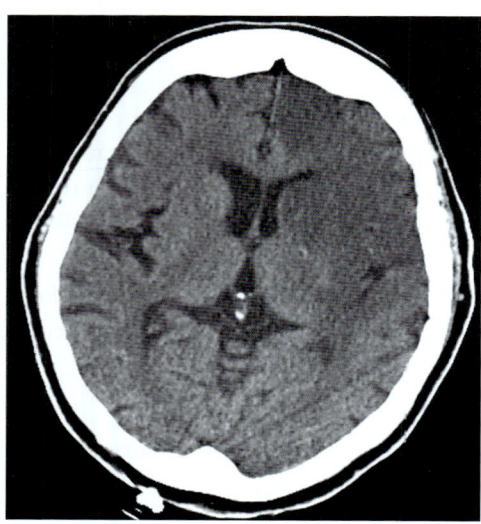

FIGURE 2   This image shows a hypodense lesion on the left consistent with an acute infarct involving the anterior and middle cerebral artery territories. There is a loss of grey–white differentiation, effacement of the sulci and mild compression of the anterior horn of the lateral ventricle

FIGURE 3   This image shows a hyperdense lesion in the right basal ganglia consistent with an acute haemorrhage. There is compression of the right anterior horn of the lateral ventricle

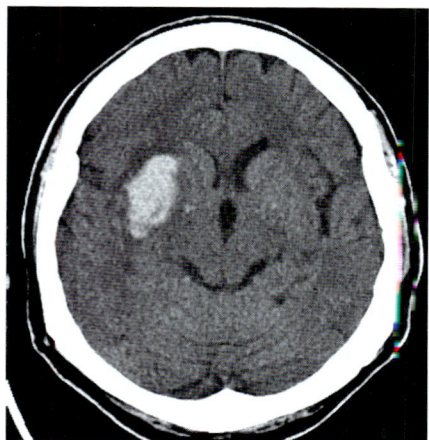

- Results of the head CT scan in these groups of patients will assist in starting appropriate medical therapy, timely neurosurgical consultation, and early prognostication. For IS patients who are candidates for thrombolysis, the goal is to complete the CT scan and have it reported within 45 minutes of presentation to the ED. In addition, a decision as to whether to or not to offer the patient thrombolysis should be made within another 15 minutes (see Tables 3 and 4 for the criteria for thrombolysis).

TABLE 3 **Criteria for intravenous thrombolysis with rTPA in patients with stroke within 3 hours**

Inclusion criteria

- Diagnosis of ischaemic stroke causing a measurable neurological deficit.
- Onset of symptoms within 3 hours:
  1. Patients whose onset of symptoms are between 3 to 4.5 hours can be considered for intravenous thrombolysis in consultation with a neurologist.
- Patients aged >18 years.

Exclusion criteria

Absolute

- Head trauma or prior stroke in previous 3 months.
- Symptoms suggesting subarachnoid haemorrhage.
- Arterial puncture at a non-compressible site within the previous 7 days.
- Elevated blood pressure (systolic >185 mmHg or diastolic >110 mmHg).
- Evidence of active bleeding on examination.
- Acute bleeding diathesis, including but not limited to:
  1. Platelet count <100,000.
  2. Heparin received within 48 hours, resulting in aPTT above upper limit of normal.
  3. Current use of anti-coagulant with INR >1.7 or PT >15 seconds.
- Blood glucose concentration that is <2.7 mmol/L.
- CT demonstrates multilobar infarction (hypodensity more than one-third of the cerebral hemisphere).

Relative

Recent experience suggests that under some circumstances – with careful consideration and weighing of risk to benefit – patients may receive fibrinolytic therapy despite ≥1 relative contraindications. Consider risk to benefit of rTPA administration carefully if any one of these relative contraindications is present:

- Only minor or rapidly improving stroke symptoms (clearing spontaneously).
- Seizure at onset with post-ictal residual neurological impairments.
- Major surgery or serious trauma within the previous 14 days.
- Recent gastrointestinal or urinary tract haemorrhage (within the previous 21 days).
- Recent acute myocardial infarction (within the previous 3 months).

TABLE 4   Additional exclusion criteria for patients in the 3–4.5-hour window

Patients >80 years.

Patients on oral anti-coagulants.

Patients with a baseline National Institutes of Health Stroke Scale (NIHSS) score of >25.

Patients with both a history of stroke and diabetes.

- rTPA should be administered at 0.9 mg/kg over 60 minutes with 10% of the total dose administered as an initial intravenous bolus over 1 minute.
- Other tests, e.g. cardiac enzymes and urea/electrolytes/creatinine, should be guided by the patient's clinical presentation but should not delay an emergent CT brain scan.

Management of elevated blood pressure in acute stroke

Refer to Chapter 39, *Hypertensive Crises* for the principles of blood pressure control and drugs used to manage elevated blood pressure.

Haemorrhagic Stroke

- Acute reduction of blood pressure (BP) may reduce rebleeding and haematoma expansion.
- However, aggressive BP control may exacerbate ischaemia in the regions immediately adjacent to the haematoma.
- Goals of BP management in patients with **acute haemorrhagic stroke** are as follows:[1]

SBP* >200 mmHg MAP** >150 mmHg	Consider aggressive reduction of BP with continuous intravenous infusion, with frequent BP monitoring every 5 minutes.
SBP >180 mmHg Or MAP >130 mmHg with possibility of elevated ICP	Consult the neurosurgeon for intracranial pressure (ICP) monitoring. Reduce BP using intermittent or continuous intravenous medications while maintaining a cerebral perfusion pressure of >60 mmHg.
SBP >180 mmHg Or MAP >130 mmHg with no evidence of elevated ICP	Consider a modest reduction of BP (e.g. MAP of 110 mmHg or target BP of 160/90 mmHg) using intermittent or continuous intravenous medications to control BP and clinically reexamine the patient every 15 minutes.

Notes: * SBP: Systolic blood pressure.
      ** MAP: Mean arterial pressure.

Ischaemic Stroke

Most consensus guidelines recommend that blood pressure not be treated acutely in the patient with ischaemic stroke. If the blood pressure is >220 systolic or 120 diastolic, cautious lowering of blood pressure by approximately 20% during the first 24 hours after stroke onset is suggested.

- **BP control is indicated on a more urgent basis** when the stroke patient has the following concurrent conditions:[1]

  1. Congestive heart failure
  2. Acute myocardial ischaemia/infarction
  3. Aortic dissection

  If the patient is a candidate for rTPA, aim to lower the blood pressure to <185 systolic and 110 diastolic.

Disposition

- All stroke patients should be admitted for further investigation, treatment, and rehabilitation. However, stable patients with a lacunar infarct of >48 hours old with non-progressive and non-disabling neurological deficits may be discharged home if close follow-up can be established.

References/Further Reading

1. Jauch EC, Cucchiara Bl, Adeoye O, et al. 2010 American Heart Association guidelines for cardiopulmonary resuscitation and emergency cardiovascular care science. *Circulation*. 2010; 122: S818–S828.

2. Adams HP, del Zoppo G, Alberts MJ, et al. Guidelines for the early management of adults with ischemic stroke: A guideline from the American Heart Association/American Stroke Association Stroke Council, Clinical Cardiology Council, Cardiovascular Radiology and Intervention Council, and the Atherosclerotic Peripheral Vascular Disease and Quality of Care Outcomes in Research Interdisciplinary Working Groups. *Stroke*. 2007; 38: 1655–1711.

3. Morgenstern LB, Hemphill JC, Anderson C, et al. Guidelines for the management of spontaneous intracerebral hemorrhage: A guideline for healthcare professionals from the American Heart Association/American Stroke Association. *Stroke*. 2010; 41L2108–2129.

69   Subarachnoid Haemorrhage

Gene Chan • Shirley Ooi

CAVEATS

- The incidence of subarachnoid haemorrhage (SAH) increases with age until it reaches a plateau at age 60 years, with the peak incidence occurring between 40 and 60 years and a 3:2 female-to-male predominance.

- The **speed of onset** of headache (**sudden**, like a **thunder-clap**) is a more useful guide than the severity of the headache or response to analgesia.

- Only 1% of emergency department patients with headache have SAH, but this figure increases to 12% in patients who report 'the worst headache of their life' or who present with pain severity of 10 (on a scale of 1 to 10).

- Approximately 10–15% of patients with SAH die before receiving medical care.

- Among those who survive to hospital presentation, 50% have an altered level of consciousness, 40% are disorientated and 25% have abnormal speech, inappropriate responses to commands, or motor deficits.

- The greater diagnostic challenge comes from patients who present with headache and a normal level of consciousness without focal neurologic signs or symptoms.

- They may have non-focal neurological symptoms and signs, e.g. nausea, vomiting, fever, syncope, confusion, migraine-like headache, or coma.

- On presentation, 20–50% of patients report a severe headache occurring days to weeks before presentation. This is known as a **warning** or **sentinel, headache**, thought to be secondary to fleeting haemorrhage from an aneurysmal sac and subsequent thrombosis.

- SAH is most commonly due to bleeding from a saccular (berry) aneurysm or arteriovenous malformation (AVM) (3–6%), but may occur with trauma as well. The history will often differentiate the two but, occasionally, the haemorrhage will precede a traumatic incident. Careful history-taking is essential. Rare causes are mycotic, oncotic and flow-related, aneurysms.

NOTE: Most (90%) spontaneous cerebral aneurysms can be found in the anterior circulation which includes the anterior and posterior communicating arteries and the middle cerebral artery.

- Various electrocardiogram (ECG) **changes**, e.g. peaked or symmetrically inverted T waves, U waves, prolongation of the QRS complex, prolonged QT interval, and dysrhythmias, may occur in association with SAH and confuse the physician into pursuing a cardiac diagnosis

PHYSICAL FINDINGS

- There are currently no validated clinical decision rules to safely rule out SAH.

- Extreme cases present with varying degrees of altered levels of consciousness, disorientation, meningismus, or focal motor deficits.

- Cranial nerve deficits are seen less frequently (12%) in SAH, but can be found in patients with expanding non-ruptured aneurysm as well.

- Third cranial nerve palsy is the commonest nerve involved in SAH.

- Patients with **posterior cerebral artery communicating aneurysms** may present with an ipsilateral dilated pupil or deviated gaze from third cranial nerve palsy.

- Patients with **middle cerebral artery aneurysms** may have contralateral hemiparesis secondary to haemorrhage in the temporal lobe or Sylvian fissure.

- Nystagmus and ataxia may be present when haemorrhage occurs in the **posterior fossa** (10% of berry aneurysms).

- Sixth cranial nerve palsy can also be seen in SAH as a result of increased intracranial pressure.

- Neck stiffness may take 2 to 3 hours to develop.

- Fundoscopic examination reveals preretinal or subhyaloid haemorrhages in up to 20% of patients and is associated with greater mortality. However, these findings do not occur in a lot of conscious patients who are neurologically intact.

- See the Hunt and Hess Classification system of SAH in Table 1 for the signs and survival rate.

TABLE 1 Hunt and Hess Classification of Subarachnoid Haemorrhage

Grade	Signs	Survival (%)
1	Normal mental state Mild headache No neurologic deficits No meningeal signs	70
2	Moderate-to-severe headache Cranial nerve palsy	60
3	Drowsy, confused Mild focal neurologic deficit	50
4	Stupor Hemiparesis, early vegetative posturing	40
5	Coma Decerebrate posturing	10

> ⇨ **SPECIAL TIPS FOR GPs**
> - The initial misdiagnosis rate for SAH is 20 to 50%. Missing the diagnosis of SAH increases the risk of rebleeding 5 fold and the risk of poor outcome 9 fold.
> - SAH is characterised by the abrupt onset of symptoms – ***thunder-clap headache*** (associated with vomiting) and rapid progression of neurological deficits.
> - Note also atypical presentations of SAH in patients who present with neck pain as a predominant symptom or in patients with headache and low-grade fever.
> - Absence of headache makes the diagnosis of SAH unlikely.
> - Beware of making a diagnosis of migraine headache in any patient above 50 years old.
> - Although rare, patients with SAH can get some relief from their headache with analgesia.
> - The initial blood pressure is usually high.
> - Patients suspected of having SAH should be referred to the emergency department by ambulance.

MANAGEMENT

Supportive measures

- Patients must be managed in the critical care area.
- Document deterioration by frequent assessment and charting the Glasgow Coma Scale.
- Ensure the necessary intubation and resuscitation equipment is available.
- Evaluate the airway. Intubate the patient to protect the airway if required.
- Provide supplemental high-flow oxygen via a reservoir mask.
- Elevate the head of the bed to a 30° angle.
- Monitoring: ECG, vital signs q 10–15 minutes, and pulse oximetry.
- Establish peripheral intravenous (IV) line at 'keep open' rate.

Investigations

- **Diagnosis**
  1. **Non-contrast computed tomography (CT)** scan of the head is the investigation of choice to detect SAH.
     a. However, the non-contrast head CT does not detect all SAHs.
     b. The sensitivity of **head CT** for detecting SAH diminishes as the time of symptom onset increases; sensitivity is 98% if the CT scan is performed within 12 hours of symptom onset. It is 93% at 24 hours after symptom onset, 73% at 5 days after symptom onset and 0% at 2 weeks from the onset of symptoms.
  2. A **lumbar puncture** is essential in the diagnostic work-up of SAH when the initial CT scan is negative. The presence of xanthochromia in a fresh cerebrospinal fluid specimen is pathognomonic for SAH.
- Labs: Full blood count, urea/electrolytes/creatinine, PT/aPTT, GXM two units.
- Others: ECG, chest X-ray (watch out for neurogenic pulmonary oedema).

Complications

- Look out for acute complications (0–48 hours after initial haemorrhage). These include:

  1. **Rebleeding**: This is the most significant acute complication after spontaneous SAH. The risk of rebleeding is 4% on the first day after spontaneous SAH and increases 1.5% with each additional day for the next 13 days. Mortality is 80% with rebleeding.

  2. **Cerebral salt wasting** causing hyponatremia.

  3. **Acute hydrocephalus** (15%).

  4. **Seizures** (6%).

  5. **Neurogenic cardiac disease** (10%).

  6. **Neurogenic pulmonary oedema**. This can occur minutes to hours after the initial haemorrhage.

Specific measures

- Non-opioid analgesia, e.g. IM diclofenac may be given for relief of the headache. Opioids are avoided since they may cause vomiting.

- Anti-emetics: IM prochlorperazine 12.5 mg or IM metoclopramide 10 mg.

- Antihypertensives, e.g. IV labetalol 10 mg stat followed by an infusion to keep systolic blood pressure under 140 mmHg. This should be administered in consultation with a neurosurgeon.

- Antihypertensives like nitroprusside and nitroglycerin, which increase intracranial pressure by cerebral vasodilatation, should be avoided.

- Consider seizure prophylaxis, e.g. phenytoin.

- **Nimodipine**, a calcium channel blocker, has been shown to reduce secondary ischaemic complications and thereby significantly reduce the frequency of poor outcomes in SAH. It has been postulated that nimodipine may have a direct neuroprotective effect or it may improve collateral circulation. It does not directly affect angiographic vasospasm, as previously thought. Use this in consultation with a neurosurgeon.

Disposition

- Admit all SAH patients under Neurology or Neurosurgery depending on institutional practice.

References/Further Reading

1   Callaway CW. Subarachnoid hemorrhage. In: Wolfson AB, eds. Harwood-Nuss. *Clinical Practice of Emergency Medicine.* 5th ed. Philadelphia, PA: Lippencott Williams & Wilkin; 2010: 757–759.

2   Birnbaum AJ, Friedman BW, Gallagher EJ. Headache. In: Wolfson AB, eds. Harwood-Nuss. *Clinical Practice of Emergency Medicine.* 5th ed. Philadelphia, PA: Lippencott Williams & Wilkin; 2010: 747–756.

3   Lipinski CA, Benz AG. Subarachnoid haemorrhage. In: Frank LR, Jobe KA, eds. *Admission and Discharge Decision in Emergency Medicine.* Philadelphia, PA: Hanley & Belfus; 2002: 152–156.

4   Manno EM, MD. Subarachnoid hemorrhage. *Neurol Clin N Am.* 2004; 22: 347–366.

5   Seibert HE, MD, FACEP. Subarachnoid hemorrhage. *Critical Decision in Emergency Medicine.* Oct 2008.

70 Temporal Arteritis

Seet Chong Meng • Shirley Ooi • Peter Manning

DEFINITION

Temporal arteritis, also known as '**giant cell arteritis**', is a common form of vasculogathy affecting patients >50 years old. Although typically affecting the superficial temporal arteritis, this inflammatory process has been shown to involve medium and large-sized vessels, including the aorta, carotid, subclavian, vertebral, and iliac arteries.

DIAGNOSIS

According to the American College of Rheumatology, the diagnosis of temporal arteritis requires the presence of three of the following criteria:

- Patients ≥50 years of age.
- New onset of localized headache.
- Temporal artery tenderness of decreased pulse.
- Erythrocyte sedimentation rate ≥55 mm per hour.
- Positive histology on biopsy.

CAVEATS

- Suspect temporal arteritis in a **woman, usually >50 years of age**, presenting with a severe throbbing, burning and unilateral temporal headache. Often, the headache has been present for several months. Associated symptoms may include malaise, anorexia, weight loss, jaw/ tongue claudication, amaurosis, muscle aches, transient ischaemic attacks, neuropathy, and stroke.
- **Sudden, painless, monocular loss of vision** (due to vascular occlusion of the ophthalmic branch of the internal ciliary artery or posterior ciliary artery with infarction of the optic nerve or retina) is the **most serious complication** since visual loss is usually permanent.
- There is increased incidence of temporal arteritis with **polymyalgia rheumatica**.

⇨ **SPECIAL TIP FOR GPs**
- Treat temporal arteritis with **prednisolone** 30–60 mg (1 mg/kg)
  PO stat once diagnosis is suspected before sending the patient to the hospital as a delay in diagnosis and treatment can result in permanent blindness.

MANAGEMENT

Supportive measures

- Patients can be managed in the intermediate care area.
- Measure and record the visual acuity.
- Labs: Full blood count and erythrocyte sedimentation rate.

Specific measures

- Start therapy immediately if history and physical examination are suspicious and erythrocyte sedimentation rate is elevated.
- Administer **prednisolone** 30–60 mg (1 mg/kg) PO stat.
- Prescribe analgesia, e.g. diclofenac IM.

Disposition

- Admit under Neurology following appropriate consultation.

References/Further Reading

1. Levine SM, Hellmann DB. Giant cell arteritis. *Curr Opin Rheumatol.* 2002; 14(1): 3–10. (Review)
2. Field AG, Wang E. Evaluation of the patient with nontraumatic headache: An evidence based approach. In: Fontanarosa PB, ed. Evidence based emergency testing: Evaluation and diagnostic testing. *Emerg Med Clin North Am.* 1999; 17(1): 139.

Lim Er Luen • Shirley Ooi

DIAGNOSIS

- Transient ischaemic attack (TIA) is **classically defined** as a neurologic deficit caused by focal brain ischaemia that completely resolves **within 24 hours**.
- However, recent studies including magnetic resonance imaging (MRI) have shown that permanent brain infarction can occur within 1 hour of symptom duration. The **current definition** of TIA is 'a transient episode of neurologic dysfunction caused by a focal disturbance of brain, spinal cord or retinal ischaemia, and without evidence of infarction'. The new definition of TIA completely eliminates the element of time and emphasizes neuroimaging instead.
- TIAs should be considered a harbinger of a potential stroke. The incidence of stroke depends on the features of the TIA and duration since the TIA occurred.
- TIAs should correspond to a discrete neurovascular territory.
- **Anterior circulation strokes** present with the following signs and symptoms:
  1. Hemiparesis.
  2. Unilateral sensory loss.
  3. Visual field deficit.
  4. Aphasia.
  5. Left-sided spatial neglect or hemi-inattention.
- **Posterior circulation strokes** usually present with the following:
  1. Hemiparesis.
  2. Disconjugate gaze, diplopia.
  3. Homonymous hemianopia.
  4. Dysarthria with dysphagia.
  5. Alexia without agraphia (inability to read without other signs of aphasia).
  6. Vertigo.
  7. Vomiting.

CAVEATS

- TIAs generally have negative symptoms such as loss of sensation or power. TIAs rarely cause positive symptoms such as tingling sensations, auras, or twitching of muscles. It is uncommon for syndromes such as syncope, isolated dizziness, drop attacks, or global amnesia to be caused by TIAs.
- Persistent neurologic deficits should be treated as a stroke, not a TIA.

- \>1 episode of TIA within 48 hours indicates a high risk of stroke. Such patients need urgent evaluation by a neurologist. Thromboembolic phenomena, e.g. atrial fibrillation and carotid stenosis must be sought.

INVESTIGATIONS

- A thorough neurological and cardiovascular evaluation, including auscultation of the carotids, is necessary.
- Blood capillary glucose and an electrocardiogram (ECG) are required.
- A computed tomography (CT) scan of the brain (non-contrast) should be done. Preferably a CT-brain angiogram should be done if no contraindications. If there are contraindications, consult Neurologist KIV alternative investigations, e.g. trans-cranial or extra-cranial Doppler.

PROGNOSTICATION

- **High-risk** patients should be admitted for further evaluation by a neurologist. These patients include:
  1. Patients already receiving anti-coagulation therapy, e.g. warfarin, or double anti-platelet agents, e.g. aspirin and clopidogrel.
  2. Patients with identifiable cardioembolic source, e.g. atrial fibrillation.
  3. Patients with recurrent TIAs.
  4. Patients with a high **ABCD2 score**.
     a. **Age**: <60 – 0 point; ≥60 – 1 point.
     b. **Blood pressure**: <140/90 mmHg – 0 point; >140/90 mmHg – 1 point.
     c. **Clinical presentation**:
        Hemiparesis – 2 points
        Speech abnormalities – 1 point
        Others – 0 point
     d. **Duration of symptoms**:
        \>1 hour – 2 points
        10 minutes to 1 hour – 1 point
        <10 minutes – 0 point
     e. **Diabetes**: Present – 1 point; absent – 0 point.
- An ABCD2 score of 6–7 is high risk; such patients have an 8.1% risk of developing a stroke within 48 hours.
- An ABCD2 score of 4–5 is moderate risk; such patients have a 4.1% risk of developing a stroke within 48 hours.
- An ABCD2 score of 0–3 is low risk; such patients have a 1% risk of developing a stroke within 48 hours.

NOTE: The ABCD2 score is a clinical score to predict stroke risk within the first two days following a TIA.

- Patients with a low ABCD2 score, normal CT brain and without high-risk features may be discharged with a neurology follow-up within 48 hours. Prior to discharge, they should be started on anti-platelet therapy (aspirin preferably) and a lipid-lowering agent. They should also be advised to return immediately if TIA symptoms recur.
- Admit high risk patients after starting **soluble aspirin** 300 mg.
- If patient is allergic to aspirin, give **clopidogrel** 150 mg stat and then 75 mg daily.

References/Further Reading

1. Transient ischaemic attack update. *Annals of Emergency Medicine*. Aug 2008: 52(2).

2. Johnston SC, Rothwell PM, Nguyen-Huynh MN, et al. Validation and refinement of scores to predict very early stroke risk after transient ischaemic attack. *Lancet*. 2007; 369: 283–292.

3. Henry GL, Little N, Jagoda A, et al. Neurologic emergencies. NY, McGraw-Hill Medical; 2010: 138–140.

72 Coping with Emerging Infectious Diseases of the 21st Century in the Emergency Department – A New Norm

Quek Lit Sin

INTRODUCTION

- Infectious diseases have been among mankind for centuries. Previous dreaded diseases such as smallpox and poliomyelitis have been and/or will soon be eliminated from the world. However, many pathogens of the past are still with us today causing human mortality and pandemics (such as the human influenza virus).

- The advent of vaccines and antibiotics in the mid-20th century gave medical professionals hope that infectious diseases would be a thing of the past. However, judging from the recent encounter with severe acute respiratory syndrome (SARS) and swine flu (H1N1 influenza), it looks like the battle will continue.

- Dealing with emerging infections will be the 'new norm' where frontline healthcare professionals must be on the alert for clustering of fever cases or any symptoms of infection, and may be the first group of people to recognize a deliberate release or other infectious disease emergency.

- Despite these uncertainties, there are some fundamental measures that we can take to strengthen and protect the frontline personnel, i.e. the general practitioners and the emergency department staff.

HOSPITAL INFECTIOUS DISEASE EMERGENCY PREPAREDNESS

- Planning for an infectious disease outbreak hospital plan is the most complex of all disaster planning.

- The overall aim of hospital preparedness for an infectious disease emergency is to be able to provide adequate medical care to those affected while at the same time continuing to provide essential medical services to the community for an extended period of time. This has implications not only on the surge capacity of the hospital infrastructure, but it also strains the manpower capacity and deployment.

- On top of the phases of the traditional disaster management cycle (preparation, response, recovery, and mitigation), infectious disease emergency management include:

  1. **Surveillance and detection**: Recognizing that an infectious disease emergency is occurring.

  2. **Control and containment**: Instituting the clinical, public health measures that reduce the health, social, and economic consequences of the incident.

INFECTION CONTROL

- McDonald et al.[1] noted that certain persons were very efficient at transmitting SARS coronavirus (SARS-CoV), and that in certain settings these so-called 'superspreaders' played a crucial role in the epidemic and transmission among healthcare workers.[2]

- Effective infection control is the key in halting the intra-hospital spread of any infectious disease and it saves lives. All healthcare workers must have knowledge and be trained in infection control precautions. Competency checks effected through the Infection Control arm of the hospital will ensure compliance to the standards.

- Frontline departments should consider the following:[3,1]

  1. Have a programme to train the staff to identify and segregate or spatially separate patients with signs and symptoms of respiratory tract infection from others.

  2. Early detection and prompt isolation of infectious cases in isolation rooms with negative pressure ensuring that the staff understands when and how it should be used.

  3. Routine fever surveillance which must be stringent at all points of entry and exit in hospitals.

  4. Hospital-wide implementation of the use of personal protective equipment in all areas where care for patients is undertaken – use of N95 mask (mask that is 95% efficient at filtering out particles of sizes 0.3 micron and above), gowns, gloves, goggles, head covers, and hand washing.

  5. Training health workers in the proper use of personal protective gear including fit testing of N95-type mask.

  6. Clusters of patients or health workers with undefined fever signal a breakdown in infection control, the immediate response must be to stop discharges and visits, and transfers between wards, clinics, and hospitals.

  7. Regular drills and simulation exercises to test departmental competency response plans.

INITIAL INVESTIGATION AND MANAGEMENT

- The aim of the initial investigation and management of a patient suspected of having a highly infectious disease is to provide medical care to the patient while ensuring staff safety.

- The following are important:

  1. Isolate the patient from the rest.

  2. Limit the number of staff exposed to the patient.

  3. Provide protection for the staff to approach and evaluate the patient.

  4. Consider transfer to a more specialized facility for better care of the patient.

  5. The laboratory must be prepared to handle samples from the infectious patient.

SURGE CAPACITY

Infrastructure Capacity

- **Surge capacity** is the ability to expand healthcare provisions to respond to an increased number of patients that exceeds usual capacity, including the provision of specialized medical care (e.g. paediatric care, intensive care requiring mechanical ventilation, haemodialysis, or haemofiltration).
- Plans for further expansion of this capacity, requires the use of alternative care facilities (e.g. schools and community halls) and/or significant changes in standards of care, sometimes referred to as '**planned degradation of care**'.

Manpower Capacity

- Parallel to infrastructure surge capacity is the availability for manpower resource to manage the additional patient load.
- Hospital emergency plans that include manpower deployment for such crises will ensure adequate patient care coverage.
- Unlike other disasters, an infectious disease outbreak crisis is slow brewing and often lasts over an extended period of time. This makes it more challenging in terms of manpower scheduling as we must take into consideration mental and physical fatigue that comes with an extended state of emergency. Often, extended shift hours and involvement of staff from other departments not affected by the crisis are required to maintain standards of care.

COMMUNICATION

- Effective communication is essential to any crisis management but is particularly important here because of the psychological impact it has on the public and hospital staff.
- The term 'communication' encompasses the provision of accurate, timely, complete, and easily understood information to the community, patients, and healthcare professionals.
- As the crisis develops, more information and new workplans become available and these have to be disseminated accurately to the ground.
- Multiple modalities of information dissemination are required so that all the staff is kept updated of the latest development, e.g. via mass emails, SMSs, Twitter, information bulletin boards, etc.
- Roll call every morning before the start of work or change of shift will ensure that the latest information is transmitted to the healthcare professionals.
- Recent international guidelines on risk communication and on communicating with the media and the public during an infectious disease emergency provide greater detail, and highlight the importance of communicating in ways that build or maintain trust, of planning and testing outbreak communications strategies, and of providing media communications training for all public officials as a part of professional development.

CARING FOR THE STAFF AND OTHERS AFFECTED BY THE EMERGENCY

- Occupational health services should be involved in hospital preparedness planning. This involvement will help to ensure that the staff is as well protected before the event as is possible (e.g. by ensuring uptake of seasonal influenza vaccine, pneumococcal vaccine and hepatitis B vaccine by all those who are eligible under existing national policies, and of vaccines specifically relevant to laboratory staff).

- An epidemiology unit should also participate in the development of systems for surveillance of infection in healthcare workers, which are needed both pre-event, as a means of detecting that an infectious disease emergency is occurring, and during an event, to monitor the outcome for potentially exposed workers, and of infection-specific protocols for post-exposure management.

- Any traumatic incident, emergency or disaster, whether natural or man-made, has a psychological impact on those involved – survivors, the bereaved, witnesses, rescuers, responders, and health professionals, and their families, relatives, friends, and workmates.[4]

- Planning should ensure that, whatever the emergency, staffing levels will be sufficient for time on duty to be limited to no more than 12 hours a day, and should make provision for staff rotation from highly taxing to less taxing functions. The staff will need somewhere 'off-scene' that is quiet, safe, and private to eat, drink and rest without interruption and the facilities will also need to be such that the staff is able to stay in touch with friends and family.

- The staff should also be made aware of other sources of support (e.g. their family doctor, hospital chaplain, and other religious and spiritual advisers), and should be provided with details of how to contact confidential listening or counselling services.[5]

- Consistent with Caplan's[6] notions of preventive psychiatry, the management of the psychosocial effects of an infectious disease threat must occur on 3 levels:

  1. Putting measures in place to protect the staff from contracting the disease.

  2. Mitigating the adverse psychological impact of the persistent threats of contracting the disease, as well as witnessing fellow workers succumb to the disease.

  3. Providing psychological treatment of the lingering adverse effects of the epidemic.

CONCLUSION

- The threat of the next pandemic is always present. It is impossible to predict which emergent infection will next threaten global public health. It is, however, possible to predict that infectious disease emergencies will continue to occur with regularity, and it is possible, with appropriate planning, to be prepared to meet them in a way that ensures that they cause as little social disruption as possible.

- The greatest danger is complacency. Thinking that a pandemic is not likely to happen and not planning for it will only result in a bad outcome.

References/Further Reading

1. McDonald LC, Simor AE, Su IJ, et al. SARS in healthcare facilities, Toronto and Taiwan. *Emerg Infect Dis*. 2004; 10: 777–781.

2. Oh VMS, Lim TK. Singapore's experience of SARS. *Clin Med*. Sep/Oct 2003; 3: 448–451.

3. Hsu LY, Lee CC, Green JA, et al. Severe acute respiratory syndrome (SARS) in Singapore: Clinical features of index patient and initial contacts. *Emerg Infect Dis*. June 2003; 9(6): 713–717.

4. Maunder R, Hunter J, Vincent L, et al. The immediate psychological and occupational impact of the 2003 SARS outbreak in a teaching hospital. *CMAJ*. 2003; 168(10): 1245–1251.

5. Dalgard OS, Lund Haheim L. Psychosocial risk factors and mortality: A prospective study with special focus on social support, social participation, and locus of control in Norway. *J Epidemiol Community Health*. 1998; 52(8): 476–481.

6. Pearlin L, Aneshensen C. Stress, coping and social supports. In: Brown P, ed. *Medical Sociology*. Prospect Heights, IL: Waveland Press; 1989: 95–102.

7. Caplan, G. *Principles of Preventive Psychiatry*. New York: Basic Books; 1964.

Gene Chan • Sim Tiong Beng

DENGUE FEVER

Definitions

- Dengue fever is an acute febrile infectious disease transmitted by infected female *Aedes aegypti* mosquitoes.
- The dengue virus, a member of the flavivirus group in the family *Flaviviridae*, is an enveloped, single-stranded RNA virus which has four anti-genetically distinct serotypes (DEN-1, DEN-2, DEN-3 and DEN-4). Since there is only transient and weak cross-protection among the 4 serotypes, persons living in an endemic area can be infected with 3, probably 4 dengue serotypes during their lifetime.
- The pathophysiology of the disease is the result of an abrupt increase of capillary permeability, with diffuse capillary leakage of plasma, haemoconcentration and, in some cases, with non-haemorrhagic hypovolaemic shock.

Caveats

- The diagnosis of dengue fever at the emergency department is clinical and often the first diagnosis that crosses the emergency physician's mind when the fever persists for >3 days and is recalcitrant to treatment.
- Abdominal symptoms like nausea, vomiting, epigastric pain, and diarrhoea often lead to a misdiagnosis of gastroenteritis or viral gastritis. This is especially true in children.
- Patients who have family members with suspected dengue infection run a higher risk of having the same infection. With this history in a symptomatic patient, it is necessary to monitor platelet counts.
- Patients with ongoing menses should not be labelled as having dengue haemorrhagic fever (DHF) unless there is a rise in haematocrit ≥20% baseline or when other DHF criteria are fulfilled.
- Take note of the following 2 features that suggest an **impending shock** in a patient with DF **haemoconcentration** and **abdominal pain**.
- **Incubation period: 4 to 7 days** after the bite of an infected mosquito. It may even be as long as **2 weeks**.

CLINICAL MANIFESTATIONS

Classic dengue fever

- The clinical symptoms of dengue fever in its early stages are similar to those of a viral infection.

- It is characterized by fever accompanied by headache, retro-orbital pain, and marked muscle and joint pains (**break-bone fever**). There may be the presence of relative bradycardia.
- Other associated symptoms include
  1. Non-specific rash (50%), e.g. petechial, diffuse erythematous, or morbilliform.
  2. Gastrointestinal symptoms, e.g. nausea and vomiting (50%) and diarrhoea (30%).
  3. Respiratory tract symptoms, e.g. cough, sore throat, and nasal congestion.
  4. Haemorrhagic manifestations (not to be confused with dengue haemorrhagic fever).
- **Laboratory findings**: Thrombocytopaenia <100,000 cells/mm^3, leucopaenia, elevated aspartate aminotransferase (AST) (2–5 times).
- When differentiating dengue fever from other viral infections, note that patients with dengue infection have fever with marked constitutional symptoms.

Dengue Haemorrhagic Fever

- Dengue haemorrhagic fever (DHF) is the most serious manifestation of dengue virus infections and may be associated with circulatory failure and shock.
- The early phase of the illness is indistinguishable from dengue fever.
- **4 cardinal features of DHF** as defined by the World Health Organization (WHO) are as follows:
  1. **Fever** lasting between 2 and 7 days.
  2. Marked **thrombocytopaenia** (<100,000 cells/mm^3).
  3. **Increased vascular permeability** (plasma leakage syndrome) resulting in haemoconcentration (>20% rise in haematocrit value), pleural effusion, or ascites.
  4. **Haemorrhagic tendency** (positive tourniquet test*) or **spontaneous bleeding**.
- *Dengue shock syndrome (DSS)* occurs when there is shock present along with these 4 criteria.

LABORATORY DIAGNOSIS

- The diagnosis of dengue fever is clinical. One should not withhold treatment if dengue is suspected, while waiting for laboratory confirmation.
- For confirmation, serum dengue antibody (serology) **IgM levels** are sent for lab analysis if the fever has been present for **>5 days**.
- If the patient is still in **day 2–3 of fever dengue viral RNA** or proteins are detected from **polymerase chain reaction** instead.

---

* A tourniquet test is performed by inflating a blood pressure cuff on the arm to a point midway between systolic and diastolic blood pressures for 5 minutes. The skin below the cuff is then examined for petechiae. A finding of more than 20 petechiae in a square inch area is considered positive.

- **Risk factors** for the development of **DHF**:
  1. **Extremes of age**. Children who are <15 years of age and the elderly.
  2. **Repeat dengue infections**. Pre-existing antibodies from an earlier infection does not prevent infection by a different serotype. These antibodies can generate an immune response which can be deleterious to the host.
  3. **Viral genotypes** with an **increase of pathogenicity**, e.g. Asian strain DEN-2.
  4. **Nutritional status**. Malnourished children are less likely to develop DHF probably due to reduced cellular immunity.
- **Clinical indicators** of impending **DSS**:
  1. Severe abdominal pain
  2. Change from fever to hypothermia
  3. Restlessness or lethargy
  4. Sweating
  5. Persistent vomiting
  6. Tender hepatomegaly

System	Manifestations	
Neurological	Encephalopathy	
	Encephalitis/aseptic meningitis Intracranial haemorrhage/thrombosis	
	Mononeuropathies/polyneuropathies/Guillaine-Barre syndrome Myelitis	
Gastrointestinal/hepatic	**Hepatitis**/fulminant hepatic failure Acalculous cholecystitis **Acute pancreatitis** **Febrile diarrhoea** Acute parotitis	
Renal	Haemolytic uraemic syndrome Renal failure	
Cardiac	**Myocarditis** Conduction abnormalities Pericarditis	
Respiratory	Acute respiratory distress syndrome Pulmonary haemorrhage	
Musculoskeletal	Myositis Rhabdomyolysis	
Lymphoreticular	Spontaneous splenic rupture Lymph node infarction	

Source: Adapted from 'Atypical manifestations of dengue', *Journal of Tropical Medicine and International Health*, 12(9): 1087–1095.

- As dengue infections are assuming global proportions, more and more atypical presentations have appeared. Refer to the following table for *atypical manifestations of dengue*.
- **Acute liver failure** with unusual change in consciousness or abnormal neurological signs (hyperreflexia) may occur. Such patients succumb quickly from severe haemorrhage, renal failure, brain oedema, pulmonary oedema, and superimposed infection. Early intervention is necessary. Diffuse capillary leakage of plasma is responsible for the haemoconcentration.

⇨ **SPECIAL TIPS FOR GPs**

- Have a high index of suspicion for dengue infections.
- Patients with dengue may not present with the classical rash. They may often appear flushed over the face. Ask for history of bleeding, e.g. from the nose and gums.
- Do **full blood count** (FBC) for all cases of fever lasting >3 days. In the FBC, look out not only for **thrombocytopaenia** (<100,000/mm³) but also an **elevation** of **haematocrit** (>50%). Elevation of the haematocrit is an indication that plasma leakage has already occurred and that fluid repletion is urgently required.
- Refer all cases of suspected or confirmed DHF or dengue shock syndrome (DSS) immediately to the hospital for inpatient management.

MANAGEMENT

- No specific treatment for dengue is available. Management is mainly supportive.
- No intramuscular injections.
- Fever and myalgias can be managed with acetaminophen. Aspirin and non-steroidal anti-inflammatory drugs (NSAIDs) should be avoided because of risk of bleeding complications, and in children because of the potential risk of Reye's syndrome. Hepatotoxic drugs and long-acting sedatives should be avoided.
- Early institution of supportive treatment (fluid replacement and correction of electrolyte imbalances) is the key to managing patients with dengue in all its forms.
- Ill patients must be managed in the critical care area where they can be monitored.
- **A full blood count is essential for any patient who presents with a persistently high fever with no definite focus of infection. Important lab findings in a patient who has dengue** are:
  1. **Leucopaenia**: The presence of leucocytosis and neutrophilia excludes the possibility of dengue, and bacterial infections must be considered.
  2. **Thrombocytopaenia** (<100,000/mm³): Leptospirosis, measles, rubella, meningococcaemia, septicaemia, malaria, and severe acute respiratory syndrome (SARS) may also cause thrombocytopaenia but rash is unusual in uncomplicated malaria.
  3. **Haematocrit** showing haemoconcentration (>50%).
  4. **Urea and electrolytes**: May show hyponatraemia.

5. **Liver function test**: Abnormal liver enzymes.

6. **Coagulation profile**.

7. **Dengue RNA polymerase chain reaction** or **serology test** is generally not indicated unless diagnosis is in doubt, i.e. other causes of thrombocytopaenia need to be considered, e.g. severe sepsis with disseminated intramuscular coagulation or idiopathic thrombocytopaenic purpura autoimmune disease. Otherwise treatment is supportive.

- It is important to manage plasma leakage in **DHF** with aggressive intravascular volume repletion, with lactated Ringer's solution or isotonic saline, to prevent or reverse DSS. Adequacy of fluid repletion should be assessed by serial determination of haematocrit, blood pressure, pulse, and urine output.

- Once the patient is stabilized, capillary leakage stops, and resorption of extravasated fluid begins rapidly. Thus, intravenous fluid supplementation should be discontinued once the patients are taking oral fluids and having normal haematocrit, vital signs, and urine output. Excessive fluid administration after this point can precipitate hypervolaemia and pulmonary oedema.

Indications for transfusion:

- Platelet transfusions are given only if significant bleeding occurs.

- There is no place for prophylactic platelet transfusion even with a count below 10,000 cells/mm^3, if there is no evidence of bleeding.

- Beware when giving large volumes of platelet concentrate as rapid transfusion may tip the patient over into fluid overload.

- Blood transfusion (packed cell transfusion or whole blood) is indicated in the presence of blood loss of >10% of total blood volume or bleeding resulting in hypovolaemic shock and the patient not responding to fluid resuscitation.

- **Disposition: Hospitalization** for intravenous fluid therapy is necessary in the following cases:

  1. Significant dehydration (>10% of normal body weight) has occurred or presence of hypotension/narrowing of pulse pressure requiring rapid intravenous volume expansion or when there is spontaneous bleeding.

  2. Clinical bleeding tendency.

  3. Severe thrombocytopaenia (i.e. platelets <50,000/mm^3).

  4. Haematocrit elevation (males >49%, females >43%).

  5. A platelet count of <20,000 will necessitate bed rest for fear of spontaneous bleeding and accidental trauma.

  6. Patients who are elderly, very young, and those with a concomitant illness (i.e. allergies, diabetes mellitus, or ischaemic heart disease), or an inability to tolerate medications orally.

NOTE: Those with a platelet count between 80,000 and 140,000 can be discharged but they have to return for serial full blood count checks until the platelet counts normalize.

References/Further Reading

1. World Health Organization (WHO). Dengue *Haemorrhagic Fever: Diagnosis, Treatment, Prevention and Control.* 2nd ed. Geneva: WHO; 1997.

2. Singapore Ministry of Health. *Clinical Guidelines on Dengue Fever/Dengue Haemorrhagic Fever;* 2002.

3. Lye DC, Chan M, Lee VJ, Leo YS. Do young adults with uncomplicated dengue fever need hospitalization? A retrospective analysis of clinical and laboratory features. *Singapore Medical Journal.* 2008; 49(6): 476.

4. Dengue fever and dengue haemorrhagic fever. A diagnostic challenge. *Australian Family Physician.* Aug 2006; 35(8).

5. Gulati S, Maheshwari A. A typical manifestations of dengue. *Tropical Medicine and International Health.* Sep 2007; 12(9): 1087–1095.

6. Rothman, AL. Clinical presentation and diagnosis of dengue virus infections – UptoDate. Jan 2008.

CHIKUNGUNYA

- Chikungunya is a viral illness almost similar in presentation to dengue fever.
- It is caused by an arbovirus, the chikungunya virus (CHIK virus in short), belonging to the genus *Alphavirus* under the *Togaviridae* family.
- The disease, first documented in Tanzania, got its name from the 'makonde' dialect which means 'that which bends up', describing the physical appearance of a patient suffering from a severe illness.
- The disease was initially endemic in most of sub-Saharan Africa, southern India and Pakistan, but is now seen commonly in Southeast Asia.
- The vectors responsible for the virus transmission are the *Aedes aegypti* and *Aedes albopictus* mosquitoes.

CLINICAL MANIFESTATIONS

- The incubation period lasts about 2 to 4 days.
- Patients develop fever with chills (92%), headache (62%), severe arthralgia (87%), backache (67%), and some have a maculopapular rash (50%) on the trunk.
- Migratory polyarthritis (70%) results in swelling and reddening of small and large joints.
- The illness may last 5 to 7 days. Complications resulting in severe haemorrhagic manifestations or death are uncommon.
- Sequelae include persistent arthralgia associated with stiffness and pain. Neurological, dermatologic, and emotional sequelae also occur.

LABORATORY DIAGNOSIS

- CHIK IgM antibodies are present after 5 days of onset.
- In the early stages, CHIK–polymerase chain reaction test results may be positive.
- There is no **pathognomonic haematological finding** – leucopaenia with lymphocyte predominance is the usual observation. Thrombocytopaenia is rare.

MANAGEMENT

Acute illness

- The disease is **self-limiting**. There is no specific treatment or anti-viral vaccine against the CHIK virus.
- Treatment is symptomatic.
- Paracetamol is used as an analgesic and anti-pyretic medication.
- Aspirin, NSAIDs and steroids are not indicated and preferably avoided for fear of adverse effects.
- Ensure adequate hydration and normal vital signs, especially blood pressure.
- Cold compression may reduce joint pain.
- Mild exercise and physiotherapy are recommended.

Chronic sequelae

- *Osteoarticular manifestations* like chronic joint pain and swelling may persist for months (in about 10% of patients) or recur with every febrile illness. Exercise and physiotherapy can prevent disability, deformity, and contractures.
- *Neurological problems* like peripheral neuropathy with a predominant sensory component may occur. Others develop entrapment syndromes, muscle weakness, seizures, or ocular/visual defects. These are treated with steroid or anti-neuralgia drugs.
- *Dermatological problems* like hyperpigmentation and papular eruptions may occur in the acute phase. However, they rarely require long-term care. Most subside with the application of zinc oxide cream or calamine lotion. Psoriatic patients may experience worsening of lesions.
- *Psycho-somatic or emotional problems* have been observed in up to 15% of cases. They are more likely to occur in persons with pre-existing mood or psychiatric disorders. Psychosocial support and reassurance may be key in rehabilitation.

PREVENTION

- Like dengue, preventive measures are adopted to control this mosquito-borne disease, e.g. using mosquito nets and repellants, searching and destroying mosquito breeding sites and spraying of insecticides to destroy mosquitoes.

References/Further Reading

1. WHO Regional Office for Southeast Asia. *Guidelines on Clinical Management of Chikungunya Fever*. Oct 2008.
2. Swaroop A, Jain A, Kumhar M, et al. Chikungunya fever. *J Ind Acad of Clin Med*. 2007; 8(2): 164–168.
3. Pialoux G, Gauzere BA, Jaureguiberry S, Strobel M. Chikungunya: An epidemic arbovirosis. *Lancet Infect Dis*. May 2007; 7(5): 319–327. Review.

74 Malaria

Toh Hong Chuen

CAVEATS

- The diagnosis of malaria should also be considered in any person with fever of unknown origin regardless of his travel history.

- The two predominant human malaria species in Southeast Asia are *P. vivax* and *P. falciparum*. Resistance to anti-malarials is emerging faster in this region than any other part of the world.

- The classical malaria attack lasts between 6 and 10 hours; onset of chills is followed by spiking fever, then defervescence with profuse sweating. These attacks occur every second day with *P. vivax*, *P. ovale* and sometimes *P. falciparum*, and every third day with *P. malariae*. Though classical, these patterns are observed infrequently.

- Relapses can occur with *P. vivax* and *P. ovale* infections (dormant liver stage parasites – hypnozoites) months to years after the primary infection.

  1. Consider malaria in those patients with fever who have recently travelled to Africa, Asia, the Middle East, Central and South America, Hispaniola, and Oceania.

- Note that the majority of patients from high-transmission areas are usually asymptomatic. This reflects a state of premunition, where infection is sufficiently contained (to be asymptomatic). The reverse is true in low-transmission areas, where patients are usually symptomatic.

- Chemoprophylaxis may not prevent malaria as a result of drug resistance and compliance (especially if the patient becomes unwell after returning from a malarious area).

- **Clinical features** are **generally non-specific**, including fever (with chills and rigors), flu-like symptoms (myalgia, lethargy, and headache) or gastroenteritis-like symptoms (nausea, vomiting, and diarrhoea). Involvement of many other organ systems can occur as well.

- **Uncomplicated malaria** is defined as symptomatic malaria without signs of severity or evidence of vital organ dysfunction.

- **Severe malaria** tends to occur in persons who have no or low immunity to malaria (i.e. those in a no or low-transmission area). It can also occur in young children and pregnant women in high-transmission areas. The diagnosis is made with the demonstration of asexual parasitaemia and any of the following clinical or laboratory findings:

  1. **Clinical manifestation**: Prostration, impaired consciousness, respiratory distress (acidotic breathing), multiple convulsions, circulatory collapse, pulmonary oedema (radiological), disseminated intramuscular coagulation, jaundice, and haemoglobinuria.

  2. **Laboratory test**: Severe anaemia, hypoglycaemia, acidosis, renal impairment, hyperlacta-taemia, and hyperparasitaemia.

- **Deterioration** can be **rapid**, particularly with *P. falciparum* infection.

- **Hypoglycaemia** can be caused by both malaria infection or treatment (e.g. quinine).

- **Mefloquine** is **not recommended** in patients with neuropsychiatric or cardiac conduction defects.

⇨ **SPECIAL TIPS FOR GPs**

- Treat with **quinine** or **mefloquine**, when malaria is diagnosed, or **chloroquine** if *P. vivax* is positively identified, before sending the patient to the emergency department as the patient may deteriorate very quickly.
- Check bedside glucose level at the clinic and treat hypoglycaemia if necessary.
- **Simple preventive measures against malaria in adults include:**
  1. Avoiding mosquito bites by utilizing repellants, e.g. 30% DEET, nets and appropriate clothing and avoiding outdoor exposure at dusk and dawn.
  2. If patients are going to a malarious area, start **chemoprophylaxis** a week before travel and continue for 4 weeks after return. Give:
     a. Mefloquine 250 mg weekly **or**
     b. Doxycycline 100 mg OM **or**
     c. Maloprim 1 tab weekly.

MANAGEMENT

- Send **blood for thin and thick film** examination for malaria in any ill patient who has been to a malarious area.
- If parasites are not visualized, repeated smears should be taken at least twice daily for 3 days to exclude malaria.
- **Admit** all patients with malaria. Patients with severe malaria should be admitted to the high dependency or intensive care unit.
- The **parasite count**, which is related to prognosis, and infecting species should be identified.
- **Labs**:
  1. Full blood count (anaemia, low or normal total white cell count, and thrombocytopaenia)
  2. Urea/electrolytes/creatinine (renal failure)
  3. Liver function test (jaundice)
  4. Blood glucose (*P. falciparum* infection or treatment with quinine)
  5. Urine dipstick for haemoglobinuria
- **Treatment**
  1. For children **<8 years old**: Use **clindamycin**; avoid doxycycline and tetracycline.
  2. **Primaquine** is used to eradicate any hypnozoite forms. Glucose 6 phosphate dehydrogenase (G6PD) deficiency must be excluded as it can cause severe haemolytic anaemia in these patients. It is also contraindicated in pregnant patients. Pregnant patients with *P. vivax* should be maintained on chloroquine prophylaxis for the duration of their pregnancy.
  3. Patients with **severe malaria** should be started on **intravenous quinine** aggressively. The following parameters should be monitored during administration:
     a. Blood pressure (for hypotension).

	Adult	Children	Pregnant
Uncomplicated malaria *P. vivax*	**Chloroquine phosphate:** 600 mg base (= 1000 mg salt) PO immediately, followed by 300 mg base (= 500 mg salt) PO at 6, 24, and 48 hours (total dose: 1500 mg base (= 2500 mg salt)) PLUS **Primaquine phosphate** 30 mg qd PO for 14 days	**Chloroquine phosphate:** 10 mg base/kg PO immediately, followed by 5 mg base/kg PO at 6, 24, and 48 hours (total dose: 25 mg base/kg) PLUS **Primaquine phosphate** 0.5 mg/kg qd PO for 14 days	**Quinine sulfate:** 542 mg base (= 650 mg salt) PO tid for 7 days
Uncomplicated malaria *P. falciparum*	**Quinine sulfate:** 542 mg base (= 650 mg salt) PO tid for 7 days PLUS one of the following: **Doxycycline:** 100 mg PO bid for 7 days; or **Tetracycline:** 250 mg PO qid for 7 days; or **Clindamycin:** 20 mg base/kg/day PO divided tid for 7 days	**Quinine sulfate:** 8.3 mg base/kg (= 10 mg salt/kg) PO tid for 3 to 7 days PLUS one of the following: **Clindamycin:** 20 mg base/kg/day PO divided tid for 7 days; or **Doxycycline:** 2.2 mg/kg PO every 12 hours for 7 days; or **Tetracycline:** 25 mg/kg/day PO divided qid for 7 days	**Quinine sulfate:** 542 mg base (= 650 mg salt) PO tid for 7 days PLUS **Clindamycin:** 20 mg base/kg/ day PO divided tid for 7 days
Severe malaria	**Quinine gluconate:** 6.25 mg base/kg (= 10 mg salt/kg) loading dose IV over 1 to 2 hours, then 0.0125 mg base/kg/min (= 0.02 mg salt/kg/min) continuous infusion for at least 24 hours. Once parasite density is less than 1% and patient can take oral medication, complete treatment with oral quinine, dose as above PLUS **Doxycycline:** 100 mg PO bid for 7 days (if patient is not able to take oral medication, give 100 mg IV every 12 hours and then switch to oral doxycycline (as above) as soon as patient can take oral medication. For IV use, avoid rapid administration) Treatment course = 7 days; or	**Quinine gluconate:** 6.25 mg base/kg (= 10 mg salt/kg) loading dose IV over 1 to 2 hours, then 0.0125 mg base/kg/min (= 0.02 mg salt/kg/min) continuous infusion for at least 24 hours. Once parasite density is less than 1% and patient can take oral medication, complete treatment with oral quinine, dose as above PLUS **Doxycycline:** 2.2 mg/kg PO every 12 hours for 7 days (if patient is not able to take oral medication, may give IV. For children weighing less than 45 kg, give 2.2 mg/kg IV every 12 hours and then switch to oral doxycycline (dose as above) as soon as patient can take oral medication.	As for adult with severe malaria

Adult	Children	Pregnant
Tetracycline: 250 mg PO qid for 7 days; or **Clindamycin:** 20 mg base/kg/day PO divided tid for 7 days (if patient is not able to take oral medication, give 10 mg base/kg loading dose IV followed by 5 mg base/kg IV every 8 hours. Switch to oral clindamycin (oral dose as above) as soon as patient can take oral medication. For IV use, avoid rapid administration) Treatment course = 7 days	Dosage in children weighing greater than or equal to 45 kg is the same as in adults. For IV use, avoid rapid administration) Treatment course = 7 days; or **Tetracycline:** 25 mg/kg/day PO divided qid for 7 days; or **Clindamycin:** 20 mg base/kg/day PO divided tid for 7 days (if patient is not able to take oral medication, give 10 mg base/kg loading dose IV followed by 5 mg base/kg IV every 8 hours. Switch to oral clindamycin (oral dose as above) as soon as patient can take oral medication. For IV use, avoid rapid administration) Treatment course = 7 days	

b. Cardiac monitor (for widening of the QRS complex and/or lengthening of the QTc interval).

c. Hourly hypocount (for hypoglycaemia).

4. Carry out an **exchange transfusion** in the following circumstances:

a. Parasite density (i.e. parasitaemia) is more than 10%

b. Cerebral malaria

c. Non-volume overload pulmonary oedema

d. Renal complications

References/Further Reading

1. White NJ. Current concepts: The treatment of malaria. *NEJM*. 1996; 335: 800–806.

2. Warrell DA, Gilles HM. *Essential Malariolgy*. London: Arnold; 2002.

3. *Treatment for Malaria (Guideline for Clinicians)*. Available at: http://www.cdc.gov/malaria/diagnosis_treatment/tx_clinicians.htm.

4. Jai P. Narain. *Indian J Med Res*. July 2008; 128: 1–3.

5. Malaria. Available at: http://www.cdc.gov/malaria/diagnosis_treatment/tx_clinicians.htm. Treatment guidelines table last updated on 24 May 2008.

6. Griffith KS, Lewis LS, Mali S, Parise M. Treatment of malaria in the United States. A systematic review. JAMA. 2007; 297(20): 2264–2277.

75 Needlestick/Body Fluid Exposure

Peter Manning • Ong Pei Yuin

DEFINITION

This type of contamination usually refers to an incident in which a patient, healthcare worker (HCW), or member of the public is contaminated with potentially infected body fluids.

CAVEATS

- In hospital, injuries happen during two-handed recapping or the transfer of a needle from one person to another during injections, venepuncture, or intravenous cannulation. Approximately one-third of injuries occur distant from the time and place of patient care, e.g. skin puncture from an uncapped needle in a garbage bag.
- HCWs have seroconverted following both parenteral and **non-parenteral exposures**.
- The risk of contracting hepatitis is much greater than that of contracting human immuno-deficiency virus (HIV).
- Typically, HIV infection in HCWs occurs secondary to accidental inoculation of blood from an HIV-positive source patient.
- A person who tests negative for anti-HIV may nonetheless harbour the virus, and seroconversion may be delayed or absent following inoculation with the virus.

> ⇨ **SPECIAL TIP FOR GPs**
> - **Post-exposure anti-retroviral chemoprophylaxis** is now the standard of care and should be implemented immediately after a known HIV-positive exposure (see later section).

MANAGEMENT

- **Patient care considerations**:
  1. **Percutaneous exposure**: Attempt to express inoculated site and wash thoroughly under running water. Then disinfect with chlorhexidine or povidone iodine and apply a dressing if deemed necessary.
  2. **Mucous membrane exposure**: Irrigate the affected area immediately with copious amounts of water.
  3. **Non-intact skin exposure**: Wash the area with soap and water or apply an antiseptic handwash. Then disinfect with chlorhexidine or povidone iodine.

NOTE: For all contacts follow your institutional policy and procedures.

- **Blood/body fluid from an identified source patient**:
  1. Send a blood sample from the exposed HCW for HBsAg, anti-HBs and anti-HIV.
  2. Send a blood sample from the source patient (only after consent has been given) for HBsAg and anti-HIV.
     a. **Identified source patient is HBV surface antigen (HBsAg) negative**:
        i. HCW with natural immunity to HBV: No further action is required.
        ii. HCW who has completed HBV immunization: No further action is required.
        iii. HCW who has not completed HBV immunization: Start/complete HBV immunization.
        iv. HCW who is HBV surface antigen (HBsAg) positive: No further action is required.
     b. **Identified source patient is HBV surface antigen (HBsAg) positive**:
        i. HCW with natural immunity: No further action is required.
        ii. HCW who has completed HBV immunization: Give booster dose of hepatitis B vaccine.
        iii. HCW who has not completed HBV immunization: Give hepatitis B specific HIG within 72 hours and start/complete HBV immunization.
        iv. HCW who is HBV surface antigen positive: No further action is required.
     c. **Identified source patient is HIV antibody negative**:
        i. Determine the hepatitis B status of the patient.
     d. **Identified source patient is HIV antibody positive**:
        i. HCW is HIV antibody positive: No further action is required.
        ii. HCW is HIV antibody negative: Implement post-exposure prophylaxis immediately (see later section) and refer the HCW to follow-up according to institutional practice.
        iii. Determine the hepatitis B virus status of the source patient and proceed as previously described.

- **Blood/body fluid from unidentified patient**:
  1. HCW who has natural immunity to HBV: No further action is required.
  2. HCW who has completed HBV immunization: Give booster dose of hepatitis B vaccine.
  3. HCW who has not completed HBV immunization: Administer hepatitis B immune globulin within 72 hours and start/complete hepatitis B immunization.

- **Post-exposure prophylaxis**: If a HCW is exposed to the blood or body fluid of a HIV-positive source patient, consider post-exposure retroviral chemoprophylaxis that may reduce the risk of seroconversion (based on animal and human studies). Studies have shown that prophylaxis administered within 24 hours of exposure reduces the transmission of HIV.
  1. Administer prophylaxis immediately: **Do not wait** for follow-up appointment in 3 days or so.

2. Prescribe **zidovudine** 300 mg PO bd and **lamivudine** 150 mg PO bd (available as combination drug combivir).

   a. Side effects: Gastrointestinal symptoms, headache, fatigue, myalgia, and seizure.

   b. Refer to an infectious disease specialist for follow-up within 3 days.

3. If the source patient's HIV status is unknown but he belongs to a high-risk group:

   a. Obtain blood specimen as above.

   b. Refer for prompt follow-up, i.e. within 48 hours.

References/Further Reading

1. CDC. Updated U.S. Public Health Service guidelines for the management of occupational exposures to HBV, HCV, and HIV and recommendations for postexposure prophylaxis. *MMWR Recommendations & Reports*. 2001; 50(RR–11): 1–42.

2. CDC. Public Health Service guidelines for the management of healthcare worker exposures to HIV and recommendations for postexposure prophylaxis. *MMWR Morb Mortal Wkly Rep*. 1998; 47(RR–7): 1–33.

3. Singapore National University Hospital. *Infection Control Manual*. 2000.

4. National University Hospital. *Hospital Administrative Policy. Sharps Injury/Body Fluid Exposure*. 2007.

76 Tetanus

Suresh Pillai • Keith Ho

CAVEATS

- A high index of suspicion must be maintained in order to detect patients presenting with tetanus.
- Wound debridement as well as management in an intensive care unit is mandatory for all suspected cases of tetanus.

⇨ **SPECIAL TIPS FOR GPs**

- Apart from ensuring adequate tetanus prophylaxis in all patients with tetanus-prone wounds, a high index of suspicion must be maintained for patients presenting with either localized or generalized muscular rigidity with or without a tetanus-susceptible wound.
- All suspected cases should be immediately referred to the emergency department for further management.

PATHOPHYSIOLOGY

- Tetanus is caused by the introduction of exotoxin liberated by *Clostridium tetani*, an anaerobic Gram-positive rod, into a wound. *Clostridium tetani* is usually introduced into a wound in the spore-forming, non-invasive state, but can germinate into a toxin-producing, vegetative form if the tissue is compromised and tissue oxygen tension is reduced.
- Tetanus originates in puncture wounds, lacerations, crush injuries as well as in parenteral drug abusers when anaerobic conditions facilitate the germination of spores.
- The clinical signs and symptoms arise because of the transport of exotoxin to the central nervous system, where it blocks the transmission at the inhibitory interneurones, leading to unopposed muscle spasm.

CLINICAL PRESENTATION

- The incubation period can vary from 3 to 21 days from the onset of infection.
- The signs of generalized tetanus include painful stiffening of the jaw and trunk muscles.
- The typical features of tetanus, including risus sardonicus, dysphagia, opisthotonus, flexing of the arms, fist clenching, abdominal muscle rigidity, and extension of the lower limbs, are caused by intermittent tonic contractions of the involved muscle groups.
- Fractures of the spine or long bones may arise from convulsive spasms of the skeletal muscles as well as from seizures.

- Consciousness is usually not lost unless laryngospasm or spasm of the respiratory muscles develops.
- Autonomic instability resulting in fever, diaphoresis, tachycardia, and hypertension are commonly present as well.

MANAGEMENT

- Management is best achieved in quiet isolation in an intensive care unit environment.
- The mainstay of therapy includes neuromuscular paralysis, orotracheal intubation, and ventilation. Tracheostomy is often indicated for prolonged ventilatory care.
- Wound debridement is essential to minimize further progression of the disease.
- A single intramuscular dose of **human tetanus immune globulin** at 3000 to 5000 IU should be administered.
- A complete course of intramuscular **anti-tetanus toxoid (ATT)** 0.5 ml should be initiated once the patient recovers from the acute phase, then at 6 weeks, and subsequently at 6 months.
- Intravenous **penicillin G** 10 million IU/day in divided doses should be initiated. Alternative antibiotics include **metronidazole** 500 mg IV q 6 hours or **doxycycline** 100 mg IV q 12 hours. If the patient is allergic to penicillin IV **erythromycin** 2 g/day or **tetracycline** 2 g/day can be substituted.
- Muscle relaxation with **diazepam** 10 mg IV q 1 to 3 hours prn is essential to control reflex painful muscle spasms.
- Prolonged neuromuscular blockade can be achieved with intravenous atracurium or pancuronium.
- Autonomic instability should be controlled with appropriate medications. Consult an intensivist for help in managing the treatment.

References/Further Reading

1. Carden DL, Joel LM. Tetanus. In: Tintinalli JE, Ma OJ, Stapczynski JS, et al, eds. *Tintinalli's Emergency Medicine: A Comprehensive Study Guide*. 7th ed. New York: McGraw-Hill; 2011: 1047–1049.

2. Applegate CN, Fox PT. Neurologic emergencies in internal medicine. In: Dunagan WC, Rindner ML, eds. *Manual of Medical Therapeutics*. 26th ed. St. Louis, MO: Little Brown Co.; 1989: 480–481.

3. CDC. Diphtheria, tetanus, and pertussis: Recommendations for vaccine use and other preventive measures. Recommendations of the Advisory Committee on Immunization Practices (ACIP). *MMWR*. 1991; 40(RR–10): 1–28.

Irwani Ibrahim • Peter Manning

CAVEATS

- It should be emphasized that blood and blood products should be administered only when they are clearly indicated and that safer alternatives should be used whenever possible. Replacement therapy should consist only of the component that the patient needs, administered in the smallest volume possible.

- The following **precautions** should be taken:

  1. The first 2 units of whole blood or red cell concentrates may be administered direct from the refrigerator. Warming is necessary when large volumes are given rapidly, i.e. at rates of >50 ml/kg/hr. In these cases, blood should only be warmed as it passes through the infusion set.

  2. Blood components must be transfused through standard blood filters designed to retain blood clots and other debris. The exceptions are platelets and cryoprecipitate that should be transfused using the respective infusion sets provided.

  3. In general, blood should **not be transfused** through infusion sets used for other fluids. Some may cause haemolysis (e.g. **5% dextrose in water**) and other clotting (e.g. **Hartmann's solution**). Only normal saline may be used for flushing infusion sets for blood transfusions. No medication or intravenous (IV) solutions other than normal saline may be added to blood or its components.

  4. Flow at high pressure or through small gauge needles may damage red cells. An 18G or 19G needle gives a good flow rate.

- During the administration of blood products a close watch must be kept on the patient for early signs of transfusion reaction (see below).

BLOOD AND BLOOD PRODUCTS

Whole Blood

- In patients with acute blood loss, the restoration of blood volume is more important than red cell replacements. Crystalloids and/or colloids can be used initially in these circumstances, reducing the need for blood transfusions.

- **Indications for whole blood transfusion**

  1. Acute haemorrhage (despite normal haemoglobin and haematocrit levels).

  NOTE: Following acute blood loss, haemoglobin (Hb) and haematocrit (Hct) may remain normal or nearly normal for ≥1 hour. Loss of approximately 20% of blood volume can safely be corrected by crystalloid solutions alone.

2. Blood loss >25% of the total blood volume.

3. At-risk patients (Table 1) developing signs and symptoms (Table 2).

TABLE 1   Patient groups at risk from intravascular volume depletion

1. Patients at risk for myocardial ischaemia
2. Coronary artery disease
3. Valvular heart disease
4. Congestive cardiac failure
5. Patients at risk for cerebral ischaemia
6. History of transient ischaemic attacks
7. Previous thrombotic strokes

TABLE 2   Signs and symptoms requiring blood transfusion in normovolaemic patients at risk

1. Syncope
2. Dyspnoea
3. Postural hypotension
4. Tachycardia
5. Angina
6. Transient ischaemic attack

Red Blood Cells

- **Indications for transfusions of red blood cells**

  1. Slow continuous blood loss.

  2. Acute and chronic leukaemia.

  3. Chronic anaemia due to bone marrow failure, uraemia, and severe symptomatic iron deficiency or megaloblastic anaemia.

- The patient's condition, **not** laboratory test result, is the most important factor in determining transfusion needs.

- Whole blood is **contraindicated in patients with chronic anaemia** because of the risk of overload.

- **One unit of red cells** should **raise** the non-bleeding **adult's Hb** by about **1 g/dl** and the **Hct** by about **3%**.

Platelets

- **Indications for platelet transfusions**

  1. A severely thrombocytopaenic patient in whom life-threatening haemorrhage is occurring or is likely, and who usually has a platelet count of $<20 \times 10^9/l$.

  2. After a transfusion of 15–20 units of whole blood or red blood cells.

NOTE: Platelet counts often fall below 80–100 × 10^9/l and platelet transfusions may be indicated for adequate haemostasis underlying major surgery or treatment of severe trauma. The decision to administer platelets should rest on the actual count and not on the replacement formula based on the number of units transfused.

- The emphasis is to treat the patient and not the laboratory result.

Fresh Frozen Plasma (FFP)

- FFP contains all the clotting factors.
- **Indications**
  1. Replacement of single coagulation factor deficiencies when specific or combined concentrates are not available.
  2. Immediate reversal of warfarin effect in patients at risk of life-threatening haemorrhage.
- In massive transfusion (defined as the replacement of a patient's total blood volume within 24 hours), there is no evidence that prophylactic replacement regimes with FFP prevent abnormal bleeding or reduce transfusion requirements. FFP is recommended only in the presence of bleeding and disturbed coagulation.

Cryoprecipitate

Cryoprecipitate is rich in factor VIII, fibrinogen, and von Willebrand factor. It is used as a replacement therapy in patients with von Willebrand's syndrome or haemophilia A when viral inactivated factor VIII concentrates are not available.

Factor VIII and Factor IX

Viral inactivated factor VIII or factor IX concentrates are used for the treatment of haemophilia A and haemophilia B, respectively. See Table 3.

Haemophilia A

Factor VIII (IU) needed = Weight (kg) × Level desired × 0.5

NOTE: One vial of factor VIII contains 250 IU.

Haemophilia B

- Factor IX (IU) needed = Weight (kg) × Level desired

NOTE: One vial of factor IX contains 500 IU.

- Haemophilia patients with inhibitors should be managed with a haematologist.

TABLE 3 **Factor concentrate level guidelines**

Mild bleeding (level desired 30%)	Moderate bleeding (level desired 50%)	Severe bleeding (level desired 75–100%)
1. Minor or single joint bleeding	1. Major or multiple joint bleeding	1. Intracranial bleeding
2. Muscle bleeding	2. Neck, tongue, pharynx bleeding (without airway compromise)	2. Major operation
3. Epistaxis		3. Major trauma
4. Dental bleeding	3. Abdominal bleeding	4. Compartment syndrome
5. Haematuria	4. Head trauma without neurological deficit	5. Neck, tongue, pharynx bleeding (with airway compromise)

Emergency Blood Transfusion

- **Emergency blood group 'O'** should not be used indiscriminately. It is safer and equally effective in emergencies to make use of crystalloids or colloids first and then matched blood.
- **Group 'O' positive** is used as emergency blood for **Chinese and Malay** patients.
- **Group 'O' negative** should be used for **Indian and Caucasian patients** especially females in the reproductive groups.
- **The following are categories of blood according to urgency**:
  1. **Unmatched emergency blood**, available instantly (no blood group match and no antibody screen).
  2. **Rapid-match blood**, available in 5 to 10 minutes (with blood group match but no antibody screen).
  3. **Full-matched blood**, available in 30–45 minutes (with blood group match and antibody screen).
- **Complications of transfusions (immediate reactions)**:
  1. **Haemolytic reaction**: The most serious immediate reaction (0.03% of all transfusions with mortality rate of 10–40%). This reaction most commonly appears before completion of the transfusion of the first unit of blood.
     a. The patient complains of fever, chills, low back and joint pain, and a sensation of chest tightness. A burning sensation is frequently felt at the IV site. It may also manifest shock.
     b. **Management** is directed towards the prevention of shock and renal cortical hypoperfusion.
        i. Terminate the transfusion immediately.
        ii. Administer vigorous IV fluid therapy and IV frusemide 80–100 mg to maintain a urine output of at least 30 ml/hr.
        iii. Give IV hydrocortisone 200 mg for adult (5 mg/kg for a child).
        iv. Obtain immediate haematology consultation in the emergency department.

2. **Febrile reaction**: The most common (3–4% of all transfusions) and least serious transfusion reaction.

NOTE: However, it is impossible clinically, in the early stages, to differentiate the febrile reaction from the more serious immediate haemolytic reaction.

    a. Patient complains of fever, chills, and malaise.

    b. **Management**:

       i. Terminate the transfusion immediately.

       ii. Administer antipyretics.

       iii. Give IV hydrocortisone 200 mg for adult (5 mg/kg for a child).

       iv. Obtain immediate haematology consultation in the emergency department.

3. **Allergic reaction**: Rare (1% of all transfusions) and occurs before 10 ml of blood has been transfused.

    a. Patient complains of chills and generalized pruritis.

    b. Clinical signs: Hypotension, skin flushing, possible urticaria, and angioedema.

    c. **Management**:

       i. Slow the transfusion rate immediately if only urticaria is present but terminate the tranfusion if fever, angioedema, and hypotension develop.

       ii. Give IV antihistamines.

       iii. Give IV hydrocortisone 200 mg (5 mg/kg for a child).

Acknowledgement

The authors thank Dr Tien Sim Leng, head of the Singapore General Hospital (SGH) Blood Transfusion Services, for providing Reference 1, the basis for most of the information in this chapter.

Reference/Further Reading

1. *Singapore General Hospital Blood Transfusion Guidelines*. 2nd ed. Singapore: SGH Internal Publication. 2nd ed. 1997.

78 Oncology Emergencies

Toh Hong Chuen • Shirley Ooi

CAVEATS

- Patients with malignancies are prone to emergencies either arising from the malignancy or related treatment.
- There are some **important principles** to follow when managing them in the emergency department:
  1. Consult the primary oncologist, especially if the patient is for discharge so as to facilitate follow-up.
  2. As these patients have been 'through the system' on numerous occasions, involving the senior clinician early with early symptom management (such as pain control) is all desirable.
  3. It is useful to find out the extent of the malignancy, the patient's response to the treatment, what the prognosis is and the treatment objectives so as to decide on palliative care versus active treatment. This is especially important if the patient presents in a critical condition and a decision must be made quickly as to whether active resuscitation should proceed.
- The **4 most common and life-threatening oncologic emergencies** are:
  1. Neutropaenic sepsis
  2. Thrombocytopaenia
  3. Hypercalcaemia
  4. Cord compression
- Reduction of mortality from neutropaenic sepsis is dependent on the speed of administration of intravenous (IV) antibiotics.

⇨ **SPECIAL TIPS FOR GPs**

- Do not attempt to treat oncology patients presenting with a fever by administering antibiotics or antipyretics in the office. Refer immediately to the emergency department, especially if the fever is >38°C.
- Afebrile patients who report a history of fever should be treated as if they are currently febrile.
- Suspect **hypercalcaemia** in all oncology patients who are generally unwell.
- Think of **bony metastases** with a possibility of **cord compression** in all oncology patients presenting with back pain. Do not dismiss it as being due to 'arthritis'.

NEUTROPAENIC FEVER

- This is an emergency and is the most common fatal side effect of chemotherapy.

Definitions

- **Neutropaenia**: A condition of an abnormally low level of neutrophils in the blood; neutrophil count is <500 cells/mm^3 or <1000 cell/mm^3 with a predicted decrease to <500 cells/mm^3. The occurrence of neutropaenia depends on the type of chemotherapeutic agent given, for periods ranging from 1 to 4 weeks. The incidence and severity of infection in cancer patients with neutropaenia are inversely proportional to the absolute neutrophil count and duration of neutropaenia.
- **Fever**: ≥38.3°C or 2 readings of ≥38°C or for ≥1 hour. The temperature should be taken orally or tympanically, not rectally. Although uncommon, immuno-compromised patients can have serious local or systemic infections without fever, manifesting as unexplained tachypnoea or tachycardia, altered mental state, metabolic acidosis or electrolyte abnormalities such as hypoglycaemia or hyponatraemia.

NOTE: Patients with neutropaenia may have few of the classic signs and symptoms of bacterial infection because of an inadequate number of circulating white blood cells.

Management

- All patients undergoing chemotherapy/radiotherapy with fever should be managed at least in the intermediate care area with high priority. Early clinical assessment with a careful search for the site of infection is important. Due to the impaired immune response, only 20% of neutropaenic patients have an identified focus of infection at presentation.
- **Investigations** include:
  1. Full blood count
  2. Urea/electrolytes/creatinine
  3. Liver function test
  4. CXR[1]
  5. Urine dipstick and culture[2]
  6. Blood culture (aerobic and anaerobic) × 2 sets.

NOTE: If the patient has an indwelling central line in place, at least one set of blood culture should be obtained through the line.

  7. Culture of any purulent drainage.

---

[1] CXR has a high false negative rate, as pneumonia is detected on high-resolution computed tomography (HRCT) in more than half of febrile neutropaenic patients with normal findings on CXR.
[2] A patient with urinary tract infection may present in a subtle fashion because white blood cells do not deposit in the urinary tract and produce the typical symptoms of dysuria and frequency. Thus, every neutropaenic patient should have a urine culture done.

- **Antibiotics**

  Early institution of broad spectrum antibiotics is critical in neutropaenic fever. The choice and route of antibiotics depend on risk assessment as indicated by the MASCC (Multinational Association of Supportive Care in Cancer) score:

  1. **Choice of antibiotics**[3]

Low risk[4] (≥21)		High risk (<21)	
On quinolone prophylaxis?		Septic shock[5] **or** colonization/infection by cephalosporin–resistant enterobacteriaceae <3 months	
Yes	**No**	**Yes**	**No**
IV piptazo **or** IV cefepime **or** IV ceftazidime	Oral augmentin **and** oral fluoroquinolone	IV imipenem **or** IV meropenem	IV piptazo **or** IV cefepime **or** IV ceftazidime

  2. **Antibiotic dosages**

Antibiotic	Creatinine clearance (ml/min/1.73m^2)			
	Normal	**>30–50**	**>10–30**	**<10**
Augmentin (oral)	625 mg tds	625 mg tds	625 mg bd	625 mg od
Ciprofloxacin (oral)	750 mg bd	500 mg bd	500 mg od	250 mg od
Levofloxacin (oral and IV)	750 mg OM	750 mg eod	500 mg eod	500 mg eod
Ceftazidime[6] (IV)	2g q8 hr	2g q12 hr	2g q24 hr	2g q48 hr
Cefepime (IV)	2g q8 hr	2g q12 hr	2g q24 hr	1g q24 hr
Piperacillin/tazobactam[7] (IV)	4.5g q6 hr	2.25g q6 hr	(20–40 ml/min)	2.25g q8 hr
Imipenem (IV)	500 mg q6 hr	500 mg q6 hr	250 mg q6 hr	250 mg q12 hr
Meropenem (IV)	1g q8 hr	1g q12 hr	(26–50 ml/min)	500 mg q24 hr
Aztreonam (IV)	2g q8 hr	2g q8 hr	1g q8 hr	500 mg q8 hr
Vancomycin (IV)	1g q12 hr	10–15 mg/kg/dose q24 hr or as determined by serum concentration monitoring.		

- **Disposition**: Admit to Haematology-Oncology isolation room with positive pressure.

---

[3] Severe penicillin/cephalosporin allergy: Use IV aztreonam **and** IV vancomycin as the empirical antibiotics of choice.

[4] A patient with an overt central line infection should be given IV vancomycin as well.

[5] A patient in septic shock with a central line in-situ should be given IV vancomycin as well.

[6] Ceftazidime monotherapy is NOT recommended in patients with severe mucositis or suspected pneumonia.

[7] Pip/tazo (piperacillin/tazobactam) administration may result in a false-positive serum galactomannan result.

NOTE:

1. There is no need for intramuscular injections, urinary catheters, or per rectal examinations unless they are critical to management.

2. For patients on chemotherapy/radiotherapy with fever but who are not neutropaenic, treat as per usual sepsis protocol. Consult the primary physician early in the course of management of these patients, especially with regard to disposition.

THROMBOCYTOPAENIA

- There is a significant chance of central nervous system bleeding if the platelet count is <20,000/µl.

Management

- GXM random platelets: 6 units
- **Precautions**:
  1. Avoid intramuscular injections.
  2. Avoid non-steroidal anti-inflammatory drugs (NSAIDs).
  3. Ensure complete rest in bed.
- Platelet transfusion may be needed if the patient has active bleeding, the afebrile patient has a count of <10,000 or the febrile patient has a count of <20,000. For the haematology patient, consult the primary haematologist with regard to the type of platelets required (e.g. irradiated platelets).
- **Disposition**: Admit to Haematology-Oncology general ward.

HYPERCALCAEMIA OF MALIGNANCY

- **Definition:** Albumin-corrected serum calcium ≥3 mmol/L.
- **Prevalance** of hypercalcaemia in malignancy ranges from 15 to 60%. This is especially common in patients with solid organ cancer involving the breast, kidney and lung, and haematological malignancies such as myeloma and lymphoma.
- Suspect hypercalcaemia in all **cancer** patients who **do not feel well**. If undiagnosed and untreated, it can be life-threatening!
- The **pathogenesis** of hypercalcaemia includes the production of parathyroid hormone (PTH) related protein[8], production of bone-resorbing cytokines (such as transforming growth factor-alpha or TGF-alpha), osteolytic effect of bone metastasis and tumour-mediated calcitriol production.

---

[8] Homologous to PTH in its 13 N-terminal amino acids, producing the effects of PTH on the PTH receptor but not subjected to the usual feedback mechanism.

- The **clinical features** of hypercalcaemia are non-specific; these include the following:
  1. **Neurological**: Fatigue, weakness, confusion, stupor or even coma (by decreasing neuronal conduction).
  2. **Gastrointestinal**: Constipation and ileus (by decreasing smooth muscle tone). Other common gastrointestinal effects include anorexia, nausea, vomiting and abdominal pain. Chronically, hypercalcaemia is associated with increased risk of peptic ulcer disease and pancreatitis.
  3. **Renal**: Polyuria, polydipsia, dehydration and electrolyte losses (acute rise in serum calcium levels impairs reabsorption of fluids and electrolytes). Chronically elevated serum calcium associated with volume depletion predisposes the patient to renal calculi.
  4. **Cardiovascular**: Hypotension from volume depletion may be masked because hypercalcaemia increases vascular tone. Electrocardiogram (ECG) changes include shortened QTc interval, prolonged PR interval and widened QRS. Remember that hypercalcaemia can potentiate the effects of digoxin.

Investigations

- Serum ionized calcium, phosphate, magnesium, urea, electrolytes and ECG

Management

- The **management** involves 4 basic steps:
  1. **Restore intravascular volume**: 2–5 litres of fluid per day are often required. The increase in glomerular filtration rate (GFR) will increase renal calcium clearance.
  2. **Enhance elimination of renal calcium**: Loop diuretics, such as IV **frusemide** (20 mg q 6 hourly) should only be used after intravascular volume has been restored.
  3. **Decrease osteoclastic activity**: Bisphosphonates, such as IV **zoledronic** acid, inhibits osteoclastic bone resorption and decreases the viability of osteoclasts. This could be started in the general ward due to its long onset of action.
  4. **Treatment of underlying malignancy**.
- **Disposition**: Admit to Haematology-Oncology general ward.

CORD COMPRESSION

- As many as 5% of all cancer patients will develop metastases to the spine and spinal cord at some point in the course of their disease.
- This complication usually signifies advanced malignancy and a limited survival.
- The ability to walk and remain independent contributes immensely to the quality of life of an oncology patient. Hence, cord compression is a **true emergency**, as the prognosis for regaining function is at least in part related to early diagnosis and institution of treatment.

- Most spinal metastases spread via haematogenous dissemination to the vertebral body, with subsequent expansion into the epidural space, causing epidural cord compression. The incidence of involvement of the cervical, thoracic and lumbar spine regions is 10%, 70% and 20% respectively. Multiple spinal levels are affected in about 30% of the cases. Metastasis to the substance of the cord is relatively rare and can present as unilateral limb weakness.
- Back pain with neurological finding, atypical features, or in patients with symptoms suggestive of undiagnosed cancer should have urgent follow-up arranged.

Presenting signs and symptoms

- >95% of patients have **back pain** (localized or radicular). Pain precedes other symptoms of spinal cord compression by 2–4 months. Back pain worsened by coughing or lying supine or is worse at night should be considered suspect.
- **Localized tenderness** on palpation.
- **Paraplegia** and **bladder/bowel incontinence** are usually late presentation (they may be an early presentation if the conus medullaris is involved). Do not wait for them to occur! However very frequently in cauda equina syndrome, the urinary incontinence is actually OVERFLOW incontinence and may not be a late sign. In other words, the main problem is urinary retention with incontinence occurring because the bladder is full and urine is therefore spilling out in small amounts; a post-void residual or bladder scan to assess for bladder distension is often helpful. Other late signs include **sensory disturbances** and **hyperreflexia**.

Management

- Do **plain X-rays of the spine** (85% sensitivity) to look for:
  1. Vertebral collapse (87% sensitivity)
  2. Pedicle destruction (31%)
  3. Lytic destruction (7%)
- **Practical approaches**:
  1. **Back pain and no neurological deficit**
     a. Do plain X-rays. If normal, perform a non-urgent bone scan.
     b. If abnormal, perform early magnetic resonance imaging (MRI) of the spine.
  2. **Back pain with neurological deficit**: Administer **steroids (IV dexamethasone 8 mg bolus)** first in patients with known history of cancer (pathology established):
     a. As soon as cord compression is confirmed or strongly suggested **or**
     b. In the presence of a collapsed vertebra **or**
     c. Absence of the pedicles is noted on plain X-rays.

Contact the oncologist immediately; keep in view urgent MRI of the spine.

NOTE: In the absence of a known diagnosis of cancer, **do not start steroids**, but contact an oncologist for further advice.

SYNDROME OF INAPPROPRIATE ANTIDIURETIC HORMONE (SIADH)

- This is usually caused by the release of anti-diuretic hormone from ectopic sites such as lung cancer. The resulting hyponatraemia may be life-threatening when serious central nervous system manifestations such as coma and seizures develop.

- **Acute symptomatic hyponatraemia (seizure or coma)** should be treated aggressively with **3% hypertonic saline** at a rate of approximately 1–2 ml/kg/hr in order to raise the serum sodium by 2.5 mEq/hr to a level above a theoretical seizure threshold, around 120 mEq/L. Once this is achieved, hypertonic saline infusion should be stopped. Frequent laboratory assessment is essential to ensure both the desired rate and the target level of correction are not exceeded, to prevent the feared complication of osmotic demyelination syndrome.

- Hyponatraemia that is chronic in nature should be corrected slowly at a rate of no more than 0.5 mEq/hr over a 24-hour period. Mild hyponatraemia secondary to SIADH includes free water restriction of 500 ml to 1 litre per day.

HYPERVISCOSITY SYNDROME AND LEUCOSTASIS SYNDROME

- The normal relative serum viscosity is between 1.4–1.8 centipoises. **Clinical symptoms** of hyperviscosity syndrome are rare unless the serum viscosity exceeds 4.0 centipoises. Directly related to microcirculatory occlusion, these include changes in mental state, unexplained dyspnoea or headache.

- This **diagnosis** must be considered in patients with haematologic malignancies, especially Waldenstrom's macroglobulinaemia, multiple myeloma, acute leukaemia with blast crisis, and polycythaemia, presenting with these symptoms.

- The **treatment** in the emergency department should be aimed at the assessment of the ABCs (airway, breathing and circulation) and the team should initiate resuscitative efforts. Begin aggressive intravenous hydration. Other efforts to lower the serum viscosity include phlebotomy and plasmapharesis. Consult the haematologist.

- **Leucostasis syndrome**, a condition defined by tissue hypoperfusion secondary to elevated white blood cells, is most commonly symptomatic when leucocyte counts approach 100,000/μl. It can also be seen in certain types of monoblastic leukaemias when the count is less elevated, at around 25,000–50,000/μl.

- As with hyperviscosity syndrome, begin treatment of leucostasis syndrome with aggressive intravenous hydration. Other key principles include rapid lowering of peripheral white blood cell counts (leucopharesis or whole blood phlebotomy) and to pre-empt the development of **tumour lysis syndrome** (hyperkalaemia, hyperuricaemia, hyperphosphataemia and renal failure). The latter can be achieved by aggressive intravenous hydration, oral phosphate binders (e.g. aluminium hydroxide 50–150 mg/kg daily), allopurinol (600 mg stat in the emergency department) and hydroxyurea (50–100 mg/kg daily), while awaiting chemotherapy.

MASSIVE PLEURAL EFFUSION CAUSING RESPIRATORY COMPROMISE

- Patients present with breathlessness, classical clinical signs of 'stony dullness', impaired vocal resonance, reduced breath sounds on auscultation and a 'white out' hemithorax on the chest X-ray. Tracheal and mediastinal deviation may be present.
- Compare current chest films with previous ones.

Management

- Prop up patient and administer supplemental oxygen to maintain oxygen saturation level (SpO_2) at more than 95%.
- Monitor patient.
- Insert chest tube size 28–32 F on the affected side.

PERICARDIAL EFFUSION CAUSING ACUTE BREATHLESSNESS

- Pericardial effusions are particularly common in lung cancers, but can occur with other malignancies such as lymphoma, due to pericardial metastases.
- Recognition of this condition may be difficult but it should be suspected on **clinical** grounds in the presence of:
  1. Sinus tachycardia
  2. Small voltages on ECG
  3. Clear breath sounds
  4. Elevated jugular venous pressure (**Kussmaul's sign**)
  5. Palpable **pulsus paradoxus** (a drop in systolic blood pressure of >10 mmHg on inspiration)
- **Diagnosis** is **confirmed** on transthoracic echocardiography.

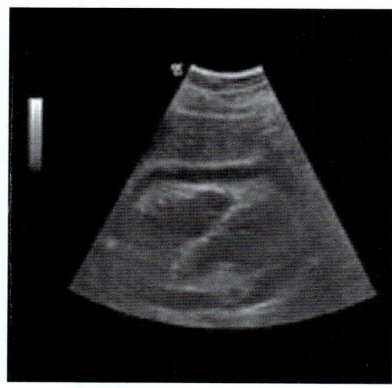

Pericardial effusion on ultrasound

Management

- In the presence of hypotension, urgent drainage is necessary. Refer to Cardiology for pericardiocentesis, which is temporary (definitive pericardial window should be performed eventually).

SUSPECTED MASSIVE PULMONARY EMBOLISM

- Refer to Chapter 41, *Pulmonary Embolism*.

SUPERIOR VENA CAVA SYNDROME

- Refer to Chapter 42, *Venous Emergencies*.

Acknowledgement

The authors would like to thank the National University Cancer Institute, Singapore, for sharing with us their protocol in the care of oncological emergency patients.

References/Further Reading

1. Hughes WT, et al. *Guidelines for the Use of Antimicrobial Agents in Neutropenic Patients with Cancer*. Infectious Disease Society of America; 2002.

2. Ugras–Rey S, Watson M. Chapter 121: Selected oucologic emergencies. In: Marx J, Hockberger RS, Walls RM, eds. *Rosen's Emergency Medicine: Concepts and Clinical Practice*. 7th ed. Philadelphia, PA: Mosby-Elsevier; 2010.

3. Huff JS. *Neoplasm, Spinal Cord*. 17 Sep 2007. Available at: http://emedicine.medscape.com/article/779872-overview.

4. Roger RL. Management of haematology/oncology patients in the ED. In: Mattu A, Goyal D, eds. *Emergency Medicine. Avoiding the Pitfalls and Improving the Outcomes*. Malden, MA: Blackwell Publishing; 2008: 93–98.

79 Overwarfarinization

Gene Chan • Shirley Ooi

CAVEATS

- The commonest cause of a falsely-elevated international normalized ratio (INR) is the presence of heparin in the blood sample. To avoid this, obtain blood from a peripheral vein instead of from the indwelling central venous catheter which might be contaminated with heparin.
- The second commonest cause is inadequate filling of the collection tubes, resulting in a higher than normal ratio of citrate anti-coagulant to patient plasma.
- Warfarin is a commonly-used oral anti-coagulant for a variety of clinical conditions.
- Patients who are on long-term oral warfarin are monitored using the **INR** aimed at a predetermined desired therapeutic range depending on clinical condition. INR provides a measurement of the extrinsic pathway of clotting cascade. INR is more reproducible and has replaced the prothrombin time (PT) ratio which varied previously due to the reagent or tissue factor used.
- The **reference range** for INR is 0.8 to 1.2 seconds while that for PT is 7 to 10 seconds.
- In general, the **target INR (range)** for deep venous thrombosis, pulmonary embolism, atrial fibrillation, mitral valve stenosis, cardiomyopathy, and ischaemic cerebrovascular disease is 2.5 (2.0–3.0) while that for mechanical heart valve is 3.0 (2.5–3.5).
- The **necessity for intervention and urgency of reversal of the INR** depends on the following:
  1. Reason the patient is anti-coagulated.
  2. Desired therapeutic INR range.
  3. Presence of local pathology or systemic disease that predisposes to bleeding tendencies.
  4. Site and severity of haemorrhage, when present.
- The **haemorrhagic complications** of anti-coagulation include:
  1. Intracranial haemorrhage.
  2. Gastrointestinal bleeding.
  3. Haemarthrosis.
  4. Compartment syndrome.
  5. Haematuria.
  6. Haemothorax.
  7. Haemopericardium.
  8. Spinal epidural haematoma.

NOTE: Consider this diagnosis in patients with midline back pain. Do a full neurological examination including a rectal examination to check for cauda equine syndrome.

9. Retroperitoneal haemorrhage.

NOTE: Consider this diagnosis in flank, back, or abdominal pain although there may be minimal or no abdominal tenderness. Paresthesias and pain may radiate along the lumbar plexus or femoral nerve distribution due to compression of these nerves. Look for ecchymoses in the periumbilical area (**Cullen's sign**), flank (**Turner's sign**), upper thigh, inferior to the inguinal ligament (**Fox's sign**), and scrotum (**blue scrotum sign of Bryant**).

10. Rectus sheath haematoma.

RISK FACTORS

- **Drug interactions**, e.g. antibiotics (sulphonamide, amoxicillin, metronidazole, fluoroquinolones including levofloxacin and doxycyline), non-steroidal anti-inflammatory drugs, paracetamol, anti-epileptics (phenytoin), amiodarone, fibrates, and proton-pump inhibitors.
- **Food interactions**, e.g. alcohol, herbal supplements (ginseng, gingko, sweet clover, evening primrose oil, vitamins A and E, garlic, or ginger).
- **Superimposed diseases**, e.g. liver disease, fever, diarrhoea, malabsorption, and worsening heart failure.
- **Vitamin K deficiency** either from poor dietary intake or malabsorption.

> ⇨ **SPECIAL TIPS FOR GPs**
> - The risk of bleeding increases dramatically with INR values of more than 4.0.
> - All patients on warfarin who have suffered a head injury have to be referred to the emergency department for intracranial imaging. This applies even to those who have sustained mild head injury and are asymptomatic at the time of presentation.

MANAGEMENT

- Degree of intervention and urgency of reversal depends on the presence of bleeding and its seriousness (refer to Table 1).
- When required, vitamin K can either be given via the oral or intravenous route. Both are effective.
- **Oral vitamin K** causes a reduction in INR within **24 hours**; **intravenous** (IV) **vitamin K** will reduce INR within **6 to 8 hours**. However, IV vitamin K may cause severe anaphylactoid reactions and cardiac or respiratory arrest despite precautions such as slow infusion and dilution. Do **NOT infuse faster than 1 mg/min**. IV vitamin K can be diluted with either NS or D5W. **Due to these potential reactions, the oral route replacement is preferred except in cases of serious or life-threatening bleeding**. The oral form is well absorbed except in gastrointestinal bleeding.

TABLE 1 **Management of supratherapeutic INR**

INR	Presence of bleeding	Recommended action			
		Warfarin	**Vitamin K**	**FFP/factor VIIa**	**Next INR check**
<5.0	No	Omit 1 dose. Resume at a lower dose when INR is in therapeutic range	–	–	1–2 days
5.0–9.0	No	Omit 1 to 2 doses. Resume at a lower dose when INR is in therapeutic range	PO 1 mg in the presence of increased bleeding risk/previous bleeding	–	1 day
>9.0	No	Withhold warfarin. Resume at a lower dose when INR is in therapeutic range	PO 1–2 mg may repeat as required	–	12–24 hours
Any value	Serious or life-threatening	Withhold warfarin	IV 10 mg via slow infusion may repeat as required	FFP 10–15 ml/kg Consider prothrombin complex concentrate or recombinant human factor VIIa	6–8 hours

- High doses of vitamin K, e.g. 10 mg, render the patient resistant to warfarin therapy. If anticoagulation is required subsequently, heparin or low molecular weight heparin should be given until vitamin K effects are reversed and the patient is responsive to warfarin again. Patients who receive oral vitamin K 1 mg are neither at risk of warfarin resistance nor increased thrombotic episodes.

- Vitamin K and fresh frozen plasma (FFP) should be given together if required because the INR may rebound if FFP is given alone.

- Type and screen must be sent to ensure compatibility of **FFP**. The thawing time for FFP is 30–45 minutes. Dose of FFP is 10–15 ml/kg, which can be a substantial fluid load. Alternatives to FFP include **prothrombin complex concentrate (PCC)** and **recombinant human factor VIIa (rFVIIa)**.

- If life-threatening haemorrhage is present, in addition to vitamin K and FFP, PCC, or rFVIIa can be given.

Special situations

- 'Superwarfarins' (coumafuryl and bromadiolone) are long-acting rodenticides which are up to 100 times more potent than warfarin.

- Their half-lives within the body can be in the order of weeks to months, compared to 40 hours for warfarin.
- Cases of poisoning with superwarfarins are normally due to accidental exposure or suicide attempts.
- Poisoned patients require massive doses of vitamin K (50–800 mg/day PO) over extended periods of time.
- Repeated monitoring of the INR and clinical status helps determine the duration of vitamin K treatment and the need for blood products with clotting factors.

Disposition

- If bleeding is not present, admit the patient to the unit that initiated warfarin and has been monitoring INR levels.
- If bleeding is present, refer to and admit to the appropriate discipline, e.g. intracranial haemorrhage to Neurosurgery and bleeding from the gastrointestinal tract to Gastroenterology or General Surgery, depending on local practice.

References/Further Reading

1. Ansell J, Hirsh J, Poller L, et al. The pharmacology and management of the vitamin K antagonists: The Seventh ACCP Conference on Antithrombotic and Thrombolytic Therapy. *Chest*. 2004; 126: 204S.

2. Chirputkar SK, Poole HJ, McNeil RC, et al. Reversal of asymptomatic overanticoagulation with oral vitamin K. *Br J Haematology*. 2006; 135: 591.

3. Hirsh J, et al. American Heart Association/American College of Cardiology Foundation Guide to warfarin therapy. *JACC*. 2003; 41: 1633–1652.

4. Lo J, Brown J, Levine M. Mild head injury, anti-coagulants, and risk of intracranial injury. *Lancet*. 2001; 357: 771.

5. Valentine KA. Hull RD. Correcting excess anticoagulation after warfarin – UptoDate. Aug 2007.

6. Jagoda AS, Bazarian JJ, Bruns JJ, et al. Clinical policy: Neuroimaging and decision making in adult mild traumatic brain injury in the acute setting. *Ann Emerg Med*. 2008; 52: 714–748. (ACEP Clinical Policy)

7. Hanlon D. An evidence-based approach to managing the anticoagulated patient in the emergency department. *Emergency Medicine Practice*. Jan 2011; 13(1).

80 Dermatology in Emergency Care

Emily Gan Yiping • Peng Li Lee • Shirley Ooi

CAVEATS

- In a febrile patient with purpuric rash, consider **meningococcaemia**.
- In an ill patient with petechial or purpuric rash, think of the possibility of **disseminated intravascular coagulation** from sepsis.
- In a hypotensive patient with joint pain and 'bruising', consider the possibility of **necrotizing soft tissue infections** which can be very deceptive in their initial presentation.
- It is still possible for a vaccinated person to have chickenpox although it is often very mild and may be mistaken for a 'viral fever'.
- Think of **varicella pneumonitis** if a patient has tachypnoea, cough, and high fever 3–5 days in the course of illness.

TABLE 1 Terminology in dermatology

Term	Description
Macule	Flat area of discoloration (can be pale, brown, black, or red) <1 cm in diameter
Patch	Large macule >1 cm in diameter
Papule	Raised lesion <1 cm in diameter
Nodule	Raised lesion >1 cm in diameter
Plaque	Raised lesion with a flat top
Vesicle	Fluid-filled lesion or blister <0.5 cm in diameter
Bulla	Larger fluid-filled lesion or blister
Pustule	Vesicle filled with neutrophils (not necessarily related to infections, e.g. pustular psoriasis comprises sterile lesions)
Annular	Ring-shaped lesion
Discoid	Flat and disc-like lesion (also called coin-like or nummular)
Erosion	Area of lost epidermis which generally heals without scarring
Ulcer	Area of skin loss involving the dermis
Fissure	A slit through the whole thickness of the skin

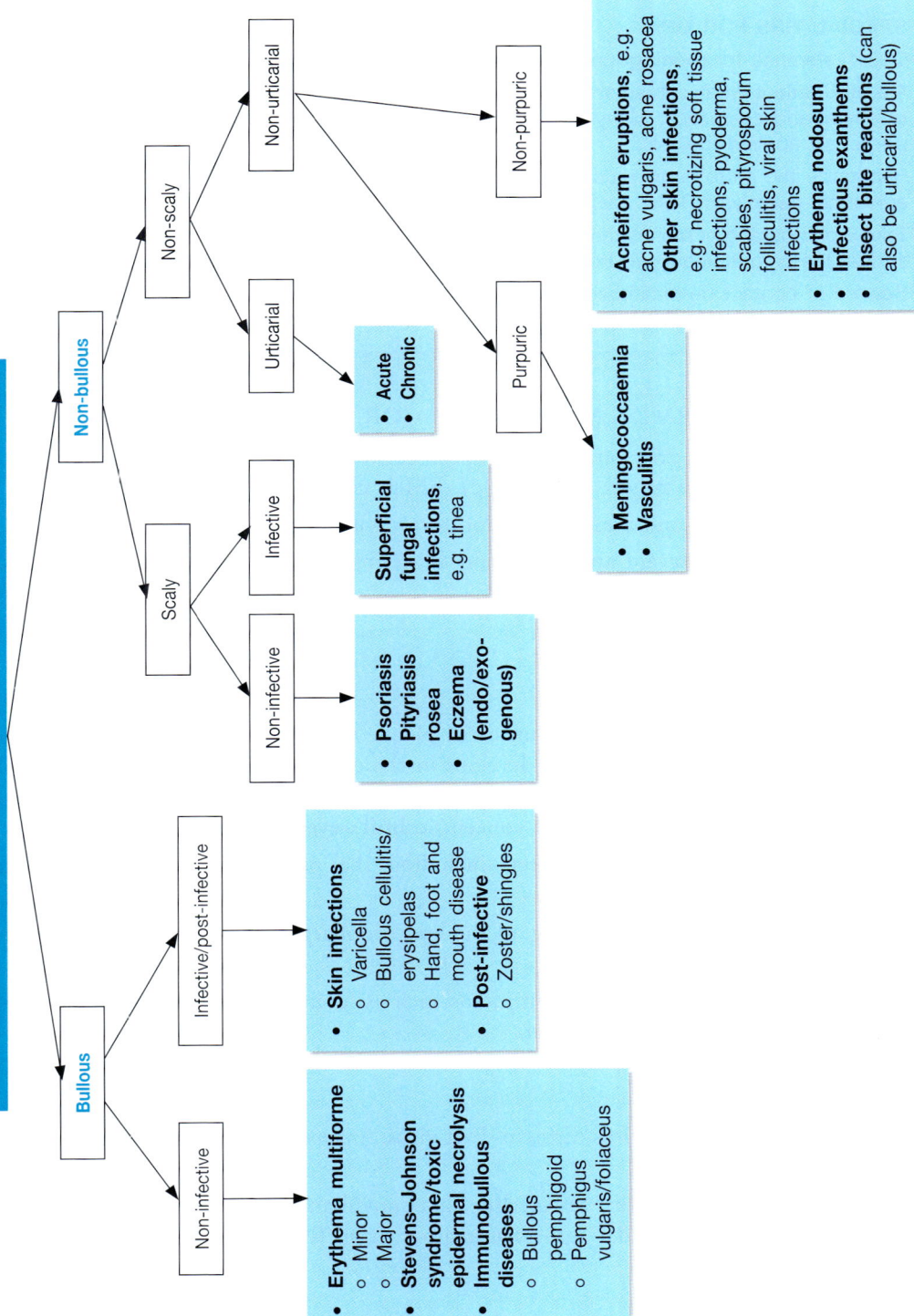

Approach to commonly-seen rashes in the emergency department

Bullous

Non-infective
- **Erythema multiforme**
  - Minor
  - Major
- **Stevens–Johnson syndrome/toxic epidermal necrolysis**
- **Immunobullous diseases**
  - Bullous pemphigoid
  - Pemphigus vulgaris/foliaceus

Infective/post-infective
- **Skin infections**
  - Varicella
  - Bullous cellulitis/erysipelas
  - Hand, foot and mouth disease
- **Post-infective**
  - Zoster/shingles

Non-bullous

Scaly

Non-infective
- **Psoriasis**
- **Pityriasis rosea**
- **Eczema (endo/exo-genous)**

Infective
- **Superficial fungal infections,** e.g. tinea

Non-scaly

Urticarial
- **Acute**
- **Chronic**

Non-urticarial

Purpuric
- **Meningococcaemia**
- **Vasculitis**

Non-purpuric
- **Acneiform eruptions,** e.g. acne vulgaris, acne rosacea
- **Other skin infections,** e.g. necrotizing soft tissue infections, pyoderma, scabies, pityrosporum folliculitis, viral skin infections
- **Erythema nodosum**
- **Infectious exanthems**
- **Insect bite reactions** (can also be urticarial/bullous)

Note: Generalized exfoliative dermatitis and **adverse cutaneous drug reactions** are separate entities which will be elaborated on in the chapter.

⇨ **SPECIAL TIPS FOR GPs**

- Quick reference for **meningococcaemia prophylaxis**: Single dose of ciprofloxacin 500 mg.
- Ask the patient what contactants he has been using, e.g. soap, topical medications, toiletries, and cosmetics. Many rashes present in cognito or in an altered form secondary to previously applied topicals.
- Recognize the more dangerous rashes, e.g. Stevens–Johnson syndrome (SJS)/toxic epidermal necrolysis (TEN), pustular psoriasis, and generalized exfoliative dermatitis.
- Take a photograph of rashes that appear unique and place the photograph in the patient's folder so that the dermatologist will be able to know what the rash looked like when it first presented.
- Beware of contact dermatitis aggravating initial lesions, especially if the patient has been treated before or has been applying over-the-counter medications or cosmetics.

ERYTHEMA MULTIFORME (EM): MINOR/MAJOR

- EM minor and major exist on a disease spectrum, distinct from Stevens-Johnson syndrome and Toxic epidermal necrolysis (see pg 532). EM is classified as follows:
  1. **EM minor**: Milder and a more common form, with minimal or no mucosal involvement.
  2. **EM major**: More severe and significant blistering and erosions of mucous membranes, potentially life-threatening.

Clinical features

- Non-pruritic and non-scaling.
- Initial lesion is a dull-red macule or urticarial plaque that expands slightly over 24–48 hours. A small papule, vesicle or bulla then develops in the centre which may clear. This is followed by the appearance of an intermediate raised pale and oedematous ring. The periphery then becomes violaceous forming a typical concentric **bull's-eye pattern** or **target lesion**.
- Usually starts in the hands and feet, including the palms and soles, before becoming generalized.
- **Erosions of mucous membranes**, e.g. of the lips, oropharynx, nasal, conjunctival, vulvar, and anal areas may be present.
- Usually preceded by constitutional symptoms such as fever, weakness, malaise, and symptoms of an upper respiratory tract infection.

Causes

- **Infections**: Herpes simplex virus, Epstein–Barr virus, *streptococcus*, and *mycoplasma* are common causes.
- **Drugs**: Sulfa drugs, penicillin, tetracycline, anticonvulsants (e.g. phenytoin, carbamazepine, and barbiturates), non-steroidal anti-inflammatory drugs (NSAIDs), allopurinol, hydrochlorothiazide, and procainamide.
- **Others**: Autoimmune causes.

Management

- Determine the **cause**:
    1. Medication review
    2. Symptomatology review for common infectious diseases
    3. Autoimmune diseases, e.g. Lupus erythematosus, Behcet's disease
- **EM minor**
    1. Provide reassurance if the cause is proven and there is no evidence of progression.
    2. Medications generally are not required as the rash is usually not pruritic or painful. Treat specific cause if found. Consider topical antiseptics for erosions.
    3. Schedule a follow-up in Dermatology/General Medicine.
- **EM major**
    1. Consider admitting the patient for inpatient care or get an urgent Dermatology consult.
    2. Provide general supportive care of fluid and electrolyte maintenance.
    3. Provide wound care.
    4. Control infection.
    5. Note that systemic steroids are controversial.

PEMPHIGOID AND PEMPHIGUS (Figures 1 and 2)*

- Both are bullous diseases due to an autoimmune process.
- The mainstay of treatment for both bullous diseases is **anti-inflammatory agents**.
- Skin biopsy is needed to confirm diagnosis.
- The differentiating clinical features are shown in Table 2.

TABLE 2   Differentiating features between pemphigoid and pemphigus

Features	Pemphigoid (prototype: Bullous pemphigoid)	Pemphigus (prototype: Pemphigus vulgaris)
Age	Elderly	Young/middle-aged
Lesions	Tense blisters	Flaccid blisters that break easily to leave erosions
	Itchy	Painful
	Mucous membrane often spared	Mucous membrane commonly involved; often the presenting feature
Prognosis	More benign	Potentially lethal

Management

- Depending on extent of involvement, both may **require inpatient management** for the following:
    1. Systemic corticosteroids ± immuno-suppressives.
    2. Local wound care.

* All images for this chapter can be found between pages 518 and 519.

3. Treatment of infection.
4. Correction of fluid and electrolyte loss from large areas of denuded skin.

VARICELLA (CHICKENPOX) (Figure 3)

- **Agent**: Varicella zoster virus (VZV).

Clinical features

- The **incubation period is** 10 to 21 days but is usually between 14 and 17 days.
- Usually preceded by prodromal symptoms that include low grade fever, malaise, and myalgia (can be absent in young children).
- Early lesions may be macular or papular before the vesicles appear, followed by crusting.
- Has a generalized distribution. The rash may appear on the scalp, genital areas, oral mucosa, and conjunctiva but predominantly on the trunk.
- Lesions appear in crops with differing stages of vesicles and crusting.
- Patients are **infectious** approximately 48 hours prior to the onset of vesicular rash, during the period of vesicle formation, generally four to five days, and until all vesicles are crusted.

Management

- Consider **acyclovir** if the patient is seen within the first 24–72 hours of the onset of the rash. Dosage:
  Children (2 years of age and older): oral acyclovir 20 mg/kg per dose 4 times daily (80 mg/kg/day) for 5 days.
  Maximum dose 3200mg/day.
  Children over 40 kg should receive the adult dose for varicella.
  Adults and Children over 40 kg: oral acyclovir 800 mg 4 times daily for 5 days
- Antihistamines for control of itch, e.g. chlorpheniramine 4 mg tds (three times daily).
- **Do not give aspirin** as an antipyretic as it may cause Reye's syndrome.
- Consider oral antibiotics if there are signs of bacterial infection, e.g. penicillin V (group A *streptococcus* is a common causative organism)/cephalexin/doxycycline (if penicillin/cephalexin allergic) or cloxacillin if *staphylococcus aureus* is suspected.
- Immuno-compromised patients should be admitted.

Complications

- Occur more commonly in adults and immuno-compromised patients: Aseptic meningitis, encephalitis, pneumonia, pneumonitis, transverse myelitis, and Reye's syndrome.
- **Foetal varicella syndrome** is associated with phocomelia; **neonatal varicella** can be fatal and can be transmitted intrapartum.
- Immunity can be rapidly determined by immunoglobulin G (IgG).

Isolation

- Advise isolation until no new vesicles erupt and all lesions are crusted.
- Pregnant women who are not immune should consider varicella zoster immune globulin (VZIg).

BULLOUS CELLULITIS/ERYSIPELA

Refer to the section on *Pyoderma*.

HAND, FOOT AND MOUTH DISEASE (HFMD) (Figure 4)

Clinical features

- Caused by **enteroviruses**, commonly coxsackievirus A16 and enterovirus 71.
- Highly contagious, spread by oral–oral and faecal–oral routes.
- **Incubation period** lasts three to six days. There is a **prodrome**, with 12–24 hours of low grade fever, malaise, abdominal pain, or respiratory symptoms.
- Cutaneous lesions begin as 2–8 mm macules or papules that quickly evolve into vesicles. Rupture of vesicles commonly occurs in the buttocks leading to the formation of erosions and crusts. Can be asymptomatic or painful and occurs together with or shortly after oral lesions.
- Mucosal lesions comprise 5–10 mm small punched out painful ulcers. These are preceded by macules which evolve into greyish vesicles and can be found on the hard palate, tongue, and buccal mucosa.

Management

- Most cases are **self-limited**.
- **Serious sequelae** include myocarditis, meningoencephalitis, aseptic meningitis, and spontaneous abortion in infections occurring in the first trimester of pregnancy. Look for signs of dehydration especially in young children who have severe oral ulcerations and food refusal.
- Symptomatic treatment includes topical lignocaine gel for oral ulcers and analgesia.
- Advise parents or patients on the importance of hand hygiene and isolation at home.
- Notify the Ministry of Health.

HERPES ZOSTER ('Shingles') (Figure 5)

Represents a reactivation of the latent varicella zoster virus.

Clinical features

- Characterized by painful vesicles in a unilateral dermatomal distribution.
- Common **sites** are the torso, scalp, and face.
- The **onset** of herpes zoster is heralded by pain within the affected dermatome that may precede lesions by 48–72 hours, followed by erythematous macules and papules which evolve rapidly to vesicular lesions.

- The total **duration** of the disease is generally between 7 and 10 days; however, it may take as long as 2 to 4 weeks before the skin returns to normal.
- **Atypical presentations**
  1. Pain unaccompanied by typical lesions.
  2. It may disseminate in immuno-compromised patients.
- **Trigeminal herpes zoster** with involvement of the opthalmic nerve (**zoster ophthalmicus**) may result in corneal ulcers and loss of vision. Always do a fluorescein staining to exclude corneal ulcers when vesicles are seen on the bridge of the nose (**Hutchinson's sign**) or around the eye and forehead.
- The most debilitating **complication** of herpes zoster is **pain** associated with acute neuritis and post-herpetic neuralgia.

NOTE: It is not possible to catch Shingles from another person. However, for a person who has never had varicella or the varicella vaccine, he can develop varicella by inhaling the virus particles.

Management

- **Pain control** with analgesia in the acute phase. Tricyclic anti-depressants, e.g. amitriptyline 10 mg ON (at night), may be considered for patients with persistent pain despite apparent healing of the lesions (**post-herpetic neuralgia**); other agents include gabapentin and narcotics (used in severe cases).
- **Antiviral agent**, e.g. acyclovir:
  1. Shown to shorten the course of herpes zoster if given within the first 48–72 hours of rash onset.
  2. Dosage: Oral acyclovir 800 mg 5 times a day for 7 to 10 days.
  3. Admit for intravenous acyclovir for immuno-compromised patients who are ill or with extensive disease.
- **Steroids** are ineffective in preventing post-herpetic neuralgia.
- Refer to Ophthalmology if there is corneal involvement.

PSORIASIS (Figures 6a and 6b)

Clinical features

- Psoriasis is usually diagnosed clinically. There are several different kinds of psoriasis, with chronic plaque psoriasis being the most common.
- In the emergency department, nail, scalp, erythrodermic, and pustular psoriasis may be encountered.
- **Chronic plaque psoriasis**: This is defined by sharply demarcated erythematous, dull-red plaques with loosely adherent, silvery-white scales. Removal of the scales results in minute blood droplets (**Auspitz's sign**). Thick scales may adhere tightly to the underlying skin, resulting in hyperkeratosis. Predilection sites include the elbows, knees, sacral–gluteal region,

scalp, hairline, palms/soles. The face is uncommonly involved. Lesions are often bilateral and symmetrical.

- **Nails**: Nail changes include pitting, subungual hyperkeratosis, ridging, onycholysis, and yellowish-brown spots under the nail plate (oil spots).
- **Scalp psoriasis**: Seen as sharply marginated pruritic plaques with thick adherent scales scattered discretely or diffusely on the entire scalp and hairline. Can occur alone or coexist with generalized psoriasis. This condition does not lead to hair loss.
- **Erythrodermic psoriasis**: Refer to the guidelines below on '**Generalized Exfoliative Dermatitis**'.
- **Pustular psoriasis (Von Zumbusch)**: This starts with a burning red erythema which spreads in hours, with the formation of clusters of pinpoint, non-follicular, and very superficial yellowish to whitish pustules. These usually become confluent, forming 'lakes of pus'. Prominent symptoms include fever, generalized weakness, and malaise.
- Potential **precipitating factors** include these:
  1. Drugs, e.g. beta blockers and anti-malarials, and the withdrawal of oral or potent topical corticosteroids.
  2. Environmental factors, e.g. heat.
  3. Trauma (**Köbner phenomenon**): Physical, chemical, electrical, surgical, infective, and inflammatory.
  4. Infections, e.g. human immunodeficiency virus (HIV) and streptococcal throat infection.
  5. Metabolic causes, e.g. hypocalcaemia (in pustular psoriasis).
  6. Stress.

Management

Refer all cases of psoriasis to Dermatology for follow-up.

CHRONIC PLAQUE PSORIASIS (PSORIASIS VULGARIS)

- **First line**: Topicals.
  1. Use **coal tar (*liquor picis carbonis*, LPC, 5%, 10%, 15%) cream ON**.
  2. Apply **topical corticosteroids OM (in the morning)** to the face, hairline, flexures, e.g. 0.025% betamethasone valerate cream.
  3. Use **salicylic acid 2% or 5%** on thick plaques. Add to LPC or topical steroids; inactivates calcipotriol.
- **Adjunctive therapy**
  1. Moisturizers, e.g. 10% urea cream, white soft paraffin, liquid paraffin 3:2, and aqueous cream.
  2. Washing agents, e.g. coal tar bath emulsion or soap and emulsifying ointment (soap substitute).

NAIL PSORIASIS

- Nail psoriasis is difficult to treat; patients are often refractory to topical therapies.
- **First line: Topical**, e.g. 0.1% betamethasone valerate ointment and calcipotriol ointment.

SCALP PSORIASIS

First line: Topicals.

- Apply coal tar shampoo (sufficient as monotherapy in mild cases).
- Add topical corticosteroids, e.g. 0.1% betamethasone valerate scalp lotion.
- For thick plaques, add cocois co ointment ON.

PUSTULAR PSORIASIS

- Admit the patient to an isolation ward.
- Give fluid replacement and order full blood count, urea/electrolytes/creatinine, corrected calcium levels, and blood cultures.
- Cover with antibiotics for any concomitant infection as patients are often febrile.
- Conduct urgent dermatology review in the ward. Rapid suppression is achieved with oral retinoids, e.g. acitretin. Systemic corticosteroids are to be avoided as withdrawal of steroids will precipitate a flare of pustular psoriasis.

PITYRIASIS ROSEA (Figure 7)

Clinical features

- A single herald patch precedes the exanthematous phase and develops over a period of one to two weeks.
- **Herald patch**: This is an oval, slightly raised salmon-red 2–5 cm plaque with a fine collarete scale at the periphery. May be multiple.
- **Exanthems**: These are fine scaling dull-pink papules and plaques with marginal collarete scattered in a '**Christmas tree**' pattern on the trunk and proximal aspects of the arms and legs. They are rarely found on the face.

Management

- **Symptomatic treatment**: Oral antihistamines for pruritus relief and reassurance are most important. Some centres advocate topical corticosteroids or a short course of systemic corticosteroids.

ECZEMA (Figure 8)

Clinical features

- Differentiate endogenous from exogenous eczema (irritant or allergic contact dermatitis). Sometimes both can exist in the same patient.

- There are several subtypes of endogenous eczema including atopic dermatitis, seborrhoeic dermatitis, hand/feet eczema, discoid eczema, stasis eczema, asteatotic eczema, and lichen simplex chronicus.

- Ask for family and personal history of atopy (allergic rhinitis, asthma, and eczema).

- Distribution of lesions varies according to different age groups in atopic dermatitis:
  1. Infants: Lesions affect the face, scalp, neck, extensor extremities, and trunk.
  2. Children: Lesions involve the flexures especially the antecubital and popliteal fossae, neck, and face.
  3. Adults: Similar distribution as in children.

- Differentiate the stages of eczema:
  1. **Acute**: Oedematous skin; erythematous patches, papules, plaques, papulovesicles, bullae, erosions; weeping, and crusting.
  2. **Subacute**: Erythema and scaling
  3. **Chronic**: Lichenification (thickening of the skin with accentuated skin markings), scaling, and fissuring (especially on the flexures, palms, fingers, and soles)

Management

- Use appropriate potency of topical corticosteroids (refer to Table 3).

- Examine for secondary bacterial infection and treat with topical or oral antibiotics.
  1. Topical antibiotics include tetracycline, fusidic acid, and mupirocin.
  2. Other topical antibiotics can be found in combination preparations with topical corticosteroids, e.g. betamethasone valerate/clioquinol 3% (has weak anti-bacterial and anti-fungal properties).
  3. Oral antibiotic options include cephalexin, cloxacillin with amoxicillin, amoxicillin–clavulanic acid, and erythromycin.

- Look for complicating factors, e.g. occupation (dishwasher), domestic causes and hobbies (gardening and cooking), topical medicament usage (concomitant contact dermatitis).

- Treat according to the stage of eczema:
  1. **Acute**: Wet compresses, e.g. potassium permanganate soaks/compresses; topical/oral antibiotics depending on a clinical suspicion of infection; and topical corticosteroids. Consider a short course of oral prednisolone with tapering doses.
  2. **Subacute**: Topical corticosteroid cream/ointment; moisturizers, e.g. aqueous cream (to face and flexures), urea 5% or 10% cream (more irritating, avoid fissured skin), white soft paraffin and liquid paraffin 3:2 (trunk and limbs); soap substitutes, e.g. emulsifying ointment; and antihistamines.
  3. **Chronic**: Topical corticosteroid ointment for thicker plaques; moisturizers; soap substitutes; and antihistamines.

- Refer to Dermatology for follow-up. More severe and recalcitrant cases may need treatment with systemic immuno-suppressives, phototherapy, etc.

TABLE 3   **Potency ranking of commonly prescribed corticosteroids**

Class	Ingredient	Brand name
I (most potent)	Betamethasone dipropionate 0.05% (optimized vehicle) Clobetasol propionate 0.05%	Diprocel Dermovate, Cloderm, Univate, Clobex lotion/spray
II	Betamethasone dipropionate ointment 0.05% Mometasone furoate ointment 0.1%	Diprosone Elomet
III	Betamethasone valerate ointment 0.1% Betamethasone dipropionate cream 0.05%	Betnovate Diprosone
IV	Fluocinolone acetonide ointment 0.025% Mometasone furoate cream 0.1%	Synalar Elomet
V	Betamethasone valerate cream 0.1% Fluocinolone acetonide cream 0.025%	Betnovate, Dermasone, Uniflex Synalar
VI	Fluocinolone acetonide cream 0.01% Desonide 0.05%	Synalar Desowen cream/lotion/ointment
VII (least potent)	Hydrocortisone acetate 1%	Dhacort, Egocort

SUPERFICIAL FUNGAL INFECTIONS

Clinical features

- **Tinea capitis**: Itchy scalp, broken hairs, scaling with pustules, swelling, and weeping.
- **Tinea corporis**: Enlarging itchy annular lesions with papules and scaling on the trunk and long limbs.
- **Tinea cruris**: Enlarging itchy annular lesions with papules and scaling in the groin region.
- **Tinea pedis**: Enlarging itchy annular lesions with papules, vesicles and scaling involving the feet. Toewebs are usually involved. Check for concomitant onychomycosis. (Differential diagnosis: hand and feet eczema.) **(Figure 9)**
- **Tinea versicolor**: Red, brown, white finely scaly itchy patches aggravated by heat and sweat. Can involve the face, trunk, and limbs. **(Figure 10)**
- **Candidal infection with underlying dermatitis**: Red papules, pustules, and scaling with signs of underlying dermatitis. **(Figure 11)**

Management

- Enquire about the previous use of topicals and over-the-counter medications as well as the duration of the disease. Many fungal infections may not be easily recognized in view of partial treatment (tinea incognito).
- Topical treatment should be commenced before oral medications.

- Refer to Dermatology before starting oral medications (a positive fungal scrape should be obtained prior to commencing therapy) as systemic medications have several side effects and significant drug interactions (cytochrome P450).

TINEA (DERMATOPHYTE) INFECTIONS OF THE SKIN

Tinea corporis/pedis (Figure 9)

- **First line**:
  1. **Topical**: 2% miconazole cream and 1% clotrimazole cream.
  2. **Oral**: Griseofulvin 500–1000 mg once daily × 4–6 weeks. A skin scrape should be done for test of cure.
- **Second line**:
  1. **Topical**: Ketoconazole cream and terbinafine cream.
  2. **Oral**: Itraconazole 100 mg once daily × 2 weeks; terbinafine 250 mg once daily × 2–4 weeks.

Tinea versicolor (Figure 10)

- **First-line topical**:
  1. **Face**: 2% miconazole cream ON × 2 weeks.
  2. **Body and limbs**: 40% propylene glycol solution ON × 2 weeks or selenium sulphide (Selsun) suspension, applied for 15–30 minutes then washed off or overnight × 2 weeks.
- **Second-line topical**:
  1. **Face**: Nizoral (ketoconazole) cream ON × 2 weeks.
  2. **Body and limbs**: Nizoral shampoo ON × 2 weeks.
- **Third-line oral**: Refer to Dermatology for review. Take an oral dose of ketoconazole 200 mg od × 10 days.

Candidal infections of the skin (Figure 11)

- **First-line topicals**: **2% miconazole cream**, 1% clotrimazole cream.
- **Second-line systemic**: Refer to Dermatology for follow-up. **Itraconazole 100 mg bd** or ketoconazole 200 mg od × 2–6 weeks.

Prevention of skin infections

- Recurrent infections: Advise on elimination or control of factors that contribute to infections, e.g. keep cool, take frequent cold showers, ventilate covered parts, use open footwear, and avoid contact with stray cats and animals.

ACUTE URTICARIA (Figure 12)

This is a fairly common condition seen at the emergency department due to the intense itching and sudden onset of a generalized rash.

Clinical features

- Pink, non-scaling, flat-topped wheals that are migratory.
- Lesions are pruritic.

Common causes

- Viral: Suggested by recent history of fever, myalgia, and upper respiratory tract infection (URTI) symptoms.
- Drugs: Penicillin, sulfa drugs, and NSAIDs.
- Food allergies.
- Environmental factors: For example, cold, sunlight, and pressure.
- Unknown: There is often no obvious cause.

Management

- Identify and eliminate causative factors if possible.
- Give symptomatic treatment.
- **Antihistamines**:
    1. Parenteral route choices:
        a. Promethazine: 25 mg intramuscular (IM) (adults) or 0.5 mg/kg (paediatrics).
        b. Diphenhydramine: 25 mg (adults) IM or 1 mg/kg (paediatrics).
    2. Oral route choices:
        a. Chlorpheniramine (Piriton®):   Tab 4 mg tds.
        b. Hydroxyzine (Atarax®):Tab 25 mg tds.
        c. Newer less sedative options: Cetirizine (Zyrtec®), loratadine (Claritin®), desloratadine (Aerius®) and levocetirizine (Xyzal®).
- **Steroids**:
    1. To be considered if the lesions are extensive and recurrent, or are associated with angiaoedema.
    2. Prednisolone tab 0.5–1 mg/kg OM × 5 days.
- **Disposition**: The patient can be discharged if the response to treatment is prompt and there is no associated angiaoedema.

CHRONIC URTICARIA (Figure 12)

Clinical features

- Single or multiple wheals (localized oedema of dermis) with erythema and itching.
- Individual wheals last less than 24 hours (except urticarial vasculitis), and resolve without staining the affected skin. Rarely affects the mucous membranes.
- **Acute:** These isolated attacks of urticaria last less than 6 weeks.

- **Chronic**: Urticaria becomes chronic when it occurs daily or almost daily for more than six weeks. It is usually associated with an impaired quality of life. Subtypes include physical urticaria, chronic idiopathic urticaria (most common), urticarial vasculitis, and autoimmune urticaria.
- Ask about triggers, e.g. physical (heat, cold, pressure, exercise, emotion, exposure to ultraviolet and/or visible light, and delayed pressure), drug/food allergies, and insect bites.

Management

- Refer chronic urticaria cases to Dermatology for follow-up.
- General measures include avoidance of NSAIDs, alcohol, stress, maintenance of a cool environment, and use of light clothing.
- Refer to Chapter 29, *Allergic Reactions/Anaphylaxis* for the management of acute urticaria.
- **Antihistamines**: Consider the combination of non-sedating antihistamines in the morning and sedating antihistamines at night. For chronic cases, a period of strict usage of antihistamines can help to 'break the cycle' of urticarial eruptions.
  1. First-generation antihistamines (sedating): Chlorpheniramine and hydroxyzine.
  2. Second-generation antihistamines (non-sedating): Loratadine, cetirizine, fexofenadine, desloratadine, and levocetirizine.

MENINGOCOCCAEMIA (Figure 13)

The causative organism is *Neisseria meningitidis* (Gram-negative diplococci on initial cerebrospinal fluid (CSF) gram stain smears).

Clinical features

- Abrupt onset of fever, malaise, myalgia, arthralgia, headache, nausea, and vomiting.
- Generally toxic with rapid progression to obtundation and signs of meningitis.
- Associated cutaneous findings: Scattered pink or purpuric papules that may become vesicular or pustular.
- May progress to **purpura fulminans**: Irregular but well-demarcated plaques of purple purpura with central grey, dusky, deep purple, or black necrosis.

Management

- The patient should be managed in the critical care area with close monitoring.
- Give fluid resuscitation and inotropic support if necessary.
- Do blood cultures.
- Antibiotics may be started before performing a lumbar puncture.
- Antibiotic of choice: **IV penicillin G 4 million units** 4 hourly (consider chloramphenicol if the patient is allergic to penicillin) or **IV ceftriaxone 2 g bd**.
- **Disposition**: High dependency or intensive care unit (request for isolation).

Prophylaxis

- **Indications**:
    1. Close contacts for at least 4 hours during the week before illness onset, e.g. housemates, day care contacts, or cellmates.
    2. Exposure to the patient's nasopharyngeal secretions, e.g. via kissing, mouth-to-mouth resuscitation, intubation, or nasotracheal suctioning.
- **Regime**:
    1. PO ciprofloxacin 500 mg single dose or PO rifampicin 600 mg bd × 4 doses (adults)
    2. PO Rifampicin 10 mg/kg bd × 4 doses (paediatrics)

VASCULITIS (Figure 14)

Clinical features

- The size of vessel involvement in cutaneous vasculitis is useful to narrow down the list of differential diagnoses.
- **Cutaneous small vessel vasculitis** differentials: Cutaneous leucocytoclastic vasculitis (secondary to drugs, infection, and idiopathic), Henoch–Schonlein Purpura, connective tissue disease-associated vasculitis (e.g. systemic lupus erythematosus, rheumatoid arthritis), antineutrophil cytoplasmic antibody (ANCA)-associated vasculitis, Behcet's disease, paraneoplastic, etc.
- **Medium vessel vasculitis** differentials: Polyarteritis nodosa, ANCA-associated vasculitis, connective tissue disease-associated vasculitis. Overlap between the two categories occurs.
- **Important history** to obtain: Comprehensive drug history, antecedent or ongoing infection, e.g. viral fever, urinary tract infection, etc. symptoms suggestive of a rheumatological condition or of systemic involvement, e.g. mononeuritis multiplex.
- **Small and medium vessel vasculitis can usually be distinguished clinically**:
    1. Small vessel vasculitis may present with palpable purpura, non-palpable purpuric macules, vesicles, pustules, urticaria, or superficial ulceration.
    2. Medium vessel vasculitis presents with one or more of the following: nodules, ulcers, livedo reticularis, digital infarcts, and papulonecrotic lesions.

Management

- Evaluate for **systemic involvement**: Full blood count, renal panel, liver function test (LFT), erythrocyte sedimentation rate (ESR), urine dipstick, and chest X-ray.
- If there are other features to suggest systemic involvement, the relevant investigations should be ordered:
    1. Myalgia or muscle weakness (creatine kinase/lactate dehydrogenase).
    2. Abdominal pain (LFT/amylase).
    3. Angina (creatine kinase/creatine kinase–myocardial band/troponin I).

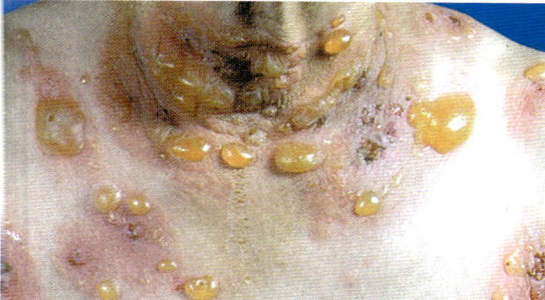

Image courtesy of National Skin Centre and Eds., Asian Skin 2005.

FIGURE 1 **Bullous pemphigoid** Multiple large tense bullae on the chest of an elderly man. Urticaria-like plaques (as shown in the figure) may precede the development of bullae. Bullae may be haemorrhagic and can arise from erythematous or non-inflamed skin. Rupture of the bullae results in erosions which may leave prominent post-inflammatory hyperpigmentation in darker-skinned Asians. Circulating antibodies against the hemidesmosomal glycoproteins BP180 and BP230 are present.

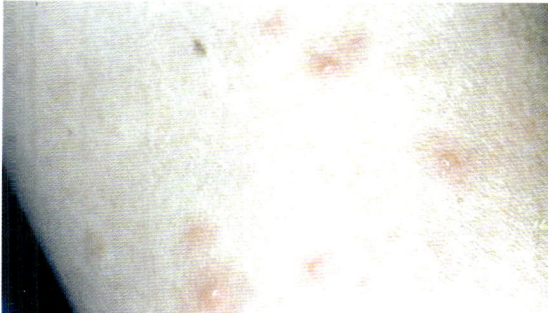

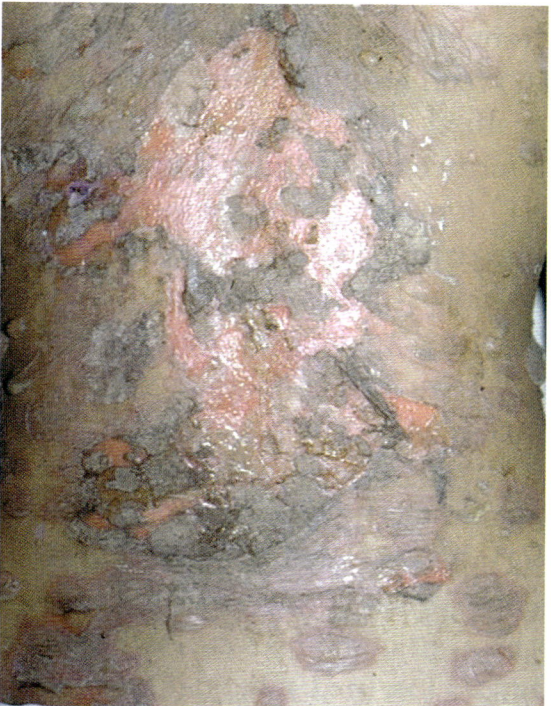

Image courtesy of National Skin Centre and Eds., Asian Skin 2005.

FIGURE 3 **Varicella** A close-up view of the characteristic vesicles, each like a dewdrop on an inflamed red base.

Image courtesy of National Skin Centre and Eds., Asian Skin 2005.

FIGURE 2 **Pemphigus vulgaris** Confluent areas of painful denuded skin secondary to flaccid blisters that are easily eroded with minimal trauma. Intact flaccid bullae are seen at the lower back and characteristically arise from normal-looking skin. Anti-desmoglein autoantibodies are responsible for the intraepidermal acantholysis of keratinocytes, which can be recognized histologically as suprabasilar cleft formation with an intact basal layer ('tombstone sign'). Lesions heal without scarring although post-inflammatory hyperpigmentation is common in Asians of darker skin.

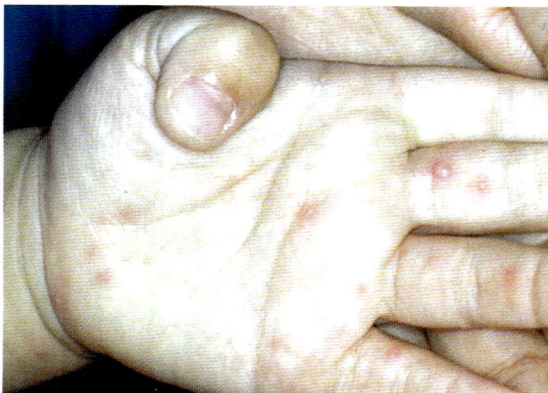

Image courtesy of National Skin Centre and Eds., Asian Skin 2005.

FIGURE 4 **Hand, foot and mouth disease** There are multiple vesicles on erythematous bases on the palm of this young child with hand, foot and mouth disease. Similar vesicles on the soles and painful oral ulcers are present as well. He is febrile with mild constitutional symptoms. This is usually a benign self-limiting infection, commonly caused by coxsackie virus and enterovirus. Outbreaks in Southeast Asia and Taiwan due to enterovirus 71 resulted in some mortality in pre-school children.

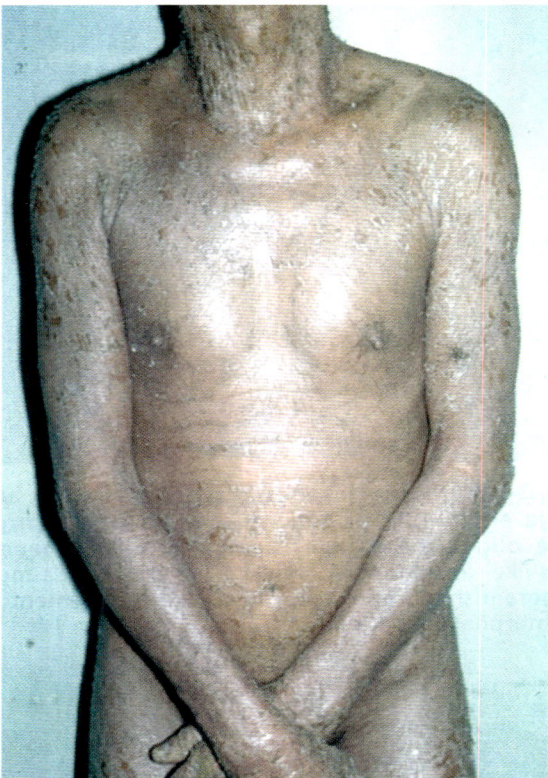

Image courtesy of National Skin Centre and Eds., Asian Skin 2005.

FIGURE 27 **Generalized exfoliative dermatitis** This 56-year-old Chinese male presents with erythroderma or generalized exfoliative dermatitis secondary to psoriasis. Erythrodermic psoriasis is associated with significant haemodynamic and temperature regulation problems. The clues to this diagnosis include a prior history of psoriasis and presence of other psoriatic lesions such as nail changes and joint involvement.

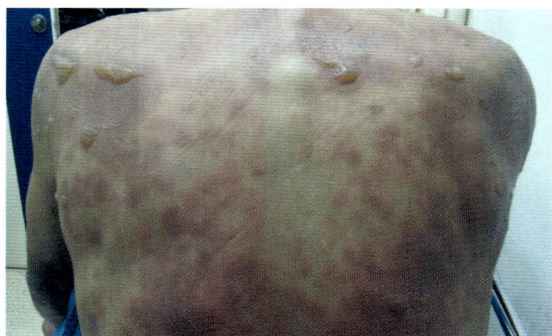

FIGURE 28a **Stevens-Johnson Syndrome** Extensive erythematous, dusky and tender patches on the back, with numerous flaccid bullae.

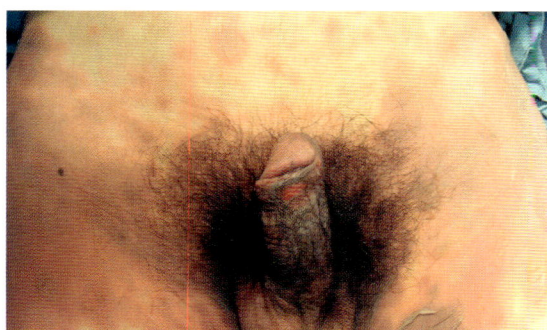

FIGURE 28b **Stevens-Johnson Syndrome – penile erosions** Erythematous and dusky atypical targets coalescing on the lower abdomen and thighs, with flaccid bullae and erosions on the penile shaft.

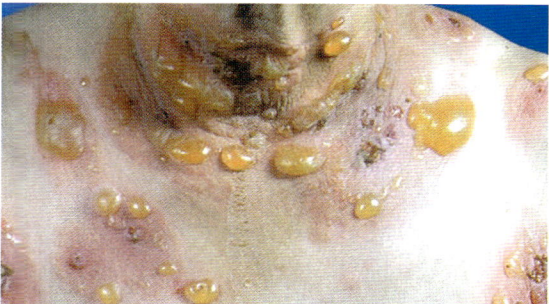

Image courtesy of National Skin Centre and Eds., Asian Skin 2005.

FIGURE 1 **Bullous pemphigoid** Multiple large tense bullae on the chest of an elderly man. Urticaria-like plaques (as shown in the figure) may precede the development of bullae. Bullae may be haemorrhagic and can arise from erythematous or non-inflamed skin. Rupture of the bullae results in erosions which may leave prominent post-inflammatory hyperpigmentation in darker-skinned Asians. Circulating antibodies against the hemidesmosomal glycoproteins BP180 and BP230 are present.

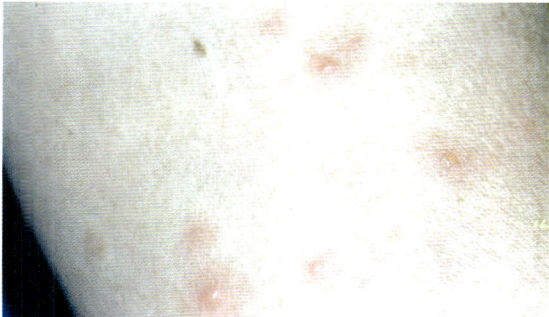

Image courtesy of National Skin Centre and Eds., Asian Skin 2005.

FIGURE 3 **Varicella** A close-up view of the characteristic vesicles, each like a dewdrop on an inflamed red base.

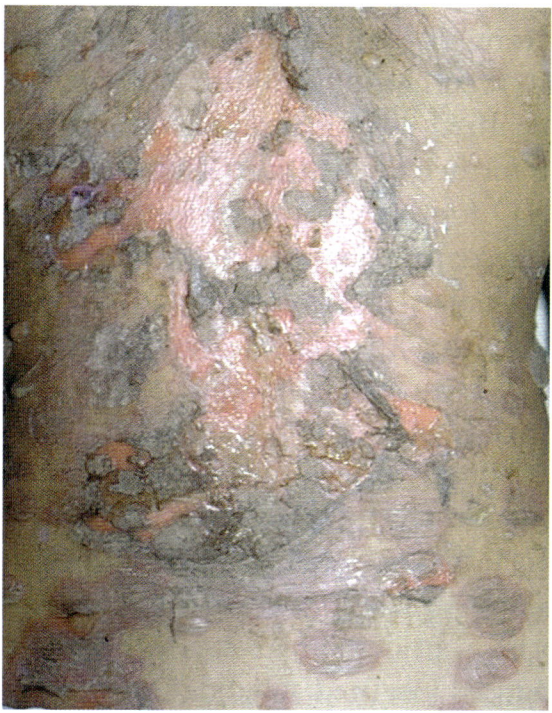

Image courtesy of National Skin Centre and Eds., Asian Skin 2005.

FIGURE 2 **Pemphigus vulgaris** Confluent areas of painful denuded skin secondary to flaccid blisters that are easily eroded with minimal trauma. Intact flaccid bullae are seen at the lower back and characteristically arise from normal-looking skin. Anti-desmoglein autoantibodies are responsible for the intraepidermal acantholysis of keratinocytes, which can be recognized histologically as suprabasilar cleft formation with an intact basal layer ('tombstone sign'). Lesions heal without scarring although post-inflammatory hyperpigmentation is common in Asians of darker skin.

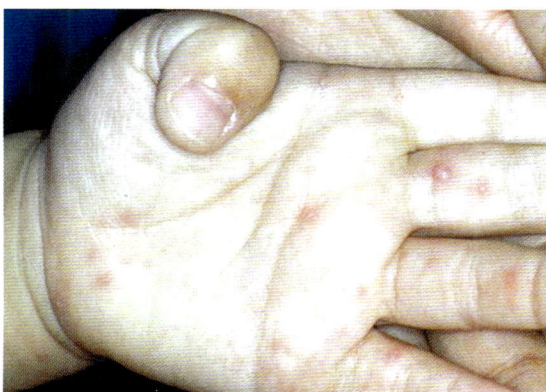

Image courtesy of National Skin Centre and Eds., Asian Skin 2005.

FIGURE 4 **Hand, foot and mouth disease** There are multiple vesicles on erythematous bases on the palm of this young child with hand, foot and mouth disease. Similar vesicles on the soles and painful oral ulcers are present as well. He is febrile with mild constitutional symptoms. This is usually a benign self-limiting infection, commonly caused by coxsackie virus and enterovirus. Outbreaks in Southeast Asia and Taiwan due to enterovirus 71 resulted in some mortality in pre-school children.

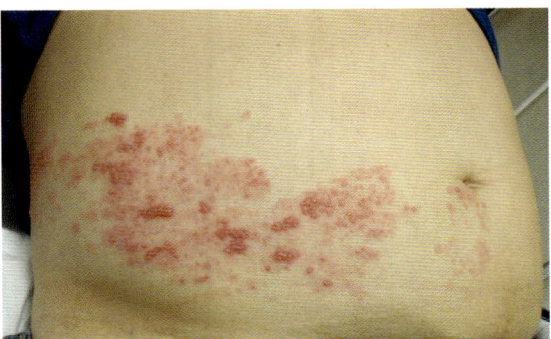

FIGURE 5 **Herpes zoster (Shingles)** Vesicles on an erythematous base in a dermatomal distribution.

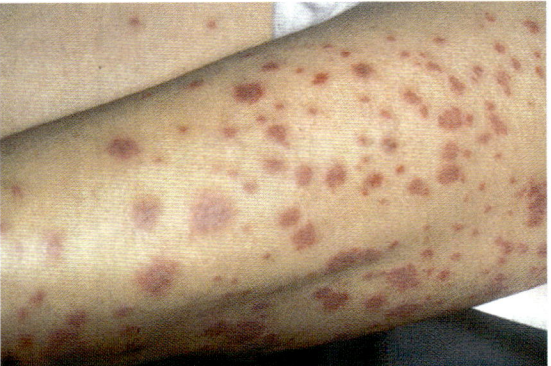

FIGURE 6a **Psoriasis** Well-demarcated, annular, scaly, erythematous plaques on the thighs. Psoriasis is more common in HIV-infected individuals than in the general population (up to 6% versus 2%). In a third of cases, it is present before HIV seroconversion (group 1). In these cases, the disease behaves as in HIV-negative individuals. In two-thirds of cases, psoriasis appears after HIV seroconversion (group 2).

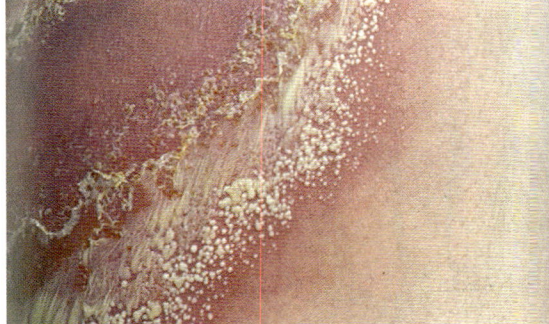

FIGURE 6b **Generalized pustular psoriasis** Generalized pustular psoriasis is one of the rare dermatological emergencies that patients may present with. The patient is usually febrile and toxic-looking. The skin is erythematous and covered with lakes of pustules. Elderly patients are particularly prone to haemodynamic instability and heat loss. Treatment includes careful management of the associated fluid and electrolyte imbalance. Systemic retinoids or methotrexate given under close monitoring can be used to hasten the resolution of the pustules.

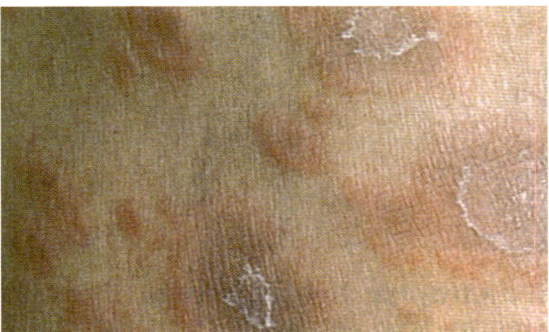

FIGURE 7 **Pityriasis rosea** Individual lesions in pityriasis rosea often have fine scales that desquamate, leaving behind fine, collarette scaling around the papular eruptions.

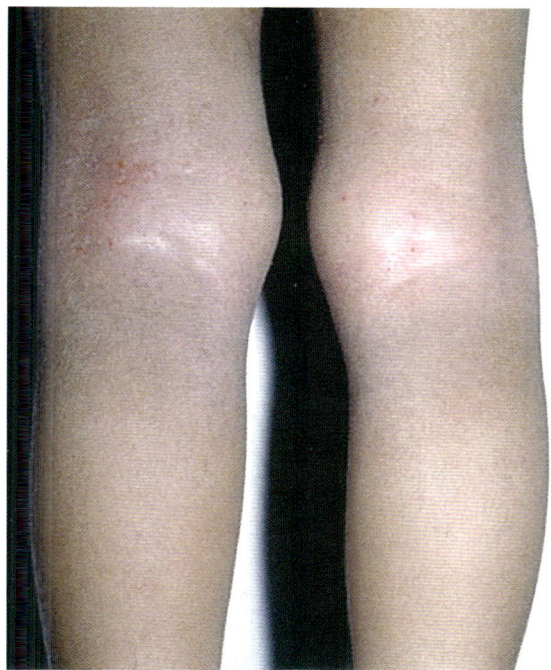

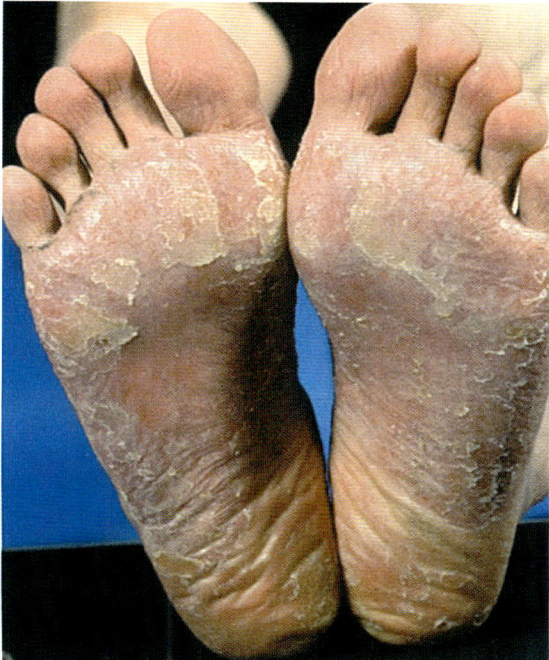

Image courtesy of National Skin Centre and Eds., Asian Skin 2005.

Image courtesy of National Skin Centre and Eds., Asian Skin 2005.

FIGURE 8 **Atopic dermatitis** This patient has chronic flexural eczema of both popliteal fossae. Note the lichenification, scaling, and pigmentation that are present. The popliteal fossae, along with other flexural areas such as the antecubital fossae, neck, wrists, and ankles, are commonly affected in atopic eczema in both childhood and adulthood. These areas are less frequently affected during infancy.

FIGURE 9 **Tinea pedis** Bilateral involvement of both soles is seen, creating a moccasin distribution. Toe nail involvement should be excluded as this can serve as a source for reinfection. Patients with tinea pedis should be advised to continue to use antifungal cream for one to two weeks after the skin appears normal.

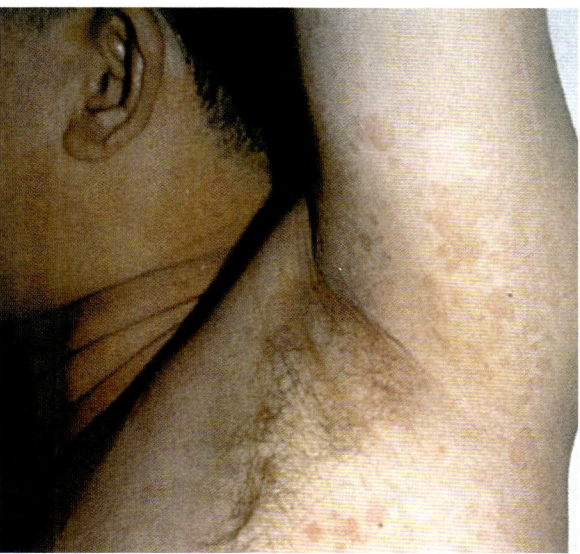

Image courtesy of National Skin Centre and Eds., Asian Skin 2005.

FIGURE 10 **Tinea versicolor** Brownish scaly macules on the arm and chest. This is a common, superficial infection by the lipophilic yeast, Malassezia furfur. Fungal scraping with potassium hydroxide (KOH) preparation was diagnostic, showing a characteristic 'spaghetti and meatballs' appearance of the hyphae.

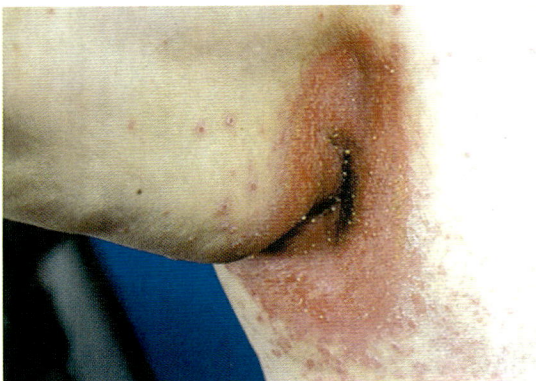

Image courtesy of National Skin Centre and Eds., Asian Skin 2005.

FIGURE 11   Candidosis There is a prominent red rash on the axilla, with numerous discrete papules and pustules. Satellite lesions are seen slightly further away. Candida intertrigo occurs more commonly in obese patients exposed to hot, humid climates, as well as patients with underlying diabetes mellitus.

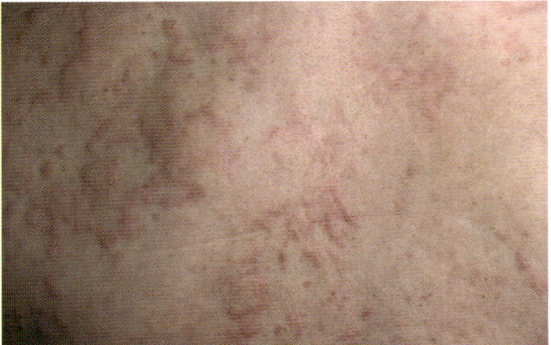

FIGURE 12   Urticaria Numerous polycyclic and annular wheals on the trunk.

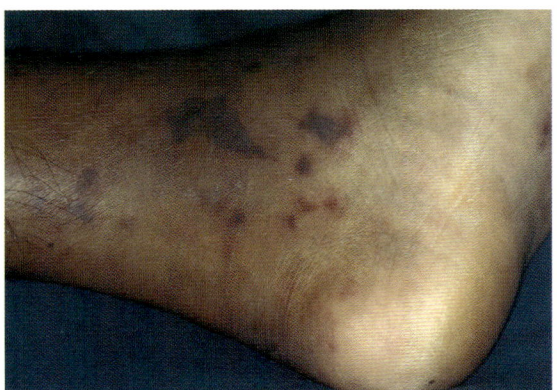

FIGURE 13   Meningococcaemia Purpuric macules and patches on the ankle and sole.

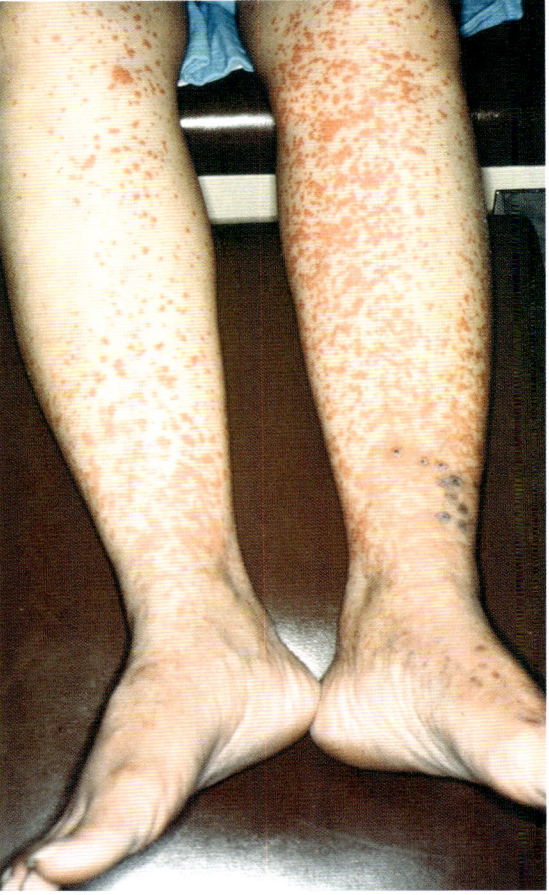

FIGURE 14   Cutaneous leucocytoclastic vasculitis Palpable purpura on both shins with several bullous haemorrhagic papules on left lower shin.

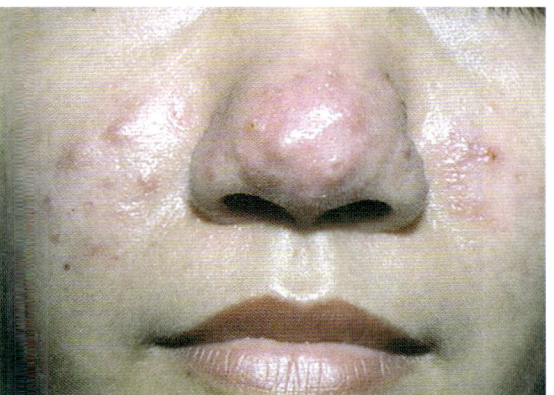

Image courtesy of National Skin Centre and Eds., Asian Skin 2005.

FIGURE 15 **Acne rosacea** The lesions of rosacea which initially occur in the central convex areas of the face consist of inflamed papules and pustules against a background of erythema, telangiectasia, oedema, and eventual permanent induration and thickening of affected skin. It may present as gross enlargement and deformity of the nose (rhinophyma) in its most extreme form. This lady has multiple inflammatory papules and pustules on a background of erythema and telangiectasia located on her cheeks and nose.

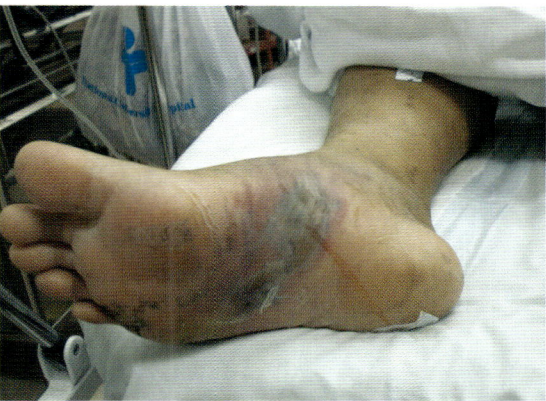

FIGURE 16 **Necrotizing fasciitis** Early involvement with deeply tender haemorrhagic bullae on the sole of the foot.

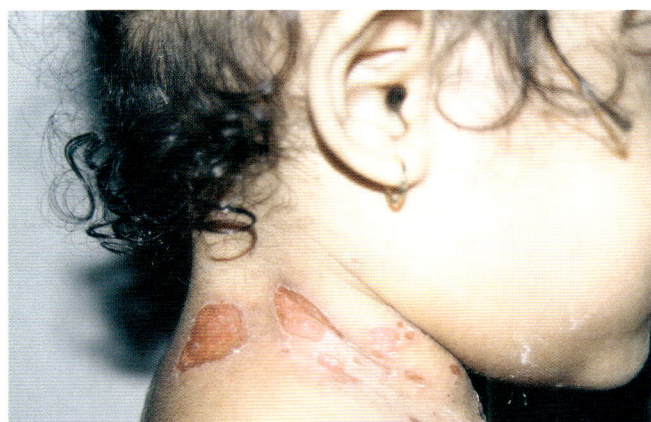

FIGURE 17 **Bullous impetigo** Raw erosions on the shoulder with some crusting.

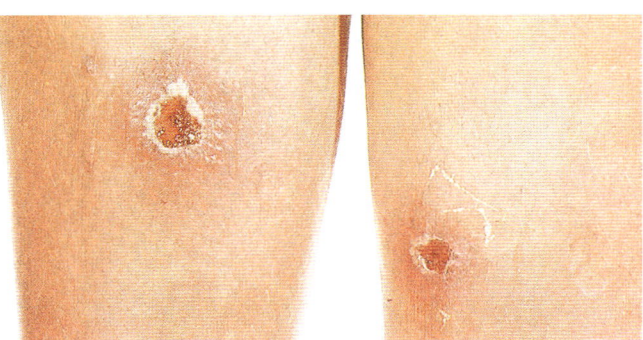

FIGURE 18 **Ecthyma** Erythematous nodules on both legs with central ulceration.

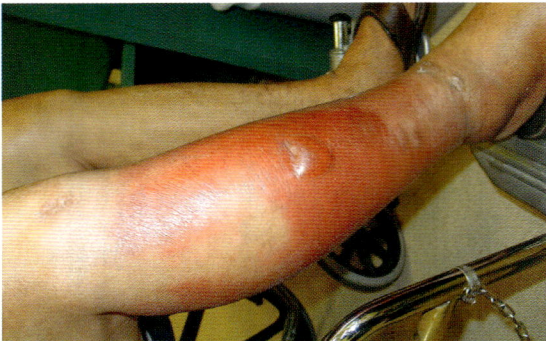

FIGURE 19 **Bullous erysipelas** Well-demarcated intense erythema on the right leg with oedema and a solitary bulla.

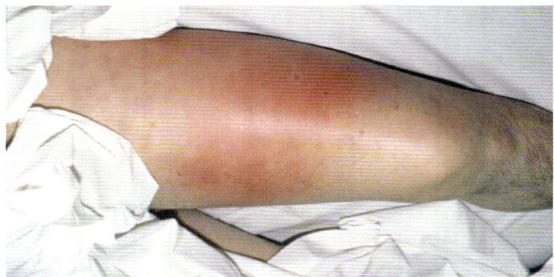

FIGURE 20 **Cellulitis** Painful, warm, tender, erythematous swelling of thigh associated with oedema. The demarcation between normal and affected skin is not as distinct as in erysipelas.

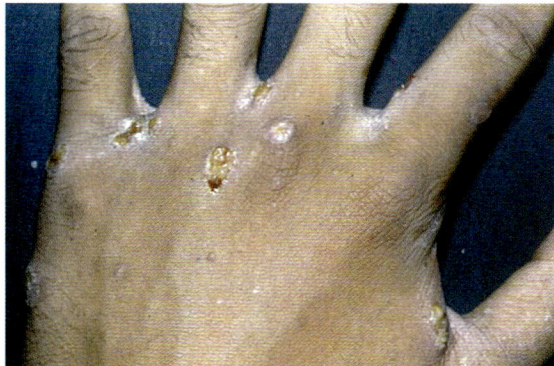

Image courtesy of National Skin Centre and Eds., Asian Skin 2005.

FIGURE 21 **Scabies** Itchy excoriated papules and crusting are seen on the dorsum of the hands and the web spaces. They are due to a mite infestation by the female Sarcoptes scabiei var. hominis. It is characterized by nocturnal exacerbation of itch, and is spread by close contact. A family history of similar complaints is usually present.

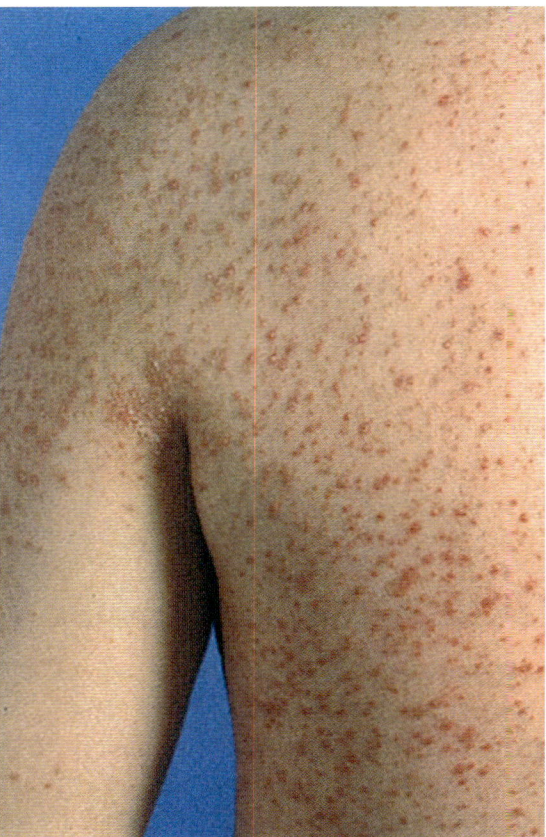

Image courtesy of National Skin Centre and Eds., Asian Skin 2005.

FIGURE 22 **Pityrosporum folliculitis** This presents as multiple scattered monomorphic papules and pustules without the presence of comedones. This condition results from a host reaction to the normal skin commensal Malassezia furfur. In Singapore, this condition is most commonly seen as a sudden eruption of monomorphic acneiform papules and pustules over the shoulders and upper trunk of healthy young adults working in a hot, humid environment or serving their National Service in the army.

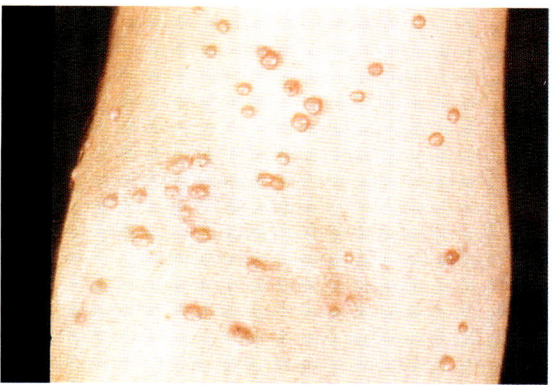

FIGURE 24 **Molluscum contagiosum** Numerous umbilicated skin-coloured papules.

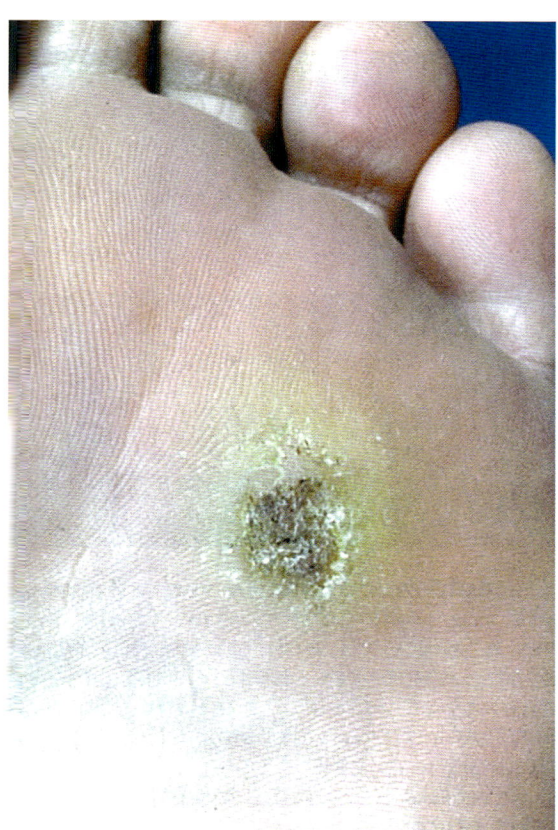

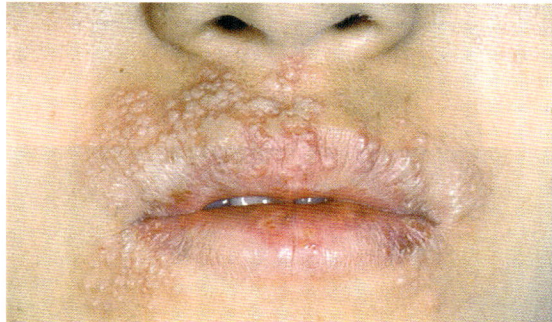

Image courtesy of National Skin Centre and Eds., Asian Skin 2005.

FIGURE 25 **Herpes gingivostomatitis** Diffuse crusting and vesiculation of the lips and perioral region are seen here. They represent a severe, primary infection of the lips by herpes simplex virus (HSV-1). After this initial bout, patients may subsequently have bouts of herpes labialis triggered by factors such as local trauma, concurrent infections, and mental stress as well as sun exposure.

Image courtesy of National Skin Centre and Eds., Asian Skin 2005.

FIGURE 23 **Plantar wart** A hyperkeratotic plaque on the sole, with multiple black dots on the surface, representing thrombosed capillaries. The normal skin lines are obscured.

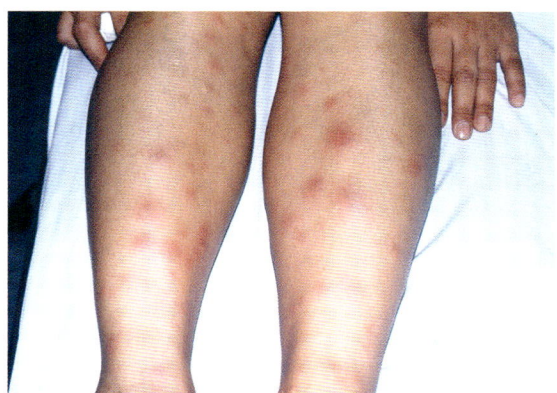

FIGURE 26 **Erythema nodosum** Erythematous tender nocules distributed mainly on the shins.

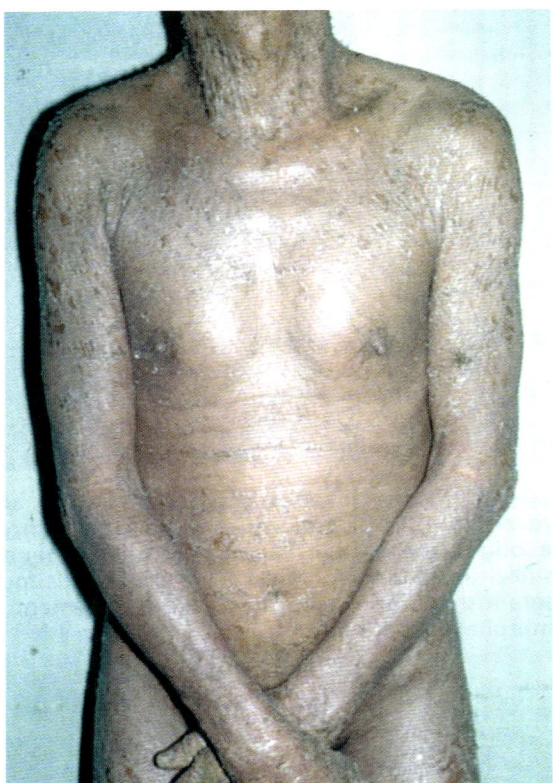

Image courtesy of National Skin Centre and Eds., Asian Skin 2005.

FIGURE 27 **Generalized exfoliative dermatitis** This 56-year-old Chinese male presents with erythroderma or generalized exfoliative dermatitis secondary to psoriasis. Erythrodermic psoriasis is associated with significant haemodynamic and temperature regulation problems. The clues to this diagnosis include a prior history of psoriasis and presence of other psoriatic lesions such as nail changes and joint involvement.

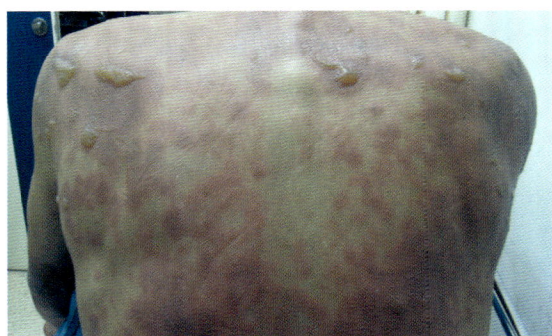

FIGURE 28a **Stevens-Johnson Syndrome** Extensive erythematous, dusky and tender patches on the back, with numerous flaccid bullae.

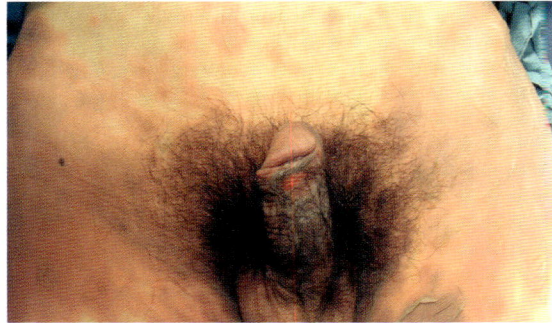

FIGURE 28b **Stevens-Johnson Syndrome – penile erosions** Erythematous and dusky atypical targets coalescing on the lower abdomen and thighs, with flaccid bullae and erosions on the penile shaft.

- Refer early to Dermatology for skin biopsy and full work-up. Alternatively, if the patient is ill-looking with systemic involvement, admit to General Medicine (with Dermatology consult) or Rheumatology depending on the suspected underlying aetiology. Systemic corticosteroids and immuno-suppressive therapy may be required.

ACNE VULGARIS

Clinical features

- Lesions can be classified as:
  1. **Non-inflammatory**: Comedones (white heads and black heads).
  2. **Inflammatory**: Red papules, pustules, nodules, and cysts.
- Hypo- and hyperpigmentation, red marks, scars, and keloids are due to past severe acne.
- Lesions can appear on the face, neck, shoulders, upper body, and arms.
- Important **red flags** in assessment:
  1. Are endocrine factors responsible for the acne? Consider polycystic ovarian syndrome, Cushing's syndrome, and 21-hydroxylase deficiency.
  2. Is the patient exposed to make-up, cosmetics, heavy oils, greases, polyvinyl chloride, or tars?
  3. Has the patient been on any medications known to cause acne? Corticosteroids, anti-epileptic drugs, isoniazid, lithium, danazol, iodides, and bromides are some drugs that can cause an acneiform eruption.
  4. Previous therapies and response.

Management

Refer all cases to Dermatology for follow-up.

TREATMENT OF COMEDONAL ACNE

- **Very mild comedonal acne**:
  1. Benzoyl peroxide (2.5%, 5%, and 10%) applied day and night if tolerable or just at night in patients with sensitive skin or
  2. Acne cream/lotion (sulphur and resorcinol).
- **Mild-to-severe comedonal acne: Topical retinoids** at the lowest strength initially, then increased as tolerated.
  1. First line: Tretinoin cream or gel (0.01%, 0.025%, 0.05%, and 0.1%).
  2. Second line: Adapalene (differin) 0.1% gel (causes less irritation and is less photo labile compared to tretinoin).

NOTE: Avoid sun exposure when using topical retinoids. Stop temporarily when the skin is irritated or if the patient is pregnant. Persistent comedones may need punctures (with a curved, pointed No. 12 blade) and expression.

TREATMENT OF INFLAMMATORY LESIONS OF ACNE

- **Very mild-to-mild inflammatory acne** (few to several papules/pustules, no nodules): Topical treatment.
    1. **First line:** Topical retinoid ON **and**:
        a. Acne lotion or acne cream (sulphur, salicylic acid, and resorcinol) or
        b. Benzoyl peroxide gel or cream (2.5%, 5%, and 10%) OM.
    2. **Second line**: Add a **topical antibiotic** (erythromycin or clindamycin) once or twice daily together with either topical retinoid or benzoyl peroxide.
- **Moderate acne** (several to many papules/pustules; few nodules): Systemic and topical treatment. Oral antibiotics are given as first line. Oral contraceptives can be considered in women of child-bearing age.
    1. **First line**: PO doxycycline 100 mg bd × 4–6/52; erythromycin 500 mg bd × 4–6/52
- **Severe/nodulocystic acne**: Refer to Dermatology for treatment and follow-up. Options include oral isotretinoin (roaccutane).

ACNE ROSACEA (Figure 15)

Clinical features

- Episodic reddening of the face (flushing) with increase in skin temperature in response to heat stimuli in the mouth, e.g. hot liquids and spicy foods.
- Aggravated by sun and heat exposure.
- May be preceded by or occur together with acne vulgaris.
- Lesions consist of tiny papules and papulopustules (2–3 mm), dusky-red nodules scattered symmetrically in the central portion of the face with characteristic red facies and episodic flushing. There are no comedones in pure acne rosacea (contrast with acne vulgaris).
- Chronic cases may show marked sebaceous hyperplasia and lymphoedema with disfigurement of the nose, forehead, eyelids, ears, and chin, e.g. formation of rhinophyma.
- Concomitant chronic blepharitis, conjunctivitis, and episcleritis can lead to red eyes.

Management

- **First line: Topical**
    1. Metronidazole gel or cream 0.75% (rozex) bd.
    2. Topical antibiotics, e.g. erythromycin gel bd (less effective).
- Refer to Dermatology for follow-up.

NECROTIZING SOFT TISSUE INFECTIONS (Figure 16)

- A group of rapidly progressive life-threatening bacterial infections of soft tissues characterized by tissue necrosis.
- Specific terms used depends on the tissues involved and causative organisms:
  1. Necrotizing fasciitis.
  2. Necrotizing myositis.
  3. Fournier's gangrene (genitalia).
- **Organisms**:
  1. Group A *streptococci*.
  2. Polymicrobial.
  3. *Staphylococcus aureus*.

Clinical features

- Toxic, febrile, and often hypotensive with or without confusion and delirium.
- The skin findings may be deceptively minor compared to the systemic toxicity of the patient.
- There is oedema and erythema initially, progressing to pallor and greyish discolouration with haemorrhagic bullae (due to ischaemia when blood vessels are destroyed) or gangrene.
- Abdominal pain is a common presenting complaint.

Differential diagnoses

- Cellulitis and other non-necrotizing soft tissue infections
- *Erysipelas* has clearly demarcated margins and streaking in lymphangitis is prominent; vesicles and bullae may develop in severe infections (common organism: Group A beta-haemolytic *streptococci*).

Management

- The patient should be managed in the critical care area with close monitoring.
- Give fluid resuscitation and inotropic support if necessary.
- Consider taking an X-ray of the soft tissue area involved to look for free air in the subcutaneous tissue.

NOTE: Absence of soft tissue gas does not rule out the diagnosis.

- Do blood cultures.
- Start broad spectrum antibiotics, e.g. IV **crystalline penicillin + clindamycin (for group A *Streptococci* + anaerobes with some *Staphylococcus* coverage) + ceftazidime (for Gram-negative rods and melioidosis)**.
- Refer to the orthopaedic/general surgeon (depending on the site involved) for immediate surgical exploration and debridement of necrotic tissue.

- **Disposition**: Admit to high dependency or intensive care unit depending on the stability of the patient.

PYODERMA

Includes impetigo, ecthyma, folliculitis, furunculosis/carbuncles, erysipelas, cellulitis, and cutaneous melioidosis.

Impetigo (Figure 17)

Clinical features

- May be **bullous** (thin-roofed fragile blisters, which break easily leaving superficial erosions; caused by *Staphylococcus aureus*) or **non-bullous** (lesions have a moist, red base with adherent honey-yellow to white-brown adherent crust; caused by *Staphylococcus aureus* or *Streptococci*).
- The lesions may be localized or widespread.
- May occur as a primary pyoderma, as a secondary phenomenon in eczema lesions or after a minor skin injury such as an insect bite. It is highly infectious and children in close physical contact are at risk.

Management

- Mild and localized cases: Topical therapy is the first line.
  1. **Fusidic acid** 2% cream/ointment tds × 5–10 days
  2. **Mupirocin** ointment bd × 5–10 days.
- The more severe cases require systemic antibiotics. The duration of treatment is 5 to 10 days. Local care, which includes cleansing, removal of crusts, and application of appropriate dressings, can be helpful.
  1. **PO cloxacillin, cephalexin, and amoxicillin-clavulanic acid (augmentin)** can be used.
  2. **PO erythromycin** is an alternative in patients who are penicillin-allergic. Locally, 8 to 18% of *Staphylococcus aureus* isolates are resistant to erythromycin and monitoring for treatment failure may be necessary.
  3. **PO cotrimoxazole** (contraindicated in glucose-6-phosphate dehydrogenase, G6PD, deficiency) can be used as a second-line agent.

Ecthyma (Figure 18)

Clinical features

- Resembles impetigo but is located deeper in the skin, producing ulceration that reaches the dermis and is often covered by adherent crusts. Heals with scarring.
- Caused by *Strep pyogenes*, *Staphylococcus aureus* or a combination of both.

Management

- **PO cloxacillin**, **cephalexin**, or **erythromycin** for 10–14 days.

Folliculitis

Clinical features

- Dome-shaped pustules with small erythematous halos arising in the centre of hair follicles.
- Most common pyoderma seen locally.
- *Staphylococcus aureus* is the primary cause. Predisposing factors include use of topical corticosteroids.

Management

- Use **chlorhexidine or triclosan wash**.
- Take oral doses of **cloxacillin**, **cephalexin**, or **erythromycin** for 7 to 10 days.
- **Cetrimide shampoo** can be used for scalp involvement.
- Very persistent scalp folliculitis may be treated with 4 to 6 weeks of **PO erythromycin** 500 mg bd or **PO doxycycline** 100 mg bd. Refer to Dermatology for follow-up.

Furuncles and carbuncles

Clinical features

- Furuncles consist of deep-seated infection of the hair follicle apparatus forming a walled-off, painful, firm or fluctuant mass enclosing a collection of pus. These often evolve from superficial folliculitis.
- Carbuncles are extremely painful, deep interconnected aggregates of several infected contiguous follicles with intense tissue inflammation.
- The predisposing factors include maceration caused by friction and sweating, diabetes mellitus, anaemia, hypogammaglobulinaemia, and neutrophil function defects.

Management

- **Incision and drainage** are indicated for larger fluctuant lesions.
- **Systemic antibiotics** (**PO cloxacillin, cephalexin, amoxicillin–clavulanic acid**, or **erythromycin**) should be considered for the following:
  1. Furuncles around the nose, within the nares, or in the external auditory canal.
  2. Large and recurrent lesions.
  3. Lesions with surrounding cellulitis.
  4. Lesions not responding to local care.

Erysipelas (Figure 19)

Clinical features

- Acute infection of the dermis and superficial subcutis with prominent lymphatic involvement. The margins are more clearly demarcated from normal skin than in cellulitis. Bullous areas may also be present. Erysipelas spreads rapidly with the affected area being hot and tender. It is often accompanied by fever.
- Erysipelas often affects the limbs and face.
- The causative agent is mostly *streptococci*.
- The predisposing factors include trauma, venous and lymphatic insufficiency, and superficial fungal infections.
- In facial erysipelas, sinus X-rays should be performed to exclude underlying sinusitis.

Management

- Patients can be treated with **PO penicillin V, penicillin V plus cloxacillin, cephalexin, erythromycin, or amoxicillin–clavulanic acid**.
- **PO cotrimoxazole and ciprofloxacin** can be used as second-line alternatives in penicillin-allergic patients.
- In severe cases where the patient is penicillin allergic and requires IV antibiotics, **IV erythromycin, or ciprofloxacin** can be used.

Cellulitis (Figure 20)

Clinical features

- Acute, subacute, or chronic infection of the dermis and subcutaneous tissue characterized by erythema, oedema, and pain.
- Most often occurs on the legs and near the sites of trauma or surgical wounds.
- Presents as an expanding, red, tender plaque with an indefinite border, usually accompanied by fever and enlarged regional lymph nodes. Some patients present with bullous lesions within the cellulitic area.
- Ask about predisposing factors, e.g. poorly-controlled diabetes mellitus.

Management

- Demarcate the area of cellulitis.
- Do full blood count, renal panel, C-reactive protein with or without blood cultures for more severe cases.
- In uncomplicated cellulitis, antibiotics against *streptococci* and *staphylococci* should be used, **PO amoxicillin, cloxacillin, amoxicillin–clavulanic acid, cephalexin, or erythromycin/ clarithromycin** for the milder cases. More severe cases require **IV cefazolin**.

- **Second-line alternatives** include PO ciprofloxacin or clindamycin for 7 to 10 days.
- In patients who are **allergic to penicillin** and require IV antibiotics, IV erythromycin, or ciprofloxacin can be used.
- Consider admission to Orthopaedics or General Medicine (if there are concomitant medical issues) for severe cases or admission to the (EDTU) for a day of IV antibiotics.

SCABIES (Figure 21)

Clinical features

- Ask about nocturnal itch exacerbation and history of similar itch among family members and close contacts.
- **Classical:** Erythematous pruritic papules and burrows with excoriations, typically in the inter-digital areas and genitalia. Can involve the trunk and limbs as well. Burrows are rarely seen.
- **Norwegian scabies** is typically NOT itchy, but thickly crusted with dense concentration of mites. It is highly contagious and close contacts often become infected and itchy. Scabies is common in institutionalized, homeless patients.
- **Definitive diagnosis** is made when the *Sarcoptes scabeii* mites, its body parts, ova, or faecal material are found on the scrape taken from a lesion or from the nail bed.

Management

Anti-scabetic treatment
- **Benzyl benzoate (EBB): 10% (children) and 25% (adults)**
  1. Apply and wash off after 24 hours. Repeat for a total of three days.
  2. Do not use in children below two years or in any patient with excoriated or infected skin as it causes irritant dermatitis, stinging, and conjunctival irritation.
  3. Use 10% formulation as 2nd-line treatment for children aged 2–12 years old.
- **Malathion 0.5% (Derbac-M®)**
  1. Apply at bedtime and wash off after 24 hours. Repeat one week later.
  2. Not to be used on children under 6 months old.
  3. First-line treatment for children aged 2–12 years old and in adults.
- **Permethrin 5%**
  1. Apply at bedtime and wash off the following morning.
  2. One application will generally suffice.
  3. First-line treatment for children younger than two years old.

Norwegian scabies should be treated in hospital. The crusts need to be removed and if unresponsive to topical treatment with repeated positive scrapes, the patient may need ivermectin as a single oral dose of 200 mcg/kg.

Concomitant treatment

- Scabies is extremely itchy. Prescribe chlorpheniramine or hydroxyzine for a week.
- Secondary bacterial infection by *Streptococcus pyogenes* and *Staphylococcus aureus* may produce frank pyodermas or subtle impetiginized lesions. If there is an infection, give antibiotics such as cloxacillin or erythromycin.
- Itch and eczematized skin can persist for up to 4 weeks after clearance of the mites. Prescribe 0.025% betamethasone valerate cream and antihistamines.
- Ask if family members have developed an itchy rash recently. Treat close contacts and symptomatic individuals with malathion or 25% emulsion benzyl benzoate.
- Laundering clothings, bedlinen, etc., is routinely advised to reduce the spread or recurrence of scabies.

PITYROSPORUM FOLLICULITIS (Figure 22)

Clinical features

- Chronic and often pruritic eruption on the back, upper arms, and chest.
- Multiple discrete 2–4 mm erythematous monomorphic papules and later pustules with a follicular pattern are present.
- Differential diagnoses include acne vulgaris and staphylococcal folliculitis.
- Caused by yeasts, specifically *Malassezia furfur* (classic spaghetti and meatballs appearance on potassium hydroxide preparation slides under the microscope).

Management

Same as for tinea versicolor.

VIRAL SKIN INFECTIONS

Warts *(Verruca vulgaris)* (Figure 23)

Clinical features

- Hyperkeratotic papules, can be filiform; present on the face, trunk/limbs, and periungual/ palmoplantar areas.
- Some patients also have plane warts. These are flat, planar erythematous macules.
- Plantar warts: Look for disruption of skin lines, thrombosed capillaries (appearing as black dots). Differentiate from calluses, which are usually found in high pressure areas of the soles.
- Cervical/vulvar warts: Refer to the DSC (Department of Sexually Transmitted Infections (STI) Control in Singapore) for treatment, further STI screen, and pap smear testing.
- Anogenital warts: Refer to the DSC for treatment and further STI screen. For extensive meatal warts, consider Urology referral.

Management

- **Face** – Refer to Dermatology for first line: Light electrocautery/cryotherapy.
- **Limbs and trunk** – First line: Salicylic acid preparations (for hyperkeratotic lesions, salicylic acid preparations may not be effective, in that case, give concomitant referral for cryotherapy).
- **Periungual and palmoplantar** – First line: Salicylic acid preparations (can be recalcitrant to topicals, refer to Dermatology for concomitant cryotherapy).

Molluscum contagiosum (Figure 24)

Clinical features

- Caused by a poxvirus.
- Average incubation period is between 2 and 7 weeks with a range extending to 6 months.
- Affects children more commonly. Self-inoculation can occur.
- It is usually asymptomatic although itch and pain may be reported in some cases. Appears as smooth skin-coloured papules initially, which later become umbilicated as the molluscum bodies begin to extrude.
- It can affect any part of the body but is predominantly found on the face, trunk, genitalia, and axillae.
- The diagnosis is clinical. Expressing the white content of the lesions, and microscopic examination to demonstrate molluscum bodies may be carried out in ambiguous cases.

Management

- Wait for **spontaneous resolution** in 6–12 months if the patient is not keen on treatment.
- If the patient is keen on treatment: refer to Dermatology. Options include topical retinoids, topical salicylic acid, topical imiquimod, liquid nitrogen, prick and express of molluscum, curettage, or electrocautery for larger lesions.

Herpes simplex virus infection (Figure 25)

Clinical features

- Genital herpes is caused by the DNA herpes simplex virus (HSV), usually HSV type 2, but type 1 infections are also possible. Transmission of the virus can occur through genital–genital, mouth–genital, genital–anal, and mouth–anal contact.
- The first episode of genital herpes is often severe, presenting with multiple grouped vesicles, which rupture easily leaving painful erosions and ulcers. In the male, lesions occur mainly on the prepuce and sub-preputial areas of the penis; in females, on the vulva, vagina, and cervix. Healing of uncomplicated lesions takes 2 to 4 weeks.
- Recurrent attacks are less severe than the first episode. Groups of vesicles or erosions develop on a single anatomical site and these usually heal within 10 days. Recurrences average 5 to 8 attacks a year and are more frequent during the first 2 years of infection. Genital herpes caused by HSV 1 generally recurs infrequently.

Management

- **Severe first-episode infection** seen within 1 to 2 days: Oral acyclovir 400 mg tds × 7–10 days, or valacyclovir 1g bd × 7–10 days.
- **Recurrent episodic** genital herpes (initiate treatment during prodrome or within a day of attack): Acyclovir 400 mg tds × 5 days or valacyclovir 500 mg bd × 3 days.
- **Topicals**: Keep clean with antiseptic wash and antibiotic ointment, e.g. tetracycline.
- Refer to DSC for follow-up including screening of other STIs. Advise the patient of the recurrent nature of HSV infections and to avoid sexual intercourse until the lesions heal.

ERYTHEMA NODOSUM (Figure 26)

This is a hypersensitivity reaction.

Clinical features

- Manifested by the acute onset of red tender nodules.
- Distributed mainly on the lower leg, especially the shins.

Causes

- Infections: *Streptococcus*, tuberculosis, infectious mononucleosis, *chlamydia,* and *yersinia*.
- Associated with sarcoidosis, Hodgkin's disease, and ulcerative disease.
- Drugs: Oral contraceptives, sulphonamides, penicillin, and tetracyclines.

Management

- Conduct systemic reviews for possible infections. Eliminate any precipitating cause.
- Give symptomatic treatment, e.g. NSAIDs for pain relief.
- Refer to Dermatology for follow-up.

INFECTIOUS EXANTHEMS

Clinical features

- These are generalized cutaneous eruptions usually associated with primary systemic infections. Etiologies include viral, bacterial, rickettsial, and parasitic infections.
- In many cases, an accurate diagnosis cannot be made based on morphology alone and relevant history needs to be asked including contact and travel history, associated prodromal symptoms, previous immunizations, or exanthematous illnesses.
- **Incubation period**: Usually lasts less than 3 weeks.
- **Prodrome**: Involves a non-specific febrile illness, e.g. fever, malaise, coryza, sore throat, diarrhoea, nausea, vomiting, abdominal pain, and headache.

- **Physical findings**: Generalized lymphadenopathy, hepato- and/or splenomegaly. Skin lesions can be:
  1. **Scarlitiniform** (diffuse to generalized erythema, may be more prominent in the skin folds or genitalia; desquamation can occur on resolution of the exanthem).
  2. **Exanthematous or morbiliform** (erythematous macules and/or papules, less frequently vesicles and petechiae; usually centrally distributed including proximal extremities).
  3. **Vesicular** (may evolve into pustules and roof sloughs resulting in erosions after a few days to a week).
  4. **Mucous membranes** (Koplik's spots in measles, palatal petechiae in Epstein-Barr (EBV) or cytomegalovirus (CMV) infections, and microulcerative lesions in herpangina due to coxsackievirus A, and conjunctivitis).

Management

- Mainly symptomatic management.
- Anti-microbial therapy in specific cases due to bacterial infections.

TABLE 4   Etiologies of infectious exanthems

Viral	Bacterial	Others
Rubella	Group A *Streptococcus* (scarlet fever)	Mycoplasmal species, e.g. *Mycoplasma pneumoniae*
Paramyxovirus (measles)	*Staphylococcus aureus* (toxic shock syndrome)	*Treponema pallidum*
Herpesviridae: CMV, EBV, human herpesvirus 6 and 7 (exanthema subitum, roseola infantum)	*Legionella*	Rickettsial infections: Rocky Mountain spotted fever, *rickettsia rickettsii*
HIV (acute symptomatic HIV syndrome)	*Leptospira*	
Enteroviruses, e.g. coxsackie viruses	Meningococci	
Parvovirus B19		

INSECT BITE REACTIONS

Clinical features

- Cutaneous reactions to arthropod bites are inflammatory and/or allergic reactions characterized by an intensely pruritic eruption at the bite sites hours or days after the bite.
- **Manifestations are varied** and include erythematous macules, solitary or grouped urticarial papules, papulovesicles and/or bullae that persist for days to weeks. Systemic symptoms can occur in some and range from mild to severe including anaphylactic shock.
- Excoriations commonly lead to **secondary infection** of the broken skin by group A *Streptococcus* and/or *Staphylococcus aureus* causing impetigo or ecthyma.

Management

- **Prevention is important**, apply insect repellant to clothing, use nets and screens at home and wear long-sleeved clothes in forested areas.
- Give **symptomatic treatment** especially antihistamines for relief of pruritus.
- Use **topical corticosteroids** for a short time to relieve intensely pruritic lesions. In some cases, a short tapering course of oral corticosteroids can be given for extensive and persistent insect bite reactions.
- Treat areas of secondary infection with **antibiotics**.

GENERALIZED EXFOLIATIVE DERMATITIS (Figure 27)

Clinical features

- Generalized exfoliative dermatitis (GED) or erythroderma is defined as an inflammatory skin disorder with erythema and scaling occurring in a generalized distribution involving more than 90% of the total body surface area.
- Etiologies are divided into five broad categories:
  1. **Pre-existing dermatoses** (53%): Atopic dermatitis, psoriasis, seborrhoeic dermatitis, contact dermatitis, pityriasis rubra pilaris, chronic actinic dermatitis, and ichthyoses (affecting primarily infants and young children).
  2. **Idiopathic** (26%).
  3. **Malignancy** (16%): Cutaneous T cell lymphoma, including Sezary syndrome (most common); Hodgkin's disease (next most common); non-Hodgkin's lymphoma; leukaemia, myelodysplasia; and visceral malignancies (rarely), e.g. prostate, thyroid, lung, liver, ovarian, rectal, and mammary.
  4. **Drug eruptions** (5%): Anti-epileptics, antihypertensives (captopril and frusemide), antibiotics (penicillins and sulphonamides), and allopurinol.
  5. **Miscellaneous disorders** (rare): Immunobullous disorders, e.g. pemphigus foliaceus; lichen planus; crusted scabies; dermatophytosis, candidiasis; acquired immunodeficiency syndrome (AIDS); and graft versus host disease (GVHD), including postoperative exfoliative dermatitis.
- Try to ascertain the aetiology and elicit complications of GED:
  1. Ask about pre-existing dermatoses, contactants, or topical medicaments, new drugs, and aggravating factors such as sunlight. Also include a systemic review (weight loss, night sweats, and bowel changes).
  2. Enquire about complications such as cardiac failure, hypoproteinaemia leading to pedal oedema, hypothermia, and hyperthermia, resulting in chills.
- The **physical examination** should document the location and percentage of body surface area affected. Lymphadenopathy occurs in up to 71% of patients; this may be due to dermatopathic lymphadenopathy (80%) or secondary to lymphoma (20%). A thorough general examination should include chest, abdominal, breast, pelvic, and rectal examination.
- Look for **complications** of erythroderma, specifically heart failure, hyper- or hypothermia, secondary impetiginization, dehydration, pallor (anaemia), and malnutrition (exacerbated by extensive scaling, oozing, or hypermetabolism).

Management

- Routine blood tests are generally not helpful in determining a specific diagnosis. Basic screening investigations include full blood count, renal panel, liver function test, urine dipstick, and chest X-ray.
- In the acute phase, treatment consists mainly of management of **complications**:
  1. Give systemic antibiotics for secondary infection, e.g. cloxacillin.
  2. Correction of fluid and electrolyte abnormalities.
  3. Provision of appropriate ambient temperature.
  4. Treatment of cardiac failure.
- Admit to General Medicine with Dermatology consult for treatment and work-up which will include a skin biopsy to rule out malignancy.

ADVERSE CUTANEOUS DRUG REACTIONS

Clinical features

- Drug eruptions can mimic virtually any skin morphological pattern and must be the first consideration in the differential diagnosis of a sudden onset symmetric eruption.
- The eruption can be caused by immunological (types I, II, III, or IV reactions) or non-immunological mechanisms.
- Adverse cutaneous drug eruptions can manifest as exanthematous rashes, urticaria/angiooedema, anaphylaxis, anaphylactoid reactions, eczematous eruptions, erythema multiforme (minor and major), exfoliative dermatitis, photosensitivity, serum sickness-like reactions, cutaneous necrosis, pigmentation, alopecia, hypertrichosis, nail changes, etc.
- **Exanthematous reactions** are the most common. The initial reaction usually occurs less than 14 days after drug intake and recurs after rechallenge. The rash is typically bright red and resolving lesions evolve into various hues of tan and purple. It is symmetrically distributed and almost always on the trunk and extremities. Confluent lesions can occur in intertriginous areas with palms and soles being variably involved.
- Drugs commonly responsible for reaction: Penicillin and related antibiotics, carbamazepine, allopurinol, non-steroidal anti-inflammatory drugs (NSAIDs), erythromycin, isoniazid, benzodiazepines, tetracyclines, and barbiturates.

Management

- Discontinue the implicated drug especially if there is urticaria (risk of anaphylaxis), facial oedema, pain, blisters, mucosal involvement, ulcers, palpable or extensive purpura, fever, or lymphadenopathy.
- Give symptomatic treatment in milder cases, e.g. antihistamines to relieve pruritus.
- Topical, oral, or IV (in severe cases) corticosteroids may help to accelerate resolution of erythema.
- If adverse drug reaction is indeed highly suspicious, give the patient a Medik Awas card.
- Recognize life-threatening manifestations, e.g. Stevens–Johnson syndrome and toxic epidermal necrolysis.

STEVENS-JOHNSON SYNDROME (SJS) AND TOXIC EPIDERMAL NECROLYSIS (TEN) (Figures 28a and 28b)

Clinical features

- These are 2 uncommon but potentially fatal adverse cutaneous drug reactions.
- Characterized by mucocutaneous tenderness, erythema and extensive exfoliation. Examine the entire skin surface and all mucous membranes including the conjunctivae, oral and anogenital mucosa.
- **Percentage BSA** affected refers to the area affected by epidermal necrolysis/death.
- **SJS**: <10% BSA affected
- **SJS-TEN overlap**: 10–30% BSA affected
- **TEN**: >30% BSA affected
- **Medications** most frequently implicated: allopurinol, NSAIDs, antibiotics and anticonvulsants. SJS and TEN usually occur 7–21 days after initiation of the responsible drug.

Management principles

- Early diagnosis is essential.
- Stop the responsible drug.
- If BSA >30%, refer to Dermatology for urgent review and arrange for transfer to the Burns Unit.
- Supportive care has to be rapidly initiated.
- Correct fluid and electrolyte imbalances.
- Maintenance of body temperature.
- Skilled nursing care is needed for wound care management to prevent infections.
- The optimum treatment modality for TEN is still controversial. Intravenous immunoglobulin or systemic cyclosporine can be considered.
- Refer to Ophthalmology for eye involvement.

References/Further Reading

1. Wolff K, Johnson RA, Suurmond D. *Fitzpatrick's Color Atlas & Synopsis of Clinical Dermatology*. 5th ed. New York: McGraw-Hill; 2005.

2. Tan HH, Chan R, Sen P, Chio M. *Sexually Transmitted Infections – Management Guidelines 2007*. DSC Clinic National Skin Centre Singapore; 2007.

3. Giam YC, Goh CL. *A Guide to Common Dermatological Disorders*. National Skin Centre Singapore; 2002.

4. Tan HH, Tay YK, Goh CL. Bacterial skin infections at a tertiary dermatological centre. *Singapore Med J*. 1998; 39(8): 353–356.

5. National Skin Centre (Singapore) Therapeutic Guidelines (as of April 2009).

6. Gilbert DN, Moellering RC, Eliopoulos GM, et al. *The Sanford Guide to Antimicrobial Therapy 2009*. 39th ed. Sperryville, VA: Antimicrobial Therapy, Inc.; 2009.

7. Sigurdsson V, Toonstra J, Hezemans-Boer M, Van Vloten WA. Erythroderma: A clinical and follow-up study of 102 patients, with special emphasis on survival. *J Am Acad Dermatol*. 1996; 35: 53–57.

8. Edwards L. *Dermatology in Emergency Care*. New York: Churchill Livingstone; 1997.

9. Buton PK, et al. *ABC of Dermatology*. London: BMJ Books; 1998.

10. Goh CL, Chua SH, Ng SK, eds. *The Asian Skin: A Reference Color Atlas of Dermatology*. Singapore: McGraw-Hill Education (Asia); 2005.

81   Geriatric Emergencies

Chong Chew Lan • Shirley Ooi • Lee Sock Koon

CAVEATS

- Vague complaints of malaise or decreased functional ability may indicate a serious illness.
  1. **Factors** that **affect diagnosis** and **treatment** of geriatric patients:
     a. **Under-reporting of signs and symptoms** by the patient and dismissal of symptoms as due to **old age** by the patient, caregiver, as well as physician.
     b. **Atypical** or attenuated **manifestation** of a serious illness in the elderly individuals makes diagnosis difficult. Be prepared to perform further diagnostic tests even with initial non-specific findings.
     c. The presence or accumulation of **multiple coexisting chronic disorders** may mask clinical symptoms of a new disease.
     d. **Polypharmacy** lowers compliance and may cause adverse effects due to drug interaction. Evaluate all medications to exclude this as a cause of symptoms for every elderly patient.
        i. Age alone is not a contraindication for diagnostic and therapeutic interventions.
     e. **Lack** of **aggressive resuscitation**:
        i. 'Normal' vital signs lead to unrecognized shock due to the following:
           - Pre-existing hypertension.
           - A lack of tachycardic response.
- Base deficit or lactate levels can help in identifying early or occult shock.

⇨ **SPECIAL TIPS FOR GPs**

- Do not dismiss complaints of functional decline as due to 'old age'.
- Vague complaints may indicate a serious illness or depression.
- Beware of atypical presentation of acute myocardial infarction (AMI) in the elderly. Have a low threshold for doing ECG and for admission.
- Fever may be absent in sepsis in the elderly. However, when **fever** is present, 90% of the time it is infectious in aetiology, most commonly **bacterial** in origin. It is only due to a viral cause in <5% of cases.
- **A temperature of ≥37.2°C** or with an **increase of 1.3°C from the baseline** should be considered to be febrile in the elderly.
- Most **predictive factors of infection** in the elderly are **delirium** and **tachypnoea**.
- Always check the patient's **feet** for a **source of infection** because of fissure and maceration on feet and between toes. If no source is found, look at organs in the **abdomen**.
- Note that the **urine nitrite test** is **specific** but **not sensitive** for **urinary tract infection**.

SPECIFIC CONDITIONS AND THEIR MANAGEMENT

- Altered mental status (AMS) manifests itself in the form of a decreased level of consciousness, an altered content of consciousness or a combination of both.
- Look for these **4 features of delirium**:
  1. Acute onset or fluctuating course.
  2. Inattention.
  3. Disorganized thinking.
  4. Altered level of consciousness.

The diagnosis of delirium requires the presence of features 1 and 2, and either 3 or 4. After making the diagnosis, focus on finding the underlying cause.

- Elderly patients with acute changes in their mental state should be assumed to have an **organic aetiology**.
- **Myoclonus** and **asterixis** when present are **pathognomonic** of delirium.
- AMS may be the sole presenting feature of **myocardial infarction**, **pneumonia**, **gastrointestinal haemorrhage**, **sepsis**, or **pulmonary embolism**.
- **Medications** are the most common reversible cause of AMS in the elderly.
- The elderly patient with delirium should be admitted to hospital for further work-up and treatment.
- Some patients who have subacute or chronic cognitive impairment (dementia) may be discharged, providing prompt medical follow-up and a safe home environment with reliable caregiver are assured.

Functional decline

- Functional decline may be defined as a **recent or progressive** difficulty in performing activities of daily living.
- There are 2 errors that the emergency physician can make with regard to functional decline:
  1. To miss it.
  2. To dismiss it as part of 'normal aging'.
- Assume that functional decline is a symptom of a **new medical illness** or established **chronic diseases** that are **decompensating**.
- The best way in assessing functional decline is the patient's history and corroborating history from a caregiver who is in a position to comment objectively on new or worsening functional impairment.

Trauma and falls

- When faced with an injured elderly patient, look beyond the injuries and consider the **cause** of the **injury**.

- Falls are the most common cause of accidental injuries. Common medical causes of falls are cerebrovascular accident (CVA) or transient ischaemic attack, giddiness, postural hypotension, and syncope.
- If there is a suspicion of a medical cause for a fall, it may be appropriate to admit the patient to a medical discipline.
- Early assessment and frequent monitoring of vital signs is important in the elderly patient.
- Also consider the impact the injury has on the patient's functional status and his ability to care for himself. A priority is to prevent further injury.
- Emergency physicians should have a heightened suspicion for elder abuse in an injured geriatric patient.

Acute myocardial infarction

- Although the elderly may present with the classical symptoms of AMI, it is **common** for them to present **atypically** (Table 1). Those older than 85 years, in fact, are unlikely to present with classic chest pain. About 60% of those >85 years old with AMI do not have chest pain. Atypical AMI is associated with greater mortality.

TABLE 1 Atypical presentation of AMI in the elderly

1. Shortness of breath
2. Acute confusion
3. Syncopal attacks
4. Strokes
5. Giddiness, vertigo, and faintness
6. Palpitations
7. Vomiting
8. Peripheral gangrene and increased claudication
9. Renal failure
10. Pulmonary embolism
11. Restlessness
12. Sweating
13. Weakness
14. Abdominal pain
15. Burning sensation or indigestion in 20% of cases

- **Dyspnoea** is the **commonest presenting complaint** of **AMI** in the elderly.
- Acute CVA and AMI are much more likely to present together in the elderly. Hence, electrocardiogram (ECG) should be done in every case of CVA in the elderly.
- As AMI may present in a myriad of ways, it is a good practice to do ECG in elderly patients presenting with seemingly unrelated complaints.
- Therapy should be based on physiological age, functional status, known risks and benefits, and the patient's wishes, if known.
- Thrombolytic therapy and anti-coagulation can be well tolerated by the elderly patient with AMI, with a significant reduction in death and disability. The small but significant risk of haemorrhage and other complications should be discussed with the patient.

Acute abdominal pain

- The elderly patient with acute abdominal pain is a great challenge to the emergency physician.
- The rate of required admission and subsequent surgery is very high in the elderly patients with acute abdominal pain.
- Pain perception and the physical examination may be altered in older patients, creating diagnostic difficulties. Abdominal guarding or muscular rigidity may be lacking in the face of serious intra-abdominal pathology with peritoneal irritation. This well-recognized phenomenon is partially attributed to the relatively thin abdominal musculature in elderly patients.
- In the elderly patient with **appendicitis**, anorexia, leucocytosis or the classic migration pattern of pain may be lacking. However, tenderness in the right lower quadrant is generally present.
- Note also that although <10% of all appendicitis patients are elderly, 50% of deaths occur in this age group. Suspect appendicitis in any patient who presents with abdominal pain. If the cause of the abdominal pain is unclear, tell the patient to have a follow-up examination within 12–24 hours.
- Half the elderly patients with **perforated peptic ulcer** do not report a sudden onset of pain. The pain may be generalized or in the lower quadrants. Epigastric rigidity and the presence of free air on plain radiography are absent in a large percentage of these patients.
- **Large bowel obstruction** may be present despite the patient's complaint of diarrhoea. Colonic pseudo-obstruction should be suspected in patients appearing to have large bowel obstruction who have a non-tender abdomen or a cavernous rectal vault.
- **Acute mesenteric ischaemia** must always be suspected in any elderly patient with abdominal pain out of proportion to the physical signs. This is particularly so if there is underlying cardiovascular disease, hypotension, peripheral vascular disease, atrial fibrillation, or with associated symptoms of chronic ischaemic bowel such as weight loss, post-prandial abdominal pain, diarrhoea, and malabsorption. These patients must undergo angiography before 'hard evidence' of mesenteric infarction develops (refer to Chapter 13, *Pain, Abdominal*).

- A **ruptured abdominal aortic aneurysm** must be considered in any elderly patient with acute abdominal or back pain. A pulsatile mass will often not be detectable on examination. Syncope may be the primary complaint.
- Suspect **cholecystitis** in any elderly patient who presents with abdominal pain or signs of sepsis.

Infections

- An aging immune system, when accompanied by chronic conditions such as diabetes (twice the rate of bacteraemia), dementia, malnutrition, cardiovascular disease, stroke, chronic lung disease, cancer, alcohol abuse, recent invasive procedure or instrumentation and indwelling catheter, places the older individual at greater risk of serious infection and secondary complications.
- The **chief presenting complaint** with infection may be altered mental state, confusion, functional decline, anorexia, excess fatigue, weakness, unexplained weight loss, new incontinence, or falls.
- The following have been shown to **fail to predict bacteraemia** in the elderly:
  1. Fever.
  2. Respiratory symptoms.
  3. Urinary symptoms.
  4. Abnormalities in vital signs.
  5. Absolute white blood cell (WBC) count.
  6. Haemoglobin.
  7. Blood urea nitrogen.
  8. Creatinine.
  9. Increased erythrocyte sedimentation rate (ESR).

NOTE: The only independent predictors of bacteraemia are **altered mental state** (odds ratio [OR] 2.88; 95% confidence interval [CI] 1.52–5.50), **vomiting** (OR 2.63, 95% CI 1.16–6.15), and **WBC band forms of >6%** (OR 3.50, 95% CI 1.58–5.27).

- Elderly patients presenting with a **temperature of 37.2°C or higher or with an increase of 1.3°C from the baseline** should be considered to be **febrile** in the emergency department. This new definition increases the sensitivity to 83%, while maintaining adequate specificity (89%) for clinically significant bacterial infection. Leucocytosis may be absent in the elderly and the neutrophil count is usually increased.
- Infections in independent, community-dwelling individuals differ from those residing in nursing homes and those who have been recently hospitalized. **Respiratory tract infections** are most common among community-living elderly and include influenza, bronchitis, and pneumonia. **Urinary tract infection** follows next in frequency and then **intra-abdominal infections**, including cholecystitis, diverticulitis, and appendicitis. In contrast, 70–80% of

infections in nursing home residents can be accounted for by the acronym **PUS**: **Pneumonia, urinary tract infection,** and **soft tissue infections**.

- Follow all the usual guidelines as in younger patients using early goal-directed therapy in managing the septic elderly patient.

- Whether to treat any elderly patient with an infection as an outpatient or an inpatient often can be a difficult decision. Consider the patient's clinical status, comorbid conditions, functional status, social support and availability of timely, appropriate support.

- In general, lower the threshold for admission in the elderly with suspected infections as their likelihood for decompensation is very high. They are also, in many cases, at risk of infection with resistant organisms, necessitating the empiric use of broad spectrum anti-microbial agents.

- **Bacteraemia** in the elderly is associated with **high mortality rates** of **20–37%** in most studies.

- One should consider admission for febrile elderly patients even if no source of infection is identified as one-third of emergency department elderly patients with bacteraemia will not have an identified local source of infection.

- Well-patients with adequate follow-up, intact functional status (i.e. the ability to adequately perform activities of daily living) and appropriate home support may be considered for discharge.

References/Further Reading

1. Sanders AB. *Emergency Care of the Elder Person*. St. Louis, MO: Beverly Cracom Publications; 1996.

2. Kingsley A. Relevance of aging issues in the emergency department. In: Yoshikawa TT, Norman DC, eds. *Acute Emergencies and Critical Care of the Geriatric Patient*. New York: M. Dekker; 2000: 1–9.

3. Fernandez-Frackelton M. Abdominal pain in elderly patients. *Foresight*. Oct 2001; 52: 1–7.

4. Caterino JM. Evaluation and management of geriatric infections in the emergency department. *Emerg Med Clin N Am*. 2008; 26: 319–343.

82 Alcohol Intoxication and Poisoning with Other Alcohols

Peter Manning

CAVEATS

- Ethanol use is associated with a significantly increased risk of serious injury due to impaired motor control and judgement.

- Depression of the level of consciousness masks many of the usual responses to pain and underlying diseases.

- Ethanol consumption is often associated with respiratory depression and a depressed gag reflex.

- There is a significant **differential diagnosis** for the alcohol-intoxicated patient (Table 1).

- Blood ethanol level falls at a rate of **20–30 mg %** **per hour**.

- **Glasgow Coma Scale (GCS)** is not statistically affected by alcohol until a blood alcohol level of >200 mg % is reached. Hence, do not attribute alterations in the conscious state to alcohol unless the patient has a minimal blood alcohol level of 200 mg %.[2,3]

TABLE 1 Differential diagnosis of altered mental state in the alcohol-intoxicated patient

Central nervous system disorders	Convulsions or post-ictal state, strokes, subdural haematoma, tumours
Environmental disorders	Hypothermia
Infectious disorders	Meningitis/encephalitis, pneumonia, sepsis
Metabolic disorders	Diabetic ketoacidosis, hepatic encephalopathy, hypercalcaemia, hypoglycaemia, hyponatraemia, uraemia
Respiratory disorders	Hypoxaemia
Toxicological disorders	Benzodiazepines, carbon monoxide, ethanol, ethylene glycol, isopropyl alcohol, methanol, narcotics, sedative hypnotics
Traumatic disorders	Cerebral concussion, cerebral contusion, epidural haematoma, hypotension, subarachnoid haemorrhage

MANAGEMENT

Philosophies of management

The goals are as follows:

- To protect the patient from hurting himself and others.

- To treat potentially **life-threatening conditions** without delay, i.e. reversible conditions such as hypoxaemia, dehydration, hypoglycaemia and hypothermia.

- To ensure appropriate disposition and follow-up.
- To examine for **injuries** that might otherwise be ignored.
- To search actively for the existence of **Wernicke's encephalopathy**: the classic triad is present in only 10% of cases. Look for mental changes of depression, apathy, confusion (80% of cases), ocular changes of horizontal nystagmus or lateral rectus palsy (30% of cases) and ataxia (20% of cases).

Goals achieved through several management principles

- Observation with frequent measurements of vital signs and neurological assessment.
- Aggressive evaluation of non-improving or deteriorating mental status.
- Continued observation until the patient is able to function independently and care for himself.
- Intravenous hydration and nutrition.
- Restraints by chemical or physical means when needed (to protect the patient and others).

Supportive care

- Evaluate drunken patients in a **monitored location**.
- Maintain airway and cervical spine evaluation.
- Use an oral pharyngeal or nasopharyngeal airway depending on the presence of a gag reflex.
- Ensure suctioning equipment is always immediately available.
- If a history of **trauma** is suspected, apply a **stiff collar with or without manual immobilization**.
- Establish peripheral intravenous access.
- Run intravenous crystalloids at a rate appropriate for volume replacement; IV D5W 500 ml over 3 to 4 hours is suitable for the normovolaemic patient.
- Use **physical restraints**: In this way the patient can be controlled without adding medications which would complicate the assessment of a patient whose level of consciousness is already depressed.
- Undress the patient.
- Measure his body temperature.
- **Labs**: The minimum, for a mildly obtunded or confused patient, is **stat capillary blood sugar testing**. Since the history and physical findings are often limited, the intoxicated patient with **altered mental state** often requires laboratory and radiological evaluation:
  1. **Essential labs**
     a. Full blood count.
     b. Urea/electrolytes/creatinine: Calculate the anion gap $[Na^+] - [HCO_3^-] - [Cl^-]$. Refer to Chapter 143, *Useful Formulae*.

2. **Optional labs**
   a. **Blood ethanol level:** The importance of this test lies in the situation where the level does not correlate as expected (e.g. where it is low or even zero), then an intensive search to explain the altered mental state is essential.

   NOTE: If you draw such a specimen do so using **non-alcohol skin preparations** and in drunk driving cases, written, signed consent of the patient to take blood is **essential**.

   b. **Urinalysis**: For blood, sugar or ketones.
   c. **Serum amylase**.
   d. **Liver function tests (including prothrombin time and partial thromboplastin time)**.
   e. **Toxicology studies**: General screening tests are of limited value but should be ordered as directed by the history and physical examination dictate.
   f. **Serum osmolality**: Useful in suggesting the presence of other alcohols, e.g. methanol and ethylene glycol (see a later section in this chapter). Normal range is 286 ± 4 mOsm/kg H_2O. Calculate the osmolal gap (should not exceed 10 mOsm/kg).
   g. **Osmolal gap** = Measured osmolality − Calculated osmolality. Refer to Chapter 143, *Useful Formulae*.
   h. **Arterial blood gas**: Not necessary if saturation of peripheral oxygen (SpO_2) is normal.

- **X-rays:**
  1. **Chest:** Useful if history is one of chest trauma, or there is fever or abnormal auscultatory finding.
  2. **Lateral cervical spine, anterior-posterior pelvis and extremities**: Need is based on history and physical examination.
  3. **Head computed tomography (CT) scan**: Indicated in cases where:
     a. There is evidence of head trauma with persistent loss of consciousness or focal neurological findings.
     b. The patient's mental state is inconsistent with the blood ethanol level (see *Caveats*).
     c. There is no improvement in, or a worsening of, neurological status with time.
- **Electrocardiogram**: Useful for the detection of a concomitant cardiac disease, e.g. ischaemic heart disease or alcoholic cardiomyopathy.

Drug therapy

- **Thiamine** 100 mg IV: Thiamine stores are often diminished in alcoholic patients.
- **D50W** 40 ml IV bolus for documented hypoglycaemia.

NOTE: Theoretically, it is important that the administration of thiamine precede the dextrose in a malnourished patient since giving dextrose first may precipitate a Wernicke's encephalopathy (triad of ataxia, global confusion and ocular abnormalities, primarily horizontal nystagmus or a bilateral sixth nerve palsy). However, this consideration is not supported by evidence. It is argued that it takes hours, if not days, for Wernicke's encephalopathy to develop clinically. Also, thiamine can be administered immediately after the dextrose dose.

- **Haloperidol** 5 mg IV: Can be repeated in 5 to 10 minutes. This drug is used in the severely agitated intoxicated patient in conjunction with physical restraints. Haloperidol produces minimal sedation with excellent behavioural control.
- If the history and physical examination suggest concomitant narcotic use, **naloxone** 2 mg IV will help to identify and reverse the central nervous system and respiratory depression.

Disposition

- **Admit the patient to a high dependency or intensive care unit setting**, after appropriate consultation, for the following:
  1. Multiple trauma.
  2. Ingestions of methanol and ethylene glycol.
  3. Sepsis.
  4. Gastrointestinal haemorrhage.
  5. Acute myocardial infarction.
  6. Major withdrawal syndromes.
- Admit to **General Medicine** for concurrent pneumonia, hepatitis or pancreatitis. Admit to **General Surgery** or **Neurosurgery** for concurrent stable head injury depending on institutional practice.

Discharge criteria

- The patient must be capable of eating or drinking, walking with a steady gait and is oriented to the surroundings.
- Availability of friends or family to accompany the patient.

SPECIAL SITUATIONS

Children

- Children are exposed to ethanol usually either by drinking alcoholic beverages or mouthwash. Respiratory depression is common even after small doses of ethanol.
- **Hypoglycaemia is common**: Treat with 2–4 ml/kg of solution of IV D25W (dilute D50W 1:1 with sterile water since D50W is very hyperosmolar).

NOTE: Repeated administration is usually not required and may result in a hyperosmolar state.

METHANOL, ETHYLENE GLYCOL AND ISOPROPYL ALCOHOL

Similarities

- Should be suspected in drunk patients who complain of abdominal pain or visual impairment, or in whom there is a high osmolar gap.
- **All** are found in a variety of household products:
  1. **Methanol**: Windshield washer fluid, model airplane fuel, photocopying fluid, perfumes, paint and illicitly-brewed alcohol or 'moonshine'.
  2. **Ethylene glycol**: Automotive anti-freeze, brake and hydraulic fluids, de-icers, fire extinguishers, lacquers and paints.
  3. **Isopropyl alcohol**: Rubbing alcohol, lacquers and as a solvent in many household, cosmetic and topical pharmaceutical products.
- All can be, and are, used as a cheap substitute for ethyl alcohol by the alcohol-addicted.
- All can produce the clinical picture of a patient who '**acts drunk, but who does not smell drunk**' – unless ethyl alcohol has been drunk concurrently.
- All are readily absorbed in the gastrointestinal tract.
- Alcohol dehydrogenase is the primary enzyme for the metabolism of all three parent compounds.
- Methanol and ethylene glycol differ in toxicity but treatment for either is essentially the same.
- None of the agents are themselves dangerous, producing only ethanol-like intoxication; it is the metabolites formed after metabolism with alcohol dehydrogenase that produce the toxicity some 6–12 hours after ingestion. This delay in onset of symptoms can be even greater with concurrent ethanol intoxication.
- Early in toxic alcohol ingestions, the ingested parent compound contributes to the measured serum osmolality, causing it to become elevated, creating an osmolal gap that is used as an early marker of toxic alcohol poisoning. Since serum levels of any of the alcohols are not readily available such an indirect measure as anion and osmolar gaps are useful.

  Osmolal gap = Measured osmolality – Calculated osmolality – **A markedly increased gap (>25 mOsm)** is pathognomonic of **toxic alcohol poisoning**.

NOTE: The osmolal gap increases first before metabolism, only for the anion gap to increase later.

Methanol and ethylene glycol toxicity

- Both undergo oxidation, via alcohol dehydrogenase, to formic acid and oxalic acid (via glycolic acid), respectively.

- In methanol toxicity, formic acid inhibits cytochrome c oxidase activity, leading to tissue hypoxia, lactate formation and metabolic acidosis.

  1. As acidosis worsens, formic acid diffuses across cell membranes leading to central nervous system depression, hypotension and further worsening of acidosis by further increases in lactate production.

  2. The undissociated formic acid targets the optic disc and optic nerve preferentially causing localized cellular hypoxia; hence, the **blindness typical of methanol toxicity**.

- The **classic triad of methanol poisoning** includes

  1. Severe metabolic acidosis.

  2. Visual disturbance.

  3. Central nervous system depression.

- Methanol also has a direct toxic effect on the pancreas leading to **pancreatitis**.

- In **ethylene glycol toxicity**, the main metabolite of oxidation is glycolic acid which is responsible for severe metabolic acidosis; this, in turn, is rapidly oxidized to oxalic acid, which chelates with calcium and is precipitated as calcium oxalate crystals in the proximal renal tubules causing **acute tubular necrosis**. The same chelation process can lead to **hypocalcaemia** of sufficient severity to cause prolongation of the QTc interval and life-threatening cardiac dysrhythmias and fits.

- Classically, three stages of ethylene glycol poisoning have been recognized:

  1. **Within 12 hours, central nervous system symptoms** of inebriation and euphoria ('act drunk but do not smell drunk'), leading to progressive lethargy and coma resulting from cerebral oedema.

  2. **Cardiovascular system** signs and symptoms of 'air hunger' due to the **severe metabolic acidosis**, **hypoxia** from aspiration, congestive heart failure or **adult respiratory distress syndrome** and ventricular dysrhythmias from **hypocalcaemia**.

  3. **Acute renal failure after 24–72 hours** that may be severe enough to need haemodialysis.

Isopropyl alcohol

- Undergoes metabolism to acetone with ketonaemia and ketonuria occurring rapidly after ingestion.

NOTE: Not an acid metabolite – **ketosis without acidosis** helps to distinguish this poisoning from that of methanol and ethylene glycol.

- Classically, poisoning from isopropyl alcohol causes **central nervous system depression (faster in onset and longer lasting than ethanol)** and gastric distress due to **haemorrhagic gastritis** from direct mucosal irritation.

MANAGEMENT OF TOXIC ALCOHOL POISONING

General points

- Focus is on the evaluation and management of immediate life-threatening complications:
  1. Attention to airway, breathing and circulation.
  2. Intravenous fluid therapy to maintain adequate urine output but to avoid fluid overload in those with impaired renal function.
  3. Administration of supplemental oxygen.
  4. Monitoring: Electrocardiogram, vital signs and oximetry.
  5. Stat capillary blood sugar for assessment of possible hypoglycaemia.
  6. Lab studies: Full blood count, serum electrolytes, blood urea nitrogen and creatinine, lipase and/or amylase, liver function tests, calcium, ketones and lactate, serum osmolality, arterial blood gases and urinalysis (with microscopy to determine the presence of calcium oxalate crystals).
  7. Determination of the osmolal gap and anion gap (see Chapter 143, *Useful Formulae*).
  8. Evidence suggests that gastric aspiration and lavage may be effective if employed within 4 hours of ingestion, especially if a large amount of alcohol has been ingested.

Specific points in the management of methanol and ethylene glycol poisoning

- Metabolic acidosis must be treated aggressively with intravenous sodium bicarbonate since the outcome correlates directly with keeping the serum pH levels >7.2–7.3.
- The inhibition of alcohol dehydrogenase (ADH) is now the mainstay of treatment of poisoning by these two agents.
- **Fomepizole** (antizol, 4-MP) is a potent inhibitor of ADH that has many advantages over ethanol, the historically preferred antidote. Its advantages are as follows:
  1. An affinity for ADH 8000 times greater than that of ethanol.
  2. A longer duration of action.
  3. Easier dosing with more predictable kinetics.
  4. A wider therapeutic index.
  5. Avoidance of the side effects seen with ethanol administration, i.e. headache, nausea and dizziness.
  6. Reduction in the need for haemodialysis.
- The principal disadvantage of fomepizole is its cost.
- **Intravenous ethanol**, though outdated, still has application if fomepizole is unavailable, or haemodialysis is not indicated, but the side effects of central nervous system depression, hypotension, hypoglycaemia and electrolyte disturbance require close monitoring in an intensive care unit setting.
  1. It is effective because ADH has an affinity for ethanol 15 times greater than its affinity for methanol and 60 to 70 times greater than its affinity for ethylene glycol.

2. A **10% intravenous solution** is administered via a central venous catheter to maintain a serum concentration of 100 mg/dl.

3. **Oral alcohol** can be used if no intravenous source is available; the goal is to give 0.7 g/kg as a loading dose and **0.12 g/kg/hr** as a maintenance dose by administering any common alcoholic beverage using the following conversion:

Grams of ethanol = Volume of beverage in ml $\times$ 0.9 $\times$ Proof/200

However, oral ethanol should not be used if the patient is obtunded or has no gag reflex.

Indications for methanol and ethylene glycol toxicity

Indications for haemodialysis (removes both parent compounds and their toxic by-products):

- Severe metabolic acidosis that is not correctable with intravenous sodium bicarbonate.
- Impending renal failure.
- End-organ toxicity, e.g. vision changes, fits and coma.
- Haemodynamic instability.
- Worsening electrolyte imbalance.

Specific points in the management of isopropyl alcohol poisoning

- A serum isopropyl alcohol level adds little to management.
- Treat as for ethanol toxicity.

Alcoholic ketoacidosis

- Seen classically in the chronic alcoholic who binges and then presents with nausea, vomiting, abdominal pain and starvation with poor caloric intake.
- Ketoacidosis results from the accumulation of acetoacetate and beta-hydroxybutarate.
- Labs reveal serum pH of about 7.1, serum bicarbonate of 10, low serum potassium phosphate and a normal or low serum glucose level.
- **Treatment:** Rehydration with 5% dextrose saline solution, anti-emetics if needed, benzodiazepines as needed for withdrawal symptoms (Table 2), potassium and phosphate replacement.

NOTE: Insulin therapy is contraindicated and bicarbonate is rarely required.

- The likelihood of developing severe withdrawal symptoms increases with concomitant infections or medical problems, a prior history of withdrawal seizures or delirium tremens and a higher intake of alcohol.
- **Withdrawal seizures** (rum fits):
  1. Usually generalized seizures and self-limited.
  2. Onset: Usually within **48 hours** of **last alcohol intake**.

TABLE 2   **Alcohol withdrawal syndrome (AWS)**

Stage	Onset	Duration	Symptoms	Signs
I The shakes	6–8 hours	2–3 days	• Anxiety • Agitation • Fear • Loss of appetite • Loss of sleep • Tremor	• Tachycardia • Hypertension • Hyperreflexia
II The horrors	0–24 hours	2–3 days	The above plus • Hallucinations	The above plus • Fever • Sweating
III Withdrawal seizures	7–48 hours	6–12 hours		The above plus • Grand mal seizures
IV Delirium tremens	3–5 days	2–5 days	The above plus • Confusion • Nightmares	The above plus • Fever • Mydriasis

3. It is usually not possible to differentiate withdrawal seizures from other aetiology from history and physical examination.

4. Suggest:

   a. **Focal seizure**: Head computed tomography (CT) scan.

   b. **Febrile seizure**: LP after head CT scan. Start antibiotics stat.

   c. **Status seizure**: Head CT scan and metabolic screen.

● **Management**

1. Provide relief from anxiety and hallucinations.

2. Halt progression of AWS.

3. **Supportive therapy**

   a. Secure the airway, breathing and circulation.

   b. Volume replacement: IV 5% dextrose saline solution alternating with dextrose 5%.

   c. Correct electrolyte and metabolic disorders: Glucose, thiamine, potassium and magnesium.

   d. IV thiamine 100 mg and IV magnesium sulphate 1–2 g may be started empirically.

4. **Drug therapy**

   a. **Benzodiazepine**: (1) IV diazepam 5–10 mg slow bolus every 5 to 10 minutes titrated clinically (maximum 20 mg). (2) PO diazepam 10–20 mg for mild cases (may be repeated after an hour).

   b. **Haloperidol**: IM haloperidol 5–10 mg for agitated patients.

   c. **Beta blockers**: (1) Indicated if multiple doses of diazepam have been used and/or significant tachyarrhythmias. (2) IV propanolol 0.5 mg every 5 to 10 minutes.

   d. **IV phenytoin has no or little role in AWS.**

5. **Disposition**

1. All cases should be admitted to General Medicine except for the mild cases who may be discharged with oral benzodiazepine and psychiatric follow-up.
2. Delirium tremens should be admitted to the intensive care unit for close monitoring.

References/Further Reading

1. Lindblad R, Galesh G. Alcohol intoxication. In: Hamilton GC, Sanders AB, Strange GR, Trott AT, eds. *Emergency Medicine: An Approach to Clinical Problem Solving*. Philadelphia, PA: WB Saunders; 1991: 20: 378–393.

2. Galbraith S, Murray WR, Patel AR, et al. The relationship between alcohol and head injury and its effect on the conscious level. *Br J Surg*. 1976; 63: 128–130.

3. Jagger J, Fife D, Vernberg K, et al. Effect of alcohol intoxication on the diagnosis and apparent severity of brain injury. *Neurosurgery*. 1984; 15: 303–306.

83   Poisoning, Benzodiazepine

Suresh Pillai • Lim Er Luen

CAVEATS

- Death from a benzodiazepine overdose is generally rare unless it is combined with other sedative agents, ethanol, or barbiturates.
- General supportive treatment measures are usually all that is required with special emphasis on the airway, breathing, and ventilation.
- The use of **benzodiazepine antagonists** like flumazenil in overdose is controversial. Do not give intravenous flumazenil to patients who are benzodiazepine-dependent and to patients with concomitant ingestion of tricyclic anti-depressants, or with an unspecified mixed overdose. Take caution in those at risk for seizures, e.g. those with head injuries and known epileptics.
- If there is associated head trauma then this must be evaluated separately with a head computed tomography scan even though the major contribution to a patient's altered mental state may be due to benzodiazepines.

PATHOPHYSIOLOGY

- Benzodiazepines cause a generalized depression of spinal reflexes as well as inhibit the reticular activating system resulting in lethargy, slurred speech, ataxia, hyporreflexia, drowsiness, stupor, coma, or even respiratory arrest.
- The **pupils** in patients with benzodiazepine overdose are usually **non-specific** and are generally not pin point as in pure opiate overdoses.
- Hypotension and cardiopulmonary arrest are possible after rapid intravenous injection of diazepam.
- The **half-lives** of benzodiazepines vary widely from 2 to 5 hours for midazolam, 5 to 30 hours for chlordiazepoxide and 50 to 100 hours for flurazepam.

> ⇨ **SPECIAL TIP FOR GPs**
> - All patients should be referred to the emergency department if there is any suspicion of a sedative-hypnotic overdose even though they may only exhibit mild drowsiness initially.

MANAGEMENT

Supportive measures

- Patients having altered mental states with impaired gag reflex and respiratory depression, haemodynamic instability or are comatose should be managed in the critical care area.
- The airway should be maintained and if necessary the patient intubated and ventilated if indicated. Otherwise, the patient should be given 100% oxygen via a non-rebreather mask.

- The patient should be placed on vital signs, cardiac and pulse oximetry monitoring q15 min.
- Maintain a peripheral intravenous infusion line.
- Take blood for full blood count, urea/electrolytes/creatinine and arterial blood gas sampling. Perform bedside blood glucose estimation.
- Chest radiography should be performed if hypoxia or aspiration is suspected. Computed tomography of the head should be considered if intracranial haemorrhage or infection is suspected.
- **Serum benzodiazepine** levels are **not necessary** during the acute management of overdoses but qualitative urine or blood-screening methods, if available, can be performed in cases where the diagnosis is in doubt.
- Induced emesis is not recommended in benzodiazepine overdose because of central nervous system depression.
- Administer **activated charcoal** if the time of ingestion is within 4 hours. **Gastric lavage** is limited to large ingestions or mixed ingestions within an hour. However, the airway must be protected and the patient intubated, if necessary, during gastric lavage or activated charcoal administration.

Antidotal therapy

- **IV flumazenil** in a dose of 0.2 mg given over 30 seconds can be administered depending on the response and repeated until a total dose of 0.5 mg is given. As its effects are generally short-lived, repeat doses may be required. However, the **contraindications** in using it are:
  1. If there is **concomitant tricyclic anti-depressant overdose** where reversal of benzodiazepine effects may precipitate status epilepticus induced by the former.
  2. Patients who are **addicted** to **benzodiazepines**, whereby flumazenil can precipitate an acute withdrawal reaction, manifested by seizures and autonomic instability.
  3. Patients who may already be predisposed to developing seizures, e.g. those who suffer head injuries or are known epileptics.
- If the history is not accurate, then the administration of IV thiamine, IV 50% dextrose and IV naloxone should be considered in patients presenting with altered mental state. IV naloxone should not be used routinely unless there are signs suggestive of opioid overdose (refer to Chapter 19, *Poisoning, General Principles*). Other causes of altered mental state should be sought, e.g. carbon monoxide poisoning, central nervous system infections, head trauma and cerebrovascular accidents.

Disposition

- All patients with benzodiazepine overdose should be admitted to the General Medical ward and if necessary to the high dependency or the intensive care unit especially if ventilatory support is required.

References/Further Reading

1. Gussow L, Carlson A. Sedative hypnotics. In: Marx JA, Hockberger RS, Walls RM, eds. *Rosen's Emergency Medicine: Concepts and Clinical Practice*. 7th ed. Philadelphia, PA: Mosby-Elsevier; 2010: 2071–2082.
2. Farrell SE. Benzodiazepines. In: Ford: Clinical Toxicology. 1st ed. Philadelphia, PA: WB Saunders; 2001.

84 Poisoning, Carbon Monoxide

Amila Punyadasa

CAVEATS

- Carbon monoxide (CO) is a colourless, tasteless, and odourless gas which acts as a respiratory asphyxiant that binds preferentially to haemoglobin (Hgb) and myoglobin, subsequently reducing the oxygen-carrying capacity of blood. Hence, its designation as a silent killer.

- **Half-life** in the body is **5 to 6 hours**.

- CO exerts its pathologic effects via different mechanisms. This results in a combination of impaired oxygen delivery, oxygen utilization and, possibly, oxidant stress injury in various susceptible tissues.

- Carbon monoxide has an affinity for Hgb 250 times greater than oxygen; it shifts the oxyhaemoglobin dissociation curve to the left, impairing the release of oxygen to the tissues.

- It binds to inactivate myoglobin (cardiac myoglobin 3 times more than skeletal myoglobin). During hypoxaemia, cardiac myoglobin takes up CO even more avidly, resulting in myocardial necrosis and depressed myocardial function.

- It causes diffuse demyelination of the brain, with autopsy findings of cerebral oedema, necrosis of superficial white matter, globus pallidus, cerebrum and hippocampus. Delayed neuropsychiatric sequlae occur in up to 40% of cases following apparent recovery. In fact, recent experimental evidence suggests that relatively intense CO exposure can trigger a cascade of events, including brain lipid peroxidation, leading to transient and irreversible neuronal dysfunction.

- CO poisoning is difficult to diagnose since there are **few pathognomonic signs and symptoms**. Mild symptoms are non-specific, e.g. headache, nausea, vomiting, and dizziness. Several members of the same family may present at the same time, seemingly indicating a flu-like illness.

METABOLISM

- CO absorption is by inhalation without further metabolism; widespread distribution by blood, with elimination via the lungs by exhalation.

- CO binds to cytochrome oxidase: Competes with oxygen for binding sites on cytochrome a_3.

- **Sources**:

  1. **Endogenous**: CO is a normal degradation product of haemoglobin and other haem-containing compounds:

     a. The carboxyhaemoglobin (COHb) level is <5% in non-smokers and <10% in smokers.

    b. In pregnant women the COHb level can be up to 2–5%.

    c. In normal infants the COHb level can be 4–5%.

    d. In haemolytic anaemia the level can rise as high as 6%.

2. **Exogenous**:

    a. Cigarette smoke: Smoke emitted by the tip of a burning cigarette contains 2½ times as much CO as the inhaled portion.

    b. Smokers often have COHb levels of 4–10%.

    c. Fires: Smoke from a major fire contains up to 10% CO (100 times the concentration needed to produce a lethal COHb level).

    d. Car exhausts contain up to 8% CO: Rear seat passengers are affected more due to their closer proximity to the exhaust system.

    e. Methylene chloride in paint removers, aerosols, and fumigants is readily absorbed through the skin and is slowly metabolized to CO. Note that the half-life of COHb due to methylene chloride exposure is twice that of inhaled CO.

ACUTE EXPOSURE

In general, organs with relatively high metabolic demands, such as the brain and heart, are most sensitive to the effects of CO exposure.

- **Central nervous system**: Headache, peripheral neuropathy, altered mental state, coma, seizure, cerebral oedema, behavioural and personality changes, ataxia, and memory impairment.
- **Respiratory**: Dyspnoea and hyperpnoea, bronchopneumonia and non-cardiogenic pulmonary oedema.
- **Cardiovascular**: Angina, ST-segment changes, tachycardia, ventricular dysrhythmias, hypotension, myocardial infarction, heart block, congestive cardiac failure, and cardiac arrest.
- **Renal**: Oliguria from acute renal failure, proteinuria, myoglobinuria, and haematuria.
- **Haematological**: Carboxyhaemoglobinaemia, tissue hypoxia, polycythaemia, haemolytic anaemia, disseminated coagulation and leucocytosis.
- **Skin**: Cyanosis is more common than the often-quoted cherry red discolouration; bullae.
- **Ophthalmologic**: Flame-shaped retinal haemorrhages, decreased visual acuity, cortical blindness, papilloedema, and scotomas.
- **Musculoskeletal**: Rhabdomyolysis, myonecrosis, and compartment syndrome.

NOTE: Arterial blood gases will typically reveal a normal partial pressure of oxygen in the blood (PaO_2) because PaO_2 is a measurement of the dissolved oxygen in arterial blood, not the amount of oxygen bound to haemoglobin. Many blood gas analyzers calculate the percentage of oxygen saturation based on the PaO_2. The calculated oxygen saturation will be falsely high when compared to those directly measured by oximetry. This '**saturation gap**' is characteristic of CO poisoning.

Potential complications

- Delayed neuropsychiatric sequela or CO-induced delayed neuropsychiatric syndrome (CO-DNS, which may occur between several days and several weeks after exposure) occurs in 10–30% of cases after apparent recovery. Its features include the following:
  1. Headache/dizziness.
  2. Memory deficits.
  3. Personality alterations.
  4. Parkinsonism.
  5. Dementia.
  6. Decrements in cognitive functioning.
  7. Decerebrate rigidity.

Studies have shown that aggressive treatment, which may include hyperbaric oxygen treatment if indicated, may prevent the occurrence of CO-DNS as well as improve its outcome. The prognosis is relatively good, with most patients recovering within a year.

- Miscellaneous
  1. Aspiration pneumonia
  2. Adult respiratory distress syndrome
  3. Myocardial ischaemia and heart failure
  4. Rhabdomyolysis and myoglobinuric renal tubular injury
  5. Skin necrosis
  6. Secondary infections

HIGH-RISK GROUPS FOR MORTALITY AND MORBIDITY

- Individuals with underlying heart disease.
- Patients with underlying chronic pulmonary disease.
- Pregnant patients – the foetus exhibits a greater sensitivity to the toxic effects of CO. Foetal haemoglobin has a greater affinity for CO, causing prolonged and severe impairment in oxygen delivery to the hypoxia-sensitive foetal tissues.

⇨ **SPECIAL TIPS FOR GPs**
- Always consider CO toxicity in patients presenting with altered mental state who were found in a confined space or who were involved in a fire or explosion some hours before.
- Remember the classic cherry red appearance described in most texts is an autopsy finding. Cyanosis is more common in a survivor.

MANAGEMENT

Supportive Measures

Management mainly consists of **supportive measures** and **supplemental oxygen therapy**.

- **Airway, breathing and circulation**:
  1. Evaluate and support the airway. Consider protecting the cervical spine, if necessary.
  2. Perform orotracheal intubation if ventilation/oxygenation is compromised.
  3. Administer **early** 100% supplemental oxygen via a tight-fitting face mask.

  NOTE: The serum elimination half-life of COHb in human adults is **320 minutes** when breathing **room air**, compared to **80 minutes** when breathing **100% oxygen**. Oxygen therapy should not be discontinued until the patient is asymptomatic and the COHb level is less than 10%.

  4. Monitoring: Electrocardiogram (ECG) showing sinus tachycardia and ST-segment changes, vital signs q 15 minutes and pulse oximetry.
  5. Consider the use of sodium bicarbonate by intravenous infusion in the face of significant metabolic acidosis (arterial pH <7.1).

Investigations

- Routine: Full blood count, stat capillary glucose, urea/electrolytes/creatinine, ABG with COHb level, 12-lead ECG.
- Optional: Chest X-ray (for severe inhalation injury, pulmonary aspiration, bronchopneumonia, or pulmonary oedema) and head computed tomography (CT) scan (in the investigation of altered mental status).

Antidote Therapy

A study by Weaver et al. (2002) shows that 3 hyperbaric oxygen treatments within a 24-hour period appeared to reduce the risk of cognitive sequelae 6 weeks and 12 weeks after acute CO poisoning. The benefit of hyperbaric oxygen is the prevention of damage caused by CO exposure rather than the removal of CO.

NOTE: Cyanide (CN) exposure from the smoke of some burning materials, e.g. nitrocellulose or polyurethane foam, may complicate CO poisoning and cause early treatment failure with high-flow oxygen. If concomitant CO and CN toxicity is suspected, cautious use of the CN antidote kit is warranted but must be limited to the administration of sodium thiosulphate. This is because the nitrite-induced methaemoglobinaemia may further impair tissue oxygen delivery.

Disposition

- Refer for **hyperbaric oxygen therapy** the following patients by contacting your local hyperbaric oxygen source, military or civilian, according to local protocols:

1. All patients with syncope, neurological abnormalities, and cardiac abnormalities with elevated levels of COHb.
2. All patients with COHb levels >25%.
3. Pregnant patients with COHb level >10%.
4. Patients with myocardial ischaemia.
5. Patients experiencing worsening symptoms despite oxygen therapy.
6. Patients whose symptoms persist after 4 hours of 100% oxygen therapy (including abnormal psychometric testing and tachycardia).
7. Neonates.

NOTE: With **hyperbaric oxygen therapy**, the elimination **half-life** of **CO** is reduced to **23 minutes**, though outside of a military setting, it is very unlikely that you would be able to implement this therapy sufficiently promptly to achieve this reduction in half-life.

- Admit to General Medicine patients with COHb levels of less than 20%, administer high-flow oxygen at 15 L/min via a tight-fitting mask for at least 4 hours until the COHb level has dropped to normal.
- Asymptomatic patients with COHb levels of less than 10% are unlikely to develop complications and may be discharged from the emergency department with advice to seek medical care promptly if any of the following symptoms develop:
  1. Difficulty breathing or shortness of breath.
  2. Chest pain or tightness.
  3. Difficulties with coordination of limbs.
  4. Memory difficulties.
  5. Prolonged headache or dizziness.
- Discharged patients should be referred for psychiatric review with a view to possible carbon monoxide neuropsychological screening battery (CONSB) to detect subtle deteriorations.
- The patient should be told to refrain from smoking for 72 hours.

References/Further Reading

1. Scheinkstel CD, et al. Hyperbaric or normobaric oxygen for acute carbon monoxide poisoning: A randomized controlled clinical trial. *Med J Aust*. 1999; 170: 203–210.
2. Gosselin RE, Smith RP, Hodge HC. *Clinical Toxicology of Commercial Products*. 5th ed. Baltimore, MD: Williams & Wilkins; 1984.
3. Weaver LK, Hopkins RO, Chan KJ, et al. Hyperbaric oxygen for acute carbon monoxide poisoning. *N Engl J Med*. 2002; 347(14): 1057–1066.
4. Seger D, Welch L. Carbon monoxide controversies: Neuropsychiatric testing, mechanism of toxicity, and hyperbaric oxygen. *Ann Emerg Med*. 1994; 24: 242–248.
5. Thom SR, Taber RL, et al. Delayed neuropsychiatric sequelae after carbon monoxide poisoning: Prevention by treatment with hyperbaric oxygen. *Ann Emerg Med*. 1995; 25: 474–480.
6. Suner S, Partridge R, Sucov A, et al. Non-invasive pulse CO-oximetry screening in the emergency department identifies occult carbon monoxide toxicity. *J Emerg Med*. May 2008; 34(4): 441–450.
7. Gorman D, Drewry A, Huang YL. The clinical toxicology of carbon monoxide. *Toxicology*. 1 May 2003; 187(1): 25–38.
8. Raub JA, Benignus VA. Carbon monoxide and the nervous system. *Neurosci Biobehav Rev*. Dec 2002; 26(8): 925–940.

85   Poisoning, Cyclic Anti-depressants

Amila Punyadasa • Peter Manning • Suresh Pillai

CAVEATS

- Commonly prescribed cyclic anti-depressants are imipramine, trimipramine, desipramine, amitriptyline, doxepin, maprotiline and amoxapine.
- Depressive illnesses are thought to be due to central neurotransmitter deficiencies including serotonin, dopamine and noradrenaline. It is postulated that tricyclic anti-depressants (TCA) work by inhibiting the reuptake of these transmitters, thereby increasing their availability within the synapse.
- Most cyclic anti-depressants have a low therapeutic index. As little as 10 times the normal therapeutic dose may cause serious intoxication.
- Heterocyclics are highly protein-bound (92% at physiological pH); forced diuresis, dialysis and haemoperfusion have no role in the management of overdose.
- The mainstay of treatment is the administration of **sodium bicarbonate** because it alters binding of the drug to the myocardial sodium channels, and may also increase protein binding of the drug, thus rendering it pharmacologically less active.
- **Drugs to avoid**:
  1. Type IA (e.g. quinidine and procainamide) and IC (e.g. flecainide) anti-dysrhythmics, which can worsen the 'quinidine-like' toxicity on the myocardium.
  2. Beta blockers and calcium channel blockers may exacerbate hypotension.
  3. Phenytoin may increase the incidence of ventricular dysrhythmias and its use is controversial.
  4. Flumazenil (Anexate®) carries the risk of precipitating fits.
  5. Physostigmine (a reversible cholinesterase inhibitor) with an almost immediate effect on reversing hallucinations and delirium in pure anti-cholinergic poisonings must NOT be used in the context of cyclic anti-depressant toxicity to treat its anti-cholinergic side effects. It has been shown to precipitate seizures and cardiac asystole.

PHARMACOLOGICAL EFFECTS

In addition to the reuptake inhibition of central neurotransmitters, the cyclics also exert secondary effects that are the cause of much of the toxic effects. These include the following:

- Sodium channel inhibition: Fast sodium channel blockade causes negative inotropy and rhythm disturbances. PR and QRS interval are prolonged.
- Potassium channel blockade: Results in QTc prolongation.
- Gamma-aminobutyric acid (GABA) receptor antagonism may cause seizures.
- Alpha receptor antagonism may cause hypotension with reflex tachycardia.
- Anti-cholinergic activity: Produces both central features (e.g. delirium, agitation, ataxia and coma) and peripheral features (e.g. dry mouth, mydriasis, diminished bowel sounds and dry skin).

CLINICAL PATHOPHYSIOLOGY

Cardiac effects

- Anti-cholinergic activity that can induce tachycardia.
- Quinidine-like activity (sodium and potassium channel blockade) that can induce intraventricular and atrioventricular blocks. Bundle branch and fascicular blocks are usually preceded by a widening QRS complex. See Figure 1. A **coexistent sinus tachycardia may simulate ventricular tachycardia**.
- Hypotension due to peripheral alpha-adrenergic blockade.
- Pulmonary oedema.

Central nervous system effects

- The patient develops confusion, agitation and hallucinations before slipping into a coma.
- Seizures are common and usually single; status epilepticus is more likely to occur with amoxapine or maprotiline.
- Physical findings may include the following:
  1. Clonus
  2. Choreoathetosis
  3. Myoclonic jerks
  4. Increased muscle tone
  5. Hyperreflexia
  6. Extensor plantar responses.

FIGURE 1   **62 yr old man presented with an overdose of amitriptyline. Fig 1 shows his ECG demonstrating broad QRS complexes and tall R waves >3 mm in aVR.**

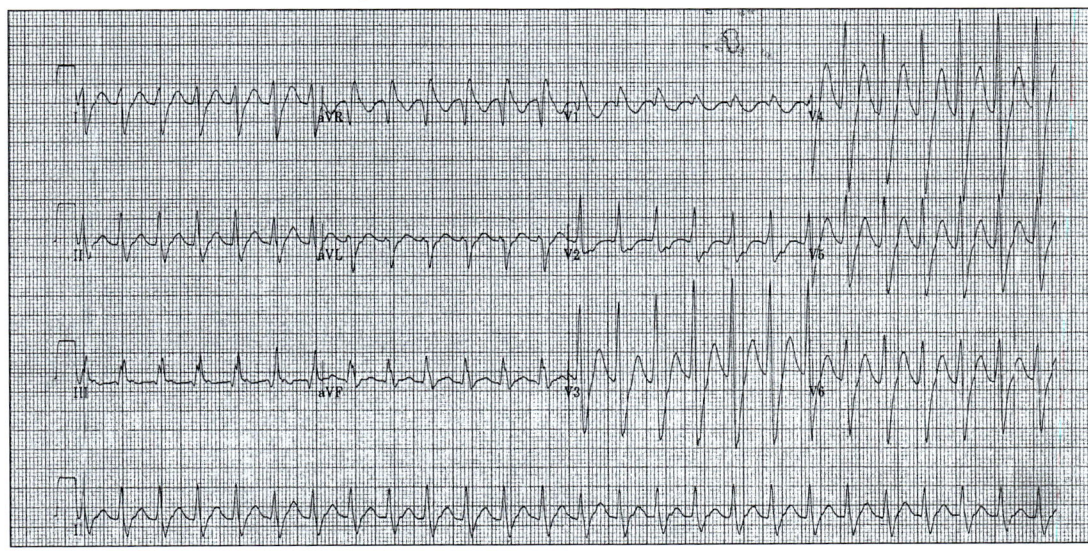

FIGURE 2   Fig 2 shows his ECG with marked QRS widening and further increased height of R waves in aVR shortly after he developed seizures.

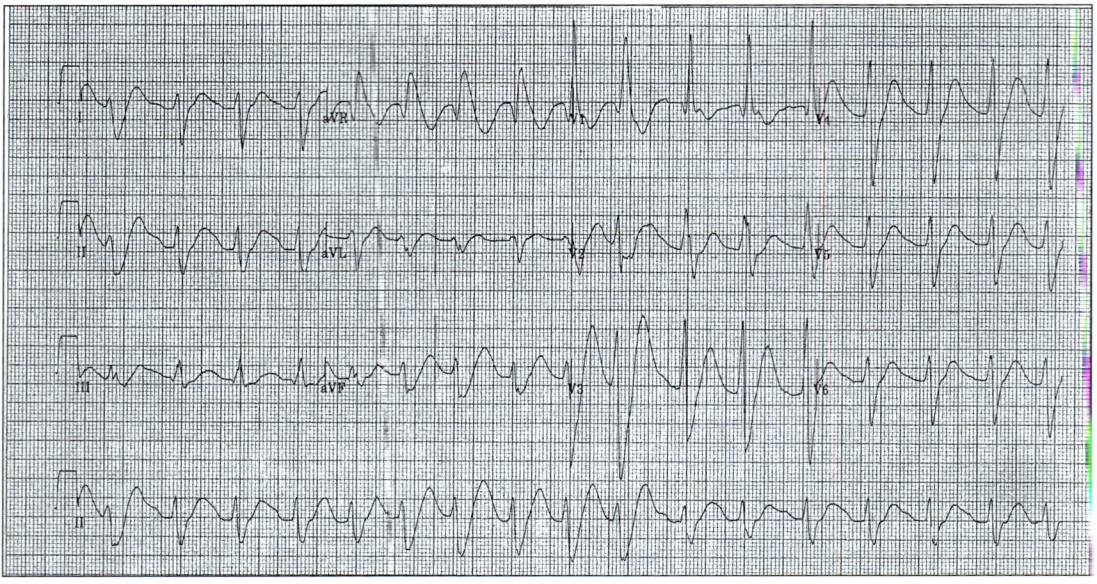

FIGURE 3   Fig 3 shows the narrowing of his QRS complexes with resolution of the tall R waves in aVR after treatment with intubation and intravenous sodium bicarbonate.

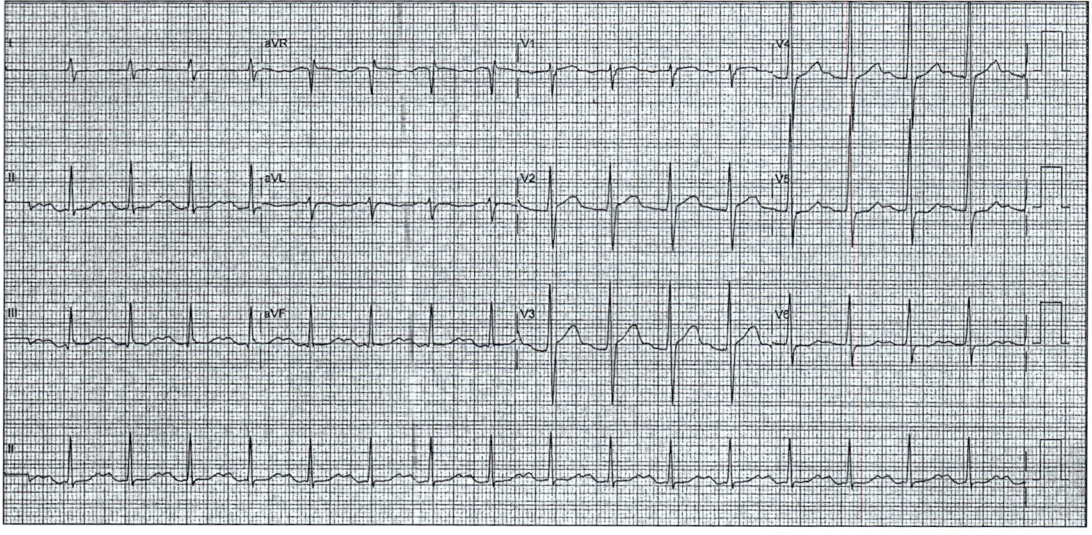

ECGs are contributed by Dr Mong Rupeng.

Anti-cholinergic effects

These may or may not occur; their absence does not exclude toxicity.

- Flushing
- Dry mouth/skin
- Dilated pupils
- Blurred vision from paralysis of accommodation
- Fever
- Absent bowel sounds
- Urinary retention

Other effects

- Skin blisters
- Rhabdomyolysis and renal failure
- Pneumonia
- ARDS

Signs that indicate a serious overdose

- Ventricular dysrhythmias
- Bradycardia and atrioventricular blocks
- Intraventricular conduction defects with a QRS complex duration of >100 milliseconds
- Fits
- Hypotension
- Pulmonary oedema
- Cardiac arrest

Clinical indicators suggestive of severe overdose

ECG is the most useful tool and the QRS interval the most sensitive indicator of a serious acute overdose.

- 30% of patients with a QRS width >100 milliseconds developed seizures.
- 50% of patients with a QRS width >160 milliseconds developed dysrhythmias.
- No patient with a QRS width <100 milliseconds had seizures or dysrhythmias.
- Consider any QRS >100 milliseconds to be abnormal in the setting of acute cyclic overdose even though 20% of normal populations have a baseline ECG with a QRS width falling between 100 and 120 milliseconds.

> ⇨ **SPECIAL TIP FOR GPs**
> - Do not induce emesis or administer activated charcoal if patients appear drowsy as they can rapidly lose consciousness, necessitating airway protection.
> - Do not administer flumazenil to reverse a concomitant benzodiazepine overdose as this may precipitate fits induced by the cyclic anti-depressants.
> - A widened QRS complex duration of >100 milliseconds on electrocardiogram (ECG) indicates serious intoxication.
> - IV **sodium bicarbonate therapy** administered in the hospital is the mainstay of therapy and is effective for TCA-induced hypotension and dysrhythmias.

MANAGEMENT

Supportive measures

- The patient must be managed in a monitored area with resuscitation equipment, including defibrillator, immediately available.
- Maintain airway; intubate the patient if a depressed level of consciousness is noted or if gag reflex is absent.
- Administer supplemental high-flow oxygen by a non-rebreather reservoir mask.
- Monitoring: ECG, vitals signs q 5–15 minutes and pulse oximetry.
- Establish peripheral intravenous line.
- Intravenous fluid of choice is normal saline.
- **Labs:** Full blood count, urea/electrolytes/creatinine, blood drug screen (send drug screen tube to the ward with the patient if a mixed overdose is suspected).

NOTE: Do not ask for plasma anti-depressant level, it adds nothing to the management.

- Perform arterial blood gases to monitor blood pH as therapy continues.
- Order a **chest X-ray** for pulmonary oedema, aspiration pneumonia and acute respiratory distress syndrome.
- Place a urinary catheter to monitor urine output/fluid status.
- Perform gastric lavage if indicated and send the first effluent specimen to the ward with the patient.

Drug therapy

- **Activated charcoal**: Dosage = 1 g/kg body weight. Administer via orogastric tube.
- Alkalinize the blood to a pH of 7.45 to 7.50. This is best achieved by a combination of **hyperventilation** and **sodium bicarbonate** administration:
  1. If intubated, mechanical ventilation at a respiratory rate of 20 breaths/min is adequate for most adults.

2. Dosage of **sodium bicarbonate** = 1–2 mmol/kg body weight in slow IV boluses, i.e. over 20–30 minutes.

3. Bicarbonate therapy is indicated if the QRS is at least 100 milliseconds wide.

SPECIFIC CLINICAL SITUATIONS

NOTE: Sodium bicarbonate is the most effective therapy for improving hypotension and abolishing dysrhythmias.

Dysrhythmias unresponsive to sodium bicarbonate

- **Lignocaine** may abolish ventricular dysrhythmias. Dosage: IV bolus of 1.0–1.5 mg/kg, then an infusion of 1–4 mg/min.
- **Magnesium sulphate** may be used to treat torsade de pointes. Dosage: IV bolus of 1–2 g over 60 seconds, then an infusion of 1–2 g/hr.
- **Synchronized cardioversion** may be used for the treatment of supraventricular tachydysrhythmias.
- **Emergency pacing** (transcutaneous pacing in the emergency department followed, if necessary, by transvenous pacing in the intensive care unit) is indicated for severe bradydysrhythmias and atrioventricular blocks.

Hypotension

- First approach is the use of **normal saline** and **alkalinization**.
- Poor or no response: Attempt **drug therapy**.
- Noradrenaline or high-dose dopamine: Both are more effective early in toxicity.
    1. **Noradrenaline**: Infusion **only** of 0.5–1.0 µg/min and titrate to effect.
    2. **Dopamine**: Infusion **only** of 10–20 µg/kg/min and titrate to effect.
- Failure of the above measures necessitates consideration of the use of an intra-aortic balloon pump.

Control of fits resistant to use of sodium bicarbonate

This is important since ensuing lactic acidosis can worsen cardiac toxicity by lowering protein binding and making more active drugs available to the susceptible tissues.

- **Diazepam**: Dosage: 2–5 mg IV bolus, repeated q 5 minutes to a total of 20 mg, **or**,
- **Lorazepam**: Dosage: 0.1 mg/kg IV bolus to a total of 8 mg.
- **Phenobarbital**:

    Dosage: IV 100 mg/min to a total of 10 mg /kg or fits are controlled; if ineffective, give
           IV 50 mg/min to a total of (including previous dose) 20 mg/kg or fits are controlled,
           IV 50 mg/min to a total of (including previous dose) 30 mg/kg or fits are controlled.

- **Paralysis/general anaesthesia**: Obtain consultation from Anaesthesia.

RISK STRATIFICATION OF PATIENTS WITH ACUTE OVERDOSE

The ADORA (AntiDepressant Overdose Risk Assessment) score has been often used. Its components are as follows:

- QRS >100 milliseconds
- Dysrhythmias
- Hypotension
- Respiratory depression
- Coma
- Seizures.

Any one or more of the above is indicative of a high-risk overdose.

POTENTIAL DISCHARGE CRITERIA

It is prudent to comply with the '6-hour' rule of observation after a potential/dubious acute overdose, as most toxic effects manifest before this time frame.

If the patient is asymptomatic, with a QRS <100 milliseconds and no dysrhythmia occurs on cardiac monitoring over this 6-hour observation period, and the psychiatrist has cleared the patient, then in general the patient may be considered for discharge from the emergency department.

DISPOSITION

- Obtain consultation from General Medicine; keep in view admission to a high dependency or intensive care unit setting for monitoring. Significant deterioration of such cases has been known to occur several hours or days after the initial ingestion.

References/Further Reading

1. Mills KC. Cyclic antidepressants. In: Tintinalli JE, Ma OJ, Stapczynski JS, et al., eds. *Tintinalli's Emergency Medicine: A Comprehensive Study Guide*. 7th ed. New York: McGraw-Hill; 2011: 1193–1198.

2. Benowitz NL. Cyclic antidepressants. In: Olson KR, ed. *Poisoning and Drug Overdose*. 2nd ed. East Norwalk, CT: Appleton & Lange; 1994: 147–150.

3. Bilden EF. Antidepressant toxicity. In: Marx TA, Hockberger RS, Walls RM, et al., eds. *Emergency Medicine: Concepts and Clinical Practice*. 7th ed. Philadelphia, PA: Mosby-Elsevier; 2010: 1964–1977.

4. Frommer DA, Kullig KW, Marx JA, et al. Tricyclic antidepressant overdose: A review. *JAMA*. 1987; 257: 521–526.

5. Brown TCK, Barker GA, Dunlop ME, et al. The use of sodium bicarbonate in the treatment of tricyclic antidepressant induced arrhythmmias. *Anesth Intensive Care*. 1973; 1: 203–210.

6. Wedin GP, Oderda GM, Klein-Schwartz W. Relative toxicity of cyclic antidepressants. *Ann Emerg Med*. 1986; 15: 797–804.

7. Sasyniuk BI, Jhamandas V. Mechanism of reversal of toxic effects of amitriptylline on cardiac Purkinje fibres by sodium bicarbonate. *Ann Emerg Med.* 1986; 15: 1052–1059.

8. Boehnert M, Lovejoy FM. Value of QRS duration versus serum frug level in predicting seizures and ventricular arrhythmias after an acute overdose of tricyclic antidepressants. *N Eng J Med.* 1985; 313: 474–479.

9. Foulke GE. Identification of toxicity risk early after antidepressant overdose. *Am J Emerg Med.* 1995; 13: 123–126.

10. Weisman RS: Cyclic antidepressants. In: Goldfrank LR, Flomenbaum NE, Lewin NA, et al, eds. *Goldfranks Toxicological Emergencies.* 6th ed. Stamford, CT: Appleton & Lange; 1998: 925–934.

11. Bailey B, Buckley NA, Amre DK. A meta-analysis of prognostic indicators to predict seizures, arrhythmias or death after tricyclic antidepressant overdose. *J Toxicol Clin Toxicol.* 2004; 42(6): 877–888.

86 Poisoning, Digoxin

Amila Punyadasa • Shirley Ooi

CAVEATS

- Digitalis and digoxin are cardiac glycosides, which are chemicals with a steroid ring, an unsaturated lactone ring and one to four sugars (or glycosides) attached. These compounds are found in plants such as foxglove and oleander.

- Digoxin is a Na-K ATPase inhibitor that increases intracellular Na and Ca and increases extracellular K. This then increases cardiac contractility by freeing cytoplasmic Ca to actin and myosin during contractions. It also causes vasodilation and thus decreases afterload.

- In **therapeutic doses**, an electrocardiogram (ECG) may show prolonged PR interval, short QT, ST scooping and depression (especially laterally – the classical '**reverse tick**' sign), and decreased amplitude of T waves.

- At higher doses digoxin suppresses the sinoatrial node (SAN), increases automaticity, and decreases conduction at the atrioventricular node (AVN). The end results are tachycardia and heart blocks.

- Digoxin is often taken for chronic atrial fibrillation. Digoxin overdose causes atrial fibrillation with complete heart block resulting in a junctional rhythm or what is termed as '**regularization of atrial fibrillation**'.

FIGURE 1 Diagram showing the different types of ST segment depression indicated by arrows. (A) Isoelectric ST segment. (B) Junctional or J type. (C) Mirror image of the pass sign (✓) ('reverse tick' sign) – 'digitalis effect'. (D) Horizontal. (E) Downsloping (Sagging).

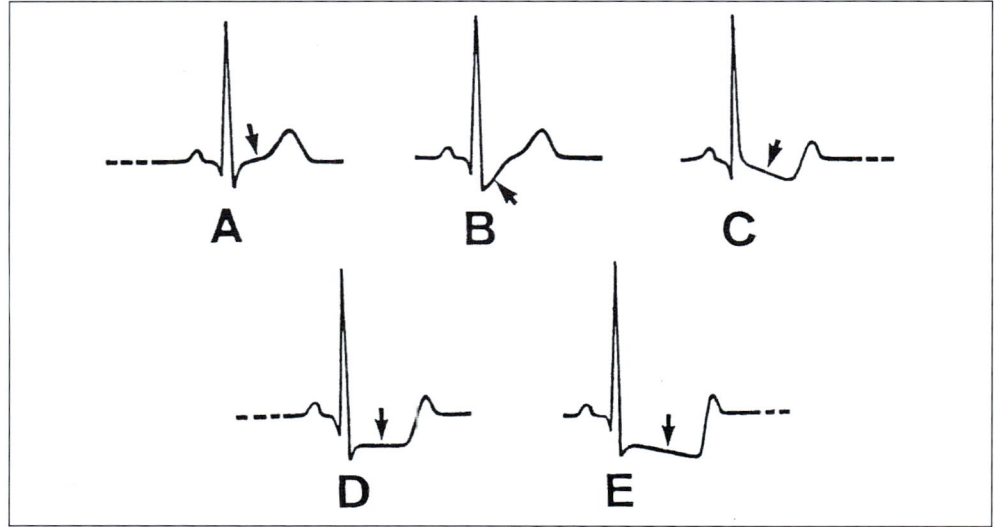

ECG CHANGES SUGGESTIVE OF DIGOXIN INTOXICATION

- Unifocal but multiform premature ventricular contractions (PVCs). (See Figure 2)
- Atrial tachycardia with block (See Figure 3)
- Mobitz type I (Wenckebach phenomenon) second degree and third degree AV block with narrow QRS complexes
- Accelerated junctional rhythm
- Sinoatrial block
- Bidirectional ventricular tachycardia (See Figure 4)

FIGURE 2   **Unifocal, multiform ventricular ectopic beats in a patient with digitalis intoxication. Note the constant coupling interval but varying morphologies of the ventricular ectopic beats (arrowheads).**

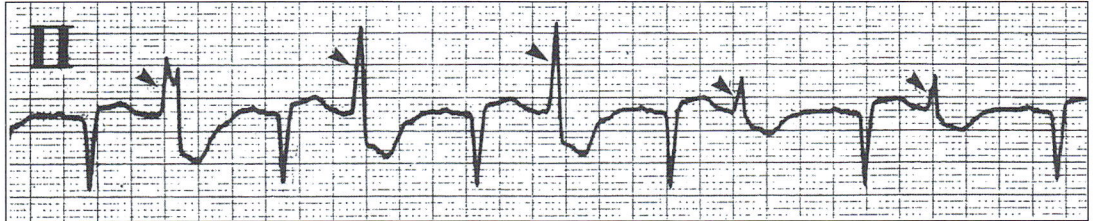

Image taken from *Clinical Electrocardiography* 3rd Edition, BL Chia, (c)1998 World Scientific. Reproduced with permission.

FIGURE 3   **Digitalis intoxication. The patient, an elderly man with previous anterior infarction, presented with deterioration of his heart failure. ECG shows atrial tachycardia with 2:1 AV block and ventricular ectopic beats (E). Arrowheads indicate atrial P waves.**

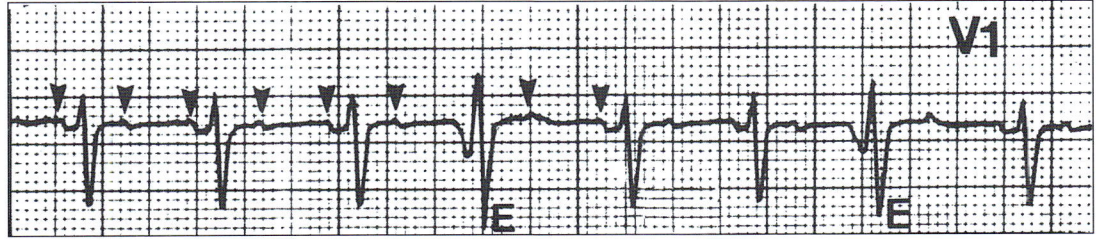

Image taken from *Clinical Electrocardiography* 3rd Edition, BL Chia, (c)1998 World Scientific. Reproduced with permission.

FIGURE 4 Bidirectional tachycardia in a 58-year-old woman with digitalis intoxication. Note that the polarity of the consecutive QRS complexes is alternately positive and negative in all the leads except for V₁ and V₂.

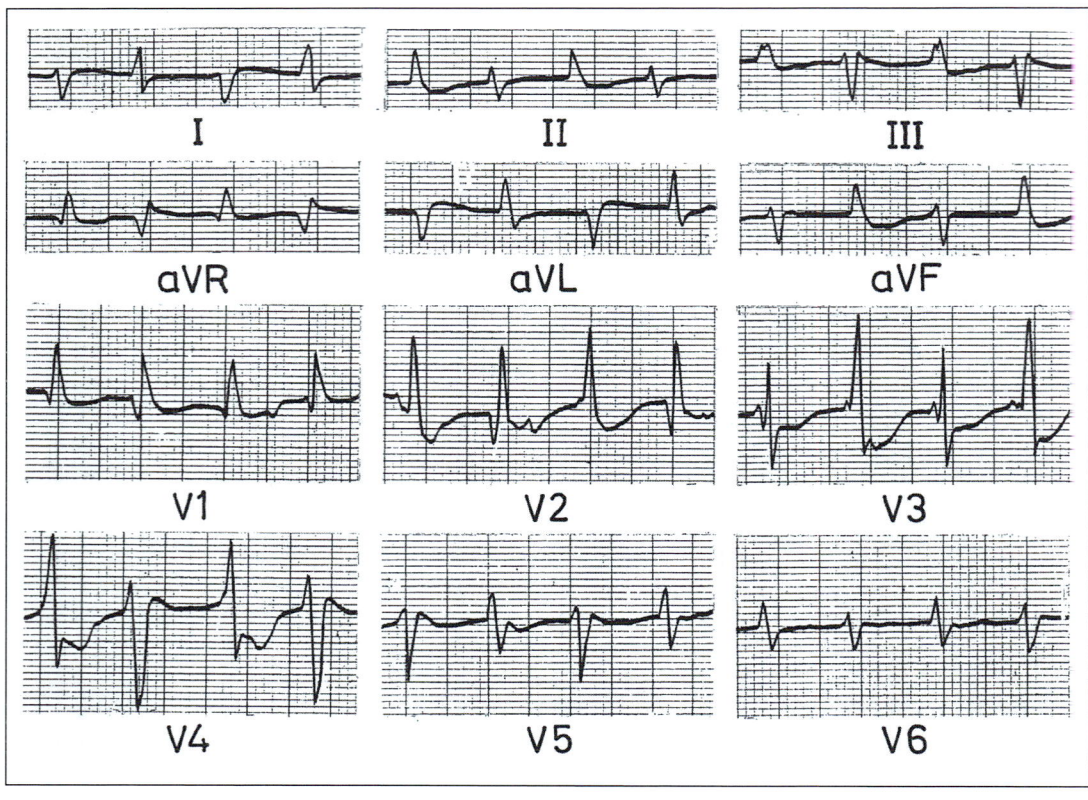

Image taken from *Clinical Electrocardiography* 3rd Edition, BL Chia, (c)1998 World Scientific. Reproduced with permission.

RISK FACTORS FOR DIGOXIN TOXICITY

- Elderly patients
- Hypoxia
- Acidosis
- Pre-existing myocardial disease
- Hypokalaemia, hypomagnesaemia, hypercalcaemia
- Concomitant calcium channel blocker or beta blocker administration
- Renal impairment
- Pulmonary disease
- Pharmacokinetic interactions with drugs such as amiodarone, quinidine, cyclosporin, and verapamil.

> ⇨ **SPECIAL TIPS FOR GPs**
>
> - It takes time for the levels of digoxin to build up in the heart and other tissues, thus symptoms do not usually occur in the first 6 hours.
> - Serious dysrhythmias occur in the first 24 hours after an acute digoxin overdose.
> - In an acute overdose, heart failure, and life-threatening hyperkalaemia are important issues.
> - Some **Chinese medications**, such as Chu An Wu, contains toad venom. Drinking tea made from plants such as **foxglove** or seeds from the **oleander plant** may cause toxicity too.
> - In an elderly cardiac patient presenting with a combination of **vague symptoms** (which may include visual, gastrointestinal and neurological symptoms) consider **chronic digoxin toxicity** in your list of differentials.

MANAGEMENT

Supportive measures

- The patient must be managed in a monitored area with resuscitation equipment, including defibrillator, immediately available.
- Maintain airway; intubate the patient if a depressed level of consciousness is noted or if gag reflex is absent.
- Administer supplemental high-flow oxygen by a non-rebreather reservoir mask.
- Monitoring: ECG, vital signs q 5–15 minutes, and pulse oximetry.
- Establish peripheral intravenous (IV) line; normal saline is suitable.
- **Labs**: Full blood count, urea/electrolytes/creatinine, blood drug screen (send drug screen tube to the ward with the patient if a mixed overdose is suspected).
- **Frequent K estimations** to detect hyperkalaemia are mandatory.
- **Plasma digoxin levels** (therapeutic range 0.5–2.0 ng/ml) should be measured at least 6 hours post-ingestion to attain steady-state levels.
- Cardiac enzymes to exclude acute myocardial infarction as a cause of increased myocardiac sensitivity to digoxin.
- Perform arterial blood gases (ABGs) as indicated.
- Do a chest X-ray for detection and confirmation of heart failure.
- Place a urinary catheter to monitor urine output/fluid status.

Drug therapy

- **Activated charcoal (AC)**: Dosage = 1 g/kg body weight. Administer via an orogastric tube, if indicated.
- As digoxin is slowly absorbed, AC is extremely useful, and in fact, multiple-dose AC actually shortens the half-life of the drug (enterohepatic circulation).
- Forced diuresis, haemodialysis, and haemoperfusion do not enhance the elimination of digoxin because of its extensive tissue binding and large volume of distribution.

- **Calcium** is **absolutely contraindicated** in the treatment of digoxin toxicity that is related to hyperkalaemia. It causes increased intracellular calcium and thus dysrhythmias.
- **Hyperkalaemia treatment** should include $NaHCO_3$, insulin, and dextrose but it is best treated with **fragment antigen-binding (Fab) antibodies**.
- Treat bradycardias in the usual way with atropine, at the usual dosages.
- All serious dysrhythmias or heart blocks greater than type I must be treated with Fab antibodies.

Fab antibodies

- Digoxin: Specific Fab antibodies are developed from sheep.
- Specific antidote for digoxin toxicity.
- Cross reacts with digitoxin and may also be used for plant and toad toxicities.
- Each vial, which will bind approximately 0.5 mg of digoxin (or digitoxin), contains 38 mg of digoxin-specific Fab fragments derived from sheep plus 75 mg of sorbitol as a stabilizer and 28 mg of sodium chloride.
- Fab binds free digoxin, thus resulting in a concentration gradient that serves to pull the tissue-bound drug into the serum where it also can then be inactivated.
- Thus, although total digoxin levels rise in the serum concentration, the free digoxin levels are almost undetectable.
- Effects commence within a few minutes to an hour. The maximum effect may take several hours.
- The advantage of Fab, rather than the entire antibody, is that it is smaller, is less immunogenic, has a wider volume of distribution (thus can target more of the offending drug) and is more easily excreted via the kidneys.
- *Indications for Fab*
  1. Severe ventricular arrhythmias.
  2. Bradycardia that is unresponsive to atropine.
  3. Rising K levels (especially K >5 mmol/L).
  4. Steady-state serum levels >10 ng/ml in adults and >0.5 ng/ml in children.
  5. Single ingestion >10 mg in adults or >4 mg in children.
  6. Co-ingestion with calcium channel blockers or beta blockers.
  7. Cardiac arrest.
  8. Poor clinical state or rapidly worsening clinical state.
- *Dose of Fab*
  Dosage may be calculated in 2 ways:
  1. If the amount of digoxin ingested is known

$$\text{Dose (in number of vials)} = \frac{\text{Total digoxin body load in mg}}{\text{0.5 mg of digoxin bound/vial}}$$

2. If the steady-state serum level of digoxin is known

$$\text{Dose (in number of vials)} = \frac{\text{(Serum digoxin concentration in ng/ml)} \times \text{(Weight in kg)}}{100}$$

- As a rough guide:
  1. **Acute overdose: 5–15 vials**
  2. **Chronic overdose: 2–4 vials**
- *Fab aftercare*
  1. In an acute overdose, as soon as Fab is given the Na-K pump starts working again and there is rapid influx of K back into the cells, which may result in **hypokalaemia**. This must be monitored for.
  2. A **rebound in free digoxin** occurs 24 hours after Fab therapy.
  3. Those patients who were digoxin-dependent (e.g. severe New York Heart Association (NYHA) class IV **heart failure** patients) may suddenly **decompensate**. This must be predicted and managed accordingly.
  4. **Idiosyncratic allergic** manifestations may occur, but are rare (less than 1% of cases). Adrenaline therapy must be readily available for possible therapy if this occurs.

GUIDES TO TREATING SPECIFIC CLINICAL SITUATIONS

Supraventricular tachycardia

- Consider diltiazem only in rapid, haemodynamically significant situations.
- Fab antibodies.

Atrioventricular block

- Atropine.
- Temporary pacing.
- Fab antibodies.

Ventricular arrhythmias

- Lignocaine or phenytoin.
- Magnesium sulphate.
- Temporary pacing.
- Fab antibodies.
- **Cardioversion only** as a last resort measure in treating life-threatening arrhythmias and even then at low energies (e.g. 10–25 J).

Chronic digoxin overdoses

- May occur especially in the elderly, in particular if renal impairment exists.

- Concomitant administration of other drugs such as calcium channel blockers or even cimetidine may increase effects of digoxin.
- Common diuretic side effects of hypokalaemia and hypomagnesaemia can induce toxicity.
- Precedent significant cardiorespiratory comorbidities, such as advanced heart disease and chronic lung disease, also make toxicity more likely.
- Presentation is very non-specific and diagnosis is difficult depending upon a high index of suspicion. Features may include the following effects:
  1. **Visual**: Perceptions of **yellow and green objects**, and halos
  2. **Gastrointestinal tract**: Anorexia, nausea, and vomiting (common)
  3. **Central nervous system**: Dizziness, fatigue, confusion, and altered mental status
- Note that the serum levels of the drug may be only marginally elevated in chronic toxicity.
- Management includes electrolyte replacements to correct possible hypokalaemia and hypomagnesaemia, and determining the need for Fab.

DISPOSITION

- Consider a psychiatric consult if indicated.
- Obtain consultation from an internist or toxicologist (if available); keep in view admission to a high dependency or intensive care unit setting for monitoring. Significant deterioration of such cases has been known to occur several hours after the initial ingestion.

References/Further Reading

1. Linden CH. Digitalis glycosides. In: Ford M, Delaney KA, Ling L, Erickson T, eds. *Clinical Toxicology*. Philadelphia, PA: WB Saunders; 2000: 379–390.

2. Antman EM, Wenger TL, Butler VP, et al. Treatment of 150 cases of life-threatening digitalis intoxication with digoxin-specific Fab antibody fragments. Final report of a multi-center study. *Circulation*. 1990; 81: 1744–1752.

3. Williamson KM, Thrasher KA, Fulton KB. Digoxin toxicity: An evaluation in current clinical practice. *Archives of Intern Med*. Dec 1998; 158(22).

4. Kinlay S, Bucklet N. Magnesium sulfate in the treatment of ventricular arrhythmias due to digoxin toxicity. *J Toxicol Clin Toxicol*. 1995; 33: 55–59.

5. Bronstein AC, Spyker DA, Cantilena LR Jr, et al. 2006 Annual Report of the American Association of Poison Control Centers' National Poison Data System (NPDS). *Clin Toxicol (Phila)*. Dec 2007; 45(8): 815–917.

6. Benowitz N. Cardiac glycosides. In: Olson KR, Anderson IB, Benowitz NL, eds. *Poisoning and Drug Overdose*. 4th ed. New York: McGraw-Hill; 2004: 155–157.

7. Jennifer SB, Kirk MA. Digitalis glycosides. In: Tintinalli JE, Ma OJ, Stapczynski JS, et al, eds. *Tintinalli's Emergency Medicine: A Comprehensive Study Guide*. 7th ed. New York: McGraw-Hill; 2011: 1260–1264.

8. Eddleston M, Rajapakse S, Rajakanthan S, et al. Anti-digoxin Fab fragments in cardiotoxicity induced by ingestion of yellow oleander: A randomised controlled trial. *Lancet*. 18 Mar 2000; 355(9208): 967–972.

9. Roberts DJ. Cardiovascular drugs. In: Marx JA, Hockberger RS, Walls RM eds. *Rosen's Emergency Medicine: Concepts and Clinical Practice*. 7th ed. Philadelphia, PA: Mosby-Elsevier; 2010; Chap 150: 1978–1988.

10. Van Deusen SK, Birkhahn RH, Gaeta TJ. Treatment of hyperkalemia in a patient with unrecognized digitalis toxicity. *J Toxicol Clin Toxicol*. 2003; 41(4): 373–376.

11. Chia BL, Clinical Electrocardiography, 3rd ed. Singapore: World Scientific; 1998; 22, 96, 97.

87 Poisoning, Organophosphates

Amila Punyadasa • Peter Manning • Suresh Pillai

CAVEATS

- Organophosphates and carbamates are two of the most commonly used classes of insecticides. Both compounds are inhibitors of carboxylic ester hydrolases, including acetylcholinesterase (AChE) and pseudocholinesterase. AChE is found in the nervous system and plays an important role in the control of synaptic neurotransmission.

- The active agent in most pesticides and insecticides is the organophosphorus compound **parathion**, which binds irreversibly with acetylcholinesterase to form a diethylphosphate bond.

- **Atropine** is a physiological anti-muscarinic antidote that acts by competitively blocking the muscarinic effects of acetylcholine.

- Atropine has no effect on the nicotinic receptors at myoneural junctions in skeletal muscle, i.e. it will not reverse paralysis.

- **Pralidoxime** is a biochemical antidote that reactivates the cholinesterase that has undergone the process of phosphorylation by the organophosphate; however, the pralidoxime must be administered within 24–36 hours after exposure, otherwise the cholinesterase molecule may be irrevocably bound and new cholinesterase will then take weeks to regenerate.

- **Classic presentation:** A patient with vomiting and diarrhoea, diaphoresis, breath smelling strongly of insecticide, and small pupils. Beware erroneous diagnosis of gastroenteritis.

PATHOPHYSIOLOGY

- Organophosphates inhibit acetylcholinesterase, which results in excess acetylcholine accumulating at the myoneural junctions and synapses.

- Excess acetylcholine initially excites, then paralyzes, neurotransmission at the motor-end plate and stimulates nicotinic and muscarinic sites:

1. **Muscarinic** effects: The mnemonic **DUMBELS** is useful to remember since these signs and symptoms develop **first**, 12–24 hours after ingestion:

   D Diarrhoea .

   U Urination.

   M Miosis (absent in 10% of cases).

   B Bronchorrhoea/bronchospasm/bradycardia.

   E Emesis.

   L Lacrimation.

   S Salivation and hypotension.

2. **Nicotinic** effects: Remembered by recalling days of the week, i.e. Monday, Tuesday, Wednesday, Thursday, Friday, and Saturday.

   a. M Muscle cramps.

   b. T Tachycardia.

   c. W Muscle weakness.

   d. H Hypertension.

   e. F Fasciculations.

   f. S Sugars (hyperglycaemia).

3. **Central nervous system (CNS)** effects

   a. Anxiety and insomnia.

   b. Respiratory depression.

   c. Convulsions and coma.

4. **Additional non-toxidromal toxic effects**

   a. Acute pancreatitis.

   b. Prolonged QTc on electrocardiogram (ECG) with or without torsades de pointes. Considered to be the result of intense and unequal sympathetic stimulation of myocardial fibres. The treatment involves magnesium sulphate and possibly pacing.

TABLE 1 Differences between organophosphates and carbamates

	Organophosphates	Carbamates
Binding at postsynaptic site	Irreversible	Reversible
Action at active site on AChE molecule	Phosphorylation	Carbamoylation
Half life	10 days	1 day
CNS actions	Yes	No
Treatment	Pralidoxime	Pralidoxime

⇨ **SPECIAL TIPS FOR GPs**

- Refer all patients with suspected organophosphate poisoning to hospital even if they are asymptomatic.
- Be aware that vomiting, diarrhoea, and hypotension can occur and can be misdiagnosed as severe GE. Look for the **DUMBELS** signs and symptoms (see the next section).
- Ensure that the implicated receptacle containing the insecticide is brought along with the patient to the hospital.

MANAGEMENT

Supportive measures

- All staff members are required to wear protective equipment since percutaneous absorption and inhalation in the course of care may cause toxicity.
- The patient must be managed in the critical care area with resuscitation equipment immediately available.
- Start detoxification by removing the patient's clothes and washing the skin thoroughly (emergency department staff should take appropriate precautions: see Chapter 19, *Poisoning, General Principles*).
- Maintain airway patency; perform orotracheal intubation if the patient is obtunded, apnoeic, or has no gag reflex.

NOTE: No neuromuscular paralyzing agent will be necessary as the patient's motor-end plates have already been blocked by the poisoning. Frequent suctioning may be required due to bronchorrhoea.

- Administer supplemental high flow oxygen via a non-rebreather reservoir mask.
- Monitoring: ECG, vital signs q 5–15 minutes, and pulse oximetry.
- Establish peripheral intravenous (IV) line.
- Administer IV fluids: Crystalloids to replace fluids lost by vomiting and diarrhoea.
- **Labs**: Full blood count, urea/electrolytes/creatinine, plasma cholinesterase gastric and serum toxicology specimens to accompany the patient to the ward (two types of cholinesterase, red blood cell (RBC) and plasma, can be measured in clinical practice. However, RBC cholinesterase levels correlate better with CNS AChE than plasma cholinesterase levels and is thus more specific for organophosphate poisonings. Yet, a single level may not help in diagnosis unless it is very low. A knowledge of the patients baseline levels and determining a trend in terms of the rate of decline of such levels would then provide additional clues in a possible toxic event.

Drug therapy

- **Activated charcoal** via gastric lavage tube.
  Dosage: 1 g/kg body weight.
- **Atropine**: First drug to be given in the treatment of symptomatic poisoning.
  1. Its major use is in the reduction of bronchorrhoea/bronchospasm.
  2. Large doses may be needed to control airway secretions.
     Dosage: Adult: 2 mg IV q 10–15 minutes as needed (prn); the dosage may be doubled q 10 minutes until secretions have been controlled **or** signs of atropinization are obvious (flushed and dry skin, tachycardia, mydriasis, and dry mouth).
     Children: 0.05 mg/kg body weight q 15 minutes prn; the dosage can be doubled q 10 minutes until secretions are controlled.

- **Pralidoxime (2-PAM® or Protopam®)**
  1. Pralidoxime should be given with atropine to every symptomatic patient.
  2. Effects will be apparent within 30 minutes and include the disappearance of convulsions and fasciculations, improvement in muscle power, and recovery of consciousness.
  3. The administration of pralidoxime usually necessitates reduction in the amount of atropine given and may unmask atropine toxicity.

     Dosage: Adult: 1 gm IV over 15–30 minutes; can be repeated in 1 to 2 hours as needed.

     Children: 25–50 mg/kg/body weight IV over 15–30 minutes; can be repeated in 1 to 2 hours.

NOTE: In very severe cases with bradycardia/hypotension and respiratory arrest, half the dosage of **pralidoxime** can be given IV over one minute.

- **Diazepam (Valium®)**: Use to reduce anxiety and restlessness and to control convulsions.
  Dosage: 5–10 mg IV for anxiety/restlessness.

NOTE: Doses up to 10–20 mg IV may be needed for the control of convulsions.

Possible Delayed Effects in Organophosphate Poisonings

- **The intermediate syndrome (IMS)**: This is a clinical syndrome that starts 24–96 hours after the onset of organophosphate poisoning. It is characterized by weakness of muscles innervated by cranial nerves (facial, extra-occular, and palatal), neck flexors, proximal extremity musculature and respiratory musculature, especially the diaphragm. The exact mechanism is unknown but its occurrence seems to correlate both with severity of the preceding acute cholinergic crisis and a high level of exposure to organophosphates. IMS is unresponsive to atropine and 2-PAM. Management involves supportive therapy including possible intubation and mechanical ventilation. The prognosis is good with the majority of cases recovering between 14 and 28 days.
- **Organophosphate-induced delayed neuropathy (OPIDN)**: This begins 1 to 3 weeks after exposure. Symptoms involve leg cramping, symmetric lower extremity weakness, and a stocking paraesthesia followed by similar symptoms in the upper limbs. Electromyographic analysis demonstrates a denervation pattern. Consequences of OPIDN include wasting of the peroneal muscles, with foot drop, and wasting of the small muscles of the hand. Again, management is only supportive. Prognosis is variable, ranging from irreversisble to slowly reversible defects over 6–15 months.

Disposition

- Obtain General Medicine consultation on high dependency or intensive care unit admission.
- Consider a psychiatric consult if deemed necessary.
- For cases of subclinical poisoning treatment is not necessary, **but** the patient should be admitted for observation for at least 24 hours to ensure that delayed toxicity does not develop.

References/Further Reading

1. Walter C. Robey III, William JM. Pesticides. In: Tintinalli JE, Ma OJ, Stapczynski JS, et al, eds. *Tintinalli's Emergency Medicine: A Comprehensive Study Guide*. 7th ed. New York: McGraw-Hill; 2011: 1297–1305.

2. Woo OF. Organophosphates: Cyclic anti-depressants. In: Olson KR, ed. *Poisoning and Drug Overdose*. 2nd ed. East Norwalk, CT: Appleton & Lange; 1994: 240–243.

3. Kurtz PH. Pralidoxime in the treatment of carbamate intoxication. *Am J Emerg Med*. 1990; 8: 68.

4. Dikart WL, Kiestra SH, Sangster B. The use of atropine and oximes in organophosphate intoxication: A modified approach. *J Toxicol Clin Toxicol*. 1988; 26: 199–208.

5. Lotti M. Treatment of acute organophosphate poisoning. *Med J Aust*. 1991; 154: 51–55.

6. Wang EIC, Braid PR. Oxime reactivation of diethylphosphoryl human serum cholinesterase. *J Biol Chem*. 1967; 242: 2683–2687.

7. Aaron CK, Howland MA. Insecticides: Organophosphates and carbamates. In: Goldfrank LR, Flomenbaum NE, Lewin NA, et al, eds. *Goldfrank's Toxicological Emergencies*. 6th ed. Stamford, CT: Appleton & Lange; 1998: 1429–1444.

8. Bleeker JD, Neucker KVD, Willems J. The intermediate syndrome in organophosphate poisoning: Presentation of a case and a review of the literature. *J Toxicol Clin Toxicol*. 1992; 30: 321–329.

9. Bleeker JD, Neucker KVD, Willems J. Neurological aspects of organophosphate poisoning. *Clin Neurol Neurosurg*. 1992; 94: 93–103.

10. Marrs TC. Organophosphate poisoning. *Pharm Ther*. 1993; 58: 51–66.

11. Liu JH, Chou CY, Liu YL, et al. Acid-base interpretation can be the predictor of outcome among patients with acute organophosphate poisoning before hospitalization. *Am J Emerg Med*. Jan 2008; 26(1): 24–30.

12. Pawar KS, Bhoite RR, Pillay CP, et al. Continuous pralidoxime infusion versus repeated bolus injection to treat organophosphorus pesticide poisoning: A randomised controlled trial. *Lancet*. 16 Dec 2006; 368(9553): 2136–2141.

13. Yurumez Y, Durukan P, Yavuz Y, et al. Acute organophosphate poisoning in university hospital emergency room patients. *Intern Med*. 2007; 46(13): 965–969.

14. He F. Neurotoxic effects of insecticides – Current and future research: A review. *Neurotoxicology*. Oct 2000; 21(5): 829–835.

88 Poisoning, Paracetamol

Peter Manning • Amila Punyadasa

CAVEATS

- Paracetamol is the commonest drug taken in overdose locally, where a single ingestion of 7.5 g is used empirically as a threshold for possible toxicity.

- **Toxicity** has been shown to occur with ingested doses **>150 mg/kg body** weight or **7.5 g (15 tablets)** in an average-sized adult.

- Toxicity may occur at lower doses in patients with hepatic enzyme induction, e.g. patients taking anti-convulsants, or anorexic patients who may have pre-existing glutathione depletion. In such cases, use the high-risk treatment line on the Rumack-Matthew nomogram (Figure 1) rather than the normal treatment line.

- The **Rumack-Matthew nomogram** is useful in determining the need for N-acetylcysteine (Parvolex®) therapy following a **single, acute ingestion only** (see *Management* section).

- **N-acetylcysteine (NAC)** is almost 100% effective if given within 8 hours of the ingestion, though it may also be used up to 24 hours after ingestion, if the history suggests a significant overdose and the serum paracetamol level is not available.

- A guiding philosophy in managing paracetamol poisoning is '**if in doubt, treat with N-acetylcysteine**'.

FIGURE 1 **Rumack-Matthew nomogram**

Figure reproduced with permission of the McGraw-Hill Companies, from Tintinalli JE, Kelen GD, Stapczynski JS, eds. *Emergency Medicine: A Comprehensive Study Guide.* New York: McGraw-Hill; 2000: 1128, Fig. 165-4.

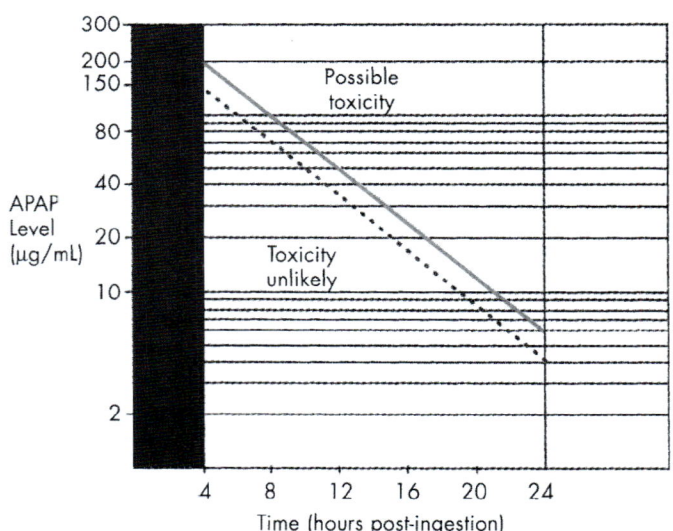

THE TOXIC EFFECTS OF PARACETAMOL

Generally, assuming normal metabolic conditions, 90% of paracetamol is conjugated in the liver with glucuronide and sulphate conjugates and is then excreted in the urine. About 2% is eliminated unchanged also by the kidneys. The remaining 8% is metabolized oxidatively by the cytochrome P450 mixed-function enzyme system in the liver. This creates an intermediate, N-acetyl-para-benzoquinoneimine (NAPQI), which is rapidly bound to glutathione and detoxified. However, if levels of glutathione fall to less than 30% of normal (e.g. in malnutrition or alcoholism) NAPQI is then free to bind to hepatocellular membranes and cause cell death and ultimately centrilobular necrosis.

THE FOUR PHASES OF PARACETAMOL TOXICITY

PHASE	TIME	CHARACTERISTICS
Phase 1 – Initial	Up to 24 hours	Anorexia, nausea or vomiting; rise in transaminases
Phase 2 – Latent	24–72 hours	Right upper quadrant pain; transaminases peaking; bilirubin and prothrombin time (PT) elevated
Phase 3 – Hepatic	72–96 hours	Hepatic necrosis characterized by jaundice, encephalopathy, coagulopathy, acute renal failure, and death
Phase 4 – Recovery	4–14 days	Resolution of hepatic dysfunction and healing of liver damage

⇨ **SPECIAL TIPS FOR GPs**
- Patients with paracetamol overdose often look well in the initial stages except for nausea and vomiting.
- If there is any doubt as to the accuracy of history or the amount ingested, patients should be referred to the emergency department (ED) for further evaluation.
- Do not induce emesis before sending patients to the ED.

MANAGEMENT

Supportive measures

- The patient should be managed in the intermediate care area, although transfer to the critical care area is mandatory if there is a significant derangement of vital signs or depressed mental state.

NOTE: Depressed mental state should trigger the search for concomitant drug ingestion since obtundation is unusual in isolated paracetamol poisoning.

- Maintain airway; perform orotracheal intubation if the patient is significantly obtunded or the gag reflex is absent (in anticipation of gastric lavage or the administration of activated charcoal, or both).
- Administer supplemental oxygen if oxygen saturation (SpO_2) is decreased.
- Monitoring: Electrocardiogram, vital signs q 15 minutes, and pulse oximetry.
- Establish peripheral intravenous line.
- Perform gastric lavage if the patient presents within an hour of ingestion of a potentially toxic dose of the drug and collect first effluent for toxicology specimen which may then be sent to the ward with the patient.

NOTE: Current evidence does **not** support gastric lavage unless the patient has ingested a potentially toxic dose of paracetamol, and has presented within the first hour. Some authors even suggest that lavage may be omitted if activated charcoal is given.

- **Labs**:
  1. Full blood count, urea/electrolytes/creatinine, liver function tests, prothrombin time.

NOTE: **Plasma alanine transaminase >5000 IU/L** is highly suggestive of hepatotoxicity due to paracetamol since such levels are seldom seen in viral hepatitis. From an evidence-based medicine standpoint, **only** a serum paracetamol level is required to be drawn in patients with paracetamol overdose who show no signs of hepatotoxicity.

  2. Serum paracetamol level (**mandatory**).
  3. If the initial level is in the toxic range when plotted on the Rumack-Matthew nomogram (Figure 1), then NAC therapy should be initiated immediately.
  4. A more precise judgement is based on the level taken 4 hours post-ingestion for those cases where NAC therapy is not indicated earlier (see the next section).

Drug therapy
- **Activated charcoal**: Administer via the gastric lavage tube.
  Dosage: 1 g/kg body weight (50 g for the average Asian – convenient as it is found in 50 g tubes).

NOTE: Activated charcoal is only useful within the first hour of ingestion and multidose charcoal therapy is no longer considered useful.

- **N-acetylcysteine (Parvolex®)**, administer if:
  1. The 4-hour serum paracetamol level lies in the toxic range on the Rumack-Matthew nomogram (see Figure 1).
  2. The initial serum paracetamol level (drawn earlier than 4 hours post-ingestion) is already in the toxic range.

3. The history is sufficiently convincing of a significant overdose, i.e. >150 mg/kg. **Do not** wait for a serum paracetamol level to return, though a specimen should still be sent from the ED to enable appropriate monitoring of the paracetamol level on the ward.

4. The liver function tests show evidence of hepatotoxicity. NAC therapy should be given in patients with hepatic failure until recovery or death.

PARVOLEX® (N-ACETYLCYSTEINE) IV INFUSION

Dosage in adults (Table 1)

TABLE 1   Treatment with Parvolex®

PATIENT'S BODY WEIGHT (kg)	Volume of Parvolex® (ml)			
	INITIAL 150 mg/kg in 200 ml of 5% dextrose in 15 minutes	SECOND 50 mg/kg in 500 ml of 5% dextrose in 4 hours	THIRD 100 mg/kg in 1 litre of 5% dextrose in 16 hours	TOTAL PARVOLEX (ml)
50	37.5	12.5	25	75
60	45.0	15.0	30	90
70	52.5	17.5	35	105
80	60.0	20.0	40	120
90	67.5	22.5	45	135
x	0.75x	0.25x	0.5x	1.5x

- Initial dosage: 150 mg/kg IV over **15 minutes**, followed by continuous infusion (50 mg/kg in 500 ml of 5% dextrose in **4 hours**), followed by continuous infusion (100 mg/kg in 1 litre 5% dextrose over **16 hours**).

- Total dosage: 300 mg/kg in 20 hours.

Mechanism of action of N-acetylcysteine (Parvolex®)

NAC is hypothesized to work in several ways:

- It acts as a precursor to cysteine, and then to glutathione. Thus, by repleting glutathione stores, it provides sulphydryl donors to which NAPQI can bind and be detoxified.

- It enhances the innate sulphation of any remaining paracetamol and thus reduces the amount of NAPQI generated.

- In patients with fulminant hepatic failure, it has been shown to improve survival presumably by (1) acting as a free radical scavenger; (2) enhancing oxygen uptake and utilization in peripheral tissues, including the brain; and (3) improving microcirculation.

Adverse effects of Parvolex® (seen most commonly in the first hour of treatment)

- Nausea, flushing, urticaria, and pruritus are the commonest manifestations and represent an anaphylactoid reaction (true anaphylactic reaction is rare). This appears to be both rate and dose related. Treatment is to stop infusion for 15 minutes and restart the infusion at the slowest rate (100 mg/kg in 1 litre 5% dextrose over 16 hours). Adjunctive treatment with anti-histaminergics (H-1 anatgonists) is also indicated.

POOR PROGNOSTIC INDICATORS FOLLOWING OVERDOSE

The King's College Hospital in London has developed a risk stratification system that is aimed at assessing the need for liver transplantation following paracetamol hepatotoxicity:

- **Serum pH <7.3** that corrects after resuscitation → mortality of 52%.
- **Normal serum pH** but with PT >100 seconds and creatinine >3.4 mg/dl, with either grade III or IV encephalopathy → mortality 81%.
- **Serum pH <7.3** which is uncorrectable with resuscitation → mortality 90%.

References/Further Reading

1. Jones AL, Volens G. Management of self poisoning. *BMJ*. 1999; 319: 1414–1417.
2. Vale JA. American Academy of Clinical Toxicology, European Association of Poison Centres and Clinical Toxicologists. Position statement: Gastric lavage. *J Toxicol Clin Toxicol*. 1997; 35(7): 711–719.
3. Bateman DN. Gastric decontamination: A view for the Millennium. *J Accid Emerg Med*. 1999; 16(2): 84–86.
4. Zed PJ, Krenzelok EP. Treatment of acetaminophen overdose. *Am J Health Syst Pharm*. 1999; 56(11): 1081–1091.
5. Chyka PA, Seger D. American Academy of Clinical Toxicology, European Association of Poison Centres and Clinical Toxicologists. Position statement: Single-dose activated charcoal. *J Toxicol Clin Toxicol*. 1997; 35(7): 721–741.
6. Jones AL. Mechanism of action and value of N-acetylcysteine in the treatment of early and late acetaminophen poisoning: A critical review. *J Toxicol Clin Toxicol*. 1998; 36: 277–285.
7. Spiller HA, Winter ML, Klein-Schwartz W, Bangh SA. Efficacy of activated charcoal administered more than 4 hours after acetaminophen overdose. *J Emerg Med*. Jan 2006; 30(1): 1–5.
8. Amato CS, Wang RY, Wright RO, Linakis JG. Evaluation of promotility agents to limit the gut bioavailability of extended-release acetaminophen. *J Toxicol Clin Toxicol*. 2004; 42(1): 73–77.

Suresh Pillai • Amila Punyadasa

CAVEATS

- Sources are multiple and include aspirin, peptobismol (salicylate content 8.8 mg/ml), sports liniments, wintergreen oil (salicylate content 530 mg/ml), and traditional Chinese medicines.
- **Mild toxicity (acute ingestions of 150–200 mg/kg)** is manifested by:
  1. Hyperpnoea with respiratory alkalosis (due to stimulation of the medullary respiratory centre).
  2. Ototoxicity as the prominent symptom (especially tinnitus).
- **Moderate toxicity (acute ingestions of 200–300 mg/kg)** is manifested by:
  1. Vomiting generally starting 3 to 6 hours post-ingestion and may cause a metabolic alkalosis.
  2. Severe hyperpnoea, hyperthermia, dehydration, abdominal pain, and diaphoresis.
- **Severe toxicity (acute ingestions of 300–400 mg/kg)** is manifested by
  1. Central nervous system (CNS) alterations with signs of stimulation initially, followed soon after by depression leading to convulsions and coma.
  2. Non-cardiogenic pulmonary oedema, dysrhythmias, haemorrhage, and acute renal failure.
  3. Metabolic acidosis.
  4. Death due to cardiovascular collapse, respiratory failure, or central nervous system failure.
- Symptoms after an acute overdose begin within 1 to 2 hours and may not peak until 12 to 24 hours later. However, if there are no clinical symptoms within 6 hours, it is unlikely that the patient will experience severe toxicity, unless a sustained-release preparation has been ingested.
- Alan Done, one of the forefathers of clinical toxicology, developed a salicylate nomogram in 1960 to correlate salicylate levels at different times post-ingestion in an acute overdose to determine the severity of toxicity. However, it is **not** used to determine treatment; thus the use of the Done nomogram is no longer recommended. Instead, the patient's clinical condition and early course, rather than the nomogram, should guide clinical therapy.
- **Serum salicylate estimations**:
  1. The first level should be drawn approximately 2 hours post-ingestion, with a repeat test drawn at 6 hours. Subsequently, serial levels (every 3 to 4 hours) should be monitored until the salicylate level is seen to have declined by about 10% from the preceding laboratory estimation.
  2. Significant toxicity can develop very rapidly in acute overdosage even before the 6-hour test is drawn.
  3. A salicylate level of <30 mg % (non-toxic range) drawn <6 hours post-ingestion **does not** rule out impending toxicity.

- There is **no** antidote for salicylate poisoning.
- **Urine alkalinization** is indicated for those patients with a rising and toxic salicylate level (>30 mg %):
  1. Salicylate is an acid whose renal excretion is increased by ionization.
  2. The kidney reabsorbs only unionized salicylate; since salicylate is an acid it ionizes in alkaline urine.
  3. If urinary pH is increased to 8 the urinary excretion of salicylate increases 10 to 20 fold.
- **Haemodialysis** is the most effective means of lowering the serum salicylate level. Indications are:
  1. An absolute overdose of >300 mg/kg
  2. Serum salicylate level of >100 mg/dl, after an acute ingestion
  3. Refractory acidosis
  4. Severe cardiac toxicity
  5. Renal failure
  6. Non-cardiogenic pulmonary oedema refractory to medical therapy
  7. Neurologic signs or symptoms, e.g. psychosis, confusion, convulsions or coma, suggestive of cerebral oedema
  8. Rising serum salicylate levels despite urinary alkalinization and multidose activated charcoal therapy.

⇨ **SPECIAL TIPS FOR GPs**
- Patients with severe salicylate toxicity may appear well initially. Always refer suspected cases to the emergency department for evaluation.
- Look out for the early signs of salicylate toxicity like tinnitus, vertigo, or hearing loss.
- Be aware that ingestion of small amounts of concentrated salicylates like methylsalicylate liniments or wintergreen oil can be lethal especially for a child.

MANAGEMENT

Supportive measures

- Patients with altered mental state or derangement of vital signs should be managed in the critical care area.
- Maintain airway; intubate if gag reflex is absent (in anticipation of gastric lavage) or patient is hypoxaemic.
- Administer 100% oxygen via a non-rebreather reservoir mask.
- Monitoring: Electrocardiogram (ECG), vital signs q 5–15 minutes, and pulse oximetry.
- Perform gastric lavage even beyond 1 hour as salicyclates delay gastric emptying.

- Establish a peripheral intravenous line.
- Treat fluid and electrolyte imbalances: Administer intravenous crystalloids at a rate sufficient to maintain adequate tissue perfusion.
- Treat coma, seizures, pulmonary oedema, and hyperthermia as you would from any cause.
- **Labs**:
  1. Serum salicylate level stat and at 2 hours post-ingestion.
  2. Arterial blood gases to determine the presence, type, and degree of acid-base derangement.
  3. Full blood count, urea/electrolytes/creatinine, and prothrombin time.

Drug therapy

- Activated charcoal via a lavage tube or orally.

  Dosage: 1 g/kg body weight (or 50 g for the average local adult).

- Sodium bicarbonate: To treat metabolic acidosis.

  Dosage: Bolus 1–2 mmol/kg 8.4% $NaHCO_3$.

  Infusion: 150 mmol $NaHCO_3$ (150 ml of 8.4% solution) in 850 ml D5W.

  Start at 1.5 to 2 times maintenance fluid rate; titrate flow rate against urine pH of 7.5 to 8.0.

NOTE: Monitor the serum potassium level (either via lab tests or by T wave morphology on an ECG monitor).

Contraindications to bicarbonate therapy

- Salicylate-induced **non-cardiogenic pulmonary oedema** as it may aggravate fluid overload.
- Concomitant **oral bicarbonate therapy** as this will increase salicylate absorption.
- The patient is already on **acetazolamide** as this will worsen systemic acidosis, thereby increasing central nervous system levels of salicylate and thus clinical toxicity.

Disposition

- For severe toxicity or those patients with rising serum salicylate levels, obtain General Medicine consultation in anticipation of admission to the high dependency or intensive care unit.
- Cases of mild toxicity can be managed by admission to a general ward.

References/Further Reading

1. Gaudreault P, Temple AR, Lovejoy F. The relative severity of acute versus chronic salicylate poisoning in children. A clinical comparison. *Paediatrics*. 1982; 70: 566.

2. Prescott LF, Balali-Mood M, Critchley JH, et al. Diuresis or urinary alkalinization for salicylate poisoning. *Br Med J*. 1982; 285: 1383.

3. Snodgrass W, Rumack BH, Petereson RG, et al. Salicylate toxicity following therapeutic doses in young children. *Clin Toxicol.* 1981; 18: 247.

4. Thisted B, Krantz T, Strom J, et al. Acute salicylate self-poisoning in 177 consecutive patients treated in ICU. *Acta Anaesthesiol Scand.* 1987; 31: 312.

5. Walters JSW, Woodring JH, Stelling CB, et al. Salicylate induced pulmonary edema. *Radiology.* 1983; 146: 289.

6. Hofman M, Diaz JE, Martella C. Oil of wintergreen overdose. *Ann Emerg Med.* 1998; 31: 793–794.

7. Krenzelok EP, Kerr F, Proudfoot AT. Salicylate toxicity. In: Haddad LM, Winchester J, eds. *Clinical Management of Poisoning and Drug Overdose.* 3rd ed. Philadelphia, PA: WB Saunders; 1998: 675–687.

8. Dargan PI, Wallace CI, Jones AL. An evidence based flowchart to guide the management of acute salicylate (aspirin) overdose. *Emerg Med J.* May 2002; 19(3): 206–209.

9. O'Malley GF. Emergency department management of the salicylate-poisoned patient. *Emerg Med Clin North Am.* May 2007; 25(2): 333–346; abstract, viii.

10. Teece S, Crawford I. Best evidence topic report. Gastric lavage in aspirin and non-steroidal anti-inflammatory drug overdose. *Emerg Med J.* Sep 2004; 21(5): 591–592.

90 Bites, Mammalian and Human

Gene Chan • Shirley Ooi

CAVEATS

- Human bites have a higher risk of infection compared to dog or cat bites.
- Think of **fight bite/**clenched fist injury in puncture wounds or infections at the fourth or fifth metacarpophalangeal joints.
- Puncture wounds may look innocuous but there is a higher risk of wound infection compared to larger wounds.
- Dogs have larger teeth and hence dog bites often cause tearing of tissues. In contrast, cats have fine, sharp teeth, and weaker biting forces, causing puncture wounds. Therefore, the infection rate for cat bite wounds is higher at 50% compared to 2–5% for dog bite wounds.

MICROBIOLOGY: DOG AND CAT BITES

- Most bite wounds are polymicrobial.

TABLE 1 **Some common microorganisms in dog and cat bite wounds**

	Dog bite (%)	Cat bite (%)
Aerobic		
Pasteurella sp. (especially *P. multocida*)	50	75
Streptococcus	46	46
Staphylococcus	46	35
Neisseria	16	19
Corynebacterium	12	28
Moraxella	10	35
Enterococcus	10	12
Bacillus	8	11
Anaerobes		
Fusobacterium sp.	32	33
Bacteroides sp.	30	28
Porphyromonas	28	30
Prevotella	28	19
Propionibacterium	20	18
Peptostreptococcus sp.	16	5

Source: Adapted from Talan et al.[4]

Pasteurella multocida

- Small aerobic, facultatively anaerobic, Gram-negative coccobacillus.
- Major pathogen isolated from cat (50–80%) and dog (25%) bites.
- Characterized by the rapid development of intense inflammatory response with prominent pain and swelling developing within 24 hours of initial injury.
- Preferred antibiotics include penicillin, augmentin, cephalosporins, tetracycline, and ciprofloxacin.

Capnocytophaga canimorsus, formerly known as 'dysgonic fermenter – 2'(DF-2)

- Fastidious, thin, Gram-negative bacillus.
- Presents with overwhelming sepsis with disseminated intravascular coagulation, acute renal failure, endocarditis, meningitis, peripheral gangrene, and cardiopulmonary failure. The clinical picture may be more severe in immuno-compromised patients, with 25% fatality.
- **Penicillin** is the drug of choice and should be used prophylactically in high-risk patients. Alternatives are cephalosporins, tetracyclines, erythromycin, and clindamycin.

MICROBIOLOGY: HUMAN BITES

- **Aerobic**: Alpha and beta-haemolytic streptococci, *S. aureus*, *S. epidermidis*, *Corynebacterium* sp., and *Eikenella corrodens*.
- **Anaerobic**: *Bacteroides fragilis*, *Peptostreptococcus*, *Fusobacterium*, and *Clostridium* sp.

Eikenella corrodens

- Fastidious, slow-growing, Gram-negative, facultatively anaerobic rod.
- Present in approximately 25% of clenched fist injuries. Frequently result in serious, chronic infections.
- Susceptible to penicillin, augmentin, bactrim, ceftriaxone, tetracycline, and ciprofloxacin.

Rare organisms transmitted by human bites

- Herpesvirus types 1 and 2
- Hepatitis B and C
- *Mycobacterium tuberculosis*
- *Treponema pallidum*
- Human immunodeficiency virus (HIV)

> ⇨ **SPECIAL TIPS FOR GPs**
> * Human bites are often unreported. Therefore, when treating cuts, scratches and lacerations to the scalp, dorsum of the hand or genitalia, consider the possibility of a human bite.
> * Remember to update tetanus status. Also, human bites can transmit organisms such as the human immunodeficiency virus, hepatitis B virus and even syphilis (refer to Chapter 75, *Needle Stick/Body Fluid Exposure*, for further details on prophylaxis).
> * Local dogs and cats in Singapore are free of rabies.
> * In Singapore, if bitten by a 'foreign dog', refer to the Communicable Disease Centre for anti-rabies prophylaxis.

MANAGEMENT

* Life-threatening injuries must be excluded first when there is a severe animal attack. However, most bite wounds are minor.

PRINCIPLES OF WOUND CARE

Diagnosis

* History
  1. Background of injury: Animal species, behaviour, provocation.
  2. Animal ownership: Location, possible rabies.
  3. Time since injury.
  4. Medical background of the patient: Immuno-suppression, peripheral vascular disease, diabetes mellitus.
  5. Medication allergy.
  6. Tetanus immune status.
* Examination
  1. **Wound**
     a. Location.
     b. Number.
     c. Type: Puncture/crush.
     d. Depth of penetration.
     e. Overt signs of infection.

  NOTE: As bite wounds are frequently punctures, they may be more extensive than they appear.

  2. **Injuries of deeper structures**
     a. Tendons.
     b. Joint spaces.

    c. Blood vessels.

    d. Nerves.

    e. Bones.

NOTE: Use local or regional anaesthesia and a proximal tourniquet to facilitate wound exploration. Use diagrams or take pictures for documentation purposes.

- Do **X-rays** if:
  1. Considerable oedema and tenderness exist about the wound.
  2. Bony penetration is suspected.
  3. Foreign bodies are suspected.
- Note the following on X-rays:
  1. Fracture.
  2. Foreign body.
  3. Tooth chips/metal pieces of dental work.
  4. Subcutaneous emphysema (necrotizing infections or air introduced during wound manipulation).
  5. Early osteomyelitis.
- Meticulous wound care is accomplished through the following ways:
  1. Thorough cleansing.
  2. Cautious debridement of devitalized tissues.
  3. Copious irrigation with normal saline solution. This markedly decreases the concentration of bacteria in contaminated wounds. To irrigate puncture wounds, use an 18-gauge needle or a plastic catheter tip with a 20-ml syringe inserted into the wound in the direction of the puncture. Care should be taken not to inflict additional trauma or to inject fluid into the tissues. If an eschar is present, it should be removed so that any abscess or exudates that have developed beneath it can be detected and treated.

NOTE: Cultures from bite wounds obtained at the time of injury are of little value because they cannot be used to predict whether infection will develop, or, if it does, the causative pathogens. Hence, aerobic and anaerobic bacterial culture should only be obtained from an infected bite wound.

Controversy: Primary closure or not

- Historically, such wounds were not closed primarily (except for face and scalp wounds). However, more recent literature supports primary closure after adequate wound preparation except for:
  1. Puncture wounds (because they cannot be cleaned adequately).
  2. Bite wounds with extensive crush injury.

3. Wounds requiring considerable amount of debridement.

4. Hand wounds (because of concerns about serious complications).

5. Bites to the arms and legs occurring more than 6–12 hours earlier.

6. Bites to the face occurring 12–24 hours earlier.

NOTE: **Delayed primary suture** should be done for the latter three situations. Subcutaneous sutures should be used sparingly because any foreign material in a contaminated wound increases the risk of infection.

Hand bite wounds

- Treatment: Always refer to Hand Surgery for early consult if in doubt.

  1. Thorough cleansing and irrigation.

  2. Debridement.

  3. Splinting with a bulky immobilization dressing: Splint in the position of function.

  4. Elevation for several days until oedema has mostly resolved: This must be emphasized to the patient.

  5. Provision of prophylactic antibiotics, especially in human bites.

  6. Administration of tetanus prophylaxis with or without rabies prophylaxis.

Drug therapy

- Whether antibiotics prevent infection in bite wounds remains controversial.

- Currently, antibiotics are not given routinely. Instead, give prophylactic antibiotics only in cases where the probability of infection is between 5 and 10%, i.e in the following circumstances:

  1. Dog or cat bites with deep full-thickness puncture.

  2. Hand or facial wounds.

  3. Lower extremity wounds.

  4. Wounds requiring surgical debridement.

  5. Wounds involving joints, tendons, ligaments, or fractures.

  6. Wounds in high-risk hosts: Immuno-compromised patients, e.g. those with diabetes mellitus and asplenia and those using immuno-suppressive drugs.

  7. Wounds adjacent to a prosthetic joint.

  8. Presentation more than 8 hours after the bite.

Give prophylactic antibiotics for 3 to 5 days. Refer to Table 2 for factors affecting the risk of infection in dog and cat bite wounds.

TABLE 2 **Factors affecting the risk of infection in dog and cat bite wounds**

Increased Risk	Increased Risk
1. Age <2 years; >50 years	1. Face and scalp wounds
2. Diabetes mellitus	
3. Chronic alcoholism	
4. Vascular disease	
5. Pre-existing oedema of affected limb	
6. Immuno-suppression: Steroids, asplenism	
7. Location: Extremities/joints	
8. Exposure >12 hours	
9. Puncture or crush wounds (40% of all infections)	

- **Choice of antibiotics**
  1. **Augmentin** has been shown in randomized controlled trials to be superior to placebo in 'uninfected wounds'. It is also cheap and easily tolerated.
  2. Give **augmentin** alone either orally 625 mg bd or intravenously 1.2 g, depending on the severity of the bite. Alternatively, intravenous ampicillin-sulbactam (unasyn 3 g) can be given. For penicillin-allergic patients, give **erythromycin** (500 mg qds) or **clindamycin** (IV 600 mg, then 300 mg orally 8 hourly) plus **ciprofloxacin** 500 mg bd or **levofloxacin** 750 mg om. In children, the fluoroquinolones can be substituted with bactrim.
- **Disposition**
  1. **Outpatient treatment** for local cellulitis only and no deep structure involvement. Arrange for early review within 24–48 hours.
  2. **Admit** for intravenous therapy and surgical consultation:
     a. Severe cellulitis.
     b. Systemic signs, e.g. fever or chills.
     c. Significant bites to the hand, complicated by tendon injuries.
     d. If infection has spread rapidly.
     e. The wound has not responded to oral or outpatient therapy.
     f. When wounds or infections are thought or known to involve a bone, joint, tendon, or nerve.
     g. Unreliable or incompetent patients.
     h. Immuno-compromised hosts, e.g. those with diabetes mellitus, receiving corticosteroids, or alcoholics.
     i. Presence of peripheral vascular disease.
     j. Injuries requiring reconstructive surgery.

- **Tetanus immunoprophylaxis**: Dog and cat bites are tetanus-prone wounds.
- **Rabies immunoprophylaxis**
  1. Local dogs and cats in Singapore are rabies free.
  2. In Singapore, if bitten by 'foreign' dogs, refer to the local health authority for rabies prophylaxis.

References/Further Reading

1. Ooi BSS. Dog, cat and human bites. *Singapore Family Physicians*. 1999; 25(4): 9–14.

2. Dire DJ. Emergency management of dog and cat bite wounds. *Emerg Med Clin North Am*. 1992; 10(4): 719–736.

3. Schwab RA, Powers RD. Puncture wounds and bites. In: Tintinalli JE, Ma OJ, Stapczynski JS, et al, eds. *Tintinalli's Emergency Medicine: A Comprehensive Study Guide*. 7th ed. New York: McGraw-Hill; 2011: 349–356.

4. Talan DA, Citron DM, Abrahamian FM, et al. Bacteriolgic analysis of infected dog and cat bite wounds. *N Eng J Med*. 1999; 340(2): 85–92.

5. Fleisher GR. The management of bite wounds (editorial). *N Eng J Med*. 1999; 340(2): 138–140.

6. Goldstein EJ. Bite wounds and infection. *Clin Infect Dis*. 1992; 14(3): 633–638.

7. Dog, cat, and human bites: A review. *Journal of the American Academy of Dermatology*. Dec 1995; 33(6).

8. Baddour LM, MD, FIDSA. Soft tissue infections due to dog and cat bites in adults – UptoDate. Jan 2008.

9. Endom EE, MD. Animal and human bites in children – UptoDate. Mar 2008.

91 Bites, Snake

Amila Punyadasa • Shirley Ooi

CAVEATS

- There are many classes of venomous snakes. They include:
    1. **Atractaspididae (burrowing asps)**: Small snakes with large maxillary fangs that are used alternately to bite their victims. They are largely found in Africa and parts of the Middle East and rarely produce fatal bites.
    2. **Colubridae**: Usually non-venomous or mildly venomous. The exceptions are the African Boomslang, Bird snake, Japanese garter snake, and red-necked keelback.
    3. **Elapidae**: These possess short fangs located anteriorly on the maxilla and the predominant characteristic of envenomation is neurotoxicity. Members include the coral snakes, the Asian and African cobras, African Mambas, Asian kraits, and the Brown and King Brown snakes of Australia.
    4. **Hydrophiidae**: Some consider the sea snakes to be part of the Elapidae family, however their taxonomy continues to evolve. They are found in the coastal waters off Australia and Southeast Asia.
    5. **Viperidae**: These possess specialized fangs which are large, generally tubular and mobile, and are attached to a relatively small maxillary bone. Viperid envenomation is characterized by tissue necrosis and haematological disturbances.
        a. Subfamily Viperinae (old world vipers): For example, Russell's viper (Asia) and Gaboon viper (Africa).
        b. Subfamily Crotalinae (pit vipers): For example, rattlesnakes. The identifying characteristics of a pit viper include these:
            i. Triangular head.
            ii. Vertical elliptical pupils.
            iii. Heat sensing pit found between the nostril and eye.
            iv. Single row of ventral scales leading to the anal plate.
            v. In the case of a rattlesnake, a caudal constellation of specialized scales arranged as the rattle.
    6. Not all bites result in envenomation. A snake bite is considered 'dry' when the snake does not inject any venom. This occurs in about 60% of coral snake and 25% of rattlesnake bites. The diagnosis of a '**dry bite**', in the case of a rattlesnake bite, can only be made after an 8-hour observation period which yields no evidence of neurotoxicity, haematological abnormalities, aberrancies in vital signs, or signs, of local tissue toxicity at any time during that period. (The same cannot be applied to other types of venomous snake bites.)
    7. Only a small minority of land snakes are venomous.

8. **All sea snakes** are **venomous**. Suspect bite by a sea snake if there is a history of **painless bite** occurring while swimming in the sea or during sorting of the fishing net. Generalized muscle aches and pains, and stiffness when the victim attempts to move, usually occur within half to 1 hour after the bite.

9. One of the most important issues in snake bites is to try to ascertain if the snake is venomous as it is usually quite difficult for the victim or bystander to be able to identify the snake.

10. In general, the best clues to a **venomous bite** are:

    a. The presence of **intense local pain**.

    b. **Oedema** surrounding a puncture wound and gradually spreading proximally.

    c. The presence of **petechiae**, **ecchymoses** and serous, or haemorrhagic **bullae**.

    d. The presence of **systemic effects** like nausea, vomiting, diarrhoea, severe abdominal pain, restlessness, hypotension, haemorrhagic manifestations (epistaxis, gum bleeding, and gastrointestinal bleeding), neurological symptoms (paralysis, ptosis, impairment of eye movements, speech and swallowing difficulty, unsteady gait, and seizures), respiratory paralysis, and dark-coloured urine (from myoglobinuria).

- If the snake is available for inspection, contact the local zoo or herpetological society, according to local practice, whose members can be asked to assist in the identification of the snake. See Figure 1 for identification of snake bites.

FIGURE 1   Identification of snake bites

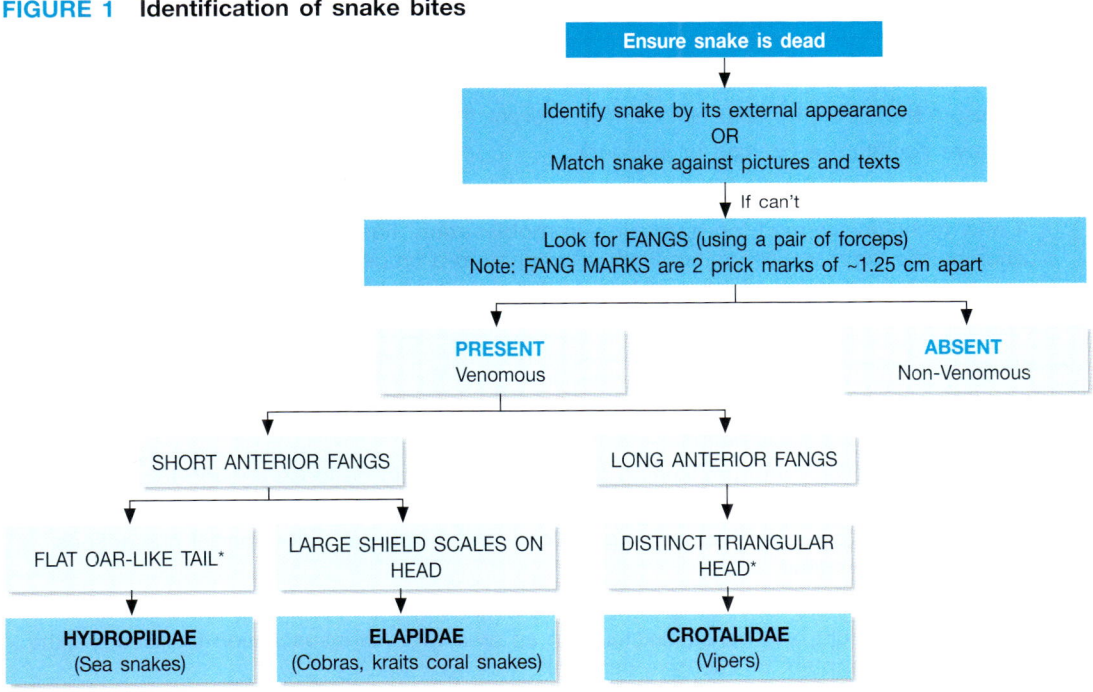

Note: * Particularly distinctive features.

- Be careful **not to handle a 'dead' snake** as reflex envenomation by a decapitated head of a snake can still occur several hours after its death.
- **Snake venom** may be broadly **classified** into:
  1. **Haematotoxins** or **cardiovascular** toxins (as in Crotalidae).
  2. **Neurotoxins** (as in Elapidae and Hydrophiidae).
  3. **Myotoxins** (as in Hydrophiidae).
- See Table 1 for grades of envenomation.
- An antivenin should only be administered in hospital if there is moderate to severe envenomation.

TABLE 1 Grades of envenomation

Grades of envenomation	
• Minimal:	No pain to moderate pain, erythema, oedema 2.5–15 cm, no systemic symptoms.
• Moderate:	Severe pain, tenderness, oedema 25–40 cm, erythema, petechiae, vomiting, fever, and weakness.
• Severe:	Widespread pain, oedema 40–50 cm, ecchymosis, and systemic signs.
• Very severe:	Rapid swelling, ecchymosis, central nervous system symptoms, visual disturbance, shock, and convulsions.

⇨ **SPECIAL TIPS FOR GPs**
- Reassure the victim to keep him calm to prevent the rapid spread of potential venom.
- Remove constrictive clothing or jewellery.
- Immobilize the bitten extremity to decrease metabolism, absorption, and the spread of venom.

  A new technique termed '**compression–immobilisation**' has been devised in Australia whereby the entire envenomated limb is wrapped in a crepe bandage and then splinted. It has been proven to be effective in treating neurotoxic snake bites. However, it is prohibited in treating envenomations by snakes with local tissue toxicity.

- Never use tourniquets.
- Squeezing or applying suction to wounds has not been proven to be effective in venom removal.
- Look for signs of envenomation.
- Apply a constricting band proximal to the wound. It should be loose enough to admit a finger between the band and the area of the wound. It is useful if applied within 30 minutes of the bite.
- Try to get the snake identified or bring it along to the hospital. Take special precautions when handling a 'dead' snake.
- Transfer to a medical centre as soon as possible.
- An antivenin should only be administered in an area with full resuscitation facilities like the emergency department or intensive care unit.

MANAGEMENT

Supportive measures

- Manage the patient in the resuscitation area. Place the patient supine and immobilize the bitten extremity in a dependent position.
- Keep the airway clear. If danger of bulbar or respiratory paralysis exists, intubate or ventilate via a surgical airway if intubation is not possible.
- Give supplemental high flow oxygen.
- Do a complete set of vital signs.
- Monitoring: Electrocardiogram (ECG), vital signs q 5–10 minutes, and pulse oximetry.
- **Labs:** Full blood count, coagulation profile, urinalysis, urea/electrolytes/creatinine, and ECG are mandatory. Severe cases: Urine myoglobin, disseminated intravascular coagulation (DIC) screen, and creatine phosphokinase. Shock or respiratory depression: Arterial blood gas (ABG).
- If the patient arrives at the hospital with a **tourniquet in place**, ensure the following before you release it, anticipating sudden envenomation from the snake bite:
  1. Peripheral intravenous (IV) line in place with normal saline.
  2. Resuscitation equipment immediately available.
  3. Full monitoring in place.
- Insert a urinary catheter to monitor the urine output (if the patient is unstable).
- Keep the patient nil by mouth: nausea and vomiting occur following haemototoxic venomous bites.
- Irrigate the eyes in cases of snake bite ophthalmia (e.g. some cobras will spit in the eyes of a victim).
- **What not to do**:
  1. **Do not** apply a tourniquet to the affected extremity.
  2. **Do not** apply ice packs to the wound since, upon removal, reflex vasodilatation may result in a more rapid absorption of venom.
  3. **Do not** incise or suck the wound.
  4. The Coghlan's Snake Bite Kit should not be used (the blade in the kit can injure digital nerves, arteries, and tendons).
  5. The use of the Sawyer Extractor suction pump to remove venom without incision is controversial and thus not advocated.
  6. Electric shock to the bite site should be condemned.

Specific measures

- **Use of an antivenin to neutralize the snake venom**: Polyvalent antivenin should be kept in the critical care area and stored in the refrigerator at 2–6°C. When used, the antivenin must be constituted quickly since it deteriorates and loses its effectiveness at room temperature.

- **Indications for use should be according to the grades of envenomation** (see Table 2).

TABLE 2   Guidelines for dosage of antivenin

Grade of envenomation	Dosage
Minimal envenomation	Antivenin **not** indicated
Moderate envenomation	20–40 ml (2–4 vials)*
Severe	50–90 ml (5–9 vials)
Very severe	100–150 ml (10–15 vials)

Note: *There is controversy over this.

- **Prevention of serum reaction**: Before injecting the antivenin, enquire about the following:
  1. Whether the patient has been given serum injections before (e.g. the old ATS, but not anti-tetanus Toxoid, ATT).
  2. Personal or family history of allergy:
     a. Test sensitivity of the patient to serum by intradermal injection of 0.1 ml of serum diluted 1:10. Observe for 30 minutes for local and general reactions. If these occur, consider giving IV diphenhydramine, IV corticosteroids and/or intramuscular (IM) adrenaline 1:1000 or IV adrenaline 1:10,000.
     b. Inject the antivenin in allergic or sensitive patients under cover of antihistamines and hydrocortisone given 15–30 minutes before the administration of the antivenin under close and experienced physician supervision. Also, consider the utility of an adrenaline infusion, to be kept as a standby in the event of anaphylaxis.
- **Complications of antivenin therapy**: This involves type I hypersensitivity reaction (5% risk of anaphylactic shock) in the short term and type III hypersensitivity reaction in the longer term.
- **Anticholinesterases**: For patients with severe neurotoxic symptoms, administer a test dose of IV edrophonium chloride (Tensilon) 10 mg with IV atropine 0.6 mg. If the response is convincing, administer IV neostigmine.
- **Analgesia/sedation**: Pain and agitation may be severe. Administer morphine or diazepam, or both, in small doses intravenously titrating to effect. Be prepared to intubate since some degree of respiratory depression may already exist due to muscular weakness resulting from toxicity from the snake venom.
- Consider the need for **fasciotomy**.
- Update **ATT** but the routine use of **antibiotics** is not evidence based.

Disposition

- Admit all cases of snake bites for observation. If severe, seek Intensive Care team consultation.

References/Further Reading

1. Gopalakrishnakone P, Chou LM, Aye MM, et al. *Snake bite and their treatment*. Singapore: Singapore University Press; 1990.

2. Gopalakrishnakone P, How J. A field guide to dangerous snakes. Headquarters Medical Services.

3. Gopalakrishnakone P, Chou LM. *Snakes of medical importance (Asia-Pacific Region)*. Venom and Toxin Research Group National University of Singapore and International Society on Toxinology (Asia-Pacific Section). Singapore: Singapore University Press; 1990.

4. Dart RC, Daly FFS. Reptile bites. In: Tintinalli JE, Ma OJ, Stapczynski JS, et al, eds. *Tintinalli's Emergency Medicine: A Comprehensive Study Guide*. 7th ed. New York: McGraw-Hill; 2011: 1354–1358.

5. Kunkel DB. Bites of venomous reptiles. *Emerg Med Clin North Am*. 1984; 2: 563.

6. Nelson BK. Snake venomation, incidence, clinical presentation, and management. *Med Toxicol*. 1989; 4: 17.

7. Podgorny G. Treatment of snake bite. In: Hadad LM, Winchester JF, eds. *Clinical Management of Poisoning and Drug Overdose*. Philadelphia, PA: WB Saunders; 1983.

8. Wythe ET. Snakebite. In: Olson KR, ed. *Poisoning and Drug Overdose*. 2nd ed. Norwalk, CT: Prentice-Hall; 1994: 285–288, 312–313.

9. Kearney TE. Antivenin, crotalidae (rattlesnake). In: Olson KR, ed. *Poisoning and Drug Overdose*. 2nd ed. Norwalk, CT: Prentice-Hall; 1994: 312–313.

10. Hurlbut KM, Dart RC, Spaite D. Reliability of clinical presentation for predicting significant pit viper envenomation. *Ann Emerg Med*. 1988; 12: 438.

11. White RR, Weber RA. Poisonous snakebite in central Texas: Possible indications for antivenin treatment. *Ann Surg*. 1991; 213: 466–471.

12. Otten, EJ. Venomous animal injuries. In: Rosen R, Barkin RM, Braen CR, et al, eds. *Emergency Medicine: Concepts and Clinical Practice*. 3rd ed. St. Louis, MO: Mosby; 1992.

13. Dart RC, Sullivan Jr. JB. Elapid snake envenomations. In: The Clinical Practice of Emergency Medicine. 2nd ed. Philadelphia, PA: Lippincott-Raven; 1996.

14. Holstege CP, Miller MB, Wermuth M, et al. Crotalid snake envenomation. *Crit Care Clin*. 1997; 13: 889–921.

15. Roberts JR, Otten EJ. Snakes and other reptiles. In: Goldfrank LR, Flomenbaum NE, Lewin NA, et al (eds). *Goldfrank's Toxicological Emergencies*. 6th ed. Stamford, CT: Appleton & Lange; 1998: 1603–1619.

16. Stewart RM, Page CP, Schwesinger WH, et al. Antivenin and fasciotomy/debridement in the treatment of severe rattle snake bite. *Am J Surg*. 1989; 158: 543–547.

17. Gold BS, Dart RC, Barish RA. Bites of venomous snakes. *New Engl J Med*. 2002; 347(5): 347–56. Review.

18. Bush SP. Snakebite suction devices don't remove venom: They just suck. *Ann Emerg Med*. Feb 2004; 43(2): 187–188.

19. Dart RC, Seifert SA, Boyer LV, Clark RF, Hall E, McKinney P, et al. A randomized multicentre trial of crotalinae polyvalent immune Fab (ovine) antivenom for the treatment for crotaline snakebite in the United States. *Arch Intern Med*. 10 Sep 2001; 161(16): 2030–2036.

20. Spiller HA, Bosse GM. Prospective study of morbidity associated with snakebite envenomation. *J Toxicol Clin Toxicol*. 2003; 41(2): 125–130.

92   Crush Syndrome

Irwani Ibrahim

DEFINITION

Crush syndrome is the systemic manifestation of muscle cell damage resulting from pressure or crushing.

CAVEATS

- Failure to recognize this condition results in full-blown crush syndrome, which has high mortality.
- Toxic metabolites released from the crush muscle result in:
  1. Blocked renal tubules leading to renal failure.
  2. Electrolyte and acid-base imbalance causing dysrhythmias followed by disseminated intravascular coagulation (DIVC).
- Injured muscles sequester fluids into their compartments upon rescue.
- **Causes**:
  1. Burns.
  2. Prolonged entrapment of >60 minutes involving large muscle mass, e.g. in crush injuries, alcoholics, or drug abusers who have laid on a limb during a period of prolonged unconsciousness.
  3. Non-traumatic neuroleptic malignant syndrome.
  4. Exertional prolonged grand mal fits.
- **Problems of crush syndrome**: Hypovolaemia, hyperkalaemia, hypocalcaemia, myoglobinuria, renal failure, adult respiratory distress syndrome, DIVC, and compartment syndrome.

> ⇨ **SPECIAL TIP FOR GPs**
> - Giving vigorous fluid resuscitation as early as possible, preferably at the scene, is beneficial.

MANAGEMENT

- Assess airway, breathing and circulation (ABCs) as in major trauma protocol.
- Establish 2 large bore intravenous lines and give vigorous fluid resuscitation immediately (at least 1.5 L/hr), preferably before extrication if possible.
- Lab: Full blood count, urea/electrolyte/creatinine, serum calcium, and coagulation profile.
- Do **urinalysis** for **myoglobin**.

- **Electrocardiogram** to detect arrhythmia as a result of hypocalcaemia and hyperkalaemia.
- **Hyperkalaemia** is often fatal and should be treated vigorously. Hypocalcaemia should be corrected only if it causes symptoms.
- Monitor **urine output** closely; consider inserting a urinary catheter. If urine output is poor (<2 ml/kg/hr), consider forced mannitol-alkaline diuresis until the urinary pH reaches a value of above 6.5. Consider dialysis if standard indications for dialysis are met.
- Consider **anti-tetanus prophylaxis** if there are open wounds.
- Inform the orthopaedic registrar who may arrange for immediate fasciotomy.

References/Further Reading

1. Sever MS, Vanholder R, Lameire N. Management of crush-related injuries after disasters. *N Engl J Med*. 9 Mar 2006; 354(10): 1052–1063.

2. Gonzalez D. Crush syndrome. *Crit Care Med*. Jan 2005; 33(1 Suppl): S34–41.

3. Smith J. Crush injury and crush syndrome: A review. *The Journal of Trauma*. 2003; 54(5): S226–230.

93 Trauma, Abdominal

Peng Li Lee • Shirley Ooi

CAVEATS

- Intra-abdominal trauma is a significant cause of preventable deaths.
- Emergency care personnel should have a high index of suspicion for its presence, and investigate and manage such cases accordingly.
- All penetrating injuries below (between) the nipple line should also be suspected of entering the abdominal cavity.
- Patients should always be log-rolled to examine the back and flanks to complete the abdominal examination in trauma cases.
- All multiple trauma patients with hypotension are presumed to have intra-abdominal injury until proven otherwise.
- Clinical examination of the abdomen may be compromised in the following setting:
  1. Change in sensorium: Alcoholic intoxication, use of illicit drugs, and head injury.
  2. Change in sensation: Injury to the spinal cord.
  3. Distracting injury to adjacent structures: Lower ribs, pelvis, and lumbar spine.
- Resuscitation and stabilization of the patient take precedence over investigations.

> ⇨ **SPECIAL TIPS FOR GPs**
> - In alert patients, the most reliable signs indicating abdominal injury are tenderness on abdominal palpation, guarding or rebound. However, the lack of such signs does not reliably exclude significant intra-abdominal injury.
> - For those with significant mechanism of injury but who present with minimal abdominal findings initially, refer to the emergency department for further evaluation.
> - For those who present to the clinic with early signs of shock, start an intravenous (IV) infusion of crystalloid and call the ambulance for transfer to hospital.

MANAGEMENT

- The patient should be managed in the critical care area.
- Physical examination and resuscitation should proceed simultaneously.
- **Principles of Advanced Trauma Life Support (ATLS)** should be followed with priorities given to:
  1. Airway: Establish and maintain the airway.
  2. Breathing: Administer high flow oxygen if the patient is conscious and spontaneously breathing. The unconscious patient may require endotracheal intubation with mechanical ventilation.

3. Circulation: Establish two large (14/16G) cannulae for venous access. In hypotensive patients, fluid should be infused rapidly. Start with normal saline (up to 2 L) followed by blood products (start group O emergency blood if available in the emergency department).

● Send blood for GXM, full blood count, and urea/electrolytes/creatinine.

● **The targeted examination** should include:

1. Chest wall: Bruising, fractured ribs, and penetrating injury.
2. Abdomen: External injuries, e.g. bruising and signs of peritonism, e.g. tenderness, guarding, and absent bowel sounds.
3. Pelvis: Tenderness and instability suggesting fracture.
4. External genitalia and rectum: Bleeding or haematoma.
5. Neurological status.

• Insert a nasogastric tube and urinary catheter unless there is a suspicion of urethral injury based on the physical examination.

• Mandatory trauma series X-rays are indicated as time permits: Chest X-ray, pelvic X-ray, cervical spine X-ray (C-spine X-rays may not be indicated in selected cases where the neck may be cleared clinically. Refer to Chapter 102, *Trauma Spinal Cord*).

• Abdominal stab wounds with implements in-situ should not be removed until the patient is in the operating room.

• Refer and consult the general surgeon early.

Indications for immediate laparotomy

• Evisceration, stab wounds with implements in-situ, and gunshot wounds traversing the abdominal cavity.

• Any penetrating injury to the abdomen with haemodynamic instability or peritoneal irritation.

• Obvious or strongly suspected intra-abdominal injury with shock or difficulty in stabilizing the haemodynamics.

• Obvious signs of peritoneal irritation.

• Rectal signs of peritoneal irritation.

• Rectal examination reveals fresh blood.

• Persistent fresh blood aspirated from the nasogastric tube if oropharyngeal injuries have been excluded as a cause for bleeding.

• X-ray evidence of pneumoperitoneum or diaphragmatic rupture.

Investigations

• In the absence of the above indications for immediate laparotomy, Figure 1 shows the modes of investigation to be considered depending on the stability of the patient.

• The patient going to the computed tomography (CT) scan room must have his vital signs **continuously monitored** and must be accompanied by a doctor.

FIGURE 1 Modes of investigation in a suspected abdominal trauma patient

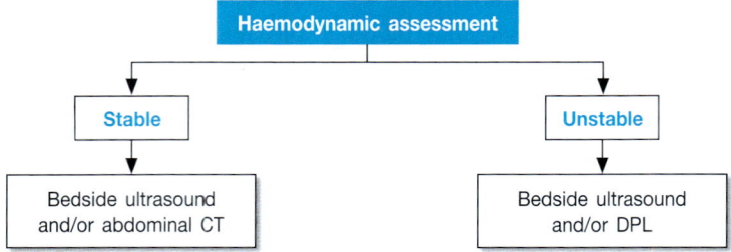

- **Abdominal CT scan**:
  1. **Indications**:
     a. Blunt trauma with stable haemodynamics and with no indication for urgent laparotomy.
     b. Further assessment for pelvic fracture, retroperitoneal, diaphragmatic and urogenital injuries.
  2. Sensitivity is consistently reported as >90%.
  3. With the advent of CT, diagnostic peritoneal lavage (DPL) is uncommonly done in stable patients due to its invasive nature.
  4. **Advantages of abdominal CT scan**:
     a. Able to precisely locate intra-abdominal lesions preoperatively.
     b. Able to evaluate retroperitoneum.
     c. Able to identify injuries that can be managed non-operatively.
     d. Not invasive.
  5. **Disadvantages of abdominal CT scan**:
     a. Expensive.
     b. Time required to perform the study.
     c. Need to transport the patient to the radiology suite.
     d. Use of contrast materials needed.
- **Diagnostic peritoneal lavage** performed by the surgical team:
  1. **Indications**:
     a. Any unstable patient in whom there is a suspicion of abdomical trauma or where clinical examination is difficult or equivocal.
     b. Unexplained hypotension in multiple trauma.
     c. The patient sustaining blunt trauma requiring immediate operation for extra-abdominal injuries.
     d. Stable patients with suspicion of intestinal injury: 'Delayed' DPL may be performed.

2. **Contraindications**: The first is an absolute contraindication but the rest are relative contraindications:

   a. Absolute indications for laparotomy already exist.

   b. Previous abdominal surgery or infections.

   c. Gravid uterus.

   d. Morbid obesity.

   e. Coagulopathy.

3. **Prerequisite**: Decompress the bladder and stomach with a urinary catheter and nasogastric tube, respectively.

4. The open technique with an infraumbilical incision. Alternatively, the percutaneous method using the Seldinger technique is also acceptable.

5. **Indicators of a positive diagnostic peritoneal lavage**:

   a. Frank blood (>5 ml) or obvious bowel contents aspirated.

   b. Lavage fluid seen to exit from the chest drain or urinary catheter.

   c. Effluent   Red blood cell count >100,000 cells per mm^3.
                    White blood cell count >500 cells per mm^3.
                    Gram stain positive for bacteria.

6. Diagnostic peritoneal lavage is exceptionally sensitive.

7. **Advantages of diagnostic peritoneal lavage**:

   a. DPL can promptly reveal or exclude the presence of intraperitoneal haemorrhage in a haemodynamically unstable patient with multiple injuries.

   b. DPL is especially valuable in the discovery of potentially lethal bowel perforations when patients are poor candidates for serial clinical observations.

8. **Disadvantages of diagnostic peritoneal lavage**:

   a. There is morbidity, although low, associated with DPL.

      i. Wound complications, including haematoma and infections occur in 0.3% of cases;

      ii. Sensitivity to intraperitoneal bleeding is more than 98%; and

      iii. Technical failure can result whereby the insertion of a catheter through an abdominal wall haematoma can create a haemoperitoneum to produce a false positive result.

   b. **False negative rate (2%)** results from the failure to recover lavage fluid, early hollow visceral injury, diaphragmatic injuries, and injuries due to retroperitoneal structures (e.g. pancreas and duodenum).

• **Focused Assessment with Sonography in Trauma (FAST)**:

1. Increasingly being used as an adjunct in the bedside assessment of abdominal trauma. The indications are the same as for DPL.

2. It is especially useful in situations where DPL is relatively contraindicated, e.g. obesity, previous laparotomy, or coagulopathy, and the patient is too unstable for transfer to the CT scan room.

3. Its accuracy is operator- as well as equipment-dependent. The amount of free fluid may be quantified based on ultrasound, which gives an idea of the degree of intra-abdominal haemorrhage. It is sensitive in detecting as little as 100 ml and more typically 500 ml of peritoneal fluid from 60–95%.

4. **Four quadrants** are looked at to detect free fluid:

   a. Subxiphoid: Pericardium

   b. Right upper quadrant: Morrison's pouch (a potential space between the liver and kidney)

   c. Left upper quadrant: Splenorenal recess and between the spleen and diaphragm

   d. Pelvis: The pouch of Douglas

5. **Advantages** of FAST:

   a. It involves the use of a portable instrument that can be brought to the bedside.

   b. Examinations can be done quickly in less than 5 minutes. Hence, it helps emergency physicians to rapidly answer whether haemoperitoneum, free pericardial fluid, and free pleural fluid are present.

   c. FAST can be used for serial examinations.

   d. Unlike CT scanning, it is not a potential radiation hazard and does not require the administration of contrast agents.

6. **Disadvantages** of FAST:

   a. FAST does not image solid parenchymal damage, the retroperitoneum, diaphragmatic defects, or bowel injury well.

   b. It is technically compromised by the uncooperative, agitated patient, as well as by obesity, substantial bowel gas, and subcutaneous air.

   c. Indeterminate studies require follow-up attempts or alternative diagnostic tests.

   d. It is less sensitive and more operator-dependent than DPL in revealing haemoperitoneum and cannot distinguish blood from ascites.

   e. FAST will not detect the presence of solid parenchymal damage if free intraperitoneal blood is absent as in subcapsular splenic injury.

7. For the haemodynamically stable blunt trauma patient with positive FAST examination results, further evaluation with a CT scan may be warranted before admission to General Surgery.

Investigations: Penetrating trauma

- In the absence of the above indications for immediate laparotomy, the following modes of investigation are considered depending on the stability of the patient:

  1. **Stab wound**: Explore the wound in the emergency department. If there is no fascial penetration, the patient can be discharged home. If there is, the patient should be examined by a surgeon.

2. **Gunshot wound**: Establish the trajectory by examining the entrance/exit wounds or using X-rays if there is no exit wound. Immediate laparotomy is required if the trajectory traverses the peritoneal cavity; if the trajectory is tangential, the wound will require surgical intervention.

References/Further Reading

1. Isenhour JL, Marx JA. Abdominal trauma. In: Marx JA, Hockberger RS, Walls RM, eds. Rosen's *Emergency Medicine: Concepts and Practice*. 7th ed. Philadelphia, PA, MO: Mosby Elsevier; 2010: 414–434.

2. Abdominal and pelvic trauma. In: Committee on Trauma of the American College of Surgeons. *Advanced Trauma Life Support Student Course Manual*. 7th ed. Chicago, IL: American College of Surgeons; 2012: 122–147.

3. Scalea TM, Boswell SA, Baron BJ, Ma OJ. Abdominal trauma. In: Tintinalli JE, Ma OJ, Stapczynski JS, et al., eds. *Tintinalli's Emergency Medicine: A Comprehensive Study Guide*. 7th ed. New York: McGraw-Hill; 2011: 1765–1771.

94 Trauma, Chest

Shirley Ooi • Victor Ong

CAVEATS

- Management of chest trauma follows standard Advanced Trauma Life Support (ATLS) protocol:
  1. Securing the ABCs (airway, breathing and circulation) is the first priority.
  2. Give immediate management for detected lesions.
  3. Early involvement of the hospital's trauma or cardiothoracic team, according to institutional practice, is important.
- During the primary survey, the clinician should watch for the following potentially **life-threatening** but salvageable conditions:
  1. Airway obstruction (e.g. due to laryngeal injury or posteriorly displaced fracture/dislocation of sternoclavicular joint).
  2. Tension pneumothorax.
  3. Open pneumothorax (sucking chest wound).
  4. Flail chest.
  5. Massive haemothorax.
  6. Pericardial tamponade.

INITIAL MANAGEMENT OF ALL THORACIC INJURIES

- Transfer the patient to the critical care or resuscitation area of the emergency department.
- Activate the in-house trauma team according to institutional protocol.
- Assess and manage the patient according to ATLS principles.
- Consider intubating the patient using rapid sequence intubation (RSI) techniques for these situations:
  1. Airway is compromised.
  2. Inadequate ventilation.
  3. Oxygen saturation (SpO_2) levels could not be maintained above 92% despite using a non-rebreather mask.

NOTE: If possible, tube thoracostomy should be performed before intubation as excessive ventilatory pressures may cause a tension pneumothorax or reduce venous return, which may induce cardiac arrest.

- Establish 2 large bore (14G/16G) intravenous lines in both antecubital fossae. Initial resuscitation fluid of choice is a crystalloid (Hartmann's or 0.9% isotonic saline).

- **Obtain blood for investigations**:
  1. GXM for 6 units of whole blood.
  2. Full blood count, urea/electrolytes/creatinine, and coagulation profiles.
  3. Arterial blood gases (hypoxia, hypercarbia, and metabolic acidosis/base excess).

Indications for chest tube insertion after a trauma

- Pneumothorax (tension and simple), haemothorax, or open chest wound.
- Rib fractures (multiple) requiring positive pressure ventilation.
- Selected patients with suspected severe lung injury, especially those being transferred by air or ground vehicles.
- Patients undergoing general anaesthesia for treatment of other injuries (e.g. cranial or extremity), who are suspected to have significant lung injury.

NOTE: The majority of thoracic pathology secondary to trauma (up to 85%) can be managed with simple measures like tube thoracostomy.

TREATMENT FOR SPECIFIC CHEST CONDITIONS

Tension pneumothorax

- Always consider the diagnosis in a patient with signs of a simple pneumothorax, haemodynamic instability, severe respiratory distress, and neck vein distension.
- The diagnosis is a **clinical** one and treatment decisions are based on a high index of suspicion.
- Immediately perform **needle thoracostomy** with a large bore (14/16G) intravenous venula at the second intercostal space along the mid-clavicular line on the ipsilateral (affected) side.
- Performing the above procedure will enable the release of raised intrathoracic pressure and allow for adequate filling of the right ventricle and hence recovery of cardiac output.
- Tube thoracostomy will need to be done soon after to resolve the open pneumothorax so created.

Open pneumothorax

- This is a large chest-wall defect with equilibration of intra-thoracic and atmospheric pressure.
- Normal breathing pattern is affected as the usual negative intra-thoracic pressure is abolished by the open chest wound.
- Cover the wound with any sterile/clean non-porous **dressing taped only** on **3 sides** leaving one side free to act as a flutter valve. Do not tape on all sides as it may create a tension pneumothorax!
- Perform tube thoracostomy 1 to 2 intercostal spaces below the open wound.
- The open chest wound would likely need exploration and closure by the cardiothoracic team.

Flail chest

- A flail chest occurs when ≥2 contiguous ribs have been fractured in ≥2 places (radiological diagnosis).
- **Clinical features include**:
  1. Paradoxical chest wall movement.
  2. Respiratory distress.
  3. External evidence of chest trauma.
  4. Pain on respiratory effort.

NOTE: Hypoxaemia in flail chest is mainly due to the underlying pulmonary contusion and resultant ventilation-perfusion (V/Q mismatch). This will affect oxygenation and ventilation. Pain from the rib fractures will result in restricted chest wall movement, further compounding the V/Q mismatch.

- **Management**
  1. Ensure adequate oxygen supplementation.
  2. Provide judicious fluid therapy.
  3. Key point is to administer adequate analgesia so that the patient will have ease of respiration.

NOTE: Patients with isolated flail chest injuries can often be managed without ventilatory support, especially if the chest pain can be adequately relieved. Fluid overloading should be prevented as it could lead to pulmonary oedema in adult respiratory distress syndrome.

- Indications for **early mechanical ventilation in flail chest**:
  1. Hypoxia and hypercarbia.
  2. Shock.
  3. >3 associated injuries.
  4. Severe head injury.
  5. Previous pulmonary disease.
  6. Fracture of >8 ribs.
  7. Patients age ≥65 years.

NOTE: When a patient requires ventilatory support, it is much safer to apply it 'prophylactically' before actual ventilatory failure develops.

- Splinting is controversial. However, in the process of transfer, it may be considered for pain relief.

Pericardial tamponade

- Diagnosis requires a high index of suspicion. Certain combinations of features point towards this possibility:

   1. Chest trauma and hypotension

   2. **Beck's triad** (hypotension, muffled heart sounds, and distended neck veins)

   NOTE: Beck's triad is seen in only 50% of cases. Neck veins in cardiac tamponade may not be distended until coexistent hypovolaemia is at least partially corrected; a muffled heart sound is the least reliable sign in Beck's triad.

   3. Chest trauma and pulseless electrical activity

   4. **Kussmaul's signs** (increased neck distension during inspiration and pulsus paradoxus)

- Other supporting evidence that may be present include:

   1. An enlarged cardiac shadow on the chest X-ray (rare).

   2. Small electrocardiogram (ECG) voltages (uncommon).

   3. Pericardial fluid demonstrated on 2D Echo or Focused Assessment Using Sonography in Trauma (FAST), which is definitive.

- **Management**

   1. Ensure adequate oxygenation of the patient (give 100% oxygen via a non-rebreather mask at 15 L/min).

   2. Establish 2 large bore intravenous lines.

   3. Give intravenous fluid bolus 500 ml stat and repeat to maintain mean arterial pressure at more than 90 mmHg.

   4. Treat pericardial tamponade by pericardiocentesis.

      a. ECG guided (with ECG lead attached to pericardiocentesis needle).

      b. 2D Echo guided. This can be diagnostic or therapeutic.

   NOTE: Aggressive fluid resuscitation helps maintain cardiac output and buys time for the patient. **Never** probe blindly with a needle as the risk of iatrogenic cardiac injury is high.

   5. The inpatient cardiothoracic/vascular team should be alerted immediately for consultation.

Massive haemothorax

- **Defined** as blood loss of >1500 ml inside the chest.

- **Management** include:

   1. Blood transfusion and correction of coagulopathy.

   2. Tube thoracostomy on the affected side (do not drain >1 litre of blood at any one time as this will lead to acute haemodynamic instability).

   3. Beware of sudden cessation of blood drainage: Check for blocked tube.

- **Indications for emergent thoracotomy** (emergent cardiothoracic consult):
  1. Initial blood drainage >1500 ml.
  2. Ongoing drainage of >500 ml/hr for the first hour, 300 ml/hr for 2 consecutive hours, or 200 ml/hr for 3 consecutive hours.
  3. Persistent blood transfusion requirements.
  4. Large retained pneumothorax especially if associated with continual bleeding.
  5. Continued haemodynamic instability.
  6. Suspicion of oesophageal, cardiac, great vessel, or major bronchial injuries.

NOTE: Think of possible damage to great vessels, hilar structures, and heart in penetrating anterior chest wounds medial to nipple line and posterior chest wounds medial to scapula.

Pulmonary contusion

- This refers to an injury resulting in the disruption of the pulmonary tissue architecture, disruption of alveolar membrane with bleeding, and extension of oedema into the alveolar spaces.
- It is usually associated with external blunt injury to the ribcage.
- Features of pulmonary contusion usually take time to develop.
- **Causes** include:
  1. Blunt and penetrating trauma.
  2. Blast injuries.
  3. Compressive injuries.
- The possible **clinical signs** are:
  1. Respiratory distress.
  2. Decreased breath sounds.
  3. Crepitations in the affected lung field.
  4. Hypoxaemia.
- **Management**
  1. Administer supplemental oxygen.
  2. Provide ventilatory support, if necessary.
  3. Provide judicious fluid therapy.
  4. Provide analgesia.

Tracheobronchial injuries

- Tracheobronchial injuries are difficult to pick up in a trauma patient. Diagnosis requires a high index of suspicion.
- The possible **aetiology**:
  1. Penetrating injuries to the neck or upper anterior torso.

2. Acceleration-deceleration force.

3. Blast injuries.

- **Clinical signs** include:

  1. Haemoptysis.

  2. Subcutaneous emphysema over the neck and chest.

  3. Tension pneumothorax.

  4. Persistent pneumothorax despite treatment.

- **Management**

  1. Administer supplemental oxygen.

  2. Provide ventilatory support.

  3. The patient may require >1 chest tube insertion.

  4. Early cardiothoracic consultation, bronchoscopic examination/thoracic computed tomography.

Blunt cardiac injury/myocardial contusion

- **Special considerations**:

  1. Clinically, there are few reliable signs and symptoms that are specific to blunt cardiac injury (BCI).

  2. The presence of a sternal fracture does not predict the presence of BCI.

  3. Neither creatine kinase-MB analysis nor bedside cardiac troponin T/I is useful in predicting which patients have or will have complications related to BCI.

  4. An abnormal ECG (ST and T wave changes) is sensitive for BCI.

- **Management**

  1. Triage the patient to the critical care area.

  2. Secure the ABCs and give oxygen if needed.

  3. Perform an ECG.

- **Management decisions**:

  1. If the **ECG is normal**, the risk of the patient having a BCI that requires treatment, i.e. a complication, is **insignificant**, and the patient may be **discharged** (assuming there is no **other** reason to admit).

  2. If the **ECG is abnormal** (**dysrhythmia, ST segment changes, ischaemic changes, atrioventricular block** or **unexplained sinus tachycardia**), the patient should be **admitted** for continuous cardiac monitoring.

  3. If the patient **is haemodynamically unstable**, an **echocardiogram** should be performed.

NOTE: Nuclear medicine studies add little when compared to Echo and are therefore not useful if an Echo has been performed.

Traumatic aortic disruption

- Most patients with traumatic aortic disruption die on site.
- Those who survive to reach hospital probably have a contained haematoma and will potentially deteriorate rapidly.
- **Telltale signs**:
  1. Blunt or penetrating injuries to the chest or acceleration/deceleration injury.
  2. Hypotension despite lack of external sources of bleeding.
  3. Massive haemothorax.
  4. Weaker or absent peripheral pulses especially on the left upper limb and both lower limbs.
  5. Principal **chest X-ray** features:
     a. Widened mediastinum.
     b. Left-sided pleural effusion.
     c. Blunting of left aortic knuckle.
     d. Depressed left bronchus.
     e. Pleural cap.
- **Management**
  1. Assess according to ATLS protocol.
  2. Perform a high resolution computed tomography (HRCT) scan of the thorax if the patient is fit enough for transport.
  3. GXM for ≥6 units of whole blood: Call Cardiothoracic and General Surgery stat.

Rib fractures

- Management is influenced by the level and number of ribs involved as well as underlying visceral injuries.

NOTE: Many clinically significant rib fractures cannot be visualized on chest X-rays (CXR). The main purpose of a CXR in patients with possible rib fractures is to eliminate associated haemothorax, pneumothorax, lung contusion, and other organ injury.

- **Upper rib (1–3) fractures and scapular fractures**:
  1. Application of a large force.
  2. Increased trauma risk to the head and neck, spinal cord, lungs, and great vessels.
  3. Mortality up to 35%.
- **Middle rib (4–9) fractures**:
  1. Most common: Significance increases if multiple. Simple rib fractures without complications can be managed on an outpatient basis.
  2. **Admit** for observation if the patient:
     a. Is dyspnoeic.

  b. Has unrelieved pain.

  c. Is elderly.

  d. Has poor pre-existing lung function.

- **Lower rib (10–12) fractures**: Associated with risks of hepatic and splenic injuries.

NOTE: Prophylactic chest tube insertion should be done for all trauma patients with multiple rib fractures who are going to be intubated. Associated injuries often missed include cardiac contusion, diaphragmatic rupture, and oesophageal injuries.

Traumatic diaphragmatic rupture

- **Indicators** of a possible diaphragmatic rupture:

  1. Persistent or progressive respiratory distress.

  2. Bowel sounds in the chest.

  3. **Chest X-ray** features:

     a. Vague and indistinct diaphragmatic shadow.

     b. Herniation of abdominal organs into the chest cavity.

     c. Displacement of a nasogastric (NG) tube into the chest cavity; the left side is more commonly affected.

- Diagnosis requires a high index of suspicion.

- All patients should be referred to General Surgery for laparotomy.

Crush injuries to the chest

- **Prognosis** depends on the duration of application of the crushing force:

  1. <5 minutes (transient force applied and prognosis is good).

  2. >5 minutes (poor prognosis).

- Crush injury to the chest produces **traumatic asphyxia**:

  1. Plethora of the upper body.

  2. Petechiae of the upper body.

  3. Cerebral oedema.

- **Management**

  1. Ensure adequate oxygenation.

  2. Provide ventilation.

  3. Treat associated injuries.

  4. Admit for observation.

Penetrating injury to the chest

- Important points to **note**:

  1. Do not remove foreign objects from the wound.

2. For penetrating injury below the nipple line, always consider intra-abdominal injuries.

3. Always secure implement with a firm doughnut-shaped roll made from bandages or towels.

Subcutaneous emphysema

- **Aetiology**:
  1. Airway injuries.
  2. Lung and pleural injuries.
  3. Oesophageal or pharnygeal injuries.
  4. Blast injuries.
- **Signs**:
  1. Crepitus.
  2. Swelling of the face, neck, or tissues involved.
- **Management**: Subcutaneous emphysema rarely requires treatment. The underlying cause should be managed instead. Assume patients with subcutaneous emphysema have an underlying pneumothorax that is not visible on chest X-rays. Hence, patients with subcutaneous emphysema after chest trauma should have a chest tube inserted before being placed on a ventilator.

Oesophageal trauma

- **Indicators** of a possible oesophageal trauma:
  1. Subcutaneous emphysema.
  2. Mediastinal air in the absence of a pneumothorax.
  3. Retropharyngeal air on a lateral neck X-ray.
  4. Left-sided pleural effusion: Drainage tested positive for amylase.
  5. Left pneumothorax or haemothorax without a rib facture.
  6. Severe blow to the lower sternum or epigastrium and the patient is in pain or shock which appears to be out of proportion to the apparent injury.
  7. Particulate water in the chest tube after the blood begins to clear.
- The patient should be referred to the general surgeon for further management.

Laryngeal trauma

- Although it is a rare injury, it can present with acute airway obstruction.
- **Diagnosis** is based on clinical triad of:
  1. Hoarseness.
  2. Subcutaneous emphysema.
  3. Palpable fracture.

- **Management**:
  1. If the patient's airway is totally obstructed or if the patient is in severe respiratory distress, attempt intubation.
  2. If intubation is unsuccessful, an emergency tracheostomy is indicated.
  3. Surgical cricothyroidotomy, although not preferred for this situation, may be life-saving if emergency tracheostomy fails.
  4. Contact an ear, nose and throat (ENT) specialist and anaesthetist early.

Indications for emergency department (ED) thoracotomy in trauma setting

- Witnessed traumatic cardiopulmonary arrest.
- Penetrating trauma with vital signs or signs of life (pupils respond to light, any spontaneous respirations, any movement to pain, or non-agonal cardiac rhythm) in the field or ED.
- Penetrating thoracic wounds even without signs of life in the field or ED (best with short duration of cardiopulmonary resuscitation (CPR)).
- Blood loss in the ED is not responsive to rapid crystalloid infusion.

ED thoracotomy not recommended

- Penetrating non-thoracic trauma without vital signs of life in the field.
- Blunt trauma without vital signs or signs of life in the ED.

References/Further Reading

1. Eastern Association for the Surgery of Trauma (EAST) Practice Parameter Workgroup for Screening of Blunt Cardiac Injury. www.east.org. 1998.

2. Thoracic Trauma. In: Committee on Trauma of the American College of Surgeons. *Advanced Trauma Life Support for Doctors (Student Course Manual)*. 9th ed. Chicago, IL: American College of Surgeons; 2004: 94–121.

3. Wilson RF, Steiger Z. Thoracic trauma: Chest wall and lung. In: Wilson RF, Walt AJ, eds. *Management of Trauma. Pitfalls and Practice*. 2nd ed. Baltimore, MD: Williams & Wilkins; 1996: 314: 42.

4. Wilson RF, Stephenson LW. Thoracic trauma: Heart. In: Wilson RF, Walt AJ, eds. *Management of Trauma. Pitfalls and Practice*. 2nd ed. Baltimore, MD: Williams & Wilkins; 1996: 343–360.

5. Hunt PA, Greaves I, Owens WA. Emergency thoracotomy in thoracic trauma – A review. *Injury*. 2006; 37: 1–19.

6. Wisbach GG, Sise MJ, Sack DI, et al. What is the role of chest x-ray in the initial assessment of stable trauma patients? *J Trauma*. 2007; 62: 74–79.

7. Velmahos GC, Karaiskakis M, Salim A, et al. Normal electrocardiography and serum troponin I levels preclude the presence of clinically significant blunt cardiac injury. *J Trauma*. 2003; 54: 45–51.

8. Weyant MJ, Fullerton DA. Blunt thoracic trauma. *Seminars in Thoracic and Cardiovascular Surgery*. 2008; 20: 26–30.

9. Bastos R, Baisden CE, Harker L, Calhoon JH. Penetrating thoracic trauma. *Seminars in Thoracic and Cardiovascular Surgery*. 2008; 20: 19–25.

Peng Li Lee • Shirley Ooi

CAVEATS

- The terms **head injury (HI)** and **traumatic brain injury (TBI)** should be used with the correct intent. They are often, but not necessarily always, related.

  1. Head injury refers to an injury that is clinically evident, e.g. scalp bruising, swelling, laceration, or skull deformity.

  2. TBI refers to an injury of the brain itself and is not always clinically evident; there is a risk of adverse outcome if it is unrecognized.

- Both HI and TBI frequently have additional injuries and patients must be managed according to Advanced Trauma Life Support (ATLS) principles, with emphasis on maintaining cervical spine immobilization until such injury is ruled out.

- The emergency physician's role is to prevent or limit the secondary brain injury following the primary insult which occurs at the point of trauma. Treatable conditions that either increase the metabolic demands of the brain or decrease the cerebral perfusion pressure must be anticipated and aggressively managed: watch for the five Hs (hypotension, hypoxia, hyercarbia, hypoglycaemia, and hyperthermia).

- **Do not** attribute **hypotension** in a trauma patient to solely head injury. Other sources of blood loss should be looked into.

- **Do not** assume that **altered mental state** in a head-injured patient is due to alcohol intoxication. It may be caused by hypoglycaemia, hypercarbia, hypotension, or other concomitant drug intoxication.

- One cannot rely on neurological assessments until adequate perfusion and oxygenation have been obtained.

- Proper observation of a head-injured patient means careful and repeated neurological examination, using **Glasgow Coma Scale (GCS)** as the standardized clinical scale to facilitate reliable inter-observer neurological assessments of head-injured patients.

- **Skull fractures** greatly increase the likelihood of an underlying brain injury (see Table 1).

TABLE 1 Risk of intracranial haematoma after head injury

		Risk of intracranial haematoma
Orientated	No skull fracture	1 in 6000
Disorientated	No skull fracture	1 in 120
Orientated	Skull fracture	1 in 30
Disorientated	Skull fracture	1 in 4

- A **lucid interval** should warrant special efforts to rule out an acute **extradural haematoma**.
- **Never sedate the restless head-injured patient** without ordering a head computed tomography (CT) scan because it may herald the development of an intracranial haematoma and should be investigated appropriately.

⇨ **SPECIAL TIPS FOR GPs**

- **Not all** patients with **mild head injury** or **scalp lacerations** need to have **skull X-rays** taken. Refer to the criteria given.
- There must be a reliable caregiver at home before any patient with head injury can be discharged. Remember to follow proper discharge instructions.

MANAGEMENT

Neuro-imaging decision in head trauma

- In the acute setting, there are only two imaging modalities to consider: Skull X-ray (SXR) and non-contrast head CT.
- For moderate and severe head injury and patients on anti-coagulants, the decision is clear – head CT is indicated.
- The variability and challenge lie in the group with mild head injury for which the following factors come into play when deciding on neuro-imaging choice:
  1. Physician's own judgement.
  2. Clinical decision rules or guidelines, e.g. Canadian CT Head Rule, New Orleans Criteria, and ATLS.
  3. Clinical policy or statement, e.g. within the institution (dependent on resource availability) or from a professional group, e.g. the American College of Emergency Physicians (ACEP).

Skull X-ray (SXR)

- The presence of a skull fracture, when seen on a SXR, increases the likelihood of an intracranial lesion. Refer to Table 1.
- Up to 50% of traumatic intracranial lesions do not have any associated skull fracture. This means that:
  1. The presence of a skull fracture raises the suspicion of traumatic intracranial lesion.
  2. The absence of a skull fracture does not rule it out (especially in the paediatric age group, likely due to a more pliable skull vault).
- **Indications of SXR**:
  1. Mild head injury with large boggy haematoma preventing accurate palpation of the underlying skull vault for depressed skull fracture, and where indication for a head CT scan is equivocal, e.g. clinically well and non-elderly patients.

NOTE: For moderate and severe head injury, a head CT scan must be considered.

2. A suspected radiopaque foreign body in scalp lacerations, e.g. broken glass.

NOTE: Simple scalp laceration is not a criterion for SXR. Careful clinical digital palpation of the scalp wound during toilet and suture (T&S) may be more sensitive than SXR for the detection of vault fracture.

- Conclusion: SXR is not recommended for the evaluation of mild TBI. Its sensitivity is not sufficient to be a useful screening test and negative findings on SXR may give a false sense of security, especially in the paediatric age group.

CT scan

- For patients with mild head injury, the variability lies in deciding which patients require a head CT scan.
- **Canadian CT Head Rule** and **New Orleans Criteria** are examples of clinical decision rules that have been validated for use in mild head injury, but clinicians using them must apply them within the limits of their inclusion criteria (refer to Table 2).
- In situations where the rules cannot be applied because patients do not fit into the inclusion criteria profile, the clinician can refer to the clinical policy and will have to make his own clinical judgement and must be able to justify his imaging decision.

TABLE 2   New Orleans Criteria vs Canadian CT Head Rule

New Orleans Criteria (NOC)	Canadian CT Head Rule (CCHR)
CT head indicated if:	*CT head indicated if:*
• Satisfy entry criteria: GCS 15 with loss of consciousness.	• Satisfy entry criteria: GCS 13–15 with loss of consciousness, amnesia, or confusion.
• And has 1 of the following:	• And has 1 of the following:
1. Symptoms of headache, vomiting, or persistent anterograde amnesia	(High risk for neurosurgical intervention)
2. Age >60 years	1. GCS <15, 2 hours after injury
3. Drug/alcohol intoxication	2. Age >65 years
4. Seizure	3. Vomiting >1 time
5. Visible trauma above clavicle	4. Base of skull fracture signs
	5. Suspected open or depressed skull
	(Medium risk for brain injury detection on head CT scan)
	6. Amnesia before impact of ≥30 minutes
	7. Dangerous mechanism of injury (pedestrian struck by vehicle, occupant ejected from vehicle, fall from a height of at least 3 feet/5 stairs)

Both rules have 100% sensitivity for predicting neurosurgical intervention but the sensitivity drops when predicting clinically important brain injury (98% for NOC versus 83% for CCHR). However, CCHR is more specific than NOC, i.e. use of CCHR would result in lower CT rates.

- Head CT scan is NOT indicated in mild head injury patients with GCS 15 (even in the presence of patients with loss of consciousness or post-traumatic amnesia) who are >60 years of age and who do NOT have:
  1. Headache/vomiting.
  2. Short-term memory loss.
  3. Drug/alcohol intoxication.
  4. Physical evidence of trauma above the clavicle.
  5. Focal neurological deficit.
  6. Coagulopathy.
  7. Seizure.
- Things to look for in **skull X-rays** (SXR):
  1. Linear or depressed skull fractures. The following radiological features may help to differentiate fractures from vascular markings on SXR. (see Table 3)

TABLE 3   How to differentiate fractures from vascular markings on SXR

Fractures	Vascular markings
More radiolucent (black)	Less radiolucent
Mostly straight but can change direction abruptly	Branching pattern
Sharply demarcated	Not sharply demarcated
Non-tapering	May taper; wide diploetic venous channels
May cross grooves and sutures	Do not cross grooves and sutures

  2. Mid-line position of calcified pineal gland (a displacement of >3 mm to one side suggests a large intracranial haematoma is present).
  3. Air-fluid levels in sinuses (including sphenoidal sinuses).
  4. Aerocoele.
  5. Facial fractures.
  6. Foreign bodies.
  7. Diastasis (widening) of sutures.

NOTE: A fluid level in a sphenoid sinus detected on a lateral SXR taken with a horizontal beam suggests a **basal skull fracture**. Recent studies have found no evidence for use of prophylactic antibiotics in basal skull fractures. This is because occult cerebrospinal fluid (CSF) leakage can continue over months and years and delayed meningitis can sometimes occur many years after the injury. Hence, there is no rational basis for an arbitrary one- or two-week course of antibiotics. Antibiotics should be given only if there is evidence of post-traumatic meningitis, usually due to *Streptococcus pneumoniae*. This is almost universally sensitive to benzyl penicillin.

Brain-specific serum biomarkers

- Among all the neuronal serum proteins that have been investigated to predict traumatic head CT scan abnormalities, **S-100B** is the best studied.
- The use of S-100B is currently not the standard of care, but it has been suggested that in mild TBI patients without significant extracranial injuries and a normal S-100B level (<0.1 mcg/L) measured within 4 hours of injury, consideration can be given to NOT performing a head CT scan (level C recommendation).
- Combining the use of S-100B with clinical variables into a clinical prediction rule can potentially help to reduce unnecessary head CT scans in mild TBI patients.

Resuscitation

The **priorities** in resuscitation are according to ATLS principles:

- Airway and cervical spine control.
- Breathing.

NOTE: Causes of **respiratory impairment** include the following: (1) Central causes such as drugs and brain stem injury and (2) peripheral causes such as airway obstruction, aspiration of blood/vomit, chest trauma, adult respiratory distress syndrome, and neurogenic pulmonary oedema.

- Circulation.
  1. Blood investigations include full blood count, urea/electrolytes/creatinine, coagulation profile and GXM ± with or without serum ethanol level.

NOTE: A blood alcohol level of <2 g/L makes it likely that altered consciousness is due to the head injury and not to alcohol consumption. However, a high alcohol level cannot be assumed to be the reason for altered consciousness in the head-injured patient.

  2. Do a bedside glucose level in all head-injured patients with an altered level of consciousness to exclude hypoglycaemia!
- Neurological assessment.
- **Indications for intubation in head injury**
  1. Coma (GCS <8).
  2. Rapidly deteriorating GCS ≥2.
  3. GCS ≤14 in the presence of a unilateral dilated pupil.

NOTE: Although a dilated or fixed pupil in an injured patient is usually due to an intracranial haematoma and/or brain damage, it may also be caused by expanding eye trauma, direct injury to the third cranial nerve, various drugs, intracranial aneurysms, hypoxia, hypotension, seizures and expanding intracranial aneurysms.

4. Clinical respiratory distress, a rate >30 breaths/min or <10 breaths/min, or an abnormal ventilatory pattern or in general, hypoxaemia not correctable by the administration of 100% oxygen by a non-rebreather mask.

5. Concomitant maxillofacial injuries.

6. Repeated convulsions.

7. Concurrent severe pulmonary oedema, cardiac, or upper abdominal injury.

Raised intracranial pressure and hernation syndromes

- Herniation is caused by raised intracranial pressure (ICP).
- Clinical manifestations include non-lateralizing signs, e.g. a decreased level of consciousness, loss of brain stem reflex, bilateral pinpoint pupils, decorticate posturing, irregular respirations, sudden death, as well as specific lateralizing neurological signs, i.e. dilatation of the pupil on the side of the lesion (due to compression of the parasympathetic fibres running with the third cranial nerve by the medial temporal lobe in uncal herniation) and hemiplegia. The side of weakness is less reliable in predicting the side of the intracranial lesion because either side of the cerebral peduncle and motor tracts can be compressed during the herniation.
- **General strategies to manage raised ICP** in the emergency department include these:
  1. Elevating the head 30 degrees to increase the outflow of cerebrospinal fluid from the skull base.
  2. Keeping the patient sedated and relaxed.
  3. Managing seizures.
  4. Maintaining cerebral perfusion by ensuring adequate volume resuscitation to a mean arterial pressure (MAP) of 80 mmHg.

NOTE: Cerebral perfusion pressure = MAP − ICP.

- Involve the neurosurgeon early in the management of the patient.
- **Hyperventilation**
  1. Used only as a temporizing measure to 'buy time' for definitive surgery in the presence of rapid neurological deterioration with raised ICP or signs of impending herniation. Examples:
     a. Cushing's reflex (hypertension with bradycardia).
     b. Comatose patient with initial normal reactive pupils but subsequently develops papillary dilatation with or without hemiparesis.
  2. Aim to achieve a **partial pressure of carbon dioxide (pCO_2) to approximately 35–40 mmHg** with intubation and hyperventilation.

NOTE: The desired effect of vasoconstriction caused by reducing carbon dioxide level also leads to cerebral ischaemia, hence, it is not recommended to be used as a prophylactic intervention in severe TBI.

3. Has an onset of action within 30–60 seconds and peaks in 8 minutes. Check arterial blood gases and titrate mechanical ventilation accordingly.

4. Brief periods of hyperventilation of 25–30 mmHg may be necessary for acute neurologic deterioration while other treatments are initiated.

- Use of mannitol

   1. **Dosage of mannitol**: 1g/kg of 20% mannitol (ml = Body weight in kg × 5) slow bolus over 15 minutes.

   2. Onset within 30–60 minutes and its effect lasts 6 to 8 hours.

   3. Acts as an osmotic agent to reduce brain oedema and ICP.

   4. **Precautions before the use of mannitol**:

      a. Insert a urinary catheter to monitor the urine output with the aim to achieve euvolaemia.

      b. Ensure the patient is not hypotensive.

      c. Ensure the patient does not have chronic renal failure.

Head injury instructions (verbal and written)

Before discharge, patients and caregivers should be advised to seek further medical advice in the event of:

- A worsening headache.
- Repeated vomiting.
- Abnormal behaviour or confusion.
- Fits.
- Fluid discharge from the nose or ears.
- Increased sleepiness or passing out.

The following images show 3 types of extra-axial traumatic intracranial haemorrhage.

FIGURE: 1   An extradural haemorrhage (on the left). Note the biconvex hyperdense lesion

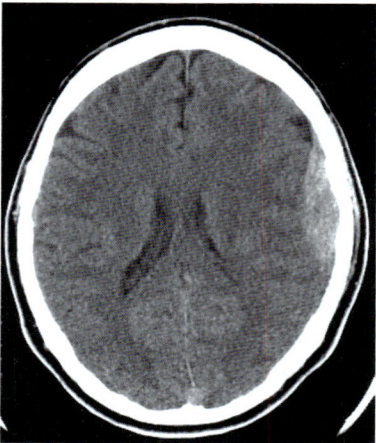

FIGURE 2 An acute-on-chronic subdural haemorrhage on the left side associated with a mid-line shift to the right and compression of the left lateral ventricle

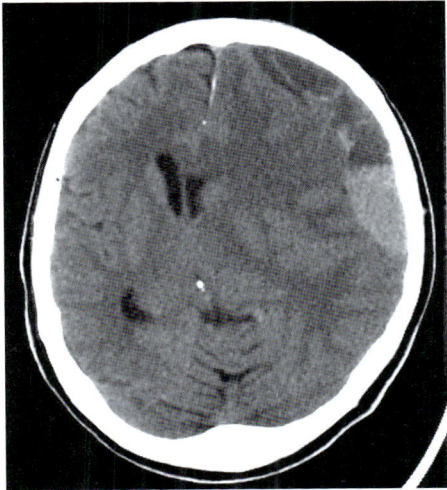

FIGURE 3 A traumatic subarachnoid haemorrhage (SAH). The blood is often seen over the cortical surfaces as opposed to non-traumatic SAH which occurs in the cisterns

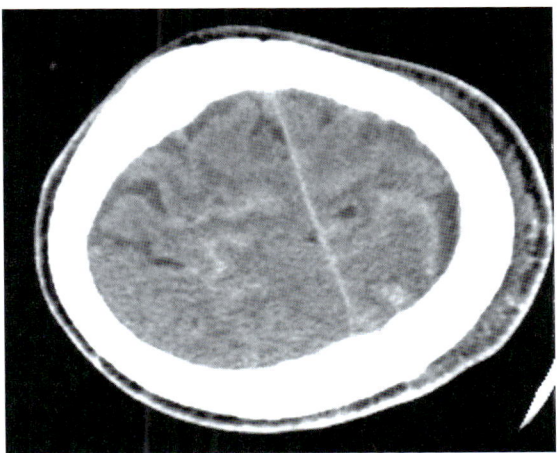

References/Further Reading

1. Jagoda AS, Bazarian JJ, Bruns JJ, et al. Clinical Policy: Neuroimaging and decisionmaking in adult mild traumatic brain injury in the acute setting. *Ann Emeg Med*. 2008; 52: 714–748.

2. Smits M, Dippel DW, de Haan GG, et al. External validation of the Canadian CT Head Rule and the New Orleans Criteria for CT scanning in patients with minor head injury. *JAMA*. Sep 2005; 294(12): 1519–1525.

3. Stiell IG, Clement CM, Rowe BH, et al. Comparison of the Canadian CT Head Rule and the New Orleans Criteria in patients with minor head injury. *JAMA*. Sep 2005; 28; 294(12): 1511–1518.

Amila Punyadasa • Peng Li Lee

'I love a hand that meets my own with a grasp that causes some sensation.'

Samuel Osgood (American politician)

CAVEATS

- The hand may be a small part of the body in terms of size but is vital to everyday functioning and hand injuries are common.
- >30% of industrial injuries involve the hand.
- Improper management of hand injuries in the acute setting can result in debilitating morbidity and time lost from work.
- Thus, the proper assessment and management of hand pathologies is essential.
- The key elements to proper management involve a focused history and detailed examination with a comprehensive knowledge of anatomy.
- Essential elements of a **hand injury/pathology history** include:
  1. Age.
  2. Hand dominance.
  3. Occupation.
  4. Special hobbies.
  5. Events pertaining to the injury/pathology (i.e. how, when, and where the injury occurred)
  6. Tetanus immunisation status, if indicated.
  7. Past history of hand injuries/pathologies.
- The basic components of a **hand examination** include:
  1. Skin and subcutaneous soft tissues.
  2. Vascular examination including Allen's test.
  3. Nerve examination (both motor and sensory).
  4. Evaluation of tendon function.
  5. Joint and ligament function and integrity.
  6. Skeletal examination.
- The key here is ***topographical anticipation*** (i.e. looking at a wound and considering what anatomical structures lie beneath) which requires a keen knowledge of anatomy.
- Do not blindly clamp bleeders. Direct pressure and elevation are keys to managing haemorrhage.
- Splinting of hand injuries is generally in the **position of function (POF)** or the **intrinsic plus position** – with the metacarpophalangeal (MCP) joint in 70 degrees of flexion, the proximal interphalangeal (PIP) joint in 20 degrees of flexion, and the distal interphalangeal (DIP) joint in 10 degrees of flexion.

⇨ **SPECIAL TIP FOR GPs**
- Preserve an amputated part by placing it in a clean piece of gauze soaked with moist saline and placing the wrapped part in a clean and dry container (e.g. a zip-lock bag). **Do not** place the amputated part directly on ice.

ACUTE NAIL BED INJURIES

- **Classifications**:
  1. Simple nail-bed lacerations and subungual haematoma.
  2. Crushing nail-bed larcerations.
  3. Avulsion laceration of the nail bed.
  4. Lacerations with associated fractures.
  5. Lacerations with loss of skin and pulp.
  6. Fingertip amputations.
- Nail-bed injuries generally do well after primary repair and less so with reconstruction, so the initial repair is vital. Hence, with the exception of (1), all other nail-bed injuries should be admitted for repair in the operating theatre where finer instruments and loupe magnification are available.
- **X-ray** is required for most fingertip and nail-bed injuries. The presence of a distal phalanx fracture adds two considerations to the management:
  1. Need for reduction: An unstable displaced fracture may require K-wire fixation.
  2. Risk of infection with open fracture: Cover with broad spectrum antibiotic.

SUBUNGUAL HAEMATOMA

- **Classification**: The percentage of area beneath the nail in which blood is visualised.
- **Treatment**: Trephination with a red-hot tip of an unfolded paper clip (Figure 1):
  1. A digital block is not required except for the most nervous patient. The nail plate (which is itself insensate) will burn and evaporate as the heated tip penetrates. The heated paper clip tip is cooled instantly upon encounter with the flush of blood and further penetration and injury to the nail bed is rare. Do not apply pressure but allow the heat to penetrate the nail plate and this avoids ramming the paper clip into the nail bed (risk of osteomyelitis).
  2. Prepare the injured finger with povidone-iodine (not alcohol as it is flammable).

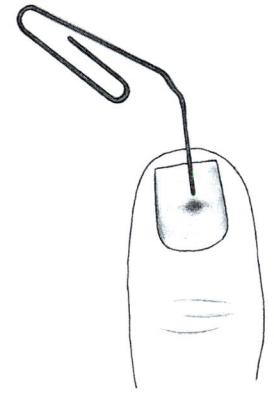

FIGURE 1 Trephining a subungual haematoma with the red-hot tip of an unfolded paper clip

3. Place 2 holes side by side to facilitate drainage. The haematoma is evacuated with gentle massaging followed by soaking in the povidone-iodine.

   a. **Follow up** with antibiotic ointment, dressing, and protective splint.

   b. For uncomplicated subungual haematomas of *any size*, without nail plate avulsion, the current hand literature supports simple trephining without the need for nail plate avulsion and nail bed repair.

LACERATION OF THE NAIL BED WITH NAIL PLATE AVULSION

- **Principles of treatment**: Minimal debridement, preservation of as much tissue as possible, and splinting with the nail plate.

  1. Perform a digital block with 1% lignocaine (allow at least 5 minutes for effect).

  2. Useful tip to attain a bloodless field: Cut off the small finger of a sterile glove and then cut a 1-mm hole at the distal tip. Place this sleave over the finger which needs repair and then roll the sleave down the finger so that it forms a band at its base (this serves to exsanguinate the finger and act as a tourniquet thus preventing the venous bleeding seen with the use of a sterile rubber band applied directly to the base of the finger in question).

  3. Cleanse and drape the finger tip.

  4. The nail plate should be gently elevated with blunt forceps and gently removed with a haemostat using continual pressure.

  5. Lacerations are repaired using a 6/0 plain catgut, dexon or vicryl suture.

  6. The nail plate is irrigated with normal saline and used as a splint over the repaired nail bed. A non-absorbable suture, e.g. Prolene, is placed through the nail plate and then through an area just proximal to the nail sulcus as an anchor (sutures to be removed in three weeks).

  7. If the nail plate is not available, the foil from the suture package may be used to keep the nail fold open.

- Advise patients: Nail plate growth takes 6–12 months and nail deformity may be unavoidable.

- Disposition: Refer to Hand Surgery for follow-up in 2 to 3 days.

FINGER TIP AMPUTATION

With skin/pulp loss only

- For a defect **<1 cm** in diameter, treat conservatively, with meticulous cleansing, and dressing with non-adherent gauze. Spontaneous epithelization is simple and cost effective.

- Refer to Hand Surgery for follow-up in 2 days.

- For a defect **>1 cm** in diameter, refer to a hand surgeon for skin-graft or free-flap reconstruction.

With bone involvement

- **A genuine hand emergency!**
- Inform the hand registrar-on-call immediately for possible replantation.
- *Never* make the decision yourself that the amputated part is not fit for replantation. This is best left to the senior hand surgeon-on-call.
- Give parenteral analgesia.
- Administer intravenous (IV) cefazolin 1 gm (or equivalent antibiotic); IM ATT 0.5 ml.
- X-ray the amputated part: Obtain two views of both the amputated and proximal portions.
- Employ digital photography to document both the proximal and amputated parts, if possible.
- Wrap the amputated portion in a saline-soaked gauze and then insert into a waterproof plastic bag which in turn is immersed in a container of ice water, after irrigation with normal saline to remove gross contamination.
- Apply a sterile, dry dressing to the proximal portion.
- Keep the patient nil by mouth (NBM) in preparation for imminent surgery.
- Perform full blood count, and urea/electrolytes/creatinine.
- Do an electrocardiogram (ECG) and chest X-ray (CXR) if the patient is more than 50 years old, or with upper or lower respiratory tract symptoms, or known cardiorespiratory comorbid factors.
- Admit to Hand Surgery for emergent surgery.

FLEXOR TENDON INJURIES

Flexor tendon injuries are frequently seen in the emergency department. The most common mechanism is laceration. The role of the emergency department physician is to make an accurate diagnosis through a thorough examination and this requires a revision and understanding of the function of the flexor tendons. Beware of subtle signs associated with partial laceration which can result in subsequent long-term disability.

Testing the integrity of flexor digitorum superficialis (FDS) and flexor digitorum profundus (FDP)

- Testing FDS function (Figure 2a). With the adjacent fingers held in full extension (prohibiting FDP motion), efforts at finger flexion produce isolated FDS motion, as indicated by solitary flexion of the PIP joint.
- Testing FDP function (Figure 2b). Isolated DIP flexion can only be accomplished with an intact FDP musculotendinous unit.

NOTE: Viewing an intact tendon through a lacerated sheath does not mean that the tendon is uninjured. The tendon may have been in a different position when the injury occurred and at the time of examination, the lacerated part of the tendon has moved proximally or distally and out of view. Test and document the integrity of the accompanying digital nerves (use the two-point discrimination test of an unfolded paper clip, approximately 5 mm apart at the finger tip and 10 mm at the base of the palm).

FIGURE 2   **Testing the integrity of (a) flexor digitorum superficialis and (b) flexor digitorum profundus functions**

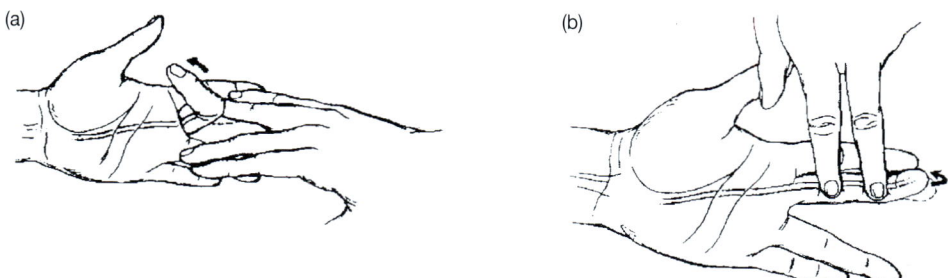

(a)   (b)

X-ray

X-ray the digit for the following reasons:

- To exclude foreign bodies in the lacerated wound.
- To exclude the avulsion of FDP insertion at the base of the distal phalanx in a closed rupture (lateral film).

Implications of zoning

- **Timing of repair**
  1. Primary repair (within 24 hours) is recommended. If this is delayed to 3 weeks, repair may require a tendon graft.
  2. Zones III, IV, and V (Figure 3) mandate urgent surgical repair because of frequent accompanying injuries to the adjacent structures.

FIGURE 3   **Classification of Verdan's flexor tendon zones**

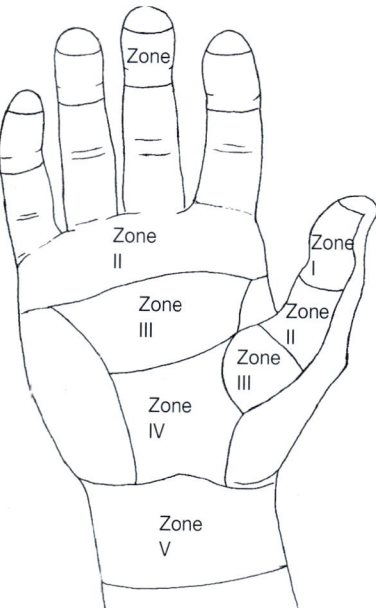

- **Outcome**
    1. Zone II: Sterling Bunnell termed this zone '**no-man's land**' because of the high incidence of poor results after attempted primary repair of a tendon laceration. The main complication is adhesion formation because of the volume contained within the tendon sheath (two FDS slips and the FDP).
    2. Zone III generally has a favourable outcome after the primary repair.

Management of flexor tendon injury at the emergency department

- Admit to Hand Surgery for primary repair.
- Administer analgesia, anti-tetanus toxoid (ATT), and prophylactic antibiotics as appropriate.

PARTIAL FLEXOR TENDON LACERATION

- **Diagnosis**: May be difficult and must be actively sought and excluded.
- **Clues**
    1. Direct visualization: If the sheath is lacerated assume the tendon is partially lacerated also (the wound should be explored with the finger in the same position as it was when the wounding occurred).
    2. Increased pain on active flexion against resistance.
- **Significance**
    1. Delayed rupture.
    2. Painful and restricting tenosynovitis.
    3. Poor healing with fibrosis and decreased function.
- All partial tendon lacerations will require exploration.
- An injury involving <25% of the cross-sectional are can be treated by trimming the lacerated ends. A laceration of ≥50% requires formal repair.
- **Management in the emergency department**: Admit for exploration by a hand surgeon.

EXTENSOR TENDON INJURY

Mallet finger

- Disruption of the insertion of the extensor tendon to the terminal phalanx.
- **Mechanism of injury**:
    1. Blunt trauma via acute flexion of the DIP joint by an axial load to the terminal phalanx, e.g. catching a ball.
    2. Laceration, which is less common.
- **Clinical presentation**:
    1. Pain, swelling, and tenderness of the DIP joint.
    2. Inability to extend the DIP joint (fixed flexion deformity at the DIP joint).
    3. Volar subluxation of the DIP joint.

- **X-ray digit**: Look for a fracture at the base of the distal phalanx (bony mallet injury).
- **Management** depends on the type of injury:
  1. Closed injury without a fracture: Mallet splint (Figure 4) for 6 weeks. Follow up with hand surgery in 5 days.
  2. Tendon avulsion with small bone fragment (<33%): mallet splint. Follow up with hand surgery in 5 days.
  3. Tendon avulsion with large bone fragment: Admit for surgical repair.
  4. Open injury: Admit for surgical repair.

FIGURE 4   A mallet finger splint

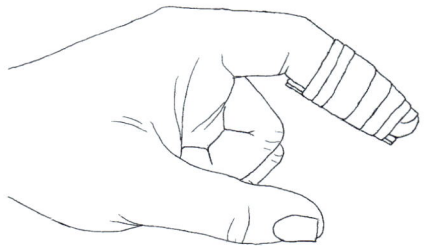

Mallet splint

- Apply a volar splint to the distal phalanx, keeping the DIP joint in slight hyperextension while allowing the PIP and MCP joints free movement.
- Mallet splint care (useful discharge advice):
  1. When removing the splint for bathing, keep the DIP joint extended by placing the finger on a flat surface, e.g. a table. Any flexion requires a further 6 weeks in the mallet splint.
  2. Gently wash, dry, and powder the finger.
  3. Then, reapply the mallet splint.

BOUTONNIERE DEFORMITY

- Disruption of the central slip of the extensor tendon over the PIP joint. The lateral bands, which normally lie dorsal to the axis of rotation and therefore extend the joint, now fall volar to this axis and become paradoxical flexors of the PIP joint and extensors of the DIP joint, thus, resulting in the characteristic deformity of the finger.
- **Mechanism of injury**:
  1. A direct blow to the dorsum of the PIP joint.
  2. Axial loading that forcefully flexes the PIP joint while the finger is held in extension.
  3. Laceration over, or distal to, the PIP joint.
- **Clinical presentation**:
  1. Pain and swelling of the PIP joint.

2. The patient may have full extension of the PIP joint initially (due to functioning of the lateral slips) though most patients with this injury demonstrate a mild weakness in the extension of the PIP joint, however full.

3. Boutonniere deformity is often not evident after acute injury but develops in 10–14 days.

4. Most have associated dislocations that have been reduced prior to arrival in the emergency department; demonstration of instability is limited by pain.

- **X-ray digit**: Typically normal but if the lateral view demonstrates an avulsion fracture at the dorsal aspect of the base of the middle phalanx, the diagnosis is confirmed.

- **Diagnosis**: Requires a high index of suspicion for any injury at the PIP joint. Diagnosis is often not apparent at once due to the acute swelling.

- **Management** depends on the type of injury:

    1. Closed injuries: Boutonniere splint. Follow up with hand surgery in 5 days.

    2. Open injuries: Admit for primary repair.

Boutonniere splint

- Apply a volar splint over the PIP joint, keeping it in full extension, and leaving the DIP and MCP joints free (Figure 5).

FIGURE 5   A boutonniere splint

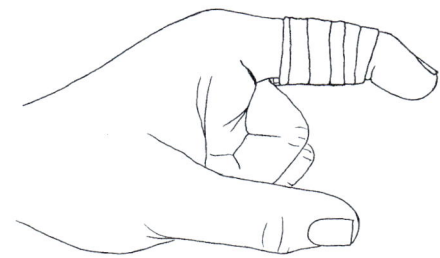

DISRUPTION TO EXTENSORS OVER THE MCP JOINT

- This is usually an open injury and thus the dreaded '**fight-bite**' must be assumed.

- The term **fight-bite** implies that the injury occurs when the patient punches an adversary in the teeth. This injury also goes by the names ***morsus humanus*** or ***closed fist injury***.

- All such wounds require formal exploration.

- It is important to **exclude** a human tooth bite/punch to the teeth (ask specifically as patients frequently deny this important part of the history).

- **Complications** of this type of injury include the following:

    1. High risk of wound infection. Frequently found pathogens include:

        a. *Eikenella corrodens*.

        b. Anaerobic *streptococci*.

      c. *Staphylococcus aureus.*

      d. *Neisseria* species.

  2. High risk of septic arthritis.

- Management principles involve the following:
  1. Aggressive wound debridement and antibiotics.
  2. Secondary closure considered versus primary closure.
- **Physical findings**: Extension of the MCP joint may still be present because of the sagittal bands at the side of the tendons.
- Take an **X-ray** of the MCP joint to look for the following:
  1. Foreign bodies, e.g. tooth fragment.
  2. Fracture of the metacarpal head or neck.
  3. If presentation is delayed, signs of advanced infection such as soft tissue emphysema and osteomyelitis.
- **Admit** for surgical debridement, wound exploration and repair.
- **Start** IV antibiotics and give tetanus prophylaxis as indicated and splint hand in position of function.

ISOLATED THERMAL BURNS OF HAND

Minor burns

- First- and second-degree (superficial and superficial partial thickness) burns.
- Administer tetanus prophylaxis.
- Provide analgesia.
- **Local therapy**:
  1. TG dressing with or without silver sulphadiazine cream (contraindicated in pregnancy and sulfa allergy).
  2. Hand dressed within a clean polythene bag to encourage mobilization.
  3. Elevate the hand in an arm-sling to reduce swelling.
- Refer to Hand Surgery for follow-up in a week.

Deep dermal burns

- Second- and third-degree (deep partial and full thickness) burns.
- Administer tetanus prophylaxis.
- Circumferential full thickness injury of the limb may induce compression injury distally: Important to check neurovascular status. Urgent escharotomy may be required.
- **Disposition**: Admit to Hand Surgery for wound care and possibly skin grafting.

NOTE: (1) Prophylactic systemic antibiotics are not routinely recommended, (2) partial thickness can be differentiated from full thickness injury by the loss of pin-prick sensations in the latter, and (3) consider non-accidental injury in the paediatric age group.

CHEMICAL BURNS OF THE HAND

- The depth of burns is directly related to the length of contact with the offending agent.
- **Document**: The chemical involved, length of exposure, and treatment initiated on-site, e.g. washing/antidote.
- **Management**:
  1. Chemical powders should be brushed off.
  2. Irrigate with copious amounts of saline/water.
  3. Elevate the hand.
- **Hydrofluoric acid burn: A hand emergency!** Refer to Chapter 113, *Burns, Minor* for further details.
  1. Very painful.
  2. Causes deep damage until fluoride ion is neutralized with calcium.
  3. For **superficial injury**, treat by **topical** application with **calcium gluconate** mixed with sterile KY gel.
  4. For **deeper or extensive injury**, consider **subcutaneous injection** of **10% calcium gluconate** into the base and around the burn using a 27G needle. Try to avoid performing a digital block as an analgesic manoeuvre since this, although will certainly remove the pain, will also eliminate the one parameter to determine the efficacy of therapy with calcium gluconate, i.e. pain.

ELECTRICAL BURNS OF THE HAND

- **Two elements** to consider:
  1. Flash burn, which causes deep dermal burn.
  2. Passage of current through the body. Possible complications are cardiac dysrhythmias and myoglobinuria with resultant acute renal failure.
- **History**: Differentiate low voltage domestic supply (240 V 50 Hz) from high voltage industrial supply.
- **Examination**:
  1. Search for the entrance and exit sites.
  2. May have thermal burns secondary to ignition of clothing.
  3. Assess the limb circulation and neurovascular status.
- **Management at the emergency department**:
  1. Perform a 12-lead ECG and cardiac monitoring for dysrhythmia.
  2. Check urea/electrolytes/creatinine, creatine kinase, and lactate dehydrogenase.
  3. Obtain an X-ray of the suspected joint dislocation from catatonic contractions of muscles secondary to high electrical voltage.
  4. Treat dermal burns as outlined above.

- **Disposition**: Admit to General Medicine for cardiac monitoring if dysrhythmia or cardiovascular collapse occurs.

HAND INFECTIONS

Paronychia

- Commonly a lateral nail fold infection with possible abscess formation.
- **Presents with** subungual tissue swelling and redness with or without frank pus.
- Screen for diabetes mellitus.
- **Treatment**:
  1. **Early** (without suppuration): Oral antibiotics, e.g. cloxacillin (activity against *Staphylococcus aureus*) and warm moist compresses daily plus elevation of the affected digit.
  2. **Late** (in the presence of suppuration): Oral antibiotics after incision and drainage of the abscess under a digital block.
  3. **Complicated**: Bilateral paronychia with subungual extension, demands removal of the proximal part of the nail plate.
- **Drainage methods** (refer to Figures 6 and 7):
  1. Slide the blade into the nail sulcus near the point of maximal tenderness.
  2. Remove a longitudinal section of nail if subungual absess is present.

FIGURE 6 **Drainage of a paronychia. The eponychial fold is elevated from the nail for a simple paronychium**

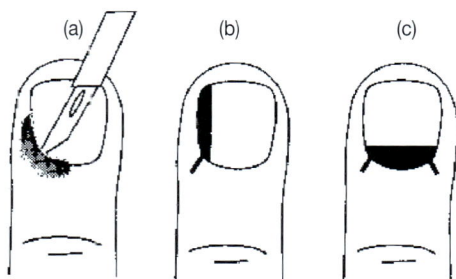

FIGURE 7 **Treatment of a proximal subungual abscess**

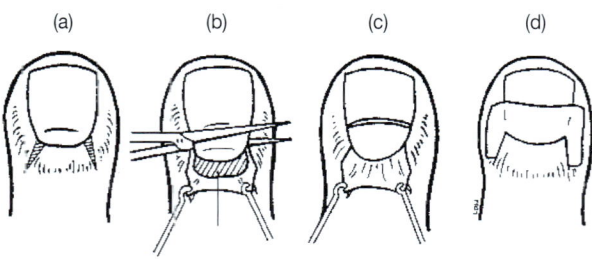

- **Disposition**: Refer to a general practitioner for follow-up if uncomplicated and to a hand surgeon in 2 days if complicated.
  a. Expose the edge of the proximal nail plate.
  b. Elevate and incise the proximal one-third of the plate and clean the nail bed.
  c. Leave the distal two-third to act as a physiological dressing. Care should be taken not to disrupt the nail matrix.
  d. Use a Bismuth impregnated gauze as a wick for approximately 48 hours.

Felon

- Infection of the distal pulp space of a digit.
- Presents with swelling, pain, and redness of the finger tip.
- **X-ray**: To exclude foreign bodies and bony involvement.
- **Treatment**: Incision and drainage under a digital block is best performed by a hand surgeon as it requires considerable expertise to do it correctly. So, refer to a hand surgeon in the emergency department.
- **Drainage methods**
  1. High lateral incision (avoid the neurovasuclar bundle): Begin 5 mm distal to the skin crease of the DIP joint and extend to the end of the nail plate.
  2. Longitudinal palmar incision; the choice of incision is based on finding the point of maximal tenderness.
  3. Fibrous septae in the finger pad should be sharply incised to provide adequate drainage of the closed space.
- **Antibiotic**: Cloxacillin (versus *Staphylococcus aureus*).
- **Disposition**:
  1. Admit to Hand Surgery for management in the presence of complications, e.g. osteitis **or** osteomyelitis of distal phalanx, pyogenic arthritis of the DIP joint, and pyogenic flexor tenosynovitis.

Suppurative flexor tenosynovitis

- Infection in the flexor tendon sheath that usually follows a penetrating injury.
- **Clinical features: Kanavel's** four cardinal signs:
  1. Fusiform swelling of the digit.
  2. Semiflexed resting position of the digit.
  3. Tenderness along the entire course of the sheath.
  4. Marked pain upon passive extension of the digit (most reliable).
- Early recognition and treatment is important to avoid tendon necrosis and proximal spread.

- **Pathophysiological progression**:
  1. Inoculation.
  2. Synovium cultures inoculums.
  3. Anatomically confined pyogenic process develops.
  4. Sheath pressure increases secondary to inflammatory process, oedema, and suppuration.
  5. Tendon ischaemia, necrosis, and rupture occur.
- **X-ray** the digit to exclude foreign bodies.
- **Disposition**:
  1. Emergent hand surgical consultation indicated.
  2. Give IV antibiotics in the emergency medical department.
  3. Elevate and splint in position of function.
  4. Admit to Hand Surgery for surgical drainage.

Acknowledgement

The authors are grateful to Dr Chong Chew Lan for drawing Figures 1, 3, 4, and 5.

References/Further Reading

1. Uehara DT, ed. The hand in emergency medicine. *Emerg Med Clin North Am.* 1993; 11(3): 758.
2. Della-Giustina DA, Coppola M, eds. Orthopaedic emergencies: Part I. *Emerg Med Clin North Am.* 1999; 17(14): 817.
3. Martin DS, Collins ED. *Manual of Acute Hand Injuries.* St Louis, MO: Mosby; 1998.
4. American Society for Surgery of the Hand. *The Hand: Primary Care of Common Problems.* New York: Churchill Livingstone; 1990.
5. Jebson Peter JL, Kasdan Morton L. *Hand Secrets.* 3rd ed. Philadelphia, PA: Mosby-Elsevier; 2006.
6. Brown RE. Acute nail bed injuries. *Hand Clin.* Nov 2002; 18(4): 561–575.
7. Bonisteel PS. Practice tips. Trephining subungual hematomas. *Can Fam Physician.* May 2008; 54(5): 693.
8. Roser SE, Gellman H. Comparison of nail bed repair versus nail trephination for subungual hematomas in children. *J Hand Surg* [Am]. Nov 1999; 24(6): 1166–1170.
9. Salter SA, Ciocon DH, Gowrishankar TR, Kimball AB. Controlled nail trephination for subungual hematoma. *Am J Emerg Med.* Nov 2006; 24(7): 875–877.

Shirley Ooi

CAVEATS

- Orthopaedic injuries may look serious, but they should not distract one from doing the Primary Survey first. They are therefore included in the Secondary Survey in a multiple trauma patient.
- Most **dislocations** are **usually not serious** and only require adequate pain relief as the immediate treatment **except** for the following **three**, which have particularly serious implications and should be reduced as soon as possible:
  1. Knee dislocations (because of popliteal artery compromise).
  2. Ankle dislocations (because of skin necrosis).
  3. Hip dislocations (because of avascular necrosis of the hip).
- For all **joint dislocations** that require manipulation and reduction at the emergency department, **do not** give **intramuscular (IM) opioids. Give intravenous (IV) opioids** instead. This is because opioids given by the IM route are erratic in their absorption. Hence, when procedural sedation is needed, one is unsure of the dosage to top up for pain relief. This may result in respiratory suppression and hypotension when the full IM dose of opioid is absorbed into the circulation.

⇨ **SPECIAL TIP FOR GPs**
- Ankle X-rays are not needed for every case of ankle injury. See the section on *Indications for ordering X-rays in ankle injury*.

HIP DISLOCATION

- **Mechanism of injury**
  1. Dashboard injury.

  NOTE: This often results in simultaneous fracture of the patella, fracture of the femoral shaft, and **posterior hip dislocation**.

  2. Falls on the foot cause **posterior hip dislocation** if the leg is flexed at the hip and adducted, **anterior dislocation** if the hip is widely abducted and **central dislocation** if the femur is in some other part of the abduction or adduction range.
  3. A weight falling on a person with legs wide apart, knees straight, and back bent forward causes **anterior hip dislocation**.
  4. Doing a 'split' causes **anterior hip dislocation**.
  5. Blow or fall on the side causes **central hip dislocation**.

- **Clinical features**
  1. **Posterior hip dislocation**: Hip held slightly flexed, adducted and internally rotated, leg appears shortened, femoral head palpable in buttock.
  2. **Anterior hip dislocation**: Hip held slightly flexed, abducted, and externally rotated. The anterior bulge of the dislocated head is seen from the side.
  3. **Central hip dislocation**: Leg in normal position, tender trochanter and hip, and some movement is possible.
- **X-ray**: Obtain an anteroposterior (AP) view of the pelvis and lateral view of the hip involved.
- **Complications**
  1. Foot drop from sciatic nerve involvement in **posterior hip dislocation**.
  2. Femoral nerve paralysis, femoral vein compression (with risks of thrombosis and embolism), and femoral artery compression in **anterior hip dislocation**.
  3. **Avascular necrosis of the femoral head (the longer the hip is dislocated, the higher the risk)**.
- **Treatment/disposition**
  1. Give pain relief in the form of IV and not IM narcotics **before** X-rays.
  2. Reduction should be performed as soon as possible under conscious sedation in the emergency department.
  3. Check X-ray after reduction and admit to Orthopaedics for further management.
  4. If unable to reduce, admit for reduction under general anaesthesia.

FIGURE 1   Views of the hip and pelvis

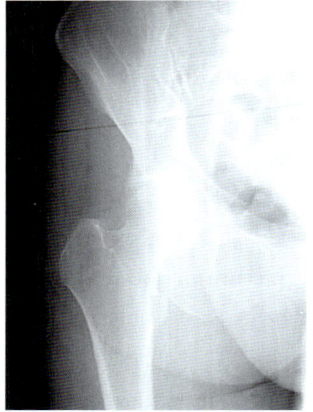
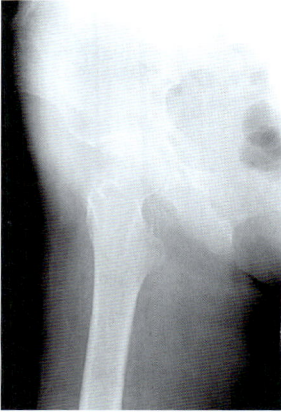
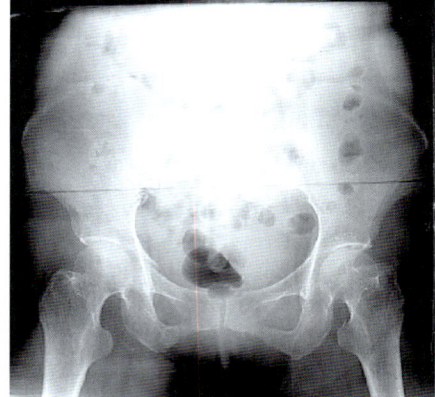

a: AP view   b: Lateral view   c: AP view of pelvis

Note: A 60-year-old lady tripped and fell and complained of pain over her right hip with limited range of movement. Figures 1a and b are the AP and lateral views of the right hip. With difficulty, a fracture of the right superior public ramus is seen. On repeating an AP pelvic x-ray (Figure 1c), besides the right superior pelvic ramus which is now shown very clearly, an impacted right inferior public ramus fracture is seen as well.

FRACTURE OF FEMORAL NECK AND TROCHANTERIC FRACTURES

- **Mechanism of injury**: Usually from falls in the elderly. (It is also important to assess the underlying cause of the fall.)
- **Clinical features**
  1. Inability to bear weight after a fall, especially in an elderly patient with or without pain in the hip. (With a non-displaced fracture, the patient may be able to bear weight with a limp.)
  2. External rotation and shortening of the lower limbs.
  3. Tenderness over the fracture site in the groin.
  4. Pain on attempted movement of the hip.
  5. Bruising is a late sign of extracapsular fractures and is absent in acute injuries.
- **X-ray**
  1. AP view of the pelvis and lateral view of the involved hip.
  2. Remember to do a chest X-ray for an elderly patient before admission.

  NOTE: It is important to bear in mind that for **all hip pains**, an **AP view of the pelvis** and the lateral view of the hip involved (Figures 1a, 1b, and 1c) should be done rather than AP and lateral views of the hip for these two reasons:

  3. Pubic rami fracture may also present with 'hip pain'. This may be missed if an AP hip instead of AP pelvis X-ray is done.
  4. An AP view of the pelvis allows comparison of Shenton's lines on both sides and helps in picking up subtle abnormalities.
- **Complications**: Femoral neck fractures are associated with avascular necrosis of the femoral head.
- **Treatment/disposition**: Give analgesia before X-rays. Admit to Orthopaedics for further management.

FRACTURE OF FEMORAL SHAFT

- **Mechanism of injury: Considerable violence** is usually required to fracture the femur except in pathological fractures. Usually seen in road traffic accidents (RTAs), falls from height, or crushing injuries.
- **Clinical features**: Weight bearing is impossible.
  1. Abnormal mobility in the limb at the level of fracture.
  2. The leg is externally rotated, abducted at the hip, and shortened.
- **X-ray**: AP and lateral views of the femoral shaft (including hip and knee joints).
- **Complication**:
  1. Haemorrhagic shock.
  2. Fat embolism syndrome.

- **Treatment/disposition**
  1. IV drip with GXM because even in a simple fracture, loss of 1/2–1 L of blood into the tissues with accompanying shock is common.
  2. Give pain relief, e.g. femoral nerve block and/or IV narcotics.
  3. Immobilise the fractured limb in a traction splint and check the distal pulses.
  4. Admit to Orthopaedics for further management.

PATELLAR FRACTURE

- **Mechanism**
  1. By direct violence, e.g. RTAs with dashboard injury, falls against a hard surface and heavy objects falling across the knee.
  2. By indirect violence as a result of a sudden contraction of the quadriceps muscle.
- **Clinical features**
  1. Inability to extend the knee.
  2. Bruising and abrasion over the knee.
  3. Presence of tenderness.
  4. A palpable gap above or beneath the patella.
  5. An obvious proximal displacement of the patella.
- **X-ray:** AP and lateral views of the knee.
- **Treatment/disposition**
  1. Give analgesia **before** X-rays.
  2. If vertical or undisplaced fractures: Apply a cylinder backslab and discharge with analgesia, crutches and Trauma Clinic referral.
  3. Where fractures are displaced >3 mm: Apply a cylinder backslab and admit for fixation.

PATELLAR DISLOCATION

- **Mechanism**
  1. Typical history: While running, the knee gets stuck and the patient falls down. The patient often notices a prominent medial bulge from the medial femoral condyle (although patella usually dislocates laterally).
  2. The dislocated patella may spontaneously reduce.
- **Clinical features**
  1. Painful knee held in flexion with a lateral displacement of the patella.

2. In cases of spontaneous reduction before assessment, there is typically tenderness at the medial aspect of the knee and possibly a mild knee effusion.

- **X-ray**: AP, lateral, and skyline views. The skyline view is to exclude associated fractures of the lateral femoral condyle.
- **Treatment/disposition**
  1. Give analgesia and reduce dislocation.
  2. If this is the first dislocation, apply a cylinder backslab and discharge with analgesia, crutches and Trauma Clinic referral.
  3. If this is a recurrent dislocation, apply pressure bandage for 1 to 2 weeks.

KNEE DISLOCATION

This is an EMERGENCY!

- **Mechanism of injury**: Usually from RTAs, especially from dashboard injury.
- **Clinical features**: Swelling, gross deformity, often with marked posterior sag.
- **X-ray**: AP and lateral views of the knee.
- **Complications**
  1. Popliteal artery injury: Look for a pale, cold, pulseless lower limb, or paresthesia of the lower limb.
  2. Common peroneal nerve palsy.
- **Treatment**
  1. Give IV analgesics.
  2. Reduce dislocation immediately, especially if there is a delay in obtaining X-rays.
  3. Apply a cylinder backslab.
  4. Call the vascular surgeon and orthopaedic surgeon and arrange for an angiogram.
- **Disposition**: Admit all patients.

KNEE HAEMARTHROSIS/EFFUSION

- **Mechanism of injury**: Usually from trauma to the knee. **Immediate haemarthrosis** is due to:
  1. Torn cruciate ligaments.
  2. Osteochondral fracture.
  3. Peripheral meniscal tear.

Delayed effusion is due to degenerative meniscal tears, inflammatory arthritis, and acute exacerbation of osteoarthritis.

FIGURE 2   **Lateral x-ray of the knee joint**

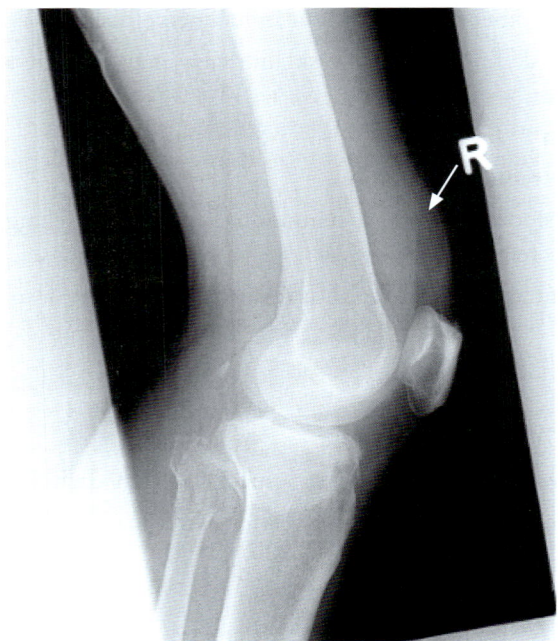

Note: Lateral x-ray of the knee joint shows fractures of tibial plateau, proximal tibia, and head of fibula. Note the fat-fluid level indicated by arrow showing lipohaemarthrosis.

- **Clinical features**: Gross swelling from haemarthrosis or effusion.
- **X-ray**:
  1. AP and lateral views of the knee. Note the fat–fluid level in the suprapatellar bursa indicates an intra-articular fracture even if a fracture is not seen (Figure 2).
  2. The skyline view is useful in subtle fractures of femoral condyles (especially in lateral dislocation of the patella) and patella.
- **Complications**: Beware that the patient is not having a knee dislocation or concomitant knee fracture.
- **Treatment**:
  1. If the knee haemarthrosis is not tense, the patient can be discharged with the **r**est, **i**ce, **c**ompression (apply crepe bandage), and **e**levation (RICE) treatment.
  2. Give analgesics.
- **Disposition**
  1. Refer to the orthopaedic clinic within 24–48 hours.
  2. In the situation of a tense haemarthrosis, the patient should be admitted for aspiration.

FRACTURE OF THE TIBIAL PLATEAU

- **Mechanism of injury**: Usually results from severe valgus stress.
- **Clinical features**:
  1. Haemarthrosis.
  2. Lateral bruising.
  3. Abrasions.
  4. Valgus deformity of the knee.
- **X-ray views**: AP and lateral views of the knee.
- **Complications**: Note that subtle tibial table fractures may be missed. If the patient continues to bear weight on it, the fracture will worsen.
- **Treatment**: Give analgesia and apply a cylinder backslab.
- **Disposition**: Admit to Orthopaedics for further management.

FRACTURE OF THE TIBIA/FIBULA

- **Mechanism of injury**: The tibia is vulnerable to a number of forces:
  1. Torsional stresses (e.g. sporting injuries).
  2. Violence transmitted through the feet (e.g. falls from height, RTAs).
     a. Direct blows (e.g. RTAs, blows from falling objects). Isolated fractures of the tibia or fibula may occur from direct violence although they are relatively uncommon.
     b. Indirect violence leads to fracture of both the tibia and fibula.
- **Clinical features**:
  1. Pain.
  2. Swelling.
  3. Deformity.
  4. Tenderness.
  5. Fracture crepitus over the shin.
  6. Very often it is an open fracture because one-third of the tibia is subcutaneous.
- **X-ray**: AP and lateral views of the tibia/fibula (must include knee and ankle joints).
- **Complications**:
  1. Early: Compartment syndrome in closed fractures, popliteal artery injury, and common peroneal nerve injury.
  2. Late: Infection in open fractures.

- **Treatment/disposition**:
  1. **Close undisplaced fracture of the tibia and fibula**:
     a. Give IM/IV analgesia before X-rays.
     b. Apply an above knee backslab.
     c. Repeat X-rays to check the final position of the fracture.
     d. Admit the patient for observation.
  2. **Close displaced fracture of the tibia and fibula**:
     a. Give IV narcotics before X-rays.
     b. Under procedural sedation with IV midazolam and narcotics, try to reduce the fracture (particularly in cases of impaired vascularity).
     c. Apply an above knee backslab.
     d. Repeat X-rays before admission.
     e Admit to Orthopaedics for further management.
  3. **Open fracture of the tibia and fibula**:
     a. Give IM/IV analgesics.
     b. Cover the wound with sterile dressing.
     c. Check the patient's tetanus immunization status.
     d. Give antibiotics (cefazolin).
     e. Apply a long leg backslab or temporary splint.
     f. Admit to Orthopaedics for further management.
  4. **Isolated closed fracture of the fibula**:
     a. Give IM analgesics.
     b. Exclude fracture of the tibia and injury to the ankle joint.
     c. Use crepe bandage to provide gentle support.
     d. Discharge the patient with oral analgesics.
     e. Refer the patient to the trauma clinic.

  NOTE: The patient can be allowed to bear weight.

ANKLE INJURY

- **Mechanism of injury**: When the ankle is very deformed, suspect ankle dislocation. This is an EMERGENCY!

NOTE: The dislocated ankle must be reduced immediately to prevent skin necrosis.

- **Clinical features**: In every suspected ankle injury, palpate 4 bony points:
  1. Medial malleolus.
  2. Lateral malleolus.

3. Whole length of the fibula.

4. Base of the fifth metatarsal.

- **X-ray**: X-rays are unnecessary for every case of sprained ankle.

  Indications for ordering X-rays in ankle injury:

  1. Age >55 years old.*

  2. Inability to bear weight both immediately *and* in the emergency department.*

  3. Bone tenderness at the posterior edge (distal 6 cm) or tip of the lateral malleolus.*

  4. Bone tenderness at the posterior edge (distal 6 cm) or tip of the medial malleolus.*

  5. In cases where there is sufficient swelling to hinder accurate palpation.

  6. In cases where there is clinical instability.

  7. For *social reasons*, e.g. an athlete.

  NOTE: The points indicated by * are known as the **Ottawa Ankle Rules**.

  X-ray views to order are:

  1. AP and lateral views of the ankle for suspected ankle fracture.

  2. Whole fibula if there is tenderness over the fibula higher up to exclude **Maissoneuve fracture**.

  3. PA and lateral views of the foot if there is tenderness over the base of the fifth metatarsal.

- **Complications**: Skin necrosis in delayed reduction of the dislocated ankle.

- **Treatment**:

  1. **Sprained ankle**:

     a. Give analgesics at the emergency department.

     b. Discharge with the RICE treatment and analgesics.

     c. Refer to a physiotherapist for ankle strapping in a severe sprain.

  2. **Ankle fracture**:

     a. Apply a below knee backslab.

     b. Admit for internal fixation except for isolated stable fractures of the lateral malleolus below the ankle mortise where it can be treated conservatively.

  3. **Ankle dislocation**:

     a. Set up a heparin plug and give IV narcotics before X-rays.

  NOTE: The dislocated ankle must be reduced as soon as possible under procedural sedation with IV midazolam and narcotics, or inhalation of entonox (nitrous oxide/oxygen) to prevent **skin necrosis**. Hence, if there is a delay in obtaining X-rays for >10–15 minutes or if there is already signs of circulatory compromise, the ankle should be relocated even before the X-rays are done.

    b. Check distal pulses before and after reduction.

    c. Apply a short leg backslab after reduction, ensuring that the ankle region is well-padded.

    d. Do post-reduction X-rays.

    e. Admit to Orthopaedics for further management.

FRACTURE OF THE CALCANEUM

- **Mechanism of injury**: Fall from a height on to the heels.

NOTE: Remember to exclude bilateral calcaneal fractures and wedge fracture of the spine.

- **Clinical features**
  1. Heel when viewed from behind may appear wider, shorter, flatter, or tilted laterally into valgus.
  2. Tense swelling of the heel.
  3. Marked local tenderness.
  4. If the patient presents later, there will be bruising which may spread to the medial side of the sole and proximally to the calf.
- **X-ray**: Lateral and axial views of the calcaneum.
- **Treatment/disposition**:
  1. If undisplaced:
     a. Apply firm bandaging over wool.
     b. Discharge with crutches, analgesics, and advice to elevate the limb at home.
     c. Refer to the trauma clinic.
  2. If bilateral fractures of the calcaneum: Admit to Orthopaedics for further management.
  3. If the calcaneum is displaced or intra-articular/crushed:
     a. Apply a well-padded bandage.
     b. Admit to Orthopaedics for further management.

FOOT INJURY

NOTE: Common ones include the following:

- Calcaneal fracture (as mentioned above).
- Tarso-metatarsal dislocations.
- Metatarsal fractures.
- Phalangeal fractures/dislocations.

Tarso-metatarsal (Lisfranc's) dislocations

- **Mechanism of injury**:
  1. Fall on the plantar flexed foot.
  2. Blow to the forefoot as in RTAs.
  3. Blows on the heel when in the kneeling position.
  4. Run-over kerb-side accidents.
  5. Forced inversion, eversion, or abduction of the forefoot.

FIGURE 3 **Views of right foot dislocation**

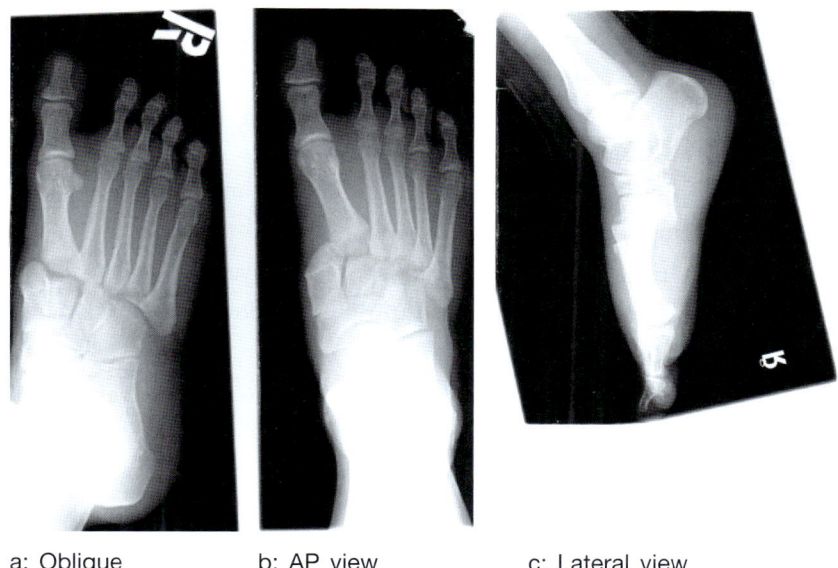

a: Oblique   b: AP view   c: Lateral view

Note: Oblique (Figure 3a) and AP (Figure 3b) x-ray views of the right foot show dislocation of the tarso-metatarsal joints with lateral displacements of all 5 metatarsals (Lisfranc's dislocations). This is further seen on the lateral view of the right foot (Figure 3c).

- **Clinical features**: Swelling and 'drifting' of the foot.
- **X-ray**: AP and oblique views of the foot (Figure 3).

NOTE: Lisfranc's dislocation is not always readily evident on radiographs and remains the most common misdiagnosed foot fracture.

- **Complications**:
  1. **Vascular injury**: Dorsalis pedis artery or medial plantar anastomosis may be in jeopardy.
  2. **Compartment syndrome**.

- **Treatment**:
  1. Give analgesics before X-rays.
  2. Apply a backslab.
  3. Admit for surgical management.

Fracture of metatarsals

- **Mechanisms**: Often due to crushing injuries.
- **X-ray**: AP and oblique views of the foot.
- **Principles of management**:
  1. **If the fracture is undisplaced without soft tissue damage**:
     a. Give analgesics before X-rays.
     b Treat symptomatically with crepe bandage or a short below knee backslab extending distally to beyond the toes.
     c. Discharge with non-weight bearing crutches (NWB) and analgesics.
     d. Refer to the orthopaedic clinic.
  2. **If fractures are multiple and undisplaced**, treat conservatively as above.
  3. **If fractures are multiple and displaced**: Apply a below knee backslab and admit to Orthopaedics for further management.

Phalangeal fracture/dislocation

- **X-ray**: AP and oblique views of the foot.
- **Principles of management**:
  1. Attend to soft tissue injuries and nail bed injuries first.
  2. Reduce dislocations using digital blocks or entonox.
  3. Immobilize fractures and dislocations using adhesive strapping to the adjacent toe.
  4. Discharge with analgesics and refer to the orthopaedic clinic.
  5. For multiple toe dislocations, admit for reduction.

Reference/Further Reading

1. McRae R. *Practical Fracture Treatment*. 5th ed. Edinburgh, UK: Churchill Livingstone; 2008.

98   Trauma, Maxillofacial

Peter Manning • Shirley Ooi

CAVEATS

- Beware the distraction of a grotesque facial injury: Principal complications are airway obstruction, haemorrhage, cervical spine, and ocular injuries.
- Since many of the injuries are due to blunt trauma, a full secondary survey examination is mandatory to exclude multisystem injury (occurs in 60% of cases of severe facial trauma).
- **Do not force** a patient with a mandibular fracture to lie supine since it may compromise the airway; permit the patient to sit up if he so feels the need.
- The absence of significant blood loss externally does not preclude internal bleeding sufficient to cause hypovolaemic shock since a supine patient may swallow the blood. Only later, upon vomiting, is the degree of blood loss evident.
- Perform a systematic examination of the face, paying particular attention to the eyes, and status of the bite.
- Given that the bones of young children are softer than that of adults, more force is needed to fracture the paediatric face with a higher incidence of associated intracranial injuries.
- The location of a facial fracture can often be inferred from a specific sensory deficit, e.g. numbness of the lip or chin suggests a fracture of the mandible, whereas numbness of the upper lip or gum suggests a maxillary fracture or an orbital floor fracture.

> ⇨ **SPECIAL TIPS FOR GPs**
> - **Do not force** a patient with a suspected mandibular fracture to lie supine since this may compromise the airway.
> - When evaluating a patient with a suspected nasal bone fracture, look particularly for a **septal haematoma**. This is a **true ear, nose and throat (ENT) emergency** requiring incision and drainage promptly.
> - Young children have an increased incidence of frontal bone injury to its prominence, whereas mid-face injuries are extremely uncommon. Always suspect non-accidental injury if a child presents with a torn frenulum, lip trauma, and mid-face bruising.
> - The **only dental** fracture that is a **true emergency** is the **Ellis Class III fracture**, identified by bleeding from the pulp.

MANAGEMENT

Broadly speaking, patients with maxillofacial injury can be divided into 2 groups:

- Those with isolated maxillofacial injury secondary to a relatively small force, e.g. punch or kick, can be managed in an intermediate or low acuity care area of the department.

NOTE: Beware ending evaluation when one obvious fracture has been identified. Evidence shows that up to 30% of patients with facial injuries have ≥2 fractures or injuries.

- Those with severe maxillofacial injury secondary to a significant blunt trauma, e.g. rapid deceleration from a road traffic accident or a fall from a height, must be managed in the critical care area of the department.

   1. Severe maxillofacial injuries must be managed in the critical care area following the tenets of Advanced Trauma Life Support (ATLS).

   2. Establish and **maintain a patent airway** with cervical spine immobilization.

      a. Sit the patient up if no spinal injury is suspected **or** if the patient feels the need to do so

      b. Perform the jaw thrust–chin lift manoeuvre.

      c. Perform the tongue traction manoeuvre by using (1) fingers, (2) 'O' silk suture, and (3) towel clip.

      d. Perform an endotracheal intubation: Awake oral intubation versus rapid sequence intubation versus cricothyroidotomy (refer to Chapter 28, *Airway Management/Rapid Sequence Intubation* for further details).

   3. Administer supplemental oxygen by a non-rebreather reservoir mask.

   4. Monitoring: Vital signs q 5 to 10 minutes, electrocardiogram (ECG), and pulse oximetry.

   5. Establish one or two peripheral large bore intravenous (IV) lines for volume replacement.

   6. Labs: GXM, full blood count, urea/electrolytes/creatinine, and coagulation profile.

   7. Facilitate the cessation of ongoing haemorrhage:

      a. Control by direct pressure.

         i. Pinching the nose.

         ii. Nasal or throat packing.

         iii. Tamponade with a Foley catheter.

      b. Use haemostatic agent tranexamic acid (Cyclokapron®).

      Dosage: 25 mg/kg body weight IV slow bolus over 5 to 10 minutes.

   8. **X-rays**: The timing of facial X-rays is **not** a priority in multiple injuries.

      See below 5 radiographic views are:

      a. Occipitomental or OM (Water's) view

      b. Posteroanterior or PA (Caldwell's) view

      c. Lateral view

      d. Submentoverical (SMV) or 'jughandle' view

      e. Towne's view

NOTE: The first 3 views above used to be the standard facial views. However, Goh, et al. (2002) showed that a **single 30-degree OM view** would be **sufficient to screen for maxillofacial trauma**. Hence, if facial fractures are suspected, a single 30-degree OM view should be ordered only and not facial views.

OM (Water's) view

See Figure 1: Good for the mid-face, showing orbital rims and floors; blood in maxillary sinus.

PA (Caldwell's) view

See Figure 2: Display the frontal bone and paranasal sinuses. Can sometimes show up the zygomaticofrontal suture diastasis in a tripod fracture better than an OM view.

Lateral view (cross-table or upright)

See Figure 3: Facilitates layering of blood in sinuses.

Submentovertical (or 'jughandle') view

See Figure 4: Displays the zygomatic arch.

Towne's view

See Figure 5: Display the mandibular rami and condyles.

FIGURE 1

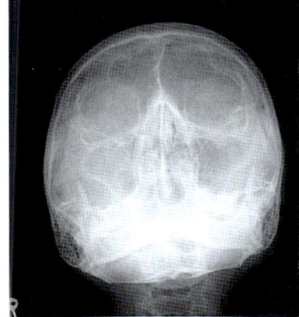

OM (Water's) view

FIGURE 2

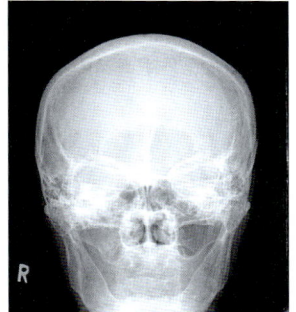

PA (Caldwell's) view

FIGURE 3

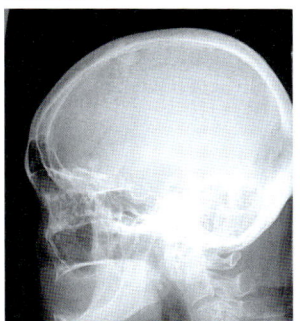

Lateral view

FIGURE 4

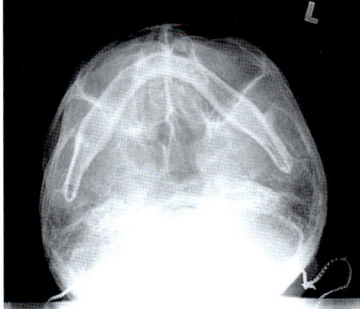

SMV ('jughandle' view)

FIGURE 5

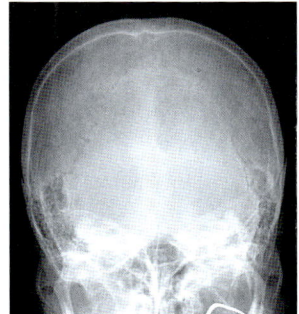

Towne's view

Systematic review of the OM view using McGrigor's lines

See Figure 6: Trace the three lines on the OM view.

- As the lines are drawn, compare the injured with the uninjured side.

- The soft tissue above and below these three lines should also be examined.

- **Line 1** (Figure 7): Start outside the face, tracing through the suture between the frontal and zygomatic bones at the lateral margin of the orbit across the forehead, assessing the superior orbital margin and the frontal sinus to the other side. Compare the injured and uninjured sides. Look for the following:
  1. Fractures
  2. Widening of the zygomatic suture
  3. Fluid level in a frontal sinus

- **Line 2** (Figure 8): Start outside the face, trace upwards along the superior border of the zygomatic arch (up the elephant's trunk), crossing the body of the zygoma, to the inferior margin of the orbit, to the contour of the nose to the other side of the face. **Compare the injured and uninjured sides.** Observe the zygomatic arch fracture, fracture through the inferior rim of the orbit soft tissue shadow in the superior maxillary antrum (tripod fracture), and 'tear-drop' sign is a blow-out fracture (see Figure 11).

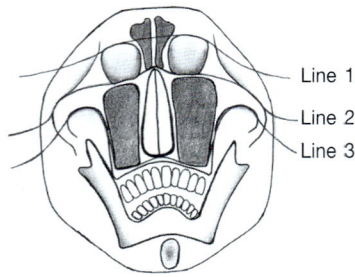

FIGURE 6 **McGrigor's 3 lines**

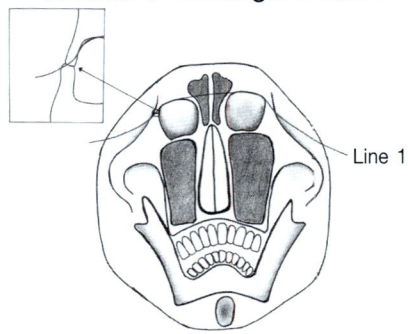

FIGURE 7 **McGrigor's Line 1**

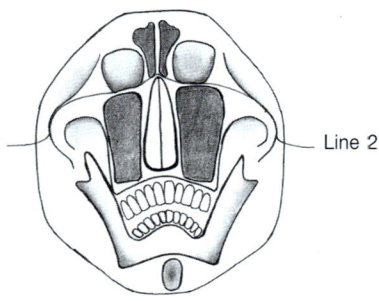

FIGURE 8 **McGrigor's Line 2**

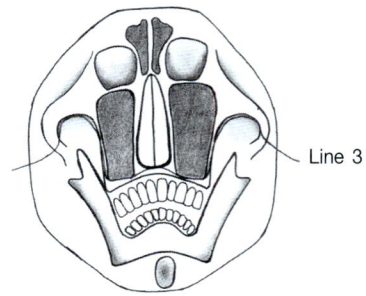

FIGURE 9 **McGrigor's Line 3**

- **Line 3** (Figure 9): Start outside the face, trace along the inferior margin of the zygomatic arch (under the elephant's trunk), and down the lateral wall of the maxillary antrum to the inferior margin of the antrum, across the maxilla along the line of the teeth to the other side.

Role of computed tomography (CT)

- Not a priority in the emergency department management.
- Most valuable for complex facial fractures, especially those involving the frontal sinus, nasoethmoid region, and the orbits.
- Standard facial X-rays are more useful for 'routine' cases, e.g. assaults, falls, etc.
- CT requires a 'cleared' cervical spine.

SPECIFIC FRACTURES

Frontal bone fracture

- **Physical examination**: Palpate periorbital rim, test for forehead anaesthesia, and test extra-occular muscles.
- **Imaging**: Skull film/Caldwell's view.
- Lacerations are frequently present in fractures involving the frontal sinus and may hide deeper injuries.
- **Disposition**: Admit for posterior table fractures and depressed fractures (treatment with IV antibiotics is controversial). Both of these fractures are likely to breach the dura with the inherent possibility of intracranial infection.

NEO (naso-ethmoidal-orbital) fracture

- **Physical examination**:
  1. Medial canthal tenderness: Easy to miss if it is thought that the patient has a simple nasal fracture; the examination should include palpation of the medial canthus to avoid missing this more serious entity.
  2. Cerebrospinal fluid rhinorrhoea.
  3. Telecanthus.
- **Imaging**: CT face.
- **Disposition**: Admit to Plastic Surgery/Maxillofacial Service (treatment with IV antibiotics is controversial).

'Blow out' orbital fracture (refer to Figures 10 and 11)

- Result from a direct compression force to the globe (e.g. from a squash ball).

NOTE: A 'blow out' fracture of the orbit does **not involve** the **orbital rim**. In fact, the finding of an orbital rim fracture should prompt close scrutiny for a 'tripod' fracture of the zygoma.

FIGURE 10 **Mechanism of injury causing a 'blow out' fracture of the orbital floor**

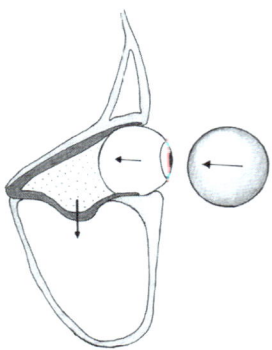

FIGURE 11 **'Blow out' fracture**

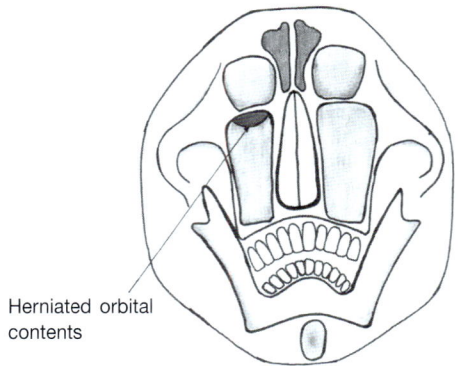

Herniated orbital
contents

Note: A frontal impact to the orbit increases intra-orbital pressure. The orbit fractures at its weakest part – the orbital walls – rather than the globe. Alternatively, a blow to the inferior orbital rim causes the orbital floor to buckle and fracture

Note: The dark shadow represents the 'tear-drop' sign

- The weakest point is the inferomedial floor of the orbit (known as the lamina papyracea).
- There is significant herniation of some orbital contents from the floor of the orbit into the maxillary antrum (known as the hanging '**tear-drop**' sign).
- **Physical examination**:
  1. Test for **infraorbital anaesthesia** by tapping for the difference in sensation between the incisor on both sides.
  2. Test the extraocular movements, looking for diplopia that is most pronounced in an upward gaze (due to entrapment of either the inferior rectus or inferior oblique muscles).
  3. Visual testing.
- **Imaging**: Water's view.
- **Disposition**: Admit for diplopia with enophthalmos; otherwise refer to plastic surgery specialist outpatient clinic.

NOTE: Diplopia alone is not an indication for admission.

- **Emergent surgical indications are:**
  1. Compressive orbital emphysema.
  2. Retrobulbar haemorrhage.
  3. Penetrating globe injury.
- **Discharge advice to patients:**
  To look out for the possible development of the following complications and to return to the ED immediately.
  1. **Compressive orbital emphysema**:
     a. Intense eye pain.
     b. Proptosis of globe.

   c. Ophthalmoplegia.

   d. Tense globe.

   e. Visual loss.

2. **Retrobulbar haemorrhage**:

   a. Those points in compressive orbital emphysema.

   b. Dilating pupil.

   c. Pale optic disc.

Nasal fracture – most common facial fracture

- **Physical examination**: Look for septal haematoma or cosmetic deformity.
- As mentioned earlier DO NOT FORGET to palpate the medial canthal region to avoid missing the NEO fracture.
- **Imaging**: Nasal view (not lateral face).
- **Disposition**: Return 4 to 7 days later to the specialist outpatient clinic for follow-up. Consult/admit for septal haematoma as failure to drain a septal haematoma will cause septal perforation.

Zygoma – 'tripod' fracture (refer to Figure 12)

- Consists of fractures of the floor AND lateral wall of the orbit, zygomatic arch and lateral wall of the maxillary antrum.
- **Physical examination**: Conduct lateral subconjunctival haemorrhage drooping lateral canthus test for intra-orbital anaesthesia. Examine for open bite.

FIGURE 12 **Fracture of the zygomaticomaxillary complex (tripod fracture)**

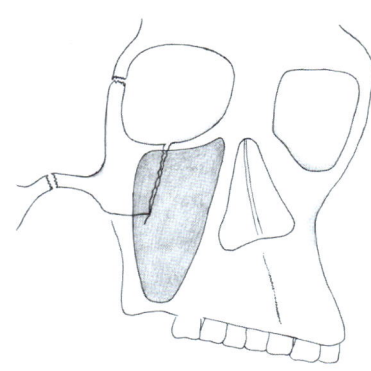

Note: There are fractures through the supporting struts of the malar bone: (1) the zygomatic arch, (2) lateral orbital rim (frontozygomatic suture), (3) inferior orbital rim and orbital floor, and (4) the anterior and lateral walls of the maxillary sinus.

- **Imaging**: OM (Water's) view.
- **Disposition**: Admit to Plastic Surgery/Maxillofacial Service

Zygoma – 'arch' fracture (an isolated arch fracture is common)

- **Physical examination**: Perform intra-oral palpation and obtain both a worm's eye view and bird's eye view.
- **Imaging**: Submental vertex (SMV) view.
- **Disposition**: Schedule specialist outpatient clinic follow-up.

LeFort fractures

- These are bilateral mid-face injuries.
- They are associated with high-energy trauma (100 times the force of gravity). Beware, many of these patients have multisystem injury.

NOTE: Fracture patterns may be mixed, e.g. LeFort II on one side and LeFort III on the other side.

- **Physical examination**: Evaluate mid-face mobility and facial lengthening. Examine for open bite.
- **Imaging**: OM/PA/lateral views (see Table 1). CT is best for operative planning.
- **Disposition**: Admit the patient to hospital (beware multisystem injury).

TABLE 1   Radiographic signs of LeFort fractures

> **Water's view**
> Bilateral mid-face fractures are characteristic of all LeFort fractures.
> Bilateral maxillary sinus air-fluid levels or opacification are usually present.
>
> **LeFort I**
> Bilateral lateral wall of the maxillary sinus fractures.
> Bilateral medial wall of the maxillary sinus fractures (can be difficult to see).
> Nasal septum fracture (inferior).
>
> **LeFort II (pyramid fracture)**
> Nasion fractures.
> Bilateral inferior orbital rim and orbital floor fractures.
> Bilateral fractures of the lateral walls of the maxillary sinuses.
>
> **LeFort III (craniofacial separation)**
> Nasion fractures.
> Bilateral lateral orbital wall fractures (frontozygomatic suture).
> Bilateral zygomatic arch fractures.

Source: Table reproduced with permission from Schwartz and Reisdorff (2001), Table 15–5, page 361.

Mandibular fractures

- These are the second most common facial fracture. Patients complain of malocclusion and pain on jaw movement associated with the rupture tympanic membrane/fracture temporal bone
- **Physical examination**:
  1. Assess for intra-oral laceration.
     a. Observe the range of motion of the jaw
     b. Conduct a **spatula test**: Place 3 wooden spatulas between the teeth and have the patient bite gently on them. Gentle rotation of the blades will produce pain in the presence of a fractured mandible.
  2. Dental examination.
  3. Lower lip anaesthesia.
- **Imaging**: Obtain Towne's, lateral oblique, and Panorex views of the mandible.
- **Disposition**
  1. Open fracture: Admit the patient for IV antibiotics.
  2. Closed fracture: Follow up at the specialist outpatient clinic or admit.

Tooth fractures (refer to Figure 13)

- Fractures of the crown are divided into categories based on the Ellis classification.
- Root fractures occur in less than 7% of dental injuries.

FIGURE 13 Tooth fractures

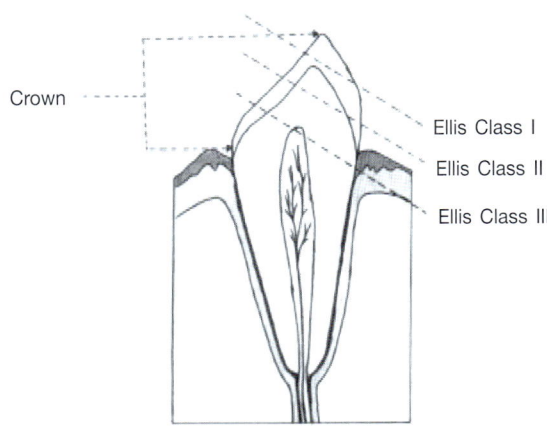

Crown

Ellis Class I
Ellis Class II
Ellis Class III

Ellis class I

- Involve only the enamel. Fractures show minimal pain.
- **Disposition**: Arrange to see a dentist the next day.

Ellis class II

- Fractures expose pinkish or yellow dentin.
- **Disposition**: Seek immediate dental opinion if the fracture occurs in a child; the next day if it occurs in an adult.

Ellis class III

- Bleeding comes from the fractured site.
- **Disposition**: Seek immediate dental opinion. These fractures are **true medical emergencies**.

Acknowledgement

The authors are grateful to Dr Chong Chew Lan for drawing Figures 6, 7, 8, 9, 10, 11, 12 and 13 in this chapter.

References/Further Reading

1. Schwartz TD, Reisdorff E. *Emergency Radiology*. New York: McGraw-Hill; 2001.

2. Hals, Gary, Sayre. The treacherous and complex spectrum of maxillofacial trauma: Etiologies, evaluation, and emergency stabilization. *Emergency Medicine Reports*. 1995.

3. Raby N, Berman L, deLacey G. *Accident and Emergency Radiology: A Survival Guide*. London: WB Saunders; 1995: 36–49.

4. Stewart C. Maxillofacial trauma: Challenges in ED diagnosis and management. *Emergency Medicine Practice*; February 2008.

5. Goh SH, Low BY. Radiologic screening for midface fractures: A single 30-degree occipitomental view is enough. *J Trauma*. 2002.

Please refer to Chapter 137.

100   Trauma, Pelvic

Irwani Ibrahim

CAVEATS

- The common pitfalls in the management of pelvic trauma include:
    1. Failure to consider pelvic fracture in the patient with multisystem trauma.
    2. Failure to give resuscitation adequately.
    3. Failure to recognize associated injuries.
- There is more severe blood loss in open pelvic fractures (as opposed to closed) because the tamponading effect of peritoneum is lost.
- Elderly women often have pelvic fractures with minimal falls because of underlying osteoporosis.
- **Mechanisms of injury**:
    1. Simple falls, avulsions from muscular attachment.
    2. Direct blows.
    3. Falls from heights, motorcycle accidents, high speed deceleration motor vehicle crashes.
- **Associated injuries**: Most mortality and morbidity with pelvic fractures occur because of associated trauma involving adjacent blood vessels and nerves, the genitourinary, and distal gastrointestinal tracts.
- **Cause of death**: Main cause of death is uncontrolled bleeding.

⇨ **SPECIAL TIP FOR GPs**
- Consider the diagnosis of pubic rami fracture in the elderly with hip pain after a fall.

MANAGEMENT

- Maintain the airway, breathing and circulation as in major trauma management.
- Correct hypovolaemia: At least 2 large bore intravenous (IV) lines should be set up.
- Send blood for full blood count, urea/electrolytes/creatinine, coagulation profile, and grooup and cross match of at least 4 to 6 units of blood.
- Do a **physical examination**. **Physical signs** associated with pelvic fractures include these:
    1. Swelling in suprapubic or groin area.
    2. Ecchymosis in external genitalia, medial thigh, and flanks.
    3. Blood from urethra.
    4. Abrasions and contusions along the bony prominence.
    5. Step-off, instability.
    6. Crepitus with bimanual palpation of the iliac wings.

NOTE: (1) **Do not** try to **spring** the **pelvis** to assess stability as this is unreliable, unnecessary, and may cause additional haemorrhage. (2) Lacerations of the perineum, groin, or buttocks after blunt trauma indicate an **open pelvic fracture** unless proven otherwise. (3) A neurological examination should be performed since **sacral plexus injury** can occur.

- **Associated injuries**:
  1. Inspect the perineum for open wounds.
  2. Perform an examination noting the position of the prostate, feeling for bony spicules, and looking for blood stains on the glove on withdrawing one's finger.
  3. Perform a vaginal examination for open wounds.
  4. If there is evidence of **urethral injury**, e.g. blood at the meatus, scrotal bruising, or a high riding prostate, look out for a pelvic fracture that can be unstable.
- Do not insert a catheter. Refer to the urologist who may decide to insert a suprapubic catheter.
- Do **pelvic X-rays** to look for disruption of the pubic symphysis and asymmetry.
- Give adequate **analgesia**.
- Start **antibiotics** in case of **open fractures**.
- Support unstable pelvic fractures using sandbags.
- Refer to Orthopaedics who may reduce and immobilize the fractures with C-clamp **external fixators**.
- If haemorrhage control fails, consider **angiography** and **embolization**.

References/Further Reading

1. In: Committee on Trauma of the American College of Surgeons. *Advanced Trauma Life Support for Doctors: Student Course Manual.* 9th ed. Chicago, IL: American College of Surgeons; 2012: 135–140.

2. Wilson RF, Tyburski J, Georgiadis GM. Pelvic fractures. In: Wilson RF, Walt AJ, eds. *Management of Trauma: Pitfalls and Practice.* 2nd ed. Baltimore, MD: Williams & Wilkins; 1996: 578–599.

3. Gillott A, Rhodes M, Lucke J. Utility of routine pelvic x-ray during blunt trauma resuscitation. *J Trauma.* 1988; 28(11): 1570–1574.

4. Kaneriya PP, Schweitzer ME, Spettell C, et al. The cost-effectiveness of routine pelvic radiography in the evaluation of blunt trauma patients. *Skeletal Radiol.* 1999; 28(5): 271–273.

5. Mackersie RC, Shackford SR, Garfin SR, et al. Major skeletal injuries in the obtunded blunt trauma patient: A case for routine radiologic survey. *J Trauma.* 1988; 28(10): 1450–1454.

6. Civil ID, Ross SE, Botehlo G, et al. Routine pelvic radiography in severe blunt trauma: Is it necessary? *Ann Emerg Med.* 1988; 17(5): 488–490.

7. Koury HI, Peschiera JL, Welling RE. Selective use of pelvic roentgenograms in blunt trauma patients. *J Trauma.* 1993; 34(2): 236–237.

8. Salvino CK, Esposito TJ, Smith D, et al. Routine pelvic x-ray studies in awake blunt trauma patients: A sensible policy? *J Trauma.* 1992; 33(3): 413–416.

9. Grant PT. The diagnosis of pelvic fractures by 'springing'. *Arch Emerg Med.* 1990; 7(3): 178–182.

101　Trauma in Pregnancy

Ong Pei Yuin • Benjamin Leong

CAVEATS

Keep in mind physiological and anatomical changes in pregnancy.

- **Airway and breathing considerations**
  1. **Difficult intubations will increase the risk of aspiration**. Pregnant patients have increased gastric pressure from uterine compression and delayed gastric emptying. All intubation should be rapid sequence intubation even in the fasted patient.
  2. **Oxygen consumption increases** by about 15%, resulting in lower oxygen reserve.
  3. **Minute ventilation increases** resulting in physiological hypocarbia. Normocarbia may indicate hypoventilation.
  4. **Diaphragmatic splinting** during pregnancy results in reduced functional residual capacity (FRC) and makes pneumothoraces and haemothoraces more life threatening.
  5. Chest tubes should be inserted **above the fourth intercostal space** due to diaphragmatic rise.

- **Circulation considerations**
  1. **Maternal blood pressure** decreases by 5–15 mmHg and **heart rate** increases by about 15–20 beats per minute during the second trimester.
  2. **Physiological hypervolaemia of pregnancy** may lead to an underestimation of blood loss. Maternal blood loss up to 30% (about 1.5 L) may be tolerated before signs of shock are evident.
  3. **Evidence of foetal compromise** may be the first sign of maternal haemorrhagic shock as uterine blood flow is diverted to support maternal circulation.
  4. **Maternal shock** is associated with up to 80% foetal mortality rate. It may also lead to infarction of the pituitary gland, which normally increases in size during pregnancy (**Sheehan's syndrome**).
  5. **Retroperitoneal haemorrhage** is more frequent due to the engorgement of pelvic organs and veins.
  6. **Supine hypotension syndrome** occurs (usually from the 20th week) when the uterus compresses the inferior vena cava (IVC) and may worsen maternal shock.
  7. **Physiological anaemia** occurs due to maternal blood volume rising by about 50% but with only a 25% corresponding increase in red cell mass.

- **Anatomical considerations**
  1. The **uterus** rises out of the pelvis from **12 weeks**, reaches the umbilicus from **20 weeks** and the xiphisternum from **36 weeks**, and may make assessment of the abdomen more difficult.

2. The **bony pelvis** is less likely to fracture due to **increased ligamentous laxity**.

3. The **symphysis pubis** and **sacroiliac joints** may be widened, **mimicking diastasis** on X-ray.

- **Injuries and complications unique to pregnancy**

  1. **Abruptio placentae**

     a. Occurs in up to 50% of severe trauma and 1–5% of minor injuries.

     b. Accounts for up to 50% of foetal loss.

     c. Symptoms of vaginal bleeding, uterine contractions, and abdominal/uterine tenderness which may be occult.

     d. Does NOT require direct abdominal trauma to occur. Rapid deceleration alone may result in shear forces that cause the abruption.

  2. **Uterine rupture**

     a. Usually caused by blunt abdominal trauma.

     b. Increased risk among women with a history of caesarean section.

     c. Clinical features include peritonism, asymmetrical uterus, and palpable foetal parts.

  3. **Preterm labour**

     a. Increased uterine irritability may occur as a result of uterine trauma.

     b. 90% of preterm labour aborts spontaneously.

  4. **Foetal injury**

     a. Occurs from direct injury or secondary to maternal shock or premature delivery.

  5. **Rh sensitization from foetal–maternal haemorrhage**

     a. Occurs when as little as 0.03 ml of blood from a Rh positive foetus enters the circulation of a Rh negative mother.

     b. Rh immunoglobulin (IM RhoGAM 50 μg for <12 weeks, 300 μg for >12 weeks) should be considered for all Rh negative mothers who sustain abdominal trauma, in consultation with the obstetrician.

  6. **Amniotic fluid embolus**

     a. Rare and carries a poor prognosis.

     b. May result in cardiovascular collapse, respiratory distress, convulsions, or disseminated intravascular coagulation (DIVC).

⇨ **SPECIAL TIPS FOR GPs**

- Prevention is better than cure.

  1. Advise pregnant patients on the **proper use of seat belts** in cars: Shoulder belts should lie above the uterus and lap belts should lie over the pelvis, below the uterus.

  2. Advise pregnant patients to use **proper footwear** to minimize falls: Flat heeled with a good grip.

3. Pregnant patients should be instructed to seek care immediately after any blunt trauma due to the potential for placental abruption.

- If the general practitioner is the first responder in a critical situation, he may perform basic measures such as these:

1. Place the patient in the left lateral position or manually displace the uterus to the left.
2. Control local bleeding.
3. Give supplemental oxygen.
4. Administer early intravenous (IV) fluids.

MANAGEMENT

General principles

- The priorities and ABCs (airway, breathing and circulation) of trauma management do not differ during pregnancy.
- There may be two patients to monitor but **stabilize the mother first**.
- **Involve the obstetrician** in addition to the **Trauma team early**.
- Manage the patient in a monitored area (high acuity or intermediate acuity care):
  1. Give supplemental oxygen.
  2. Monitoring: Electrocardiogram (ECG), pulse oximetry, vital signs q 5 to 10 minutes, and continuous cardiotocography (CTG) monitoring for pregnant patients beyond 20 weeks' gestation.
- **Patient position (for those beyond 20 weeks' gestation)**:
  1. If spinal injury is suspected, **tilt the patient or spinal board 15–30 degrees to the left or displace the uterus to the left manually**.
  2. Otherwise, manage the patient in the **left lateral position**.

Initial management

- Identify and stabilize maternal condition first. Manage airway and resuscitate as indicated.
- Check the foetal heart sounds by Doppler tone or ultrasound. If absent, the foetus is unlikely to survive; resuscitate the mother only.
- Determine the gestational age by using LMP (last menstrual period), fundal height (cm) (approximate weeks of gestation after 16 weeks), or ultrasonography.
- Perform a speculum examination to rule out rupture of membranes and vaginal bleeding.
- Perform a sonography to check for placenta abruption. Small abruptions can be missed.
- For an unborn child of 24 weeks' gestational age (viable foetuses), perform continuous foetal tocography, and maternal monitoring for at least 4 hours for uterine contractions, and foetal heart rate decelerations. Normal tracing with normal physical examination has negative predictive value of nearly 100%.

Investigations

- Full blood count and electrolyte panel.
- Coagulation profile and arterial blood gas.
- Group and cross match (note the Rh status of the mother).
- **Kleihauer** test (in Rh negative mothers).
- Necessary **X-rays** and computed tomography (**CT) scans** should not be withheld, using lead shields as appropriate, although alternatives such as ultrasound or diagnostic peritoneal lavage (DPL) may be considered.
- X-rays: No adverse effects are expected with radiation up to 5–10 rads. Risk is higher in the first trimester.

Estimated rad exposure:

Chest X-ray, cervical spine X-ray	<0.005 rad
Femur	<0.012 rad
Pelvis, spine, kidney, ureter, and bladder X-rays	<0.5 rad each
CT abdomen and pelvis	3–9 rad

- **Diagnostic peritoneal lavage**, if necessary, should be supraumbilical with the open technique.
- **Triple contrast CT** is advocated for penetrating injuries in stable patients.
- **Ultrasound** is very useful for detecting haemoperitoneum, foetal heart tones and movement, placenta location, and amniotic fluid index. However, up to 50% of placental abruptions can be missed by ultrasound.
- **Continuous foetal tocography** is more sensitive in detecting placental abruption than ultrasonography, Kleihauer test or physical examination. It is best used for reassurance in foetal status and in discharging the patient.

Definitive care

- Decisions for definitive treatment for respective injuries should be made between the respective surgeons and the obstetrician.
- **Situations which may require emergent delivery** of the foetus include:
  1. **Abruptio placentae** (also known as placenta abruption).
  2. **Foetal distress**.
  3. **Maternal cardiac arrest. Perimortem caesarean delivery** is performed for a patient with a viable foetus of >24 weeks' gestation within 5 minutes of maternal cardiac arrest. This carries the best chance of both foetal and maternal survival as maternal perfusion can improve after the caesarean delivery. In advanced pregnancy, external cardiac massage may be ineffective. In that situation, **anterior thoractomy (without aortic cross-clamping) with open cardiac massage** should be considered to improve oxygenation to the foetus and mother while awaiting caesarean delivery.

- Even if no obvious maternal injury has occurred, the patient should have **continuous cardiotocograph monitoring for 4 hours**. Even seemingly trivial injuries may result in placental separation.

Disposition

- Patients with major trauma should generally be admitted to the general surgical intensive care or high dependency unit.
- Patients may also be admitted to the respective surgical subspecialities depending on the spectrum of injury to the mother (e.g. isolated traumatic brain injury under neurosurgery or isolated limb fracture under Orthopaedics).
- If there has been no obvious significant injury, the patient may be admitted to the labour ward for monitoring.

References/Further Reading

1. Trauma in pregnancy and intimate partner violence. In: Committee on Trauma of the American College of Surgeons. *Advanced Trauma Life Support for Doctors: Instructor Course Manual.* 9th ed. Chicago, IL: American College of Surgeons; 2012: 286–297.

2. Wyatt JP, Illingworth RN, Graham CA, et al., eds. *Oxford Handbook of Emergency Medicine.* 3rd ed. Oxford, UK: Oxford University Press; 2006: 588–589.

3. Scaletta TA, Schaider JJ, eds. *Emergent Management of Trauma.* 2nd ed. New York: McGraw-Hill; 2001: 359–368.

4. Schaider JJ, Hayden SR, Wolfe RE, et al., eds. Pregnancy, trauma. In: *Rosen & Barkin's 5-Minute Emergency Medicine Consult.* Philadelphia, PA: Lippincott Williams & Wilkins; 2007.

5. Grossman N. Blunt trauma in pregnancy. *Am Fam Physician.* 1 Oct 2004; 70(7): 1303–1310.

6. Desjardins G. *Management of the Injured Pregnant Patient;* 2004. Available at: www.trauma.org/archive/resus/pregnancytrauma.html. Last accessed 23 Apr 2014.

102   Trauma, Spinal Cord and Cervical Spine Clearance

Peng Li Lee • Toh Hong Chuen

MECHANISMS OF SPINAL CORD INJURY

• Penetrating injury.
• Blunt trauma with disruption of the vertebral column causing transection or compression of neural elements.
• Primary vascular damage to the spinal cord, e.g. compression by extradural haematoma.

CAVEATS

• **Spinal cord injury** should be suspected and cervical immobilization maintained from the time of injury in the following:
  1. The unconscious trauma patient.
  2. Survivors of high velocity accidents.
  3. Presence of associated injuries:.
     a. Significant head or facial trauma: 4–20% incidence of associated cervical injury.
     b. Scapula contusion: May suggest flexion and rotation of the thoracic spine.
     c. Seat belt injuries: May be associated with thoracic and lumbar injuries.
     d. Injury to feet/ankle from a fall from a height: May be associated with compression injury to the lumbar spine.
• **Signs of spinal cord injury**:
  1. Vital signs: **Neurogenic shock** (hypotension with relative bradycardia).

  NOTE: Although neurogenic shock should be considered in trauma patients with hypotension in the absence of tachycardia, hypovolaemia from blood loss must still be excluded first (some patients may not mount a tachycardia response, especially if they are on beta blockers).

  2. On **inspection**:
     a. Diaphragmatic breathing.
     b. Flexed posture of the upper limbs suggests a high cervical cord injury.
     c. Spontaneous muscle fasciculations.
     d. Priaprism.
  3. On **testing**:
     a. **Myotomic pattern of power loss**: See Table 1.
     b. **Dermatomic pattern of sensory loss**: See Figure 1.

TABLE 1 Nerve function

Nerve root	Motor/function	Sensory	Reflex
C4	Diaphragm/ventilation	Suprasternal notch	
C5	Deltoid/shoulder shrug	Below clavicle	Biceps
C6	Biceps/elbow flexion and wrist extension	Thumb	Biceps
C7	Triceps/elbow extension	Middle finger	Triceps
C8	Flexor digitorum/finger flexion	Little finger	
T1	Interossei/spread fingers	Medial forearm	
T4	Intercostal/ventilation	Nipples	
T8		Xiphoid	
T10	Abdominal musculature	Umbilicus	
T12		Pubic symphysis	
L1/L2	Iliopsoas/hip flexion	Upper thigh	
L3	Quadriceps/knee extension	Medial thigh	Patellar
L4	Quadriceps/knee extension	Big toe	Patellar
L5	Extensor hallucis longus/great toe dorsiflexion	Middle toe	
S1	Gastrocnemius and soleus/ankle plantar flexion	Little toe	Achilles
S2/S3/S4	Anal sphincter/bowel and bladder	Perianal area	Bulbocavernosus

Table reproduced with permission of the McGraw-Hill Companies, from Scaletta TA, Schaider JJ. *Emergent Management of Trauma*. Boston, MA: McGraw-Hill; 2001, Table 10.1.

FIGURE 1 Sensory function

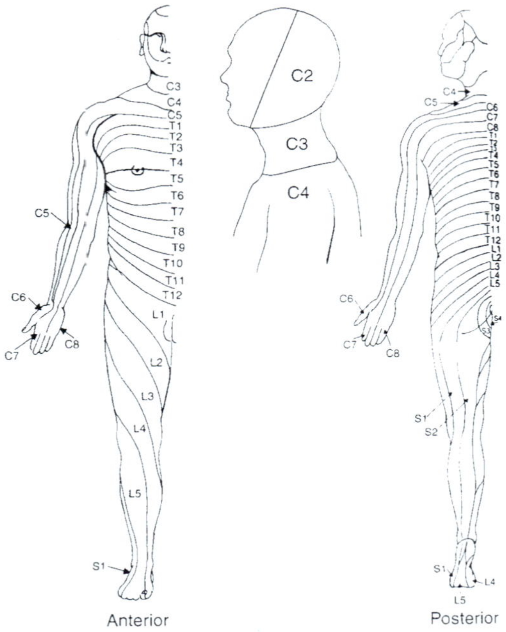

Anterior   Posterior

Figure reproduced with permission from Scaletta TA, Schaider JJ, Figure 10.11.[1]

c. **Complete spinal cord lesion**: Complete loss of motor power and sensation distal to the site of spinal cord injury. Look for **sacral sparing** (prognosticate for functional recovery, i.e. intact perianal sensation, intact rectal sphincter tone, and flexor toe movement).

Spinal shock is a transient spinal concussion with loss of all motor and sensory function below the cord lesion. It usually lasts <24 hours and rarely beyond 48 hours. The return of spinal reflexes below the cord lesion, e.g. bulbocavernosus reflex[1] indicate the end of spinal shock.

d. **Incomplete cord lesions**: Classified into three main types:

   i. **Central cord syndrome** (Figure 2), commonly seen in degenerative arthritis of the cervical spine.

FIGURE 2   Central cord syndrome

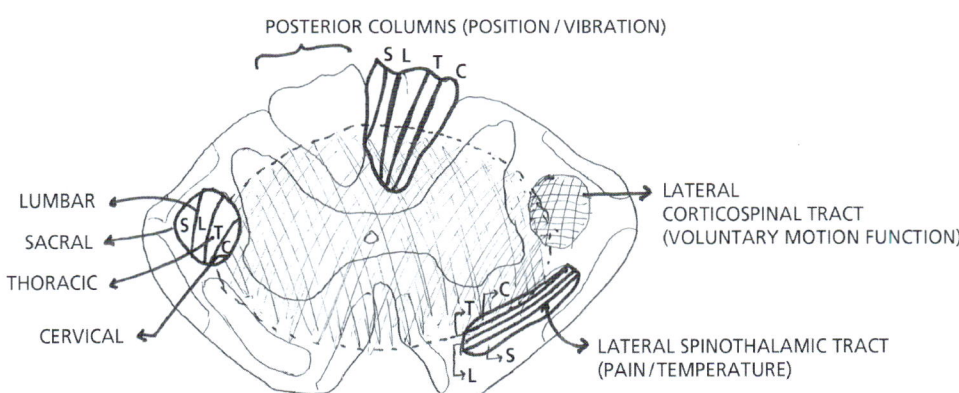

- Characterized by a disproportionately greater loss of motor power in the upper limbs than lower limbs.
- Sensory loss may occur in varying degrees.
- Fibres controlling voluntary bowel and bladder function are centrally located and often affected, although 'sacral sparing' is usually present.
- Mechanism: Hyperextension, e.g. typically a forward fall onto the face in an elderly person.

---

[1] Bulbocavernosus reflex: External anal sphincter contraction felt with a gloved finger when the glans penis/clitoris is squeezed or the in-situ Foley's catheter is gently tugged. This reflex is NOT a sign of sacral sparing. Absence of this reflex is seen during spinal shock while the return of this reflex indicates the end of spinal shock. Persistent absence of this reflex indicates damage to the sacral reflex arc itself, i.e. conus medullaris or cauda equina injury.

   ii. **Brown–Sequard syndrome** (Figure 3).

- Ipsilateral motor paralysis.

- Ipsilateral loss of position and vibration (test with tuning fork) sense (posterior column).

- Contralateral sensory loss of pain and temperature (spinothalamic tract).

- Mechanism: Penetrating injury or lateral mass fractures of the vertebrae resulting in hemisection of the cord.

  iii. **Anterior cord syndrome** (Figure 4).

Paraplegia.

- Dissociated sensory loss: Loss of pain and temperature sensation but preservation of position sense/vibration (posterior column).

- Mechanism: Cervical flexion injury causing cord contusion or disruption of the anterior spinal artery (e.g. in complications of descending aorta injury or repair), acute disc herniation, or protrusion of bony fragments.

FIGURE 3   Brown–Sequard syndrome

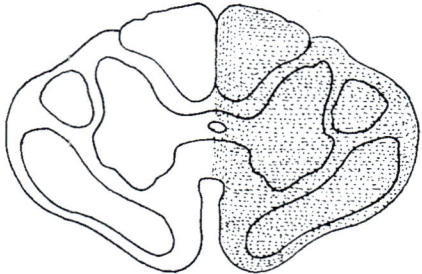

Figure reproduced with permission from Scaletta TA, Schaider JJ, Figure 10.13.

FIGURE 4   Anterior cord syndrome

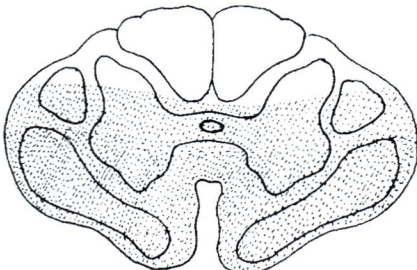

Figure reproduced with permission from Scaletta TA, Schaider JJ, Figure 10.14.

MANAGEMENT

- Attend to life-threatening injuries first while minimizing movement of the spinal column.
- Immobilize the spine in a neutral position.
- Document neurological deficits.
- **Radiological investigations**:
  1. Cervical spine X-ray: Mandatory anteroposterior (AP)/lateral/open mouth view.

     The patient's shoulders may have to be pulled down during lateral view to ensure adequate visualization of the C7/T1 junction. Consider the swimmer's view if the C7/T1 junction is not seen on lateral view.
  2. Thoracic and lumbar spine X-ray: AP/lateral views.
  3. CT scan is indicated in the following:
     a. Good visualization of the lower cervical spine not obtained on X-ray.
     b. Suspicious abnormality seen on X-ray.
  4. Magnetic resonance imaging (MRI):
     a. Provides the most accurate data in the presence of neurological deficits.
     b. The limitation is its availability in the urgent setting.
- **IV fluids**:
  1. Avoid overzealous fluid administration as it may precipitate pulmonary oedema.
  2. Insert a urinary catheter to monitor the urinary output.
  3. For neurogenic shock, consider vasopressors if the blood pressure does not improve after fluid challenge.
- The use of **IV methylprednisolone** is a treatment option, NOT the standard of care. The evidence of harm may be more consistent with the available evidence (from the National Acute Spinal Cord Injury Studies (NASCIS) I, II, and III) than evidence of benefit.
  1. **Indications**:
     a. Proven non-penetrating spinal cord injury.
     b. Within 8 hours post injury.
  2. **Dosage**: 30 mg/kg over 15 minutes followed by 5.4 mg/kg/hr. For patients in whom the drug is administered within 3 hours post injury, continue infusion for 24 hours; if administered between 3 and 8 hours, continue for 48 hours.

3. **Contraindications**:
   a. Children under 13 years of age.
   b. Pregnancy.
   c. Mild injury limited to the cauda equina/nerve roots.
   d. Presence of abdominal trauma.
   e. Major life-threatening morbidity.
- **Disposition**: Refer to the orthopaedic surgeon and/or neurosurgeon depending on local practice.

References/Further Reading

1. All the figures and Table 1 in this chapter were reproduced with permission of the McGraw-Hill Companies, from Scaletta TA, Schaider JJ. *Emergent Management of Trauma*. Boston, MA: McGraw-Hill; 2001.

2. Stahmer SA, Raps EC, Mines DI. Carotid and vertebral artery dissection. In: Neurologic emergenices. *Em Med Clin North Am*. 1997; 15: 677–698.

3. Chong CL, SBS Ooi, Neck pain after minor neck trauma: Is it always neck sprain? *Eur J Em Med*. 2000; 7: 147–149.

4. Spine and spinal cord trauma. In: Committee on Trauma of the American College of Surgeons. *Advanced Trauma Life Support Program Student Course Manual*. 9th ed. Chicago, IL: American College of Surgeons; 2012: 174–205.

5. Nesathurai S. Steroids and spinal cord injury: Revisiting the NASCIS 2 and NASCIS 3 trials. *J Trauma*. Dec 1998 45(6): 1088–1093.

6. Beattie LK, Choi J. Acute spinal injuries: Assessment and management. *Emergency Medicine Practice*. May 2006; 8: 5

7. Hockberger RS, Kaji AH, Newton EJ. Spinal Injuries. In: Marx JA, Hockberger RS, Walls RM, eds. *Rosen's Emergency Medicine: Concepts and Clinical Practice*. 7th ed. Philadelphia, PA: Mosby Elsevier; 2010: 337–376.

CERVICAL SPINE CLEARANCE

Cervical Spine (C-spine) Clearance refers to the initial assessments done to rule out unstable bony injuries to the cervical spine and / or cord injuries in blunt trauma. It can be cleared either clinically or with the aid of imaging.

Clinical Clearance of C-spine	*Radiological* Clearance of C-spine
Best aided by use of clinical decision rules e.g: 1) Canadian C-spine rule 2) NEXUS criteria	Selection of appropriate initial imaging modality involves understanding the pros / cons of each modality, as well as the adherence to the local practice guidelines.
Main intent is to enable physician to exercise prudence & judgment in order to avoid unnecessary spine imaging in low risk (<0.5%) patients for C-spine injury.	**C-spine (plain) X-ray (AP / Lat / odontoid views)** • Generally adequate to identify or raise suspicion of clinically important cervical injuries if all 3 views are done with optimal visualisation of C7-T1 junction. • A single lateral view of C-spine can identify up to 90% of bony and ligamentous injuries. • Limitations: body habitus may prevent visualisation of all 7 vertebral bodies; C1-C2 may not be well seen on plain X-ray.

C-spine CT
- CT is more sensitive & specific than plain X-ray for C-spine injuries.
- Imaging strategy: C-spine CT may be used as the initial imaging modality (current trend in most trauma centres) or as a supplement to plain X-rays.
- May be used as the initial imaging modality for: patients with associated head injury for which emergent CT head scan is to be performed, high clinical suspicion of cervical spine injury, obtunded trauma patients.
- May be used as a supplement to plain X-rays for suspicious or inadequately visualised areas on plain X-ray.

C-spine MRI
- Not done as part of the initial 'C-spine clearance' in ED.

Canadian C-spine rule	NEXUS criteria
Intended for patients who are alert, stable and with no neurological deficits.	Intended for patients who are alert, stable and with no neurological deficits.
Reported sensitivity 100%, specificity 42.5% for clinically important C-spine injuries. NPV 100%, PPV 2.9%.	Reported sensitivity 99.6%, specificity 12.9% for clinically significant C-spine injuries. NPV 99.9%, PPV 2.7%.
If patients meet the 3 criteria, no imaging is indicated.	If patients meet the 5 criteria, no imaging is indicated.

NEXUS criteria

C-spine imaging is NOT necessary in patients meeting ALL 5 criteria:

(1) No evidence of intoxication
(2) Normal level of alertness and consciousness
(3) Absence of midline cervical tenderness
(4) Absence of distracting injury
(5) Absence of focal neurological deficit

Canadian C-spine rule

C-spine imaging is NOT necessary in patients meeting ALL 3 criteria:

(1) No high risk factors	i) Age < 65 yrs ii) No dangerous mechanism: • Fall from height > 3ft • Axial loading injury • High speed motor vehicle accident, roller over or ejection.

| (2) At low risk of C-spine injury and therefore allows for safe assessment of range of motion of cervical spine. | i) Patient ambulatory at any time (including pre-hospital).
ii) Absence of midline cervical tenderness.
iii) Delayed onset of neck pain.
iv) Simple rear-end collision.
v) Patient able to sit up in ED. |
| (3) Patient is able to actively rotate his/her neck. | Can rotate 45 degrees to the left and right. |

References/Further Reading

1. Baron BJ, McSherry KJ, Larson JL Jr, Scalea TM. Spine and Spinal Cord Trauma. In: *Tintinalli's Emergency Medicine: A Comprehensive Study Guide*. 7th ed. NY; McGraw-Hill; 2011: 1709–1729.

2. Hoffman JR, Wolfson AB, Todd K, Mower WR. Selective Cervical Spine Radiography in Blunt Trauma: Methodology of the National Emergency X-Radiography Utilization Study (NEXUS). *Ann Emerg Med*. 1998 Oct; 32(4): 461–469.

3. Hoffman JR, Mower WR, Wolfson AB, et al. Validity of a set of clinical criteria to rule out injury to the cervical spine in patients with blunt trauma. National Emergency X-Radiography Utilization Study Group. *N Engl J Med*. 2000 Jul 13; 343(2): 94–99.

4. Stiell IG, Wells GA, Vandemheen KL, et al. The Canadian C-spine rule for radiography in alert and stable trauma patients. *JAMA* 2001; 286: 1841–1848.

5. Stiell IG, Clement CM, McKnight RD, et al. The Canadian C-spine rule versus the NEXUS low-risk criteria in patients with trauma. *N Engl J Med* 2003; 349: 2510–2518.

6. Dickinson G. et al. Retrospective application of the NEXUS low-risk criteria for cervical spine radiography in Canadian emergency departments. *Ann Emerg Med*. 2004 Apr; 43(4): 507–514.

103 Trauma, Upper Extremity

Peter Manning • Rakhee Yash Pal • Shirley Ooi

CAVEATS

- Orthopaedic injuries may look serious, but should not distract one from doing the primary survey first. They are therefore included in the secondary survey in a multiple trauma patient.

- For all joint dislocations that require manipulation and reduction at the emergency department, do **not** give **intramuscular (IM) opioids**. **Give intravenous (IV) opioids** instead. This is because opioids given by the IM route are erratic in absorption. Hence, when procedural sedation is needed, one is unsure of the dosage to top up for pain relief. This may result in respiratory suppression and hypotension when the full IM dose of opioid is absorbed into the circulation.

- For all orthopaedic injuries, always remember to record the neurovascular status before and after manipulation/reduction or application of a plaster splint.

> ⇨ **SPECIAL TIPS FOR GPs**
> - Remember to give analgesia and splint the fracture or dislocation before referring the patient to the emergency department. Remember that splinting is a form of pain relief.
> - Do not give IM opioids if you are unsure whether the patient requires manipulation and reduction (M&R) for the fracture or dislocation.

CLAVICULAR FRACTURES

- **Mechanism of injury**:
  1. Most commonly due to a direct blow on the point of the shoulder, e.g. a fall on the side.
  2. May also be due to a fall on an outstretched hand.
- **Clinical features**:
  1. Tenderness at the fracture site.
  2. Deformity with local swelling.
- **X-ray view**: A single anteroposterior (AP) view of the shoulder is usually adequate.
- **Complications**: In rare cases, the fracture fragments may endanger the subclavian neurovascular structures.
- **Treatment/disposition**:
  1. Patients should be placed with a broad arm-sling and review at the orthopaedic clinic.
  2. Patients with open fractures, skin tenting, or neurovascular compromise should be admitted to Orthopaedics.

STERNOCLAVICULAR JOINT INJURIES

- **Mechanism of injury**: Usually due to a fall or blow to the front of the shoulder.
- **Clinical features**:
  1. Tenderness and swelling over the sternoclavicular joint.
  2. Pain with movement of the arm and on lateral compression of the shoulders.
  3. With dislocations, the medial clavicle is displaced relative to the manubrium.
  4. Dyspnoea, dysphagis, or choking (in patients with posterior dislocations due to compression of mediastinal structures).
- **X-ray views**: AP and oblique views are difficult to interpret. The diagnosis is essentially a clinical one. Tomograms or computed tomography (CT) may be needed.
- **Complications**: Rarely, the dislocation may endanger the great vessels posterior to the clavicle.
- **Treatment/disposition**:
  1. Contusion: Broad arm-sling/analgesics and an early review at the orthopaedic clinic.
  2. Dislocation: Admit to Orthopaedics for exploration/reduction under general anaesthesia.

NOTE: Life-threatening injuries to adjacent structures occur in up to 25% of posterior dislocations.

ACROMIOCLAVICULAR JOINT INJURIES

- **Mechanism of injury**: Usually due to a fall in which the patient lands on the shoulder with the arm adducted or due to a fall on an outstretched arm.
- **Clinical features**: Unusual prominence of the lateral end of the clavicle and local tenderness.
- **X-ray view**: An AP view of the acromioclavicular or AC joint (inferior aspects of the acromion and clavicle should form a straight line).

NOTE: An AC joint X-ray should be done with the patient standing instead of in the normal recumbent position in which AP radiographs are taken as spontaneous reduction tends to occur.

- **Treatment/disposition**: Broad arm-sling, analgesia, and review at the orthopaedic clinic.

SCAPULAR FRACTURES

- **Mechanism of injury**: Usually due to significant direct trauma to the posterolateral chest.
- **Clinical features**: Local tenderness and swelling and associated injuries.
- **X-ray view**: An AP view of the shoulder with or without scapular views.
- **Complications**: Scapular fractures are commonly associated with significant thoracic injuries such as rib, clavicular and vertebral fractures, injuries to the pulmonary vessels and brachial plexus, pneumothorax and lung contusion.

- **Treatment/disposition**
  1. Isolated scapular fractures: Broad arm-sling, analgesics, and early review at the orthopaedic clinic.
  2. Coexistent thoracic injuries: Admit under General Surgery for either observation or definitive care of the individual injuries.

SHOULDER DISLOCATIONS

Statistically, 96% of shoulder dislocations are anterior, 3–4% are posterior, and 0–1% are inferior (luxatio erecta) dislocations.

Anterior dislocation

- **Mechanism of injury**: Usually due to a fall leading to external rotation of the shoulder.
- **Clinical features**
  1. It is typical for the patient to be sitting up and holding the injured arm at the elbow with the other hand.
  2. The injured arm is held in slight abduction.
  3. Contour appears 'squared off'.
  4. The glenoid fossa is palpable using the index and middle fingers (**Shirley's glenoid sign**). This is a useful sign in patients whose squaring of the contour of shoulder is not obvious.[2]
  5. This dislocation is extremely painful.
- **X-ray views**: AP (Figure 1a) and axillary (Figure 1b) or Y-scapular views assist in differentiating anterior from posterior dislocations.

FIGURE 1b Axial view of shoulder showing the anatomy of the shoulder

FIGURE 1a AP view of shoulder showing anterior shoulder dislocation in the subcoracoid region

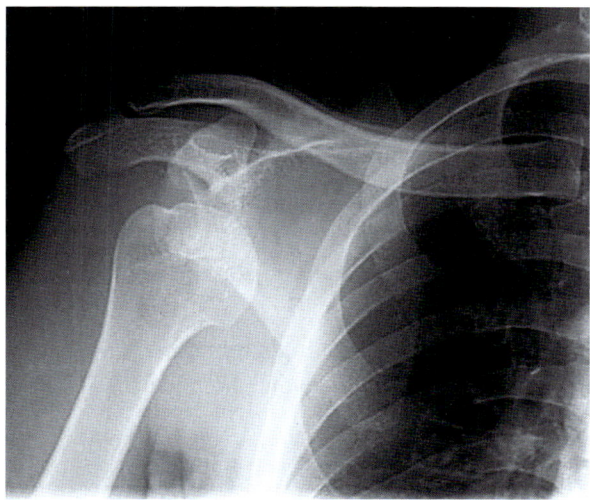

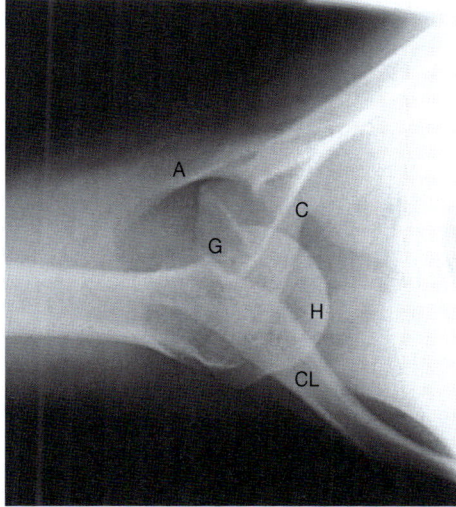

Note the locations of the acromion (A); coracoid (C); glenoid (G); clavicle (CL), head of humerus (H). The acromion is posterior while the coracoid is anterior. Hence, this x-ray confirms anterior dislocation of the head of humerus.

NOTE: (1) A **Hill–Sachs lesion** (compression fracture of the posterolateral aspect of the humeral head) may be seen in patients with previous anterior dislocation. (2) X-rays are essential from a medicolegal standpoint to exclude a coexisting fracture **prior to** manipulation and reduction (M&R). There is increasing evidence to suggest that atraumatic recurrent shoulder dislocations **do not need** pre-M&R X-rays. However, this is not widely accepted in orthopaedic circles.

- **Complications**
  1. Recurrence.
  2. Avulsion of the greater tuberosity (more common in patients who are >45 years old).
  3. Fractures of the anterior glenoid lip.
  4. Axillary nerve palsy.
  5. Rarely, axillary artery transection and brachial plexus injuries.

  NOTE: Must examine the following:

  6. Axillary nerve function by checking pin-prick sensation in the '**regimental badge**' area of the deltoid.
  7. Pulses at the wrist.
  8. Radial nerve function.
- **Treatment**
  1. Isolated anterior dislocation: M&R (for which there are multiple techniques available) under procedural sedation.
  2. Anterior dislocation with fracture of the greater or lesser tuberosities of the humerus: M&R under procedural sedation.
  3. Anterior dislocation with fracture of the proximal humeral shaft: Admit for M&R under general anaesthesia; keep in view open reduction and internal fixation (ORIF).
- **Sequence of management**: IV analgesia, **not** IM (place plug in anticipation of M&R), then X-ray, followed by M&R under procedural sedation.
- **M&R:** Traction techniques are preferred and some of the previously popular manipulation techniques are no longer favoured, e.g. Hippocratic and Kocher's manoeuvres. Traction should be performed in the critical or intermediate care area where full monitoring can be achieved, with the patient under procedural sedation (refer to Chapter 140, *Pain Management*).
  1. **Cooper–Milch technique**
     a. Under procedural sedation, place the patient in the supine position with his elbow flexed at 90 degrees.
     b. Extend the elbow and very slowly move the arm into full abduction with sustained inline traction while an assistant applies gentle pressure on the medial and inferior aspect of the humeral head.

   c. Following relocation of the head of humerus, which can be almost imperceptible on occasions, adduct the arm gradually.

   d. Place the arm in a collar and cuff and order post-reduction X-ray.

2. **Stimson's technique**: A method that employs gravity and which is particularly useful when the emergency department is very busy.

   a. Administer IV analgesia with the patient lying in the prone position with the injured arm hanging over the side of the trolley with a 2.5 kg to 5 kg weight attached to the arm.

   b. Slowly, over a period of 5 to 30 minutes the gravitational force overcomes the muscle spasm and the shoulder relocates.

   c. Apply collar and cuff and order post-reduction X-ray.

3. **Countertraction technique**: Useful as a back-up manoeuvre when either of the above fails.

   a. Under procedural sedation, place the patient in the supine position and place a rolled sheet under the axilla of the affected shoulder.

   b. Abduct the affected arm to 45 degrees and apply sustained inline traction while an assistant applies traction in the opposite direction using the rolled sheet.

   c. After relocation, apply collar and cuff and order post-reduction X-ray.

4. **Spaso technique**: Although this is not a widely known technique, it is one of the easiest methods to use and has high success rates.

   a. Under procedural sedation, bring the affected arm close to the chest wall.

   b. Forward flex the arm at the shoulder and externally rotate it simultaneously. Most of the time even before the shoulder reaches 90-degree forward flexion, a 'clunk' is heard and the head of the humerus relocates.

   c. Adduct the arm.

   d. Apply collar and cuff and order post-reduction X-ray.

NOTE: Recheck neurovascular status post-reduction.

- **Disposition**: Early review at the orthopaedic clinic.

Posterior dislocation

- **Mechanism of injury**
  1. Usually due to a fall on an outstretched internally rotated hand or a direct blow to the front of the shoulder.
  2. Associated with violent muscle contractions (called convulsions) or electrical contact injuries.
- **Clinical features**
  1. The arm is held in internal rotation and adduction.
  2. The patient experiences pain and a greatly decreased range of shoulder movement.

• **X-ray views**: AP (Figure 2a) and Y-scapular views (Figure 2b).

NOTE: It is very easy to miss a posterior shoulder dislocation on the AP view (Figure 2a). Suspect posterior shoulder dislocation if the '**light-bulb sign**' due to internal rotation of the shoulder and the lack of overlap between the head of humerus and the glenoid labrum on the AP shoulder view are seen. The latter is called the '**rim sign**' and it refers to the distance between the medial border of the humeral head and anterior glenoid rim >6 mm.

FIGURE 2a   Posterior dislocation of right shoulder

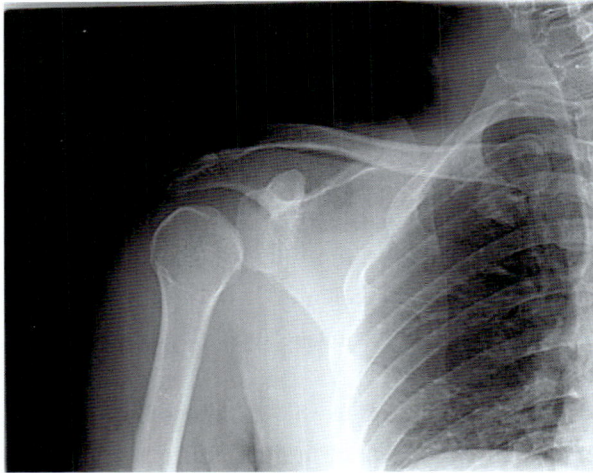

This view shows the 'light-bulb sign' due to internal rotation of the head of humerus. Note the lack of overlap between head of humerus and glenoid labrum on the AP shoulder view.

FIGURE 2b   Y-scapular view

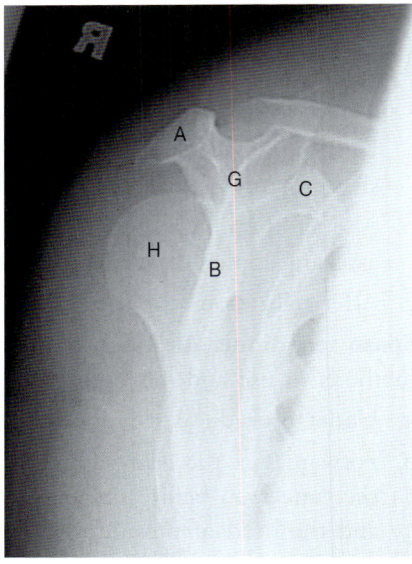

The humeral head (H) is displaced away from the coracoid/chest and is hence a posterior dislocation. The Y is formed by the junction of the scapular blade (B), coracoid (C) and the acromion (A). Normally, the head of humerus should sit at the junction of the Y, which is the glenoid fossa (G).

• **Complications**: Damage to the axillary nerve and brachial plexus.
• **Treatment**: The principles of management are the same as for anterior dislocations.
  1. For isolated posterior dislocation, attempt M&R under IV procedural sedation.
  2. For posterior dislocation with fracture of the tuberosities, attempt M&R under procedural sedation.
  3. For posterior dislocation with humeral shaft fracture, admit for M&R under general anaesthesia, keeping in view open reduction and internal fixation.
• **Technique**
  1. Under conditions of IV procedural sedation, apply traction to the arm in a position of 90 degrees' abduction.

2. Sometimes countertraction by an assistant using a rolled sheet under the axilla is required.

3. Then gently externally rotate the arm.

4. After relocation in the first time dislocation in the young adult, apply strapping together with collar and cuff.

5. After relocation in the elderly, apply collar and cuff keeping in view early mobilization.

6. Order post-reduction X-ray.

7. Recheck neurovascular status.

- **Disposition: Early** review in the orthopaedic clinic.

Inferior dislocation

- **Mechanism of injury**: Usually due to a fall with the arm in an abducted position.
- **Clinical features**
  1. Upper arm abducted with 'hand over head' position.
  2. Loss of the usual rounded contour of the shoulder.
- **X-ray view**: The AP view is sufficient to make the diagnosis.
- **Complications**: Damage to the axillary nerve and brachial plexus.
- **Treatment**: The principles of management are the same as for the other dislocations.
  1. For dislocation with or without fracture of the tuberosities, attempt M&R under IV procedural sedation.
  2. For dislocated fractures of the humeral neck, admit to Orthopaedics for M&R under general anaesthesia, keeping in view open reduction and internal fixation.
- **Technique**
  1. Under conditions of IV procedural sedation, apply steady traction to the abducted arm.
  2. Sometimes countertraction by an assistant using a rolled sheet placed over the acromion is needed.
  3. After relocation, apply collar and cuff.
  4. Order post-reduction X-ray.
  5. Recheck neurovascular status.
- **Disposition: Early** review in the orthopaedic clinic.

PROXIMAL HUMERAL FRACTURES

These fractures may involve the anatomical and surgical necks, either tuberosity or various combinations.

- **Mechanism of injury**: Usually due to a fall on the side, a direct blow to that area or a fall on an outstretched hand.

- **Clinical features**
  1. Tenderness and swelling over the proximal humerus.
  2. Later, gross bruising gravitating down the arm.
- **X-ray views**: AP and lateral views of the humerus.
- **Complications**
  1. Adhesive capsulitis (frozen shoulder).
  2. Injury to neurovascular structures.
  3. Avascular necrosis of the humeral head.
- **Treatment**: Apply collar and cuff.
- **Disposition**
  1. Severely displaced fractures of the greater tuberosity may require admission for open reduction and internal fixation under general anaesthesia.
  2. Mildly displaced fractures can be discharged, to be reviewed early in the orthopaedic clinic.

HUMERAL SHAFT FRACTURES

- **Mechanism of injury**: Usually due to indirect forces, such as a fall on an outstretched hand or a direct blow to the area.
- **Clinical features**
  1. Local tenderness and swelling.
  2. Deformity may be present.
- **X-ray views**: AP and lateral views of the humerus.
- **Complications**: Radial nerve palsy (drop wrist) and vascular compromise.
- **Treatment/disposition**
  1. For minimally angulated fractures, apply a **U-slab**; this can be more easily done with the patient seated on the trolley rather than in the supine position, followed by collar and cuff and review in the orthopaedic clinic early.
  2. For severely displaced fractures, perform M&R under IV procedural sedation; apply a U-slab and collar and cuff, and review in the orthopaedic clinic early.
  3. For cases complicated by neurovascular damage, admit to Orthopaedics.

Supracondylar humeral fractures

- **Mechanism of injury**: A fall on an outstretched hand usually occurring in a child.
- **Clinical features**
  1. Tenderness and swelling over the distal humerus and elbow.
  2. Deformity may be present.

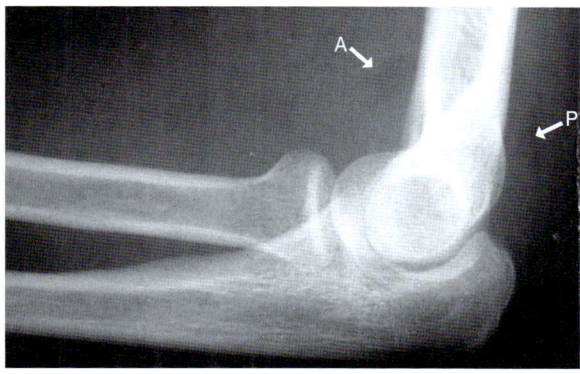

FIGURE 3 **Lateral view of elbow showing anterior (A) and posterior (P) fat-pad sign**

A visible anterior fat pad is normal, but the *displacement* of the anterior fat pad as is shown in (A) raises the strong possibility of a fracture. A visible posterior fat pad (P) is always abnormal because the posterior fat pad lies within the olecranon fossa. The 2 commonest causes are a supracondylar fracture of the humerus in a child or a radial head fracture in an adult although any intraarticular fracture can cause a 'fat-pad' sign.

3. The olecranon and medial and lateral epicondyles preserve their equilateral triangle relationship.

- **X-ray views**: AP and lateral views of the elbow (**beware lateral condylar fracture: Admit for open reduction and internal fixation**). Look for the 'fat-pad' sign (Figure 3).

- **Complications**
    1. **Brachial artery damage**.
        a. Check radial pulse and capillary refill.
        b. Look for pallor and coolness of the extremity, pain, paraesthesia, or paralysis of the forearm.
    2. Check the fingers and thumb for neurological deficit due to radial, ulnar, and median nerve involvement.

NOTE: Document the presence or absence of these features.

- **Treatment/disposition**
    1. For undisplaced fracture, apply a long arm back slab and review in the orthopaedic clinic early. Give clear written instructions pertaining to signs of developing **compartment syndrome**.
    2. If there is considerable swelling in the region of the elbow with a minimally angulated fracture, consider erring on the side of safety and admit a child overnight for observation of the circulation.
    3. If the fracture is angulated with posterior cortical contact, apply a long arm back slab and admit to Orthopaedics for closed reduction under general anaesthesia.
    4. If the fracture is displaced, apply a long arm back slab and admit to Orthopaedics for closed reduction and wiring.

MEDIAL EPICONDYLAR FRACTURES OF THE HUMERUS

- **Mechanism of injury**
  1. May be avulsed by the ulnar collateral ligament when the elbow is forcibly abducted.
  2. Avulsion due to a sudden contraction of the forearm flexor muscles.
  3. Direct trauma.
- **Clinical features**: Local swelling and tenderness.
- **X-ray views**: AP and lateral views of the elbow.
- **Complications**: Ulnar nerve injury.
- **Treatment/disposition**:
  1. If the fracture has minimal or no displacement, apply a long arm back slab and review in the orthopaedic clinic early.
  2. If the fracture is widely displaced or with an intra-articular fragment or with an ulnar nerve injury, admit for surgical management.

LATERAL CONDYLAR FRACTURES OF THE HUMERUS

NOTE: This type of fracture is commonly missed as it could be confused with a supracondylar fracture!

- **Mechanism of injury**: Adduction injury of the elbow.
- **Clinical features**: Local tenderness and swelling.
- **X-ray views**: AP and lateral views of the elbow.
- **Complications**: No acute complications. The delayed complications are:
  1. Malunion and non-union causing cubitus valgus and tardy ulnar nerve palsy.
  2. Elbow stiffness especially in adults.
- **Treatment/disposition**
  1. If the fracture is undisplaced or minimally displaced, apply a long arm back slab and review in the orthopaedic clinic early.
  2. If the fracture is displaced >2 mm or rotated, admit to Orthopaedics for M&R under general anaesthesia, keeping in view open reduction and internal fixation.

ELBOW DISLOCATIONS

- **Mechanism of injury**: Usually due to a fall on an outstretched hand; posterolateral dislocation is the commonest.
- **Clinical features**
  1. Elbow deformity with tenderness and swelling.
  2. The equilateral triangle relationship between olecranon and medial and lateral epicondyles is disrupted (compared with supracondylar fracture).

- **X-ray views**: AP and lateral views of the elbow.
- **Complications**: Injury to the brachial artery, ulnar nerve, or medial nerve.
- **Treatment/disposition**: M&R under IV procedural sedation.
  1. For a supine patient, apply traction in the line of the limb.
  2. Slight flexion of the elbow may be necessary while maintaining traction.
  3. After relocation, apply a long arm back slab.
  4. If no evidence of neurovascular damage exists, review in the orthopaedic clinic early.
  5. If even the mildest hint of neurovascular damage exists, admit to Orthopaedics for observation.
  6. Ensure the joint is truly reduced; X-rays can be really tricky.

'PULLED ELBOW' (subluxed radial head)

- **Mechanism of injury**: Usually occurs in a child aged between 9 months and 6 years, due to an abrupt pull on an outstretched hand, i.e. an axial or distracting force which pulls the annular ligament over the radial head.
- **Clinical features**
  1. The affected arm hangs limply.
  2. The child either complains of pain in the arm or refuses to use the arm.
  3. Local tenderness is evident over the proximal forearm.
  4. Pain is elicited by flexion of the elbow or supination of the forearm.
  5. No swelling or deformity is seen.
- **X-ray view**: Not required in the classic scenario; **however**, if there is a history of a fall or a direct blow to the forearm, then order AP and lateral views of the elbow and forearm as clinically indicated.
- **Treatment/disposition**: Manipulation without anaesthesia is the norm.
  1. Hold the hand of the affected arm in a 'hand-shaking' position with your other hand behind the elbow with thumb over the head of the radius.
  2. Gently, but firmly, impact the forearm in to the elbow, and forcibly supinate the arm or rapidly alternately pronate and supinate the forearm until an audible or palpable 'pop' is felt. No sling is required since the child will start to use the arm normally within 5 to 10 minutes.
  3. Should the above manoeuvre be unsuccessful, the arm should be rested in a sling, when spontaneous reduction usually occurs within 48 hours.
  4. **No referral** to the orthopaedic clinic is required; simply, the parents and other family members need to be educated as to how to lift the child properly and to not pull the child by the hand or play 'helicopter' with him.

OLECRANON FRACTURES

- **Mechanism of injury**: Usually due to a fall on the elbow, but may also result from a violent contraction of the triceps muscle.
- **Clinical features**: Local tenderness and swelling/bruising over the olecranon.
- **X-ray views**: AP and lateral views of the elbow.
- **Treatment/disposition**
  1. If there is minimal or no displacement of the fracture, apply a long arm back slab with the patient's elbow in extension and refer to the orthopaedic clinic for early review.
  2. If the fracture is displaced, apply a long arm back slab with the patient's elbow in extension and admit for M&R under general anaesthesia, keeping in view open reduction and internal fixation.

RADIAL HEAD/NECK FRACTURES

- **Mechanism of injury**: Due either to a fall on an outstretched hand or due to a direct blow on the forearm.
- **Clinical features**: Local pain and tenderness, with swelling over the lateral elbow.
- **X-ray views**: AP and lateral views of the elbow.

NOTE: (1) Occult fractures of the radial neck/head may **only** show a '**positive posterior fat-pad sign**' on the lateral film (Figure 3); always look specifically for this sign!
(2) An oblique view X-ray of the radial head may sometimes reveal the fracture not seen on the standard AP and lateral views of the elbow.

- **Treatment/disposition**
  1. If the fracture is undisplaced, apply a long arm back slab and review in the orthopaedic clinic early.
  2. If the fracture is displaced, apply a long arm back slab and admit to Orthopaedics for M&R under general anaesthesia, keeping in view open reduction and internal fixation.

FOREARM FRACTURES

- **Mechanism of injury**: Usually due to direct trauma, but may also result from a fall on an outstretched hand.
- **Clinical features**: Tenderness and swelling of the forearm, with deformity if the fracture is displaced.
- **X-ray views**: AP and lateral views of the forearm.

NOTE: Ensure that the film includes the elbow and wrist so that a Monteggia or a Galeazzi fracture can be excluded. **Never** treat a single forearm bone fracture until you have excluded the above fracture dislocations.

1. A **Monteggia** fracture dislocation refers to **a fracture of the ulna** with dislocation of the radial head.

NOTE: Many legal suits have resulted from a missed bowed (greenstick) ulna!

2. A **Galeazzi** fracture dislocation refers to **a fracture of the radius** with dislocation of the inferior radio-ulnar joint.

- **Complications**: Vascular injury or compromise with possible development of compartment syndrome.
- **Treatment/disposition**
  1. For fractures with minimal or no displacement, apply a long arm back slab and refer to the orthopaedic clinic early.
  2. For displaced fractures, apply a long arm back slab and admit to Orthopaedics.

COLLES' FRACTURE

NOTE: Colles' fracture traditionally refers to an extraarticular fracture of the distal radius within 2.5 cm from the wrist in middle-aged and elderly women with osteoporotic bones.

- **Mechanism of injury**: Usually due to a fall on an outstretched hand.
- **Clinical features**: Characteristic 'dinner fork' deformity with local tenderness.
- **X-ray views**: Lateral (Figure 4a) and AP views (Figure 4b) of the wrist. It classically shows an impacted fracture of the distal radius with dorsal tilt and dorsal displacement, radial tilt and radial displacement and fracture ulnar styloid.

FIGURE 4a Lateral view of wrist showing Colles' fracture

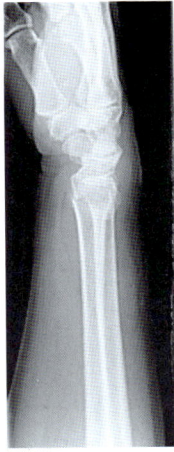

Note the posterior displacement of the distal fragment.

FIGURE 4b AP view of wrist showing Colles' fracture

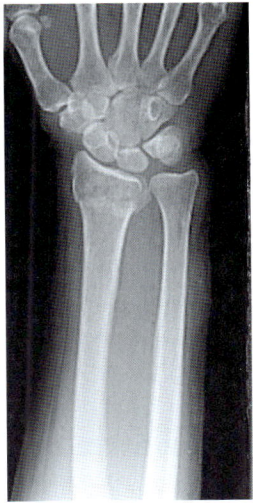

- **Complications**: Malunion, delayed rupture of the extensor pollicis longus, median nerve compression, post-traumatic carpal tunnel syndrome, and Sudeck's atrophy.
- **Treatment**
  1. Reduce under Bier's block (refer to Chapter 140, *Pain Management*) if the fracture is closed and not intra-articular.
  2. Requires monitoring of the vital signs and electrocardiogram (ECG) rhythms.
- **Reduction technique**
  1. Apply longitudinal traction to disimpact the fracture.
  2. Consider hyper-extending the distal fragment, then translating it distally (while in extended position) until it can be 'hooked over' proximal fragment.
  3. Then apply flexion and ulnar deviation force to the fragment using the fingers and thumb or the ball of your thumb.
  4. Following reduction, apply a short arm back slab with the forearm in pronation and ulnar deviation and slight flexion at the wrist.
  5. If re-X-ray shows satisfactory reduction, apply a sling and advise the patient to mobilise the shoulder, elbow, and fingers of the affected arm.
- **Disposition**
  1. If reduction is satisfactory, refer to the Hand Surgery outpatient clinic within 1 week.
  2. If the fracture is open, admit to Hand Surgery for surgical management.
  3. The following fractures may require operative fixation unstable fracture (refer to Hand Surgery Outpatient Clinic early).
     a. Unstable fracture.
     b. Younger patients with involvement of dominant side.
     c. Moderately high functional demands.

SMITH'S (OR REVERSE COLLES') FRACTURE

- **Mechanism of injury**: Usually due to a fall on the back of the hand, with the distal fragment being tilted anteriorly.
- **Clinical features**: Local tenderness, swelling, and deformity.
- **X-ray views**: AP (Figure 5a) and lateral views (Figure 5b) of the wrist.

FIGURE 5a   X-ray of the wrist showing Smith's (reverse Colles') fracture

FIGURE 5b   Lateral view of the same fracture

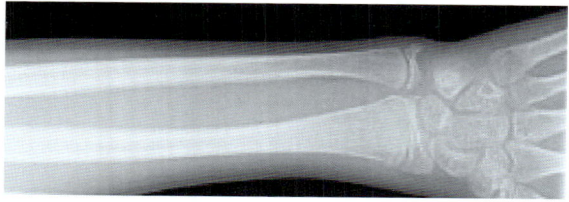
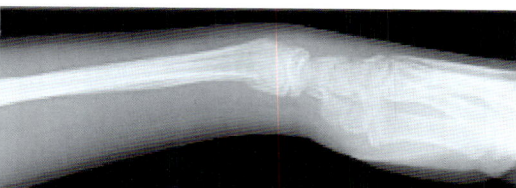

Note the anterior displacement of the fracture fragment.

- **Treatment**
  1. Reduce under Bier's block (refer to Chapter 140, *Pain Management*) if the fracture is closed and not intra-articular.
  2. Requires monitoring of the signs and ECG rhythms.
- **Reduction technique**
  1. Apply traction to the arm in supination until disimpaction is achieved.
  2. Apply dorsally-directed pressure to the fragment.
  3. Apply a short arm volar slab with the forearm in full supination, wrist in dorsiflexion, and the elbow in extension first. As this fracture is difficult to hold, a long arm back slab is applied after this with the elbow at 90-degree flexion.
- **Disposition**
  1. If reduction is satisfactory, refer to the Hand Surgery clinic early.
  2. If the fracture is open or intra-articular, admit to Hand Surgery for surgical management.

BARTON'S FRACTURE

This is a form of Smith's fracture in which only the anterior portion of the radius is involved.

FIGURE 6   Lateral view of wrist showing Barton's fracture

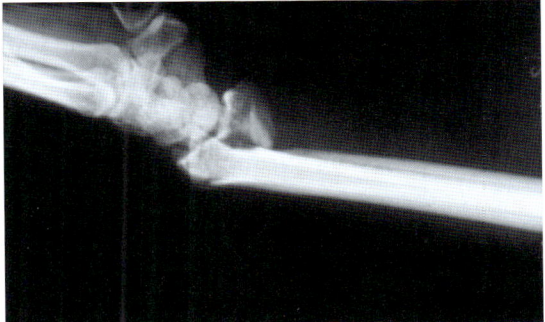

- **Mechanism of injury**: Usually due to a fall on an outstretched hand.
- **Clinical features**: Local tenderness, swelling, and deformity.
- **X-ray view**: Lateral view of the wrist (Figure 6).
- **Treatment/disposition**: Apply a short arm volar slab and admit to Hand Surgery for open reduction and internal fixation.

SCAPHOID (CARPAL NAVICULAR) FRACTURES

- **Mechanism of injury**
  1. Usually due to a fall on an outstretched hand.
  2. Occasionally due to 'kickback' when using a starting handle, pump, or compressor.
- **Clinical features**
  1. Pain in the radial border of the wrist.
  2. Tenderness in the anatomical snuffbox and dorsal and ventral aspects of the scaphoid.
- **X-ray views: Scaphoid views** (Figure 7a) and AP and lateral views (Figure 7b) of the wrist.

NOTE: Scaphoid views should be ordered in any patient with tenderness around the 'snuffbox' area.

FIGURE 7a   **Scaphoid views**   **FIGURE 7b**   **AP and lateral views of the wrist**

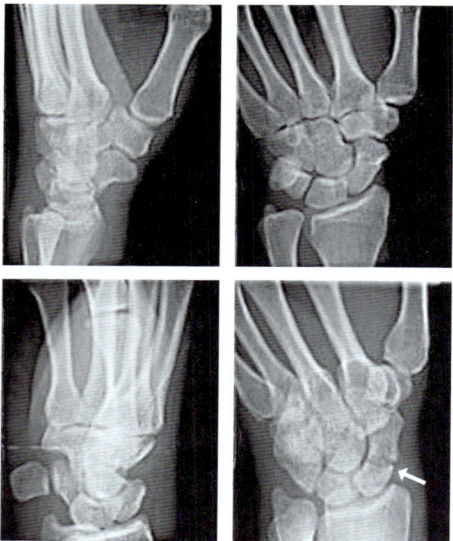   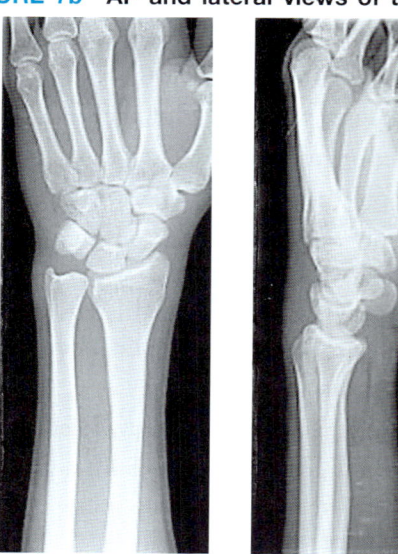

Scaphoid views (a) showing fracture at waist of scaphoid indicated by arrow. Note that the fracture is not obvious on the standard AP and lateral views (b) of the wrist.

- **Complications**: Avascular necrosis, non-union, osteoarthritis, and Sudeck's atrophy.
- **Treatment/disposition**
  1. If a scaphoid fracture is identified, apply a scaphoid spica splint and review in the Hand Surgery clinic early.
  2. If there is clinical suspicion of a scaphoid fracture but there is no X-ray substantiation of a fracture, apply a scaphoid spica splint and review in the Hand Surgery clinic.

LUNATE DISLOCATIONS

- **Mechanism of injury**: Usually due to a fall on an outstretched hand.
- **Clinical features**: Local tenderness and swelling.
- **X-ray view**: Lateral view of the wrist (Figure 8).
- **Complications**: Median nerve palsy, avascular necrosis, and Sudeck's atrophy.
- **Treatment**
  1. Reduction under Bier's block (refer to Chapter 140, *Pain Management*).
  2. Requires monitoring of the vital signs and ECG rhythms.

FIGURE 8   **Lateral view of wrist x-ray showing lunate (L) dislocated anteriorly**

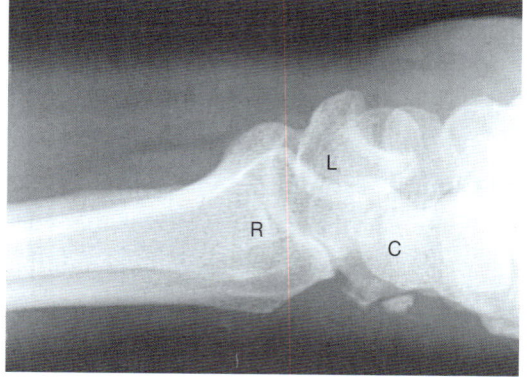

The concavity of the lunate is empty. The radius (R) and capitate (C) remain in a straight line.

- **Reduction technique**
  1. Apply traction to the supinated wrist.
  2. Extend the wrist, maintaining traction.
  3. Apply pressure with the thumb over the lunate.
  4. Flex the wrist as soon as you feel the lunate slip into place.
  5. Apply a short arm back slab in a position of moderate flexion.
- **Disposition**
  1. If the reduction is successful, review in the Hand Surgery clinic early.
  2. If reduction attempts are unsuccessful, apply a back slab and admit to Hand Surgery for open reduction and internal fixation.

PERILUNATE DISLOCATIONS

- **Mechanism of injury/clinical features/ X-ray views**: As above.
- Often associated with fractures of the scaphoid bone (Figure 9).
- **Treatment/disposition**: Admit to Hand Surgery for open reduction and internal fixation.

FIGURE 9   X-ray of the wrist showing a trans scapho-perilunate dislocation

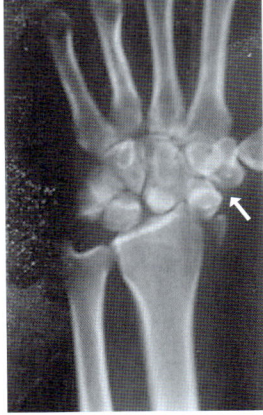 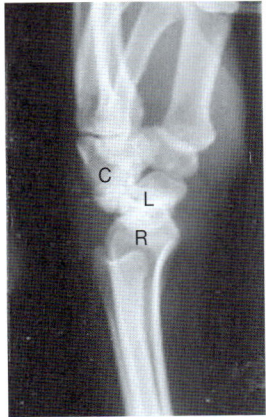

The scaphoid fracture is indicated by an arrow. The whole carpus except the lunate (L) is displaced posteriorly. The concavity of the lunate is empty but the radius (R) and lunate remain in a straight line. The capitate (C) lies posteriorly and out of line.

METACARPAL FRACTURES

- **Mechanism of injury**: Due either to a fall on an outstretched hand or due to a direct blow to the hand.
- **Clinical features**: Local tenderness, swelling, and deformity.
- **X-ray views**: AP and oblique views of the metacarpal.
- **Treatment/disposition**:
  1. If the fracture is undisplaced, apply a short arm back slab and review in Hand Surgery clinic early.
  2. If the fracture is displaced, attempt reduction under Bier's block, followed by application of a back slab. Review in Hand Surgery clinic early.
  3. If the fracture involves the metacarpal neck, the splint should extend beyond the proximal interphalangeal (PIP) joint with the metacarpophalangeal (MCP) joint flexed at 90 degrees. Review in Hand Surgery clinic early.

BENNETT'S FRACTURE

This is a fracture of the thumb metacarpal, where there is a small medial fragment of bone which may tilt, but which maintains its relationship with the trapezium.

- **X-ray views**: AP and lateral views of the thumb metacarpal.

NOTE: The vertical fracture line involves the trapezo-metacarpal joint and there is proximal and lateral subluxation of the thumb metacarpal.

- **Treatment/disposition**: Apply a scaphoid thumb spica back slab and admit to Hand Surgery for open reduction and internal fixation.

FRACTURES OF THE PROXIMAL AND MIDDLE PHALANGES OF FINGER(S)

- If the fracture is displaced, perform M&R under Entonox or a digital block first.
- Then apply an aluminium splint, extending from the wrist to the tip of the finger at volar aspect, with the MCP joint flexed at 90 degrees and the PIP joint extended.
- If the fracture is undisplaced, apply the aluminium splint without the M&R.
- Review in Hand Surgery clinic.

FRACTURES OF THE TERMINAL PHALANGES

- Treatment of soft tissue injury takes precedence.
- **Closed fractures**: No M&R is required; just apply a short aluminium splint to the volar aspect of the digit.
- **Open fractures (terminal tuft only)**
  1. Irrigate with a minimum 500 ml sterile saline.
  2. Administer IV cefazolin 1 g within an hour of the patient's arrival in the emergency department, before X-ray when possible.
  3. Apply a short aluminium splint to the volar aspect of the digit and review in Hand Surgery clinic early.
- **Open fracture (shaft or base)**: Administer IV antibiotics as above, apply dressing or an aluminium splint and admit to Hand Surgery clinic for open reduction and internal fixation.

References/Further Reading

1. McRae R. *Practical fracture treatment*. 5th ed. Edinburgh, UK: Churchill Livingstone; 2008.
2. ZJ Daruwalle, Ooi SB. Diagnosing anterior shoulder dislocation in the not-so-slim and obese: A novel examination technique. *Am J Emerg Med* 2013 Feb; 31(2): 406.

Amila Punyadasa • Irwani Ibrahim • Shirley Ooi

DEFINITIONS

- **Laceration**: Indicates blunt force trauma to soft tissues producing wounding with typically irregular wound edges.
- **Incised wound**: Indicates trauma to soft tissues produced by a cutting instrument as in the case of wounding produced by a knife or other cutting instruments.
- **Dirty wound**: Such as 'road rash' (an abrasion, resulting from the epidermis skidding tangentially across the hard ground usually after a road traffic accident) resulting from predominantly contact with the gravel may be 'dirty' but has a low bacterial count and thus do not have high rates of infection.
- **Contaminated wound**: Such as that exposed to, say, faecal matter in drains, has a high bacterial count and is considered contaminated. This type of wound experiences higher rates of wound infection and demands the use of prophylactic antibiotics.

CAVEATS

- **Good history** of event is important to determine possible associated injuries and the degree of contamination, e.g. punch bite, high pressure injection injuries, and crush injuries.
- A thorough examination for foreign bodies (FB), tendon function, neurovascular function, contamination, and infection is essential.
- Wounds should be explored under **appropriate anaesthesia** for thorough assessment.
- **Do not** explore neck wounds in the emergency department, no matter how superficial they may appear. There is a possibility of uncontrollable haemorrhage and those lacerations transgressing the platysma should be explored in the operating theatre.
- Document abnormalities or their **absence**. Photographs are an important tool in the documentation process.
- The following cases should be **X-rayed (anteroposterior/lateral views)**:
  1. All cases of wounds produced by glass.
  2. Selected cases to exclude open fractures, joint involvement, and foreign bodies.
- Radiopaque markers (useful tip – use two paperclips) taped to the wound in planes at 90 degrees to each other, may help identify the foreign body in relation to the wound.
- Wound swabs are **not** needed in fresh injuries unless they are associated with fractures.
- Haemorrhage should be controlled by direct pressure and elevation of the limb: **Do not** use artery forceps or tourniquets. However, in potentially exsanguinating haemorrhage, one may use an inflatable cuff (useful tip – use a Bier's block cuff) as a temporary and temporizing measure until emergent surgical intervention can be arranged.

- **Never** shave an eyebrow.
- **Do not remove** a large foreign body embedded in the wound.
- **Do not** prescribe antibiotics in patients with normal immune status with little wound contamination.
- Antibiotics **cannot** substitute for good wound debridement.
- Take the opportunity to update the patient's tetanus status.

> ⇨ **SPECIAL TIPS FOR GPs**
> - Refer cases to the emergency department if unable to achieve a good wound debridement due to time constraint or non-sterile conditions.
> - Beware of innocuous wounds which look 'benign' but may have extensive tissue destruction, e.g. **pressure jet injuries** or crush injuries.
> - Beware the so-called 'simple' **plantar puncture wound**. It is anything but simple (see page 698).

MANAGEMENT

- If haemorrhage is severe
  1. Secure the airway, breathing and circulation.
  2. Establish large bore intravenous (IV) line(s) and initiate fluid resuscitation.
  3. Group and cross match 2 to 4 units of blood.
  4. Elevate and compress.

NOTE: Although sterile techniques such as the routine use of sterile gloves have been adopted as the standard surgical practice, a multicentre, prospective, single-blinded, randomized trial suggests that the use of non-sterile clean gloves for treating single lacerations in a patient with no pre-existing risk factors is acceptable.

- **Technique**
  1. Wound cleaning is the most important part of wound care. Wounds should be cleaned with chlorhexidine solution **except** facial wounds (sterile normal saline).
  2. Wounds in hair-bearing areas should have the adjacent hair trimmed with scissors: Shaving may predispose the wound to infection through epidermal damage.
  3. Remove all dirt and foreign materials that are visible; deep wounds should be irrigated copiously with sterile normal saline. Irrigation with normal saline is the single most important step in preventing wound infection in traumatic wounds. For most wounds, 8 to 10 pounds per square inch (psi) is considered adequate and this can be attained using a 19G needle and a syringe with a 30-ml capacity. As a guide, the optimal volume of irrigant is 60 ml per cm of wound length.

4. Published evidence[13] has shown that tap water appears to be a viable, cost-effective alternative to sterile normal saline for wound irrigation in the emergency department. Despite the fact that published trials have inconsistent methods (e.g. differences in temperature, volume, and irrigation pressure), there appears to be no benefit of sterile over clean tap water.

5. The local anaesthetic drug of choice is **1% buffered plain lignocaine**, used for direct infiltration and nerve blocks.

NOTE: Evidence has shown that buffering of local anaesthetics to minimize the pain of infiltration appears to provide minimal benefit.[14] Topical antibiotic ointments should not be applied on tissue adhesives as they may result in dehiscence.

6. **Explore the wounds** when the presence of a foreign body is suspected and history is suggestive of deep damage with no clinical confirmation.

- There are 3 different types of wound closure:

  1. **Primary closure**: Involves closure of the wound margins within 24 hours of wound occurrence. More specifically this technique is used in closing any clean wound >6 to 8 hours old anywhere on the body.

NOTE: Wounds on the face and scalp have an excellent blood supply and thus may be closed primarily up to 24 hours post-wounding.

  2. **Secondary closure**: Allows the wound to heal by granulation without any mechanical approximation of the wound margins.

  3. **Delayed primary closure**: Involves closure of a dirty wound 3 to 5 days after wound occurrence to decrease the risk of infection from possible early wound closure. In the interim period the wound should be irrigated copiously and debrided judiciously and then packed with ribbon gauze soaked with a non-irritative antiseptic solution. A review of the wound in 3 days is essential to elicit signs of infection (erythema of wound edges or suppuration) which would preclude this type of wound closure.

- **Methods of closure**: If in doubt, suturing is always the best option:

  1. **Steristrips**

     a. Less painful to apply and less likely to cause tissue ischaemia.

     b. Fast and easy to use; saves time.

     c. Suitable for children, flap lacerations in the elderly, and skin closure where deep layer sutures have been placed.

     d. Inappropriate to apply over joints.

  2. **Tissue glue**

     a. Suitable for small cuts and lacerations in children and most suitable for lacerations which gape <3 mm. Tissue glue should especially be considered in those patients who are not likely to return for follow-up for suture removal or who cannot tolerate the pain of traditional sutures.

    b. Technique: Clean the wound and achieve good hameostasis. Oppose the wound edges and place the glue along the wound in a continuous line. Hold the edges together for at least 30 seconds to allow the glue to set. Do not place the glue into the wound as it acts as a foreign body.

    c. If one inadvertently gets tissue glue on the eye lids use 1% tetracycline ointment to break the adhesive bonds and remove the glue. Inadvertent application on less sensitive sites may be removed with the application of petroleum jelly.

3. **Staples**

    a. Very useful for long and superficial wounds in view of ease of and rapidity of application.

    b. It is not suitable for cosmetic wounds or deep wounds, as staples will not approximate deeper tissue planes.

    c. Advantages of this technique include low tissue reactivity of the staples and low risk of needlestick injuries.

4. **Suture technique**

    a. Generally, use a 2-layer technique (subcutaneous and skin) in deep wounds to promote better wound healing.

    b. Use absorbable sutures, e.g. Dexon or Vicryl for subcutaneous tissues:
       Trunk and extremities: 4/0 and face: 5/0.

    c. Use non-absorbable sutures for the skin, e.g. Prolene or Silk:
       Scalp: 2/0 Silk; trunk and extremities: 4/0 Prolene; and face: 6/0 Prolene.

    d. In general, one can use one size smaller sutures in children and can remove them earlier.

- **Disposition**: Consider **admission or referral**.

1. If the wound extends into the muscle, is heavily contaminated, is inadequately debrided or there is evidence of sensory or motor damage, admit to Orthopaedics.

2. Admit all wounds with tendon damage. Those with injuries distal to the wrist should be admitted to Hand Surgery. Admit all others to Orthopaedics.

3. Immuno-compromised, e.g. diabetic, chronic renal failure, and oncology patients.

4. Large wounds: Surgery requires 30–60 minutes of theatre time.

5. Refer special wounds, e.g. eyelid lacerations to Plastic Surgery.

WOUNDS NOT SUITABLE FOR PRIMARY CLOSURE

- Bites, except facial bite wounds.
- Heavily contaminated wounds.
- Infected wounds.
- Wounds that are >12 hours old except facial/scalp wounds.

Wound care

- Remember the mnemonics **LACERATE**.

  1. **L** Look at the wound (the planning phase includes setting up the necessary closure devices and equipment).
  2. **A** Anaesthetize.
  3. **C** Clip and clean the wound.
  4. **E** Evaluate for wound repair.
  5. **R** Repair the wound.
  6. **A** Assess the adequacy of the wound repair and revise as necessary.
  7. **T** Anti-tetanus toxoid is given to the patient.
  8. **E** Educate (give wound care advice and provide dates for suture removal).

- Wounds should be dressed with a non-adherent dressing, e.g. Tulle-gras.
- Dressing is not necessary for facial and scalp wounds.
- The wound should be kept clean and dry for at least 48 hours after primary closure.
- **Suture removal**:

  1. Scalp: 7 days
  2. Face: 3–5 days
  3. Limbs: 10–14 days
  4. Trunk: 10 days

- Review contaminated wounds daily; clean wounds can be reviewed at 3 to 5 days.
- Consider **antibiotics prophylaxis** in the following:

  1. All contaminated wounds.
  2. Compound fingertip fractures.
  3. Bite wounds.
  4. Wounds in those at risk, e.g. valvular heart disease and post-splenectomy.
  5. Penetrating injuries not properly debrided.
  6. Wounds that are >6 hours old.
  7. Complex intra-oral wounds.
  8. Workers at high risk, e.g. agricultural workers and fishermen.
  9. Consider in selected patients with conditions such as immuno-suppression (e.g. diabetes mellitus) and those with poor predisposition to wound healing (e.g. patients with peripheral vascular disease with a foot laceration).
  10. Choice of antibiotics: Cloxacillin and penicillin (commonest infecting organisms are *Staphylococcal aureus* and *Beta-haemolytic streptococcus*) are cost-effective choices; Augmentin®.

NOTE: There is evidence to show that topical antibiotics in traumatic wounds are recommended.

SPECIAL WOUNDS AND ANATOMICAL SITES

Plantar puncture wounds

- These wounds look innocuous but remember that the joints of the foot are not deep. Hence joint penetration is a possibility with potential for serious infectious complications. The area from the metatarsal neck to the distal toes is at highest risk for infection.
- The **complications** include:
  1. *Staph* and *Strep* soft tissue infections in the majority of patients.
  2. Osteomyelitis (90% of osteomyelitis is due to *Pseudomonas aeruginosa*).
- Perform an X-ray to exclude foreign bodies and joint penetration.
- The **management** of puncture wounds is **controversial**. The following are **guidelines** based on different clinical presentations:
  1. **Simple punctures**

     Usually with clean objects such as tacks, needles, and small non-rusty exposed nails. If none of the following is seen, i.e. indications of a retained foreign body, dirty and devitalized wound edges or an indurated or excessively tender puncture site, skin cleansing and a small application of an antibiotic ointment, followed by a Band-Aid should suffice.
  2. **Puncture with retained material**
     a. The puncture is often larger than the above mentioned. The wound edges are contaminated, stellate, or shredded appearing.
     b. Usually due to old nails, exposed bolts, and unclean puncturing objects that broke during the puncture or possibly has forced sock or shoe fragment in the wound.
     c. After providing anaesthesia, a transverse incision parallel to the wrinkle line of a curled foot is made through the puncture site and any foreign body is removed.
     d. Thorough irrigation is carried out.
     e. Do not suture the wound. Just apply an antibiotic ointment and a Band-Aid.
     f. Administer tetanus prophylaxis.
     g. Advise the patient to use crutches for 2 to 3 days.
     h. Discharge with antibiotics, e.g. Augmentin®.
     i. Advise the patient to look out for signs of infection.
     j. Review the wound early.
  3. **Complicated punctures**
     a. Suspect the presence of a retained foreign body if the puncture site is infected.
     b. Do X-rays to exclude the presence of a radiopaque foreign body.
     c. Give IV broad spectrum antibiotics, e.g. Unasyn® or Augmentin®.
     d. Administer tetanus prophylaxis.
     e. Admit for further management, i.e. surgical debridement.

NOTE:

- The use of **prophylactic antibiotics** in uninfected puncture wounds is not supported by clinical studies. They should only be considered in high risk patients and wounds.
- Extensive coring or debridement of vital tissues, high pressure irrigation, or deep probing has not been shown to improve outcome.
- In prescribing antibiotics, remember about possible **pseudomonal infection** and consider ciprofloxacin therapy.

Pretibial flap wounds

- The blood supply of the flap wounds may be compromised, especially distally based flaps.
- Flap wounds are suitable for primary suturing if they occur in the region of the face or in a young patient where quality of the skin is good.
- The skin in the elderly is thin, hence the flap may die if sutured under even minimal tension.
- Consider the use of a corner stitch and tagging steristrips or loose sutures to approximate such a flap. Advise the patient that there is a high risk of wound closure failure necessitating plastic surgical intervention later and then document clearly in your clinical notes. Wound failure in this case scenario has been a relatively common source for litigation.
- Consideration must be given to primary excision and grafting, especially if the flap is large.

Scalp wounds

- Lacerations of the scalp have the propensity to bleed to a degree sufficient to cause hypovolaemia requiring fluid resuscitation and even death. This bleeding is due to both (1) the high vascularity of the scalp and (2) the integrity of the dense connective tissue (CT) layer of the scalp, which although is protective against infection, tends to hold vessels open in the context of a scalp laceration.
- The best way to secure scalp wound haemostasis is to apply a pressure bandage.
- In the preparation for wound closure, remove any gross contaminants, and briefly cleanse the wound. Subsequently, use a 2/0 Silk suture to take deep bites of all five layers of the scalp. This will almost invariably stop the bleeding. It is not necessary to suture or diathermize the bleeding point.
- It is not uncommon for scalp lacerations to be accompanied by large haematomas underlying the wound. These haematomas are potential sources for infection and must be removed prior to closure.
- Do not shave any hair. Rather, trim it flush with the scalp. Shaving damages the epidermis and hair follicles and may predispose the wound to infection.

- **Hair Apposition Technique (HAT)** where hair on both sides of the laceration (Figure 1a) is apposed with a single twist (Figure 1b) and held with tissue adhesives (Figure 1c) is a useful technique for treating scalp lacerations, especially in children.

FIGURE 1   Hair Apposition Technique

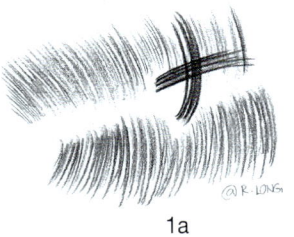
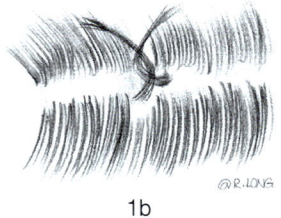
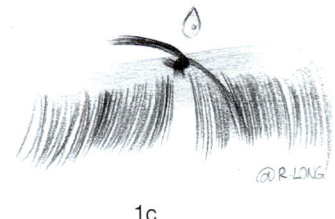

| 1a | 1b | 1c |

1. **Advantages**
   a. Reduced pain.
   b. Increased speed.
   c. Simplicity.
   d. No follow up necessary.
   e. No chance of needlestick injuries.
   f. Reduced costs.
   g. No hair removal necessary.
   h. Reduce scarring by 69% (6.3% versus 20.4%).
   i. A decreased rate of any complication with respect to suturing by 66% (7.4% versus 21.5%).
2. **Disadvantages**
   a. Apposition of only the outermost layers of the skin, allowing for the creation of a potential dead space, especially in deep scalp wounds.

Eye wounds

- A complete eye examination including visual acuity is mandatory.
- X-ray examination of the orbits is needed if the presence of an intra-ocular foreign body is suspected, such as when there is a history of foreign body entry or metal-on-metal episode but no foreign body is seen on the surface of the cornea or when there is a distortion of the shape of the iris.
- The **'no-go' areas** are as follows:
  1. Intramarginal eyelid lacerations.
  2. Lacerations to the lacrimal gland or its drainage mechanism (the tear duct apparatus).
  3. Lacerations to the medial canthal ligament.
  4. Lacerations to the tarsal plate.
  5. Lacerations that may involve the globe.
  6. Lacerations involving the levator palpebrae superioris.

- Lid lacerations which cross the lid margins, those through both surfaces of the lid and those that may have damaged the lacrimal gland or duct must be referred to Ophthalmology or Plastic Surgery, depending on institutional practice.

Nasal wounds

- Examine for septal haematoma. If present, urgent drainage will be needed.
- Caveats for closure of uncomplicated lacerations:
  1. Suture simple lacerations over undisplaced fractures only.
  2. Use 6/0 monofilament non-absorbable sutures.
  3. Remove sutures in 3 to 5 days.
  4. No antibiotics necessary.
- Full thickness lacerations will need careful layered suturing. If severe, should be referred to Plastic Surgery.
- The main principle is to **accurately** appose the junction between the skin and the mucosa.
- In the context of an open fracture, the decision to close depends on fracture morphology.
  1. Uncomplicated laceration of the skin over an undisplaced nasal fracture may be **closed**.
  2. Complex lacerations with fracture displacement, mucosal injury from bone fragmentation, **or** extensive cartilaginous involvement should be **referred for formal closure**.

Lip wounds

- It is of **utmost importance** to accurately align the **vermillion border** if the wound *crosses the junction of the lip and the skin.*
- The next most important step is to align the **mucosal border** between the intra-oral and extra-oral mucosa.
- The above two steps are vital for cosmesis.
- Through and through wounds should be repaired in layers.
- **Aftercare of lip lacerations**:
  1. Do not bring excessive pressure to bear on the suture line while the sutures are in place.
  2. Mouth rinsing after eating to prevent small particulate matter from penetrating the suture line.
  3. STO extra-oral sutures 4 to 5 days in adults and between 3 and 5 days in children.
  4. For intra-oral lacerations, studies have demonstrated a benefit from penicillin V or erythromycin prophylaxis.

Tongue wounds

- Must check for embedded teeth.
- May consider X-rays to exclude the presence of foreign bodies.
- Minor wounds need not be repaired.
- Refer large bleeding wounds to Dental Surgery or Plastic Surgery.
- Use absorbable sutures with short resorption time, e.g. catgut 5/0.

Ear wounds

- Give a ring block around the ear to provide anaesthesia.
- If some cartilage is lacerated, generally, percutaneous skin closure alone affords enough tensile repair that allows adequate healing.
- Always apply pressure (with ribbon gauze) bandage, termed *Mastoid dressing*, after toilet and suture to prevent perichondral haematoma formation. If this important step is omitted, the patient may develop fibrosis and scarring with intolerable cosmetic sequelae (i.e. the dreaded 'cauliflower ear').
- Always give antibiotics and review in 1 to 2 days. Its utility is to prevent chondritis with subsequent wound breakdown. Suture removal in 4 to 5 days is ideal.

Acknowledgment

Figure 1 of this chapter was drawn by Ms Rebecca Long.

References/Further Reading

1. Trott A. *Wounds and Lacerations: Emergency Care and Closure*. St. Louis, MO: Mosby; 1991.
2. Wardrope J. *The Management of Wounds and Burns*. New York: Oxford University Press; 1992.
3. Wedmore IS, Charette J. Emergency department evaluation and treatment of ankle and foot injuries. In: Della-Giustina D, Coppola M, eds. *Emerg Med Clin North Am*. 2000; 18(1): 108–109.
4. Ong MEH, Ooi SBS, Saw SM, et al. A randomized controlled trial comparing the hair apposition technique with tissue glue to standard suturing in scalp lacerations (HAT study). *Ann Emerg Med*. 2002; 40: 19–26.
5. Howell JM, Chishholm CD. Wound care. *Emerg Med Clin North Am*. 1997; 15: 417–425.
6. Singer AJ, Hollander JE, Quinn JV. Evaluation and management of traumatic lacerations. *N Eng J Med*. 1997; 337: 1142–1148.
7. Brown DJ, Jaffe JE, Henson JK. Advanced laceration management. *Emerg Med Clin North Am*. Feb 2007; 25(1): 83–99.
8. Baurmash HD, Monto M. Delayed healing human bite wounds of the orofacial area managed with immediate primary closure: Treatment rationale. *J Oral Maxillofac Surg*. Sep 2005; 63(9): 1391–1397.
9. Patel A. Tongue lacerations. *Br Dent J*. 12 Apr 2008; 204(7): 355.
10. Perry JD, Aguilar CL, Kuchtey R. Modified vertical mattress technique for eyelid margin repair. *Dermatol Surg*. Dec 2004; 30(12 Part 2): 1580–1582.
11. Section Six: Emergency Wound Management. In: Tintinalli JE, Ma OJ, Stapczynski JS, et al., eds. *Tintinalli's Emergency Medicine: A Comprehensive Study Guide*. 7th ed. New York: McGraw-Hill; 2011: 299–360.
12. Perelman VS, Francis GJ, Rutledge T, et al. Sterile versus nonsterile gloves for repair of uncomplicated lacerations in the emergency department and randomized controlled trial. *Ann Emerg Med*. 2004; 43: 362–370.
13. Fernandez R, Griffiths R, Ussia C. Water for wound cleaning. *Cochrare Database Syst Rev*. 2002; 4: CD 00386.
14. Pire D, Coppola M, Dwyer DA, et al. Prospective evaluation of topical antibiotics for preventing infections in uncomplicated soft-tissue wounds repaired in the ED. *Acad Emerg Med*. 1995; 2: 4–10.

Peng Li Lee • Shirley Ooi

⇨ **SPECIAL TIPS FOR GPs**

- Suspect **foreign bodies (FB)** in the nose in a child who presents with foul smelling nasal discharge.
- Enquire about the **ingestion of foreign bodies** in patients who present with chest pain not suggestive of angina.
- Do **not** use the **syringing technique** to remove **organic FB** (e.g. pea, sponge, and tissue paper) in the ear as it may swell up rending removal difficult, and there may also be a danger of tympanic membrane perforation.
- Suspect **epiglottitis** in a sick patient with severe sore throat, muffled voice, and an absence of significant findings from an examination of the oral cavity.

BELL'S PALSY (IDIOPATHIC FACIAL NERVE PARALYSIS)

- The most common cause of facial paralysis worldwide.
- A diagnosis of exclusion.
- **The role of the emergency physician** is to
  1. Exclude other causes of facial paralysis.
  2. Begin appropriate treatment.
  3. Protect the eye.
  4. Arrange appropriate follow-up.
- **Clinical features**
  1. Sudden onset: A partial paralysis of gradual onset is likely to have an underlying aetiology (e.g. tumour).
  2. Unilateral paralysis/weakness on one side of the entire face: Eyebrow sagging, inability to close the eyes, decreased nasolabial fold, and downwards slanting of the corners of the mouth.
  3. Pay particular attention to sparing of the forehead muscles (orbicularis and frontalis), which is indicative of a central (upper motor neuron) lesion.
  4. Other symptoms include drooling, decreased tearing, altered taste, hyperacusis, and pain behind the ear.
  5. Look into the ear for vesicles or scabs (indicative of herpes zoster – **Ramsay Hunt Syndrome**) and examine the parotid gland for a mass lesion.
  6. Association with a recent upper respiratory tract infection/viral syndrome.

- **Differential diagnosis** of Bell's palsy may be considered in relationship to the course of the seventh nerve.
  1. Intracranial: Meningioma and acoustic neuroma
  2. Intratemporal: Acute/chronic ear disease, herpes zoster, temporal bone fracture, or tumour
  3. Extratemporal: Parotid malignancy and facial laceration

A careful history and ear, nose and throat (ENT)/parotid gland/neurological examination should be able to differentiate the above causes.

- **Management**

  Up to 70% of untreated patients with Bell's palsy have good recovery, while about 15% have poor or no recovery. **Poor prognostic factors** include complete facial paralysis, older age, diabetes, hypertension, taste impairment, and an absence of nerve excitability in nerve conduction study.

  Current evidence suggests that steroid is probably effective and acyclovir is possibly effective in improving functional facial outcome. We recommend early treatment (within 3 days of onset of symptoms) of all patients with Bell's palsy on combination of prednisolone and acyclovir, unless the risk of treatment, e.g. deranged sugar control, outweighs the benefit.

  1. **Steroids**
     a. Dosage: 1 mg/kg (60–80 mg) for 1 week.
     b. Precautions: To be used with caution in patients with diabetes, peptic ulcer disease, hepatic dysfunction, hepatitis B, and pre-existing psychiatric conditions.
  2. **Acyclovir (Zovirax®)**
     a. Dosage: 800 mg 5 times daily for 1 week.
     b. Precautions: To be used with caution in patients with renal impairment.
  3. **Eye care**
     a. Artificial tears and eyeglasses/shields/taping of eyelids at night to decrease the risk of corneal drying and ulceration.
  4. **Referrals**
     a. Neurology: Atypical presentation of Bell's palsy or other neurological signs found.
     b. ENT: All typical Bell's palsy.
     c. Eye: Unexplained ocular pain or abnormal eye findings.

EPISTAXIS

- Priorities are to:
  1. Assess and **stabilize** the haemodynamic status.
  2. **Identify the site** and cause of bleeding.
  3. **Stop the bleeding.**

- Most nose bleeds come from ruptured blood vessels on the nasal septum. Absence of anterior bleeding site, presence of bilateral nose bleed, or blood draining down the oropharynx is suggestive of a posterior source.
- **Differential diagnosis**: Blood dyscrasias, local vascular malformation, e.g. hereditary telangiectasia, nasal tumour, and trauma.
- Institute **stabilization** efforts upon arrival at the emergency department:
  1. Pinch the nostril between a finger and the thumb for at least 10 minutes.
  2. Apply ice packs to the bridge of the nose.
  3. Have the patient sit up and hold a bowl into which the blood can drip. Swallowing, which may displace the accumulating clot, must be discouraged.
  4. If the patient is **unstable haemodynamically**:
     a. Transfer the patient to the critical care area.
     b. Establish a peripheral intravenous (IV) line and administer crystalloids at a rate sufficient to maintain perfusion.
     c. Take blood for group and cross matching, full blood count, urea/electrolytes/creatinine, and coagulation profile.
     d. Monitoring: Electrocardiogram (ECG), vital signs q 5–15 minutes, and pulse oximetry.
- Proceed **to identify the source of bleeding** (good illumination with a headlight is required).
  1. Remove clotted blood with Tilley's forceps or sucker.
  2. As each part of the nasal septum comes into view, it may be sprayed with cophenylcaine (constricts the blood vessels and anaesthetizes the mucosa).
- **Upon cessation of haemorrhage**
  1. Bleeding points seen may be cauterized with a bead of silver nitrate on a stick (avoid cauterizing both sides of the nasal septum due to a small risk of septal perforation) or packed with gauze soaked in adrenaline 1:10,000 for 15–30 minutes.
  2. If there is no further bleeding after a short period of observation, the patient may be discharged with bed rest advice and an early ENT clinic review.
  3. **If bleeding persists**, anterior nasal packing is required:
     a. Options: Merocel (8 or 10 cm pack for adults) lubricated with tetracycline ointment, BIPP (bismuth subnitrate and iodoform paste) using a Tilley's nasal dressing forceps.
     b. Admit the patient for observation and oral antibiotics.
  4. **If bleeding persists despite the presence of an effective anterior nasal pack**, posterior nasal packing is required:
     a. Reassess haemodynamic stability: Monitor the vital signs, take blood for full blood count, coagulation profile, GXM, and urea/electrolytes/creatinine.
     b. A Foley catheter (size 12) is inserted via the nostril (choose the side from which more bleeding is suspected) until the tip is seen in the oral pharynx.

- Inflate the balloon of the Foley catheter with 8 ml of water and withdraw the Foley catheter until the balloon sits snugly at the postnasal space, at which point, further inflate the Foley catheter with another 8 ml of water.
- Secure the catheter at the nose with an umbilical clamp and guard the ala from pressure of the catheter. **Tip:** Cut the proximal end of the Foley catheter and thread the clamp through the catheter to act as a cushion for the ala.

- **Disposition**: Admit the patient for observation and oral antibiotics **after** ENT consultation. **Always refer to an ENT medical officer** for review:
  1. If epistaxis is prolonged.
  2. In the event of repeat visits.
  3. If recurrent epistaxis presents.
  4. If the patient is elderly.

FRACTURE OF NASAL BONES

- **Caused** by direct trauma to the nose.
- **Clinical features**:
  1. Distorted nose shape.
  2. Soft tissue swelling.
  3. Tenderness over the nasal bone area.
- **Important to exclude**
  1. Injuries to other parts of the facial skeleton.
  2. **Septal haematoma** (bluish swelling on both sides of the nasal septum visible from the front of the nose): If present **urgent ENT referral** is required for haematoma aspiration/incision and drainage, in order to prevent the development of septal ischaemia or abscess, which may lead to necrosis, collapse, and deformity of the cartilaginous structure of the nose.
- Nasal X-ray is done more for medicolegal reasons. It does not affect the clinical management.
- The need for **manipulation and reduction (M&R)** should be assessed 5 to 7 days post-injury, when the soft tissue swelling has subsided. M&R is usually done within 7 to 10 days of injury before the nasal bones become firmly set.

FOREIGN BODY: EAR

- Generally, a foreign body can be removed using microforceps or a blunt hook (under otoscopy) or syringing.
- In an uncooperative child, removal under general anaesthesia is advised.
  1. If the foreign body is an insect: Kill it with a few drops of 1% lignocaine or olive oil before removing it with microforceps.
  2. Organic foreign bodies (e.g. pea, tissue paper, and sponge): **Do not** use the syringing technique as they may swell up, rendering removal difficult.

- If removal of the foreign body is deemed difficult under otoscopy, refer to the ENT clinic (during office hours) where a microscope is available.
- One attempt by an emergency department staff is recommended, failing which the patient should be referred to the ENT clinic.

FOREIGN BODY: NOSE

- Usually occurs in a child, presenting with unilateral, foul smelling nasal discharge.
- There is the danger of inhalation and obstruction of the respiratory tract during removal, especially if the patient is supine during the removal attempt. **Tip**: Secure the child in a papoose restrainer held vertically against the assistant's legs for the removal attempt.
- If the foreign body is of an irregular shape, use small alligator forceps for removal.
- If it is a round or smooth foreign body, use a blunt hook (e.g. Jobson-Horne's probe) to engage the posterior end of the foreign body before removing it.
- A cophenylcaine nasal spray may be used to aid the removal of the foreign body by causing mucosal shrinkage.
- One attempt at removal by an emergency department staff is recommended, failing which, the ENT medical officer should be informed for keep in view removal of the foreign body under general anaesthesia.

FOREIGN BODY: THROAT

- Ask about the nature of the foreign body: Fish bone, chicken bone, etc.
- Ask the patient to identify the exact site of pain: Pain over the lower part of the neck or chest may suggest an oesophageal foreign body which is not easily visualized clinically and radiologically (lateral neck X-ray).
- Enquire about the presence of haemoptysis or haemetemesis and migratory pain, e.g. from the throat to the neck, or the neck to the chest.
- Inspect the tonsillar region carefully. Options are:
  1. Indirect laryngoscopy (IDL).
  2. Fibreoptic nasopharyngoscopy.
  3. Direct pharyngolaryngoscopy using a laryngoscope with the patient lying supine after the throat has been sprayed with cophenylcaine. The advantage of this technique is that a foreign body can be removed easily with Magill's forceps. It allows a quick look and this should only be done for children as they are often uncooperative. For an adult, it is better to use IDL or fibreoptic nasopharyngoscopy to visualize.
- Inspect closely for foreign bodies at the tonsillar poles, base of the tongue, vallecular region and pyriform fossae.
- If no foreign body can be seen, proceed with lateral (soft tissue) X-ray of the neck.
- If the X-ray shows the presence of a foreign body, inform the ENT medical officer.

- If the **X-ray and IDL** are **negative** for foreign bodies **and the patient is comfortable**, reassure and treat symptomatically with lozenges and gargle. Oral antibiotics (e.g. amoxicillin, formerly amoxycillin) may be considered if an ulcer or abrasion is seen. Refer to the ENT clinic in 1 to 2 days for review. The discharge advice should be to return immediately if there is dyspnoea, fever, chest pain, or haemetemesis.
- If the X-ray and IDL are **negative** for foreign bodies but the **patient is still symptomatic**, inform the ENT medical officer for review and keep in view the barium swallow test (especially for the lower neck pain and chest pain) or rigid oesophagoscopy under general anaesthesia.
- See Figure 1 for the algorithm showing the management of foreign bodies in the throat.

FIGURE 1   A practical algorithm showing the management of foreign bodies in the throat

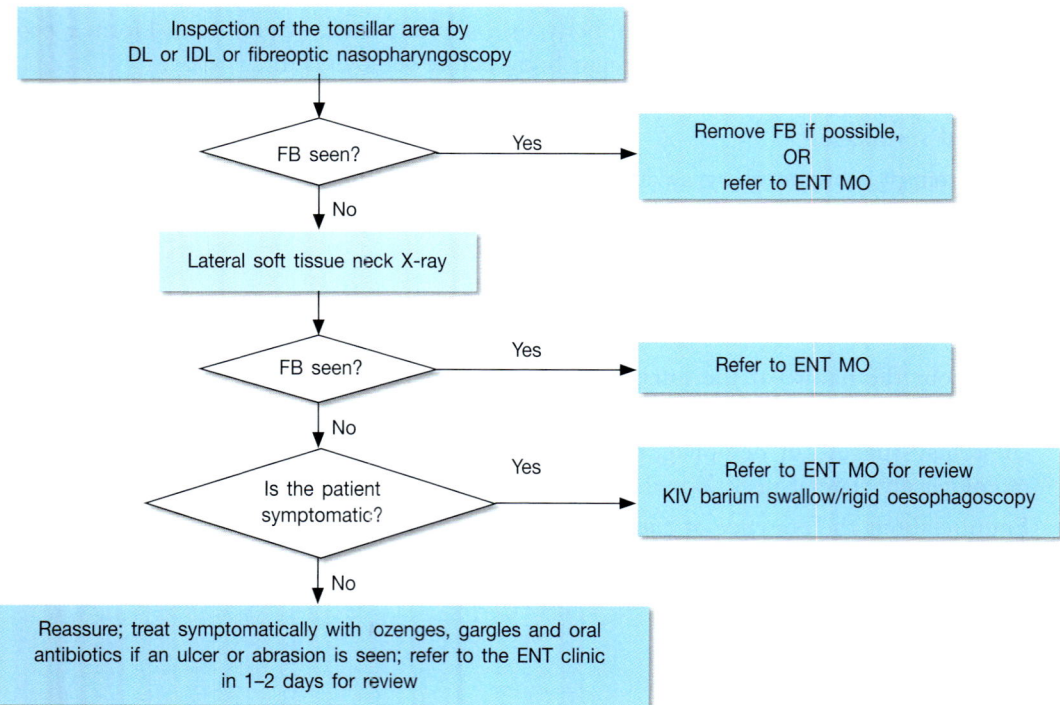

HEARING LOSS: SUDDEN, SENSORINEURAL HEARING LOSS (SSNHL)

- This is a medical emergency.
- Definition: A sudden hearing loss in a period of less than 72 hours. The ear examination typically reveals a sensorineural hearing loss.
- Differentiate from:
  1. Bilateral progressive sensorineural hearing loss (SNHL): Presbyacusis is a common cause.
  2. Unilateral progressive SNHL: Ménière's disease and acoustic neuroma.

- **Clinical features**

  1. Usually unilateral.

  2. Weber test: Lateralizes away from the affected ear.

  3. Rinne test may be positive (in the partially deaf ear: Air conduction is still better than bone conduction in SNHL) or falsely negative (in a totally deaf ear: Bone conducted sound from the deaf ear will be heard by the intact cochlea on the unaffected side).

- **Causes**

  1. Trauma to head or ear: Traumatic tears of the intralabyrinthine membranes (perilymph fistula).

  2. Infection: For example, herpes viruses, mumps, measles, rubella, syphilis, tuberculosis, mycoplasma, etc.

  3. Vascular: Sudden impairment of cochlear blood flow.

  4. Autoimmune causes.

  5. Neoplasm: For example, acoustic neuroma, which usually presents as unilateral progressive SNHL.

  6. Ototoxic drugs: Aminoglycosides, anti-malarials, vancomycin, erythromycin, and loop diuretics.

  7. Idiopathic (i.e. there is no apparent cause).

- **Treatment** is empirical if no obvious cause is found.

- Oral steroids have been considered to be the standard therapy for SNHL. Antiviral drugs have also been used empirically despite the lack of conclusive evidence.

  1. Systemic steroids: Prednisolone in a reducing dose over 5 days (1 mg/kg).

  2. Vasodilator drugs: For example, Tanakan® (ginko biloba) 1 tab 3 times a day (tds).

  3. Antiviral drugs: Acyclovir (400 mg 5 times daily for 1 week).

OTITIS MEDIA: ACUTE

- Common childhood illness: Common causative organisms are *Streptococcus pneumoniae*, *Haemophilus influenzae*, and *Moraxella catarrhalis*.

- **Clinical features**:

  1. Fever.

  2. Earache.

  3. Ear discharge if the tympanic membrane is perforated.

- **Examination findings**: The tympanic membrane appears red and bulging or perforated with a mucopurulent discharge on otoscopy.

- **Treatment**:

  1. Oral antibiotic options: Amoxicillin, augmentin, cefaclor, co-trimaxazole, and erythromycin.

  2. Topical nasal decongestant, e.g. Iliadin® (oxymetazolin) 3 times daily for 5 days.

3. Oral antihistamines, e.g. promethazine, Clarityne®, Clarinase®, and Zyrtec®.
4. Analgesia.
5. Antibiotic ear drops are indicated only if the tympanic membrane is ruptured (this differs from the treatment of traumatic rupture of the tympanic membrane).

- Refer to the ENT clinic for follow-up.

OTITIS MEDIA: CHRONIC

- Chronic otitis media (COM) refers to a chronic non-healing tympanic membrane perforation, usually associated with a conductive hearing loss.
- The patient often presents with an acute super-infection with a mucopurulent discharge; otalgia is unusual.
- Treat with topical antibiotics and refer to the ENT clinic for aural toilet.

NOTE: Oral antibiotics are only indicated if concurrent pharyngitis/sinusitis is suspected.

OTITIS EXTERNA: ACUTE

- **Presents** with itching, ear pain, and ear discharge.
- **Clinically** there may be diffuse inflammation or a furuncle.
- **Treatment** is with topical antibiotics (with steroid combination), e.g. otosporin or sofradex 2 drops 3 times daily and analgesia.
  1. Oral antibiotics are indicated **only** when there is a **systemic illness with fever and lymphadenitis**.
  2. Refer to ENT for follow-up.
- **Suspect 'malignant' otitis externa** if the pain is excessive of clinical signs, especially in the elderly/diabetic patients.
  1. Requires admission for IV antibiotics.
  2. Risk of spread of infection to the base of the skull and adjacent soft tissues.

PERITONSILLAR ABSCESS (QUINSY)

- **Presents** with a typical picture of tonsillitis but
  1. Is almost always unilateral.
  2. Is associated with increasing difficulty in swallowing (dysphagia).
  3. Is associated with painful swallowing (odynophagia).
  4. There is limited ability to open the mouth fully (trismus).
- **Clinical examination**: The involved tonsil is often obscured by a swollen soft palate and the uvula is displaced contralaterally.
- **Treatment**: Incision and drainage under local anaesthesia; refer to the ENT medical officer.

SINUSITIS

- **Classically divided into**:
  1. Acute: Symptoms lasting less than 3 weeks.
  2. Subacute: Symptoms lasting for 3 weeks to 3 months.
  3. Chronic: Symptoms lasting more than 3 months.
- **Commonly presents with**:
  1. A persistent cold.
  2. Nasal congestion.
  3. A purulent discharge.
  4. Facial pain with headache.
- **Clinical findings**:
  1. Purulent secretions in the middle meatus may be seen using a nasal speculum and a direct light.
     NOTE: Purulent secretions may be seen better if the nasal mucosa is first decongested with a cophenylcaine nasal spray.
  2. Facial tenderness on palpation.
- **X-rays**:
  1. Uncomplicated sinusitis is often a clinical diagnosis and imaging is not mandatory.
  2. Plain sinus films have a high (40%) false negative rate. Radiographic signs of infection: Air-fluid levels are present in the affected sinus on the paranasal sinus X-ray.
- Exclude **complications**: Intracranial extension of infection, osteomyelitis, and orbital cellulitis in children.
- **Goals of treatment** in uncomplicated sinusitis is:
  1. To relieve obstruction of the sinus ostia.
  2. Avoid antihistamines as they thicken secretions.
     a. **Nasal decongestant**: Oxymetazoline (Iliadin®) nose drops.
        Dosage: Adult 0.05%; paediatric 0.025%; and infants 0.01% for 3 to 5 days.
     b. **Systemic decongestant**: Pseudoephedrine (Sudafed®).
     c. **Antibiotics**: Empiric coverage for *Haemophilus influenzae and Streptococcus pneumoniae*; in addition *Moraxella catarrhalis* in children.
        Dosage: Take the following for a minimum of 10–14 days:

	Augmentin	**Bactrim**
Adult:	625 mg bd (twice daily)	2 tabs bd
Child: 6 years	5 ml bd	
Child: 7–12 years	10 ml bd (228 mg/5 ml)	

If the patient is allergic to penicillin, alternative antibiotics are cephalosporins or azithromycin.

- Refer to the ENT clinic for follow-up.

TONSILLITIS: ACUTE

- The patient presents with sore throat and fever.
- **Clinical examination**: The tonsils are injected, swollen, and may show purulent exudates.
- **Differentials** to consider: Diphtheria and infectious mononucleosis.
- **Treat** with antibiotics (penicillin is the antibiotic of choice), gargles, lozenges, and anti-pyretic agents.
- Consider **admission** for IV antibiotics/hydration if
  1. Tonsillitis is prolonged.
  2. The patient has a prolonged fever.
  3. The patient has difficulty swallowing.
  4. The patient is clinically dehydrated.
- The patient can be discharged with oral antibiotics for 10 days with a referral for review by a general practitioner if the infection is non-recurrent. Refer to the ENT clinic if there are recurrent episodes over several years or multiple episodes per year.

TYMPANIC MEMBRANE: ACUTE, TRAUMATIC PERFORATION

- Usually caused by a slap or punch to the side of the head.
- Other causes: Foreign body insertion, forceful ear irrigation, barotrauma (air travel or scuba diving), and sudden negative pressure (suction applied to ear canal).
- **Clinical features**
  1. Unilateral otalgia, hearing loss, tinnitus, vertigo, and bleeding from the affected ear.
  2. Perforation of the tympanic membrane seen on otoscopy (often blood-stained).
  3. A variable degree of conductive hearing loss depending on the size of the perforation (the Weber test lateralizes to the side of the TM perforation; negative Rinne test).
  4. Rarely sensorineural hearing loss is found. If present, suspect injury to the connection of the third ossicle (the stapes) with the inner ear (the Weber test lateralizes away from the side of the TM perforation; positive Rinne test).
- **Management**
  1. Give analgesics.
  2. **Do not** prescribe ear drops.
  3. Give prophylactic broad spectrum oral antibiotics e.g. amoxicillin in a dirty injury.
  4. Important to instruct the patient to **keep the affected ear dry**:
     a. No swimming.
     b. Use vaseline-soaked cotton-ball in the affected ear if necessary during baths/showers.

There is generally an excellent chance of spontaneous complete healing within 3 months (>90%) in traumatic perforation.

- **Disposition**
    1. If there is **hearing loss**, refer the patient to the ENT clinic on the **next** working day for documentation of the hearing loss.
    2. If there is **no hearing loss**, refer the patient to the ENT clinic within a week.

References/Further Reading

1. Ludman H. *ABC of Otolaryngology*. 4th ed. London: BMJ Books; 1997.

2. Salinas RA, Alvarez G, Ferreira J. Corticosteroids for Bell's palsy (idiopathic facial paralysis). *Cochrane Database Syst Rev*. 2004; CD001942.

3. Grogan PM, Gronseth GS. Practice parameter: Steroids, acyclovir, and surgery for Bell's palsy (an evidence-based review). Report of the Quality Standards Subcommittee of the American Academy of Neurology. *Neurology*. 2001; 56: 830.

4. Allen D, Dunn L. Aciclovir or valaciclovir for Bell's palsy (idiopathic facial paralysis). *Cochrane Database Syst Rev*. 2004; CD001869.

5. Rauch SD. Clinical practice. Idiopathic sudden sensorineural hearing loss. *N Engl J Med*. 2008; 359: 833.

6. Slattery WH, Fisher LM, Iqbal Z, Liu N. Oral steroid regimens for idiopathic sudden sensorineural hearing loss. *Otolaryngol Head Neck Surg*. 2005; 132: 5.

Please refer to Chapter 4, *Blurring of Vision* and Chapter 20, *Red Eye*.

107 Assault (non-sexual)

Peter Manning

DEFINITION

- **Abrasion**
  1. The most superficial type of injury, i.e. scratch or graze.
  2. Confined to the epidermis or most superficial of dermis.
- **Contusion, i.e. bruise**
  1. Blunt injury to the tissues damaging blood vessels beneath the surface, allowing blood to extravasate (leak) into the surrounding tissues.
  2. May be associated with overlying lacerations or abrasions.
  3. May be flat or elevated.
- **Laceration, i.e. cut, gash, or tear**
  1. A splitting or tearing wound caused by **blunt** injury that passes through the full thickness of the skin and thus bleeds profusely.
  2. Should **not** be confused with an incised wound.
- **Incised wounds**, i.e. 2 types of sharply-cut wounds caused by an object with a **cutting edge**.
  1. Slash wound in which the length is greater than the depth.
  2. Stab wound in which the depth is greater than the length.

CAVEATS

- Assume that all assault cases will come to court and that you may be called upon to give evidence, whereupon your opinion becomes public knowledge. The case may come to court several years after the attack. You will have to rely on your written notes taken at the time of the examination in addition to any diagrammatic or photographic evidence that you obtained.
- Therefore, your medical records should be thorough and accurate.
- There is no such thing as a 'medicolegal' X-ray. X-rays should be ordered, or not ordered, based on clinical grounds only. It is the documentation that is critical medicolegally.

History

- Record accurately in, wherever possible, the patient's own words, including:
  1. **Time** of the assault.
  2. **Method** of the assault, i.e. kicking, punching, beating with a weapon, etc.
  3. **Weapon(s)** used, e.g. knife, *parang* (machete), gun, etc.

4. Remember, the patient may not be the victim of the assault but, rather, the assailant presenting typically with a 'fight-bite', i.e. abrasions or lacerations over the dorsal aspects of the metacarpophalangeal joints of the index and/or middle fingers.

Examination

- Record all major and minor injuries.
- Include shape, size, depth, colour, and diameters (see comments below on the use of cameras).
- Photograph all lesions; the best images are now obtained with digital cameras:
  1. Place a linear scale next to the lesion being photographed to enhance the accuracy of your documentation.
  2. Use the photos as an *aide-mémoire* so that you can accurately record all injuries without wasting your time making multiple trips to the patient.
  3. Label and date all photos with the initials of the person who took them using an addressograph label.
  4. File the photos with the emergency department record.

Post-examination

- Fill in all details required in any requested **police report**, including whether or not the lesion(s) is/are consistent with the mode and time of injury. If requested to give an opinion on 'fitness for detention', state 'don't know' since you are probably unaware of the conditions that prevail when a prisoner is detained. You should not make yourself legally responsible for committing a patient to detention, especially if that patient suffers morbidity or mortality.
- If your department's workflow permits, recall the patient for **review in approximately 24–48 hours** (your next shift would be ideal). This serves for reevaluation and photography of previously injured areas which might have changed in appearance **and** for evaluation of areas which only at the time of the review are showing signs of injury.

Reference/Further Reading

1. Knight B. *Simpson's Forensic Medicine*. 11th ed. London: Arnold; 1997: 44–45.

108   Eclampsia

Peter Manning • Gene Chan

DEFINITIONS

- **Pre-eclampsia:** Elevation of the systolic or diastolic blood pressure that occurs after the 20th week up until the 24th week of pregnancy in a previously normotensive or hypertensive woman, in association with proteinuria (0.3 g/24 hr) with/without oedema.
- **Eclampsia:** Grand mal seizures (fits) or coma superimposed on pre-eclampsia.
- **Clinical features** of severe pre-eclampsia (in addition to hypertension and proteinuria) are:
  1. Symptoms of severe headache.
  2. Visual disturbances.
  3. Epigastric pain and/or vomiting.
  4. Signs of clonus.
  5. Papilloedema.
  6. Liver tenderness.
  7. Platelet count falling to $<100 \times 10^9$/L.
  8. Abnormal liver enzymes (alanine transaminase, ALT, or aspartate transaminase, AST >70 IU/L).
  9. HELLP syndrome (see below).

CAVEATS

- The **aim of management** is, first of all, to stabilize the mother and then deliver the baby:
  1. Management of the maternal airway.
  2. Prevention and control of convulsions with magnesium sulphate therapy.
  3. Restoration of intravascular volume.
  4. Control of blood pressure.
- Delivery of baby: How and when the baby is delivered is a decision to be made by an obstetrics and gynaecology (O&G) specialist.
- Immediate O&G consultation to be made when diagnosis is evident.
- HELLP syndrome is a very severe form of pre-eclampsia characterized by:
  1. Haemolysis.
  2. Elevated liver enzymes.
  3. Low Platelets ($<100,000$/mm^3).

- **Symptoms**: pain in the right hypochondrium (RHC) with nausea and vomiting are the most common.
- **Signs**: commonly include generalized oedema, RHC tenderness, jaundice, gastrointestinal bleeding, and haematuria.

⇨ **SPECIAL TIPS FOR GPs**

- 60% of cases occur during the first pregnancy.
- Primagravidas at the extremes of age (<17 or >35 years old) are at increased risk.
- Patients with a history of chronic hypertension are more prone to develop pre-eclampsia and eclampsia.
- There is no way to adequately predict who will progress to eclampsia, thus, all pregnant women with pre-eclampsia should be considered for admission.
- **New onset seizures** that occur between 48 hours to 4 weeks after delivery should be considered **late onset eclampsia** until proven otherwise.

MANAGEMENT

Supportive measures

- The patient must be managed in the critical care area.
- Airway management equipment must be immediately available.

NOTE: The patient who does not require intubation should be nursed in the left lateral position.

- Resuscitation drugs must be immediately available.
- Calcium gluconate (the antidote for magnesium toxicity) must be immediately available.
- Administer supplemental high flow oxygen via a reservoir mask.
- Monitoring: Electrocardiogram (ECG), vital signs q 5 minutes, and pulse oximetry.
- Establish a peripheral intravenous (IV) line and commence Hartmann's solution: Give bolus of 250 ml stat followed by infusion at 100 ml/hr.
- Labs: Full blood count, urea/electrolytes/creatinine, liver function tests, group and cross match and prothrombin time/partial thromboplastin time.
- Perform ECG tests (optional).
- Insert a urinary catheter to measure the hourly urine output.

Drug therapy for convulsion

- **Magnesium sulphate** (the MAGPIE study demonstrated a reduction in the risk of progression to an eclamptic seizure).

1. **Dosage**
   a. **Loading dose**: An initial loading dose of 4 g IV over 5 to 10 minutes via an infusion pump.
   b. **Maintenance dose**: IV infusion of magnesium sulphate at a rate of 1 g/hr until 24 hours after the last seizure.
   c. Recurrent seizure can be treated with a further bolus of 2 g magnesium sulphate or an increase in the infusion rate to 1.5 g or 2 g/hr.

NOTE: The drug should only be given if these criteria are satisfied: (1) The patellar reflex is present (**most important**) and (2) the respiratory rate is not depressed, i.e. the rate is >16 breaths per minute.

2. **Side effects**: Flushing, nausea, and epigastric discomfort.
3. **Clinical signs of magnesium toxicity**: Diminished deep tendon reflexes, muscle weakness manifesting as ptosis, slurred speech, respiratory depression, and oliguria/anuria.
4. **Management of magnesium toxicity**:
   a. Administer 10 ml (1 g) calcium gluconate IV over 10 minutes.
   b. **Stop magnesium sulphate infusion** if.
      i. Patellar reflexes are absent.
      ii. Respiration rate is <16 breaths per minute.
      iii. Oxygen saturation (SpO_2) levels fall below 90% in spite of supplemental oxygen.
      iv. Anuria (or oliguria with a urine output of <20 ml/hr) persists beyond 2 hours.
   c. If oliguric, do serum magnesium levels and stop the infusion if the level >3 mmol/L.

- **Diazepam (Valium®)**: The second choice anti-convulsant, which is indicated if magnesium sulphate therapy is contraindicated or magnesium toxicity is evident.
  1. **Dosage**: 10 mg slowly IV over 2 minutes; can be repeated to a total of 20 mg.

NOTE: A dose of 5 mg is too low for pregnancy.

  2. **Infusion**: 1 mg/min.
  3. **Management of recurrent convulsions**:
     a. Repeat magnesium sulphate 2.5–5.0 g IV.
     b. Administer diazepam 10 mg IV.
     c. If there is no response, or the patient has a prolonged period of obtundation after only being given magnesium sulphate, then the possibility of intracranial haemorrhage exists, and a head computed tomography (CT) scan should be sought at an appropriate juncture.
     d. Consider consulting Anaesthesia regarding phenytoin/thiopentone infusion.

Drug therapy for hypertension

Women with blood pressures >110 mmHg diastolic or >160 mmHg systolic risk arterial damage and should be treated. The aim of therapy is smooth reduction of blood pressure over 20–30 minutes, to a level of 90–100 mmHg diastolic or 140–150 mmHg systolic. Too rapid or too great a reduction in blood pressure may have adverse effects on both the mother and baby.

NOTE: Antihypertensive therapy **should not be given** before IV fluid administration. Due to vasoconstriction, eclamptics usually have a low intravascular volume which may predispose to renal shutdown and precipitous falls in blood pressure when antihypertensive therapy is commenced.

- **Hydralazine (Apresoline®)**

  Dosage: 5 mg IV or oral (PO) bolus and repeated in doses of 5–10 mg IV or PO every 20 minutes as needed (prn) or

- **Labetalol (Trandate®/Normadyne®)**: See **Note** below.

  Dosage: 20 mg over 5 minutes, followed by increasing doses of 20–80 mg by IV bolus q 10 minutes until the desired effect is achieved, or to a maximum cumulative dose of 300 mg.

NOTE:

1. Avoid felodipine or nifedipine if magnesium sulphate is being used for control of convulsions since a synergistic hypotensive effect may be seen.

2. If there is no response to hydralazine or the patient is unconscious, the drug of choice is labetalol. Experience suggests a smoother control of blood pressure and there is published evidence suggesting that it may be of benefit to the foetus by accelerating lung maturity.

References/Further Reading

1. Schwab, R. Pre-eclampsia/eclampsia: Establishing the diagnosis and providing prompt, effective treatment. *Emerg Med Rep.* 25 Nov 1996: 237–244.

2. Tuffnell DJ, Shennan AH, Waugh JJS, Walker JJ. *The Management of Severe Pre-eclampsia/Eclampsia: Green Top Guideline No. 10 (A).* London: RCOG Press. March 2006.

3. Keadey M, Houry D. Complications in pregnancy (Part II): Hypertensive disorders of pregnancy and vaginal bleeding. *Emergency Medicine Practice.* May 2009; 11:5.

109 Ectopic Pregnancy

Gene Chan • Irwani Ibrahim

CAVEATS

- Any sexually active woman presenting with abdominal pain and vaginal bleeding with or without amenorrhoea has an ectopic pregnancy until proven otherwise.
- Diagnosis is easily missed unless suspected. Hence, consider ectopic pregnancy in all females of child-bearing age.
- The absence of cervical motion tenderness does not exclude ectopic pregnancy.

⇨ **SPECIAL TIPS FOR GPs**

- Ectopic pregnancy must be suspected in all females of child-bearing age presenting with abdominal pain.
- Most presentations are atypical (see below).
- A history of tubal ligation does not exclude an ectopic pregnancy.
- The urine pregnancy test is a simple tool that can be used but beware of its limitations.

MANAGEMENT

Risk factors

Degree of risk	Risk factors	Odds ratio
High	Previous ectopic pregnancy	9.3–47
	Previous tubal surgery	6.0–11.5
	Tubal ligation	3.0–139
	Tubal pathology	3.5–25
	In utero diethylstilbestrol (DES) exposure	2.4–13
	Current intrauterine device (IUD) use	1.1–45
Moderate	Infertility	1.1–28
	Previous cervicitis (gonorrhoea, chlamydia)	2.8–3.7
	History of pelvic inflammatory disease	2.1–3.0
	Multiple sexual partners	1.4–4.8
	Smoking	2.3–3.9
Low	Previous pelvic/abdominal surgery	0.93–3.8
	Vaginal douching	1.1–3.1
	Early age of intercourse (<18 years)	1.1–2.5

Sources: Adapted from data in ref 8 Ankum WM, Mol BWJ, Van Der Veen F, Bossuyt PMM, Fertil Steril. Title of Publication 1996;65:1093; ref 9 Murray H, Baakdah H, Bardell T, Tulandi T. *CMAJ.* 2005;173:905; and ref 10 Bouyer J, Coste J, Shojaei T, et al. *Am J Epidemiol.* 2003;157:185.

Presentation

Classic triad of abdominal pain, amenorrhoea, and vaginal bleeding.

* Usually around 8 weeks of amenorrhoea.
* However, the spectrum of clinical symptoms ranges from pelvic pain and vaginal bleeding indistinguishable from spontaneous abortion, ovarian accident or pelvic inflammatory disease to catastrophic intra-abdominal haemorrhage.
* The patient may present with syncope.

Typical presentation: Sudden onset of unilateral severe abdominal pain accompanied by collapse and fresh vaginal bleeding. Commonest presenting symptom is abdominal pain with or without vaginal bleeding.

Atypical presentation: Chronic recurrent lower abdominal pain combined with irregular vaginal bleeding, gastrointestinal symptoms (vomiting or diarrhoea), and urinary symptoms such as dysuria or shoulder tip pain.

Diagnosis

Urine HCG

* Most urine human chorionic gonadotrophin (HCG) kits have almost 100% specificity but sensitivities vary (generally still around 90%).
* All females of child-bearing age with abdominal pain should have a urine pregnancy test done to exclude ectopic pregnancy. In one study, the percentage of potentially missed cases dropped from 40% when based on history alone, to 3% when urine HCG was negative, to 2% when serum HCG was negative, and to 1% when ultrasound was negative.
* A urine pregnancy test becomes positive between the fourth and fifth weeks after conception and serum HCG becomes positive from the third to the fourth week post-conception.
* Different urine pregnancy test kits give different sensitivities. Some can detect as low as 10 IU/L, e.g. the Abbott Test Pack Plus detects urine HCG of 25 IU/L.
* **False positive results** can be due to trophoblastic diseases (hydatidiform moles or choriocarcinoma), HCG producing pituitary tumours as well as drugs such as anti-convulsants and phenothiazines.
* **False negative results** occur if the urine specimen is too dilute (the best specimen is the first morning specimen) and in patients who are on diuretics.
* According to a recent article in HCG-based urine pregnancy test has a sensitivity of 90% only if conducted on the first day of a missed period, as 10% of women may not have implanted yet. Sensitivity rises to 97% if a test is conducted within a week after the first day of a missed period.

Management of the unstable patient

- The patient must be managed in the critical care area.
- Maintain the airway and give supplemental high flow oxygen.
- Monitoring: Electrocardiogram (ECG), vital signs every 5 minutes, and pulse oximetry.
- Establish 2 large bore intravenous (IV) lines.
- Give fluid challenge of 1 L crystalloid. Reassess parameters.
- Labs (mandatory):
  1. Full blood count.
  2. Urea/electrolytes/creatinine.
  3. Goup and cross match 2 to 4 units of blood.
  4. Urine HCG.
  5. Disseminated intravascular coagulation (DIVC) screen.
- Insert a urinary catheter to monitor the urinary output.
- Inform the obstetrics and gynaecology registrar stat.

Management of the stable patient

- Keep the patient nil by mouth.
- Put the patient in a monitored bed.
- Monitor the vital signs every 5 to 10 minutes.
- Establish at least 1 large bore peripheral line (14G/16G).
- Administer crystalloids at maintenance rate.
- Labs:
  1. Mandatory: Group and cross match 4 units of blood.
  2. Optional: Full blood count and urea/electrolytes/creatinine.
- Inform the obstetrics and gynaecology registrar who may arrange for immediate ultrasound scan.

NOTE: The choice of best management ranging from expectant, to outpatient medication (methotrexate), to conservative versus radical surgery is based on the patient's clinical condition, evidence of rupture, size of the ectopic, rate of HCG rise, and the patient's wishes for future fertility.

References/Further Reading

1. Carson SA, Buster JE. Ectopic pregnancy. *N Engl J Med*. 1993; 329(16): 1174–1181.

2. Ankum WM. Diagnosing suspected ectopic pregnancy: HCG monitoring and transvaginal ultrasound lead the way. *BMJ*. 2000; 321; 1235–1236.

3. Wong E, Ooi SBS. Ectopic pregnancy: A diagnostic challenge in the emergency department. *Eur J Emerg Med*. 2000; 7(3): 189–194.

4. Brennan DF. Ectopic pregnancy (Part 1): Clinical and laboratory diagnosis. *Acad Emerg Med*. 1995; 2(12): 1081–1089.

5. Wilox AJ, Baird DD, Dunson D, et al. Natural limits of pregnancy testing in relation to the expected menstrual period. *JAMA*. 2001; 286(14): 1759–1761.

6. Current management of ectopic pregnancy. *Obstetrics and Gynaecology Clinics*. Sep 2007; 34: 3.

7. The management of tubal pregnancy. *RCOG Guideline No. 21*. May 2004.

8. Ankum WM, Mol BW, Van der Veen F, Bossuyt PM. Risk factors for ectopic pregnancy: a meta-analysis. *Fertil Steril* 1996 Jun; 65(6): 1093–1099.

9. Bouyer J, Coste J, Shojaei T, et al. Risk factors for ectopic pregnancy: a comprehensive analysis based on a large case-control, population-based study in France. *Am J Epidemiol*. 2003 Feb 1; 157(3): 185–194. Review.

110   Emergency Delivery of the Newborn

Peter Manning

Peter Manning

CAVEATS

- If the patient is multiparous and she says 'It's coming!', then believe her. You will have no time to transfer her to the labour ward since she is probably about to deliver.
- Activate the staff of Obstetrics and Gynaecology (O&G) and Neonatology or Paediatrics (if available at your institution) as soon as possible, but be prepared to initiate delivery of the newborn pending their arrival.
- 'Crowning', i.e. bulging of the perineum by the foetal head as it moves through the birth canal, indicates imminent delivery; **do not** transfer the patient to the labour ward.
- If there is ANY history of **vaginal bleeding** in the **last few weeks**, **do not** perform a **vaginal examination** since she may have a placenta praevia. Disruption of the placenta by a digital or speculum examination could lead to exsanguinating haemorrhage.
- During delivery of the newborn, prevent tearing of the perineum by supporting it with one hand until the baby has been delivered. Hopefully, this will prevent the need for an episiotomy.
- **Newborns** are **obligate nasal breathers**; suction both mouth *and* nostrils after delivery of the head – do not delay until delivery of the baby before suctioning.

Stages of Labour and Delivery

- **Stage 1**: The cervix dilates as a result of progressive rhythmic uterine contractions. Typically, this is the longest stage of labour. During this stage the cervix thins (cervical effacement).
- **Stage 2**: The time between complete cervical dilatation and delivery of the newborn. This phase lasts minutes to hours.
- **Stage 3**: The delivery of the placenta. Typically this occurs within 30 minutes of the delivery of the newborn. As the uterus contracts, a plane of separation develops at the placenta–endometrium interface. As the uterus contracts further, the placenta is expelled.

Emergency delivery of the newborn

- The assumption is that 'crowning' is present and, therefore, you do not have time to transfer the patient to the labour ward.
- Activate O&G staff and Neonatology or Paediatrics (if available at your institution) as soon as possible, but be prepared to initiate delivery of the newborn pending their arrival.
- Take a ***brief and focused obstetric history*** if time permits:
  1. Parity: If multiparous, labour is likely to be very rapid.
  2. Any vaginal bleeding in recent weeks.
  3. Gestational age.
     a. By last normal menstrual period (pregnancy wheel).

   b. By estimated day of delivery or Naegle's rule of 'LNMP + 9 months + 7 days'.

   c. Fundal height: Falsely high in obese patients.

4. Prenatal care.

5. Complications in this and other pregnancies.

6. Past medical history, e.g. hypertension/eclampsia.

- Perform a *focused physical examination*:

   1. Look for 'crowning' (Figure 1).

FIGURE 1   'Crowning'

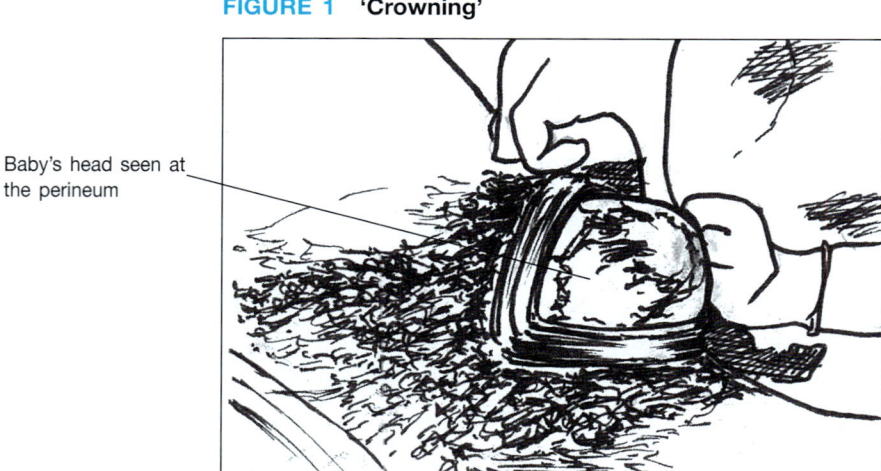

Baby's head seen at the perineum

2. If there is no vaginal bleeding in the history, perform a sterile speculum and bimanual examination to determine presentation.

   a. A vertex presentation is best confirmed with palpation of the cranial sutures, whereas palpation of the feet or hands represents a malpresentation.

3. If in doubt about the presentation, bedside ultrasound will reveal the presenting part of the foetus.

- **Delivery steps**

   1. Position of the patient: She may choose the delivery position that is most comfortable. Most commonly, women assume a partially sitting position, with the knees flexed and the back supported. The gravity advantage of being at least partially upright can help during delivery.

   2. Drape the perineum and prepare the delivery equipment for imminent delivery.

      a. Drapes and gowns protect the staff from fluid ejected during the delivery; however, sterile preparation is not required.

   3. Support the perineum with one hand. This minimizes the risk of a perineal tear. Use the other hand to support and maintain the head in the flexed position as it delivers (Figure 2).

FIGURE 2 **Right hand supports perineum. Left hand supports and maintains head in flexed position**

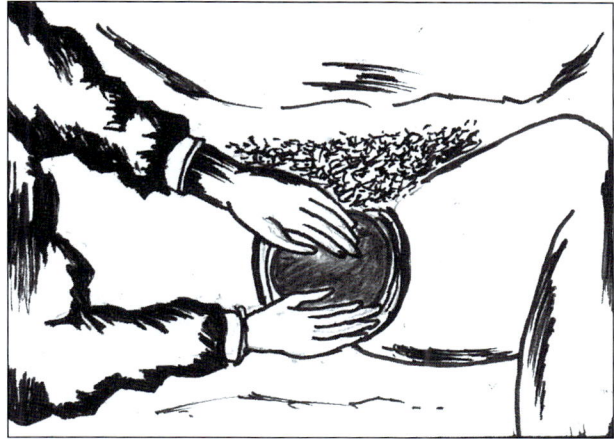

4. Control the pace of the delivery of the head to prevent tearing of the perineum.

5. Once the baby is delivered, encourage the mother to withhold pushing and check that the umbilical cord is not wrapped around the baby's neck (Figure 3).

FIGURE 3 **Check that umbilical cord is not wrapped around baby's neck**

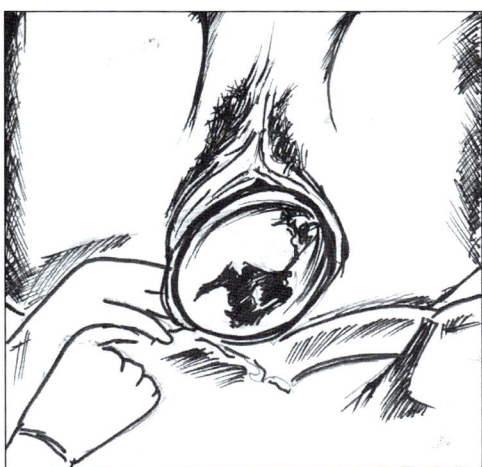

    a. If the cord is around the neck, then unwrap it and free it from the neck.

    b. If the cord cannot be freed, then clamp the cord in two places and divide the cord between the clamps using sterile scissors.

6. Suction the mouth and nares of the baby (remember, newborns and infants are obligate nasal breathers).

7. **Delivery of the shoulders**:

a. With both hands on the head, support delivery of the shoulders one at a time as the mother pushes with a contraction; with gentle traction lower the head to facilitate delivery of the anterior shoulder (Figure 4) **Do not make** jerky or forceful movements.

FIGURE 4   Gentle traction to lower the baby's head to facilitate delivery of the anterior shoulder

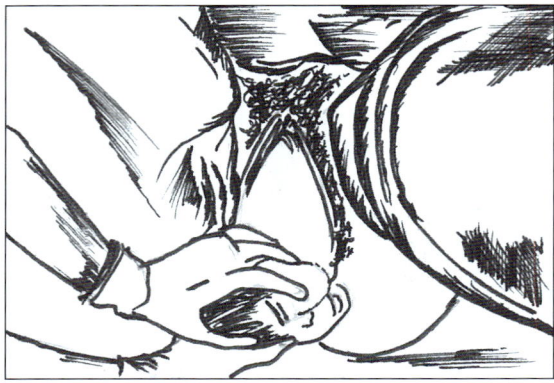

b. Once the anterior shoulder has been delivered, intramuscular (IM) syntometrine 0.5 mg should be administered.

8. **Delivery of the body**:

a. While supporting the head and shoulders, control the pace of the delivery of the baby's body (Figure 5).

FIGURE 5   Baby delivered

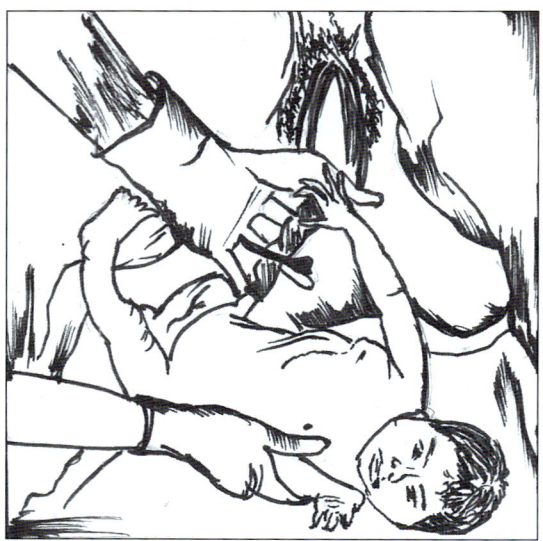

b. Suction the nares again and perform an initial assessment of the newborn (see the section on APGAR).

c. After drying and wrapping the baby in warm towels and/or a blanket, double clamp the umbilical cord 2 inches apart (1 inch and 3 inches from the baby); divide the cord with sterile scissors and collect appropriate blood specimens according to your departmental or hospital protocol.

9. If the neonatologist is unavailable, initiate neonatal resuscitation if a cyanotic/apnoeic or unresponsive (to stimulation) baby has been delivered.

- **Episiotomy**
  1. The decision to perform an episiotomy is often made as the newborn crowns. Evidence does not support the routine practice of episiotomy.
  2. When indicated (imminent tearing of the perineum at the fourchette), episiotomies are made in a midline or mediolateral position using sterile scissors with two fingers of the clinician's non-dominant hand behind the fourchette and between the scissors and the baby's head.
  3. The cut is made at the height of a contraction and requires no local anaesthetic. The depth of the cut is directly proportional to how precipitous the delivery is and to the stiffness of the perineum.

FIGURE 6   Episiotomy

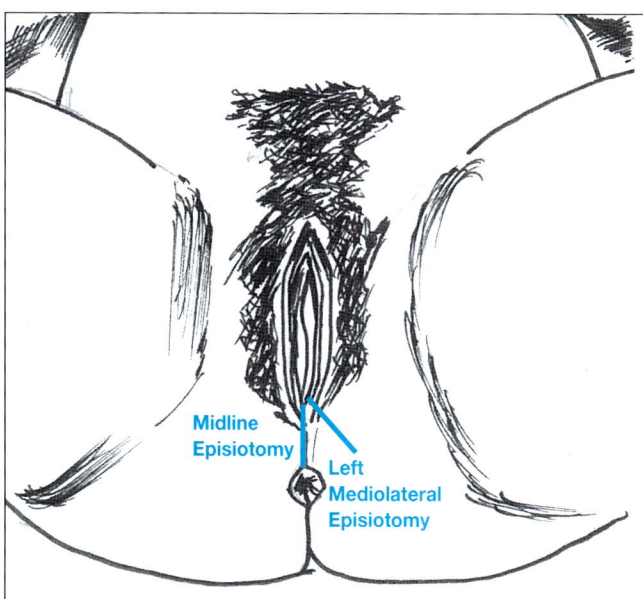

- **Delivery of the placenta**
  1. Occurs 15–20 minutes after the infant is delivered.
  2. Allow spontaneous separation with *gentle* traction.

NOTE: Aggressive traction on the cord can lead to:

    a. Uterine inversion.

    b. Cord tearing.

    c. Placental disruption $\rightarrow$ severe vaginal bleeding.

3. Massage the uterus after delivery of the infant to promote contraction of the uterus.

4. While one hand is looped around the cord to facilitate gentle traction, the other hand should be placed superior to the symphysis pubis with vertical pressure to prevent inversion of the uterus.

5. **Placental separation** is shown by any of the following:

    a. Increase in umbilical cord slack.

    b. A bolus of blood from the uterus.

    c. Superior migration of the uterus within the abdomen with an increase in uterine firmness.

6. Inspect the placenta after delivery.

    a. Open the sac and confirm that all segments (cotyledons) are present.

    b. Retained placental fragments increase the risk of postpartum haemorrhage (PPH).

- **Postpartum haemorrhage (PPH)**

1. An essential part of the third stage of labour is assessing the integrity of the placenta to exclude a retained placental fragment.

2. Blood loss in excess of 500 ml from vaginal delivery is abnormal. The most common causes of PPH are uterine atony and deep tears within the vagina/perineum; hence, the importance of a peripheral intravenous (IV) line for volume replacement.

- **APGAR (American Pediatric Gross Assessment Record) assessment of the newborn**: To be performed at 1 and 5 minutes after delivery (at 10 minutes too if the first 2 sets of scores are low).

Sign	Score		
	0	**1**	**2**
A – activity	Absent	Limbs flexed	Active movement
P – pulse	Absent	<100/min	>100/min
G – grimace	No response	Grimace	Sneezes, coughs and pulls away
A – appearance	Blue-grey or pale all over	Normal colour except at extremities	Normal colour entire body
R – respiration	Absent	Slow, irregular	Good, crying

Acknowledgement

All illustrations in this chapter were drawn by Dr Swati Jain.

Reference/Further Reading

1. Gabbe SG, Niebyl JR, Simpson JL. *Obstetrics: Normal and Problem Pregnancies*. 4th ed. Philadelphia, PA: Churchill & Livingstone; 2002.

111   Pelvic Inflammatory Disease (PID)

Gene Chan

CAVEATS

- Consider ectopic pregnancy and pelvic inflammatory disease (PID) in any pregnancy-capable female patient with lower abdominal pain.

- **Criteria for the clinical diagnosis of acute PID**: The **classic triad** of lower abdominal pain/tenderness, cervical motion tenderness, and bilateral adnexal tenderness, detected on either a vaginal or rectal examination is present in most cases. Other symptoms include vaginal discharge, vaginal bleeding, and dyspareunia. Fever (a temperature above 38°C), nausea, and vomiting may be present. On speculum examination, a purulent discharge is seen in about 95% of women with PID. If an adnexal mass is palpated and a tubo-ovarian abscess is suspected, pelvic ultrasonography should be performed.

- **Predisposing factors**:
  1. Multiple sexual partners.
  2. Young age at sexual debut.
  3. History of sexually transmitted diseases.
  4. Recent instrumentation to lower genital tract (e.g. dilation and curettage, hysterosalpin-gography, etc.).
  5. Recent abortion, miscarriage, or delivery.
  6. Presence of a foreign body (e.g. IUCD, intrauterine contraceptive device).
  7. Frequent douching.
  8. Smoking.

- **Classical presentation** is that of subacute lower abdominal pain that is dull in nature and usually bilateral. Unilateral lower abdominal pain and adnexal tenderness are probably not PID. On the other hand, bear in mind other possible diagnoses in the face of bilateral lower abdominal pain and adnexal tenderness (e.g. ectopic pregnancy, tubo-ovarian abscess, and adnexal torsion).

- Generally, women with appendicitis have been symptomatic for a *shorter* period of time and have more pronounced gastrointestinal symptoms. They are clinically more unwell, with signs localizing to the right iliac fossa.

- It is mandatory to **exclude a pregnancy**. Other investigations include full blood count and urine dipstick.

⇨ **SPECIAL TIPS FOR GPs**

- Admit following Obstetrics and Gynaecology (O&G) consultation if the following apply: toxic patient, poor response to outpatient treatment, pregnancy, presence of vomiting, surgical emergency causing the pain cannot be excluded, suspected tubo-ovarian abscess, immunodeficiency, and a poor likelihood of outpatient follow-up.
- Have a low threshold for empirical treatment of suspected PID. This can decrease the risk of long-term sequelae such as ectopic pregnancy, subfertility, and chronic pelvic pain.

MANAGEMENT

- Manage in the intermediate acuity care area.
- Take high vaginal swabs for culture/sensitivity and endocervical swabs for *chlamydia* and *gonococcus*.
- Establish intravenous (IV) access and take blood for full blood count and urea/electrolytes/creatinine.
- Initiate IV rehydration if needed and pain should be controlled.
- Consider the removal of an IUCD, if present.
- In acute PID, consider **admission** for **IV antibiotics**.
- The following antibiotic regimes can be used:
  1. Oral **ofloxacin** 400 mg bd (twice daily) and oral **metronidazole** 400 mg bd for 14 days.
  2. Intramuscular **ceftriaxone** 250 mg stat followed by oral **doxycycline** 100 mg bd and oral **metronidazole** 400 mg bd for 14 days (substitute **erythromycin** 500 mg PO qd (orally every day) for 10–14 days if the patient is allergic to doxycycline).
  3. Intravenous **clindamycin** 900 mg tds (three times daily) and intravenous **gentamycin** 2 mg/kg loading dose followed by 1.5 mg/kg tds; followed by either oral **clindamycin** 450 mg qds 4 times daily or oral **doxycycline** 100 mg bd and oral **metronidazole** 400 mg bd for 14 days.
- If the patient is discharged, complete discharge instructions should be given, with the following advice: Arrange close follow-up in the next 48–72 hours, and get sexual partner to seek medical attention.
- The patient should be counselled to avoid sexual contact until the patient and partner have completed treatment. They should also be advised about condom use.
- Patients should be encouraged to be tested for syphilis, hepatitis, and the human immunodeficiency virus (HIV).
- Patients who are HIV positive should be treated with the same antibiotic regimens.

References/Further Reading

1. Moors A, Bevan CD, Thomas EJ. Pelvic inflammatory disease. In: Shaw RW, Soutter WP, Stanton SL, eds. *Gynaecology*. London: Churchill-Livingstone; 1997: 813–825.
2. *Management of Acute Pelvic Inflammatory Disease: Guideline No. 32*. London: Royal College of Obstetricians and Gynaecologists; May 2003.

112   Burns, Major

Francis Lee • Victor Ong • Shirley Ooi

CAVEATS

- **Definitions of major burns** requiring admission to a **burns centre**:
  1. Full thickness burns are those that destroy >5% of the total body surface area (BSA) in any age group.
  2. Mixed partial and full thickness burns are those that affect >10% of the body surface area in the elderly (>50 years) and children (<10 years).
  3. Mixed partial and full thickness burns involve >20% of the total body surface area in victims aged 10–50 years.
  4. These burns involve special areas such as the eyes, ears, face, hands, buttocks and perineum, and feet.
  5. Inhalation injury.
  6. Circumferential burns of body parts like limbs and trunk.
  7. Electrical injury and chemical burns.
  8. Burns in patient with coexisting chronic medical illnesses.
- Assessment of a patient with major burns follows Advanced Trauma Life Support (ATLS) principles. The primary survey stage screens for life-threatening injuries, such as airway problems and respiratory difficulties. The secondary survey involves a thorough examination of the patient. It is at this juncture that the extent of burns is assessed and fluid regime calculated.

INITIAL MANAGEMENT

- The burns patient should be managed in the critical or resuscitation care area with close monitoring.
- During the primary survey (which assesses the airway, breathing, circulation, disability, and exposure or ABCDEs), airway risk assessment is carried out and a decision made for prophylactic intubation. The **risk factors** (in increasing probability) for **upper airway obstruction** are:
  1. Burns and scalds around the nose or mouth.
  2. Soot in the nostrils or singed nasal hairs.
  3. Burns of the tongue.
  4. Swelling of the buccal mucosa.
  5. Voice becoming hoarse.
  6. Laryngeal oedema visible on laryngoscopy.
  7. Inspiratory stridor.

- Consider intubation **early** if the airway is at risk. Progressive swelling of the oral/ pharynx and larynx may make delayed intubation more difficult (refer to Chapter 28, *Airway Management/Rapid Sequence Intubation*):

  1. The patient shall be closely monitored (blood pressure/cardiac activity/oxygen saturation/ end-tidal carbon dioxide) before rapid sequence induction (RSI) is commenced.

  2. As it is a potentially difficult airway, the 'awake intubation technique' may be used first before RSI.

  3. Suxamethonium is **not** contraindicated in acute burns.

  4. Equipment necessary for a surgical airway, e.g. cricothyroidotomy set, should be close at hand in case intubation fails.

  5. Intubation should be carried out in the presence of a senior emergency physician or anaesthetist.

- Oxygen supplementation via a non-rebreather mask at 15 L/min should be provided to those patients who do not require intubation.

- Establish intravenous (IV) access and initiate crystalloid infusion.

- **Investigations** are ordered:

  1. Mandatory blood investigations: Group and cross match (GXM), full blood count, urea/ electrolytes/creatinine, coagulation studies, arterial blood gas, and capillary blood glucose.

  2. Other relevant blood investigations: Carboxyhaemoglobin level.

  3. Electrocardiograms (ECG) and chest X-ray should be performed.

- The patient should be catheterized to assess the urine output.

- Care should be taken to prevent hypothermia.

BURNS ASSESSMENT AND FLUID REGIME

- The **severity** of burns should be assessed. The severity is based on the

  1. Depth of the burns.

  2. Extent of the burns.

  3. Location of the burns.

- The **depth** of burn is documented as superficial, partial, or full thickness (refer to Chapter 113, *Burns, Minor*).

- The **extent** of burns is commonly assessed using **Wallace's rule of nines** in adults (see Figure 1). For children, the differences in body proportion according to age make assessment with a **Lund–Browder chart** (see Figure 2) more appropriate. Only partial to full thickness burns are considered in the calculation of extent of burns.

- Based on the size of burn wounds assessed, the fluid regime is calculated. Generally, any patient with burns that involve more than 20% of the total BSA needs circulatory volume support. Establish a large bore (at least 16G) IV catheter in a peripheral vein. If the extent of burn precludes catheter placement through unburned skins, overlying burned skin should not

FIGURE 1   Wallace's rule of nines

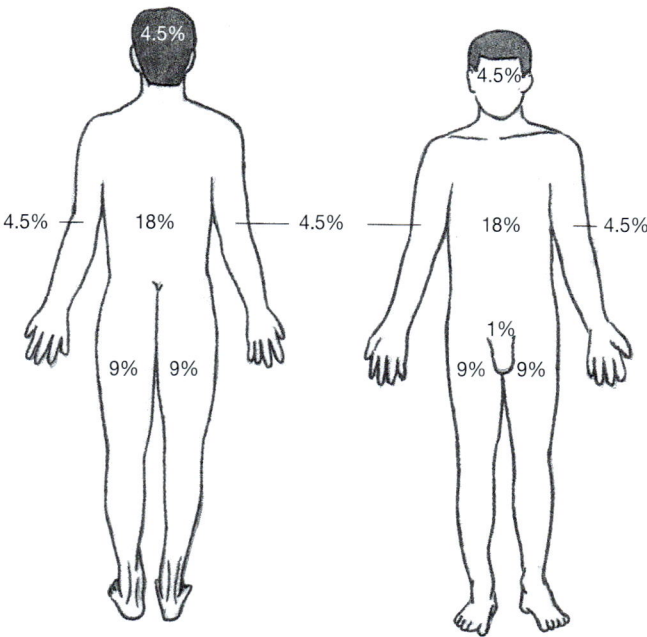

FIGURE 2   Lund–Browder chart

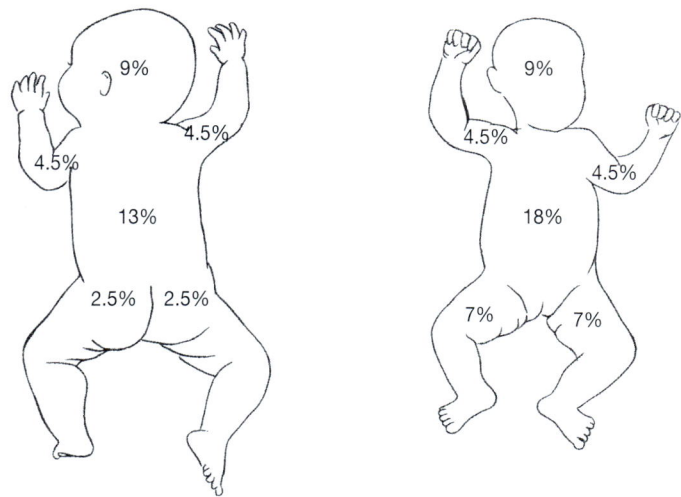

deter catheter placement in an accessible vein. The upper extremities are preferable to lower extremities for venous access because of the high incidence of phlebitis and septic phlebitis in the saphenous veins. Many formulae have been developed using various combinations of crystalloids and colloids. Parkland's formula in Table 1 is an example.

TABLE 1   Parkland's formula

Total replacement fluid requirements in the first 24 hours = 2–4 ml/kg/% of the total BSA:
- Divide total volume into two halves.
- Infuse the first half in the first 8 hours.
- Infuse the rest in the next 16 hours.

Start time = Time of actual burn injury occurrence.

(Hence, if the burn victim starts to receive fluid replacement 2 hours after injury onset, then the first half of the calculated fluid will need to be infused over 6 hours instead of the 8 hours as stated.)

Fluid of choice could be either Hartmann's solution or normal saline.

Other formulae such as the Muir and Barclay and Galveston have been used in various countries in the world.

Remember that these formulae calculate the amount of fluid needed to replace fluids lost as a result of burn injuries. This is on top of the daily fluid requirements in a normal average person.

PAIN RELIEF

- Adequate pain relief should be given:
  1. IV fentanyl 2–3 µg/kg, or
  2. IV morphine 1–2 mg every 10–15 minutes, or
  3. IV tramadol 50 mg followed by an infusion.
  4. Entonox inhalation may be used during wound dressings.

Bear in mind that opioids, though the ideal first choice for analgesia in this setting, can cause hypotension, hence the need for adequate appropriate fluid replacement.

BURN WOUND MANAGEMENT

- The burns should be cooled with copious amounts of clean water, then covered with a non-adherent clean sterile dressing (refer to Chapter 113, *Burns, Minor*).

NOTE: Do **NOT** apply cold water to a patient with extensive burns (>10% body surface area) as it may cause hypothermia.

- **Escharotomy** should be performed for full thickness circumferential burns of the trunk and limb:

FIGURE 3 Emergency Escharotomy

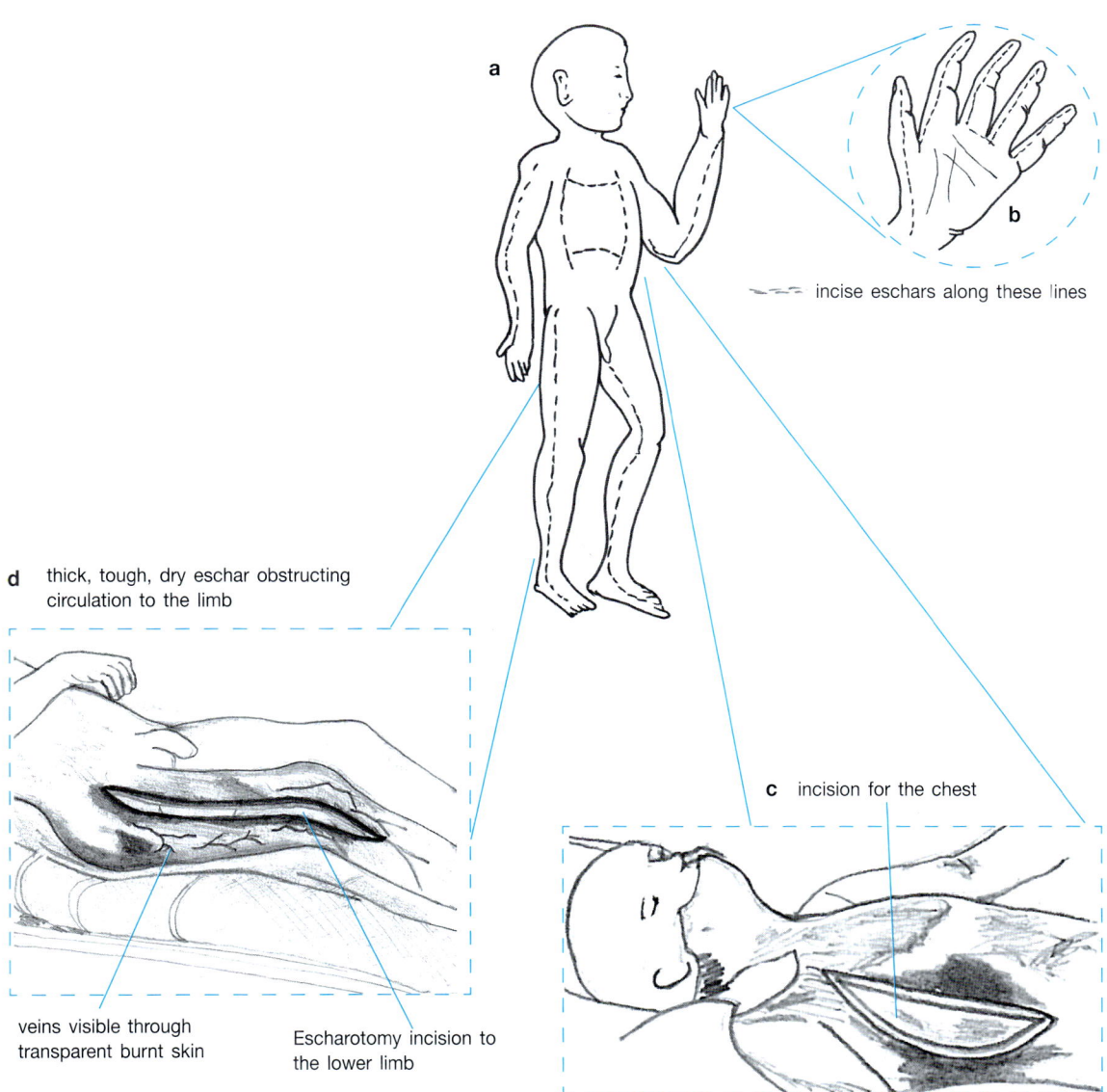

a

b

incise eschars along these lines

d thick, tough, dry eschar obstructing circulation to the limb

veins visible through transparent burnt skin

Escharotomy incision to the lower limb

c incision for the chest

1. Escharotomy can be carried out without analgesia.
2. A sterile knife is used.
3. Incision should be carried out along anatomical lines, starting with a few lines and increasing when necessary. The incision must extend across the entire length of the eschar in the lateral and/or medial line of the limb including the joints. For circumferential burns of the thorax, bilateral escharotomy incisions in the anterior axillary lines should be considered if respiratory excursions are limited.

4. The end point is that the depth of incision should reach the fat layer. Cutting until bleeding is seen is not recommended.

Acknowledgements

Figures 1 and 2 were drawn by Dr Chong Chew Lan, Figures 3a and 3b by Dr Swati Jain, and Figures 3c and 3d by Ms Sandra Han.

References/Further Reading

1. Settle J, ed. *Principles and Practice of Burns Management*. New York: Churchill Livingstone; 1996.

2. Masellis M, Gunn SWA, eds. *The Management of Burns and Fire Disasters. Perspectives 2000*. Dordrecht, The Netherlands: Kluwer Academic Publishers; 1995.

3. Herndon DN. *Total Burns Care*. Philadelphia, PA: WB Saunders; 1996.

4. Thermal Injuries. *Advanced Trauma Life Support for Doctors Manual*. 9th ed. Chicago, IL: American College of Surgeons Commitee on Trauma. 2012: 230–235.

5. Guidelines for the operation of burns center (pp. 79–86). In: Resources for Optimal Care of the Injured Patient 2006. Committee on Trauma. Chicago, IL: American College of Surgeons.

6. Singer AJ. Thermal burns: Rapid assessment and treatment. *Emergency Medicine Practice*. Sep 2000; 7.2(9); 1–20.

113 Burns, Minor

Francis Lee • Victor Ong • Peter Manning

DEFINITIONS

- **Superficial or first-degree burns** (e.g. sunburn) are characterized by erythema, pain, and the absence of blisters. They are not life-threatening, and generally do not require intravenous fluid replacement.
- **Partial thickness or second-degree burns** are characterized by a red or mottled appearance with associated swelling and blister formation. The surface may have a weeping, wet appearance, and is painfully hypersensitive, even to air current.
- **Full thickness or third-degree burns** usually appear dark and leathery, translucent, or waxy white. The surface may be red and does not blanch with pressure. The surface is painless and generally dry.

CAVEATS

- Burn wounds can be managed on an outpatient basis provided they do not fall into the following categories:
  1. Burns that involve >15% of the total body surface area (BSA) in adults, >10% in children.
  2. Burns involving special areas such as the eyes, ears, face, hands, buttocks, and perineum.
  3. Suspected inhalation injury.
  4. Circumferential burns.
  5. Electrical injury.
  6. Full thickness burns.
- **Cooling** is an important facet in the management of burns that is seldom remembered. This action limits the damage caused by heat that is retained in the skin tissues, reduces swelling, and relieves pain.
- **Alkali burns** are generally of greater significance than acid burns due to the former's tendency to penetrate into deeper tissues by liquefactive necrosis.

INITIAL MANAGEMENT OF MINOR BURNS

- Ensure that the airway, breathing and circulation are secured and vital signs are stable.
- Remove all burning objects from the wound.
- Remove all potentially constricting objects from the affected body region, e.g. bangles and rings.

> ⇨ **SPECIAL TIPS FOR GPs**
> - Very often burn injuries warrant a referral to the emergency department. The quick management steps include these:
>   1. Quick assessment of the patient's conscious state, airway, breathing and circulation to determine whether ambulance transport is needed.
>   2. Quick cooling of the burn wounds, as described below.
>   3. If dressing could not be performed, the burn area can be protected with a clean dry sheet of cloth or plastic wrap (cling film is a possible improvisation) and bandaged.
> - **Hydrofluoric acid (HF) burns** are highly significant, regardless of the size, and must be referred to the emergency department.

- **Cooling** burns. This could be achieved using a **'10–15' rule**:
  1. Cool the burns within 10–15 minutes of the incident.
  2. Use cold water (approximately 10–15°C).
  3. Run water or immerse the burnt part in cool water for 10–15 minutes.
- The wound size should be documented for the purpose of follow-up (refer to Chapter 112, *Burns, Major*).
- A **dressing** is then applied to the skin. There are various commercial preparations but a good burn dressing should consist of three layers:
  1. An inner non-adherent layer (e.g. Tulle-gras and Opsite)
  2. Middle absorbent layer (e.g. cotton wool and Gamgee)
  3. Outer protective layer (e.g. plastic wrap and bandage)
- A suitable alternative to commercial dressing is polyvinyl chloride film (cling film) as it is impermeable, transparent for inspection, and non-adherent.
- Analgesia should be given. Opioids may be required initially, but subsequent to first-aid treatment, non-steroidal anti-inflammatory drugs (NSAIDs) and paracetamol will often suffice.
- **Blisters** should be left alone unless they are large and tense. These should be aspirated using a clean needle. Blisters should not be de-roofed as the skin layer acts as a good protective cover and natural dressing.
- **Minor facial burns** could be managed without the need for a dressing. The good circulation of the face contributes to the good healing and low risk of infection:
  1. Cold saline is applied to the burn areas for 1 to 2 hours.
  2. Wounds are washed with a mild antiseptic solution and then left to air.
  3. The patient is advised to wash his face twice daily with soap and water.
  4. Avoidance of sun exposure for 15 days is necessary to prevent hyperpigmentation.
  5. The patient should also be warned of possible swelling occurring in the first 3 days.
  6. Cover the burn areas with a bland ointment or cream, e.g. liquid paraffin on a 1- to 4-hourly basis to minimize crust formation.

- **Antibiotic cream** is helpful but oral prophylaxis is unnecessary. A commonly used topical preparation is 1% silver sulfadiazine that can be applied to the wound before dressing.
  1. Covers Gram-negative bacteria including *Pseudomonas*.
  2. The dressing needs to be changed every 24–48 hours.
  3. Avoid the use of silver sulfadiazine in the following situations:
     a. Known allergy to sulfa drugs.
     b. G6PD (glucose-6-phosphatase dehydrogenase) deficiency.
     c. Late pregnancy.
     e. Children under 2 years old.
     f. Sun-exposed areas, e.g. face and neck. Silver tarnishes and leaves a black stain (arguria), especially, if the treated area is exposed to ultraviolet.

NOTE: It is unnecessary to use 1% silver sulfadiazine in superficial partial thickness burns.

- The patient's **tetanus immunization status** should be checked and updated with additional boosters when needed.

FOLLOW-UP CARE OF PATIENTS

- All patients treated as outpatients should be seen again in 24–48 hours. At this point, the wound is checked for the extension of burn injury.
- Check for the presence of **exudate seepage** through the dresssing. If exudate is present, the following could be done:
  1. If excessive oozing occurs, another layer of dressing could be applied onto the existing one.
  2. If Opsite is the primary dressing, any exudate could be aspirated with a clean needle. An additional layer of Opsite is then applied onto the existing one.
- **Signs of infection** include:
  1. Seroanguinous, pus-like, or foul-smelling discharge.
  2. Inflamed wound margins.
  3. Wound tenderness.
  4. Fever and chills.
- Dressing changes for burns should initially be within the first 48 hours (during the initial wound review) and then subsequently at an interval of 3 to 5 days. Attempts to remove the dressing for the purpose of changing may affect wound healing as the peeling action disrupts newly formed epithelium and granulation tissues.
- Aseptic techniques should be used for the change.
- During the follow-up, a change of the outer layer and middle absorbent layer of the dressing may be necessary. A partial thickness burn wound generally heals in 10–15 days and the inner layer separates from the wound when new epithelium is formed.

SPECIAL BURNS

Tar or asphalt burns

- Superficial black tar can be removed 30–45 minutes after applying a layer of white paraffin or Neosporin ointment.
- Embedded tar should be left alone as attempts at removal often result in more damage.
- The embedded tar will separate when new epithelium is formed.

Acid/alkali burns

- **Hydrogen fluoride (HF)** is primarily an industrial raw material. It is used in separating uranium isotopes, as a cracking catalyst in oil refineries, and for etching glass and enamel, removing rust, and cleaning brass and crystal. It is also used in manufacturing silicon semi-conductor chips.
- Consumer products that may contain HF include automotive cleaning products, rust inhibitors, rust removers, and water-spot removers.
- HF **acts like alkalis** and will cause progressive tissue loss including bony destruction.
- HF is one of the **strongest inorganic acids**, causing tissue damage by two mechanisms: A **corrosive burn** from the free hydrogen ions and a **chemical burn** from tissue penetration of the fluoride ions.
- Fluoride ions penetrate and form insoluble salts with calcium and magnesium and poison cellular enzymatic reactions.
- Soluble salts are also formed with other cations but dissociate rapidly, releasing the fluoride ions, and causing further tissue destruction.
- Absorption of fluoride ions can result in hypocalcaemia, hypomagnesaemia, hyperkalaemia, and cardiac arrest.
- Hypocalcaemia should be considered in all instances of inhalation and ingestion exposure and whenever skin burns exceed 60 cm^2.
- Patients exposed to solutions of 7% or less may take 12–24 hours to produce symptoms.
- The adverse action of the fluoride ions may progress for several days.
- **Potential sequelae**:
  1. Fingertip injuries cause persistent pain, bone loss, and nail bed injury.
  2. Skin burns heal slowly with extensive scarring.
  3. Eye exposure can lead to prolonged or permanent visual defects, blindness or total eye destruction.
  4. Ingestion exposure may lead to oesophageal strictures.
- **Exposure to skin**:
  1. HF burns are a unique clinical entity; burns to the fingers and nail beds may leave the overlying nails intact.

2. Contact with solutions of ≤7% produces no immediate pain on contact. Delayed serious injury may occur up to 24 hours later.

3. Contact with solutions of 12% causes a throbbing pain and swelling, often delayed up to 8 hours.

4. Contact with solutions of ≥14% causes immediate severe throbbing pain and a whitish skin discolouration and blisters.

- **Exposure to the eyes** results in problems ranging from eye irritation to the death of superficial cells leading to permanent clouding.

MANAGEMENT OF HF BURNS

- Consist of supportive care and the use of specific antidotes in the form of calcium-containing medications. **Calcium gluconate** is given to bind the enzyme-poisoning fluoride ion and curtail its toxic effects. It can be given topically, subcutaneously, intradermally, by intra-arterial infusion or by an intravenous regional perfusion technique based on Bier's method.

NOTE: A hydrogen fluoride antidote should be kept in the emergency department pharmacy. Liberal consultations with multiple specialities are encouraged.

- Decontamination: Rapid skin decontamination is critical.
- Airway, breathing and circulation:
  1. Evaluate and support the airway.
  2. Intubate orotracheally if ventilation/oxygenation is compromised.
  3. Keep a cricothyroidotomy set as standby in case intubation is not achieved.
  4. Administer 100% supplemental oxygen in patients with respiratory symptoms.
  5. Monitoring: Electrocardiogram (ECG), vital signs q 5–15 minutes, and pulse oximetry.

NOTE: Hypocalcaemia may cause a prolonged QT interval and dysrhythmias.

- **Inhalation exposure**: Administer calcium gluconate nebuliser therapies (25 ml of calcium gluconate diluted to 100 ml of water) for patients with severe respiratory distress.
- **Blisters**:
  1. Open and drain, and debride of the necrotic tissue before treatment.
  2. Then, continuously massage the burn area with calcium gluconate gel until the pain is relieved.

  NOTE: The main limitation of topical therapy is the impermeability of the skin to calcium.

  3. The gel is available in the hydrogen fluoride antidote kit or can be constituted by dissolving 10% calcium gluconate solution in 3 times the volume of water-soluble lubricant, e.g. KY gel.

4. Ensure that the medical staff wears rubber gloves during this procedure.

5. If some pain relief is not obtained within 30–60 minutes, consider calcium gluconate injections.

- **Large burns or deeply penetrating burns**:
   1. Inject sterile aqueous calcium gluconate into and around the burn area.
   2. Technique: Inject 5% calcium gluconate using a small gauge needle (No. 27–30G). Do not inject more than 0.5 ml per cm^2.
   3. **Do not inject calcium chloride** to treat skin burns. It will cause extreme pain and cause further tissue injury.

- **Hand exposure**:
   1. Subungual burns often do not respond to immersion treatment.
   2. Consider nail avulsion to expose the area in contact with the acid.

NOTE: It may be necessary to give a digital block but be aware that it may interfere with determining the adequacy of therapy.

   3. Calcium gluconate may be injected in very small amounts into the involved digit using a very small gauge needle (No. 27–30G). Care must be taken since multiple injections into the fingers can lead to tissue ischaemia.
   4. An alternative to digital block is intravenous (IV) regional calcium gluconate. Technique: Using a Bier's ischaemia arm block technique, infuse an IV solution of 10–15 ml of 10% calcium gluconate plus 5000 units of heparin diluted up to 40 ml in 5% dextrose saline. End point is:
       a. Pain relief in the digit(s).
       b. The cuff is more painful than the burn.
       c. Twenty-minute ischaemic time point has elapsed.
   5. Consider intra-arterial infusion of calcium gluconate for large burns and digital burns. Place a catheter in the brachial or radial artery and infuse a solution of 10 ml of 10% calcium gluconate in 40 ml of 5% dextrose over 4 hours. This can be repeated after 4 hours until the pain subsides.
   6. Consult Hand Surgery for all cases except those where pain disappears completely with treatment.

- **Eye exposure**:
   1. **Do not use oils, salves, or ointment** for the injured eyes.
   2. Give continuous irrigation with sterile water or saline for 15 minutes.
   3. If the pain persists, irrigate with 1% solution of calcium gluconate (50 ml of 10% solution in 450 ml of sterile saline).

NOTE: Do **not use** the **10% solution for eye irrigation**.

4. Test visual acuity:

   a. Instil fluorescein stain and perform slit-lamp examination.

5. Obtain Ophthalmology consultation if corneal defects are noted.

- **Ingestion**:

  1. DO NOT induce vomiting.

  2. May consider insertion of a nasogastric tube for gastric lavage with 10% calcium gluconate within an hour of ingestion.

     CAUTION: Risk of oesophageal and gastric perforation exists.

  3. Milk or calcium containing beverages may be consumed by the patient to bind the fluoride and dilute the acid.

  4. Consult the gastroentetologist regarding further intervention.

- **Disposition**: Admit all cases of HF acid burns.

References/Further Reading

1. Richter F, Fuilla C, et al. The early cooling of burns. In: Masellis M, Gunn SWA, eds. *The Management of Mass Burn Casualties and Fire Disasters.* London: Kluwer Academic Publishers; 1992: 273.

2. US Department of Health and Human Services. Public Health Service Agency for Toxic Substances and Disease Registry. Hydrogen fluoride. In: *Medical Management Guidelines for Acute Chemical Exposure.* 1994; III: 11–15.

3. Hudspith J, Rayatt S. ABC of burns: First aid and treatment of minor burns. *BMJ.* 19 June 2004; 328: 1487–1489.

4. Makarovsky I, Markel G, Dushnitsky T, Eisenkraft A. Hydrogen flouride: The protoplasmic poison. *Israel Med Assoc J.* May 2008; 10: 381–385.

114 Diving Emergencies

Gene Chan • Francis Lee

- The majority of diving-related medical conditions are related to the behaviour of gases, which are governed by two basic gas laws:
  1. **Boyle's law** states that at a constant temperature, the volume of a gas varies inversely with the pressure to which it is subjected. (This helps to explain the principles behind diving-related barotraumas and air embolisms.)
  2. **Henry's law** states that at a constant temperature, the amount of a gas that is dissolved in a liquid is directly proportional to the partial pressure of that gas. (This helps to explain the principles behind decompression sickness and nitrogen narcosis.)

CAVEATS

- Two major diving emergencies may be seen in the emergency department:
  1. Decompression sickness (DCS).
  2. Arterial gas embolism (AGE).
- When making the diagnosis of a dive injury, it is helpful to think of the injuries in terms of occurring during descent, while at depth or during ascent.
  1. **Descent**: Middle, inner, and external ear barotraumas, facial barotraumas, and sinus barotraumas.
  2. **Depth**: Nitrogen narcosis, hypothermia, oxygen toxicity, and contaminated gases.
  3. **Ascent**:
     a. **Rapid ascent**: Pulmonary barotraumas, e.g. pneumothorax, pneumomediastinum, pulmonary haemorrhage, AGE, barodentalgia, and gastrointestinal barotrauma.
     b. **Long/deep** near limit: Decompression sickness DCS, I or II.
- **DCS** refers to a spectrum of clinical illnesses that result from the formation of small nitrogen bubbles in the blood and tissues.
- **DCS I**: Include cutaneous manifestations and minor joint pain, or 'pain only'.
  1. **Musculoskeletal**: Bubbles accumulate in the periarticular tissues causing impaired blood flow and non-compliant tissues to stretch. Pain is most common in the elbow and shoulder joints (**the bends**).
  2. **Cutaneous**: Pruritus, local erythema, and marbling (cutis marmorata).
  3. **Lymphatic**: Localized oedema (peau d'orange effect), lymphadenopathy, or occasionally pain.
- **DCS II**: Severe symptoms related to cardiopulmonary and neurologic systems.
  1. **Neurologic**: Cerebral or spinal DCS. Spinal DCS includes limb weakness, paraesthesia, paralysis, or back pain – commonly at the lower thoracic to upper lumbar regions. Cerebral DCS includes headache, diplopia, dysarthria, unusual fatigue, or inappropriate behaviour.

2. **Inner ear**: Nausea, dizziness, vertigo or nystagmus with or without ataxia (**the staggers**).

3. **Pulmonary**: Chest pain, cough, wheezing, dyspnoea, or eventually cyanosis (**the chokes**).

- **AGE**:

  1. This is the second leading cause of mortality in divers after drowning. It results when air bubbles are forced across the alveolar-capillary membrane, escape into the pulmonary venous circulation, proceeding through the left atrium and ventricle into the arterial circulation. Embolizations into the coronary and cerebral arteries are associated with most severe consequences.

  2. Emboli to the coronary arteries may cause cardiac ischaemia, myocardial infarction, dysrhythmias, or cardiac arrest. Emboli to the cerebral arteries cause a variety of symptoms and signs similar to a stroke.

  3. Any diver who surfaces unconscious or loses consciousness within 10 minutes of reaching the surface should be assumed to be suffering from AGE.

- **DCS III**: A combination of AGE and DCS with neurologic symptoms.

⇨ **SPECIAL TIP FOR GPs**
- Think of diving emergencies in patients presenting with new vague symptoms but with a history of recent (<24 hours) participation in compressed air diving.

MANAGEMENT

- Immediate: If the patient is **stable** (most common presentation),

  1. Place the patient in the intermediate care area.

  2. Nurse in the left lateral decubitus and mild Trendelenburg position.

  3. Give 100% oxygen.

  4. Set up intravenous (IV) drip.

  5. Run IV normal saline 500 ml over 1 hour followed by 500 ml over 4 hours.

  6. If the patient is unstable, management should be carried out in the critical care area. The patient's airway, breathing and circulation (ABCs) should be assessed and monitoring is required. In very severe cases with cardiopulmonary complications or arrest, management is according to standard Advanced Cardiac Life Support (ACLS) regime.

  7. The patient should also be checked for any physical trauma sustained concomitant to diving complications.

- **Investigations**:

  1. **Chest X-ray** to look for pneumothorax or pneumomediastinum.

  2. **Electrocardiogram (ECG)** to exclude cardiac cause of chest pain if this is a primary symptom.

  3. **Arterial blood gas** if the patient is breathless or has low oxygen saturation.

- **Definitive**: The definitive treatment for diving emergencies is **immediate** recompression therapy.

  1. If you suspect that a patient has DCI or AGE, you should seek advice from a diving medicine specialist, after initial stabilization of the patient. Definitive treatment includes hyperbaric oxygen therapy in a recompression chamber initiated as quickly as possible.

  2. **If the diagnosis of a diving injury is certain, do not admit such patients to neurological or medical units 'for investigation':**

     a. These departments have no recompression facility.

     b. Delay in treatment of DCS and AGE increases morbidity or even mortality.

COMPARISONS BETWEEN DCS AND AGE

- Generally, the characteristics of **AGE** can simply be described as '**fast, short, and shallow**' and that of **DCS** as '**slow, long, and deep**' (Table 1).

TABLE 1   Characteristics of AGE and DCS

Factors	AGE	DCS
Precipitating factors	Panic underwater, resulting in rapid uncontrolled ascent	Poor dive profile. Diving longer and deeper than recommended safety limits
Diving depth	Generally shallow. Can occur with depth as shallow as 3 metres	Usually deep, beyond limits
Time course/onset of symptoms	A rapid event, seconds to minutes. Tends to be immediate, after surfacing	A slow event, few minutes to hours. Delayed
Loss of consciousness	Frequent	Infrequent
Non-specific symptoms	Infrequent	Frequent
Joint pains	Uncommon	Very common
Neurological symptoms	Tends to be unilateral like a cerebrovascular accident	Tends to be bilateral and patchy
Sensory loss	Unilateral, focal	Common, patchy

References/Further Reading

1. Bennett P, Elliot D. *The Physiology and Medicine of Diving*. 4th ed. London: WB Saunders; 1993.

2. Edmonds C, Lowry C, Pennefather J. *Diving and Subaquatic Medicine*. 3rd ed. Boston, MA: Butterworth-Heinemann; 1992.

3. Kindwall E, Whelan T. *Hyperbaric Medicine Practice*. 2nd ed. Flagstaff, AZ: Best Pub Co.; 1999.

4. Schilling CW, Carlston CB, Mathias RA. *The Physician's Guide to Diving Medicine*. New York: Plenum Press; 1984.

5. Chandy D, Weinhouse GL. Complications of scuba diving: UptoDate. Feb 2008.

6. Byyny RL, Shockley LW. Scuba diving and dysbarism. In: Marx JA, Hockberger RS, Walls RH. *Rosen's Emergency Medicine: Concepts and Clinical Practice*. 7th ed. Philadelphia, PA: Mosby Elsevier; 2010: 1903–1916.

7. www.scuba_doc.com/decosknss.htm

115 Electrical and Lightning Injuries

Peter Manning • Gene Chan

CAVEATS

- Low voltage injuries (<1000 volts) are less frequently serious than high voltage injuries. As the voltage increases, the likelihood of extensive burns increases.
- Resistance varies from tissue to tissue, with bones being the most resistant.
- The longer the duration of contact, the more severe the injury.
- Dry skin takes 3000 volts to induce ventricular fibrillation, whereas wet skin only requires household current (220–240 volts).
- Alternating current is more dangerous than direct current, causing flexor muscle tetanic contractions, 'freezing' the victim to the point of electrical contact.
- Direct current will cause a single muscle contraction that can throw the victim from his current source; lightning does the same.
- Pathway: Once the skin is breached, current passes through the least resistant tissues (nerves, vessels, and muscles) with damage being inversely proportional to the cross-sectional diameter of the affected tissue.
- True electrical conduction injuries are more like crush injuries than thermal in that the total amount of damage is often not apparent.
- **Good fluid management** is **essential** to avoid acute renal failure.

NOTE: Fluid replacement cannot be calculated based on Wallace's rule of nines as in thermal burns.

- Traditional rules of mass casualty triage do not apply to lightning victims. Victims without signs of life are treated first. Victims who are breathing are likely to survive the incident with supportive management.
- Never forget to address possible **associated injuries**:
  1. Cervical spine injuries.
  2. Toxic inhalations.
  3. Falls with fractures/dislocations.
  4. Thermal burns with possible inhalation injury.
  5. Foetal injury during pregnancy.

⇨ **SPECIAL TIP FOR GPs**
- If called to the scene first, ensure the electricity supply is switched off before approaching the victim.

TYPES OF ELECTRICAL INJURY

- **True electrical injuries (direct strike)** occur when current actually passes through the body to the ground.
- **Flash burns**:
  1. Current does not involve internal body. It only strikes the skin.
  2. Wounds are characterized by central blanching with surrounding erythema; these are simple thermal burns and are treated as such.
- **Flame burns**:
  1. Caused by ignition of clothing and are **not** considered true electrical injuries.
  2. Managed as thermal burns once electrical injury is excluded.
- **Lightning injury**: See Table 1 for details of complications.
  1. High voltage (in the millions) direct current.
  2. Cardiac injury results in asystole: Treated via Advanced Cardiac Life Support (ACLS) guidelines with delayed recovery possible.
  3. The skin around the entry site may have a spidery or pine tree appearance (**Lichtenberg figures**).

TABLE 1   Complications of electrical and lightning injuries

Body system affected	Shared complications	Unique features
Cardiovascular system	Ventricular dysrhythmias, low blood pressure (fluid loss), high blood pressure (catecholamine release), and myocardial ischaemia	Myocardial infarction is rare and tends to be a late finding in both types of injury
Neurologic	Loss of consciousness, altered mental state, convulsions, aphasia, amnesia, and peripheral neuropathy. Transient paralysis (keraunoparalysis): Peripheral vasoconstriction and sensory disturbance (specific form following a lightning injury)	Respiratory centre paralysis, intracerebral haemorrhage (ICH), cerebral oedema and infarction, and Parkinsonism are features of lightning injuries. Neuralgias are a late feature
Skin	Electrothermal contact burns, non-contact arc, and 'flash' burns, secondary thermal burns of varying depths (clothing ignition and heating of metal jewellery)	Scars and contractures are late features
Vascular	Thrombosis, coagulation necrosis, intravascular necrosis, intravascular haemolysis, delayed vessel rupture, and compartment syndrome	Disseminated intravascular coagulation in lightning injuries
Respiratory	Respiratory arrest, aspiration pneumonia, and pulmonary contusion	Pulmonary infarction and pneumonia are late features

Body system affected	Shared complications	Unique features
Renal/metabolic	Myoglobinuria, haemoglobinuria, metabolic acidosis, hypokalaemia, hypocalcaemia, and hyperglycaemia	Renal failure is uncommon
Gastrointestinal tract	Gastric atony and intestinal ileus, bowel perforation, intramural oesophageal haemorrhage, hepatic and pancreatic necrosis, and gastrointestinal bleeding	
Muscular	Compartment sydrome, clostridial myositis, and myonecrosis	
Skeletal	Secondary blunt trauma common in both types including vertebral compression fractures (from falls), long bone fractures (from victim being flung or violent muscle contractions), large joint dislocations, aseptic necrosis, periosteal burn, osteomyelitis, and osteonecrosis	
Eye	Corneal burns, intra-ocular haemorrhage or thrombosis, uveitis, retinal detachment and orbital fracture. Fixed and dilated pupils may result from autonomic dysfunction	Late injuries are delayed cataracts, macular degeneration, and optic atrophy
Ear	Hearing loss (temporary), tinnitus, haemotympanum and cerebrospinal fluid rhinorrhoea	Tympanic membrane rupture is rare
Oral burns	Delayed labial artery haemorrhage (in children who bite electrical cords) with subsequent scarring and facial deformity, delayed speech development and impaired mandibular/dentition development	These injuries are almost always seen in electrical injuries only
Foetal	Spontaneous abortion, foetal death, oligohydramnios, intrauterine growth retardation, and hyperbilirubinaemia	
Psychiatric	Hysteria, anxiety, sleep disturbance, depression, storm phobia, and cognitive dysfunction	These features tend to be more common in lightning injuries

MECHANISM OF INJURY

- Injuries due to electricity occur by 3 mechanisms:
    1. **Direct effect** of **electrical current** on body tissues.
    2. **Conversion** of **electrical to thermal energy**. This results in superficial or deep burns.
    3. **Blunt mechanical injury** caused by a fall or being thrown from an electrical source by an intense muscular contraction or explosive force.

MANAGEMENT

Supportive measures

- Patients with altered mental state or cardiac dysrhythmias should be managed in the critical care area.
- Maintain the airway with cervical spine immobilisation.
- Monitoring: Electrocardiogram, vital signs q 5–15 minutes, pulse oximetry, and cardiac monitoring.
- Establish peripheral intravenous access (2 lines if the patient is haemodynamically unstable).
- **Labs**: Full blood count, urea/electrolytes/creatinine, disseminated intravascular coagulation screen, urinalysis including myoglobin, cardiac screen, creatinine kinase, arterial blood gases (ABGs) and carboxyhaemoglobin levels in associated inhalation injury, and GXM if the injury warrants it.
- ECG in all electrical injuries.
- Administer IV crystalloid at a rate to maintain peripheral perfusion and urine output of 1–1.5 ml/kg/hr. Those with lightning injuries typically require less volume. Aim for a urine output of more than 100 ml/hr in rhabdomyolysis.
- **X-rays**: Cervical spine; then as indicated by injuries. Chest X-ray in associated inhalation injury.
- **Pain management**:
  1. Pethidine® 50–75 mg intramuscularly (IM) or 25 mg IV, **or**
  2. Diclofenac sodium (Voltaren®) 50–75 mg IM
- Insert a Foley catheter.
- Consider alkalinisation of urine to prevent renal tubular necrosis if myoglobin is demonstrated in the urine.

  Dosage: IV sodium bicarbonate 1 mmol/kg/body weight over 2 hours (1 ml of 8.4% sodium bicarbonate = 1 mmol).
- Consider placement of Ryle's tube if paralytic ileus is suspected.
- Administer anti-tetanus toxoid (ATT) 0.5 ml IM according to standard protocols.
- Cutaneous burns should be treated and dressed with a barrier/antibiotic cream, such as silver sulfadiazine.
- Consider the need for **fasciotomy/escharotomy** and consult Hand Surgery or Orthopaedics in the case of:
  1. Muscle tightness.
  2. Sensory loss.
  3. Circulatory compromise.
  4. Rapid tissue swelling.

- In case of cardiac arrest, follow standard ACLS protocols except that prolonged resuscitative efforts should be made since recovery from prolonged asystole is possible.

Special situations

- **Paediatric considerations**:
  1. **Oral commissure burns** are almost exclusively found in children and can involve considerable morbidity. There is a high likelihood of cosmetic deformity.
  2. Fatalities are rare since the electrical circuit is completed locally in the mouth.
  3. There is **local sloughing of tissue** on the 7th to 10th days and this may lead to brisk bleeding from the labial artery when the eschar separates.
  4. **Admit** all such burns on the day of presentation.

- **Obstetric considerations**:
  1. Foetal injury depends on the flow of current through the mother's body.
  2. Significant foetal injury (death or intrauterine growth restriction) may occur following even minor degrees of electrical shock to the mother, especially in cases of oligohydramnios.
  3. Placental abruption is the most common cause of foetal death after blunt trauma. In early pregnancy, spontaneous abortion may occur.
  4. Obtain Obstetrics and Gynaecology consultation in all cases of electrical injuries during pregnancy and keep in view foetal monitoring.

- **Electronic weapons**:
  1. Law enforcement and security personnel are using electronic weapons, e.g. stun gun (Tasers) to provide less lethal alternatives to conventional weapons.
  2. These devices deliver brief bursts of high voltage, low amperage direct current that incapacitate the subject.
  3. There have been no deaths directly attributable to the electrical discharge, however, the Tasers are capable of inducing fatal arrhythmias and cardiac arrest.
  4. Evaluation and treatment should focus on wounds caused by the probes and secondary injuries associated with any induced fall.

Disposition

- **Admission criteria**:
  1. All patients with high voltage injury (>1000 volts).
  2. All patients with specific organ system involvement.
  3. All patients with suspected neurovascular compromise to the extremities.
  4. All patients with oral commissure burns.
  5. Deep hand burns.

- **Discharge criteria**:

  1. Patients without evidence of burns.

  2. Patients with minor injuries including feathering burns (Lichtenberg figures) with appropriate referral to an outpatient setting.

References/Further Reading

1. Fish RM. Electrical injuries. Lightning injuries. In: Tintinalli JE, Ma OJ, Stapczynski JS, et al., eds. *Tintinalli's Emergency Medicine: A Comprehensive Study Guide*. 7th ed. New York: McGraw-Hill; 201: 1386–1394.

2. Price TG, Cooper MA. Electrical and lightning injuries. In: Marx JA, Hockberger RS, Walls RH. *Rosen's Emergency Medicine: Concepts and Clinical Practice*. 7th ed. Philadelphia, PA: Mosby Elsevier; 2010: 1893–1902.

3. Duane SP, Peter FC. Environmental electrical injuries – UptoDate Mar 2008. Lit Review version: Jan 2011.

Keith Ho • Francis Lee

CAVEATS

- **Hyperthermia** is a rise in body temperature above the hypothalamic set point when heat dissipating mechanisms are impaired or overwhelmed.
- **Heat injuries** span a spectrum from **heat cramps** and **heat syncope** to **heat exhaustion** and **heat stroke**. Heat stroke can lead to multi-organ dysfunction with acute respiratory distress syndrome (ARDS), disseminated intravascular coagulation (DIVC), hepatic dysfunction, shock, rhabdomyolysis, renal failure, cerebral oedema, and seizures.
- Other causes of hyperthermia include **malignant hyperthermia** (following treatment with anaesthetic agents) and **neuroleptic malignant syndrome** (an idiosyncratic reaction to anti-psychotic agents).

HEAT STROKE

- The **classic triad** for heat stroke is:
  1. Rectal temperature of >40.5°C.
  2. Altered mental state.
  3. Hot dry skin.

  This triad represents an advanced stage of the condition and should be used with caution. If followed too rigidly, one may miss many cases of early heat stroke.
- Diagnosis requires a high index of suspicion as many of the symptoms and signs are non-specific. Altered mental state, delirium, convulsions and syncope with an exposure to environmental heat (classical heat stroke) or strenuous physical exercise (exertional heat stroke) should alert one to the diagnosis of heat stroke.
- Central nervous system infections, sepsis, neuroleptic malignant syndrome or malignant hyperthermia should be excluded prior to making the diagnosis of heat stroke.
- Prolonged activity or incarceration in an enclosed space (e.g. a nursing home, sauna, boiler room, etc.) without proper ventilation or air-conditioning is a significant risk factor for heat stroke.

HEAT EXHAUSTION

- Heat exhaustion is a precursor of heat stroke caused by either salt or water depletion.
- **Clinical features**:
  1. Anxiety, irritability, malaise, and fatigue.
  2. Polydipsia, nausea, and vomiting.
  3. Hyperventilation and carpopedal spasm.

4. Raised rectal temperature (<40°C).

5. Tachycardia and orthostatic hypotension.

6. Mild liver enzyme abnormalities.

7. Raised creatine kinase levels.

- There is no clear distinction between heat exhaustion and heat stroke and the 2 conditions share some common features, making diagnosis difficult. As a general guide, patients with **heat exhaustion** usually have **no history of altered mental state**.

RISK FACTORS FOR HEAT STROKE

- Several factors may predispose a person to heat injuries:
  1. Lack of acclimatization and poor physical fitness.
  2. Obesity.
  3. Extremes of age.
  4. Concurrent diseases such as ischaemic heart disease, diabetes mellitus, skin disorders, infectious disease.
  5. States of dehydration such as alcohol use, diarrhoea, and vomiting.
  6. Drugs such as anticholinergics, antihistamines, diuretics, and beta blockers.
  7. Recreational drugs such as amphetamines and cocaine.
  8. Preceding pyrexia.
  9. Prior history of heat injuries.

DIFFERENTIAL DIAGNOSES

- Many conditions producing altered mental state with pyrexia, mimic heat stroke:
  1. Intracranial infections such as meningitis and encephalitis.
  2. Infections such as typhoid and malaria.
  3. Malignant hyperthermia and neuroleptic malignant syndrome.
  4. Neurologic disorders such as stroke and epilepsy.
  5. Metabolic conditions such as thyroid storm.

⇨ **SPECIAL TIPS FOR GPs**
- Call for the ambulance for transport to the emergency department.
- Institute early cooling by undressing the patient as much as possible and sponging or spraying with water to wet the skin. Direct a fan at the victim to aid cooling by evaporation.
- Hydration is important. Oral fluids could be given if the patient is alert and able to tolerate it. An intravenous (IV) drip treatment would be ideal.

MANAGEMENT

- The **initial steps** in the **management of heat injuries** are as follows:
  1. Transfer the patient to the resuscitation or critical care area of the emergency department.
  2. Secure the airway, breathing and circulation.
  3. Provide supplemental oxygen.
  4. Set up large bore IV in both cubital fossae and infuse cool fluids.
  5. Set up cardiac and vital signs monitoring.
  6. Assess rectal temperature.

- **Cooling** of the patient must be carried out next:
  1. Remove all clothing.
  2. Use body cooling unit (evaporative cooling method) or sponge and spray with cold water and fan the patient.
  3. Cooling should be carried out until rectal temperature reaches 38.5°C.

- **Perform an ECG** to look for cardiovascular problems. In acute heat disorders, tachycardia is almost always present. Other features may include non-specific ST and T changes and conduction abnormalities. ECG may indicate any pre-existing cardiovascular disorders.

- Perform a **chest X-ray** to look for evidence of pulmonary oedema or ARDS. Pulmonary infarctions have been described in heat stroke.

- Order a **stat capillary blood glucose** to look for hypoglycaemia so that treatment can be instituted. However, hyperglycaemia may be seen in heat stroke and does not necessarily indicate the presence of diabetes mellitus.

- **Blood investigations**:
  1. Full blood count: Leucocytosis is common without infection. Thrombocytopaenia may be seen.
  2. Electrolytes: Sodium and potassium levels may be elevated, normal, or low, depending on many factors. Hypomagnesaemia and hypocalcaemia may occur.
  3. Muscle enzymes are commonly raised.
  4. Liver function test: Abnormalities of hepatic enzymes are almost always present.
  5. Arterial blood gas test may indicate alkalosis from hyperventilation or metabolic acidosis from tissue injury and hypoxia.
  6. A coagulation profile may indicate the onset of coagulopathy.

- **Urine dipstick** to look for blood and myoglobin. Alternatively, a sample may be sent to the lab to measure urine myoglobin.

- During cooling, shivering may occur, countering efforts in lowering the body temperature. This can be controlled with IV diazepam 5 mg or IV chlorpromazine 25–50 mg.

- Insert a nasogastric tube to manage acute gastric distension.

- Give IV cimetidine 400 mg stat to prevent acute gastritis.
- The patient must be catheterized to measure the urine output.
- **Precautions**
  1. The mechanism for heat stroke does not involve a shift in the 'physiological thermostat' and therefore **antipyretics** are **not helpful**. Aspirin must be avoided as it may cause coagulation problems while the use of paracetamol may aggravate hepatic injury.
  2. **Alcohol cannot be used** for body cooling despite a higher specific heat for vaporization because skin absorption may cause progressive drowsiness and obtundation.
  3. **Hypotension must be corrected** before effective cooling can be carried out.
  4. Beware of **rebound pulmonary oedema** when vasoconstriction occurs after the heat stroke is controlled.

DISPOSITION

- Admit all heat stroke patients.
- Recovered heat exhaustion without end-organ damage can be observed in the emergency department and then discharged.

References/Further Reading

1. Waters TA, Al-Salamah MA. Heat emergencies In: Tintinalli JE, Ma OJ, Stapczynski JS, et al., eds. *Tintinalli's Emergency Medicine: A Comprehensive Study Guide*. 7th ed. New York: McGraw-Hill; 2011: 1339–1343.

2. Gaffin SL, Gardner JW, Flinn SD. Cooling method for exertional heatstroke victims. *Ann Intern Med*. 2000; 132: 678.

3. Bouchama A, Knochel JP. Heat stroke. *N Engl J Med*. 2002; 345(25): 1978–1988.

117   Submersion Injuries

Keith Ho • Francis Lee

DEFINITIONS

- **Drowning**: Submersion injuries resulting in death within 24 hours.
- **Submersion injury**: Survival, at least temporarily, for >24 hours after aspiration of fluid into the lungs, or after a period of asphyxia secondary to laryngospasm.

CAVEATS

- **Immediate rescue** (<5 minutes) and **early on-site resuscitation** (cardiopulmonary resuscitation, and rescue breathing) are the keys to patient survival.
- An important part of assessment is to look for a **cause** (e.g. trauma, suicide, poisoning, and sea creature envenomation).
- **Hypothermia** is a potential complication, especially in the younger age group.

INITIAL PREHOSPITAL MANAGEMENT

- Immediate rescue from water.
- Assessment of the airway, breathing and circulation (ABCs).
- Routine stabilization of the cervical spine during resuscitation is unnecessary unless the circumstances leading up to the submersion event suggest trauma (e.g. history of diving, use of a water slide, alcohol intoxication, or signs of injuries).
- The pulse may be difficult to palpate in patients with submersion injuries due to hypothermia or dysrhythmias. Initiate CPR promptly if a pulse is not felt within 10 seconds.
- Provide high flow oxygen via a face mask (if the patient is breathing) or via bag-valve-mask (if the patient is apnoeic).
- Establish intravenous (IV) access (if the necessary equipment is available).

MANAGEMENT

- The management of near drowning focuses on securing the ABCs and correction of hypoxia.
- The duration and severity of hypoxia are the most important determinants of outcome. The distinction between **fresh water** and **salt water drowning** has been deemphasized as it has not been shown to be clinically significant.
- **Lung drainage procedures**, e.g. the Heimlich manoeuvre or abdominal thrusts, are controversial. These are **not** recommended because their effectiveness is not concretely proven, the execution of the manoeuvres could potentially cause more harm than good to the victim and distracts the care provider from more urgent goals of resuscitation.

- **Antibiotics** and **steroids** have **no proven benefit** in near-drowning victims.
- **Diuretics** are of **no help** in non-cardiogenic pulmonary oedema.

Initial hospital management

- Transfer the patient to a high acuity area of the department.
- **Primary survey**:
  1. Check the ABCs. Consider intubation if the airway is not secured.
  2. Stabilize the cervical spine and avoid neck movements.
  3. Give 100% oxygen. Assist ventilation if breathing is inadequate.
  4. Provide positive end-expiratory pressure (PEEP); this will often improve oxygenation.
  5. Establish an IV line and draw blood for full blood count, urea/electrolytes/creatinine, and arterial blood gas.
  6. Put the patient on full monitoring: Electrocardiogram (ECG), parameters, and pulse oximetry.
  7. Perform a **chest X-ray** to assess the severity of aspiration.
  8. Keep the patient warm at all times.
  9. Treat **hypothermia** (in the tropics, hypothermia is uncommon and if it occurs, it is usually mild: 32–35°C):
     a. Remove all the wet clothing and dry the patient.
     b. Provide adequate insulation (wrap the patient in a clean dry blanket or aluminium foil).
     c. Apply external warming if necessary (warming blanket).
     d. Warm all the fluids for the patient.
- **Secondary survey**:
  1. Do a head-to-toe examination for possible causes or effects of the near-drowning incident.
  2. Pay special attention to the following:
     a. Altered sensorium after resuscitation: Possible alcohol and drug use.
     b. Head injury: Look for signs on the scalp and face.
     c. Cervical spine injury may be the cause or effect of the near-drowning incident.
     d. Epilepsy: Abrasions and injury to the tongue is a clue.
     e. Cardiac dysrhythmias: ECG assessment and monitoring is important.
     f. Diving injuries: For example, decompression illness (DCI) or cerebral arterial gas embolism (CAGE).
  3. Perform serial Glasgow Coma Scale (GCS) assessment.

Disposition

- **Generally all** victims with submersion injuries should be **admitted**.
- Those who look well can be managed in an observation ward for at least 12 hours and subsequently be **discharged** if:
  1. The patient looks well and alert.
  2. There are no abnormal vital signs.
  3. The chest X-ray is normal.
  4. There is a reliable guardian or caregiver at home.
- A patient should be admitted to the **intensive care unit** if:
  1. The patient is intubated.
  2. There is continued altered mental state.
  3. There are unstable parameters despite resuscitation.

Prognosis

- Patients with the following factors have a **poor prognosis**:
  1. Children <3 years old.
  2. Estimated submersion time is >10 minutes.
  3. No resuscitation was provided within 10 minutes of the rescue.
  4. Glasgow Coma Scale score of <5.
  5. Delayed respiratory gasp only occurred 20 minutes after the rescue.
  6. Persistent apnoea and requirement of cardiopulmonary resuscitation in the emergency department.
  7. Resuscitation attempts lasted >25 minutes.
  8. Arterial blood pH is <7.1 upon presentation.

References/Further Reading

1. Causey AL, Nichter MA. Drowning. In: Tintinalli JE, Ma OJ, Stapczynski JS, et al., eds. *Tintinalli's Emergency Medicine: A Comprehensive Study Guide*. 7th ed. New York: McGraw-Hill; 2011: 1371–1374.

2. 2005 American Heart Association Guidelines for Cardiopulmonary Resuscitation and Emergency Cardiovascular Care: Part 10.3 Drowning. *Circulation*. 2005; 112(suppl I): IV–133–IV–135.

3. Bierens JJ, Knape JT, Gelissen HP. Drowning. *Curr Opin Crit Care*. 2002; 8: 578.

118 Emergency Ultrasound

Toh Hong Chuen • Peng Li Lee • Sim Tiong Beng

CAVEATS

- Emergency ultrasound can be thought of as a procedural skill that yields the fruits of a point of care test.

- It differs from formal ultrasound fundamentally in that it is performed by the bedside and focused in nature, directed to look for the presence or absence of a particular sonographic finding. In addition, it is usually one single clinician provider who orders, performs, interprets and intervenes based on the scan. The entire clinical decision making process can thus be shortened, and strengthened with the ultrasound findings.

- Emergency ultrasound is particularly useful in the assessment and management of the critically ill patient.

- Being focused in nature, it does not replace formal ultrasound when indicated. It is also not an extension of the stethoscope, and should not be used as a replacement for good physical examination.

- Be familiar with the knobs, probes and presets of the ultrasound machine in your department (or work area), and learn how to optimize its image. It will yield dividends on the accuracy and efficiency of your scans.

- Always save your scans: it is important for clinical documentation, competency assessment, credentialing, accreditation and quality audit purposes.

IMAGE OPTIMIZATION

- **Gel**: Gel facilitates the transmission of the ultrasound beam into the patient's body. Use it well.
- Use the **correct probe**, with the **correct presets**.
  1. **Liner probe**: high frequency but poor penetration, for superficial structure e.g. localizing foreign body in skin/soft tissue.
  2. **Curvilinear probe**: low frequency but good penetration, for deep structure e.g. abdominal aorta
  3. **Sector probe**: low frequency probe but small foot print, allow scanning in-between ribs e.g. cardiac ultrasound.
- **Depth**: Maximize the view by bringing the target tissue/organ to the least depth required for visualization
- **Focus**: Set the focus at the level of the organ/tissue of interest. It will improve the spatial resolution at that level.
- **Time gain compensation (TGC)**: Set it neutral first; get the image, then apply TGC.
- **Angle the beam at 90 degrees to the long axis of organ/tissue of interest**: This will maximize returning echoes, hence generating a clearer image.

- **Respiratory maneuvers**: Abdominal organs such as the liver and spleen moves with respiration. Deep inspiratory hold, for example, often allows a better visualization of the gallbladder.

Lung ultrasound for pneumothorax/tension pneumothorax

- **Image acquisition**:
  1. Patient: supine
  2. Preset: lung
  3. Probe: curvilinear, in B and M mode. (if indicated, the linear probe could be used to identify other pleural-based pathologies)
  4. Position: anterior chest wall mid clavicular line, sagittal plane; or the highest point on the anterior chest wall when the patient is lying supine.

- **Identification of pleura** (bat's sign):
  1. On the B mode: identify the 2 ribs (two bright curves facing posteriorly, each casting an acoustic shadow). The bright line/curve facing upward just below and in between the ribs is the pleura: the 2 ribs being the 'bat wings' and the pleura being the body of the 'bat'. (Figure 1)

- **Interpretation**:
  1. The outer parietal pleura normally slides over the visceral pleura during respiration, producing a shimmering effect on the pleural on B mode called **lung sliding** and a **sea-shore appearance** on M mode: the horizontal lines above the pleura is the *sea* and granular sandy appearance below the pleura is the *shore* (Figure 2). On M mode, when the 2 pleurae are not sliding against each other (e.g. pneumothorax, pleurodesis), the 'sandy' pattern below the pleura is lost, replaced by straight horizontal lines. This pattern is termed the '**stratosphere**' sign. The term 'bar-code' sign may not be appropriate given the varying configurations of day bar-codes nowadays.
  2. **A line**. A-lines are repetitive **horizontal** artifacts that recur at regular intervals that are equal to the distance between the probe-skin interface and the pleural-subpleural air interface. This is a form of reverberation artifact. This artifact in itself does not denote any pathology.

FIGURE 1   **Bat's wing, for identification of the pleura (B mode)**

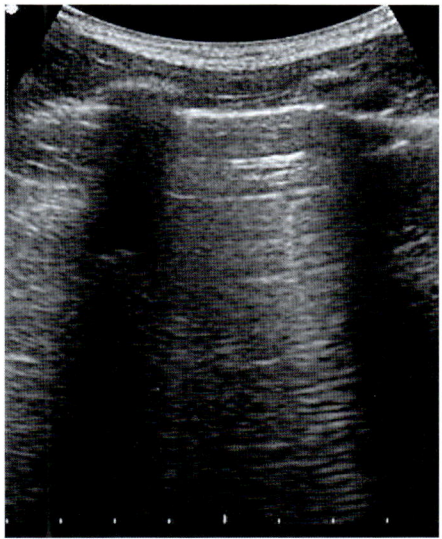

FIGURE 2   **Seashore sign (M mode)**

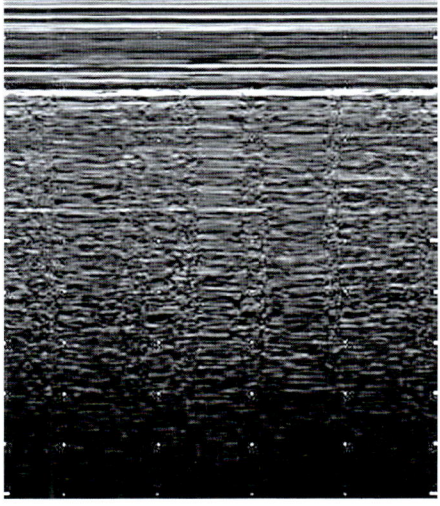

3. **B line**. B-lines are defined as discrete laser-like **vertical** hyperechoic reverberation artifacts that arise from the pleural line, extending to the bottom of the screen **without fading**, and moves synchronously with lung sliding if lung sliding is present. The anatomic and physical basis of B-lines is not known with certainty at this time. They are thought to arise from sub-pleural interlobular septa thickening, usually from fluid. B lines confined laterally to the last intercostal space just above the diaphragm, if not associated with alveolar consolidation, is considered normal, equivalent of Kerley B line on Chest X-ray. Multiple and diffuse B lines, however, is pathological and indicates an interstitial syndrome. (Figure 3). As the visceral pleura must touch the parietal pleura for B lines to be generated, the presence of B line excludes pneumothorax at that site.

4. **Pneumothorax** is *suggested* in the appropriate clinical context if there is **absence of lung sliding/sea shore sign** (i.e. no lung sliding). It can be diagnosed with 100% specificity if **lung point** is demonstrated: the lung point is the interface between the normal lung and pneumothorax, where there is alternating presence and absence of lung sliding with respiration. On the M mode, the lung point is where 'sea-shore' sign alternates with the 'stratosphere' sign. (Figure 4). As both visceral and parietal pleura must be touching for B lines to be seen, the **presence of B lines excludes pneumothorax**.

• **Pitfalls**:
1. Absence of lung sliding can be observed whenever there is no parietal and visceral pleura sliding on each other, e.g. non-ventilated left lung in right mainstem bronchus intubation or pleurodesis.

FIGURE 3   Multiple B lines from the pleura (B mode)

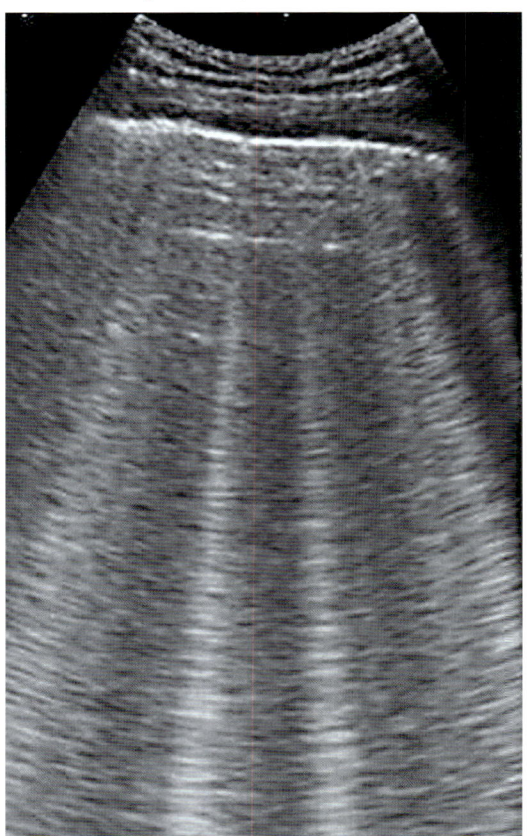

FIGURE 4   Lung point, where the 'seashore' sign transits into the 'barcode' sign

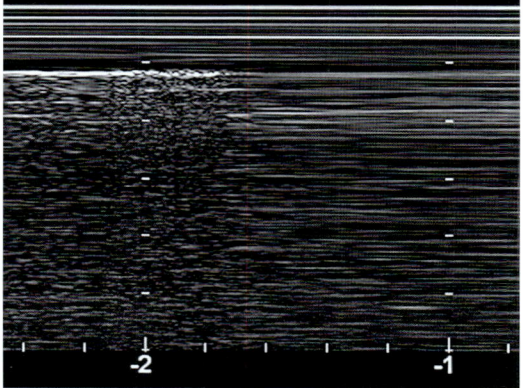

2. **Z-lines**. They are vertical hyperechoic artifact arising from the pleura, but unlike the B lines, they fade away before reaching the bottom of the screen. They are of unknown clinical significance, and must not be mistaken for B lines.

- **Comments**

   1. The presence of either B lines or lung sliding rules out pneumothorax. This can be done very quickly and the search for other causes of shock can be initiated.

Inferior vena cava assessment as a surrogate marker for right atrial pressure

- **Image acquisition**:

   1. Patient: Supine

   2. Preset: Abdominal

   3. Probe: Curvilinear probe, B mode

   4. Position: Right costal margin, start with the transverse view for identification of the IVC, then examine it in the longitudinal view

- **Identification**:

   1. The IVC is identified on the transverse view on B mode, as a round structure resting on the right side of the spine (as opposed to the aorta on the left) then rotate 90 degrees clockwise to get the longitudinal view. Measurement of the IVC diameter should be made at end-expiration and just proximal to the junction with the middle hepatic vein. (Figure 5)

FIGURE 5   Measuring the size of the IVC, 1–2 cm distal to the middle hepatic vein

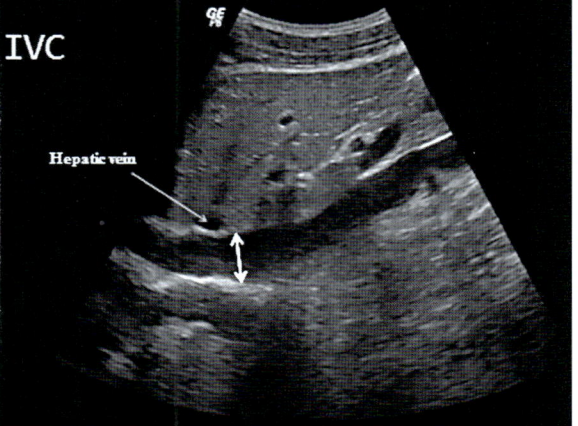

- **Interpretation**:

IVC diameter (cm)	Respiratory collapse with sniff (%)	Right atrial pressure (mmHg)
≤2.1	>50	Normal: 0–5 [3]
≤2.1	<50	Intermediate: 5–10 [8]
>2.1	>50	Intermediate: 5–10 [8]
>2.1	<50	High: 10–20 [15]

- **Pitfalls**:

   1. While applying pressure on the probe may be needed to displace bowel gas interference, take note that excessive pressure can compress the IVC giving a erroneously small diameter

   2. The IVC moves in the cranial-caudal direction with respiration. Therefore, the measurement of IVC size and collapsibility is preferably made using B mode rather than M mode.

- **Comments**:

1. The IVC size and collapsibility are affected by both the **volume status** and **right atrial pressure**. Like the CVP, it does not accurately reflect the pre-load to the left ventricular, i.e. the left ventricular end-diastolic pressure.

2. The above values apply spontaneously breathing patients. In patients who are unable to perform a sniff, an IVC that collapses <20% with quiet respiration suggests an elevated right atrial pressure.

Cardiac ultrasound for cardiac tamponade

- **Image acquisition**:
  1. Patient: Supine
  2. Preset: Cardiac
  3. Probe: Sector probe, B mode
  4. Position: Apical 4 chamber view (place the probe at the apex beat, tilt the probe toward the right shoulder and scan the heart in the coronal plane that depicts the 4 chambers)
     a. Alternatively, use the subcostal 4 chamber view as per the FAST protocol.

- **Identification of heart/pericardial fluid**:
  1. The 4 chambers of the heart are easily recognized. Pericardial fluid appears as a hypoechoic rim surrounding the heart.

- **Interpretation**:
  1. **Cardiac tamponade** (Figure 6) is diagnosed if there is haemodynamic instability with a pericardial effusion that causes
     a. Right atrial systolic collapse (early)
     b. Right ventricle diastolic collapse (late)
     c. Distension and lack of respiratory variation in the IVC.

- **Pitfalls**:
  1. Pericardial fluid first accumulates in the most dependent area of the heart, usually at the atrio-ventricular groove, best appreciated in the parasternal long axis view. Pericardial fluid in this groove is considered physiologic (normal) if seen only in systole, and disappears in diastole.

FIGURE 6 **Pericardial tamponade. Large pericardial effusion as shown by arrow with collapsed chambers**

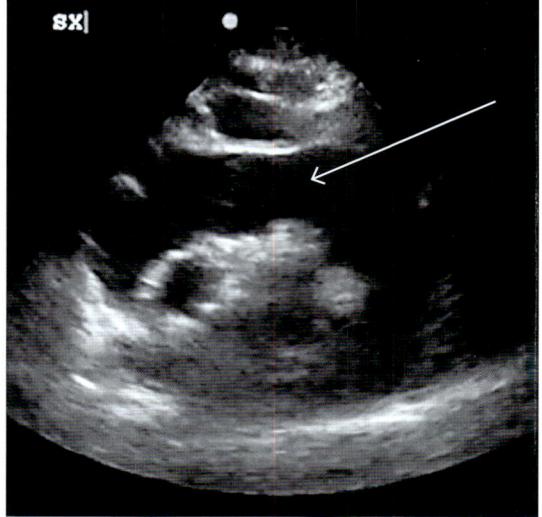

2. It may be difficult to *time* (systole-diastole) the atrial/ventricle collapse. If the right sided chambers are grossly collapsed in the presence of pericardial effusion *and* hypotension, treat as for a cardiac tamponade.

3. Epicardial fat that is usually located in the anterior precordial space may sometimes be mistaken for a pericardial clot. Closer examination usually reveals echogenicity characteristic of fat. Being epicardial in location, the fat will move in tandem with the cardiac contraction, with equal vigor; unlike pericardial clot.

4. It is the **rate, rather than the volume**, of pericardial fluid accumulation that tips the heart into the tamponade physiology.

5. Patients who are not able to mount a tachycardia response, e.g. on beta-blockers, are more prone to go into cardiac tamponade.

Cardiac ultrasound for estimation of left ventricular ejection function

- **Image acquisition**:
  1. Patient: supine (or ideally left lateral decubitus position with left arm above head)
  2. Preset: cardiac
  3. Probe: sector probe, B mode
  4. Position: 4 standard cardiac views (Parasternal long axis: 2–4th left intercostal space just next to the sternum, parallel to the long axis of the left ventricle/parasternal short axis: rotate 90 degrees clockwise from the parasternal long axis view to get the short axis/apical 4 chamber – as above/subcostal 4 chamber – see below)

- **Identification of heart**:
  1. The chambers of the heart are easily identified in the parasternal and apical views. In the subcostal 4 chamber view, the right ventricle and atrium are adjacent to the diaphragm/liver, while the left sided chambers are away.

- **Interpretation**:
  1. Make a visual estimation of the **ejection fraction** (how well the endocardial border is moving towards the centre of the LV) and the filling status of the left ventricle:
     a. Contractility: normal (≥EF 55%), mildly depressed (45–54%); moderately depressed (EF 30–44%), severely depressed (EF < 30%)
     b. Filling status: well filled or under filled.

Cardiac Ultrasound	Suggested clinical entity
Well filled hyperdynamic LV	Distributive shock
Well filled hypodynamic LV	Cardiogenic shock (ischemic or metabolic, toxidromes)
Under filled hyperdynamic LV	Hypovolemic shock, obstructive shock

- **Comments**:
  1. To appreciate the global systolic function of the LV, visualize it in at least 2 out of the 4 standard views.

2. With training, visual estimation of ejection fraction is as good as the calculated ejection fraction. Both tend to be more accurate when the ventricle is regularly shaped and contracts in a symmetric fashion.

3. Other visual estimate of a normal systolic function include a good swing of the mitral valve during diastole (the anterior mitral valve leaflet should nearly touch the interventricular septum during early diastolic filling) and a shortening of the LV internal diameter at the level of the papillary muscle by at least 25%.

4. Always assess the IVC and the lung (in particular for B lines) together with cardiac ultrasound to assess for the patient's hemodynamic status.

5. Identification of regional wall motion abnormality and valvular pathologies are typically not within the scope of basic emergency cardiac ultrasound.

Cardiac ultrasound for massive acute pulmonary embolism

- **Image acquisition**:
  1. Patient: supine
  2. Preset: cardiac
  3. Probe: sector probe, B mode
  4. Position: apical 4 chamber view, parasternal short axis view
- **Identification**:
  1. The 4 chambers of the heart, shape and movement of the interventricular septum
- **Interpretation**:
  1. Massive pulmonary embolism with acute right heart strain

     a. **Large** (approaching or even exceeding the size of LV in diastole) **right ventricle**, with blunting of the RV apex (which is normally sharp)

     b. The **RV wall** is **thin** (<5mm, as measured in the subcostal 4 chamber view). The combination of RV dilatation with normal thickness suggests that an acute RV pressure overload. (Figure 7)

     c. Paradoxical bowing of septum into the left ventricle during diastole, causing a **"D" shaped LV** (Figure 8). Normally, the interventricular septum is round during both systole and diastole, as the LV pressure is always higher than the RV. In a massive acute PE, however,

FIGURE 7   **An enlarged right ventricle as shown by arrow**

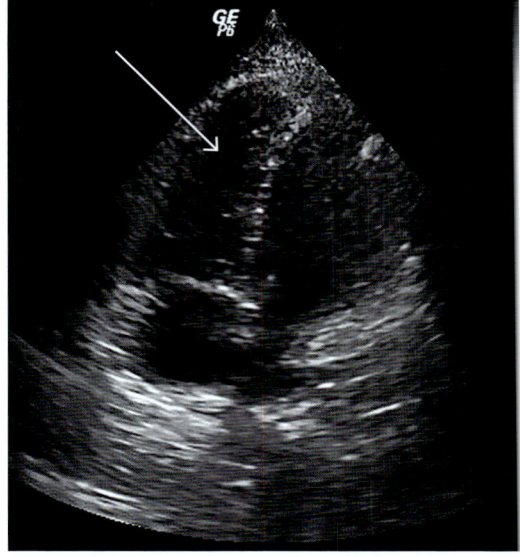

there is sudden rise in right ventricular pressure. Coupled with reduced left ventricular filling, this increased RV pressure deforms the septum during diastole. During systole, however, the LV pressure exceeds the RV pressure again, restoring the shape of the septum.

d. This diastolic paradoxical septal movement can also seen in patients who are volume overloaded. This, however, can be usually distinguished clinically.

e. In patients with chronic pulmonary hypertension, the RV hypertrophies and could raise the RV pressure high enough during both systole and diastole, resulting in a D-shaped septum throughout the cardiac cycle.

FIGURE 8 **'D' shaped LV due to increased right ventricular pressure as shown by arrow**

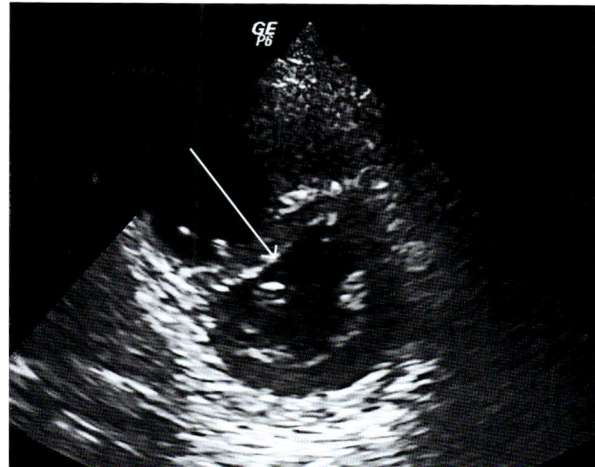

- **Pitfall**:

1. The above mentioned changes may not be detectable if the PE load is small and does not produce significant right heart strain.

- **Comments**:

1. The **McConnel sign** (hypomotility of RV free wall with relative apical sparing) is no longer considered a reliable sign for pulmonary embolism.

2. Proceed to search for deep vein thrombosis if pulmonary embolism is suspected.

Focused Assessment with Sonography in Trauma (FAST)

- **Image acquisition**:

1. Patient: Supine
2. Preset: Abdominal
3. Probe: Curvilinear, B mode
4. Position:

   a. **Right upper quadrant view (Morrison's pouch)**.

      i. Start on the right mid-axillary line in the coronal plane, at the level of the xiphisternum.

   b. **Left upper quadrant view (Spleno-renal angle)**

      i. Start on the left posterior axillary line in the coronal plane, at the level of the xiphisternum.

c. **Suprapubic**

i. Transverse and longitudinal view, just above the pubic symphysis.

d. **Subcostal**

i. Over the epigastrium, almost in the coronal plane, using liver as acoustic window.

- **Identification**:

1. **RUQ/LUQ view**: identify hypoechoic collection in hepato-renal and spleno-renal space respectively (Figure 9)

2. **Suprapubic view**: identify hypoechoic collection in the rectovesical or rectouterine pouch. (Figure 10)

3. **Subcostal view**: identify the presence of hypoechoic collection in the pericardial sac.

- **Pitfalls**:

1. **False negative**:

a. Not completing the 4 standard views. A single view of Morrison's pouch has sensitivity of only 51%, compared to 87% with all 4 views.

b. Not enough blood (yet). With infusion of fluid via DPL, the mean amount of free fluid that results in a positive RUQ scan is 619 ml. But, when patient is *hypotensive* from intraperitoneal bleed, ultrasound is nearly 100% sensitive. Use the trendenlenburg position for RUQ/LUQ view and reverse trendenlenburg position for pelvic view to increase sensitivity.

c. Clotted blood could have similar echogenicity as parenchymal tissue, and thus could be easily missed.

d. In patients with peritoneal/pleural adhesions, the free fluid may not develop in the expected locations.

2. **False positive**:

a. Hypoechoic/anechoic areas with small amounts of internal echos: perinephric fat/epicardial fat pads, pericardial cysts.

b. Anechoic areas without any internal echoes: urine, ascites, pleural-pericardial effusion, fluid-filled hollow viscus (stomach/bowel)

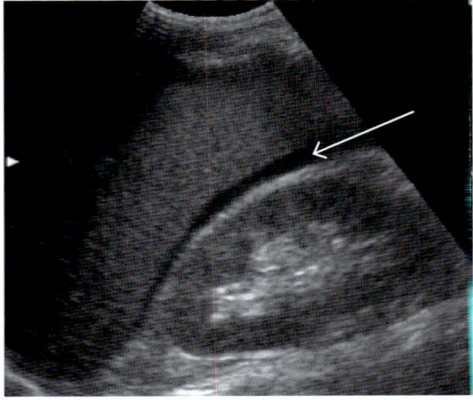

FIGURE 9   **Free fluid in the Morrison's pouch as shown by arrow**

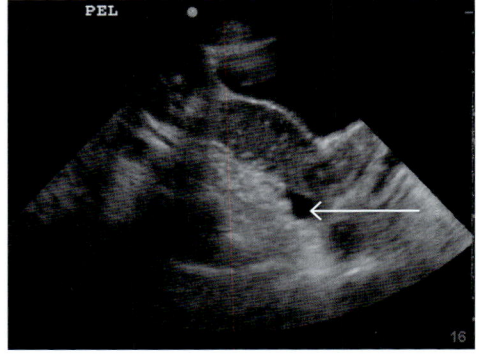

FIGURE 10   **Free fluid in the pouch of Douglas as shown by arrow**

c. Small amount of pelvic fluid in children and woman of reproductive age may be physiological.

- **Comments**:

  1. The diaphragm is visualised by sliding the probe up 1–2 rib spaces OR by asking the patient to inhale deeply. Pay attention to the left subdiaphragmatic space, which is often where blood first accumulates on the LUQ.

  2. Similarly, the paracolic gutters are visualised by sliding downward from the RUQ/LUQ view towards the iliac crest, looking for hypoechoic collections on which the large bowel is usually seen 'floating' on.

  3. **Extended FAST** is variably defined. It usually involved pulmonary ultrasound to assess for pneumothorax, with or without IVC assessment.

Abdominal ultrasound for abdominal aortic aneurysm:

- **Image acquisition**:

  1. Patient: supine

  2. Preset: abdominal

  3. Probe: curvilinear, B mode

  4. Position: transverse and longitudinal view – from epigastrium to umbilicus

- **Identification**:

  1. First identify the spine on the transverse view (bright C shaped line facing posteriorly and casting an acoustic shadow). The tubular structure just above spine on the patient's left is the aorta. Trace the course of the abdominal aorta from just above the celiac axis (in the epigastrium) to its bifurcation (at the umbilicus) into the iliac arteries. Take measurement from outer wall to outer wall of the abdominal aorta and iliac arteries.

- **Interpretation**:

  1. Abdominal aortic aneurysm = diameter of ≥ **3cm**

  2. Iliac artery aneurysm = diameter of ≥ **1.5cm**

- **Pitfalls**:

  1. Failing to distinguish the IVC from the aorta. (See table.)

  2. **False negative**: measuring the inner diameter of aortic aneurysm underestimate the size of aneurysm, especially if there is a flap or mural thrombus. (Figure 11)

  3. **False positive**: occurs when the imaging plane is oblique to the long axis of the aorta; especially in tortuous aorta. So align the probe perpendicular to the long axis of the aorta.

FIGURE 11 **An abdominal aortic aneurysm of approximately 5cm in outer diameter**

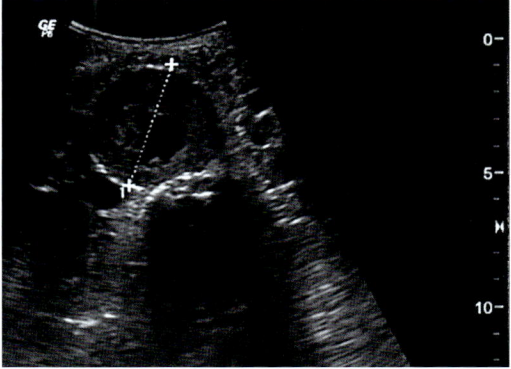

4. **Difficulty in visualising the entire abdominal aorta**

   a. Usually due to overlying bowel gas. Often, all that is needed is patience, for peristalsis to 'disperse' the gas away. Consider applying gentle pressure, if at all. Alternatively, slide the probe to laterally, away from the gas until a soft tissue window is obtained, then angulate the probe towards the aorta. Consider using the kidneys as windows to visualise the aorta in the coronal plane.

   b. Flex the patient's hip as for a standard abdominal physical examination, to relax the rectus abdominis muscles. This could bring the probe nearer to the deep abdominal aorta.

   c. Consider CT scan if clinically indicated.

5. Abdominal ultrasound does not reliably exclude the presence of complications from the aneurysm, such as retroperitoneal leakage.

Differentiating the aorta from the IVC

	Aorta	IVC
Position	Left	Right
Wall	Thick	Thin
Compressibility	No	Yes Walls may collapse with deep inspiration (ask the patient to take a sniff)
Pulsatile	Yes	May be transmitted from aorta
Colour flow	Flow away from heart	Flow towards heart

Abdominal ultrasound for cholecystitis

- **Image acquisition**:
  1. Patient: Supine or left lateral decubitus
  2. Preset: Abdominal
  3. Probe: Curvilinear probe, B mode
  4. Position: Right costal margin in mid clavicular line at 90 degrees, tilted to Rt shoulder. Scan through the entire gallbladder, in 2 planes.

- **Identification**:
  1. The gallbladder is identified as a cystic structure.

- **Interpretation**:
  1. With appropriate clinical setting, cholecystitis is diagnosed in the presence of gallstones (bright masses casting an acoustic shadow within the gall bladder, Figure 12) and the following

FIGURE 12 Gallstone casting an acoustic shadow

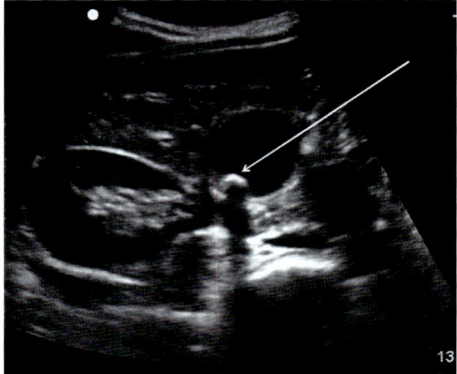

a. **Wall thickness greater than 3mm** (measure only the anterior wall, as the posterior wall may be difficult to visualise due to acoustic enhancement or from apposition with the bowels) (Figure 13)

b. **Pericholecystic fluid** (Figure 14)

c. **Sonographic murphy's sign** (tenderness elicited with the probe in pressing on the sonographically identified gall bladder)

| FIGURE 13 | Normal gallbladder wall thickness | FIGURE 14 | Thickened gallbladder wall with pericholecystic fluid |

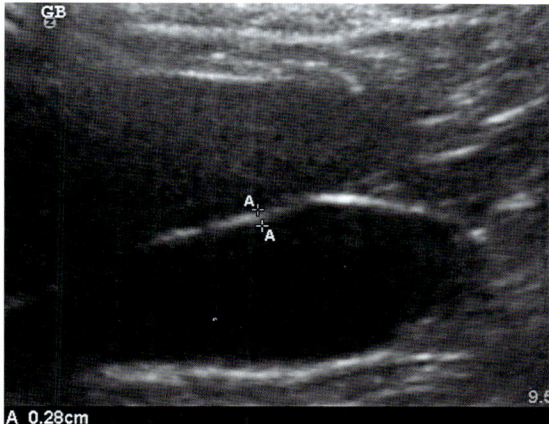

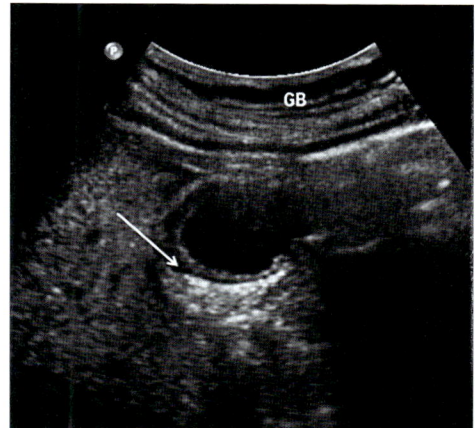

- **Pitfalls**:
  1. Spiral valves, polyps and sludge may be mistaken for stones
  2. Gallbladder wall thickening occurs in other conditions, including hepatitis, pancreatitis and ascites.
  3. Small stones <4mm may not generate an acoustic shadow and hence may be missed.

References/Further Reading

1. Lichtenstein DA, Meziere GA. Relevance of lung ultrasound in the diagnosis of acute respiratory failure: the BLUE protocol. *Chest* July 2008; 134(1): 117–125

2. Lichtenstein DA. Chapter 16: pneumothorax and introduction to ultrasound signs in the lung. In: *General ultrasound in the critically ill*. New York: Srpinger. 2007: 105–115.

3. Ma OJ, Mateer JR, Blaivas N. *Emergency Ultrasound* 2nd ed, New York:McGraw-Hill; 2008.

4. Weekes AJ, Zapata RJ, Napolitano A. Symptomatic Hypotension: ED Stabilization and the Emergency Role of Sonography. *Emergency Medicine Practice* Nov 2007.

Shirley Ooi

SKULL VIEWS

X-ray views	Indications	Remarks
Standard views		
• Anteroposterior (AP)	Suspected vault fracture	Refer to Chapter 95, *Trauma, Head* for indications for ordering skull X-rays.
• Lateral (right or left according to the side of the injury)	Suspected vault fracture Fluid in the sphenoidal sinus in the base of the skull fracture	*Note:* Skull X-rays are very rarely done nowadays.
Additional views		
• Towne's	Suspected occiput fracture	Can only be taken if cervical spine injury has been excluded
• Tangential	To evaluate suspected depressed skull fracture	

FACIAL VIEWS

Refer to Chapter 98, *Trauma, Maxillofacial* for illustrations of the X-rays.

X-ray views	Indications	Remarks
• 30-degree occipitomental (OM) view	Suspected maxilla, zygomatic complex, and orbital floor fracture	This single view is enough as a radiologic screening for mid-face fractures. Refer to Chapter 98, *Trauma, Maxillofacial* for further explanation. Need to exclude cervical spine injury first.
• Submentovertical ('jug handle') view	Suspected zygomatic arch fracture	Need to exclude cervical spine injury first.
• Nasal bone (lateral view)	Suspected nasal bone fracture	This X-ray may not be necessary as management is based on clinical evaluation of deformity.
• Orthopantomogram (OPG) view	To visualize the whole of the mandible for suspected fracture	If OPG view is not available at the emergency department, 3 plain films, i.e. a PA and 2 oblique views of the mandible can be done instead.

CERVICAL SPINE X-RAYS

• This is one of the 3 standard X-rays done in a multiple trauma victim.

NOTE: Following trauma, there is **no need** for **cervical spine X-rays** in any patient who meets the NEXUS criteria or the Canadian c-spine rule. (see Chapter 102, *Trauma, Spinal Cord and Cervical Spine Clearance*).

- An important neck injury may still be present despite normal plain cervical spine X-rays. Clinical history and examination must always take precedence over apparently normal X-rays.

X-ray views	Remarks
• Lateral (to include the top of the T_1 vertebral body)	In a multiple trauma patient, a lateral cervical spine X-ray is the only view required in the initial phase.
• Swimmer's view	Done if the C_7/T_1 junction is not visualized on the lateral cervical spine X-ray.
	Sensitivity of the lateral view alone with or without the swimmer's view is 85%.
	NOTE: If X-ray is done to exclude **foreign bodies** (FB), the request should be '**X-ray neck (soft tissue lateral)**'.
• Anteroposterior	Sensitivity of lateral, AP and open mouth views combined is 92%.
• Open mouth AP	To show the C_1–C_2 articulation.

ABDOMEN AND PELVIS VIEWS

X-ray views	Indications	Remarks
Standard view		
• Supine abdominal X-ray (AXR)	To identify 'free' air/pneumoperitoneum To identify air/fluid interfaces To identify ectopic calcifications	**The erect CXR is a fundamental part of the examination of an acute abdomen as it is the most sensitive X-ray for detecting a small pneumoperitoneum.** As little as 1 ml of free air can be demonstrated.
Additional views		
• Erect AXR	Air-fluid levels	Air-fluid levels are not pathognomonic of intestinal obstruction. Causes of air-fluid levels on erect AXR: • Ileus • Intestinal obstruction • Gastroenteritis
• Left lateral decubitus	To visualize air-fluid levels or pneumoperitoneum in patients who are unable to sit upright or stand	

CHEST VIEWS

X-ray views	Indications	Remarks
Standard view		
• Posteroanterior (PA) or anteroposterior (AP) chest X-ray (CXR)		**PA CXR** should be obtained whenever possible as it enables a more accurate diagnosis of heart size and mediastinal width.
		AP films can be done supine or sitting.
		NOTE: Pneumothorax and pleural effusions are difficult to see on supine or upright portable CXR.
		In general CXR should be done in **full inspiration**.
		The only **exception** is when small pneumothorax or diagnosis of inhaled foreign body ('gas trapping') is suspected when an **expiratory film** is requested instead.
Specialized views		
• Lateral CXR	Useful to confirm and localize: • Intrapulmonary opacities • Hilar abnormalities (adenopathy, masses, and increased vascularity) • Cardiomegaly, heart chamber enlargement, and aortic abnormalities • Small pleural effusions	Rarely useful in an emergency situation. *NOTE:* Retrosternal and retrocardiac regions are better seen on the lateral than on PA CXR.
• Oblique CXR	Rib fractures	
• Lateral decubitus CXR	Small pleural effusion and to differentiate from pleural thickening	PA CXR taken with patient lying on his side (usually abnormal side down).
4. Sternal view	Suspected fractured sternum	

THORACIC AND LUMBAR SPINE VIEWS

X-ray views	Indications
Standard views	
• Lateral	Suspected malignancy with possible metastases to the spine. History of significant trauma to the spine.
• Anteroposterior	Fever and tenderness suggesting osteomyelitis. Acute, unexplained neurological deficit.

UPPER LIMB VIEWS

Refer to Chapter 103, *Trauma, Upper Extremity* for X-ray examples.

X-ray views	Indications	Remarks
Shoulder		
● AP	Standard view to evaluate shoulder pathology	
● Axial view		Equivalent to looking up into the patient's armpit.
		Disadvantages:
		• Abducting the injured arm may be painful.
		• Pain may make it difficult to obtain a technically optimal film.
		• The head of the humerus sits on the glenoid.
		Orientation is easy; the fingers (the acromion and coracoid processes) always point anteriorly.
● Y-scapular view		For patients who cannot abduct arm. Anterior is on the side of the rib cage.
● Lateral transthoracic view	Only useful for assessing humeral fractures and not dislocations	
Humerus		
● AP	Standard view for humeral injuries	
● Lateral	Standard view for humeral injuries	
Elbow		
● AP	Standard view for elbow injuries	
● Lateral	Standard view for elbow injuries	In normal patients, the posterior fat-pad is never visible as it is within the olecranon fossa, but the anterior fat-pad may be seen closely applied to the humerus.
		Whenever a posterior **fat-pad sign** or '**sail sign**' is present, but there is no obvious fracture, look carefully for a radial head fracture in adults or supracondylar fracture of the humerus, especially in children.
● Oblique	Only for subtle injuries of the radial head and distal humerus	
Radius and ulna		
● AP	Standard views for forearm injuries	
● Lateral		

X-ray views	Indications	Remarks
Wrist		
• AP	Standard views for wrist/distal forearm	
• Lateral		
• Scaphoid views	When scaphoid fracture is suspected	These include PA and AP oblique with wrist in ulnar deviation besides the above two standard views.
Hand		
• PA	Standard views for hand injuries	
• PA oblique		
• Lateral	To visualise foreign bodies	The standard radiographic projections of the whole hand are required to evaluate the base of the proximal phalanges and metacarpals.
Digits		
• PA	Standard views for injury to the digits	When the injury is confined to the distal end of a single digit, radiography should be limited to that digit.
• Lateral		

LOWER LIMB VIEWS

X-ray views	Indications	Remarks
Hips		Do not order AP and lateral X-rays of the hip. Instead order AP X-ray of the pelvis and lateral of the hip. AP view of pelvis:
• AP pelvis	Standard views for hip injury	• Allows assessment and comparison of the pelvic rami on both sides.
• Lateral view of that symptomatic joint		• A pubic ramus fracture can mimic signs and symptoms of a neck of femur fracture and may be missed on an AP view of the hip.
Femur (shaft)		
• AP	Standard views for femoral shaft injuries	
• Lateral		
Knee		
• AP	Standard views for knee injuries	A fat-fluid level within the suprapatellar bursa should be regarded as indicating an intra-articular fracture.
• Lateral		

X-ray views	Indications	Remarks
• Skyline view	Special view; use in subtle fractures of: • Femoral condyles (especially in lateral dislocation of the patella) • Patella	
Tibia/fibula		
• AP	Standard views for tibia/fibula injuries	
• Lateral		
Ankle		
• AP	Standard views for ankle injuries	
• Lateral		
• Axial view of the calcaneum	Special views for calcaneal injuries (in addition to AP and lateral views of the ankle)	
Foot		
• AP	Standard views of foot injuries	
• Oblique		

120 Commonly Used Emergency Drugs in Adults

Ong Pei Yuin, Shirley Ooi

Drug	Route	Dose	Indications	Contraindications	Remarks/precautions
Resuscitation (Advanced Cardiac Life Support drugs)					
Adrenaline	IV	1 mg q 3–5 minutes	Asystole, pulseless electrical activity (PEA)		
	IV	0.1 mg over 5 minutes, then infusion 1–4 μg/min	Anaphylactic shock		
	SC/IM	0.3 mg (0.3 ml of 1:1000) q 15–20 minutes prn	Anaphylaxis/allergic reaction		
	IV	0–0.2 μg/kg/min	Shock		Must give through central line
Atropine	IV	2.4 mg, 2x dose if via ETT	Asystole, PEA		
	IV	0.6–1.2 mg, repeat every 3 minutes up to a maximum of 3 mg	Symptomatic bradycardia with hypotension		
Sodium bicarbonate 8.4%	IV	1–2 mmol/kg	Severe metabolic acidosis, severe hyperkalaemia		
Calcium chloride 10% (1 g = 6.8 mmol elemental calcium)	IV	10 ml over 10 minutes	Hyperkalaemia with electrocardiographic (ECG) changes, hypocalcaemia		Can cause extravasation, give into large vein
Calcium gluconate 10% (1 g = 2.2 mmol elemental calcium)	IV	10–20 ml over 10–20 minutes	Hyperkalaemia with ECG changes, hypocalcaemia		Less risk of extravasation than calcium chloride, lower than calcium concentration of calcium chloride

Drug	Route	Dose	Indication	Notes
Dopamine	IV	0–20 µg/kg/min	Inotropic support	Give into large vein
Dobutamine	IV	0–20 µg/kg/min	Inotropic support	Give into large vein
Noradrenaline	IV	0–0.2 µg/kg/min	Shock state, good for septic shock	Must give through central line
Mannitol 20%	IV	0.25–2 g/kg over 30–60 minutes	Cerebral oedema, raised intracranial pressure, raised intra-ocular pressure	Osmotic diuresis, caution in hypotensive patients
Amiodarone	IV	300 mg bolus	Ventricular fibrillation (VF), pulseless ventricular tachycardia VT)	Iodine allergy
	IV	150 mg in 100 ml D5W over 10 minutes	VT with pulse, atrial fibrillation	
Dextrose 50%	IV	40 ml combined with IV insulin 10 U	Hyperkalaemia	
Magnesium sulphate	IV	1–2 g in 100 ml D5W over 15 minutes	Torsades	
Induction/sedative agents				
Etomidate	IV	0.2–0.6 mg/kg, usually 0.3 mg/kg	Induction, sedation	Onset 60 seconds, duration 3–5 minutes, haemodynamically stable
Fentanyl	IV	Induction: 2–10 µg/kg Sedation: 2–3 µg/kg	Analgesia, sedation	Onset 60 seconds, duration 30–60 minutes
Midazolam	IV	Induction: 0.15–0.2 mg/kg (maximum 0.35 mg/kg) Sedation: 0.1 mg/kg in divided doses	Procedural sedation	Onset 2 minutes, duration 1–2 hours
Ketamine	IV	2.0 mg/kg	Sedation, especially in asthmatics and hypotensive patients	Onset 30–60 seconds, duration 15 minutes. Contraindicated in raised intracranial pressure, glaucoma

(Continued)

Drug	Route	Dose	Indications	Contraindications	Remarks/precautions
Thiopentone	IV	3–5 mg/kg	Cerebroprotective		Onset 20–40 seconds, duration 5–10 minutes
Propofol	IV	Induction: 2 mg/kg, 0.5–1 mg/kg over Procedural sedation: 5 minutes	Induction for general anaesthesia, procedural sedation	Allergy to soybean, caution in epilepsy, liver disease. Monitor for hypotension	Onset 30–60 seconds, duration 3–5 minutes
Atropine	IV/IM	0.6 mg	Adjunct to ketamine in procedural sedation		Useful to decrease salivation, particularly in paediatric patients
Neuromuscular blocking agents					
Succinylcholine	IV	1–2 mg/kg for rapid sequence induction (RSI)		Hyperkalaemia, burns >24 hours, neuromuscular disease	Onset 30–60 seconds, duration 4–6 minutes
Atracurium	IV	0.4 mg/kg for maintenance			Onset 3–5 minutes, duration 30 minutes, useful in renal dysfunction
Rocuronium	IV	0.6–1.2 mg/kg for RSI 0.6 mg/kg for maintenance			Onset 2 minutes, duration 30 minutes
Pancuronium	IV	0.1 mg/kg for maintenance			Onset 3–5 minutes, duration 60 minutes
Analgesics					
Paracetamol	PO	1 g tds–qds prn	Fever, mild pain		
	Suppository	2 tds prn	Fever, pain		Useful when oral intake is not possible
Panadeine® (Paracetamol 500 mg + Codeine phosphate 8 mg)	PO	2 tabs tds	Moderate pain, dysmenorrhoea, myalgia		Can cause mild sedation
Anarex® (Paracetamol 450 mg + Orphenadrine 35 mg)	PO	2 tabs tds	Mild to moderate pain, muscular spasm		Can cause dry mouth, thirst, constipation, vomiting, mild giddiness

Drug	Route	Dose	Indication	Contraindications	Notes
Mefenamic acid (Ponstan®)	PO	500 mg tds	Mild to moderate pain	Non-steroidal anti-inflammatory drugs (NSAIDs), aspirin allergy, gastrointestinal (GI) bleeding, active peptic ulcer disease	Caution in asthmatics, renal impairment
Ibuprofen (Brufen®)	PO	400 mg tds–qds	Mild to moderate pain	NSAIDs, aspirin allergy, GI bleeding, active peptic ulcer disease	Caution in asthmatics, renal impairment
Diclofenac (Voltaren®)	PO	50 mg tds or SR 75 mg bd	Mild to moderate pain	NSAIDs, aspirin allergy, GI bleeding, active peptic ulcer disease	Caution in asthmatics, renal impairment
	IM	50–75 mg bd–tds	Moderate pain	NSAIDs, aspirin allergy, GI bleeding, active peptic ulcer disease	Caution in asthmatics, renal impairment
Naproxen (Synflex®)	PO	550 mg bd	Mild to moderate pain	NSAIDs, aspirin allergy, GI bleeding, active peptic ulcer disease	Caution in asthmatics, renal impairment
Ketorolac (Toradol®)	PO	10 mg tds–qds	Moderate pain	NSAIDs, aspirin allergy, GI bleeding, active peptic ulcer disease	Caution in asthmatics, renal impairment
	IV/IM	10–30 mg q 4–6 hours	Moderate to severe pain	NSAIDs, aspirin allergy, GI bleeding, active peptic ulcer disease	Caution in asthmatics, renal impairment
Celecoxib (Celebrex®)	PO	100–200 mg OM–bd	Moderate pain	NSAID allergy, active peptic ulcer, GI bleeding	COX-2 inhibitor, less risk of GI side effects than NSAIDs
Meloxicam (Mobic®)	PO	7.5 mg od	Moderate pain, arthritis	NSAID allergy, active peptic ulcer, GI bleeding	COX-2 inhibitor, less risk of GI side effects than NSAIDs
Etoricoxib (Arcoxia®)	PO	60–90 mg od	Moderate pain, arthritis	NSAID allergy, active peptic ulcer, GI bleeding	COX-2 inhibitor, less risk of GI side effects than NSAIDs

(Continued)

Drug	Route	Dose	Indications	Contraindications	Remarks/precautions
Codeine phosphate	PO	15–60 mg tds	Moderate to severe pain		Can cause drowsiness, confusion, constipation
Tramadol (Tramal® or Acugesic®)	PO/IM/IV	50 mg tds	Moderate to severe pain		Can cause drowsiness or nausea/giddiness
Pethidine	IM/IV	0.5–2 mg/kg bolus	Severe pain		Causes drowsiness, sedation
Morphine	PO (mist)	0.2–0.4 mg/kg q 4 hours	Chronic severe pain		
	IM/IV	0.1–0.2 mg/kg titrated up to 15 mg	Severe pain		Causes drowsiness, sedation. Useful for acute coronary syndrome
Antibiotics					
PENICILLINS					5–10% cross hypersensitivity between penicillins and cephalosporins
Amoxicillin	PO	500 mg tds	Bacterial respiratory tract infections, streptococcal infections	Causes rash in infectious mononucleosis	GI side effects
Amoxicillin + Clavulanate (Augmentin®)	PO	625 mg bd–tds	Respiratory, urinary, skin infections, streptococcal infections	Causes rash in infectious mononucleosis	GI side effects
Penicillin V	PO	500 mg tds–qds	Skin and soft tissue infections		
Crystalline penicillin	IV	2–4 MU 6 hourly	Skin and soft tissue infections		
Cloxacillin	PO	500 mg qds	Skin infections		
	IV	500 mg–1 g qds	Skin infections, endocarditis		

CEPHALOSPORINS

Drug	Route	Dose	Uses	Notes
Cephalexin (Keflex®)	PO	500 mg tds	Skin, soft tissue, urinary, respiratory infections	5–10% cross hypersensitivity between penicillins and cephalosporins
Cefuroxime (Zinnat®)	PO	500 mg bd	Urinary tract infections	
Cephazolin®	IV	1g 8 hourly	Skin infections	
Ceftriaxone (Rocephin®)	IV	1g OM–bd, 2g bd for meningitis	Broad spectrum against respiratory tract, urinary, skin infections, meningitis	
Ceftazidime (Fortum®)	IV	1–2 g 8 hourly	Broad spectrum antibiotic for respiratory, urinary infections. Effective against pseudomonas, meliodosis, hospital acquired infections	

MACROLIDES

Drug	Route	Dose	Uses	Notes
Erythromycin	PO	500 mg qds	Respiratory, urinary infections	GI side effects
Erythromycin ethinyl succinate (EES®)	PO	800 mg bd	Respiratory, urinary infections	GI side effects

LINCOSAMIDES

Drug	Route	Dose	Uses	Notes
Clindamycin	PO	300–600 mg tds	Cellulitis, pelvic inflammatory disease	
Clindamycin	IV	450–900 mg tds	Cellulitis, necrotizing fasciitis, streptococcal infections, pelvic inflammatory disease	

(Continued)

Drug	Route	Dose	Indications	Contraindications	Remarks/precautions
QUINOLONES					
Ciprofloxacin (Ciprobay®)	PO	250–500 mg bd	Respiratory, urinary, GI infections		Can cause nausea
	IV		Respiratory, urinary, GI infections		Can cause nausea
Levofloxacin (Cravit®)	PO	500 mg OM	Respiratory infections		
	IV	500 mg OM			
Gatifloxacin (Tequin®)	PO/IV	400 mg OM	Gonorrhoea, urinary tract infections (UTIs)	Pregnancy, diabetes, concurrent use of class 1A and III anti-arrhythmics	May prolong QT interval
Moxifloxacin (Avelox®)	PO/IV	400 mg OM 7–14 days	Respiratory infections	Impaired liver function, concurrent use of drugs that prolong QT interval, heart failure	May prolong QT interval
AMINOGLYCOSIDES					
Gentamicin	IV/IM	3 mg/kg/day in 3 divided doses 8 hourly	Gram −ve infections, biliary, meningitis, endocarditis, serious respiratory and urinary tract infections	Neonates, lactating mothers, myasthenia gravis, ototoxicity, or nephrotoxicity from previous use of gentamicin	Can cause ototoxicity, nephrotoxicity, purpura, leucopaenia, and thrombocytopaenia
ANTIFUNGALS					
Nystatin	PO	5 ml qds	Oral candidiasis	Pregnancy	
Fluconazole	PO	150 mg once weekly × 4 weeks	Dermatophytosis		Can cause nausea, vomiting, diarrhoea, rash, abdominal pain, and flatulence. Potentiates effect of warfarin

CHAPTER 120 Commonly used Emergency Drugs in Adults 787

Drug	Route	Indication	Dose	Notes
	PO	Candidiasis (UTI, vaginal candidiasis, peritonitis)	50–200 mg od	Can cause nausea, vomiting, diarrhoea, rash, abdominal pain, and flatulence. Potentiates effect of warfarin
	IV	Cryptococcal and candidal infections	400 mg loading dose, then 200–400 mg daily	Can cause nausea, vomiting, diarrhoea, rash, abdominal pain, and flatulence. Potentiates effect of warfarin. May be proarrhythmic
Ketoconazole	PO	Vaginal candidiasis	200 mg bd × 5 days	Caution in underlying liver disease
Amphotericin B	IV	Life-threatening fungal infections	Test dose 1 mg over 20–30 minutes, then 0.25 mg/kg/day over 2–6 hours if well tolerated	Causes fever, chills, phlebitis, nausea, vomiting, diarrhoea, haematological disorders, decreased renal function
ANTIVIRALS				
Acyclovir	PO	Chickenpox, Bell's palsy of presumed viral aetiology, herpes simplex infection	400–800 mg 5x/day for 5 days	Can cause rash, GI effects, headache
	IV	Herpes simplex encephalitis	10 mg/kg 8 hourly × 10 days	Decrease dose in renal impairment. IV use can cause neurotoxicity
Oseltamivir (Tamiflu®)	PO	Influenza	Treatment: 75 mg bd for 5 days Prophylaxis: 75 mg OM for 10 days	Causes nausea and vomiting. To decrease dosing in renal impairment. Caution in pregnancy. Increased risk of behavioural disturbances

(Continued)

Drug	Route	Dose	Indications	Contraindications	Remarks/precautions
Zanamivir (Relenza®)	PO	Treatment: 10 mg bd for 5 days Prophylaxis: 10 mg OM for 10 days	Influenza	Caution in underlying airway disease, psychiatric history, and lactose intolerance	Contains lactose. Increased risk of bronchospasm in underlying airway disease, increased risk of neuropsychiatric events (seizures, confusion, abnormal behaviour)

ANTIHELMINTICS

Drug	Route	Dose	Indications	Contraindications	Remarks/precautions
Albendazole	PO	400 mg single dose	Intestinal parasites	Teratogenic in pregnancy	
Mebendazole	PO	100 mg bd × 3 days	Threadworms, whipworms, hookworms, roundworms	Pregnancy, <2 years	

Cardiovascular drugs

ANTIPLATELETS

Drug	Route	Dose	Indications	Contraindications	Remarks/precautions
Aspirin	PO	300 mg loading dose, 100 mg OM maintenance	Unstable angina, acute myocardial infarction (AMI), acute coronary syndrome (ACS)	GI bleeding, active peptic ulcer disease	Caution in asthmatics
Clopidogrel (Plavix®)	PO	600 mg	Loading dose for primary percutaneous coronary intervention (PCI) for ST-elevation myocardial infarction (STEMI) who cannot be given Prasugrel, non-ST elevation ACS with no dynamic ST changes or negative cardiac markers Onset 30 minutes		Less risk of GI haemorrhage than aspirin

Drug	Route	Dose	Indication	Contraindication/Caution	Notes
	PO	75 mg OM	Ischaemic heart disease (IHD), maintenance		May cause bleeding
Prasugrel	PO	60 mg loading, 10 mg OM maintenance	STEMI for PCI	Age >75 yrs Body wt <60 kg h/o stroke/transient ischaemic attack or intracranial haemorrhage (ICH)	
Tricagrelor	PO	180 mg loading dose, 90 mg bd maintenance	Non-ST elevation ACS with dynamic ST changes or positive cardiac markers	GI bleeding, h/o ICH, reduced liver function	Risk of bleeding
Ticlopidine (Ticlid®)	PO	250 mg bd	If aspirin/plavix contraindicated		Can cause neutropaenia
THROMBOLYTICS					
Streptokinase	IV	1.5 MU in 100 ml normal saline over 1 hour	AMI, STEMI if primary PCI not available	Streptococcal infection in past 6 months, any other contraindications for thrombolysis including bleeding disorders, aortic dissection, stroke, pregnancy	
Recombinant tissue plasminogen activator (rTPA)	IV	15 mg bolus, then 0.75 mg/kg (maximum 50 mg) over 30 minutes, then 0.5 mg/kg (maximum 35 mg) over 60 minutes	AMI, STEMI if primary PCI not available	Any contraindication for thrombolysis including bleeding disorders, aortic dissection, stroke, pregnancy	Higher risk of bleeding than streptokinase, Caution in elderly patients
ANTIHYPERTENSIVES					
GTN	IV	0–300 µg/min	Acute pulmonary oedema, hypertensive emergencies, unstable angina		Can cause headache due to vasodilatation

(Continued)

Drug	Route	Dose	Indications	Contraindications	Remarks/precautions
Labetalol	IV	10–20 mg q 10 minutes to lower blood pressure rapidly, then infusion 0.5–2.0 mg/min	Hypertensive emergencies, intracranial bleeding	Heart failure, asthma exacerbation, heart blocks	β-blocker effects
Propranolol	PO	20–40 mg bd	SVT, AF, thyrocardiac disease	Heart failure, asthma exacerbation, heart blocks	β-blocker effects
Metoprolol	PO	12.5–25 mg bd-tds	Hypertension, AMI	Heart blocks	β-blocker effects
Atenolol	PO	25–100 mg OM	Hypertension, AF	Heart blocks	β-blocker effects
Esmolol	IV	Loading dose: 500 μg/kg over 1 minute Maintenance dose: 0–200 μg/kg/min	Hypertension Tachydysrhythmia		Primarily used when there is concern that β blockade will not be well tolerated because it is very short acting so that if an adverse reaction occurs, the drug will wear off quickly
Felodipine	PO	2.5–5 mg OM–bd	Hypertensive urgency		Calcium channel blocker, onset about 2 hours
Amlodipine	PO	2.5–10 mg OM–bd	Hypertension		Calcium channel blocker, onset about 2 hours
Captopril	PO	12.5–25 mg bd-tds	Hypertension	Renal impairment, hyperkalaemia	ACE inhibitor, can cause cough and ACE inhibitor induced angiooedema
Enalapril	PO	2.5–10 mg OM	Hypertension	Renal impairment, hyperkalaemia	ACE inhibitor, can cause cough and ACE inhibitor induced angiooedema
Frusemide (Lasix®)	PO	20–80 mg OM-tds	Hypertension, heart failure		Can cause hypokalaemia, may need potassium supplementation

Drug	Route	Dose	Indication	Contraindication/Caution	Comments
	IV	40–160 mg	Heart failure, fluid overload, pulmonary oedema		Can worsen renal function, caution in patients with kidney transplant
Bumetamide (Burinex®)	IV	0.5-1.0 mg	Fluid overload secondary to liver, renal, cardiac cause	Concurrent use of lithium, anuria	Diuretic effect inhibited by probenecid
Hydralazine	IV	5-10 mg q 15 minutes	Eclampsia		
ANTIARRHYTHMICS					
Adenosine	IV	6-12 mg rapid IV push, can repeat to maximum 30 mg	SVT		Purine nucleoside, causes transient flushing, nausea, shortness of breath; use a proximal vein
Verapamil	IV	2.5-10 mg over 30 minutes	SVT, fast AF, narrow complex tachycardia	Heart failure, decreased cardiac function	Calcium channel blocker
Diltiazem	IV	0.25 mg/kg (usual adult dose 20 mg) over 2 min. After 15 min, 0.35 mg/kg (usual adult dose 25 mg) if 1st dose tolerated but response inadequate. Additional doses q 15 min. Continuous infusion: 10 mg/h initially, increased to ≤15 mg/h for up to 24 hours.	Fast AF, narrow complex tachycardia	Heart failure	Calcium channel blocker
Digoxin	IV	Loading: 0.125- 0.5 mg over 15 minutes	Fast AF, atrial flutter		Useful in decreased cardiac function. Limited by slow onset of action. Narrow therapeutic window. Increased risk of toxicity in elderly
	PO	0.0625-0.25 mg OM	Maintenance for AF		

(Continued)

Drug	Route	Dose	Indications	Contraindications	Remarks/precautions
Procainamide	IV	Load: 20 mg/min to maximum of 17 mg/kg Infusion: 1–4 mg/min	Wide complex tachydysrhythmias		
Lignocaine	IV	1.0–1.5 mg/kg bolus, can repeat to maximum of 3.0 mg/kg	Ventricular tachycardia		Overdose can lead to lignocaine toxicity causing seizures
Respiratory drugs					
Chlorpheniramine (Piriton®)	PO	1 tab tds prn	Nasal congestion, rhinitis, urticaria		Can cause drowsiness, dry mouth
Loratidine	PO	5–10 mg od	Nasal congestion, rhinitis, urticaria, pruritus		Less drowsy side effects than chlorpheniramine
Cetirizine	PO	5–10 mg od	Nasal congestion, rhinitis, urticaria, pruritus		
Pseudoephedrine	PO	60–120 mg od	Nasal and bronchial congestion	Severe coronary artery disease, severe hypertension	Can cause tachycardia, palpitations, sympathomimetic effects
Promethazine	PO	10 ml tds prn	Dry cough, vomiting, allergic reactions	Narrow angle glaucoma, prostatic hypertrophy, urinary retention	Causes drowsiness
Procodin	PO	10 ml tds prn	Dry cough	Narrow angle glaucoma, prostatic hypertrophy, urinary retention	Causes drowsiness, can cause constipation
Diphenhydramine	PO	10 ml tds prn	Dry cough	Narrow angle glaucoma, prostatic hypertrophy, urinary retention	Causes drowsiness
Bromhexine	PO	4–8 mg tds prn	Mucolytic		
Dextromethorphan	PO	10 ml tds prn	Mucolytic		

Drug	Route	Dose	Indication	Comments
Acetylcysteine (Fluimucil®)	PO	1 satchet OM	Mucolytic, bronchitis, asthma, chronic obstructive pulmonary disease (COPD)	
Salbutamol (Ventolin®)	Inhaled	Metered dose inhaler (MDI): 4–12 puffs prn; Neb: 1 ml (5 mg) salbutamol: 1 or 2 ml atrovent: 2 ml saline	Asthma/COPD exacerbation	Asthma reliever
Ipratropium (Atrovent®)	Inhaled	MDI: 4–12 puffs prn; Neb: 1 ml salbutamol: 1 or 2 ml atrovent: 2 ml saline	Asthma/COPD exacerbation	Asthma reliever
Salmeterol/fluticasone (Seretide®)	Accuhaler (50/100, 50/250, 50/500 µg) Evohaler (25/50, 25/125, 25/250 µg)	1–2 puffs od–bd depending on severity, increase during exacerbations	Asthma/COPD	Combination β-agonist and steroid inhaler
Budesonide/formoterol (Symbicort®)	Turbuhaler (160/4.5 µg)	1–2 puffs od–bd depending on severity, increase during exacerbations	Asthma/COPD	Combination β-agonist and steroid inhaler
Budesonide (Pulmicort®, Inflammide®)	MDI, turbuhaler	200–400 µg bd depending on severity	Asthma	Asthma preventer
Beclomethasone	MDI	1–4 puffs (50–200 µg) od–bd	Asthma	Asthma preventer
Prednisolone	PO	0.5–1 mg/kg OM	Asthma/COPD exacerbation	
Hydrocortisone	IV	200–400 mg	Asthma/COPD exacerbation	
Magnesium sulphate	IV	1–2 g infusion over 15–20 min	Asthma exacerbation	Second-line therapy for asthma exacerbation

(Continued)

Drug	Route	Dose	Indications	Contraindications	Remarks/precautions
Gastrointestinal drugs					
Montelukast (Singulair®)	PO	10 mg ON	Asthma		
Antacids: Magnesium trisilicate, magnesium carbonate, aluminium hydroxide, sodium alginate various combinations (MMT, Mist carminative, Mylanta, Gaviscon®)	PO	10–20 ml tds prn or 1–2 tabs tds prn	Gastritis, heartburn, reflux, flatulence	Hypophosphataemia, renal failure	Can cause constipation or diarrhoea in excess, interferes with absorption of iron and tetracycline
Metoclopramide (Maxolon®)	PO	1 tds prn	Vomiting, nausea	Intestinal obstruction	Can cause oculogyric crisis
	IV	10 mg tds prn	Vomiting	Intestinal obstruction	Can cause oculogyric crisis
Charcoal	PO	2 tabs tds prn	Diarrhoea, flatulence		Interferes with absorption of other drugs, take 2 hours apart
Loperamide (Imodium®)	PO	4 mg stat or 2 mg tds prn	Diarrhoea		
Diphenoxylate-atropine (Lomotil®)	PO	1–2 tabs tds prn	Diarrhoea		Can cause mouth dryness
Kaolin Pectin Mixture	PO	10 ml tds prn	Diarrhoea		Oral rehydration therapy should be given
Lacteol Fort	PO	1–2 satchets daily	Diarrhoea		
Hyoscine (Buscopan®)	PO	10–20 mg tds prn	Gastrointestinal, biliary, urinary tract spasm	Intestinal obstruction, narrow angle glaucoma, retention of urine, pregnancy	

Drug	Route	Dose	Indications	Contraindications	Notes
	IV/IM	Up to 40 mg stat, 10–20 mg tds	Gastrointestinal, biliary, urinary tract spasm	Intestinal obstruction, narrow angle glaucoma, retention of urine, pregnancy	
Lactulose	PO	10–20 ml tds prn	Constipation, portal encephalopathy	Galactosaemia, intestinal obstruction	Can cause flatulence
Senna	PO	2 tabs ON prn	Constipation	Intestinal obstruction	
Bisacodyl (Dulcolax®)	PO/suppository	1–2 tabs ON prn	Constipation	Intestinal obstruction, inflammatory bowel diseases	
Fleet enema	Suppository	1 fleet	Constipation	Intestinal obstruction	Caution in renal failure, heart disease, electrolyte disturbances
Mebeverine (Duspatalin®)	PO	1 tab tds prn	Abdominal pain, cramps, spasm, irritable bowel syndrome		
Debridat	PO	100–200 mg tds	Irritable bowel syndrome, functional digestive disorders		
Cimetidine	PO	200 mg tds	Peptic ulcer disease, reflux oesophagitis, gastritis		Can cause diarrhoea, gynaecomastia, reversible liver function changes
Famotidine	PO	20 mg bd	Peptic ulcer disease, reflux oesophagitis, gastritis		
Ranitidine	PO	150 mg bd	Peptic ulcer disease, reflux oesophagitis, gastritis		
Omeprazole	PO	20 mg OM–bd	Peptic ulcer disease, reflux oesophagitis, gastritis, combination therapy for helicobacter pylori infection		Interacts with warfarin, phenytoin, diazepam, drugs metabolized by cytochrome P450

(Continued)

Drug	Route	Dose	Indications	Contraindications	Remarks/precautions
Esomeprazole (Nexium®)	IV	40–80 mg OM–bd	Gastrointestinal haemorrhage, active peptic ulcers, gastritis		
Somatostatin	IV	250 µg stat then 250 µg/hr	Variceal bleeding, severe gastric/duodenal haemorrhage		Also works as adjuvant treatment for diabetic ketoacidosis, caution in insulin-dependent diabetics
Hesperidin (Daflon®)	PO	1–2 tabs bd–tds	Haemorrhoids, chronic venous insufficiency		
Ispaghula Husk (Fybogel®)	PO	1 satchet daily	Constipation, haemorrhoids, irritable bowel syndrome	Intestinal obstruction	Can cause flatulence
Neurological drugs					
Lorazepam	IV	1–4 mg prn to a total of 8 mg in adults	Seizures		Causes sedation
Diazepam (Valium®)	IV	5–10 mg prn to a total of 20 mg in adults	Seizures		Causes sedation
Phenytoin	PO	Loading: 300 mg 1 hourly × 3 Maintenance: 200–360 mg ON	Epilepsy/seizures		
	IV	Loading: 17 mg/kg over 30 minutes	Seizures, status epilepticus		Proarrhythmic effects, Requires cardiac monitoring during loading
Phenobarbitone	IV	20 mg/kg	Status epilepticus, second-line therapy after phenytoin		Causes respiratory depression, consider intubation to protect airway

Drug	Route	Dose	Indication	Contraindication	Comments
Benztropine (Cogentin®)	IM/IV	2 mg	Acute dystonia, extrapyramidal side effects		
	PO	2 mg tds	Dystonia		
Prochlorperazine (Stemetil®)	PO	5 mg tds prn	Vertigo, giddiness		
	IM	12.5 mg tds prn	Vertigo, giddiness		
Chlorpromazine	PO	25–50 mg tds × 3 days	Severe headache, Intractable hiccups	Central nervous system (CNS) depression, phaeochromocytoma	Potentiates anticholinergic effect of antiparkinson medications. Additive sedative effect. Prolonged use may cause tardive dyskinesia
Amitryptyline	PO	10 mg ON	Severe headache		Tricyclic anti-depressant
Caffeine 100 mg, ergotamine 1 mg (Cafergot®)	PO	2 tabs stat then 1 tab 6 hourly, maximum 6 tabs/day	Migraine	Peripheral vascular disease, hemiplegic/basilic migraine	Avoid concomitant use with macrolides
Sumatriptan	PO	50 or 100 mg single dose	Migraine	IHD, peripheral vascular disease, uncontrolled hypertension	
Endocrine drugs					
HYPER/HYPOGLYCAEMIC AGENTS					
Dextrose 50%	IV	40 ml	Hypoglycaemia		Risk of extravasation, give via larger vein
Dextrose 20%	IV	500 ml 4–8 hourly	Hypoglycaemia		Give via larger vein
Dextrose 10%	IV	500 ml 4–8 hourly	Maintenance for hypoglycaemia		

(Continued)

Drug	Route	Dose	Indications	Contraindications	Remarks/precautions
Soluble insulin	SC	4–12 units stat	Hyperglycaemia		Short acting
	IV	0.15 U/kg infusion	Hyperglycaemia, diabetic ketoacidosis (DKA), hyperosmolar non-ketotic state (HHNK)		
Mixtard (30% soluble insulin, 70% isophane insulin)	SC	Individualised	Insulin-dependent diabetes mellitus (IDDM)		
Metformin	PO	500 mg or 850 mg bd–tds	Non-insulin-dependent diabetes mellitus (NIDDM)		
Insulatard	SC	Individualised	IDDM		Long acting
Tolbutamide	PO	250 mg–1g bd–tds	NIDDM		Short acting
Glipizide	PO	2.5–10 mg OM–bd	NIDDM		
Gliclazide	PO	30–120 mg OM	NIDDM		
Glibenclamide	PO	2.5–15 mg OM	NIDDM		Prolonged duration of action, avoid in elderly
Acarbose	PO	50–100 mg tds	NIDDM	Severe renal impairment	Can cause flatulence and diarrhoea
THYROID DRUGS					
Thyroxine	PO	50–100 µg OM	Hypothyroidism		
Propranolol	PO	60 mg q 4 hours or 80 mg q 8 hours	Thyrotoxicosis induced tachycardia		
	IV	1 mg q 5 minutes	Severe tachycardia in thyroid storm		
Propylthiouracil	PO	200 mg q 4–6 hours for 24 hours	Thyroid storm		

Drug	Route	Dose	Indication	Contraindications	Notes
	PO	300–600 mg loading, then 50–150 mg od	Thyrotoxicosis		Risk of agranulocytosis
Carbimazole	PO	5–20 mg tds	Thyrotoxicosis, Graves' disease	Contraindicated in pregnancy	
Lugol's iodine	PO	5 drops	Thyroid storm		Must give 1–2 hours post-propylthiouracil therapy
ADDISONIAN CRISIS					
Hydrocortisone	IV	100 mg	Addisonian crisis		Measure cortisol levels prior to administration, if required
Dexamethazone	IV	2–8 mg	Addisonian crisis		
Obstetric, gynaecological, urological drugs					
Nystatin	Vaginal tab	1–2 tabs daily × 5 days	Vaginal candidiasis		
Clotrimazole	Vaginal tab	100 mg bedtime × 6 days	Vaginal candidiasis, vaginal trichomoniasis		Avoid menstrual period
Premarin vaginal cream (conjugated oestrogens)	Vaginal cream	2–4 g intravaginally × 3 weeks	Atrophic vaginitis	Oestrogen-dependent neoplasias, thromboembolic disease	Systemic absorption occurs, can cause weight changes, migraine, breast tenderness
Norethisterone	PO	5–10 mg tds × 10 days	Functional uterine bleeding, menorrhagia	Pregnancy (causes virilization of female foetus), complete/missed abortion	Can cause acne, oedema, weight gain
Depot Proluton (hydroxyprogesterone)	IM	500 mg	Threatened abortion		
Syntometrine (oxytocin 5 IU, ergometrine 0.5 mg)	IM	1 ml	Immediately post-delivery or for postpartum haemorrhage	Severe hypertension, peripheral vascular disease, severe renal/liver/cardiac disease	

(Continued)

Drug	Route	Dose	Indications	Contraindications	Remarks/precautions
Levonorgestrel (Postinor-2®)	PO	0.75 mg stat and 12 hours later	Emergency contraception		To be taken within 72 hours following intercourse
Terazosin (Hytrin®)	PO	1 mg ON, then increase every week until 5 mg ON	Benign prostatic hyperplasia		May caused blurred vision, giddiness, asthenia
Eye/ear/nose/throat drugs					
Normal saline eye drops	Eye drops	prn	Irritation of eyes		
Hypromellose eye drops	Eye drops	prn	Dry eyes, irritation		
Waxsol	Ear drops	2–3 drops ON × 2 nights before syringing	Earwax	Perforated tympanic membrane	
Olive oil	Ear drops	2–3 drops ON	Earwax	Perforated tympanic membrane	
Chloramphenicol eye drops	Eye/ear drops	2 drops tds	Bacterial conjunctivitis, otitis externa	Viral infections of ear, perforated tympanic membrane	
Ciprofloxacin eye and ear drops	Eye/ear drops	Corneal ulcer: 2 drops q 15 minutes × 6 hours, then q 30 minutes × 1 day. Bacterial conjunctivitis: 2 drops q 2 hours × 2 days, then q 4 hours × 5 days. Otitis externa: 3 drops qds × 5–10 days	Corneal ulcer, bacterial conjunctivitis, otitis externa		
Sofradex® (framycetin, gramicidin, dexamethasone)	Eye/ear drops	1–2 drops tds–qds	Inflammatory infections of eye/ear	Viral infections of cornea, conjunctiva, fungal infections of eye	

Drug	Route/Form	Dose	Indication	Contraindication	Notes
Timolol	Eye drops	1 drop bd affected eye	Glaucoma, intra-ocular hypertension	Acute heart failure	
Pilocarpine	Eye drops	1 drop q 5 minutes until miosis	Emergency treatment for acute closed angle glaucoma	Iritis, uveitis, secondary glaucoma, acute heart failure	
Phenylephrine	Eye drops	1 drop	For mydriasis in diagnostic and therapeutic procedures	Closed angle glaucoma, thyrotoxicosis, hypertension	
Tropicamide	Eye drops	1–2 drops	For mydriasis and cycloplegia	Closed angle glaucoma	Causes transient stinging effect
Oxymetazoline 0.025% (Iliadin®)	Nasal drops	2–3 drops affected nostril bd × 5 days	Allergic rhinitis, sinusitis		Not for use >5 days to prevent rebound effect
Fluticasone (Flixonase®)	Nasal spray	2 sprays each nostril od	Allergic rhinitis	Untreated bacterial or fungal infection of nose	
Triamcinolone (Nasocort®)	Nasal spray	2 sprays each nostril od	Allergic rhinitis	Untreated bacterial or fungal infection of nose	
Topicals					
Voltaren gel (Fastum®, Emugel®)	Topical	bd–tds prn	Topical analgesic, NSAIDs		
Ketoprofen plaster	Plaster	prn	Topical analgesic, NSAIDs		
Liniment methyl salicylate (LMS)	Topical liniment	tds prn	Topical analgesic, contains salicylate		
Chlorhexidine wash	Wash	prn	Antiseptic wash for infected wounds, burns		
Chlorhexidine cream	Topical	bd–tds prn	Antiseptic cream for skin disinfection		
Potassium permanganate	Wash	tds	Wound disinfectant or cleansing bath		

(Continued)

Drug	Route	Dose	Indications	Contraindications	Remarks/precautions
Miconazole 2% cream	Topical	bd	Fungal skin infections		Continue for 2 weeks after rash resolves to ensure spore eradication
Miconazole 2% powder	Topical	bd, dust inside clothing or sock to keep skin dry	Fungal skin infections		Continue for 2 weeks after rash resolves to ensure spore eradication
Hydrocortisone 1%	Topical	bd-tds	Mild steroid cream, can use for face. For eczema, dermatitis		Not to be used by itself for skin infections. Can cause skin atrophy, avoid prolonged use
Betamethasone 0.025%	Topical	bd-tds	Mild steroid. For eczema, dermatitis		Not to be used by itself for skin infections. Can cause skin atrophy, avoid prolonged use
Betamethasone 0.1%	Topical	bd-tds	Intermediate strength steroid, not for face. For eczema, dermatitis		Not to be used by itself for skin infections. Can cause skin atrophy, avoid prolonged use
Mucopuricin (Bactroban®)	Topical	tds	Bacterial skin infections		
Fusidic acid	Topical	bd	Staphylococcal and streptoccal skin infections		
Fucicort (Fusidic acid 2%, Betamethasone 0.1%)	Topical	bd	Eczema with superimposed staphylococcal and streptoccal infections		Can cause skin atrophy, avoid prolonged use
Combiderm, Triderm (Betamethasone 0.05%, Gentamicin 0.1%, Clotrimazole 1%)	Topical	bd-tds	Combination cream with steroid, antibacterial, antifungal effect		Can cause skin atrophy, avoid prolonged use

Tri-Micon cream (Betamethasone 0.1%, Gentamicin 0.1%, Miconazole 2%)	Topical	bd–tds	Combination cream with steroid, antibacterial, antifungal effect	Can cause skin atrophy, avoid prolonged use
Acyclovir cream	Topical	5 times/day × 10 days	Herpes simplex skin infections	
Aqueous cream	Topical	tds prn	Moisturising for dry skin	
Urea cream	Topical	tds prn	Moisturizing for dry, scaly or peeling skin	
Silver sulfadiazine	Topical	bd	For second- and third-degree burns	Can stain skin, do not use on face
Selenium sulphide	Detergent solution	Twice weekly for seborrhoiec dermatitis and dandruff. Apply to affected areas for 10 minutes before rinsing for pityriasis versicolor	Pityriasis versicolor, dandruff, seborrhoeic dermatitis	
Malathion	Shampoo	Shampoo and leave on for 10 minutes before rinsing. Apply weekly × 2 weeks.	Head lice	

Antidotes				
Poison	**Toxic level**	**Antidote**	**Dose**	**Special precautions**
				Remarks
Paracetamol	140 mg/kg	N-acetylcysteine (Parvolex)	Initial 150 mg/kg in 200 ml D5W over 15 minutes, then 50 mg/kg in 500 ml D5W over 4 hours, then 100 mg/kg in 1000 ml D5W over 16 hours	Monitor for anaphylactoid reaction
				Check levels 4 hours after ingestion, use Rumack–Mathew nomogram

(Continued)

Poison/Toxic level	Antidote	Dose	Remarks	Special Precautions
Salicylate	Sodium bicarbonate	1–2 mmol/kg bolus then infusion titrated against urine pH	Check levels 2 hours and 6 hours post-ingestion, use Done nomogram	Contraindicated in salicylate induced pulmonary oedema
Tricyclic anti-depressant	Sodium bicarbonate	1–2 mmol/kg over 20–30 minutes	Indicated if QRS >100 ms, achieve alkalinization to pH 7.45–7.50	Other drugs may be needed to control dysrhythmias and fits
Benzodiazepines	Flumazenil (Anexate®)	0.2 mg, can repeat every minute until maximum dose of 1.0 mg		Toxic dose varies for individual. Reversal required when significant respiratory depression occurs Contraindicated if concomitant tricyclic anti-depressant overdose or chronic benzodiazepine use
Opioids, e.g. morphine	Naloxone	0.4–2 mg q 2–3 minutes		
Cholinergics, e.g. organophosphates, paraquat	Atropine	2–4 mg q 10–15 minutes prn until atropinization		
	Pralidoxime	25–50 mg/kg over 15–30 minutes, can repeat after 1–2 hours		

NOTE: Information in this chapter is selective rather than comprehensive; not all indications, contraindications, and precautions are included.

References/Further Reading

1. Wong WM, Ho R, eds. *Medi-Bank.* 2nd Singapore edition. Singapore: Vital Base Company Pte Ltd; 2007.

2. *MIMS Singapore.* Singapore: CMP Medica; 2009. Available at: www.mims.com. Accessed June to September 2009.

3. *National University Hospital Department of Pharmacy Drug Administration Guidelines.* Available at: National University Hospital Intranet. Accessed August 2009.

4. Schaider JJ, Hayden SR, Wolfe RE, et al., eds. Rosen & Barkin's 5-Minute Emergency Medicine Consult. Philadelphia, PA: Lippincott Williams & Wilkins; 2007.

Irwani Ibrahim • Lim Er Luen

ANALGESICS

- Acetylsalicylic acid (Aspirin)
- Acetophenetidin (Phenacetin)

SULPHONAMIDES AND SULFONES

- Sulphanilamide
- Sulphapyridine
- Sulphadimidine
- Sulphacetamide
- Sulphafurazone
- Dapsone
- Sulphoxone
- Glucosulfone sodium
- Co-trimoxazole

OTHER ANTI-BACTERIAL COMPOUNDS

- Nitrofurans: Nitrofurantoin, furazolidone, nitrofurazone
- Nalidixic acid
- Chloramphenicol
- Fluoroquinolones, e.g. ciprofloxacin, ofloxacin, moxifloxacin

ANTI-MALARIALS

- Primaquine
- Pamaquine
- Chloroquine

CARDIOVASCULAR

- Procainamide
- Quinidine

MISCELLANEOUS

- Vitamin C
- Vitamin K analogues
- Naphthalene (mothballs)
- Probenecid
- Dimercaprol (BAL)
- Methylene blue
- Glibenclamide
- Phenylhydrazine
- Toluidine blue
- Doxorubicin
- Phenytoin
- Mepacrine
- Phenazopyridine (Urogesic)

References/Further Reading

1. Lin Yijun. Glucose-6-phosphate dehydrogenase deficiency. *National University Hospital Allergy and Adverse Drug Reaction Bulletin*. August 2007; 3.

2. Hoffman R, Benz Jr. EJ, Shattil SJ, et al., eds. Hematology: Basic Principles and Practice. 4th ed. Philadelphia, PA: Churchill Livingstone; 2005.

Lim Er Luen

CAVEATS

Before prescribing in pregnancy, always consider the benefits of the treatment which should outweigh the risks. This is especially so during the first trimester, when teratogenic risk is the highest. The list below applies to available drugs commonly used in the emergency department only. Many drugs are known to have adverse effects in pregnancy and only some are safe. In a critical situation the welfare of the mother takes priority over that of the foetus.

Safe	Avoid	Unclear/special precautions	Serious cases only
Antibiotics			
Penicillins	Tetracycline	Metronidazole (teratogenic in the first trimester)	
Amoxicillin–clavulanate potassium (Augmentin®)	Co-trimoxazole, sulphonamides		
Cephalosporins	Aminoglycosides		
Erythromycin, clarithromycin			
Anti-tuberculosis drugs: Rifampicin, isoniazid, ethambutol	Fluoroquinolones		
For pain			
Codeine	Cafergot (caffeine 100 mg ergotamine tartrate 1 mg per tablet)	Hyoscine-N-butylbromide (Buscopan®; its safety has not been established)	Ibuprofen
Paracetamol		Pethidine® (not before labour)	Indomethacin (Indocid®)
Fentanyl		Aspirin (avoid in last trimester)	Diclofenac (Voltaren®)
		Bisacodyl (stimulates gravid uterus)	Mefenamic acid (Ponstan®)
		Morphine/pethidine (care in perinatal period)	Naproxen

(Continued)

Safe	Avoid	Unclear/special precautions	Serious cases only
For vomiting and diarrhoea			
Metoclopramide		Prochloperazine (Stemetil®)	
Promethazine			
Ondansetron			
Loperamide			
Epigastric pain/ulcer			
Antacids			
Cimetidine, ranitidine			
Omeprazole			
Cardiopulmonary			
Digoxin	ACE inhibitors (captopril, enalapril)		Felodipine
Magnesium	Adrenaline (occasionally used in asthma)		Hydralazine (neonatal thrombocyto-paenia)
	Warfarin		
Heparin	Verapamil		GTN/ISDN (safety not established/SP lactation)
Hydrocortisone			Atenolol/propranolol (long-term use retards foetal growth)
Salbutamol nebulizer			Procainamide (safety not established)
Prednisolone			Amiodarone (not in perinatal period)
Inhaled steroids			Frusemide (Lasix®)
			Adenosine
			Adrenaline

Safe	Avoid	Unclear/special precautions	Serious cases only
Neurological and anti-epileptics			
	Midazolam		Phenytoin
	Sodium valproate		Phenobarbitone (teratogenic)
			Diazepam
			Chlorpromazine (Largactil®)
			Haloperidol
Immunizations			
Anti-tetanus toxoid (killed vaccines)	Measles, mumps, rubella, smallpox (live attenuated)		

Reference/Further Reading

1. Gabbe SG, Niebyl JR, Simpson JL, eds. *Obstetrics: Normal and problem pregnancies*. 5th ed. Philadelphia, PA: Churchill Livingstone; 2007.

123 Child, Abdominal Pain

Peter Manning

CAVEATS

- The duration of pain is useful since a surgical diagnosis is less likely in a child with chronic abdominal pain.
- The presence of fever suggests an infective course or peritonitis.
- Children under 5 years old usually have an organic cause for their pain.
- The possibility of functional abdominal pain should be considered in older children.
- The age of the child is useful since the diagnosis is narrowed accordingly.
- Bilious vomiting or persistent vomiting in the presence of abdominal pain is always an ominous sign and should be considered due to a mechanical obstruction until proven otherwise.

THE MOST COMMON LIFE-THREATENING CAUSES OF ABDOMINAL PAIN

Table 1 lists the most common life-threatening causes of abdominal pain for 4 age groups.

TABLE 1 Common life-threatening causes of abdominal pain

Neonatal	Infancy (<2 years)	Childhood (2–10 years)	Adolescence
Severe gastroenteritis	Severe gastroenteritis	Appendicitis	Toxic overdose
Sepsis	Toxic overdose	Trauma	Trauma
Incarcerated hernia	Sepsis	Intussusception	Appendicitis
Malrotation/volvulus	Intussusception	Toxic overdose	Ectopic pregnancy
Pyloric stenosis	Appendicitis	Sepsis	Peptic ulcer disease
Hirschsprung's disease	Incarcerated hernia	Diabetic ketoacidosis	Pancreatitis
Trauma	Meckel's diverticulum	Megacolon	Diabetic ketoacidosis
	Trauma		Aortic dissection/aneurysm
	Diabetic ketoacidosis		Megacolon

⇨ **SPECIAL TIPS FOR GPs**
- The physical examination is especially important given that the history may be inconclusive, and up to one-third of children display atypical presentations of specific diseases.
- Palpation should be left until last in the examination so as not to lose the trust of the child.
- Do not forget to examine the genital area and perform a rectal examination.

MANAGEMENT

- Most children with abdominal pain can be managed in the ambulatory area.
- Assess the child's airway, breathing and circulation (ABCs) and transfer him to the intermediate or critical care area if necessary to implement supplemental oxygen therapy, monitoring of vital signs and oximetry and administration of crystalloids via peripheral intravenous (IV) lines.

HISTORY

- However thorough, this may be inconclusive.
- Characteristics of the pain are useful for differentiating disease processes.

Onset

- **Sudden onset** of pain is more likely associated with perforation, intussusception, torsion, and ectopic pregnancy.
- **Slow** or **insidious** onset occurs in appendicitis, pancreatitis, and cholecystitis.
- **Colicky** pain characterizes hollow viscus irritation or obstruction.
- Chronic severe pain is more likely associated with inflammatory bowel disease.

Location of pain at the onset

- **Periumbilical** pain suggests pathology in the small bowel or proximal colon.
- **Epigastric** pain suggests proximal gastrointestinal tract disease including pancreatic disease.
- **Hypogastric** pain correlates with disease of the distal colon and pelvic pathology including incarcerated hernia.
- **Referred** pain to the shoulder pain suggests diaphragmatic irritation.

Associated symptoms

- Vomiting preceding or coincidental with the onset of pain suggests intussusception, gastroenteritis, or ureteric colic.
- Vomiting following well after the onset of pain is more suggestive of peritoneal irritation as in appendicitis, bowel obstruction, or cholecystitis.
- Bilious vomiting is always significant and indicates mechanical obstruction.
- **Diarrhoea** suggests gastroenteritis **but can be seen in surgical conditions too**.
- Fever and vomiting are non-specific in children, occurring in both intra-abdominal and extra-abdominal causes of abdominal pain as well as various viral infections.

Past medical history

- Episodes of previous abdominal pain and outcome should be noted as should recent illnesses in the household or day care. It is important to note and document chronic medical illnesses such as diabetes mellitus, nephritic syndrome, and sickle cell disease in Afro-Americans.

PHYSICAL EXAMINATION

- The importance of a physical examination is underlined by the fact that the history may be inconclusive and up to one-third of children display atypical presentations of specific diseases. It also requires a great deal of patience starting with observation from a distance while the parents are giving the history.
- Note the child's:
  1. Activity level.
  2. Interaction with his parents.
  3. Apparent degree of discomfort.
- Generally:
  1. A writhing, rocking, or moaning child has a colicky pain.
  2. An ill-appearing and lethargic child suggests dehydration or sepsis.
  3. A motionless child lying with knees drawn up suggests peritoneal irritation.
- A complete set of vital signs should be reviewed and documented.
- Perform the abdominal examination last following complete physical examination.
  1. **Inspection**: Is the abdomen scaphoid or distended? Look for scars, abdominal wall defects, and peristaltic waves.
  2. **Auscultation**: In all four quadrants:
     a. Hypoactive bowel sounds suggest peritonitis or bowel obstruction (ileus).
     b. Hyperactive bowel sounds suggest gastroenteritis or early bowel obstruction (mechanical).
  3. **Percussion**: Avoid the most tender area; an alternative is to shake the couch/trolley to assess for peritoneal irritation.
  4. **Palpation**: This is the most informative part of the examination but should be done last due to the pain likely to be induced. Distraction techniques or palpating the abdomen over the child's own hand may be useful.
     a. Involuntary guarding or rebound tenderness suggests peritoneal irritation.
     b. Rigidity usually indicates perforation.
     c. Do not forget to examine the genital area and perform a rectal examination.

INVESTIGATIONS

Investigations are useful in patients with an unclear diagnosis, a history suggestive of a surgical aetiology and signs of peritoneal irritation.

- **Full blood count**: Useful to identify an infectious process or blood loss. Note that the total white cell count may be elevated in any intra-abdominal or febrile condition and so the interpretation may be difficult.
- **Urea/electrolytes/creatinine and blood sugar**: Useful in patients requiring IV fluid resuscitation as in bowel obstruction, peritonitis, or gastroenteritis.
- **Others**: Liver function tests and amylase should be obtained if indicated clinically.

- **Urinalysis** is indicated in patients of any age with abdominal pain looking for pyuria, haematuria, and ketonuria with or without glycosuria.

- **A urine pregnancy test** is indicated in any teenage girl who is capable of pregnancy regardless of her menstrual or sexual history.

- **Plain abdominal X-rays** are most likely to be significant in the following cases:
  1. Prior abdominal surgery.
  2. Foreign body ingestion.
  3. Abnormal bowel sounds.
  4. Abdominal distention.
  5. Signs of peritoneal irritation.

  Abnormalities to be sought include these:
  1. Air-fluid levels.
  2. Decreased intestinal gas.
  3. Sentinel loops.
  4. Facecoliths.
  5. Free air.
  6. Foreign bodies.
  7. Masses.
  8. Constipation.
  9. **Abdominal ultrasonography**: A sensitive method to detect intra-abdominal pathology including intussusception, appendicitis, pyloric stenosis, masses, and abscesses. It is particularly useful in the adolescent female with lower abdominal pain to differentiate appendicitis from other pelvic pathology.

SPECIFIC ENTITIES ACCORDING TO AGE OF CHILD

The most common causes of abdominal pain, both surgical and non-surgical are presented in Table 2.

NON-ABDOMINAL CAUSES OF ADBOMINAL PAIN

Table 3 presents non-abdominal causes of abdominal pain.

DISPOSITION

- Any child with a probable surgical abdomen requires an immediate surgical consultation.

- A liberal policy regarding admission is suggested for children with equivocal signs and symptoms. If the parents insist on taking the child home, a full documentation of advice given must be recorded.

TABLE 2 Common causes of abdominal pain

Neonatal	Infancy (<2 years)	Childhood (2–10 years)	Adolescence
Non-surgical			
Colic	Gastroenteritis	Gastroenteritis	Gastroenteritis
Milk allergy	Viral syndromes	Constipation	Viral syndrome
Gastroenteritis	Constipation	Functional pain	Functional pain
Gastroesophageal reflux	Urinary tract infection	Viral syndrome	Pneumonia
	Sepsis	Urinary tract infection	
		Pneumonia	
Surgical			
Volvulus/malrotation	Intussusception	Appendicitis	Appendicitis
Incarcerated hernia	Incarcerated hernia	Trauma	Trauma
Pyloric stenosis	Trauma	Meckel's diverticulum	Ectopic pregnancy
Intestinal anomalies	Meckel's diverticulum	Intussusception	Testicular torsion
Hirschsprung's disease	Appendicitis	Tumour	Tumour
Intestinal perforation	Tumour (Wilm's)		
Trauma			

TABLE 3 Extra-abdominal causes of abdominal pain

Inflammatory	**Toxicological**
Viral illness	Heavy metal poisoning
Streptococcal pharyngitis	Ingestions of alcohol, aspirin, and insecticides
Henoch–Schonlein Purpura	
Sepsis	**Referred from extra-abdominal sources**
Acute rheumatic fever	Pneumonia
Collagen vascular disease	Pyelonephritis
	Urolithiasis
Metabolic/haematologic	Testicular torsion
Diabetic ketoacidosis	Epididymitis
Leukaemia	Abdominal migraine
Sickle cell crisis	Myocarditis and pericarditis
	Functional abdominal pain

Reference/Further Reading

1. Singer AJ. Acute abdominal conditions. In: Strange G, Ahrens W, Schafermeyer R, Wiebe R, eds. *Paediatric Emergency Medicine*. 3rd ed. New York: McGraw-Hill; 2009: Chap 9: 57–70.

124   Child with Breathlessness

Elizabeth Khor • Peter Manning

CAVEATS

- Remember the airway, breathing and circulation (ABCs): **Do not** delay the transfer of an acutely dyspnoeic child to the critical care area of the emergency department by asking the parents to give the child's medical history.

- A **breathless child with no audible cry** is in imminent danger of respiratory arrest: Transfer to the critical care area of the emergency department.

- A child crying vigorously and screaming volubly is demonstrating good lung function.

- A breathless child could be in severe pain from, e.g. biliary colic (choledochal cyst) and acute abdomen (peritonitis and intussusception). Anyone in pain can be breathless!

- A breathless child with a normal chest examination and a normal chest X-ray could have diabetic ketoacidosis (findings include typical air hunger, raised stat capillary blood sugar and ketones in the breath and urine).

- When attempting to auscultate the chest of a child you may need to distract the child first since it is very easy to miss physical findings in a screaming child.

- In auscultating the chest of a child, **pay attention to the degree of air entry**, not only the crackles and wheezing: Diminished air entry over one lobe or one lung may be the only clue to the diagnosis of lobar consolidation **before** the development of localized crackles or bronchial breath sounds, the presence of a pleural effusion, or pneumothorax.

- Aspirin or other drug overdose may present with breathlessness as a reflection of metabolic acidosis.

- Always consider cardiac causes of breathlessness such as heart failure due to congenital heart disease, myocarditis, or supraventricular tachycardia (SVT).

⇨ **SPECIAL TIPS FOR GPs**

- Place a breathless child in a position of comfort (the position he finds most comfortable): **Do not force** him to lie flat.
- If the child is frightened by the application of an oxygen mask, then administer 'blow by' oxygen by having the mother hold the mask a short distance from the child's face directing the flow on to the face.
- Effective bag-valve-mask ventilation is the most important skill in managing respiratory failure in a child.

THINGS TO ASK PARENTS OR CAREGIVERS

- **Onset of breathlessness.**
  1. Is breathlessness abrupt while playing with a toy or while eating?
  2. Did the child become breathless while vomiting? Vomiting and cyanosis suggest aspiration.
     a. Vomiting, chest pain, and dyspnoea may suggest lower lobe pneumonia.
     b. Vomiting, dyspnoea, and wheezing may indicate sticky phlegm, e.g. in bronchitis.
- **Exposure of family members to pulmonary tuberculosis (PTB), recent pneumonia or chest infections, or viral illnesses.**
- **History of asthma or previous wheeze.**

EXAMINATION

NOTES:

1. A breathless child could be in **cardiac failure**, yet presents like bronchiolitis with wheezing; the heart sounds may be difficult to hear.
2. The breathless child with **head retractions** may have signs of **meningeal irritation:** Remember to look for signs of increased intracranial pressure in a drowsy, breathless, or apnoeic child.
3. A breathless child with **failure to thrive** could have gastroesophageal reflux, tracheoesophageal fistula, cystic fibrosis, or be immuno-compromised.

- The **most important sign** to recognize is the mental state: This is an early indicator of hypoxaemia or hypercarbia. Beware irritability, drowsiness, inability to recognise parents, and inappropriate social responses.
- Look for presence of **central cyanosis**: If noted, transfer the child immediately to the critical care area of the emergency department and administer 100% supplemental oxygen by a face mask.
- Look for **signs of respiratory distress such as** cyanosis, head retractions, use of accessory muscles, tracheal tug, retractions, grunting or flaring of the nostrils, or stridor. If noted, transfer immediately to the critical care area of the emergency department: place the child in a position of comfort and administer 100% supplemental oxygen by a face mask.
- Count the **respiratory rate** of the child.
- Do the signs suggest upper or lower respiratory tract disease?
  1. **Upper respiratory tract obstruction** is suggested by snoring and stridor (presence of the latter demands transfer to the critical care area).
  2. **Grunting** suggests alveolar pathology requiring positive end-expiratory pressure (PEEP) to clear the alveoli as in consolidation of pneumonia, pulmonary oedema, or sepsis.
- **Observe the chest** for signs of unequal expansion. First, palpate the trachea for position. Then palpate for subcutaneous emphysema: Vocal resonance is best evaluated by asking the child to repeat the names of their favourite cartoon characters.
- Complete the examination by evaluating the **ear, nose and throat (ENT) system**.

MANAGEMENT

- **X-ray considerations**

  1. A clinical diagnosis should be made before ordering a chest X-ray for any breathless child.

  2. A chest X-ray is useful in dyspnoeic infants since pulmonary findings as well as cardiac size can be ascertained.

  3. Not all asthmatic patients need chest X-rays but they are useful to exclude foreign body aspiration, presence of pneumonia, or atelectasis.

  4. A chest X-ray is indicated in all first wheezes, and the clinical triad of fever, cough, and dyspnoea.

  5. It may be dangerous to send a child (e.g. a child with croup and epiglottitis) to the X-ray room to have his X-ray taken rather than have it done in the critical care area.

- **Severely dyspnoeic child**

  1. Manage the child in the critical care area.

  2. Evaluate and support the airway.

  3. Administer 100% supplemental oxygen by mask.

  4. Monitoring: Electrocardiogram (ECG), vital signs every 5–15 minutes, and pulse oximetry.

  5. Perform a careful examination of the chest.

  6. Perform a chest X-ray as needed (see above).

  7. Give nebulized salbutamol therapy for the wheezing child.

     Dosage: **0.5 ml: 1.5 ml saline for those under one year**

     1 ml: 3 ml saline for those aged more than one year; can be repeated every 20 minutes.

     Obtain paediatric consultation and transfer the child to the paediatric intensive care unit.

  8. Set heparin plug in a peripheral vein: Obtain venous blood gas since this is useful in assessing the pH and pCO_2.

- **Mildly or moderately dyspnoeic child**

  1. Can be managed in the intermediate care area of the emergency department.

  2. Monitor pulse oximetry.

  3. Administer supplemental oxygen if the oxygen saturation level (SpO_2) falls below 96%.

  4. In asthmatics

     a. Give nebulised salbutamol therapy as needed every 20 minutes.

     b. Start oral prednisolone 1–2 mg/kg **early** if discharge from the emergency department is likely.

DISPOSITION

- **Admit**
  1. Children who are intubated, following appropriate paediatric consultation.
  2. Children who do not improve with therapy.
  3. Children whose SpO_2 on room air is below 96%.
  4. Children whose parents/caregivers do not seem competent to follow instructions.
- **Discharge to outpatient care**
  1. Children who respond appropriately to therapy.
  2. Children with competent parents/caregivers who will/can follow instructions.

Reference/Further Reading

1. Cohen J, Brown KM. Respiratory distress. In: Strange G, Ahrens W, Schafermeyer R, Wiebe R, eds. *Pediatric Emergency Medicine*. 3rd ed. New York: McGraw-Hill; 2009: Chap 4: 23–36.

125   Child/Baby, Crying

Elizabeth Khor • Peter Manning

CAVEATS

- A crying baby/child refers to the child who cries continually and refuses to be pacified.
- Be cognizant that this is a situation that is fraught with anxiety, since the caregivers cannot tolerate the crying and have brought the child to the emergency department out of sheer desperation.
- **Avoid** prescribing sedating agents: **Do not** accede to the parents' request for such treatment. The crying is a symptom of a problem, and sedating the child will simply mask the underlying cause.

⇨ **SPECIAL TIPS FOR GPs**

- Remember to undress the child totally to expose the abdomen, perineum, and extremities fully.
- A crying infant who is not interacting with the parents probably has a serious reason for the crying. Review the vital signs for abnormalities consistent with age.

MANAGEMENT

Is the child in pain?

- **Abdominal conditions**

  1. Acute **intussusception**: Non-stop screaming, vomiting, and refusal to feed.

  NOTE: Do a rectal examination to look for blood or red currant jelly stools.

  2. **Volvulus**: Abdominal distension.
  3. **Obstructed inguinal herniae** (baby boys and girls): Remember to look at the groin and feel the testes in boys for acute **torsion**.
  4. **Ureteric colic**, **biliary colic**, or acute **urinary tract infection** (UTI): Carry out a urine dipstick test for leucocytes, blood, and nitrites.

- **Head, Eyes, Ears, Nose, Throat conditions**

  1. Acute **otitis media**: Beware the 'normal' injected tympanic membrane of the crying infant.
  2. Check the oropharynx for scalds or burns and herpangina or gingivostomatitis (characterized by mouth ulcers).

3. Look for **corneal abrasions** or a foreign body under the eyelid.

4. Examine the head for **bulging fontanelles** (for those <15 to 18 months old).

- **Extremity conditions**

  1. **Circumferential ligature** ('pseudoainhum'): The infant's toes, fingers, or even the penis (in the case of a boy) can be strangulated by a loose thread from a mitten, blanket, or maternal hair.

  2. **Long bone injury or bruising in extremities**: Think of non-accidental injuries.

  3. **Osteomyelitis**: Examine the extremities for local tenderness, swelling, and redness.

- **Chest pain** (rare, but possible)

  1. Cardiac **ischaemia**: Kawasaki's disease or pericarditis.

  2. **Supraventricular tachycardia** may present with crying and poor perfusion: **Remember** to count the pulse rate.

- Consider **meningeal irritation**

  1. A crying child with a high-pitched cry.

  2. The patient may show head retraction, drowsiness, a bulging fontanelle, or stiff neck.

  3. Paradoxical irritability is worrisome and suggests meningeal irritation. This type of irritability occurs when the infant cries when held but is calm and quiet when left alone.

- Consider **shaken baby syndrome**: Suspect this if the child is pale and drowsy with unexplained physical injuries and/or retinal haemorrhages.

Disposition

- Admit the child to hospital: This is prudent since the caregivers are probably sleep-deprived and too weary to cope with the incessant crying. This allows caregivers to sleep. This also permits further investigation of the cause, e.g. possible non-accidental injury (NAI).

Reference/Further Reading

1. Marrinal JM. The crying infant. In: Strange G, Ahrens W, Schafermeyer R, Wiebe R, eds. *Pediatric Emergency Medicine*. 3rd ed. New York: McGraw-Hill; 2009: 91–95.

Elizabeth Khor • Peter Manning

CAVEATS

- Refer to the child with diarrhoea only, without vomiting.
- Consider the possibility that the **diarrhoea** is 'spurious' and caused by:
  1. Constipation (can palpate faecal masses in the abdomen).
  2. Laxatives, antacids, or antibiotics.
  3. Too much sorbitol-containing fruit juices (e.g. apple juice).
- Most cases are due to **acute gastrointestinal infections**:
  1. **Viral**: For example, rotavirus. Urinary tract infection symptoms followed by non-bilious vomiting, then profuse, and watery diarrhoea.
  2. **Invasive**: *Salmonella*, *Shigella*, *Campylobacter jejuni* or *E. coli*: Blood-stained mucoid stools, high fever, tenesmus, and 'sick' appearance.
  3. **Toddler's diarrhoea**: Often begins after a bout of acute gastroenteritis but child looks well without fever, weight loss, or tenesmus; parents are concerned about frequent passage of soft, pasty stools with undigested vegetables in the stool.
- **Do not** prescribe Lomotil® or Imodium®-type products in children under 6 years of age as these medications may cause paralytic ileus.
- Teach parents that **even with treatment, some diarrhoea should be expected**: The aim of therapy is to prevent dehydration in their child.

> ⇨ **SPECIAL TIP FOR GPs**
> - Remember to perform a focused hydration history and examination (see below).

QUESTIONS TO ASK PARENTS OR CAREGIVERS

- **What has been the recent bowel habit?** For example, constipation.
- **What are in your child's diet?** For example, fibre and sorbitol-containing fruit juices.
- **Has your child recently been prescribed laxatives, antacids, or antibiotics?**

EXAMINATION ESSENTIALS

- **Quick hydration check**:
  1. Is the diaper dry or wet? If dry, ask when the child last passed urine; no urine for more than 8 hours is a symptom of dehydration.
  2. Beware the crying child who sheds no tears.

- **Focused hydration check** (Table 1):
  1. Look for sunken eyes, dry mouth, poor peripheral perfusion, and reduced skin turgor.
  2. If the patient is severely dehydrated, there is a danger of hypovolaemic shock: Start intravenous (IV) resuscitation in the emergency department prior to admission.
- **Tachypnoea** may indicate hyperpyrexia or the air hunger of metabolic acidosis.
- **Head, Eyes, Ears, Nose, Throat conditions**:
  1. Examine the ears for acute otitis media.
  2. Auscultate the bases of the lungs for basilar pneumonia.
  3. Check the throat for signs of pharyngitis or tonsillitis: Absence of these signs makes diagnosis less likely.

TABLE 1   **Clinical assessment of the severity of dehydration**

Signs and symptoms	Mild dehydration (5%)	Moderate dehydration (7%)	Severe dehydration (10%)
General appearance and condition			
Infants and young children	Thirsty, alert, restless	Thirsty, restless, lethargic but irritable or drowsy	Drowsy, limp cold, sweaty, cyanotic extremities, may be comatose
Older children and adults	Thirsty, alert, restless	Thirsty, alert, postural hypotension	Cold, sweaty, muscle cramps, cyanotic extremities, conscious
Radial pulse	Normal rate and strength	Rapid and weak	Rapid, sometimes impalpable
Respiration	Normal	Deep ± rapid	Deep and rapid
Anterior fontanelle	Normal	Sunken	Very sunken
Systolic blood pressure	Normal	Normal or low	<90 mmHg; may be unrecordable
Skin elasticity	Pinch retracts immediately	Pinch retracts slowly	Pinch retracts slowly (>2 seconds)
Eyes	Normal	Sunken (detectable)	Grossly sunken
Tears	Present	Absent	Absent
Mucous membranes	Moist	Dry	Very dry
Urine flow	Normal	Reduced amount, dark	None for several hours
Body weight loss (%)	4–5	6–9	10 or more
Estimated fluid deficit (ml/kg)	40–50	60–90	100–110

Source: Table adapted with permission of the McGraw-Hill Companies, from Powell EC, Reynolds S. Gastroenteritis. In: Strange GR, Ahrens W, Lelyveld S, et al., eds. *Paediatric Emergency Medicine: A Comprehensive Study Guide*. New York: McGraw-Hill; 1995: 291.

- **Examine the abdomen for**:
  1. Tenderness (appendicitis or peritonitis).
  2. Hepatomegaly (may have sepsis).
  3. Masses (intussusception).
  4. Distension (intestinal obstruction or paralytic ileus).
- **Perform a rectal examination** (you may be able to disimpact faecal masses): Any blood should already be obvious on the diaper.

MANAGEMENT

- **Stool cultures** have no place in emergency medicine.
- **Urinalysis** for **ketonuria**: Useful, particularly in the obese child in whom signs of dehydration are difficult to assess.
- **Urinalysis** for nitrites/white blood cells: For presumptive diagnosis of urinary tract infection (UTI).
- **X-rays**: Perform a kidney, ureter and bladder (KUB) X-ray if the child has abdominal distension or is passing bloody diarrhoea.
- **Stat capillary blood sugar** if altered mental status exists.
- **Rehydration of the severely dehydrated child (10% dehydration)**: Refer to Chapter 133, *Fluid Replacement in Paediatrics*.
  1. Establish a peripheral IV line.
  2. Administer crystalloid (normal saline or Hartmann's solution) at 20 ml/kg body weight as bolus over 20–30 minutes.
  3. Labs: Full blood count, urea/electrolytes/creatinine, and stat capillary blood sugar.
  4. Obtain paediatric consultation and transfer the child to the paediatric intensive care unit.

DISPOSITION

- **Admit** the following for IV fluid therapy:
  1. A neonate or young infant with profuse diarrhoea.
  2. The child with signs of moderate/severe diarrhoea and who refuses oral fluids.
  3. The child with pathological chronic diarrhoea with failure to thrive, or signs of colitis and possible electrolyte, and water deficiencies.
- **Discharge to outpatient care** the child who is not toxic-looking and whose urinalysis shows the absence of ketones or trace ketones.
  1. Oral rehydration solutions (ORS), e.g. Servidrat or diluted rice cereal.
  2. Continue breastfeeding when possible.
  3. If the duration of diarrhoea is longer than 24 hours, the child may be offered lactose-free milk, e.g. O-Lac or any soy-based milk formula or Milupa HN25 for 48–72 hours.

4. Allow the child to eat solid foods as soon as they can be tolerated and appetite has returned: most solids are acceptable.

5. Kaolin products are not useful. Instead, Smecta will reduce, but not eliminate totally, the number of bowel movements by 30–40%.

6. Toddler's diarrhoea: Avoid lactose and sorbitol-containing products and reduce dietary fibre intake for 1 week.

Reference/Further Reading

1. Powell EC, Reynolds S. Vomiting diarrhoea and gastroenteritis. In: Strange GR, Ahrens W, Schaefermeyer R, et al., eds. *Pediatric Emergency Medicine: A Comprehensive Study Guide*. 3rd ed. New York: McGraw-Hill; 2009: 73–78.

127　Child with Fever

Ng Kee Chong • Petrina Wong • Wong Chin Khoon

CAVEATS

- Fever is a normal response.
- Fever is a symptom, not a disease.
- Fever persists until the disease process resolves.
- Fever determination need not always be exact.
- Fever is often a useful body defence.
- Fever, especially a low grade fever, need not always be treated.
- Clinical appearance is usually more important than the height of the fever.

PHYSIOLOGICAL EFFECTS OF FEVER

- Fever appears to increase:
  1. The phagocytic and bactericidal activity of neutrophils.
  2. The cytotoxic effects of lymphocytes.
- For each 1°C elevation of body temperature there is:
  1. A 13% increase in oxygen consumption.
  2. Tachycardia (10 beats per minute for every 1°C increase in body temperature).
  3. Tachypnoea (2.5 breaths per minute for every 1°C increase in body temperature).
- The increased metabolic demand may stress foetuses as well as patients with marginal cardiac or cerebral vascular supply.

POTENTIAL COMPLICATIONS OF FEVER

- Dehydration.
- Fits.
- Delirium (especially in younger children).
- Hyperpyrexia (>41.1°C): Must consider serious bacterial infection (SBI).

NOTE: **SBI** are meningitis, pneumonia, sepsis, osteomyelitis, urinary tract infection, *Salmonella enteritis*, *Listeria*, *E. coli*, and *Staphylococcus/Streptococcus* infections. **Symptoms and signs** are irritability, decreased activity, weak cry, poor feeding, diarrhoea and vomiting, abdominal distension, drowsiness, respiratory distress, hypothermia, or hyperthermia, and poor peripheral perfusion. Rate of SBI = 9.5% (<40°C) versus 36% (>40°C). SBI occurs in 9.5% of children with a temperature <40°C compared to 36% with a temperature of >40°C.

⇨ **SPECIAL TIPS FOR GPs**

- There is little evidence that low grade or moderate fever is harmful or that antipyretic therapy for such fever is beneficial. Exceptions are children with febrile fits and children with impaired cardiac, pulmonary or cerebral function.
- **Red flags!**
  1. Young baby
  2. Clueless fever (no cough/running nose/diarrhoea, etc.)
  3. Danger clues
     a. Prolonged fever.
     b. Child looking sicker than should be.
     c. Pallor, bruises, weight loss, irritability, lethargy, weak cry, poor feeding, hypothermia, and poor perfusion.
     d. Height of fever is greater than 40°C.
- **Low risk infants**:

Clinical
  1. Appears well.
  2. Previously healthy.
     a. Born at term.
     b. No prior antibiotics.
     c. No previous hospitalisation.
     d. No chronic or underlying illness.
  3. No evidence of skin, soft tissue, bone, joint or ear infection.

Lab values
  1. White blood cells 5–15 $\times$ 10^9/L.
  2. Absolute band form ≤1.5 $\times$ 10^9/L.
  3. Normal urinalysis.

MANAGEMENT: POINTS TO CONSIDER

Does the child have a fever?

- **Definition of fever**: Body temperature of 1°C or greater above the mean standard deviation at the site of recording.
- Normal baby body temperature according to the site of recording:
  1. Rectal route: ≤38.0°C.
  2. Oral route: ≤37.5°C.
  3. Axillary route: ≤37.5°C.
  4. Tympanic route: ≤38.0°C.

What is the age of the child?

- The age of the child correlates with the risk of SBI. See Table 1.

TABLE 1   Risk of SBI in the different age groups

<1 month	12%
1–2 months	6%
<3 months versus >3 months	21 times the risk

NOTE: Assume infection between day 2 and day 3 unless otherwise proven.

What is the duration of the fever?

- Table 2 shows the three main groups of fever encountered in paediatric practice and their usual duration.

TABLE 2   Groups of fever encountered in paediatric practice and usual duration

Group	Commonest cause	Usual duration
Fever with localising signs	Upper respiratory tract infection	<2 weeks
Fever without localising signs	Viral infection, urinary tract infection, bacteraemia, malaria and pneumonia (maximum temperature >39°C and total white blood cells >20,000)	<2 weeks
Pyrexia of unknown origin (PUO)	Infection and rheumatoid arthritis	>2 weeks

Is there a focus of infection?

- **Fever without localising signs**
  1. Occurs in 20% of all febrile episodes.
  2. The most common cause is a viral infection (22.5%).
  3. Bacterial infection: Urinary tract infection, bacteraemia, and pneumonia.
  4. Incidence of bacteraemia in children 3–24 months old is 3–4%.
  5. Incidence of bacteraemia according to the height of the fever:
     a. 40–40.4°C = 1.7%
     b. 40.5–40.9°C = 2.4%
     c. >40.9°C   = 2.8%
  6. Septicaemia: Meningitis, pneumonia, and otitis media due to group B *Streptococcus*, *E. coli*, *Listeria* (neonate), *Streptococcus pneumonia*, and *Haemophilus influenzae*.

- **Pyrexia of unknown origin (PUO)**
    1. Fever higher than 38.3°C on several occasions.
    2. Diagnosis is still uncertain after more than 1 week of investigations.
    3. Infection occur in 50–60% of cases (viral 15%).
    4. Collagen disease 20%.
    5. Malignancy 5%.
    6. Miscellaneous 5–10%.
    7. Undiagnosed 5%.

Are there any red flags?

See *Special Tips for GPs*.

MANAGEMENT: TO TREAT OR NOT TO TREAT?

- Antipyretics **do not** shorten the duration of the febrile episode or interfere directly with pyrogen formation or heat loss.
- **Indications for antipyretics**:
    1. Fever >38.5°C associated with painful or unpleasant symptoms, e.g. otitis media, myalgia and discomfort.
    2. Fever >39°C without obvious symptoms.
    3. Poor nutrition, cardiovascular diseases, burns, or postoperative state.
    4. History of fits or delirium secondary to fever.

NOTE: In the Singaporean context, it may be difficult to convince parents to give antipyretics only if the fever is >38.5°C, so 37.5°C is a practical threshold.

- **Antipyretics**
    1. **Paracetamol**
        a. Dosage: 10–15 mg/kg dose every 4 to 6 hours by oral or rectal routes.
        b. Maximum daily dosage: 65 mg/kg/day.
        c. Onset of action at 30 minutes, nadir of fever 3 hours later and has a duration of 3 to 6 hours.
        d. Improves activity and alertness but not mood or appetite.
        e. Side effects are rare (gastrointestinal upset, rash, thrombocytopaenia, hypoglycaemia, and bronchospasm).

NOTE: Use with caution in patients with liver disease or jaundice.

2. **Ibuprofen (Brufen®)**
   a. The *only* non-steroidal anti-inflammatory drug (NSAID) approved as an antipyretic in the United States (1984) and the United Kingdom (1990).
   b. Dosage: 5–10 mg/kg/dose every 6 hours.
   c. Earlier onset of action, more potent, and lasts longer than that of paracetamol.

NOTE: There is no documented evidence that alternating paracetamol with NSAIDs provides better control of fever, but NSAIDs can be used together with paracetamol at different intervals because the mechanism of action is different. It is recommended that ibuprofen be given at least an hour after the last dose of paracetamol (to allow paracetamol time to work).

   d. Side effects are few (platelet inhibition and reduced renal blood flow are both extremely rare).

NOTE: Use with caution in patients with bleeding diathesis and asthma as NSAIDs have anti-platelet effects and may cause bronchospasm.

3. **Diclofenac (Voltaren®)**: Although commonly used as an antipyretic it is not indicated as such, but can be useful for the myalgias sometimes associated with fever.

NOTE: Prescribing information provided by the manufacturer (Novartis) states '*Fever alone is not an indication*'.

- **Adjunctive measures for fever**:
  1. Tepid sponging (appropriate water temperature is 27–34°C).
     a. Useful if the temperature is >41°C or 40°C with discomfort.
     b. Start after giving antipyretic.
  2. Bed rest has no significant effect on temperature control.
  3. Total body cooling, ice packs, and air-conditioning are indicated only for hyperthermia.
  4. Alcohol sponging is contraindicated in children.

DISPOSITION

- Children **under 3 months** of age: Admit for full septic work-up.
- Children between **3 and 36 months** of age:
  1. Clear-cut focus: Treat focus as appropriate; if discharged, to follow up within 24–48 hours.
  2. No clear-cut focus:
     a. Non-toxic and low risk: Discharge with follow-up within 24 hours.
     b. Toxic or high risk: Admit for full septic work-up and antibiotics.

NOTE: Urinalysis for all and full blood count if the fever lasts longer than 3 days.

Other admission criteria

- Life-threatening infections, e.g. meningitis.
- Severe soft tissue infections, e.g. septic arthritis, buccal, or orbital cellulitis.
- Hypoxia due to a lower respiratory tract infection.
- Electrolyte imbalance due to gastroenteritis.
- Impression of parental competence:
  1. Can the parents provide adequate care?
  2. Will antibiotics, if indicated, be given as recommended?
  3. Can the parents be trusted to return to hospital if needed?
  4. Can follow-up be ensured?

References/Further Reading

1. Fauci AS, et al., eds. *Harrison's Principles of Internal Medicine*. 14th ed. New York: McGraw-Hill; 1998.

2. Bachur R, Perry H, Harper M. Occult pneumonias: Empiric chest radiographs in febrile children with leukocytosis. *Ann Emerg Med*. 1999; 33(2): 166–173.

3. Lee GM. Risk of bacteraemia in the post Hib era. *Arch Pediatr Adolesc Med*. 1998; 152: 624–628.

4. Waldrop RD, Felter RA, et al., eds. The febrile or septic appearing infant or child. In: Strange G, Ahrens W, Schafermeyer R, Wiebe R, eds. *Pediatric Emergency Medicine*. 3rd ed. New York: McGraw-Hill; 2009: 15–22.

Peter Manning • Saumya • Wong Chin Khoon

CAVEATS

- The **objectives** for the emergency department **management** are:
  1. Maintenance of adequate airway, breathing and circulation.
  2. Termination of convulsive activity and prevention of recurrence.
  3. Diagnosis and initial therapy of life-threatening causes, which includes the reversal of physiological changes that may have taken place.
  4. Arrangement for the appropriate disposition of the child (e.g. investigations, admission, or referral).
- For the purpose of **subsequent management**, there is a need to differentiate between febrile seizure (simple or complex) and non-febrile seizure, both of which can present as status epilepticus.
- When the exact onset of seizure is unknown, any fitting patient arriving at the emergency department should be managed as though he is having status epilepticus.
- Always consider the following important **differential diagnoses** in Table 1.

TABLE 1   Differential diagnoses of seizure

1.	Rigors
2.	Hypoglycaemic seizure
3.	Meningitis/meningoencephalitis
4.	Reye's syndrome
5.	Drug intoxication, e.g. oculogyric crisis
6.	Breath-holding attacks
7.	Gastroesophageal reflux
8.	Syncope
9.	Pseudoseizure

⇨ **SPECIAL TIPS FOR GPs**

- Neck stiffness may be absent in children younger than 18 months old or it is difficult to elicit in uncooperative children.
- Opisthotonic posturing in a drowsy child suggests increased intracranial pressure.
- An irritable child who is difficult to examine may have meningeal irritation.
- Bradycardia, hypotension, and poor perfusion in a fitting child are ominous signs and imply severe hypoxia and an immediate need to establish the airway and ventilate the child.
- Before giving any medication, always get a brief history on seizure disorder, medication usage and chronic disease, or drug allergies.

- Monitor **bedside blood sugar** level in all fitting children.
- Metoclopramide-induced oculogyric crisis may mimic a febrile seizure and has a totally different management, i.e. intramuscular (IM) or intravenous (IV) diphenhydramine (for those under 3 years old) or benztropine (for those more than 3 years old).
- A recognized source of infection (e.g. otitis media) does not exclude the presence of meningitis.

MANAGEMENT OF A FITTING CHILD

- Most seizures are brief and do not require any specific treatment.
  1. Position the child semi-prone to minimize the chance of aspiration.
  2. Secure the airway: If necessary clear the airway with gentle suction.

NOTE: Put a padded gag between the teeth to prevent the biting of the tongue **only if** the jaw is relaxed; otherwise more damage is done with the use of force.

Administer supplemental oxygen by face mask and keep the oxygen saturation level above 95%.

- **If the seizure continues**
  1. Give **rectal diazepam** 0.5 mg/kg (maximum dose 10 mg; good guide: infant 2.5 mg, older than 1 year old 5 mg, may repeat twice) only if unable to insert intravenous (IV) plug. Otherwise give **IV diazepam** 0.1–0.25 mg/kg no faster than 2 mg/min; may repeat twice every 5 minutes if the seizure is not controlled.
     a. An alternative is IV lorazepam (0.1 mg/kg), limited to a maximum of 4 mg per dose. The half life is 12–24 hours compared with 15–25 minutes of diazepam).
  2. Monitor carefully for respiratory depression.
  3. Establish a peripheral intravenous line.
  4. Take blood for bedside blood glucose and electrolytes.
  5. Measure and record the vital signs and temperature.
  6. If the seizure continues, treat as for status epilepticus (see below).
- **After the seizure stops**
  1. Continue to monitor respiratory function and neurological status.
  2. If the child is febrile, bring the temperature down with **tepid sponging** and **antipyretics**.
  3. Measure the vital signs, temperature, and oxygen saturation.
  4. Continue to give supplemental oxygen if the oxygen saturation level falls below 95%.
  5. Consider investigations: Anti-convulsant level, full blood count, urea/electrolytes/creatinine, liver function test, ionized calcium, magnesium, lumbar puncture, chest X-ray, and urinalysis (depending on clinical suspicion).

- Admit all patients with a first non-febrile seizure. In a child with a **first non-febrile seizure**,
  a. Lumbar puncture is of limited value and is used primarily when there is concern about possible meningitis or encephalitis.
  b. Electroencephalogram (EEG) is recommended as a part of the neurodiagnostic evaluation.
  c. If a neuroimaging study is obtained, magnetic resonance imaging (MRI) is the preferred modality as it can better demonstrate small tumour vascular malformation and atrophy.

STATUS EPILEPTICUS

Definition

Continuous seizure activity or intermittent seizure activity with failure to regain consciousness between seizures for more than 30 minutes.

MANAGEMENT

- The initial management of a fitting child is discussed below.
- When setting up an IV line, take blood for:
  1. Stat capillary blood sugar. Consider full blood count, urea/electrolytes/creatinine, liver function tests, ionized calcium, magnesium, phosphate, and blood gases in selected cases.
  2. Include anti-convulsant level(s) in all patients on long-term therapy.
- If the patient is hypoglycaemic, give IV glucose bolus: 25% dextrose 1–2 ml/kg and 10% dextrose 2–3 ml/kg. Maintain IV 10% dextrose infusion at 5–10 mg/kg/min to retain normoglycaemia.
- Prepare intubation equipment in case of inability to maintain airway and adequate oxygenation.
- **If the seizure continues**:
  1. Administer **IV phenytoin** 20 mg/kg diluted in **normal saline** at a rate of 1 mg/kg/min (maximum dose 50 mg/min). Additional 5 mg/kg increments of phenytoin may be given up to a maximum dose of 30 mg/kg (maximum dose 1000 mg) if the seizure continues (monitor electrocardiogram and blood pressure as it may cause cardiac arrhythmias).

  NOTE: The use of dilution with saline is dependent on institutional policy. Phenytoin can be administered without dilution though the precautions regarding the rate of administration still apply.

  2. **IV phenobarbitone** 20 mg/kg may be given at a rate of 2 mg/kg/min (maximum dose 30 mg/min) after the loading dose of phenytoin if the seizure continues. Additional 5 mg/kg increments may be given, up to a maximum total dose of 30 mg/kg (maximum dose 600 mg) if the seizure continues (may cause respiratory depression, hypotension, and sedation at high doses).

- If the seizure continues despite the above measures taken, consider rapid sequence intubation: Paralysis and intubation by an individual skilled in airway management.
- **Disposition**:
  1. Admit the child to the paediatric intensive care unit and obtain an immediate paediatric neurological consult.
  2. All children with status epilepticus should have a **computed tomography (CT) scan of the head** done. The CT scan may be undertaken after the convulsion has terminated and the airway, breathing and circulation are stabilized.
  3. Start **maintenance therapy of anti-convulsant** (phenytoin or phenobarbitone or both, depending on what has been used in the initial therapy).

Isolated fit in an epileptic

- Measure the **blood levels of every anti-convulsant**:
  1. If *low*, administer a double dose of medication.
  2. If the patient is *non-compliant*, strongly encourage compliance.
  3. If the patient is *already compliant* with his medication, increase the dose if the maximum dose has not been reached.
  4. If the *maximum dose* has already been reached, consult the paediatric neurologist for further anti-convulsants.
- **Disposition**: Observe in the emergency department for 2 to 3 hours, discharge if there is no further seizure and refer to the paediatric neurologist in the specialist clinic.

References/Further Reading

1. Practice parameter: Evaluating a first non-febrile seizure in children. Report of the Quality Standards Subcommittee of the American Academy of Neurology, the Child Neurology Society and the American Epilepsy Society. *Neurology*. 2000; 55: 616–629. Also available at: www.aan.com/professional/practice/pdfs/g10081.pdf.

2. Fuchs S. Seizure. In: Strange G, Ahrens W, Schafermeyer R, Wiebe R, eds. *Pediatric Emergency Medicine*. 3rd ed. New York: McGraw-Hill; 2009; 39–50.

4. Management of the Paediatric Patient with Generalized Convulsive Status Epilepticus in the Emergency Department. Position Statement from the Emergency Paediatrics Section, Canadian Paediatric Society, January 2002. Available at: www.cps.ca/english/statement/EP/ep95-01.htm. Accessed 13 August 2002.

129 Child, Vomiting

Elizabeth Khor • Peter Manning • Angelina Ang

CAVEATS

- Not every child who vomits has an acute gastrointestinal problem: Be aware of meningitis, increased intracranial pressure, otitis media, acute asthma, lower lobe pneumonia or urinary tract infection, which also present with vomiting.

- Beware the infant or neonate who vomits: The diagnosis of 'overfeeding' or 'mild reflux' is made only after medical or surgical conditions have been excluded. Be aware that **vomiting** is **often** the **presenting symptom** of a **septic** neonate, a neonate with inborn error of metabolism, an infant with acute **appendicitis**, **meningitis**, or **pyloric stenosis**.

- **Avoid** prescribing metoclopramide and prochlorperazine to children under 12 years old since oculogyric crises are a distressing and undesirable side effect.

- Oral promethazine syrup is a safe and mild anti-emetic.

- Avoid prescribing Prepulsid in young children since one must be absolutely certain that there are no signs of an acute surgical abdomen.

> ⇨ **SPECIAL TIP FOR GPs**
> - Remember to perform a focused hydration history and examination (see below).

QUESTIONS TO ASK PARENTS OR CAREGIVERS

- **What is the colour of the vomitus?**
  1. **Bile** (malrotation of the gut) or **blood** points towards an acute surgical condition that warrants admission for further investigation.
  2. Examine the vomitus itself or vomit-stained clothing.

NOTE: Bile often resembles sugar cane juice and blood may look like Milo (a chocolate malt beverage).

- **What medication has been prescribed? How many doctors have they consulted?** Be aware that certain prescribed medications may cause gastric irritation and vomiting, e.g. macrolide antibiotics, oral theophylline, oral non-steroidal anti-inflammatory drugs (NSAIDs), and oral prednisolone.

- **When did you last note a wet diaper or when did your child last urinate?** No urine for more than 8 hours is a symptom of dehydration.

- **Did your child sustain a recent head injury?**

- **Is there a history of family members/siblings suffering from similar symptoms?** For example, rotavirus gastroenteritis usually starts with upper respiratory tract infection symptoms followed by vomiting and profuse diarrhoea; there is a high risk of dehydration in children under 3 years of age.

EXAMINATION ESSENTIALS

- **Quick hydration check**:
  1. Is the child's diaper dry or wet? If dry, ask the above questions.
  2. Beware the crying child who sheds no tears.
- **Focused hydration check**: Refer to Table 1 in Chapter 126, *Child with Diarrhoea* for the clinical assessment of the severity of dehydration.
  1. Look for sunken eyes, dry mouth, poor peripheral perfusion, and reduced skin turgor.
  2. If the patient is severely dehydrated, there is a danger of hypovolaemic shock: Start intravenous (IV) resuscitation in the emergency department prior to admission.
- **Tachypnoea** may indicate hyperpyrexia or the air hunger of metabolic acidosis.
- **Tachycardia** may indicate impending shock in the young child.
- **Head, Eyes, Ears, Nose, Throat conditions**:
  1. Examine the ears for acute otitis media.
  2. Auscultate the lung bases for basilar pneumonia.
  3. Check the throat for signs of pharyngitis or tonsillitis: Absence of these signs makes diagnosis less likely.
  4. Check for bulging fontanelles (for children under 18 months or for those between 15 and 18 months of age).
- **Examine the abdomen** for:
  1. Tenderness (appendicitis or peritonitis).
  2. Hepatomegaly (may have sepsis).
  3. Masses, e.g. pyloric stenosis or intussusception.
  4. Distension, e.g. intestinal obstruction or paralytic ileus.
  5. Perform a rectal examination to check for blood or red currant jelly stools of intussusceptions.
- If there is a history of **head injury**, examine for:
  1. Any boggy scalp swelling.
  2. Pupillary response.
  3. Fundus.
  4. Gait and symmetry of neurological parameters.

MANAGEMENT

- **Urine dipstick** for **ketonuria**: Useful, particularly in the obese child in whom signs of dehydration are difficult to assess.
- **Urine dipstick** for **nitrites/leucocytes** for a presumptive diagnosis of urinary tract infection.
- **X-rays**:
  1. **Chest X-ray** for vomiting children with respiratory symptoms or abdominal pain/epigastric tenderness.
  2. **Kidney, ureter, and bladder X-ray** if the child is vomiting bile or blood.
  3. **X-ray** of the **skull** is still medically and culturally the norm in Singapore, particularly in younger children in whom the calvarium is very thin.
- **Stat capillary blood sugar** if altered mental status exists:
  1. The drowsy child with low blood sugar and hepatomegaly could have acute sepsis or Reye's syndrome.
  2. The drowsy child with hyperglycaemia and 'air hunger' could have acute diabetic ketoacidosis.
- **Rehydration of the severely dehydrated child (10% dehydration)**: Refer to the *Fluid Replacement in Paediatrics* chapter.
  1. Establish a peripheral IV line.
  2. Administer crystalloid (normal saline or Hartmann's solution) at 20 ml/kg body weight as bolus over 20–30 minutes.
  3. Labs: Full blood count and urea/electrolytes/creatinine.
  4. Obtain paediatric consultation and transfer the child to the paediatric intensive care unit.
- **Disposition**:
  1. **Admit the following**:
     a. Children who are still vomiting or have diarrhoea, show anorexia or dehydration in spite of outpatient care (i.e. outpatient treatment fails) with anti-emetics or antispasmodics.
     b. Children who have signs of epigastric tenderness with even mild dehydration, since this child is less likely to be able to drink and retain oral rehydration solutions (ORS).
     c. Children with a history of head injury with several episodes of vomiting (after skull X-rays: see Chapter 95, *Trauma, Head* chapter for the criteria): Admit to Paediatric Surgery.
  2. **Discharge to outpatient care**:
     a. Children in whom you are certain of the diagnosis with no or very mild dehydration.
     b. Parents to administer clear fluids like porridge water or ORS (Servidrat, Gastrolyte, or Pedialyte) in small, frequent volumes for the next 6 to 8 hours.
     c. Oral promethazine syrup is a safe and mild anti-emetic.
     d. In viral gastroenteritis, symptoms subside after 24–48 hours: Advise parents to return the child for a review if no improvement is noted after 8–12 hours of oral rehydration therapy at home.

Reference/Further Reading

1. Ahrens WR. Diarrhoea and gastroenteritis. In: Strange G, Ahrens W, Schafermeyer R, Wiebe R, eds. *Paediatric Emergency Medicine*. 3rd ed. New York: McGraw-Hill; 2009: 73–78.

130 Paediatric Asthma

Peng Li Lee

CAVEATS

- Not all wheezers are *asthmatic*.
- Consider the following age-specific differentials in a paediatric wheezer:
  1. **Infancy**: Tracheoesophageal fistula, bronchomalacia, broncho-pulmonary dysplasia, recurrent aspiration, heart failure, acute bronchiolitis, pneumonia, inhaled foreign bodies, and infantile asthma.
  2. **Children between 1 and 5 years of age**: Acute bronchiolitis/bronchitis, inhaled solid objects, e.g. peanut (causing a ball-valve obstruction), croup, and asthma.
  3. **School-age children**: Asthma, adenovirus bronchitis, and extrinsic compression from mediastinal mass.
- Role of the **chest X-ray**:
  1. Generally indicated in all first-time wheezers.
  2. Doubt about diagnosis of asthma, e.g. suspected foreign body inhalation.
  3. Clinical signs suggest pneumonia or pneumothorax.
  4. Response to treatment is abnormally slow or there is clinical deterioration.
  5. Persistent hypoxia or need for intensive care.
- Use of **steroids** in acute exacerbations
  1. Early systemic (oral or parenteral) steroids given within an hour of presentation in the emergency department in acute asthma to reduce airway inflammation have been shown to be effective in reducing admission rates.
  2. General guidelines for the use of steroids:
     a. Moderate or severe exacerbations.
     b. History of life-threatening asthma.
     c. Patients already on high dose inhaled steroids or low dose oral steroids.
     d. Patients requiring frequent β_2-agonist therapy in this current exacerbation.
     e. Exacerbations that last for more than 48 hours.

     Dosage: **1–2 mg/kg/day** (maximum dose 60 mg), for a duration of 3 to 5 days.

MANAGEMENT

See Figure 1 for the management of acute asthma.

FIGURE 1 Emergency management of acute asthma

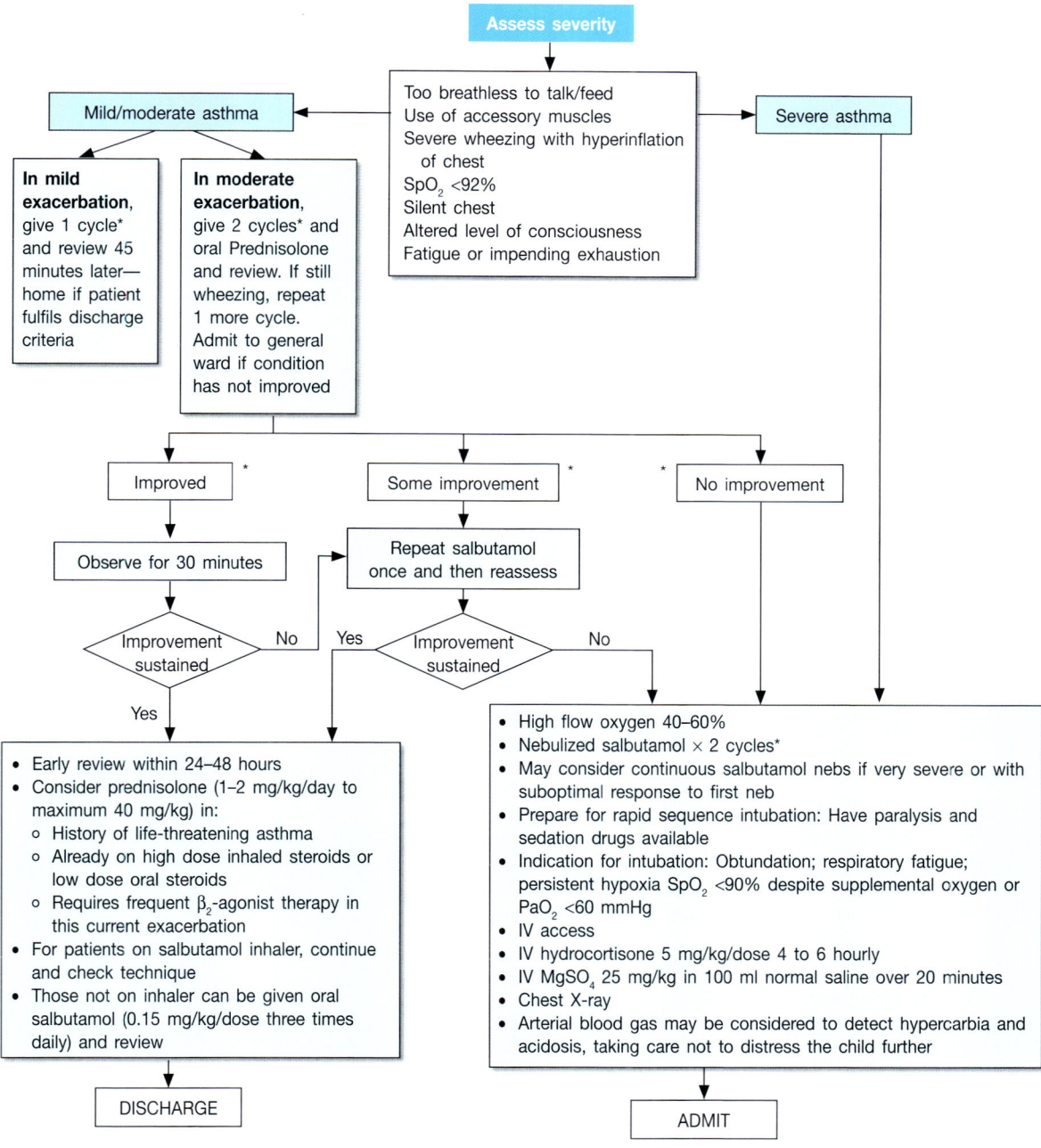

* For salbutamol inhalation: Either inhaler with spacer chamber or nebulization. Dosage of 1 cycle:
For children <1 year old and <10 kg
Salbutamol 5 puffs: Ipratropium bromide 2 puffs OR Salbutamol 0.5 ml: Ipratropium bromide 0.5 ml: 1 ml normal saline
For children >1 year and >10 kg
Salbutamol 10 puffs: Ipratropium bromide 4 puffs OR Salbutamol 1 ml: Ipratropium bromide 1 ml: 2 ml normal saline

---

Chest X-ray indicated if

Diagnosis is uncertain.
Clinical sign suggests pneumonia/pneumothorax.
Atypical features are present or there is poor response to therapy.

Severity of Asthma Exacerbation

Mild

Breathless when walking

Talks in sentences

Conscious

Slight increase in respiratory rate

No use of accessory muscles/retraction

No physical exhaustion

Variable wheeze (end expiratory)

Heart rate <100 beats per minute

SpO_2 more than 95%

Moderate

Breathless when talking, short cry, and difficulty feeding

Talks in phrases

With or without agitation

Moderate increase in respiratory rate

Minimal use of accessory muscles/retraction

No physical exhaustion

Loud wheezing throughout expiratory phase

Heart rate: 100–200 beats per minute

SpO_2 91–95%

Severe

Breathless at rest/infant stops feeding

Talks in single words

Agitated

Marked increase in respiratory rate

Moderate to severe use of accessory muscles/retraction

Physical exhaustion

Loud wheezing throughout respiration

Heart rate >200 beats per minute

SpO_2 <91%

Respiratory arrest imminent

Drowsy/confused

Paradoxical

Thoraco-abdominal movement

Absence of wheezing

Bradycardia

Cyanosed

⇨ **SPECIAL TIPS FOR GPs**

- For all **first onset paediatric wheezers**, be vigilant in looking for the differentials other than asthma, e.g. **exclude foreign body ingestion** in a toddler with atypical presentation of 'asthma' such as first onset of sudden wheezing, no preceding or accompanying upper respiratory tract infection symptoms and no known history of atopy.
- **Not all asthmatics are wheezers**. Consider the diagnosis and treatment of asthma in patients who present with a **persistent cough** that is especially worse at night, but who are otherwise well.
- Patients should be referred to hospital for further management if they do not respond after two ventolin nebs given in the clinic.

Discharge Criteria

- Wheezing: end-expiratory or not present.
- Respiratory retractions: mild or not present.
- The patient is not tachypnoeic on 4 hourly inhaled bronchodilators or 6 hourly oral bronchodilators.
- SpO_2 falls below 95% on room air.
- The patient is well hydrated.

References/Further Reading

1. Murphy S, Kelly HW, eds. *Paediatric Asthma*. New York: M Dekker; 1999.

2. Hall JB, Corbridge T, Rodrigo, et al., eds. *Acute Asthma: Assessment and Management*. New York: McGraw-Hill; 2000.

3. Putucheary J, Tan TH, Tan CL, Phua KB, eds. *The Baby Bear Book: A Practical Guide on Paediatrics*, 2nd ed. Singapore: Red Cells; 2010.

4. Kleigman. Nelson Textbook of Pediatrics, 19th ed. Philadelphia, PA: Saunders Elsevier; 2011.

131 Bronchiolitis

Peng Li Lee • Shirley Ooi

CAVEATS

- The term 'bronchiolitis' refers to a viral syndrome in infants (under two years of age) that is characterized by:
    1. A preceding history of common cold symptoms with e.g. cough or coryza for 2 to 3 days.
    2. Followed by lower respiratory tract symptoms: dyspnoea, wheezing, difficulty feeding, and agitation from airway obstruction.
    3. **Clinical findings** include tachypnoea, nasal flaring, intercostal or subcostal retractions, prolonged expiration with rhonchi and creps, and cyanosis.
- **Causative organisms**:
    1. Respiratory syncytial virus (RSV) is the most common cause (50–90%).
    2. Parainfluenza, influenza, mumps, adenovirus, echovirus, rhinovirus, *Mycoplasma pneumonia*, and *Chlamydia trachomatis*.

NOTE: Mycoplasma is the principal agent in school-age children with bronchiolitis.

- **Differential diagnosis**:
    1. Pneumonia.
    2. Foreign bodies.
    3. Gastroesophageal reflux.
    4. A previously undiagnosed congenital heart disease with heart failure.
    5. Previously undiagnosed anatomic abnormalities of the airway, e.g. tracheoesophageal fistula.
    6. Early asthma.
- Identify the **high risk group** for complications of apnoea and acute deterioration, e.g.
    1. Premature infants with associated chronic lung disease or bronchopulmonary dysplasia.
    2. Congenital heart disease.
    3. Cystic fibrosis.

⇨ **SPECIAL TIPS FOR GPs**
- Bronchiolitis is a short-lived, self-limited disease lasting a few days. If the patient is discharged, a follow-up within 24 hours is recommended.
- Refer all patients with a history of prematurity, congenital heart disease, bronchopulmonary disease, underlying lung disease, and compromised immune function for admission.

MANAGEMENT

Most bronchiolitis cases are self-limiting. Careful monitoring for apnoea and hypoxia and good supportive care remain the cornerstone of management.

- Mandatory **oxygen saturation** (SpO$_2$) readings of less than 92% indicate moderate to severe distress.
- Assess **hydration**: Poor oral intake from breathlessness and cough-induced vomiting result in dehydration.
- Assess the severity of **respiratory distress**:
  1. Mild: No retractions.
  2. Moderate: Intercostal retractions, no cyanosis.
  3. Severe: Cyanosis, apnoea, hypoxia (<92%), dehydration, and severe intercostal retractions.
- **Chest radiography** is indicated in the very ill, atypical patients, and difficult respiratory examination in crying infants.
- Indications for hospital **admissions**:
  1. Infants in high risk group (unless symptoms are very mild and parents are confident of managing the patients at home).
  2. Infants younger than four months of age who are at risk of apnoea and rapid progression to more severe disease.
  3. Poor feeding, dehydration, and agitation.
  4. Previously seen by several general practitioners during this current illness with potential worsening of condition especially within 3 to 4 days of the onset of illness.
- Patients for **discharge**:
  1. If they are not in moderate or severe distress, able to feed and are well hydrated.
  2. Parents are able to understand and recognize the signs of deterioration, i.e. poor feeding and agitation.
- Schedule a follow-up review in the paediatric clinic in a day or two.

Supportive treatment

- Humidified oxygen therapy.
- Hydration (taking care not to overhydrate as well).

Specific treatment

- **Bronchodilators**:
  1. Often used but their efficacy is debatable.
  2. No convincing evidence that they are effective, and in some cases may be associated with detrimental effects (hypoxia from increased ventilation–perfusion (V/Q) mismatch especially if nebulized without oxygen).

3. In older infants in whom it may be difficult to distinguish bronchiolitis from other forms of virus-induced wheeze, a trial of bronchodilators is reasonable because a proportion of these patients do respond.

4. Generally, avoid prescribing for patients who are discharged (Alternatively mucolytics, e.g. bisolvon, may be a better choice.)

- **Steroids**: No consistent role in bronchiolitis management in the acute stage.

- **Antibiotics**:

1. Not indicated routinely unless dual infection is suspected (e.g. RSV and a bacterial infection) but this is uncommon.

2. Avoid the empirical use of outpatient antibiotics. For patients in whom antibiotics are required, hospital admission should be considered.

- **Ribavirin** is not routinely used but may have a role in selected high risk patients.

References/Further Reading

1. Everard ML. Acute bronchiolitis and pneumonia in infancy resulting from RSV. In: Taussig LM, Landau LI, LeSouef P, et al., eds. *Pediatric Respiratory Medicine*. St. Louis, MO: Mosby; 1998: 585–590.

2. Finberg L. Lower respiratory infections. In: Finberg L, Kleinman RE, eds. *Saunders Manual of Pediatric Practice*. 2nd ed. Philadelphia, PA: WB Saunders; 2002: 315.

3. Brown KM. Bronchiolitis. In: Strange GR. Ahrens W, Schaefermeyer RW, Wiebe R. *Paediatric Emergency Medicine*. New York: McGraw-Hill; 2009: 373–378

Elizabeth Khor • Peter Manning

DEFINITIONS

Diagnostic criteria for febrile fits

- First fit experienced by the child is associated with a temperature of more than 38°C and is usually within the first 24 hours of illness, often as the temperature is rapidly increasing.
- The child is between 6 months and 6 years old.
- No evidence of central nervous system infection or inflammation.
- No acute systematic metabolic disorder.

Benign febrile fit

- The fit lasts less than 15 minutes.
- The fit does not have significant focal features.
- The fit does not occur in a series with a total duration of more than 30 minutes.

Complex febrile fit

- The febrile fit is longer in duration than a benign febrile fit and has focal features.
- The fits occur in prolonged series.

CAVEATS

- About 4% of normal children between 6 months and 6 years of age will experience a febrile fit.
- Recurrent fits are more likely if a family history exists of febrile fits or if the first febrile fit occurs at more than 1 year of age.
- Drug history: A Maxolon®-induced oculogyric crisis may mimic a febrile seizure and has a totally different management, i.e. intramuscular (IM) or intravenous (IV) benztropine (Cogentin®).
- Remember to note the allergy history prior to the administration of rectal panadol or Voltaren®.
- Note the child's posture and temperament:
  1. Opisthotonic posturing in a drowsy child suggests increased intracranial pressure.
  2. An irritable child who is difficult to examine may have meningeal irritation: Note that there is a difference between true irritability and the 'crankiness' exhibited by a child who feels unwell.
  3. A child with postictal paralysis is more likely to have abnormal neurological signs.

- Remember that **neck stiffness may be absent** in infants or is difficult to elicit in uncooperative children.
- Cyanosis may indicate airway obstruction or aspiration.
- Remember to palpate the **fontanelle** in infants and record the findings.
- Remember to assess for hepatomegaly, which is common in children with sepsis or Reye's syndrome.

⇨ **SPECIAL TIPS FOR GPs**
- Refer all cases of first febrile fit to the emergency department.
- Give antipyretic and do tepid sponging before referring the patient to the emergency department.

MANAGEMENT

Child actively fitting

- Secure the airway.
- Administer supplemental oxygen by mask.
- Administer IV diazepam 0.1–0.25 mg/kg at a rate no faster than 2 mg/min **or** administer rectal diazepam (Valium®/Stesolid®). This route is more suitable in a general practice setting:
  1. A dose of 5 mg for those older than 1 year.
  2. A dose of 2.5 mg for infants.

NOTE: If the fit exceeds 30 minutes in duration treat as febrile status epilepticus; give IV phenytoin infusion in normal saline at 20 mg/kg/body weight at a rate not to exceed 50 mg per minute under electrocardiogram (ECG) monitoring.

- Monitoring: ECG and pulse oximetry.
- Establish a peripheral IV line.
- Labs: Stat capillary blood sugar, screen urea/electrolytes/creatinine, ionized calcium, and magnesium.
- Measure and record the temperature and pulse rate.

Child not fitting

- Measure the pulse rate and temperature: If the temperature is more than 38.5°C, administer antipyretics or tepid sponge.
- Administer supplemental oxygen by mask if cyanosis is present.
- Consider performing a urinalysis (UC9) to exclude occult urinary tract infection.

DISPOSITION

Admission criteria

- First febrile fits since most parents or caregivers are too 'stressed out' to cope at home.
- Suspicion of intracranial or metabolic disease.
- The child has had more than one fit during the current illness.
- The child has had febrile status epilepticus.
- A history of recent head injury (within 72 hours).

Discharge criteria

- Hospitalisation may not be necessary if **all** the following criteria are met:
  1. Brief (<15 minutes) simple febrile seizure with full recovery and no abnormal neurological signs. This means that when you review the child 1 hour later, the child behaves normally and can talk, walk or run about the room.
  2. The child is above 2 years of age (it is easier to examine older children, and you are more confident of your clinical signs).
  3. The seizure occurred within the first 24 hours of fever.
  4. You are confident that the cause of the fever is viral in origin (i.e. you have excluded meningitis, otitis media, and pneumonia and the child is not septic).
  5. The parents are trustworthy, calm and willing to observe the child closely at home, and outpatient follow-up has been arranged within the next 24–48 hours.
  6. You have given clear instructions on how to administer antipyretics and rectal Stesolid.

NOTE: Do not prescribe non-steroidal anti-inflammatory drugs (NSAIDs) for more than 48 hours.

Occasionally, a parent who reports that the patient or siblings have had similar febrile seizures in the past may choose not to admit the child. It is your responsibility to ensure that the above six criteria are met before you discharge the patient.

References/Further Reading

1. Green M, Haggerty RJ, Weitzman M, eds. *Ambulatory Paediatrics*. 5th ed. Philadelphia, PA: WB Saunders; 1999.
2. Barkin RM, Caputo GL, Jaffe DM, et al., eds. *Paediatric Emergency Medicine: Concepts and Clinical Practice*. 2nd ed. St. Louis, MO: Mosby; 1997.
3. Reisdorff EJ, Roberts MR, Wiegenstein JG. *Paediatric Emergency Medicine*. Philadelphia, PA: WB Saunders; 1993.

IV THERAPY FOR PATIENTS NOT IN SHOCK

- Total amount of fluid required (ml per 24 hours)

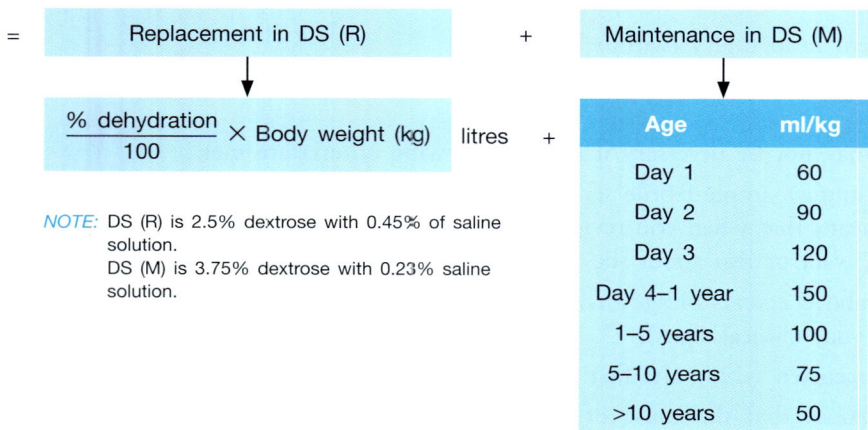

= | Replacement in DS (R) | + | Maintenance in DS (M)

$$\frac{\% \text{ dehydration}}{100} \times \text{Body weight (kg)} \quad \text{litres} \quad +$$

NOTE: DS (R) is 2.5% dextrose with 0.45% of saline solution.
DS (M) is 3.75% dextrose with 0.23% saline solution.

Age	ml/kg
Day 1	60
Day 2	90
Day 3	120
Day 4–1 year	150
1–5 years	100
5–10 years	75
>10 years	50

- Give half the calculated replacement and maintenance volume over the first 8 hours.
  Example: 3% dehydration in a 10 kg, 1-year-old child
  Replacement volume = (3/100 × 10) L   = 300 ml
  Maintenance volume = 10 kg × 100 ml/kg = 1000 ml
  Order at Accident and Emergency = 300 ml DS (R) + 350 ml DS (M) over 8 hours

NOTE: Both DS (R) and DS (M) can either be run concurrently or consecutively.

RESUSCITATION FOR SHOCK

- Crystalloids (Hartmann's or normal saline) = 10–20 ml/kg as quickly as possible over 15 minutes to rapidly expand extracellular volume. Repeat as required.

METHODS FOR CALCULATING MAINTENANCE FLUID RATES

- 4 methods are commonly used to calculate maintenance fluid requirements:
  1. Body surface area (BSA) method: 1500 ml/BSA (m²)/day
     For estimation of body surface area refer to Chapter 136, *Paediatric Drugs and Equipment.*

2. 100/50/20 method:

Weight (kg)	Fluid
0–10	100 ml/kg/day
11–20	100 ml + 50 ml/kg/day for every kg >10 kg
>20	1500 ml + 20 ml/kg/day for every kg >20 kg

3. Insensible and measured losses method:

400–600 ml/BSA (m²)/day + urine output (ml) + Other measured losses (ml)

4. 4/2/1 method:

Weight (kg)	Fluid
0–10	4 ml/kg/h
11–20	40 ml + 2 ml/kg/h for every kg >10 kg
>20	60 ml + 1 ml/kg/h for every kg >20 kg

Reference/Further Reading

1. Kecstes SA. Fluid and electrolyte disorders. In: Strange G, Ahrens W, Schaefermeyer R, Wiebe R, eds. *Pediatric Emergency Medicine*. 3rd ed. New York: McGraw-Hill; 2009: 657–667.

134 Newborn Resuscitation in the Emergency Department

Lee Jiun

CAVEATS

- Newborn resuscitation almost always results in a spontaneously breathing infant, as opposed to resuscitation in other age groups.
- **Ventilation** is the key to successful newborn resuscitation.
- **Goldilocks principle:** The aim of ventilation is to deliver an appropriate tidal volume (as evidenced by an adequate chest rise) that is neither too much nor too little.
- Most newborns require only **warming**. Some may need stimulation and airway suctioning. Routine airway suctioning is not recommended.
- Bag-and-mask ventilation is the most important skill to acquire. Ventilate at a rate of 40–60 inflations per minute. Endotracheal intubation to deliver positive pressure ventilation is seldom required.
- For successful endotracheal intubation, **neck positioning** is critical. It must be in a **neutral** or **slightly extended** position. If the neck is extended too much, the glottis will disappear anteriorly out of view. For orotracheal intubation, the marking of the endotracheal tube at the lips should be 7, 8, or 9 cm for infants who weigh 1, 2, or 3 kg, respectively.
- Chest compressions should be coordinated with ventilation for both to be effective. The ratio of **compressions to inflations** is **3:1**.
- **Adrenaline** (1:10,000) is often the only drug needed in newborn resuscitation. The dose is 0.1–0.3 ml/kg via the intravenous route and 0.5–1 ml/kg via the endotracheal route.
- Newborn infants' blood oxygen levels do not normally reach extrauterine values until about 10 minutes after birth. Pulse oximetry should be used during neonatal resuscitation to guide supplemental oxygen usage. At 5 minutes of age, the recommended pulse oximetry range is 80–85%, and at 10 minutes of age it is 85–95%. Blended oxygen should be used to achieve these targets. If blended oxygen is unavailable, room air should be used. Administration of 100% oxygen is indicated if the heart rate remains at less than 60 beats per minute (bpm) after 90 seconds of resuscitation with a lower concentration of oxygen.
- In the presence of thick meconium-stained liquor, tracheal suctioning is indicated only for a depressed infant. It is not required if the infant is vigorous.
- Food-grade polyethylene sheets are recommended to be used for wrapping very preterm infants to preserve body heat.

⇨ **SPECIAL TIP FOR GPs**
- In the unlikely event that a delivery occurs in the general practitioner's clinic, the most important step in resuscitation is effective ventilation.

MANAGEMENT

Preparation

- Get ready all the equipment (bag-and-mask, intubation, suction and meconium aspirator), overhead warmer, warm towels, polyethylene wrap, drug cards, and medications.

Quick history

- Twins? Two persons may be needed to do resuscitation.
- Meconium-stained liquor? There is a need to do tracheal toilet if the infant is depressed.
- Is the baby premature? If a baby is born preterm, there is a higher likelihood that some degree of resuscitation will be needed.

Actual resuscitation

This should follow the algorithm shown below (Figure 1). The main steps are these:

- Maintain normal body temperature.

FIGURE 1 Neonatal Resuscitation Algorithm

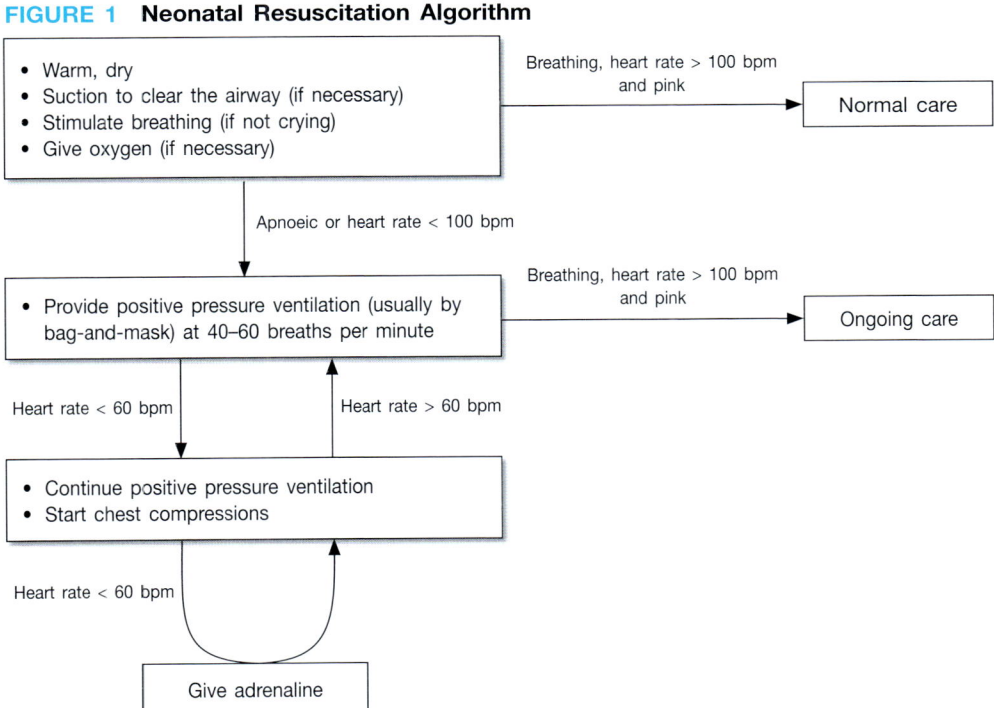

Note:
1. The intervals between the boxes are approximately 30 seconds.
2. Always evaluate the newborn's heart rate, respiration, and colour before deciding on the next step.

- Decide what further intervention is needed in a stepwise manner.
  1. Suction/clear the airway (only if there is obvious obstruction to spontaneous breathing, not routinely).
  2. Stimulate breathing.
  3. Apply positive pressure ventilation.
  4. Perform chest compressions.
  5. Give medications (rarely).

NOTE: Endotracheal intubation may be considered at any point.

Reference/Further Reading

1. Neonatal Resuscitation: 2010 American Heart Association Guidelines for Cardiopulmonary Resuscitation and Emergency Cardiovascular Care. *Paediatrics*. Nov 2010; 126: e1400–1413.

Chong Chew Lan • Darryl Lim • Peter Manning

CAVEATS

- According to the **World Health Organization**, child abuse or maltreatment constitutes all forms of physical and emotional ill-treatment, sexual abuse, neglect or commercial or other exploitation, resulting in actual or potential harm to the child's health, survival, development, or dignity in the context of a relationship of responsibility, trust or power.
- There is a need to consider the culture, attitudes, and values prevalent in the society at a given time to diagnose non-accidental injury (NAI). The following are the various types of NAI:
  1. Physical abuse.
  2. Emotional abuse.
  3. Neglect and negligent treatment.
  4. Sexual abuse.
  5. Exploitation.

DIAGNOSIS

Diagnosis requires a **high index of suspicion** and is based on a combination of medical findings that are unexplained, implausible and inconsistent with the history obtained, patterns of injury that suggest abuse and certain characteristics and behaviour of the child and family.

Social indicators of NAI

- **Abused child**
  1. Was unwanted.
  2. Was separated from the mother soon after birth.
  3. Poor bonding with parents.
  4. Is a disappointment, whether because of sex or a defect.
  5. Is highly irritable and demanding.
  6. Is difficult to manage because of illness.
  7. Is different from the rest of the family.
- **Abusive parents**
  1. Were abused or experienced family disruption in their childhood.
  2. Lack family support and are unreasonably fearful of caring for their child.
  3. Lack parenting skills and/or knowledge of child development, having unrealistic expectations.
  4. Have poor impulse control and are generally rigid and authoritarian.

5. Were teen parents.

6. Abuse alcohol and/or other substances.

7. Have physical or mental illness.

- **The family**

  1. Has employment and financial stress.

  2. Has marital conflict and domestic violence.

  3. Experiences crises due to stressful events, e.g. death in the family, recent move, fighting, etc.

  4. Loneliness or isolation of mothers when their partners left or are working away from home; heavy child care responsibility.

  5. Experiences geographic isolation, lack of transportation, and lack of social support.

Clinical features

- Vague, inconsistent, contradictory, inadequate or implausible story when explaining the cause of the child's injury.
- Delay in seeking medical attention.
- Inappropriate parent or caregiver response.
- The child is not immunized.
- Failure-to-thrive with or without developmental delay.
- Child with poor hygiene, dental and gum disease, and untreated sores.
- Sexual behaviour beyond the child's years and supposed knowledge.
- Multiple injuries of various types and of different ages.
- Bruises or burns with patterns, e.g. 3 or 4 oval bruises suggestive of a slap on the face or a grasp around a limb.
- Bruises to padded areas like the buttocks, breasts, lower abdomen, or medial aspect of both thighs.
- Circular marks around the wrists or ankles suggestive of use of physical restraints.
- Genital injuries associated with a vague history.
- Head injuries with a vague history.
- Subdural haematoma associated with bilateral retinal haemorrhages in an infant, suggestive of **shaken baby syndrome**.
- Metaphyseal corner fractures, sternal fractures, posterior rib fractures, and spiral fractures of the long bones in a non-ambulatory child.
- Scalds of the lower limbs and abdomen with no splash marks or a glove and stocking distribution or doughnut pattern, suggestive of immersion burns.
- Cigarette burn marks.
- Sexually transmitted disease in children.
- Need to exclude diseases which may present like NAI, e.g. osteogenesis imperfecta, haemophilia and idiopathic thrombocytopaenia, and Ehlers–Danlos syndrome.

Munchausen syndrome by proxy (MSP)

- Warning signs:
    1. Illness is unexplained, prolonged, or extremely rare.
    2. Signs and symptoms have a temporal association with the mother's presence.
    3. Treatment prescribed is ineffective and not tolerated.
    4. Other siblings may be similarly affected and there has been NAI or unexplained deaths of other children in the family.

⇨ **SPECIAL TIPS FOR GPs**

- Maintain a very high index of suspicion for these injuries and refer early.
- Knowledge of the developmental milestones of a child is useful in detecting suspicious history, e.g. a one-month-old infant rolling off the bed (and sustaining a skull fracture). This event seems to conflict with the developmental level of the child.

MANAGEMENT

- When child abuse is suspected, the child should be referred to a paediatric specialist centre according to local protocols.
- **Admission** is recommended. This gives an opportunity for a more thorough history taking and physical examination while the child is in a safe environment. Admission facilitates appropriate investigations and thorough assessment of the child and the family.
- Be firm and polite, and be honest with the parents about the concerns raised by the child's injuries and his future well-being.
- If the child's safety is in danger or the parents are uncooperative and insist on discharging the child against medical advice, the medical staff can seek social services or police assistance to authorize the detention of the child in the hospital (gazetted as a place of safety).
- Admit the child to the department responsible for treating his presenting medical problem, e.g. Orthopaedic Surgery for fracture. These children should then be referred to the paediatrician-on-call on the day of admission of the child. The paediatrician and his team of doctors will be responsible for the overall management of the child in the hospital and the subsequent follow-up medical care.
- **Alleged child sexual abuse**:
    1. The female victim will be referred to the gynaecologist-on-call and be seen at the emergency department as soon as possible. A paediatric surgeon will usually examine the male victim, though evaluation should follow local protocols.
    2. Keep the interview and medical examination to a minimum to avoid contamination of evidence and traumatisation of the child.

- The police have the primary responsibility in documenting the photographic evidence of all injuries. They should be informed as soon as possible.
- **Keep good notes**.

References/Further Reading

1. Bechtel K. Identifying the subtle signs of paediatric physical abuse. *Ped Emerg Med Reports*. 2001; 6(6): 57–67.

2. Singapore Ministry of Health. Responding to Child Abuse and Neglect: Guidelines for the Recognition and Management of Child Abuse and Neglect. Oct 2000; 1–31.

Chong Chew Lan • Peter Manning

FORMULAE FOR ESTIMATION OF NORMAL VALUES

- **Weight (kg)** is estimated by:
  1. [2 × Age (year)] + 9   for children <9 years old
  2. 3 × Age (year)   for children >9 years old
- **Surface area (m²)** is the square root of (Height in cm × Body weight in kg/3600)
- **Lowest systolic blood pressure** in:
  1. Neonate ~ 60 mmHg
  2. Infant ~ 70 mmHg
  3. Thereafter = [70 + (2 × Age in years)] mmHg

Age (years)	Heart rate (in beats per minute)	Respiratory rate (per minute)
<1	110–160	30–40
2–5	95–140	20–30
5–12	80–120	15–20
>12	60–100	12–16

NOTE: In children <5 years: If the heart rate is >180 bpm, consider sinus tachycardia.
- In children >5 years: If the heart rate is >160 bpm, consider sinus tachycardia.
- All ages: If the heart rate is >220 bpm, consider supraventricular tachycardia.
- Paediatric estimated **total blood volume** (ml) = **80 × Body weight in kg**

EQUIPMENT

- **Paediatric endotracheal tube size (ETT) size (mm)** is estimated by **4 + Age (year)/4** (from age 2 years).
- **Paediatric ETT length (cm) from mouth** is estimated by **12 + Age (year)/2**. Add 3 cm for distance from the nose (from age 2 years). Alternatively, **(ETT size × 3) cm at the mouth** can be used.
  1. **Cardioversion for atrial arrhythmia**: 1 J/kg
  2. **Cardioversion for ventricular arrhythmia**: 2–4 J/kg

Age	Newborn	1 month	3 months	6 months	1 year
ETT size	3 mm	3 mm	3.5 mm	4 mm	4 mm
ETT length (oral)	9 cm	10 cm	10.5 cm	11 cm	12 cm
Chest tube	8F	8F	10F	10F	10F
Urine catheter	5F	5F	8F	8F	8F

DRUGS

Resuscitation

Drug type	Concentration	Dosage (in mg/kg)	Dosage (in ml/kg)
Adenosine (IV/IO)		0.1 Repeat 0.2 Rapid IV/IO dose	
Amiodarone		5 mg/kg IV/IO (maximum 300 mg/dose)	
Adrenaline (IV/IO)	1:10,000	0.01 (up to 0.3 mg/kg/dose if no response)	0.1 (up to 1 ml/kg/dose if no response)
Adrenaline (via ETT)	1:1000	0.1	0.1
Atropine (minimum of 0.1 mg/dose to avoid paradoxical bradycardia; maximum of 0.6 mg/dose)	0.6 mg/ml	0.02	0.03
Calcium gluconate	10%		0.2 ml/kg IV/IO
Magnesium sulphate		25–50 mg/kg IV/IO 10–20 minutes	
Naloxone		0.1 if <5 years or ≤20 kg IV/IO/ETT 2.0 if ≥5 years or > 20 kg IV/IO/ETT	
Bicarbonate	4.2%	1–2 mmol/kg	1–2 ml/kg
Lignocaine	10 mg/ml (1%)	1	0.1
Dextrose	25%	0.5	2
Volume expansion	Crystalloid/ colloid		10 Repeat 2–3 times if needed

Antifungals

Drug type	Dosage	Remarks
Nystatin Oral	Neonates: 200,000 U 6–8 hours Child: 500,000 U 6–8 hours	
Amphotericin B IV	0.5–1.0 mg/kg/day over 6 hours	Test dose: 0.1 mg/kg. Protect from light
Fluconazole Oral and IV	3–6 mg/kg/day 12–24 hours	Not recommended for infants

Antivirals

Drug type	Dosage
Acyclovir (Zovirax)	
Oral	*Varicella in normal children* 20 mg/kg/dose (maximum 800 mg) 4x/day × 5 days
	Herpes simplex virus (HSV) in normal children >2 years: 200 mg 5x/day × 5 days <2 years: 100 mg 5x/day × 5 days
IV	*Varicella or zoster in the immuno-compromised/pneumonia/encephalitis* <1 year: IV 10 mg/kg/dose 8 hourly >1 year: IV 500 mg/m^2/dose 8 hourly Duration: 7 days or until no new lesions have appeared for 48 hours
	HSV encephalitis IV 10 mg/kg/dose 8 hourly × 14–21 days (neonates 21 days)
	Neonatal HSV infections IV 10–20 mg/kg/dose 8 hourly × 14–21 days

Antibiotics

Drug type	Dosage	Remarks
Ampicillin Oral IV	 50–100 mg/kg/day 6 hourly 100–200 mg/kg/day 6 hourly (severe) 200–400 mg/kg/day 4 hourly (meningitis)	Rubella-like rash common with many viral infections which may not equate to ampicillin allergy
Amoxicillin Oral	50 mg/kg/day 8 hourly	
Amoxicillin + Clavulanic acid (Augmentin®) Oral IV	 50 mg/kg/day 12 hourly (up to 90 mg/kg/day) 50 mg/kg/dose 8 hourly	

Antibiotics (Cont'd)

Drug type	Dosage	Remarks
Amoxicillin + Sulbactam (Unasyn®) Oral IV	50 mg/kg/day 12 hourly 100–200 mg/kg/day 6 hourly	
Penicillin V Oral	50 mg/kg/day 6 hourly (treatment) 250 mg bd (rheumatic fever prophylaxis)	
Crystalline penicillin IV	100,000–400,000 U/kg/day 6 hourly	
Cloxacillin Oral IV	50–100 mg/kg/day 6 hourly 50–200 mg/kg/day 6 hourly	
Cephalexin (Keflex®) Oral	50 mg/kg/day 6–8 hourly	First-generation cephalosporin
Cefuroxime (Zinacef®, Zinnat®) IV Oral	50–100 mg/kg/day 6 hourly 15 mg/kg/dose 12 hourly	Second-generation cephalosporin. Good activity against *Haemophilus influenzae*
Ceftazidine (Fortum®) IV	50–100 mg/kg/day 8 hourly 150 mg/kg/day for meningitis	Third-generation cephalosporin. Good for *Pseudomonas*. Adjust dosing interval in renal failure
Ceftriaxone (Rocephine®) IV	50mg/kg/day 12–24 hourly 100 mg/kg/day 12 hourly for meningitis	Third-generation cephalosporin
Erythromycin Oral	30–50 mg/kg/day 6 hourly (twice daily for erythromycin ethyl succinate, EES)	
Clarithromycin Oral	15 mg/kg/day bd	
Gentamicin IV	(<1/52 old) 2.5 mg/kg/dose 12 hourly (1/52–1/12 old) 2.5 mg/kg/dose 8 hourly (>1/12 old) 2 mg/kg/dose 8 hourly	Can be given at 8, 12- or 24-hourly intervals as long as total dose per day remains the same. Nephrotoxic and ototoxic
Metronidazole Oral	30–50 mg/kg/day 8 hourly	
Trimethoprim Oral	4 mg/kg/dose 12 hourly	Not to be used in G6PD (glucose-6-phosphate dehydrogenase) deficiency or in infants <2 months of age. Every 6 mg bactrim contains 1 mg of trimethoprim

Antibiotics (Cont'd)

Drug type	Dosage	Remarks
Nalidixic acid Oral	50 mg/kg/day 6 hourly	
Nitrofurantoin Oral (>12 years)	5 mg/kg/day 6 hourly	

Analgesics/antipyretics/anti-inflammatory

Drug type	Dosage	Remarks
Paracetamol Oral	10 mg/kg/dose 6 hourly	Not to be used in infants <3 months of age
Ibuprofen Oral	20 mg/kg/day 6 hourly (antipyretic) 20–50 mg/kg/day 4–6 hourly (anti-inflammatory)	Not to be used in children <1 year old
Diclofenac (Voltaren®) Oral/rectal	0.5–3 mg/kg/day bd (maximum 50 mg per dose)	Not recommended in children <1 year old
Pethidine® IV/IM	0.5–1 mg/kg/dose (maximum dose 75 mg)	
Morphine IV Oral	0.1–0.2 mg/kg/dose (maximum 15 mg) 0.01–0.04 mg/kg/hr infusion in normal saline 0.2–0.4 mg/kg/dose 4 hourly	

Sedatives

Drug type	Dosage	Remarks
Chloral hydrate Oral	30–50 mg/kg/day 6–8 hourly or stat	Contraindicated in hepatic or renal failure
Midazolam (Dormicum®) IV/IM	0.1–0.2 mg/kg/dose (up to 0.5 mg/kg/dose)	
Diazepam (Valium®) IV/IM Oral Rectal	0.1–0.25 mg/kg/dose (≤0.6 mg/kg in 8 hours) 0.2–0.5 mg/kg/day bd or tds <10 kg: 2.5 mg 12 hourly >10 kg: 5.0 mg 12 hourly	

Sedatives   (Cont'd)

Drug type	Dosage	Remarks
Cardiac cocktail Promethazine IV	0.5 mg/kg/dose	To be given for sedation 30 minutes before procedure
Pethidine® IV/IM	1 mg/kg/dose	
Chlorpromazine (Largactil®) IV/IM	0.5 mg/kg/dose	
Conscious sedation Ketamine IV IM	1–2 mg/kg/dose 3–6 mg/kg/dose	
Atropine IV/IM	0.02 mg/kg/dose (minimum 0.1 mg, maximum 0.6 mg)	
± midazolam IV/IM	0.1–0.2 mg/kg/dose	

Asthma drugs

Drug type	Dosage	Remarks
Hydrocortisone IV	4–5 mg/kg/dose 4–6 hourly	
Prednisolone Oral	1–2 mg/kg/day, usually OM × 5 days	
Salbutamol Oral Nebulized MDI	0.1 mg/kg/dose tds/qds 0.03 ml/kg/dose 0.15 × 0.2 puff/kg/dose, i.e. 2 × 6 puffs 4 hr/as needed	Continuously q 1/2 hourly q 6 hourly (1 puff = 100 mg)
Beclotide® MDI	2–6 puffs bd	
Ipratropium bromide (Atrovent®) Nebulized	0.3–1 ml 4–6 hourly	
Theophylline (Neulin®) Oral	15–20 mg/kg/day 6 hourly (for sustained-release formulations bd)	

Respiratory drugs

Drug type	Dosage	Remarks
Dexamethasone Oral	For croup: 0.2 mg/kg 12 hourly × 3 doses	
Adrenaline Nebulized	For croup: 0.5 ml/kg/dose (1:1000) (maximum 5 ml)	
Acetylcysteine (Fluimucil) Oral	<1 year: 1/2 satchet bd 1–2 years: 1/2 satchet tds 2–6 years: 1 satchet tds 6–10 years: 2 satchets bd >10 years: 2 satchets tds	
Bisolvon Oral	0.1 mg/kg/dose tds	
Chlorpheniramine Oral	0.1 mg/kg/dose tds to qds	
Promethazine Oral	<6/12: Not recommended 6–12 months: 0.125–0.25 mg/kg/dose bd >12–24 months: 0.125–0.25 mg/kg/dose tds	Antihistamines, antitussives and anti-emetics
Loratidine Oral	0.2 mg/kg daily (maximum 10 mg daily)	

Anti-emetics

Drug type	Dosage	Remarks

Metoclopramide
(Maxolon®)
  IV/IM
  Oral
	0.1 mg/kg/dose bd or tds	Safety not established in children
		Can cause extrapyramidal reactions usually of the dystonic type

Prochlorperazine
(Stemetil®)
  IM
  Oral
	0.2 mg/kg/day qds
	0.4 mg/kg/day tds or qds
		May cause oculogyric crisis
		Do not use in children <2 years=

Ondansetron
(Zofran®)
  IV
  Oral
	0.2 mg/kg/dose 8 hourly	Maximum per dose: 10 mg

Antidiarrhoeal drugs

Drug type	Dosage
Lacteo Fort®/Smecta® Oral	<1 year: 1 satchet/day 8–12 hourly 1–2 years: 1–2 satchets/day 8–12 hourly >2 years: 2–3 satchets 8–12 hourly
Kaopectate Oral	<1 year: 5 ml tds 2–3 years: 10 ml tds >3 years: 15 ml tds

Antispasmodic drugs

Drug type	Dosage	Remarks
Hyosine N-butylbromide (Buscopan®) Oral IM	0.5 mg/kg/dose tds (maximum 40 mg)	Might cause functional ileus in younger children
Propantheline Oral	1.5 mg/kg/dose tds	
Infacol Wind Drops (Simethicone®) Oral	<2 years: 0.2 ml per dose (maximum × 2) >2 years: 0.4 ml per dose	
Trimebutine maleate (Debridat®) Oral	1 ml/kg/day bd–tds or 24 mg/5 kg/day	72 mg/15 ml

Laxatives

Drug type	Dosage
Glycerin Suppository	Neonate: 1/4–1/2 stat Infant: 1 stat
Lactulose Oral	0.5 ml/kg/dose 12–24 hourly 1 ml/kg/dose hourly until bowel cleared, then 6–8 hourly for hepatic coma
Liquid paraffin Oral	1 ml/kg daily (maximum 45 ml/day)

Antacids and anti-ulcerants

Drug type	Dosage	Remarks
Cimetidine IV Oral	20–40 mg/kg/day 4–6 hourly (maximum 200 mg)	
Ranitidine IV Oral	1 mg/kg/day 6–8 hourly 2 mg/kg/dose (maximum 150 mg) 12 hourly	
MMT Oral	1–5 years: 2.5 ml qds 6–12 years: 5ml qds	
Mylanta Oral	0.25 ml/kg/dose 4–6 hourly	
Omeprazole (Losec®) IV Oral	2 mg/kg stat (maximum 80 mg) then 1 mg/kg/dose 12 hourly (maximum 40 mg) 0.4–0.8 mg/kg/day	

Muscle relaxants

Drug type	Dosage	Remarks
Succinylcholine IV	2 mg/kg/dose 1 mg/kg/dose for older children and adolescents	Duration of action: 10 minutes
Atracurium IV	0.5 mg/kg bolus	Useful in patients with renal dysfunction
Pancuronium IV	0.05–0.1 mg/kg/dose 1–2 hourly	
Vecuronium IV	0.1 mg/kg/dose 1–2 hourly	
Rocuronium IV	0.6 mg/kg/dose	

Anti-convulsants

Drug type	Dosage	Remarks
Diazepam	100–300 mg/kg slow IV 100–400 mg/kg/hr IV infusion Under 1 year: 2.5 mg rectal 1–3 years: 5 mg rectal 4–12 years: 10 mg rectal	
Phenobarbitone	15 mg/kg by slow IV – no more than 1 mg/kg/min	Must be diluted
Phenytoin	15 mg/kg loading dose by slow IV at no more than 1 mg kg/min	Monitor electrocardiogram and blood pressure

References/Further Reading

1. Singapore Ministry of Health. *A Guide on Paediatrics*. 1997: 126–157.

2. Shann F. *Drug Doses*. 10th ed. Melbourne: Collective Pty Ltd; 1998: 1–69.

Chong Chew Lan • Darryl Lim • Peter Manning

CAVEATS

- Children with multisystem injuries can deteriorate rapidly and develop serious complications.
- The unique anatomical characteristics of children require special consideration in assessment and management.
- The paediatric skeleton is more pliable and therefore internal organ damage is often noted without overlying fractures. For the same reason, the presence of rib fractures in a child suggests a high impact injury and multiple, serious organ injuries should be suspected.
- Be aware of the possibility of **non-accidental injury** as a cause of the injuries seen.

⇨ **SPECIAL TIPS FOR GPs**

- Remember the airway, breathing and circulation (ABCs). Open and maintain the airway **with cervical control**. Then give high flow oxygen if the child is spontaneously breathing. Otherwise, start bag-valve-mask ventilation.
- Call for an ambulance as soon as possible.
- If possible, obtain venous access with a 22G canula before the arrival of the ambulance.

MANAGEMENT

Airway

- Perform orotracheal intubation under direct vision with adequate immobilization and protection of the cervical spine.
- Preoxygenate before attempting to intubate.
- Use **uncuffed endotracheal tubes (ETT)** for intubation in children. The size of the ETT can be estimated by approximating the diameter of the external nares or the child's little finger. Refer to Chapter 136, *Paediatric Drugs and Equipment* for further details.
- **Atropine** (0.1–0.5 mg) should be given prior to intubation to prevent bradycardia during intubation.
- When airway access and control cannot be accomplished by bag-valve-mask or orotracheal intubation, needle cricothyroidotomy is the preferred method. Surgical cricothyroidotomy is rarely, if ever, indicated.

Breathing

- Respiratory rate (RR) in the child decreases with age:

  Infant: 40–60 breaths per minute
  Older child: 20 breaths per minute

- Overzealous ventilation with high tidal volume and airway pressure can result in iatrogenic bronchoalveolar injury. **Tidal volume** is **7 to 10 ml/kg**.
- Pleural decompression is done with tube thoracostomy, as in the adult, at the fifth intercostal space, anterior to the mid-axillary line. Chest tubes are placed into the thoracic cavity by tunnelling the tube over the rib above the skin incision site.

Circulation

- The increased physiological reserve of the child allows the maintenance of most vital signs in the normal range, even in the presence of severe shock. **The earliest sign of hypovolaemic shock is tachycardia and poor skin perfusion**. A 25% decrease in circulating blood volume is required to manifest the minimal signs of shock:
  1. Tachycardia.
  2. Poor skin perfusion.
  3. Decrease in pulse pressure.
  4. Skin mottling.
  5. Cool extremities compared to torso skin.
  6. Decreased level of consciousness with dulled response to pain.
  7. Decrease in blood pressure.
  8. Poor urine output.
- Hypotension in the child represents a state of uncompensated shock and indicates severe blood loss of more than 45% of the circulating blood volume. Tachycardia changing to bradycardia often accompanies this hypotension and is an ominous sign.

  Systolic blood pressure (SBP) = 70 + (2 × Age in years)
  Diastolic blood pressure = 2/3 × SBP

Fluid resuscitation

- Fluid resuscitation in the child is based on the child's weight. The quickest and easiest method of determining the appropriate fluid volume and drug dosages is with the **Broselow resuscitation measuring tape**.
- For **shock**, a **fluid bolus of 20 ml/kg of warmed crystalloid** solution is given. It may be necessary to give a total of three boluses of 20 ml/kg of fluid to replace the lost 25% blood volume. **When giving the third bolus of fluid, consider giving 10 ml/kg of type specific blood. Refer stat to a surgeon if there is no improvement after the first bolus of fluid.**
- The **sites** for **venous access** in children, in order of preference, are:
  1. Percutaneous peripheral (two attempts).
  2. Intraosseous (children ≤6 years of age).
  3. Venous cutdown: The saphenous vein at the ankle.
  4. Percutaneous placement: Femoral vein.

Intraosseous infusion should be discontinued when suitable peripheral access has been established. The preferred site for intraosseous cannulation is the anteromedial surface of the proximal tibia, 2 cm below the tibial tuberosity. This site is unsuitable if it is distal to a fracture site; cannulation can then be performed at the distal femur. Urinary output in adequately resuscitated patients should be 1–2 ml/kg/hr.

MANAGEMENT OF SPECIFIC INJURIES

Chest trauma

- Chest injury is a marker for other organ injury since more than two-thirds of children with chest injury also have other organ system injury.
- Rib fractures represent an additional marker for a severe injuring force.
- The specific injuries and their management are identical to those for adults.

Abdominal trauma

- Penetrating abdominal injuries dictate the prompt attention of the surgeon.
- Abdominal assessment in children with blunt trauma may be difficult as they are unlikely to cooperate, especially when frightened by the preceding trauma.
- Gastric and urinary decompression may facilitate evaluation.
- Diagnostic aids include:
  1. **Computed tomography (CT)**
     a. Useful in the haemodynamically normal or stabilizing child.
     b. Should be done with double or triple contrast.
     c. Usually requires sedation.
     d. Should not delay further treatment.
     e. Allows for precise identification of injuries.
  2. **Diagnostic peritoneal lavage (DPL)**
     a. Used to detect intra-abdominal bleeding in the haemodynamically abnormal child.
     b. Warmed saline solution in volumes of 10 ml/kg (up to 1000 ml) is run in over 10 minutes.
     c. Retroperitoneal organ injuries cannot be reliably detected.
     d. Definition of positive lavage is the same for children and adults.
     e. The presence of blood in the peritoneum does not by itself mandate laparotomy.
     f. Should be performed by a surgeon.

3. **Focused Assessment with Sonography in Trauma (FAST)**
    a. Few studies on the efficacy of ultrasound in the child have been reported.
    b. Selective, non-operative management of children with blunt abdominal injuries is performed in many trauma centres. It has been well demonstrated that bleeding from an injured spleen, liver, and kidney is generally self-limiting.
    c. These children should be monitored closely in an intensive care unit with frequent, repeated examination by the surgeon.

Head trauma

- Management is the same as in adults. The Glasgow Coma Scale is useful. However, the verbal score component must be modified for children. Paediatric verbal score:

Verbal response	V score
1. Appropriate words or social smile, fixes and follows objects with eyes	5
2. Cries, but consolable	4
3. Persistently irritable	3
4. Restless, agitated	2
5. None	1

- As in the adult, hypotension is rarely, if ever, caused by head injury alone, and other causes of hypotension should be excluded. Infants may, albeit infrequently, become hypotensive from blood loss into either the subgaleal or epidural space. This occurs because of open cranial sutures and fontanelle in infants.
- Adequate and rapid restoration of an appropriate circulating blood volume is imperative and hypoxia must be avoided.
- In a young child with open fontanelle and mobile cranial suture lines, signs of an expanding mass may be hidden until rapid decompensation occurs. Therefore, an infant who is not in coma, but who has a bulging fontanelle or suture diastasis, should be treated as having severe head injury.
- Vomiting, seizures and even amnesia are more common in children after head injury. Investigate the child with persistent or worsening vomiting or recurrent seizures with CT scans.
- **Drugs** frequently used in children with head injury include:
    1. **Phenobarbital** 2–3 mg/kg.
    2. **Diazepam** 0.25 mg/kg, slow IV bolus.
    3. **Phenytoin** 15–20 mg/kg, administered at 1 mg/kg/min as a loading dose, then 4–7 mg/kg/day for maintenance.
    4. **Mannitol** 0.5–1.0 g/kg (rarely required). This may worsen hypovolaemia and should be withheld early in the resuscitation of the child with head injury.

Spinal cord injury

- Spinal cord injury in children is fortunately uncommon.
- Children suffer **s**pinal **c**ord **i**njury **w**ith**o**ut **r**adiographic **a**bnormalities (**SCIWORA**) more commonly than adults. Normal spine radiographs can be found in up to two-thirds of children with spinal cord injury. Therefore, **normal spine X-rays do not exclude significant spinal injury**.
- Spinal cord injury is treated the same way as injuries occurring in adults.

References/Further Reading

1. *Advanced Trauma Life Support Student Course*. 9th ed. Chicago, IL: American College of Surgeon; 2012: 246–271.

2. Singapore Ministry of Health. *A Guide on Paediatrics*. 1997: 181.

138 Commonly Used Scoring Systems

Chong Chew Lan • Shirley Ooi • Victor Ong

USES OF INJURY SEVERITY SCORING SYSTEMS

- Allow us to quantify the severity of an injury, enabling comparison of injuries between patients.
- This, in turn, allows us to predict and compare outcomes. Hence, they are useful in clinical audit and research.
- Trauma scoring is useful in triage, especially in the field. It augments the clinical judgement of the prehospital personnel, facilitating the transfer of patients to the appropriate facility and the allocation of resources.

PHYSIOLOGIC SCORES

Glasgow Coma Scale (GCS)

- The GCS is widely used to assess a patient's level of consciousness. It is computed as the sum of coded values for three behavioural responses, eye opening, best verbal response, and best motor response (Table 1).

TABLE 1 Glasgow Coma Scale

	Score
Eye opening (E)	
• Spontaneous	4
• To calling	3
• To pain	2
• None	1
Verbal response (V)	
• Oriented	5
• Confused	4
• Inappropriate words	3
• Incomprehensible sounds	2
• None	1
Motor responses (M)	
• Obeys commands	6
• Localises pain	5
• Withdraws (pain)	4
• Flexion (pain)	3
• Extension (pain)	2
• None (pain)	1
Total GCS points (1 + 2 + 3)	*Lowest 3, highest 15*

TABLE 2   Paediatric verbal score

Verbal response	Score
Appropriate words or social smile, fixes and follows objects with the eyes	5
Cries, but consolable	4
Persistently irritable	3
Restless, agitated	2
None	1

- The GCS itself can be used to categorise patients:
  1. **Coma**: A patient in coma is defined as having no eye opening (E = 1), no ability to follow commands (M = 1 to 5) and no word verbalizations (V = 1 to 2). This means that all patients with a GCS score <8 and most with a GCS = 8 are in coma. Patients with a GCS score >8 are not in coma.
  2. **Head injury (HI) severity**: On the basis of the GCS, patients are classified as having:
     a. Severe HI: GCS is ≤8 points.
     b. Moderate HI: GCS score 9–13 points.
     c. Mild HI: GCS score 14–15 points.
- The GCS can be applied to the paediatric age group. However, the verbal component must be modified for children under 4 years of age (Table 2).
- GCS has been correlated with mortality and with the Glasgow Outcome Scale, which measures the level of ultimate brain function. It is widely used for prehospital triage and for determining the level of consciousness after hospital admissions.

Revised Trauma Score (RTS)

The RTS (Table 3) is based on the GCS score, systolic blood pressure (SBP), and respiratory rate (RR). It is widely used in triage. Variables are assigned coded values from 4 (normal) to 0. The coded values of GCS, SBP, and RR are weighted and summed to yield the RTS, which takes values from 0 to 7.84. Higher values are associated with better prognoses.

TABLE 3   Revised Trauma Score

GCS	SBP	RR	Coded value
13–15	>89	10–29	4
9–12	76–89	>29	3
6–8	50–75	6–9	2
4–5	1–49	1–5	1
3	0	0	0

Note: RTS = 0.9368 GCS_c + 0.7326 SBP_c + 0.2908 RR_c where the subscript c refers to a coded value.

ANATOMIC SCORES

Abbreviated Injury Scale (AIS)

The AIS attributes a score between 1 and 6 to each individual injury (see Table 4). It has been revised several times since it was first introduced in 1971.

TABLE 4   Abbreviated Injury Scale

Scale	Attributes of injury
AIS 1	Minor injury
AIS 2	Moderate injury
AIS 3	Serious injury
AIS 4	Severe injury
AIS 5	Critical injury
AIS 6	Fatal injury

Injury Severity Score (ISS)

- ISS considers the body to comprise six regions:
  1. Head/neck
  2. Face
  3. Thorax
  4. Abdomen or pelvic contents
  5. Extremities or pelvic girdle
  6. External structures (skin)
- It is computed as the sum of the squares of the three highest AIS for injuries from the different body regions. Possible ISS scores range from 1 to 75. Any patient with AIS 6 scores 75 for ISS. The ISS correlates with mortality but has limitations in that it incorporates only the greatest AIS value from each body region, takes into account 3 injuries at most and considers injuries with the same AIS values to be of equal severity regardless of the body region. As a result, some ISS values or interval cohorts contain data on patients with heterogenous injuries, who have substantially different prognoses and are poor bases for prediction of outcome. Nonetheless, it remains the most frequently used summary measure of severity of anatomic injury.

OTHER SCORING SYSTEMS

The **Trauma and Injury Severity Score (TRISS) methodology** is used to quantify the probability of survival (Ps) as a function of injury severity and hence is widely used to compare 'performances' (e.g. one hospital against another). The Ps is calculated by combining ISS with RTS and adding a weighting factor according to the age of the patient. Patients who survive with Ps <0.5 are 'unexpected survivors' while patients who die with Ps >0.5 are 'unexpected deaths'.

References/Further Reading

1. Wyatt JP, Illingworth RN, Graham CA, et al., eds. *Oxford Handbook of Accident and Emergency Medicine.* Oxford, UK: Oxford University Press 3rd ed.; 2006: 321.

2. Head trauma. In: *Advanced Trauma Life Support: Student Course Manual.* 9th ed. Chicago, IL: American College of Surgeons; 2012: 148–173.

URETHRAL CATHETERISATION

- **Indications**
  1. Monitoring of the urine output.
  2. Relief of urinary retention.
  3. Collection of uncontaminated urine sample for analysis.

- **Contraindications**
  1. Urethral injury, e.g. trauma patients with blood at the urethral meatus.
  2. Tight urethral stricture that prohibits the insertion of a Foley's catheter.

- **Equipment**
  1. Prepacked catheter pack.
  2. Sterile lignocaine gel with nozzle.
  3. Foley's catheter, usually 12F–16F.
  4. Drainage bag.

- **Procedure**
  1. Place the patient in a supine position. Female patients should have their knees flexed and thighs apart.
  2. Check the balloon of the urinary catheter first by inflating it with 8 ml of water to ensure there is no leak and then completely deflating it.
  3. Locate the urethral meatus and cleanse with chlorhexidine or sterile saline solution. See Figures 1 and 2.

     Males: The foreskin should be retracted.

     Females: The labia should be held apart with one hand.

FIGURE 1 Insertion of a catheter into a female

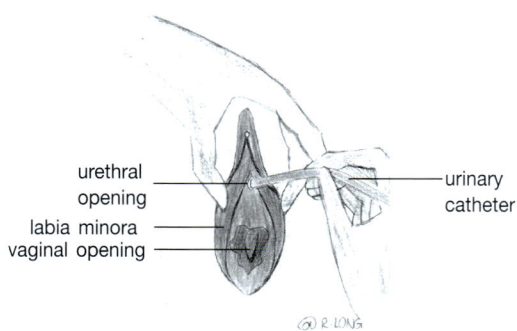

FIGURE 2 Insertion of a catheter into a male

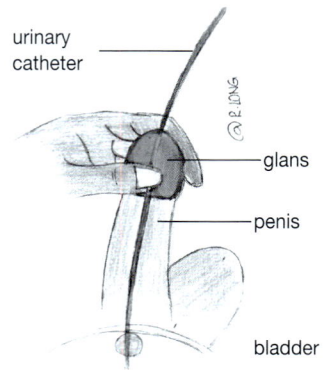

4. Connect the nozzle to the lignocaine gel and apply to both the tip of the Foley's catheter and the urethra.

5. Gently insert the lubricated catheter into the urethra. For males, the penis should be held perpendicular to the body. Insert all the way until the side arm. Confirmation of placement is indicated by drainage of urine.

6. Inflate the balloon with 8 ml of sterile water and withdraw the catheter until it reaches the bladder neck.

7. Connect to the drainage bag and secure the catheter with tape.

- **Complications**
  1. Urethral trauma.
  2. Infection.
- **Special tips/precautions**
  1. Always reposition the foreskin after urethral catheterization; otherwise it may result in paraphimosis.
  2. Use a larger-sized catheter or Coude catheter if prostatic obstruction is suspected.
  3. Use a smaller-sized catheter in cases of urethral strictures.
  4. Do not force the catheter if there is resistance for fear of creating a false passage or causing urethral trauma. Consider Urology consult.
  5. Do not use saline to inflate the balloon for fear of crystallization.

Chest Tube Insertion

- **Indications**
  1. Drainage of large pneumothorax.
  2. Drainage of fluid, e.g. haemothorax and pleural effusion.
  3. Prophylaxis in trauma patients with pulmonary contusions needing positive pressure ventilation.
- **Relative contraindications**
  1. Uncontrolled bleeding diasthesis.
  2. Infection at the insertion site.
- **Equipment**
  1. Prepacked surgical set (including forceps, artery clamp, blade holder, and scissors).
  2. Scalpel blade.
  3. 1% lignocaine for local anaesthesia.
  4. An appropriate size chest drain ranging from 24F to 32F (use a larger drain for drainage of fluid and a smaller one for air drainage).

5. Underwater-seal bottle and connection tubing.

6. 2/0 Prolene and 2/0 Silk.

7. Dressings.

- **Procedure**

  1. Place the patient supine or in a 45-degree sitting position and have the ipsilateral arm over the head.

  2. Determine the insertion site which should be within the triangle of safety bordered by the mid-axillary line, the 5th intercostal line and lateral border of pectoralis major (to avoid injury to the long thoracic nerve).

  3. Clean and drape the chest at the predetermined site of the tube insertion.

  4. Apply 1% lignocaine over the site of insertion above the rib border (to avoid the neurovascular bundle). Then infiltrate the skin, muscle tissues, rib periosteum, and pleura.

FIGURE 3   Incision made at 5th intercostal space

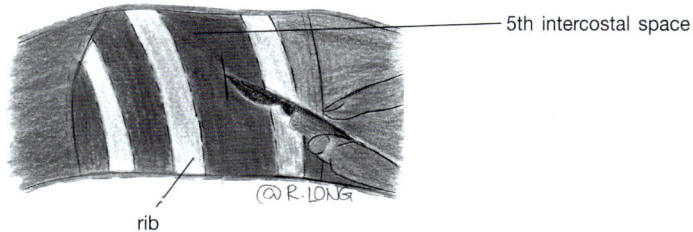

  5. Make a 2–3 cm horizontal incision at the predetermined site (Figure 3) and bluntly dissect through the skin and subcutaneous tissues down to the pleura (Figure 4).

  6. Insert the artery clamp through the incision and open the jaws widely to create a track. Entry into the pleural space is indicated by a gush of air.

  7. Clamp the proximal end of the chest tube.

FIGURE 4   Blunt dissection through skin and
subcutaneous tissues down to pleura

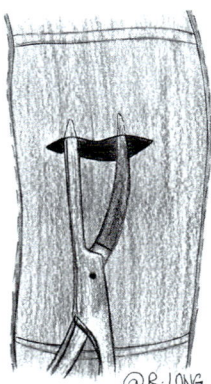

8. Insert a gloved finger into the incision and slowly guide the tube into the chest cavity. The sharp end of the trocar should be withdrawn from the end of the tube at the point of insertion. The trocar should be slowly withdrawn as the thoracostomy tube is being inserted (Figure 5).

9. Once the desired length of the chest tube is inserted, unclamp the tube, and connect it to the underwater seal. Watch for bubbling and oscillations.

10. Suture the tube in place with 2/0 Silk followed by purse-string using 2/0 Prolene.

11. Apply dressing and tape the tube to the chest.

12. Obtain a chest X-ray.

- **Complications**
  1. Bleeding.
  2. Infection (usually delayed).
  3. Inadvertent puncture of other organs such as the liver, spleen, and heart.
  4. Passage of the tube along the chest wall instead of into the chest cavity.

- **Special tips/precautions**
  1. The patient must be placed on supplemental oxygen and on close monitoring.
  2. A precautionary intravenous plug should be placed before insertion of the chest tube.
  3. Always insert a finger into the incision before inserting the chest tube and remove the trocar early to avoid injury to other organs.

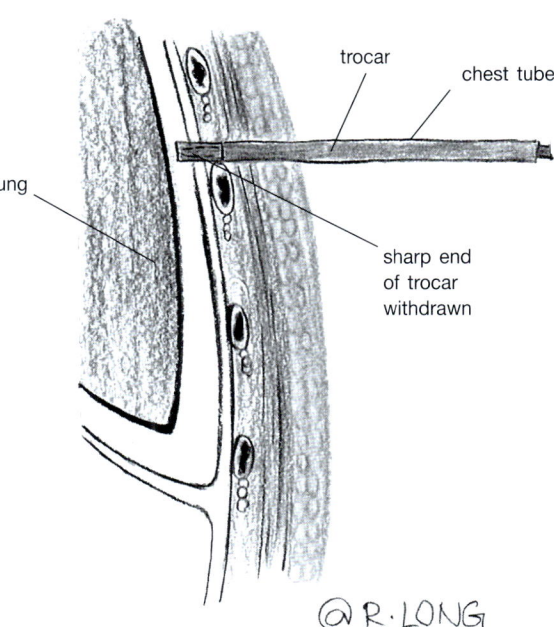

FIGURE 5   **Insertion of chest tube through incised and dissected wound**

trocar

chest tube

lung

sharp end of trocar withdrawn

@ R·LONG

Needle Aspiration/Thoracocentesis

- **Indication**
  1. Relief of tension pneumothorax.

- **Contraindication**
  1. None as indication is a life-threatening condition.

- **Equipment**
  1. Simple dressing set.
  2. 1% lignocaine for local anaesthesia.
  3. A 14G or 16G cannula with or without a 10-ml syringe containing saline connected to it.
  4. Dressings.

- **Procedure**
  1. Determine the site of insertion which is the second intercostal space in the mid-clavicular line on the side of the tension pneumothorax.

FIGURE 6　**Thoracocentesis of tension pneumothorax**

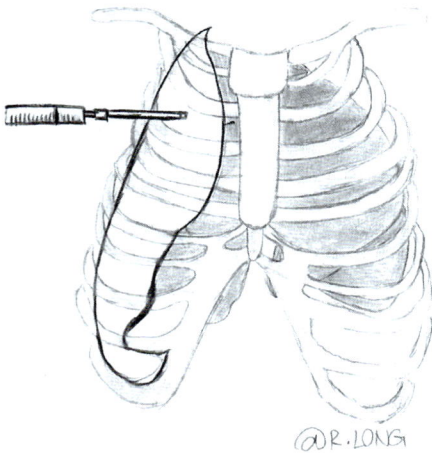

  2. Clean and drape the chest at the site of insertion.
  3. Apply local anaesthesia to the skin if the patient is conscious or time allows.
  4. Insert the cannula with the attached 10-ml syringe containing 1–2 ml normal saline above the rib border into the intercostal space.
  5. Puncture the parietal pleura and aspirate. There should be bubbling of air in the normal saline indicating that the tension pneumothorax has been relieved.
  6. Remove the needle and leave the plastic catheter in place.
  7. Apply dressing to the insertion site.
- **Complications**
  1. Local haematoma.
  2. Lung injury.
  3. Pneumothorax.
- **Special tips/precautions**
  1. The patient should be placed on closed monitoring with supplemental oxygen.
  2. A precautionary intravenous cannula should be placed.
  3. A chest tube should be inserted immediately after relief of a tension pneumothorax. The plastic catheter can then be removed.

Incision and Drainage of Abscesses

- Definition: A cutaneous abscess is a localized collection of pus that results in a painful, fluctuant soft tissue mass.

- **Indication**
  1. An abscess that is palpable on the skin.
- **Contraindications**
  1. Very large abscesses will require extensive incision and debridement and local anaesthesia may not be adequate.
  2. Special areas:
     a. Deep space abscesses of the groin and head and neck region due to their proximity to major neurovascular structures.
     b. Supralevator or ischiorector abscesses due to the need for general anaesthesia to obtain proper exposure as well as associated fistulas that may need treatment.
     c. Palmar or deep plantar spaces will require more extensive exploration and referral to specialities for drainage.
- **Equipment**
  1. Dressing set.
  2. 1% lignocaine for local anaesthesia with or without adrenaline. Will probably need some procedural sedation with eg. IV ketamine (see Chapter 140, *Pain Management* and Chapter 141, *Procedural Sedation*).
  3. A No. 11 scalpel blade with handle.
  4. Haemostat, scissors, and packing.
- **Procedure**
  1. Cleanse the site over the abscess with skin preparation and drape to create a sterile field.
  2. Consider procedural sedations.
  3. Infiltrate local anesthetic; allow 2 to 3 minutes for the anesthetic to take effect.
  4. Make a wide incision over the abscess with the blade and into the abscess cavity (Figure 7).

FIGURE 7 Incision and drainage of abscess
Incise over abscess with blade

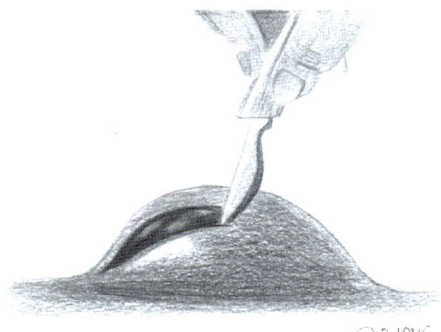

5. Allow the pus to drain. Use the haemostat to break up any loculations within the cavity and allow further drainage if need be.

6. Pack the cavity with a ribbon gauze soaked with chlorhexidine (Figure 8).

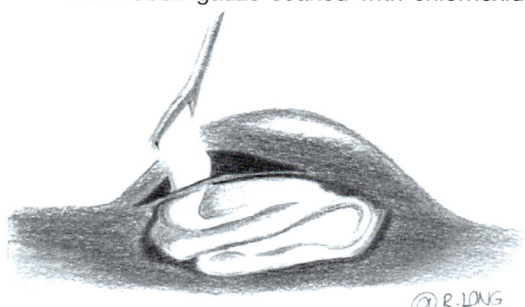

7. Apply dressing.
- **Complications**
  1. Inadequate local anaesthetic.
  2. Incomplete drainage of abscess.
- **Special tips/precautions**
  1. Infiltrate sufficient lignocaine and wait until enough time has passed before performing the procedure.
  2. Make as wide an incision as possible to ensure complete drainage.

Intra-arterial Line Insertion (**Figure 9**)

- **Indications**
  1. Need for close blood pressure monitoring, e.g. patients on inotropes.
  2. Need for frequent blood taking.
- **Contraindications**
  1. Severe bleeding diasthesis or coagulopathy.
  2. Poor collateral circulation at the proposed insertion site.
- **Sites of insertion**
  1. Radial artery (most common and preferred).
  2. Other sites include the dorsalis pedis, brachial, and femoral arteries.

NOTE: Long catheters are required for intra-arterial line insertion at the femoral artery. Try to avoid insertion in the brachial artery as it is the main artery supplying the upper limb circulation.

- **Equipment**
  1. Simple dressing set.
  2. Arterial line monitoring equipment.
  3. Arterial catheter.

- **Procedure**
  1. Perform Allen's test to confirm adequate collateral flow from the ulnar artery.
  2. Flush the arterial line tubing with normal saline to reduce the risk of air embolism during placement.
  3. Ask the patient to hold his hand in front with the palm up and wrist in dorsiflexion. Support the patient's hand with a rolled towel or normal saline pack under the wrist.
  4. Clean and drape the area at the site of insertion.
  5. Apply 1% lignocaine at the puncture area for local anaesthesia.
  6 Use one hand to palpate the artery and the other to hold the artery cannula. Puncture the skin with a needle bevel at 30 degrees.

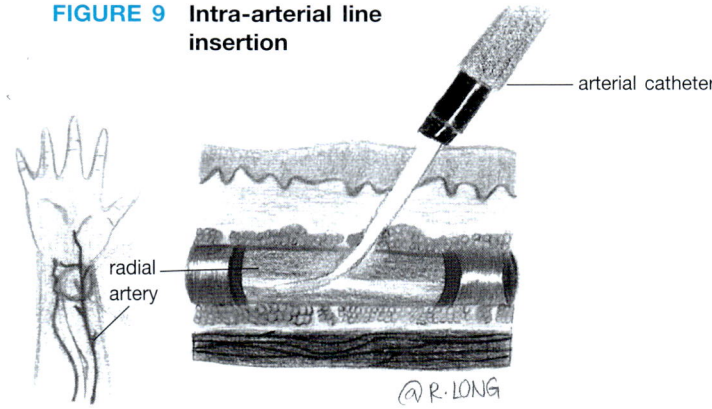

FIGURE 9   Intra-arterial line insertion

arterial catheter

radial artery

@ R·LONG

  7. Advance the needle until a flash is obtained and slowly push forward the catheter while removing the stylet.
  8. Connect to the arterial line tubing and watch the waveform to ensure that the reading is accurate.
  9. Apply dressing to secure the intra-arterial line.
- **Complications**
  1. Radial nerve injury.
  2. Local haematoma.
  3. Infection (usually delayed).
  4. Arterial vasospasm.
- **Special tips/precautions**
  1. Avoid prolonged dorsiflexion of the wrist to avoid radial nerve injury.
  2. Apply adequate compression to the puncture site to avoid haematoma formation in failed attempts.
  3. Consider using ultrasound guidance when pulses are not well-felt or in vasospasm.

Central Venous Line Insertion

- **Indications**
  1. Monitoring of central venous pressure.
  2. For venous access when peripheral sites are inaccessible or unavailable.
  3. For administration of:
     a. Rapid infusion of fluids/blood products in emergency situations.
     b. Sclerosing agents, e.g. TPN (total parenteral nutrition).
     c. Inotropes, e.g. noradrenaline and adrenaline.
  4. Insertion of a transvenous pacemaker.
- **Contraindications**
  1. Bleeding diasthesis or coagulopathy.
  2. Infection over the site of insertion.
  3. Distorted anatomy from any cause (relative).
- **Equipment**
  1. Central venous catheter set.
  2. Prepacked surgical set (including forceps, artery clamp, blade holder, and scissors).
  3. Scalpel blade.
  4. 1% lignocaine for local anaesthesia.
  5. Heparinized saline.
  6. Dressings and tape.
  7. Central venous line tubing.
  8. Sutures made from prolene or silk.
  9. Ultrasound machine, gel and sterile plastic sheath for probe.
- **Procedure**
  1. Positioning.
     a. Place the patient in the Trendelenburg position (30 degress head down) to reduce risk of air embolism.
     b. Position the patient's head to the side contralateral to the site of insertion.
     c. Place a rolled towel between the shoulder blades to make the clavicles more prominent.
  2. Flush the central venous line tubing with normal saline and attach it to intravenous fluids.
  3. Flush the 3 ports of central venous catheter with heparinized saline.
  4. Clean and drape the area over the sternocleidomastoid and upper chest wall.
  5. **Landmarks:**
     a. **Subclavian vein**
        i. Located just deep to the middle third of the clavicle and runs parallel to it.
        ii. Point of entry:
            - 1 cm caudal to the junction of the middle and medial third of the clavicle. Direct the needle medially, slightly cephalad, and posteriorly behind the clavicle towards the suprasternal notch.

FIGURE 10   Central venous line insertion into subclavian vein

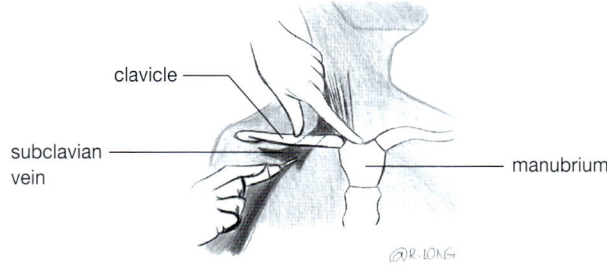

clavicle

subclavian vein

manubrium

@R.LONG

b. **Internal jugular vein**
   i. Located lateral to the carotid artery within the triangle bordered by the clavicle and two heads (clavicular and sternal) of the sternocleidomastoid muscles (Figure 11a) but landmark is best located with ultrasound.
   ii. Point of entry:
       ▪ Apex of triangle and direct the needle 30–45 degrees to the skin caudally towards the ipsilateral nipple (Figure 11b).

FIGURE 11a   Relation of internal jugular vein to carotoid artery

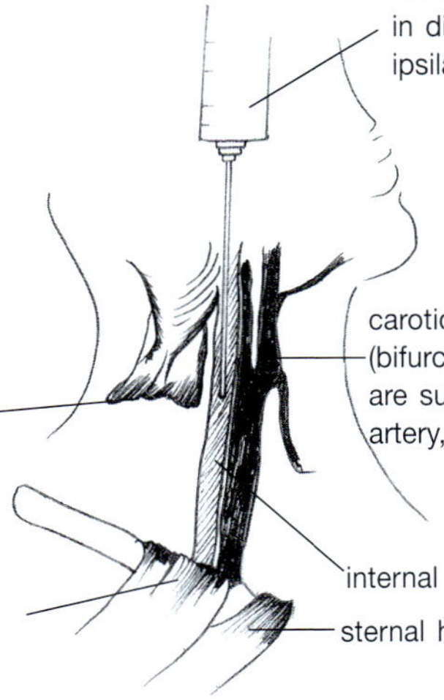

FIGURE 11b   Needle is injected into the apex of triangle formed by clavicular and sternal heads of sternocleidomastoid

needle pointing in direction of ipsilateral nipple

carotid artery (bifurcations shown are superior thyroid artery, facial artery)

cut end of sternocleidomastoid (SCM)

clavicular head of SCM

internal jugular view

sternal head of SCM

sternocleidomastoid (SCM)

internal jugular vein

apex of triangle

clavicle

clavicular head

sternal head of SCM

internal jugular vein

manubrium

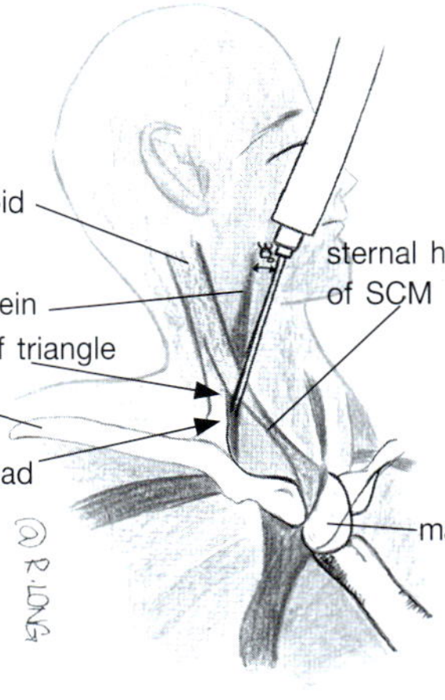

6. Apply 1% lignocaine for local anaesthesia at the selected site of insertion.
7. Attach a syringe filled with 1 ml of saline to the introducer needle. Locate the vein as described by the landmarks and apply gentle aspiration while advancing the needle.
8. Once the introducer needle enters the vein, ensure that blood can be withdrawn easily into the syringe.
9. Stabilize the needle and remove the syringe. Occlude the hub with a finger.
10. Insert the guidewire through the introducer needle until about 15 cm and remove the introducer needle while keeping the guidewire still.

11   Use the scalpel blade to enlarge the puncture site of the vein.

12. Pass the dilator through the guidewire to dilate the entry point of the vein.

13. Pass the distal tip of the venous catheter over the guidewire. Ensure the length of the guidewire at the proximal end is sufficient so that it protrudes out of the catheter.

Hold the proximal end of the guidewire and slowly remove it while advancing the catheter until the desired length (usual length is 13–15 cm at the skin level).

1. Check for free flow of blood in all three lumens and flush each port with heparinized saline to prevent clotting of blood.

2. Connect the catheter to the intravenous tubing.

3. Discontinue the Trendelenburg position.

4. Suture the catheter to the skin and apply dressing.

5. Check the chest X-ray.

- **Complications**
  1. Pneumothorax.
  2. Arterial puncture.
  3. Catheter embolization.

NOTE: Do not withdraw a catheter past a needle bevel which can shear off the catheter.

1. Infection.
2. Cardiac dysrhythmia.
3. Air embolism.

- **Special tips/precautions**
  1. The patient should always be placed on cardiac monitoring to watch for cardiac arrhythmias during insertion of the guidewire.
  2. Consider ultrasound guidance if there is difficulty locating the vein, e.g. distorted anatomy.
  3. Apply adequate compression in the event of arterial puncture to avoid haematoma formation.
  4. Never push the guidewire through if resistance is met. Remove the guidewire and introducer together and re-attempt. Do not withdraw the guidewire through the introducer needle as this may cause severance of the wire.

Acknowledgements

Figure 11a was drawn by Dr Swati Jain. All other illustrations in this chapter were drawn by Ms Rebecca Long.

Shirley Ooi • Peng Li Lee • Chong Chew Lan

ANALGESIA/SEDATION FOR SHORT PROCEDURES

Joint dislocation, incision and drainage of abscesses, and removal of foreign body

First choice	Second choice
IV **propofol** 40 mg every 10 sec until onset of sedation. Dose required is 2 to 2.5 mg/kg or IV **fentanyl** 2–3 µg/kg to a total of 150 µg, given as small serial doses alternating with small serial doses of intravenous (IV) **midazolam** 0.1–0.2 mg/kg (not to exceed 10 mg)	For I&D of abscesses consider IV **ketamine** at dose of 0.5–1.0 mg/kg body weight

Notes:
1. The options given are used as adjuncts to local anaesthetics whenever appropriate.
2. Consider adjunct with **Entonox** self-administered through a valve system if fear of respiratory suppression (e.g. in the elderly and those with respiratory problems) exists.
3. For patients >55 years old, give lower IV **propofol** dose 20 mg every 10 sec until onset (1–1.5 mg/kg).

Emergency cardioversion

First choice	Second choice
IV **midazolam** 0.1–0.2 mg/kg and IV **fentanyl** 25 mcg	IV **etomidate** 0.1 mg/kg followed by IV **ketamine** 1–2 mg/kg

Paediatric patient with forearm fracture, joint dislocation, and laceration in anatomically challenging sites, e.g. face

First choice	Second choice
IM **ketamine** 2.4 mg/kg and atropine 0.02 mg/kg, or IV **ketamine** 1 mg/kg and atropine 0.02 mg/kg, or IV **fentanyl** 0.5–3 µg/kg and midazolam 0.05–0.1 mg/kg	Oral **midazolam** 0.4 mg/kg

Notes:
1. Refer to Chapter 141, *Procedural Sedation*.
2. Local anaesthetics are preferably buffered (1% lignocaine 9 ml to 1 ml 8.4% sodium bicarbonate) to minimize pain on infiltration.

ANALGESIA/SEDATION FOR SEVERE PAIN OF LONGER DURATION

Orthopaedic fracture

First choice	Second choice
IM **tramadol** 50–75 mg	IV **morphine** 3–5 mg initially, repeat every 10 minutes if necessary.

Notes:
1. Proper splintage is a form of pain relief.
2. IV metoclopramide 10 mg can be given as an anti-emetic if required.

Special cases of fracture

- **Humeral shaft/tibial shaft/radius** and **ulna shaft fractures** before application of plaster

First choice	Second choice
Entonox	IV **fentanyl** 2–3 µg/kg slow bolus and IV **midazolam** 0.1–0.2 mg/kg

Note: Allows gross manipulation of the fracture prior to plaster application.

- **Femoral shaft fracture**

First choice	Second choice
Femoral nerve block	IV **morphine** 2–5 mg

Notes:
1. Allows application of a traction splint.
2. The femoral nerve block is useful if sedation is not indicated, e.g. concomitant head injury.

- **Forearm/wrist fracture** for manipulation and reduction

First choice
Bier's block with 20 ml 0.5% lignocaine

Note: Allows accurate manipulation and reduction of the fracture.

- **Palm**

First choice	Second choice
Ulnar, median, or radial nerve blocks depending on the site involved	**Bier's block**

Notes:
1. Do not use Bier's block in children below 8 years old.
2. For Bier's block, **minimum** time between injection and first deflation of cuff should be **20 minutes**. For children and the elderly this interval should be 30 minutes.

- **Fingers**

First choice	Second choice
Metacarpal block with 1% lignocaine	**Digital nerve block** with 1% lignocaine

- **Foot**

First choice
Ankle block

- **Orthopaedic fractures** in the presence of **head injury**

First choice	Second choice
IV **tramadol** 50–100 mg	IV or IM **ketorolac** 30–60 mg

Note: 1. Tramadol has fewer sedative effects than Pethidine®/morphine.

Non-traumatic neck/back pain

First choice	Second choice
IM non-steroidal anti-inflammatory drugs (NSAIDs), e.g. **diclofenac** 75 mg and IV **diazepam** 10 mg (in the presence of muscle spasm)	IM **tramadol** 50–75 mg

Notes:
1. Discharge with:
   a. Oral analgesics.
   b. Anarex®/Beserol® two tablets three times daily (tds) or diazepam 2.5–5 mg three times/4 times daily (qds).
   c. Soft cervical collar for cervical strain but not for tension myalgia.
   d. Heat treatment.
   e. Referral for physiotherapy.

Abdominal pain

- **Acute abdomen**

First choice	Second choice
IV **fentanyl** 25–50 µg slow bolus	IV **morphine** 2–5 mg slow bolus

Notes:
Fentanyl has certain advantages over morphine:
- it does not release histamine
- it enters the CNS faster than morphine
- it has no intermediate metabolites and, hence, is the opiate of choice in chronic kidney disease and chronic liver disease.

- **Renal/ureteric colic**

First choice	Second choice
IM **NSAIDs**, e.g. **diclofenac** 50–75 mg	IM **tramadol**® 50–75 mg

- **Abdominal colic from gastroenteritis**

First choice
IM or IV hyoscine-N-butylbromide (**Buscopan**®) 40 mg

Chest pain

- **Ischaemic chest pain**
  1. Angina

First choice
Glyceryl trinitrate (GTN): Sublingual (SL), patch or intravenous

  2. Myocardial infarction

First choice	Second choice
SL **GTN** and IV **morphine sulphate** 2–5 mg, repeat every 10 minutes IV metoclopramide 10 mg as anti-emetic if needed	If pain is unrelieved after 2–3 doses of IV morphine, and especially if the patient is hypertensive or in heart failure, consider IV **GTN infusion** starting at 5–15 mcg/min with the dose doubled every 5 minutes 1. as tolerated or 2. until blood pressure/pulse changes or 3. until pain relief is obtained. Alternatively, give Entonox as an adjunct.

  a. Refer to Chapter 36, *Coronary Syndromes, Acute*.
  b. **Caution:** GTN is contraindicated in right ventricular infarct, hypovolaemia, or pericardial tamponade.

- **Non-ischaemic chest pain:** Pericarditis

First choice	Second choice
IV **dexamethasone** 15 mg	**NSAIDs**

Facial pain

- **Trigeminal neuralgia**

First choice	Second choice
Carbamazepine 100–200 mg bd (twice daily) PO (orally). Increase dosage gradually until pain free or side effects occur (drowsiness, dizziness, and unsteadiness)	**Baclofen** 10 mg tds PO

Notes:
1. Do full blood count before starting carbamazepine.
2. A combination therapy of carbamazepine or phenytoin with Baclofen® may be tried.

- ## Postherpetic neuralgia

First choice	Second choice
Prednisolone 60 mg/day PO × one week, then 30 mg/day × one week, then 15 mg/day × one week	**Amitryptyline** 25–75 mg ON (at night) and **fluphenazine** 1–3 mg ON PO once postherpetic neuralgia is established

Note: 1. Prednisolone given during the acute phase of trigeminal herpes will prevent postherpetic neuralgia.

- ## Temporal arteritis

First choice
Prednisolone 30–60 mg/day or 1 mg/kg/day PO

Headaches

- ## Migraine

First choice	Second choice
IM or oral NSAIDs, e.g. IM **diclofenac** 75 mg or **naproxen** 550 mg PO IV **metoclopramide** 10 mg	Subcutaneous (SC) **sumatriptan** 6 mg Repeat a second dose of 6 mg at least 1 hour after the first dose if symptoms recur; total dose = 12 mg/24 hr, or oral **sumatriptan** 100 mg. If no response, do not give second dose during the same attack. **Ergotamine tartrate** 1–2 mg PO, repeat half an hour later. 1. Dosage: ≤4–6 mg/24 hr 2. Dosage: ≤10–12 mg/wk

Notes:
1. **Sumatriptan** is **contraindicated** in:
   a. Uncontrolled hypertension.
   b. Ischaemic heart disease.
   c. Myocardial infarction.
   d. Prinzmetal angina.
2. Do not give sumatriptan with ergotamine.
3. Ergotamine is contraindicated in:
   a. Severe hypertension.
   b. Peripheral vascular disease.
   c. Ischaemic heart disease.
   d. Impaired hepatic and renal function.
   e. Pregnancy.

- ## Tension headache

First choice	Second choice
Paracetamol 1 g PO	IM or oral **NSAIDs**, or oral narcotic type of analgesics, e.g. codeine, codeine with paracetamol (Panadeine®and Viocodin®)

BIER'S BLOCK (IV REGIONAL ANAESTHESIA)

- **Indication**
  1. Manipulation and reduction (M&R) of forearm fractures, e.g. Colles' fracture.
- **Contraindications**
  1. Uncooperative patient.
  2. Known hypersensitivity.
  3. Patient is under 8 years of age or weighs <25 kg.
  4. Epilepsy.
  5. Severe hypertension and obesity (risk of leakage under tourniquet).
  6. Severe peripheral vascular disease.
  7. When pulse needs to be monitored as a guide to reduction, e.g. M&R of severe supracondylar fracture.
  8. Sickle cell disease.
- **Preparation**
  1. Medical history.
  2. Examination: Note the baseline blood pressure, cardiovascular, and respiratory systems.
  3. Baseline investigation: Electrocardiogram (ECG) for patients aged 60 years or more.
  4. Inform the patient of the procedure; no formal consent is required.
- **Technique**
  1. Place the patient on monitors: Blood pressure, pulse oximetry (SpO_2), and cardiac monitors.
  2. Get the resuscitation equipment ready.
  3. Insert an IV cannula on the hand of the affected limb.
  4. Elevate the affected arm above the heart level for 3 minutes to exanguinate the limb before inflating the tourniquet.
  5. **Place the tourniquet on the affected limb 50–100 mmHg above the systolic blood pressure** (about 250–300 mmHg for adults).
  6. Check that the tourniquet is not leaking and confirm the disappearance of the radial pulse before injecting a local anaesthetic (LA) such as **lignocaine**.
  7. Note the time of LA injection.
  8. Blanching of skin is expected and is indicative of the success of anaesthesia.
- **Dilution and dosage**
  1. Dilution of LA.
     a. Dilute **10 ml of 1% lignocaine with 10 ml of normal saline.**
     b. 20 ml of 0.5% solution contains 100 mg lignocaine, i.e. **1 ml = 5 mg.**
  2. Dosage: **0.4 ml/kg (= 2 mg/kg)** of 0.5% lignocaine solution.

3. Suggested dosage schedule:

Adult	20 ml
Elderly	15 ml
Child >10 years	10–15 ml
Child <10 years	8 ml

Weight (kg)	ml
25	10
30	12
35	14

a. **Toxic** dose of lignocaine: **3 mg/kg**.

b. **Tip**: If anaesthesia is incomplete after 20 ml of 0.5% lignocaine, inject 10–15 ml normal saline to flush more lignocaine peripherally.

c. **Onset**: 3 minutes.

NOTE: Prilocaine is the drug of choice as it has a proven track record of efficacy and safety. However, lignocaine is widely used locally.

- **Deflation**: **Do not deflate** the cuff if injection time is **<20 minutes** as this will result in a high concentration entering the circulation. Lignocaine fixes to tissues after 20 minutes and cuff release usually produces no adverse effects.
- **Complications**
  1. Lignocaine allergy.
  2. Lignocaine toxicity due to inadvertent systemic bolus injection.
     a. Early: Cicumoral numbness, lightheadedness, tinnitus, and slurred speech.
     b. Late: Unconsciousness, seizures, bradydysrhythmias, hypotension, and respiratory arrest.
- **Discharge**
  1. The patient may be discharged after a 2-hour observation period.
  2. Check limb circulation prior to discharge.

SUPRAORBITAL AND SUPRATROCHLEAR NERVE BLOCK (FOREHEAD BLOCK)

- **Anatomy**:
  1. The supraorbital nerve divides into two branches and leaves the orbit through two notches in the superior orbital margin, about 2.5 cm from the midline. It supplies the sensation to most of the forehead and the frontal region of the scalp.
  2. The supratrochlear nerve emerges from the upper medial corner of the orbit and supplies sensation to the medial part of the forehead.
- **Dosage**: 1% lignocaine 3–5 ml with or without adrenaline.

- **Technique** (Figure 1):
  1. Insert the needle in the midline between the eyebrows and direct it laterally.
  2. Inject the lignocaine subcutaneously from the point of insertion along the upper margin of the eyebrow.

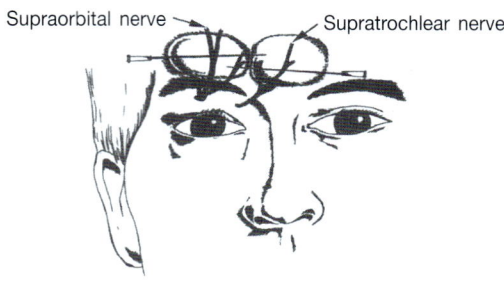

FIGURE 1 **Supraorbital and supratrochlear nerve blocks**

Supraorbital nerve —   — Supratrochlear nerve

  3. If the wound extends into the lateral part of the forehead, subcutaneous infiltration of lignocaine may be needed lateral to the eyebrow to block the zygomaticotemporal and auriculotemporal nerves.
- **Onset**: 5 minutes.
- **Duration**: 30–45 minutes.

AURICULAR BLOCK

- **Anatomy**:
  1. The auricle derives its sensory innervation from branches of the auriculotemporal, greater auricular, and lesser occipital nerves. The vagus nerve supplies sensory nerves to the meatus as well.
  2. The auriculotemporal nerve lies anterior to the pinna while both the greater auricular and lesser occipital nerves lie posteriorly.
- **Dosage**: 1% lignocaine 8–12 ml without adrenaline.
- **Technique** (Figure 2):
  1. Insert the needle just beneath the labule and direct it behind the ear, parallel and just superficial to the bone. Inject lignocaine along this track.
  2. Without reinserting the needle, redirect the needle anterior to the lobule and tragus. Leave a similar trace of lignocaine while withdrawing the needle.
  3. To complete the field block, insert the needle at a point above the superior portion of the helix. Similarly, leave a track of lignocaine anteriorly and posteriorly to the superior portion of the ear.
- **Onset**: 15 minutes.
- **Duration**: 30–45 minutes.

FIGURE 2 **Field anaesthesia of the ear**

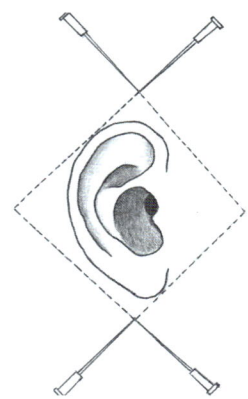

DIGITAL NERVE BLOCK

- **Anatomy**: There are 4 digital nerves to each finger or toe, i.e. 2 palmar digital nerves and 2 dorsal digital nerves. They lie close to the phalanges and these bony structures are used as landmarks for locating the nerves.
- **Dosage**: 1% lignocaine 4 ml maximum (**without adrenaline** added).
- **Technique** (Figures 3 and 4):
  1. **Web space approach**:
     a. A needle (e.g. 27G) is inserted into the web space just distal to the metacarpal-phalangeal joint and advanced adjacent to the phalanx and directed towards the volar surface of the digit: 1 ml of lignocaine is deposited near the palmar nerve.

FIGURE 3   Digital nerve block at the base of the finger and at the metacarpal level

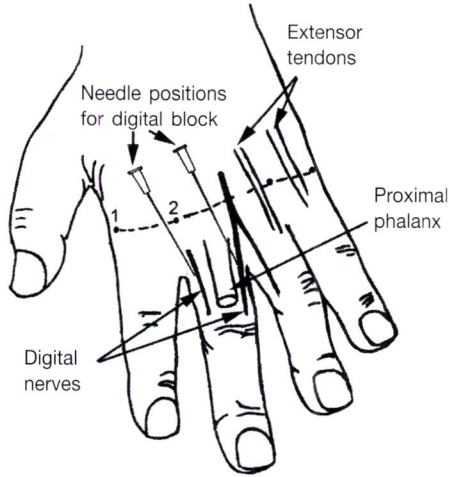

1 and 2 = Needle positions for metacarpal block

FIGURE 4   Cross-section of the finger/toe

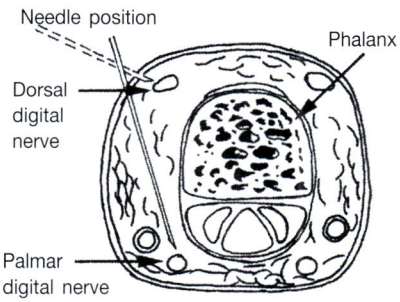

b. The needle is then withdrawn and (without leaving the original puncture site) advanced towards the dorso-lateral aspect of the phalanx until it touches the bone: 0.5 ml of lignocaine is deposited near the dorsal nerve.

c. The procedure is repeated on the opposite side of the digit.

2. The basic procedure for the digital block described above may be used for the thumb and the great toe. For the **thumb**, the injections are **near** the **mid-point** as the neurovascular bundle runs in the midline of the thumb.

3. **For the second to fifth toes**: A single midline dorsal needlestick can be used to anaesthetize both sides of the toes.

4. **Metacarpal approach**:

a. Digital nerves can be blocked where they run in the interspaces between the metacarpals.

b. Insert a needle into the palm through the distal palmar crease, between the flexor tendons of adjacent fingers. Inject 3–4 ml of plain 1% lignocaine. This will anaesthetize the adjacent sites of these two fingers. Alternatively, inject 3–4 ml of 1% lignocaine through the distal palmar crease at the mid-point of the base of the finger. This single injection will anaesthetize the finger involved.

- **Onset**: 5 minutes.
- **Duration**: 45–60 minutes.

WRIST BLOCK

- **Indications**: Minor surgery to areas of the hand innervated by the median, ulnar, and radial nerves.

Median nerve

- **Anatomy**: At the level of the proximal palmar crease, the median nerve lies superficially between the palmaris longus and flexor carpi radialis (or medial to the flexor carpi radialis if the palmaris longus is absent).
- **Contraindications**: History of carpal tunnel syndrome.
- **Dosage**: 1% lignocaine 4–6 ml is used (with or without adrenaline).
- **Technique**:

1. Insert a 23G or 25G needle at the proximal skin crease of the wrist, between the tendons of the palmaris longus and flexor carpi radialis (the two tendons may be made more apparent by asking the patient to flex the wrist).

2. Move the needle fanwise up and down until paraesthesia is elicited; withdraw the needle and slowly inject 2–4 ml of lignocaine.

- **Onset**: 5–10 minutes.
- **Duration**: 1.5 hours.

Ulnar nerve

- **Anatomy**:
  1. The ulnar nerve divides into a dorsal and a palmar branch about 5 cm proximal to the wrist.
  2. At the wrist, the palmar branch lies between the flexor carpi ulnaris and the ulnar artery.
- **Dosage**: 1% lignocaine 7–10 ml (with or without adrenaline).
- **Technique** (Figure 5):
  1. **Palmar branch**: Insert a 23–25G needle between the flexor carpi ulnaris and the ulnar artery at the same level with the ulnar styloid process. If paraesthesia is elicited, withdraw the needle and inject 2–4 ml of 1% lignocaine.
  2. **Dorsal branch**: 5 ml of 1% lignocaine is injected subcutaneously from the tendon of the flexor carpi ulnaris around the ulnar aspect of the wrist.
- **Onset**: 5–10 minutes (the dorsal branch blockade has a faster onset of action).
- **Duration**: 1.5 hours.

FIGURE 5 **The wrist block showing median and ulnar nerve blocks**

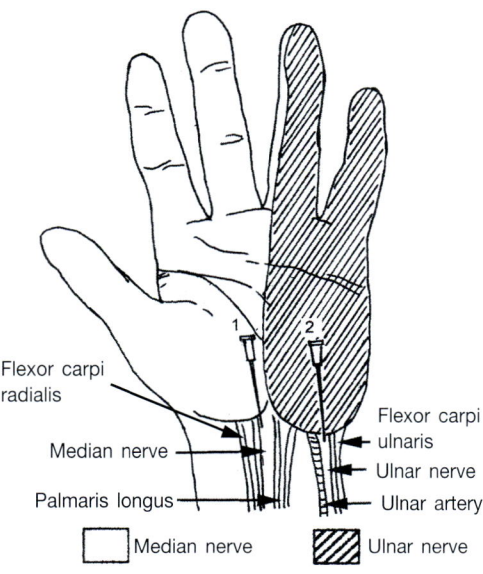

1 = Position of needle in median nerve block
2 = Position of needle in ulnar nerve block

Radial nerve

- **Anatomy**: At the level of the wrist the radial nerve gives off superficial branches which lie subcutaneously on the extensor aspect.
- **Dosage**: 1% lignocaine 5 ml (with or without adrenaline).
- **Technique** (Figure 6): Subcutaneous infiltration starting from the radial styloid to the ulnar styloid at the level of the wrist.
- **Onset**: 2 minutes
- **Duration**: 1 hour

FIGURE 6   Radial nerve block

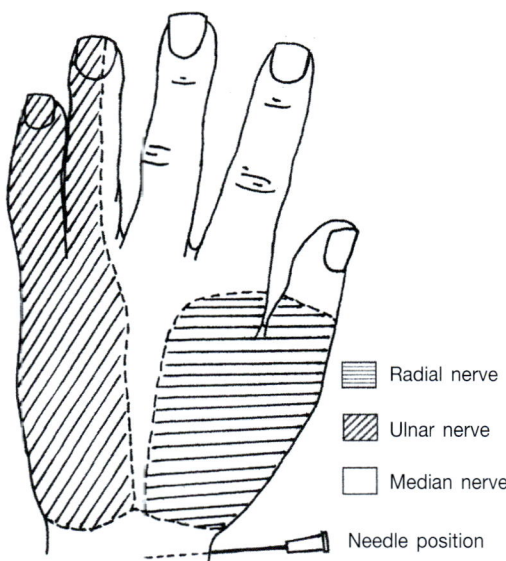

- Radial nerve
- Ulnar nerve
- Median nerve
- Needle position

NERVE BLOCKS AT THE ANKLE

- Lignocaine blocks at the ankle are particularly useful for anaesthetizing the sole of the foot, where local infiltration is very painful and unsatisfactory.
- **Anatomy:**
  1. Sensation in the ankle and foot is supplied by five main nerves (Figure 7):
     a. **Saphenous nerve** (medial side of the ankle).
     b. **Superficial peroneal nerve** (front of the ankle and dorsum of the foot).
     c. **Deep peroneal nerve** (lateral side of the great toe and medial side of the second toe).

FIGURE 7   Sensory supply of the foot and ankle

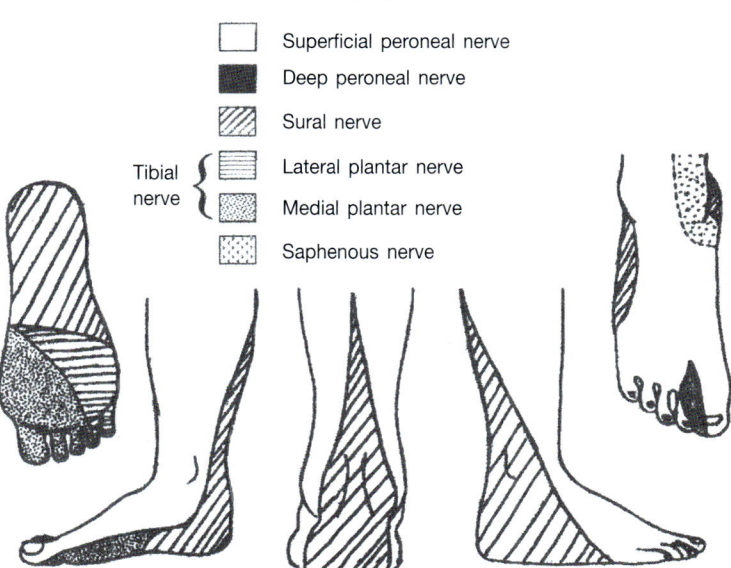

d. **Sural nerve** (heel and lateral side of the hind foot).

e. **Tibial nerve** (which forms the medial and lateral plantar nerves, providing sensation to the anterior half of the sole).

2. There is significant overlap between the areas supplied by the different nerves, especially on the sole of the foot. It is often necessary to block more than one nerve.

● **Dosage**: 1% lignocaine (with or without adrenaline) 5 ml or 0.5% bupivacaine. Do not use adrenaline in patients with peripheral vascular disease.

● **Technique**:

1. **Saphenous nerve**: Infiltrate LA subcutaneously around the great saphenous vein, anterior to and just above the medial malleolus. Aspirate carefully because of the risk of IV injection.

2. **Superficial peroneal nerve**: Infiltrate LA subcutaneously above the ankle joint from the anterior border of the tibia to the lateral malleolus.

3. **Deep peroneal nerve**: Insert the needle above the ankle joint between the tendons of the tibialis anterior and the extensor hallucis longus. Inject 5 ml of LA.

FIGURE 8 **Sural nerve block**

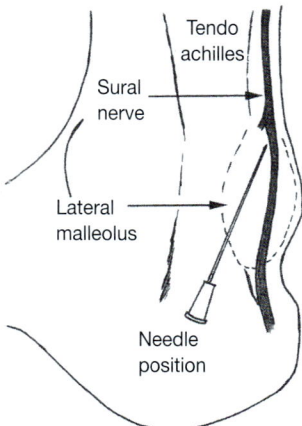

FIGURE 9 **Tibial nerve block**

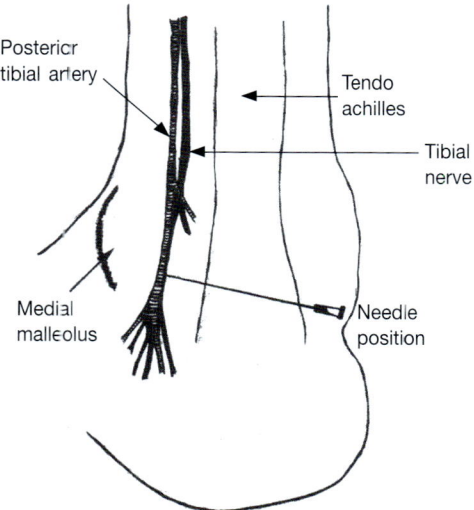

4. **Sural nerve** (Figure 8): Get the patient to lie in the prone position. Insert the needle lateral to the Achilles tendon and infiltrate subcutaneously to the lateral malleolus.

5. **Tibial nerve** (Figure 9): Get the patient to lie in the prone position. Palpate the posterior tibial artery. Insert the needle medial to the Achilles tendon and level with the upper border of the medial malleolus, so the needle tip is just lateral to the artery. Withdraw slightly if paraesthesia occurs. Aspirate. Inject 5–10 ml LA.

FEMORAL BLOCK

- **Anatomy**: The femoral nerve passes under the inguinal ligament to enter the thigh and lies lateral to the femoral artery (mnemonics: VAN: vein lies most medial).
- **Dosage**: 1% lignocaine 10–15 ml.
- **Technique** (Figure 10):
  1. Use a 21–23G needle at least 4 cm long.
  2. Palpate the femoral artery.
  3. Insert the needle perpendicular to the skin and just lateral to the artery as it emerges under the inguinal ligament.
  4. When paraesthesia is elicited, withdraw the needle slightly, and inject 10 ml of lignocaine while moving the needle 4 cm up and down, gradually moving laterally to about 2–3 cm from the artery.
- **Onset**: 5–15 minutes.
- **Duration**: 1.5 hours.

FIGURE 10   Right femoral nerve block

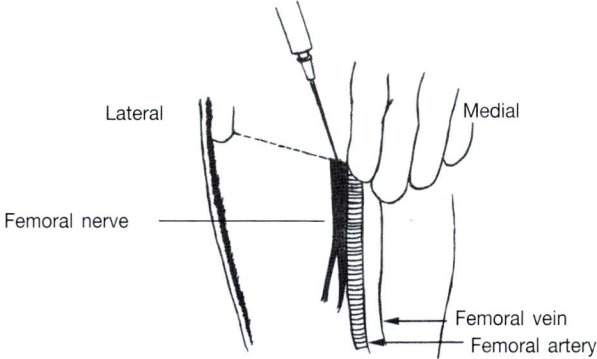

Acknowledgement

All illustrations in this chapter were drawn by Dr Chong Chew Lan.

References/Further Reading

1. Nolan JP, Baskett PJF. Analgesia and anaesthesia. In: Skinner D, Swain A, Peyton R, et al., eds. *Cambridge Textbook of Accident and Emergency Medicine*. Cambridge, NY: Cambridge University Press; 1997: 183–205.

2. Illingworth KA. Anesthesia and pain control. In: Rutherford WH, Illingworth RN, Marsden AK, et al., eds. *Accident and Emergency Medicine*. 2nd ed. Edinburgh, UK: Churchill Livingstone; 1989: 83–106.

3. Smith DW, Peterson MR, DeBerard SC. Infiltration and nerve block anesthesia. In: Trott AT. *Wounds and Lacerations: Emergency Care and Closure*. 2nd ed. St. Louis, MO: Mosby; 1997: 53–89.

4. Analgesia and anaesthesia. In: Wyatt JP, Illingworth RN, Graham CA, et al., eds. *Oxford Handbook of Accident and Emergency Medicine*. 3rd ed. Oxford, UK: Oxford University Press; 2006: 269–316.

141 Procedural Sedation

Ian Mathews • Peter Manning

DEFINITION

The use of a short acting sedative with or without an analgesic, to induce a minimally depressed level of consciousness that retains the patient's protective airway and cardiac reflexes, and the ability to respond appropriately to physical stimulation and/or verbal commands

CAVEATS

- It is assumed that the patient has been assessed for suitability for sedation, which includes the documentation of allergies, current medications and abnormal airway patency.
- In the absence of a senior emergency physician or anaesthetist, consider admitting for general anaesthetic children under the age of 5 years.
- The use of procedural sedation requires at least 2 operators. One performs the procedure, while the other performs the sedation, and is responsible for the constant monitoring of the patient's cardiorespiratory status. The physician performing the sedation should not supervise the procedure.
- The physician performing the sedation should be sedation trained, or supervised by a sedation trained emergency physician.

INDICATIONS

- Any patient undergoing a procedure in which the patient's pain or anxiety may be excessive and impede performance of the procedure. Some examples include:
  1. Closed joint dislocations
  2. Incisions and drainages of abscesses
  3. Complicated or anatomically challenging laceration repair
  4. Lumbar punctures
  5. Electrical cardioversions.

CONTRAINDICATIONS

- There are no absolute contraindications to procedural sedation.
- Relative contraindications include:
  1. The elderly (>65 years old)
  2. Patients with potentially difficult airways (expected difficulty in ventilation and oxygenation)
  3. Patients with American Society of Anaesthesiologists (ASA) III and greater

> ⇨ **SPECIAL TIP FOR GPs**
> - Procedural sedation is not a procedure that you should consider undertaking in the clinic, unless your clinic set-up includes haemodynamic monitoring capability and **immediate** anaesthesia assistance.

MANAGEMENT

Preparation

- ALL patients must be managed in a monitored area, regardless of age and medical fitness status. Idiosyncratic and allergic reactions are difficult to predict.
- Informed consent – verbal, then documented clearly in case notes thereafter.
- Pre-sedation fasting is not required.
- Peripheral IV cannula (preferably minimum 20G) with IV normal saline at slow rate for flushing.
- Supplemental oxygen via nasal cannulae.
- Monitoring: Continuous cardiac rhythm and pulse oximetry monitoring. Vital signs q 5 min.
- Immediately available resuscitation equipment to include:
  1. Oral airway.
  2. Bag-valve-mask (BVM) devices.
  3. Endotracheal tubes.
  4. Defibrillator.
  5. Reversal agents naloxone (Narcan®) and flumazenil (Anexate®).

Drug Therapy

A variety of sedatives and analgesics are available, each with their own advantages and disadvantages. Level of consciousness is assessed based on the Modified Ramsay Scale (Table 1), aiming for a level of 2–3. Refer to Table 2 for dosages of sedating agents and analgesia.

Choice of sedatives:

- **Propofol** is advantageous as it has both sedative and amnesic effects, and has a rapid onset and recovery. However, its lack of analgesic property *may* require the concurrent use of an opioid agonist analgesic.
- **Etomidate** is advantageous in that it maintains cardiovascular stability. Like propofol, it has sedative and amnesic, but no analgesic properties.
- **Midazolam** is a benzodiazepine which, together with its amnesic and sedative effect, also has anxiolytic properties. However, it does not have analgesic effect and may cause significant hypotension.
- **Ketamine** is a dissociative amnesic and sedating agent with profound analgesic properties.

TABLE 1   Modified Ramsay Scale

Awake States

1. Patient anxious, agitated or restless
2. Patient cooperative, oriented, tranquil
3. Patient asleep, brisk response to loud auditory stimulus

Sleep States

4. Patient asleep, sluggish response to loud auditory stimulus
5. Patient has no response to loud auditory stimulus but does respond to painful stimulus
6. Patient does not respond to painful stimulus

Source: Ramsay M, Savege T, Simpson B, et al. Controlled Sedation with alphaxalone-alphadolone. *Britiish Medical Journal* 2: 555 (1974).

Choice of analgesic:

- **Fentanyl** is an opiate analgesic which has the significant advantages of not producing histamine release (anaphylactoid reaction), and, the absence of intermediate metabolites making fentanyl the ideal analgesic for moderate to severe pain in patients with chronic liver and chronic renal disease.

Complications of procedural sedation

- **Respiratory depression** due to propofol, midazolam and opioid agonists. Management by:
  1. Supplemental oxygen.
  2. Bag-valve-mask ventilation.
  3. Reversal agents – flumazenil and naloxone.
- **Laryngospasm** due to ketamine. Management by:
  1. Positive pressure ventilation (PPV).
  2. Succinylchonline (IV 1–2mg/kg or IM 4mg/kg) if laryngospasm persists after PPV.
  3. Airway management with BVM or intubation after paralysis.
- **Hypotension** due to midazolam and opioid agonists. Management by:
  1. Trendelenburg position.
  2. Normal saline infusion 20ml/kg.
- **Chest wall rigidity** due to fentanyl. Management by:
  1. Naloxone.
  2. If naloxone fails: Succinylcholine (IV 1–2mg/kg or IM 4mg/kg).
  3. Airway management after paralysis.
- **Allergic reaction**. – refer to Chapter 29, *Allergic reactions/Anaphylaxis*.

TABLE 2 Doses of Drugs used in Procedural Sedation

Drug	Dosage		Onset	Duration	Advantages	Disadvantages	Remarks
	Adult	Paeds					
				Sedative agents			
Propofol	IV 0.5–1mg/kg; repeat q 1–2 minutes until desired effect.	N/A	40sec	6 min	Rapid onset and recovery	Respiratory and CNS depression, especially when used with opioids. No analgesic properties.	Contraindicated in soy/egg allergies. Suggest half dose in elderly (>65 years of age)
Etomidate	IV 0.1–0.2mg/kg followed by 0.05mg/kg q 3–5 mins until desired effect.	N/A	30–60 sec	5–15 min	Maintains cardiovascular stability. Rapid onset and recovery.	No analgesic properties	Prolonged effect in elderly, renal/hepatic impairment.
Midazolam (Dormicum®, Versed®)	IV 0.1mg/kg in divided doses	IV 0.05mg/kg in divided doses, (max dose of 2mg if <70kg)	2–5 min	30–60 min	Anxiolytic properties	Respiratory and CNS depression, especially when used with opioids. No analgesic properties.	
Ketamine	IV 1–2mg/kg; followed by 0.25 to 0.5 mg/kg q 5–10 mins	IM use: 3mg/kg and round up to multiples of 5, but ensure final dose is <4mg/kg. IV use: 1mg/kg slow bolus	30sec	10–20min	Fairly safe, side effects rare. Both sedative and analgesic properties.	Laryngospasm with large doses (uncommon)	Useful in asthmatics due to bronchodilator effect. In paediatrics, use in conjunction with atropine to decrease secretions.
Atropine	N/A	IV or IM 0.02mg/kg (min 0.1mg, max 0.6mg)					

(Continued)

Drug	Dosage		Onset	Duration	Advantages	Disadvantages	Remarks
	Adult	**Paeds**					
				Sedative agents			
Fentanyl	IV 0.5–1µg/kg q 2 mins till appropriate level of analgesia achieved (up to max 2µg/kg)	IV 0.5µg/kg q 2 mins (up to max of 2µg/kg)	2–3min	30–60min	Rapid analgesic effect. Short duration. Minimal histamine release.	Respiratory depression with concurrent use of sedatives. Chest wall rigidity with large doses. Hypotension (uncommon).	For use in combination with propofol and midazolam, suggest dose 15 mins before sedative. Half dose in elderly.
Morphine	IV 0.1–0.2mg/kg in divided doses	IV 0.01–0.04mg/ kg in divided doses	>5min	3–4 hours	Titratable	Respiratory and CNS depression. Also an emetic. Slow onset with prolonged action. Causes histamine release.	For use in combination with propofol and midazolam, suggest dose 15 mins before sedative. Half dose in elderly.
				Reversal agents			
Naloxone	IV 0.2mg over 15 sec; repeat with 0.3mg if no response after 1 min; repeat with 0.5mg if no response after 1 min. Repeat till max cumulative dose of 5mg/hr.	IV 0.01mg/kg q1h	1min	45 mins	Fairly safe		Opioid agonist antidote
Flumazenil	100 µg q 2–3 mins till reversal	IV 0.1mg	1–2min	10–15min	Fairly safe	Half-life shorter than benzodiazepine half-life.	Benzodiazepine antidote

Use of reversal agents.

- **Appropriate use**: Naloxone and/or flumazenil should only be administered should the patient become bradypnoeic or apnoeic, or deeply unconscious during the sedation.
- **Inappropriate use**: It is preferable to permit the patient to regain full consciousness naturally without the use of antidotes since the half-life of the agents used in conscious sedation is longer than that of their respective antidotes. Indiscriminate use of the antidotes could therefore lead to fluctuating levels of consciousness.
- **Dosages**: Refer to Table 1.

Post-procedure

- **Position patient** in recovery position with mild Trendelenburg tilt.
- **Monitor** vital signs q15 min until patient is discharged.
- **Documentation** of procedure, including drugs used and dosages, and any adverse effects and corrective treatment.

Discharge

- Discharge only when patient is fully awake, can breathe deeply, cough and drink, and able to stand and walk as per pre-sedation baseline.
- The doctor administering sedation must review and authorise discharge.
- Patient should be escorted home by a friend or family member.
- Discharge instructions: For the next 24 hours, patient should not:
  1. Drive an automobile or operate heavy machinery.
  2. Climb to heights.
  3. Swim.
  4. Take alcohol, or other medications that may produce drowsiness.

References/further reading

1. American College of Emergency Physicians. Clinical Policy: Procedural Sedation and Analgesia in the Emergency Department; 2014.
2. National University Hospital, Singapore. Paediatric Sedation Protocol, 2003.

142 Simple Statistics

Shirley Ooi • Irwani Ibrahim

DESIGN ISSUES

- **Random allocation/sampling**
    1. In random allocation/sampling, each individual has a known chance (usually equal) of being allocated a treatment/being selected.
    2. For random sampling, use either random number tables or a computer-generated sampling plan.
    3. For random allocation, use a block-randomization design for a balanced allocation.
    4. Both random sampling and allocation deal with possible **bias** at treatment allocation.
- **Bias**: This is the error related to the ways the targeted and sampled populations differ. It is also called the **measurement/systematic error** and it threatens the validity of a study. Examples of bias include:
    1. Volunteer bias: Subjects may have a vested interest to enter trial.
    2. Selection bias: Subject selection may affect the outcome (choose from one group type only).
    3. Response bias: Placebo effect and desiring to please doctor!
    4. Assessment bias: The assessor should not be the investigator (blind) or subject (double blind).
- **Confounder**: A variable more likely to be present in one group of subjects than another that is related to the outcome of interest and thus potentially confuses or 'confounds' the results, e.g. age or gender in a study on treatment of ischaemic heart disease.
- **Blinding/masking**: This is a technique to increase objectivity and decrease subjectivity of assessing the efficacy of a treatment. Types of blinding:
    1. **Single blind**: Only the patient is unaware of whether he is in the treatment or control group.
    2. **Double blind**: Both the patient and investigator are unaware of the group assignment.
    3. **Triple blind**: The patient, investigator, and assessor are unaware of the group assessment.

However, the current trend is to report on who were blinded rather than use terms like single, double, or triple blind.

- **Sample size**: Sample size increases with
    1. Bigger power.

NOTE: **Power** is the ability of test statistics to detect a specified alternative hypothesis or difference of a specified size when the alternative hypothesis is true. More loosely, it is the ability of a study to detect an actual effect or difference.

    2. Smaller effect size.

DATE ISSUES

Data types

- **Quantitative/numerical data** for which the differences between the numbers have meaning on a numerical scale.

  1. **Continuous scale** has values on a continuum, e.g. age.

  2. **Discrete scale** has values equal to integers, e.g. number of fractures.

- **Qualitative (categorical) data**

  1. **Nominal scales** have no ranking order (e.g. gender).

  2. **Ordinal scales** have an inherent order or ranking among the categories (e.g. stages I and IV of disease X).

Summarizing data

- **Measures of the middle (central tendency)**: The decision on which measure of central tendency is to be used depends on 2 factors: (1) Scale of measurement (ordinal or numerical) and (2) shape of the distribution of measurement.

  1. **Mean** (arithmetic): The sum of the observations divided by the number of observations, e.g. 2, 5, 8, 3, 4 is 22/5 = 4.4 (used if the variable is normally distributed). This is used for numerical data and for symmetric (not skewed) distributions.

  2. **Median** is the central value of the distribution (used if the variable is skewed), i.e. half of the observations are smaller and half are larger. For 1, 3, 4, 7, 8, 12, 13, 20, 30 the median is 8 but the mean is 10.88. It is also equal to the 50th percentile. This is used for ordinal data or for numerical data when the distribution is skewed.

  3. **Mode** is the value that occurs most frequently. For example, the mode for 2, 2, 2, 3, 3, 4, 5 is 2. Mode is used primarily for bimodal distribution.

- **Measures of spread (dispersion)**

  1. **Range** is the difference between the largest observation and the smallest observation. This is used with numerical data when the purpose is to emphasize extreme values.

  2. **Degrees of freedom**: Total number of observations (n) made − 1 or ($n − 1$).

  3. **Variance**: The sum of the deviations from the mean for all observations (n) made in a sample group will always be 0 (i.e. +2 mmHg, +1 mmHg, 0 mmHg, −1 mmHg, −2 mmHg = 0 mmHg). Therefore, we have to square this sum to produce a +ve value (this gets rid of the minus sign, +4, +1, 0, +1, +4). If we divide this sum by the degrees of freedom ($n − 1$), we obtain the variance (10/4 = 2.5). So if the deviations from the mean are large and the number of observations (n) is small, then the variance will be large! The **variance is a numerical unit only and not descriptive**, i.e. 2.4 and not 2.4 mmHg). To change it back to descriptive, we use the standard deviation.

FIGURE 1   A bell-shaped or normal distribution

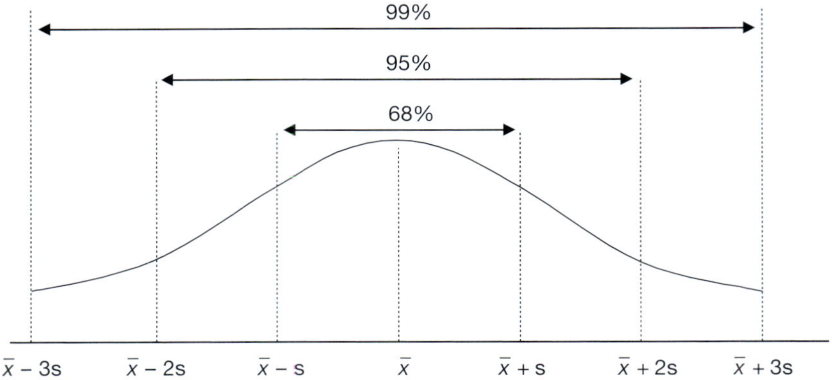

Source: 95% of the observations lie between $\bar{x} - 2s$ and, $\bar{x} + 2s$ where $\bar{x}$ is the mean of the observations.

4. **Standard deviation (s)** is a measure of the spread of data about their mean (Figure 1). This is used with symmetric (not skewed) numerical data. It is this square root of the variance and it is a way of reverting to descriptive terms.

$$s = \sqrt{\frac{\sum(x - \bar{x})^2}{n - 1}}$$

Where $\bar{x}$ = mean

n = number of observations

s^2 = variance

5. **Standard error** provides an estimate of how far the calculated true value of the mean of the sample population is from the unknown value of the mean of the parent population. The larger the sample size, the closer the sample mean to the parent population mean and the smaller the standard error. Therefore, the sample is more representative of the parent.

6. **Percentile** is a number that indicates the percentage of distribution less than or equal to that number. This is used, in the following two situations:

a. When the median is used, i.e. with ordinal data or with skewed numerical data.

b. When the mean is used but the objective is to compare individual observations with a set of norm.

HYPOTHESIS TESTING

- **Null hypothesis**: This hypothesis states that there is no difference or no effect between the groups under study.
- **Alternative hypothesis**: This is the opposite to the null hypothesis. It is the conclusion when the null hypothesis is rejected.

- **Type I error**: This is the error that results if a true null hypothesis is rejected or if a difference is concluded when there is no difference.
- **Type II error**: This is the error that results if a false null hypothesis is not rejected or if a difference is not detected when there is a difference.
- **Probability *p***: This is the number of times an outcome occurs in the total number of trials. *p* is the probability that the difference obtained between two groups is due to chance (usually taken as significant if the probability is less than 5% or less than 1 in 20).
- **A 95% confidence interval** means that you are 95% confident that the unknown parameter such as the mean or proportion is contained within the interval.

TEST TYPES

Figure 2 summarizes the decision making on statistical test usage.

FIGURE 2   **How to decide on types of statistical tests to use**

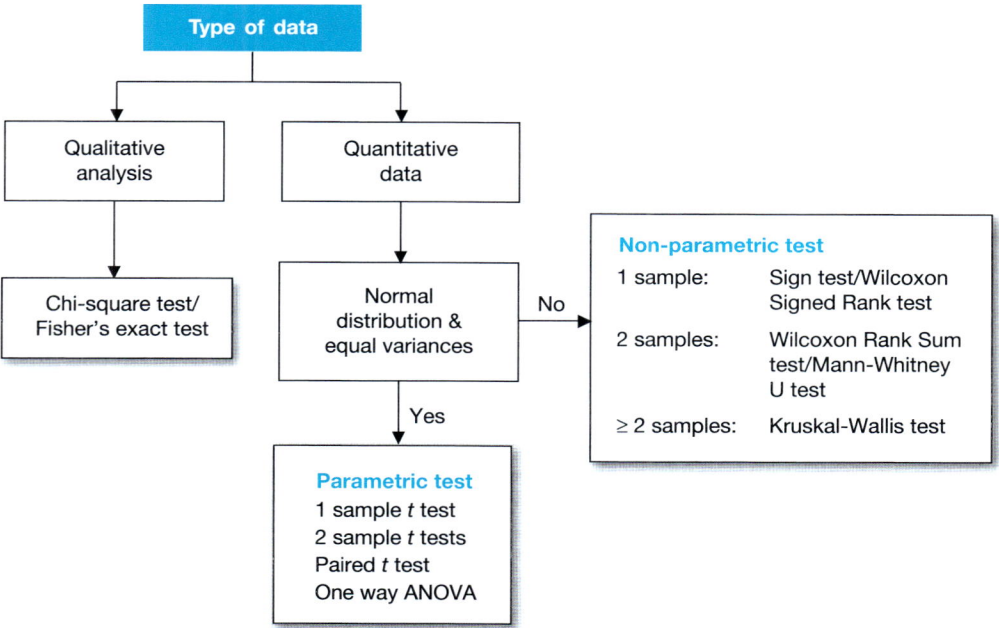

Qualitative data

For evaluating categorical versus categorical variables (when there is any association between two categorical variables), use the **Chi-square** test. If the Chi-square test assumptions are not satisfied (usually if the sampling size is small), use **Fisher's exact** test.

Quantitative data

- **Parametric tests or student's *t* test**

  1. Ideal for comparing between two groups of data in 'before and after' studies (**paired *t* test**) or between two groups with **similar normal distribution**. A *t* test is used to determine if the mean from one group is significantly different from the mean of another group. The larger the *t* value, the more significant is the difference, e.g. $t = 7.8$ at $p <0.05$ means that the probability of obtaining a *t* value of this magnitude due to chance is less than 5%.

  2. **One-tailed *t* test** is used if a treatment is assumed to be always better than the control.

  3. **Two-tailed *t* test** is used if a treatment could be better or worse than the control.

  4. **One-sample *t* test** is used to determine whether the mean of a single variable differs from a specified constant.

  5. **Two-sample or independent-sample *t* test** is used to compare means for 2 groups of cases. The assumption is that the 2 groups are independent random samples, the population variances are equal, and the observations are normally distributed in each population.

  6. **Paired-samples *t* test** compares the means of 2 variables for a single group. The assumption is that the difference between the 2 paired variables follows a normal distribution.

  7. **Analysis of Variance (ANOVA).**

     a. One-way ANOVA produces a one-way analysis of variance for a quantitative dependent variable by a single (independent) variable. The assumptions are that the observations are normally distributed in each population, all the population variances are equal, and all the groups are independent random samples.

     b. If used for 3 or more group comparisons, ANOVA will only show **if there is a difference between the groups** but will not identify where the difference(s) is/are. If a difference is found, then a post-hoc test (usually Bonferroni correction) is used to identify where the differences are between the groups.

- **Non-parametric tests such as the Mann–Whitney U test or Wilcoxon rank sum test** is used when normality assumptions are not satisfied.

- **Correlation analysis** is used to establish if there is a linear relationship between 2 quantitative or ordinal variables, e.g. rising examination score versus intelligence quotient (IQ) score. If normality assumptions are satisfied for the 2 variables, use Pearson correlation. Otherwise use Spearman correlation.

- **Regression analysis** is used to quantify a linear relationship between a continuous outcome variable and a continuous/qualitative independent variable (e.g. comparing increasing age versus rise in serum cholesterol; this is a **simple linear regression. Multiple linear regression** is used when more than one continuous/qualitative independent variables are being used (e.g. gender, race, and cholesterol levels).

STATISTICS USED IN DIAGNOSTIC TESTS

	Definition	Based on Table 1
Sensitivity	Population of people with a target disorder in whom a test result is positive, i.e. **PID** = **P**ositive (test) **i**n **D**isease	$= \dfrac{a}{a + c}$
Specificity	Proportion of people without target disorder in whom a test result is negative, i.e. **NIH** = **N**egative **i**n **H**ealth	$= \dfrac{d}{b + d}$
Positive predictive value (PPV)/predictive value of a positive test	The proportion of time that a patient with a positive diagnostic test result has the disease being investigated	$= \dfrac{a}{a + b}$
Negative predictive value (NPV)/predictive value of a negative test	The proportion of time that a patient with a negative diagnostic test result does not have the disease being investigated	$= \dfrac{d}{c + d}$
Likelihood ratio of a positive test [LR(+)]	The relative likelihood that a positive test would be expected in a patient with (as opposed to one without) a disorder of interest	$= \dfrac{a/(a + c)}{b/(b + d)}$ $= \dfrac{\text{sensitivity}}{1 - \text{specificity}}$
Likelihood ratio of a negative test [LR(−)]	The relative likelihood that a negative test would be expected in a patient with (as opposed to one without) a disorder of interest	$= \dfrac{c/(a + c)}{d/(b + d)}$ $= \dfrac{1 - \text{sensitivity}}{\text{specificity}}$

TABLE 1 Probable outcomes of test results

Test	Disease	
	Present	**Absent**
+ve	True positive (a)	False positive (b)
−ve	False negative (c)	True negative (d)

CONCEPTS USED IN THERAPY ARTICLES

	Definitions	Formula
Control risk (Rc)	Risk of the event among control patients	
Treatment risk (Rt)	Risk of the event among treated patients	
Relative risk reduction (RRR)	Percentage of risk lost	$\dfrac{R_c - R_t}{R_c} \times 100\%$
Relative risk (RR)	Percentage of risk remaining	$\dfrac{R_t}{R_c}$
Absolute risk reduction (ARR)	Absolute risk lost	$R_c - R_t$
Number needed to treat (NNT)	The number of patients who need to be treated over a specific period of time to prevent one bad outcome	$\dfrac{1}{\text{ARR}}$

References/Further Reading

1. Bland M. *An Introduction to Medical Statistics*. Oxford, UK: Oxford University Press; 1993.

2. Byrne D. *Publishing Your Medical Research Paper*. Baltimore, MD: Lippincott Williams & Wilkins; 1998.

3. Dawson-Saunders B, Trapp RG. *Basic and Clinical Biostatistics*. 2nd ed. Norwalk, CT: Appleton & Lange; 1994.

4. Guyatt G, Rennie D, eds. *Users' Guide to the Medical Literature: A Manual for Evidence-based Clinical Practice*. Chicago, IL: AMA Press; 2002.

5. Chan YH. Randomized controlled trials (RCTs): Essentials. *Singapore Med J*. 2003; 44(2): 60–63.

6. Chan YH. Randomized controlled trials (RCTs): Sample size—The magic number? *Singapore Med J*. 2003; 44(2): 172–174.

7. Chan YH. Biostatistics 101: Data presentation. *Singapore Med J*. 2003; 44(6): 280–285.

8. Chan YH. Biostatistics 102: Quantitative data: Parametric and non-parametric tests. *Singapore Med J*. 2003; 44(8): 391–396.

143 Useful Formulae

Chong Chew Lan

Many clinical problems may be deciphered with the aid of 'mathematical equations'. When appropriately applied, these can help in the formulation of differential diagnosis, interpretation of laboratory data, and clinical management. The following are useful formulae for daily practice.

- **Calculated serum osmolality in mmol/L = (2 × Na + Urea + Glucose)**

  1. Serum osmolality has to be >350 mOsm/kg H_2O (water) for diagnosis of hyperosmolar non-ketotic coma. **Normal range is 286 ± 4 mOsm/kg H_2O.**

  2. Calculated serum osmolality can also be used to calculate the **osmolal gap**.

  3. **Osmolal gap** = Measured serum osmolality − Calculated serum osmolality.

  4. The '**normal**' osmolal gap is arbitrarily set at **10 mOsm/kg H_2O**. In the emergency department setting, an elevated osmolal gap usually represents the presence of ethanol or other toxic alcohols such as methanol, ethylene glycol, isopropyl alcohol, proteins, or lipids.

- **AG (anion gap) = Na (mmol/L) − [Chloride (mmol/L) + Bicarbonate (mmol/L)]**

  The **normal range is 7 ± 4 mEq/L**. The reference range for the AG has shifted 'downwards'. Historically, the 'normal' AG has been 12 ± 4. The newer 'normal' range is 7 ± 4, which reflects the current methods for measuring Na^+, Cl^-, and HCO_3^-. This downward shift in the normal AG value is primarily due to an upward shift in the chloride value that has accompanied changes in laboratory assessment methods. AG is useful in the evaluation of patients with metabolic acidosis. See Chapter 57 Tables 1 and 2, for causes of high and normal AG.

- **Acid base disorders**: For more details, refer to Chapter 57, *Acid Base Emergencies* chapter.

  1. The diagnosis of acid base disorders can be complicated and the recognition of mixed **acid base disorders** (Figure 1) often proves elusive. Unless the clinician knows what degree of compensation is expected of a disorder, he may not recognize the existence of an overlapping second disorder.

  2. **Rules of compensation** in acid base disorders (pCO_2 in mmHg; HCO_3^- in mmol/L):

Primary disturbance	Normal compensatory response
Metabolic acidosis	$pCO_2 = (1.5 \times HCO_3^-) + 8 \pm 2$
Metabolic alkalosis	$pCO_2 = [(0.6 \times HCO_3^- - 24)] + 40$
Acute respiratory acidosis	$\Delta HCO_3^- = (0.1 \times \Delta pCO_2)$
Acute respiratory alkalosis	$\Delta HCO_3^- = (0.2 \times \Delta pCO_2)$
Chronic respiratory acidosis/alkalosis	$\Delta HCO_3^- = (0.4 - \Delta pCO_2)$

FIGURE 1 **Algorithm for determination of type of acidosis and mixed acid-base disturbances when the pH indicates acidaemia**

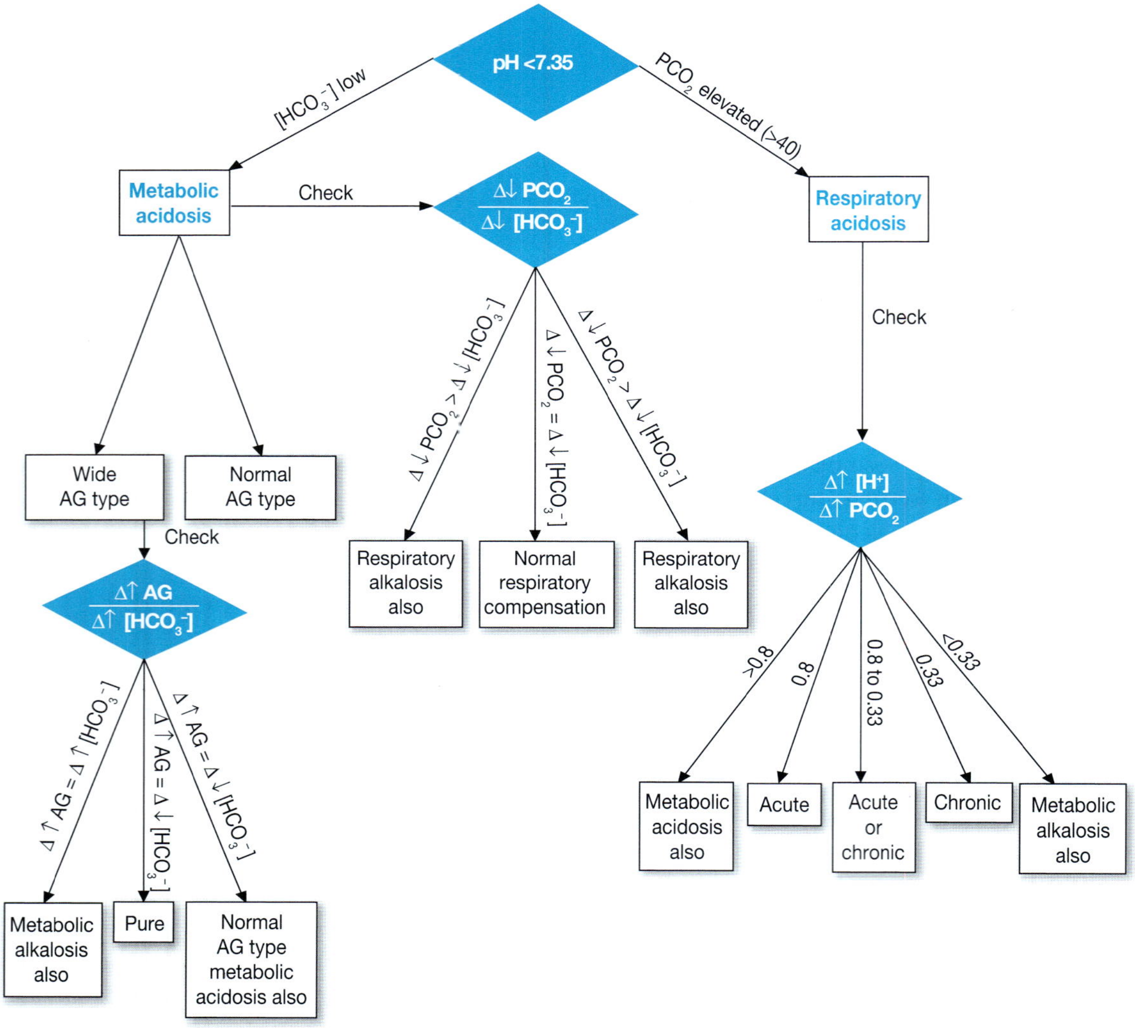

Figure reproduced with permission of the McGraw-Hill Companies, from Tintinalli JE, Kelen GD, Stapczynski JS, et al., eds. *Emergency Medicine: A Comprehensive Study Guide*. 5th ed. New York: McGraw-Hill; 2000: 133: Figure 21–2A.

- **Bicarbonate deficit (mEq) = 0.5 × Weight (kg) × (Desired – Measured) bicarbonate**

  In the absence of superimposed respiratory acid base disorder, a serum bicarbonate level of 15 mEq/L can be used to calculate the bicarbonate deficit. One-half of the bicarbonate deficit is replaced immediately and the rest is infused over the next 4 to 6 hours.

- **Alveolar–arterial (A–a) oxygen gradient**: The A–a gradient is not discussed there.

1. The A–a oxygen gradient can be used to assist the physician in differentiating between hypoxia caused by hypoventilation alone, in which the A–a gradient is normal, and that caused by ventilation–perfusion mismatch, right to left shunt and diffusion abnormalities, in which the A–a gradient is abnormal. For arterial blood gas taken in room air at sea level (partial pressures expressed in mmHg),

$$\text{A–a gradient} = \left[(760 - 47) \times FiO_2 - \frac{PaCO_2}{0.8} \right] - PaO_2$$

where FiO_2 is expressed in decimal.

2. To account for age-dependent variations,

A normal A–a gradient is defined as $\leq$ (age/4 + 4).

3. The A–a gradient can assist the emergency physician in determining the causes of hypoxia but literature remains unclear as to how to interpret a normal A–a gradient in the setting of a suspected pulmonary embolus.

- **QT interval**

  1. Useful rule of thumb: The QT interval should be less than one-half the RR interval. More precisely,

     Corrected QT interval (QTc) = $\dfrac{\text{QT}}{\sqrt{\text{RR}}}$.

  2. Normal QTc = 0.42 seconds.

  3. See Table 3 for the causes of prolonged QT interval.

TABLE 3 Causes of prolonged QT interval

Acquired long QT syndrome

• Drugs	1. Class 1A, 1C, and III antiarrhythmics (e.g. quinidine, procainamide, disopyramide, sotalol, and amiodarone) 2. Psychotropic agents (e.g. tricyclic anti-depressants, phenothiazines, tetracyclic agents, and haloperidol) 3. Others: Organophosphates, erythromycin, pentamidine, astemizole, and terfenadine
• Electrolyte abnormalities	1. Hypokalaemia 2. Hypomagnesaemia 3. Hypocalcaemia
• Cardiac abnormalities	1. Myocardial ischaemia 2. Myocarditis 3. Complete atrioventricular block 4. Sinus node dysfunction
• Intracranial disease	1. Subarachnoid haemorrhage
• Altered nutritional state	1. Liquid protein modified fast diet 2. Starvation (anorexia nervosa)

Congenital
- Jervell and Lange–Nielsen syndrome (autosomal recessive with congenital deafness)
- Romano–Ward syndrome (autosomal dominant)
- Sporadic type

FIGURE 2 **PEFR nomogram for adult Chinese in Singapore (Use height and age)**

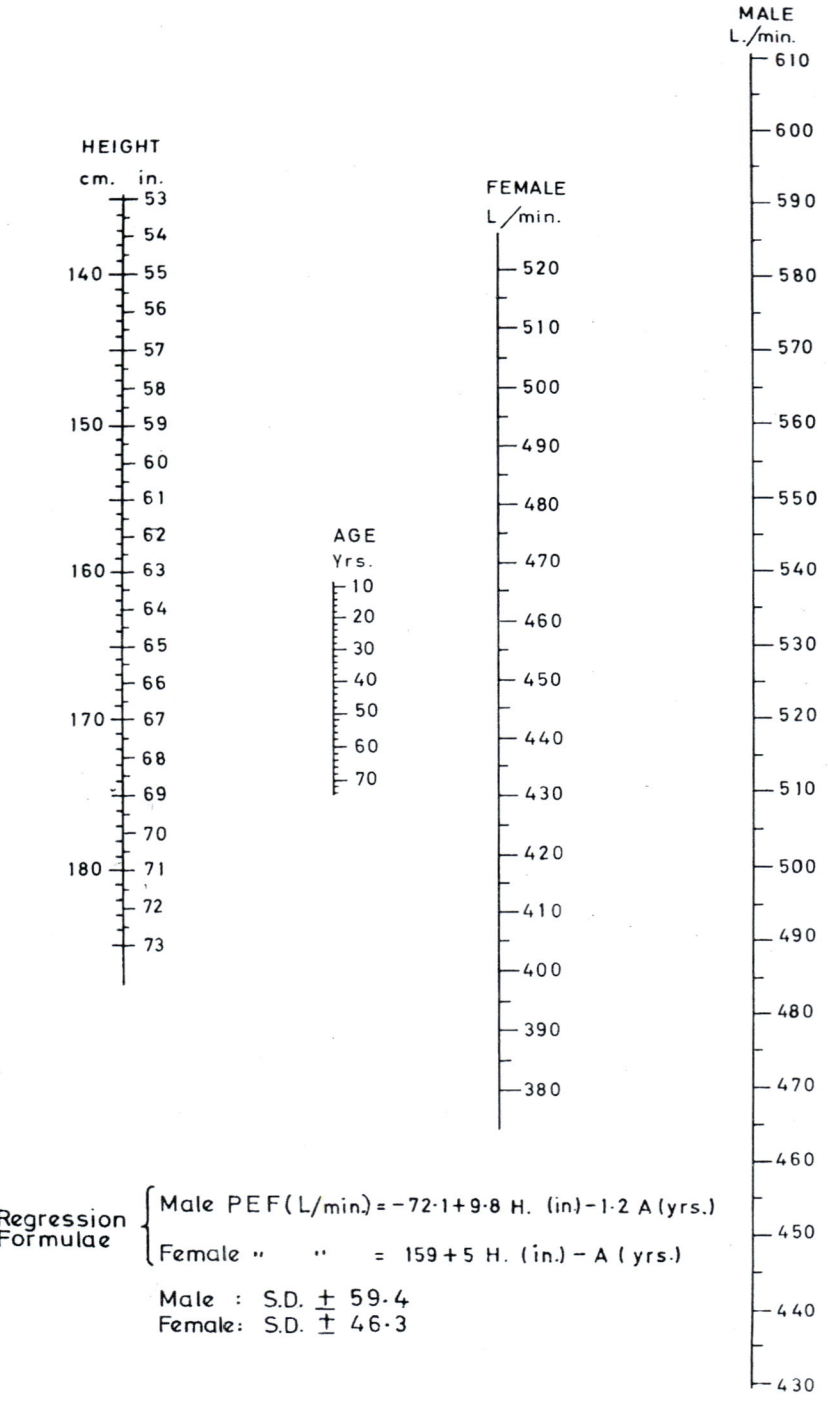

Regression Formulae

Male PEF (L/min.) = $-72 \cdot 1 + 9 \cdot 8$ H. (in.) $- 1 \cdot 2$ A (yrs.)

Female " " = $159 + 5$ H. (in.) $-$ A (yrs.)

Male : S.D. $\pm$ 59.4
Female: S.D. $\pm$ 46.3

- **Diagnostic tools for the evaluation of azotaemia**
  1. **Fractional excretion of sodium**:

  $$FE_{Na} = \frac{Urine\ (Na)/Plasma\ (Na) \times 100}{Urine\ (Cr)/Plasma\ (Cr)}$$

  2. **Renal failure index (RFI)**: $RFI = \dfrac{Urine_{Na+} \times Plasma_{Cr}}{Urine_{Cr}}$

  3. **Urine findings in prerenal azotaemia and acute tubular necrosis (ATN)**

Diagnostic tool	Prerenal Azotaemia	ATN
Urine osmolality U_{osmo} (mOsm/kg)	>500	<350
Urine sodium U_{Na} (mEq/L)	<20	>40
Urine/plasma creatinine (U/P Cr)	>40	<20
Renal failure index (RFI)	<1	>1
Fractional excretion of sodium FE_{Na+}	<1%	>1%
Blood urea nitrogen/Cr ratio (mg/dL)	>20	≤10

- **Peak flow**: See Figure 2.
- **Peak flow for men** (l/min) = **[3.95 − (0.0151 × Age)] × Height** (cm).
- **Peak flow for women** (l/min) = **[2.93 − (0.0072 × Age)] × Height** (cm).
- **Conversion factor between different units**:

  kPa = 0.133 × mmHg; **mmHg** = 7.5 × kPa
  °F = (9/5°C) + 32; **°C** = 5/9(°F − 32)
  Serum creatinine, mg/dL = mmol/L × 88.4
  Serum urea, mg/dL = mmol/L × 2.8
  Serum glucose, mg/dL = mmol/L × 18

References/Further Reading

1. Hope RA, Longmore JM, McManus SK, et al. *Oxford Handbook of Clinical Medicine*. 4th ed. Oxford, UK: Oxford University Press; 1998: 630–633.

2. Marino PL. *The ICU Book*. 2nd ed. Baltimore, MD: William & Wilkins; 1998: 340–342.

3. Nacouzi V. Fluids, electrolytes and acid-base disorders. In: Cline DH, Ma OJ, Tintinalli JE, et al., eds. *Emergency Medicine: A Comprehensive Study Guide Companion Handbook*. 5th ed. New York: McGraw-Hill; 2000: 46–52.

4. James JH, Bosker G. Mathematical Formulas, Equations, and Diagnostic Aids in Emergency Medicine: Practical and Systematic Approaches to Solving Complex Clinical Problems. *Emerg Med Rep*. 1995; 16(26): 255–266.

5. David DN, Kelen GD. Acid-base disorders. In: Tintinalli JE, Stapczynski JS, Ma OJ, et al., eds. *Tintinalli's Emergency Medicine: A Comprehensive Study Guide*. 7th ed. New York: McGraw-Hill; 2011: 102–112.

Index

Page numbers in **bold** print refer to main entries.

A

Abbreviated Injury Scale (AIS), **874**
ABCD$_2$ score, 463–4
ABCD survey, 233–4
  primary, **197–200**
  secondary, **200–2, 204**
  tachydysrhythmias, 304
abciximab, 245
abdominal aortic aneurysm (AAA), 55,
  225–8
abdominal bleeding, 869
abdominal colic, 24, 890
abdominal CT imaging, 51–2
abdominal examination, 11
abdominal films, 227
abdominal migraine, 814
abdominal pain, **51–7**
  in children, **810–14**
  colicky central, 57
  epigastric, 56–7
  flank pain, 55
  in haemodynamically stable patient,
    53
  in haemodynamically unstable
    patient, 52–3
  imaging for, 51–2
  life-threatening causes of, 51
  lower, 56
  pain management, 889–90
  right hypochondrial (RHC) pain,
    54
abdominal trauma, 118, 369, 600,
  600–5, 663, 672, 869–70
abdominal ultrasound
  for abdominal aortic aneurysm,
    771–2
  for cholecystitis, 772–3
abdominal x-ray view, 52, 775
abnormal vaginal bleeding, 11–13
abortion, 722, 731, 751, 753, 799
abrasions, 344, 643, 660, 715–16, 760,
  820
abruptio placentae, 663, 665
acarbose, 798

accelerated idioventricular rhythm
  (AIVR), 94
acceleration/deceleration injury, 612
acetaminophen, 118–19, 253, 473,
  580, *see also* paracetamol;
    paracetamol poisoning
acetazolamide, 18, 386, 583
acetophenetidin, 805
acetylcholine, 319, 571
acetylcysteine (Fluimicil®), 792
acetylralicylic acid, 805
achlorhydria, 388
acidaemia, 403, 916
acid base balance, 404, 406
acid base disorders, 141, 382–91
acid base emergencies, 293, 382–91
  acid base disorders, **382–91**
  alveolar–arterial (A–a) oxygen
    gradient, 916–17
  bicarbonate deficit (mEq), 916
  metabolic acidosis, **385–7**
  metabolic alkalosis, **387–9**
  respiratory acidosis, **387**
  respiratory alkalosis, **389**
  rules of compensation in, 915
acid burns, 739, 742–3
acid loss, 388
acidosis, 4, 20–1, 23, 45–6, 107, 112,
  120, 133, 136, 141, 202,
  216, 235, 320, 340, 358,
  360, 365, 371, 382–7, 390,
  393, 406, 414, 418, 422–3,
  425–6, 428, 477, 492, 543–6,
  554, 561, 565, 581–3, 607,
  751, 757, 780, 815, 822,
  836, 839, 915–16
ACLS Universal Algorithm, 198
acne rosacea, **520**
acne vulgaris, **519–20**
  comedonal acne, treatment for,
    519–20
  inflammatory lesions, treatment for,
    520
acoustic neuroma, 32, 704, 708–9

acquired immunodeficiency syndrome
  (AIDS), 530
acromioclavicular joint injuries, 676,
  676
activated charcoal, 5, 24, 113, 117–18,
  120, 188, 550, 560, 567, 573,
  578, 582–3, 794
acute abdomen, 51, 53–4, 429, 775,
  815, 889
acute adrenal insufficiency ('Addisonian
  crisis'), **392–4**
acute angle-closure glaucoma, 18, 122,
  124
acute arterial occlusion, 286
acute cardiogenic pulmonary oedema,
  262
acute cholangitis, 355, **357–8**
acute cholecystitis, **355–6**
acute coronary syndrome (ACS), 20–1,
  30, 36, 58, 61, 64, 147, 151,
  238–9, 242, 262, 267, 273,
  277, 282, 358, 368, 784,
  788
  clinical features of patients, 59
  intermediate likelihood of, 59
  -related heart failure, 262
acute decompensation of chronic left
  heart failure (ADHF), 262
acute epididymo-orchitis, **77**
acute heart failure, 36, **251–69**
  admission to observation units,
    268
  non-specific complaints, 262
  pharmacological management,
    264–7
  precipitating causes of, 263
  raised BNP or NT-proBNP, 263
acute hydrocephalus, 459
acute ischaemic stroke (AIS), 275
acute laryngo-tracheo-bronchitis (ALTB),
  142
  in paediatrics, 143
acute left ventricular failure, 276–7
acute liver failure, 473

acute myocardial infarction (AMI), 240, 277, 392
    atypical, 240
    criteria for diagnosis of, 240
    in elderly, **535–6**
acute pancreatitis, 400
acute respiratory distress syndrome (ARDS), 342, 371, 472, 560, 755
acute tonsllllltis, 712
acute tubular necrosis (ATN), 544, 919
acute urticaria, **515–16**
acyclovir, 508, 510, 528, 704, 709, 787, 802, 859
adapalene, 520
Addison's disease, 386, 393
Adenitis, 345
adenopathy, 145, 295, 776
adenosine, 90, 98, 101, 106, 133, 306–7, 309, 311, 314, 791, 808, 858
adenovirus infection, 125
adhesion colic, 57
adhesions, 57, 361, 429, 770
Adhesive capsulitis, 682
ADORA (AntiDepressant Overdose Risk Assessment) score, 562
adrenaline, 84, 139–40, 143–4, 188–91, 201, 204–5, 233–4, 320, 380, 569, 596, 705, 780, 808, 850–1, 858, 863, 881, 883, 893–9
adrenal insufficiency, 132, 136, 220, 386, 392–5, 401, 411, 413, 419
adrenocorticotropin (ACTH), 393
adult respiratory distress syndrome, 20, 218, 544, 553, 598, 608, 620
advanced airway devices, 194
advanced cardiac life support (ACLS), 194–7, 229, 303
Advanced Trauma Life Support (ATLS), 600–1, 620
adverse cutaneous drug reactions, **531–2**
Aedes aegypti, 470, 475, **475**
Aedes albopictus, **475**
aerocoele, 619
afebrile patient
    flank pain, 55
    right hypochondrial (RHC) pain, 54
Agarol®, 378

aged patients, *see* geriatric emergencies
age-related macular degeneration, 17
agitation, 21, 146, 168–70, 396, 416, 547, 556–7, 596, 840, 842–3
air embolism, 156, 427–8, 746, 882, 884, 886
airway, breathing and circulation (ABCs), 399, 664
airway management, 114, 129, 136, 142, 172–85, **172–85,** 188, 190, 320, 340, 650, 718, 734, 834, 904
airway obstruction, 20, 22, 116, 139, 145–6, 187, 199, 301, 606, 614, 620, 649, 733, 842, 846
albendazole, 788
alcohol, 446
alcohol abuse/alcoholism, 7, 69, 126, 128, 151, 328, 398, 413, 537, 577, 590
alcohol dehydrogenase (ADH), 543, 545
alcoholic ketoacidosis, 112, 386, 546, **546–8**
alcohol intoxication, 539–48
    altered mental state in, 539
    children exposed to, 542
    differential diagnosis, 539
    discharge criteria, 542
    drug therapy, 541–2
    evaluation and management of immediate life-threatening complications, 545
    indications for haemodialysis, 546
    management principles, 539–40
    methanol, ethylene glycol and isopropyl alcohol toxicity, 543–4
    renal failure in, 544
    supportive care, 540–1
    withdrawal seizures in, 546–7
alcoholism, 69
alcohol withdrawal syndrome (AWS), 547
A-lines, 763
alkali burns, 19, 739, 742–3
alkaline diuresis, 120, 599
alkalinisation of urine, 752
alkalinization, 114, 120, 561, 582–3, 803
alkalosis, 46, 134, 156, 339, 352, 382, 385–90, 403, 424, 426, 581, 757, 915

see also metabolic alkalosis; respiratory alkalosis
allergic reactions, 20, 52, 140, 186–9, **186–92**, 191, 517, 529, 792, 903–4
allopurinol, 71, 435, 497, 506, 530–1
alopecia, 531
Alphavirus, **475**
alprazolam, 46
altered mental state (AMS), 2–5, **2–5**, 23, 46, 107, 111, 114, 120, 159–60, 172, 187, 211, 217, 264, 267, 273–4, 328, 330, 350, 382, 390, 392, 398–9, 409, 413, 416, 419, 425, 436–7, 492, 534, 537, 539–41, 549–50, 552–3, 582, 616, 750, 752, 755–6, 761
    in alcohol intoxication, 539
    approach to differential diagnosis of, 3
    causes, 4
    cocktail, 4
    due to suspected structural causes, 5
    due to suspected toxic-metabolic causes, 5
    suspicion of drug overdose (DO), 107
altered nutritional state, 917
alternative hypothesis, 910
aluminium hydroxide, 374, 497, 794
Alvarado scoring system, 347
alveolar–arterial oxygen gradient, 340, 342
amaurosis, 18, 460
amaurosis fugax, 18
aminoglycosides, 33, 53, 219, 709, 786, 807
aminophylline, 325
amiodarone, 101, 104, 106, 201, 204, 260, 311–15, 419, 501, 566, 781, 808, 858, 917
amitriptyline, 43, 444, 446, 510, 556–7, 797
amlodipine, 283, 790
amnesia, 462, 618–19, 750, 870
amniotic fluid embolus, 663
amoebiasis, 25
amorolfine, 515
amoxapine, 556–7
amoxicillin, 70, 324, 332, 432, 501, 513, 522–4, 708–9, 712, 784, 807, 859–60

amoxicillin + clavulanate (Augmentin®), 324, 522–4, 784
amoxicillin plus cloxacillin, 524
amphetamines, 108–11, 118, 263, 272, 278, 756
amphotericin B, 787, 859
ampicillin, 253, 440, 590, 859
ampicillin-sulbactam, 590
AMPLE, 154, 161
amyl nitrite pearls, 119
anaemia, 6, 11, 20, 33–4, 245, 255–6, 263, 339, 373–5, 389, 420, 428, 477–8, 487, 523, 531, 552, 662
anaerobic microorganisms, 53, 55
anaerobic respiration, 133
anaesthesia, regional, 214, 588, 892–3
anal fissures, 378, **378**
anal fistula, 379
Analysis of Variance (ANOVA), 912
anaphylactoid reactions, 186, 192, **192,** 501, 531
anaphylaxis, 20–1, 140–1, 146, 186–92, **187–9**, 295, 517, 531–2, 596, 780, 904
Anarex®, 782
anatomic scores, 874
Anexate, 4, 115, 119, 556, 803, 903
angina, 58–60, 64, 222, 239–40, 244, 249, 400, 487, 518, 552, 703, 788–9, 890
angioedema/anaphylaxis, 20, 135, 143–4, 146, **146**, 186, **190–1**, 490, 531
    drug-induced, 190
    hereditary, 191
angiotension converting enzyme inhibitor, 269
animal bite, 132
    see also snake bites
ankle block, 899
ankle dislocation, 645
ankle fracture, 645
ankle injury, 637, **644–5**, 644–6
ankylosing spondylitis, 67
anogenital warts, 526
anorectal sepsis, 378–9
anorexia, 251, 328, 345, 347, 355, 392, 396, 399, 407, 411, 442, 460, 495, 536–7, 569, 577, 837, 918
anorexia nervosa, 411, 917
antacids., 373, 794, 808, 821, 865
antepartum haemorrhage, 14, 152
anterior cord syndrome, 670

anterior hip dislocation, 637–8
anti-bacterial, 513
antibiotics, 324
antibiotics, IV, 53
anticholinergics, 5, 17, 108–9, 111, 756
anticholinesterase drugs, 108, 596
anticoagulants, 11, 42, 312
anticonvulsants, 26, 33, 108, 506
anti-depressant poisoning, 107
anti-depressants, 110, 132, 166, 413, 446, 510, 549, 556–7, 559–61, 563, 575, 917
antidiarrhoeal drugs, 864
antidotes for toxins, 119
antidysrhythmics, 33, 104
antiemetic, 24, 890
anti-epileptic drug (AED), 126, 501, 530, 809
anti-fungal, 513
antihistamines, 33, 108–9, 111, 125, 165, 188–92, 490, 508, 512–13, 516–17, 526, 530, 532, 596, 711, 756, 863
antihypertensive, 31, 33, 108, 272, 275, 459, 530, 720, 789
anti-inflammatory agents, 33, 507
anti-malarials, 413, 477, 511, 709, 805
antineutrophil cytoplasmic antibody (ANCA)-associated vasculitis, 518
antipyretics, 26, 209, 416, 439, 490–1, 758, 828, 832, 846–7, 861
antispasmodics, 54, 354, 837
anti-tetanus toxoid (ATT), 485, 596, 628, 697, 752, 809
antithrombin deficiency, 289
anti-ulcerants, 865
antivenin, 594–6
antivirals, 787, 859
anuria., 223, 719, 781, 790
anxiety, 30, 59 87, 111, 115, 152, 217, 240, 244, 277, 351, 389, 547, 572, 574, 751, 755, 819, 902
aortic disruption, traumatic, 612
aortic aneurysm, abdominal, 8, 52–3, 55–6, 72, 81, 147, 225, 368, 374, 434, 537, 771
aortic aneurysm (aortoenteric fistula), 6
aortic aneurysms, 225
aortic arch syndrome, 148
aortic dissection, 20–1, 51–2, 55–6, 58–60, 64, 73, 147–8, 180,

211, 221–5, 246, 264, 273, 276, 279–82, 368, 374, 450, 455, 789, 810
aortic stenosis, 34, 139, 148, 152, 245, 266
aortobronchial fistula, 39
aortoenteric fistula, 6, 8
apathy, 351, 540
APGAR (American Pediatric Gross Assessment Record) assessment of the newborn, 730
aphasia, 443, 449, 451, 462, 750
apnoea, 172, 179–80, 761, 842–3
apnoeic oxygenation, 179–80
appendicitis, 23, 27, 51–2, 56, 81, 345–8, 358, 375, 431, 433–4, 536–7, 731, 810–11, 813–14, 823, 835–6
    acute, **345–8**
    by the Alvarado score and management strategies, 348
    borderline cases of, 347
    clinical probability of acute, 346
    differential diagnosis of, 345
appetite loss, 359, 375, 547
Apresoline, 720
aqueous cream, 802
'arch' fracture, 656
arrhythmogenic ventricular dysplasia, 152
arsenic, 109, 118–19
arterial blood gas, 21, 28, 128, 146, 158, 160, 218, 259, 267, 293, 318, 323, 325, 328, 331, 339–40, 342, 358, 365, 382, 391, 393–4, 404, 406, 420, 425–6, 428, 438, 541, 545, 549, 552, 560, 567, 583, 595, 607, 622, 665, 734, 747, 752, 757, 760, 839, 917
arterial gas embolism (AGE), **746–8**
arteritis, temporal, 17–18, 41, 44, 460–1, 891
arthralgia, 475, 517
arthritis, 26, 47, 60, 66–71, 179, 250, 437, 491, 518, 632, 635, 641, 669, 783, 827, 830
arthrocentesis, 68
articular pain, 66
ascites, 251, 254, 258, 352, 471, 604, 770, 773
aseptic meningitis, 472, 508–9
aseptic necrosis, 751
asphalt burns, 742

asphyxiation, 38–9
aspiration, 7–8, 20, 39, 69, 83, 117,
        145, 158, 172, 182, 328,
        332, 336–8, 343, 405, 544–5,
        550, 553–4, 560, 620, 643,
        662, 706, 750, 759–60,
        816–17, 832, 838, 846, 879,
        885
aspiration pneumonia, 20, 328, 553,
        560, 750
aspirin, 24, 43, 61, 64, 118, 191–2,
        241–5, 252, 287, 312, 416,
        444, 451, 463–4, 473, 476,
        508, 581, 758, 783, 788–9,
        805, 807, 814–15
assault, non-sexual, **715–16**
astemizole, 917
asterixis, 534
asthma, 184, **316–21**, 816
    aims of emergency department
            therapy, 318–19
    bronchodilators, 319
    in children, **838–40**
    classification of severity, 317
    clinical assessment, 316
    definition, 316
    drugs, 862
    investigations, 318
    levels of control, 318
    magnesium sulphate, 319
    risk factors of death from, 317
    steroids, 319
asystole, 195, 200, 202, 204–6, **205**,
        234, 309, 556, 750, 753,
        780
    algorithm, 206
Atarax, 516
ataxia, 32, 399, 443, 457, 540–1, 549,
        552, 556, 747
atelectasis, 293, 817
atenolol, 244, 446, 790, 808
atherosclerosis, 57, 221, 227, 286, 364
atopic dermatitis, 530
atractaspididae, 592
atracurium (Tracium®), 185, 485, 782,
        865
atrial fibrillation (AF), 36, 57, **91**, 101,
        106, 213, 258–60, 263, 267,
        286, 288, 305, 307, 310, 364,
        416, 449, 463, 500, 536, 564,
        781
    with pre-excitation (WPW), 311
    rhythm control in, 311
atrial flutter, **90**, 307, 791
    with variable block, 307

atrial tachycardia, **88–9**
atrial thrombus, 312
atropine, 11, 109, 119, 195, **195**, 202,
        215, 232–4, 567, 569, 571,
        571, 573–5, 596, 780, 782,
        804, 858, 862, 867, 887,
        905
Atroven, 793, 862
atypical chest pain syndrome, 64
augmentin, 219, 493, 522, 586, 590,
        590, 697–8, 709, 711, 784,
        807, 859
auricular block, **894**
Auspitz's sign, 510
autoimmune disorders, 250, 253, 392
automated external defibrillator (AED),
        197
automated implantable cardiac
        defibrillator, 103
autonomic neuropathy, 148, 240
avascular necrosis, 66, 637–9, 682, 690,
        750
AV blocks, 231, 234, 238, 565
AV nodal re-entrant tachycardia
        (AVNRT), 306
AV re-entrant tachycardia (AVRT), 306
awake intubation technique, 734
azithromycin, 25, **25**, 219, 325, 332,
        711
azotaemia, 919
azotemia, 352, 363

B

Bacillus, 438, 585–6
back pain, 72–3, 226, 430, 491, 496,
        500, 537, 746, **889**
baclofen, **890**
bacteraemia, 3, 216–17, 537–**8**, 827
bacterial infections, 473, 521, 529
bacterial meningitis, 438
Bacteroides sp., 585
bactrim, 25, 436, 586, 590, 711, 860
Baker's cyst, 47
BAL, 119, 806
balanoposthitis, **81**
barbiturates, 26, 109–11, 120, 129, 506,
        531, 549
Barton's fracture, **689**
Bartter's syndrome, 388
basal pneumonia, 358
basal skull fracture, 619
basic cardiac life support (BCLS), 194
basilar pneumonia, 53–4, 822, 836
bat's sign, 763
Bazett's correction for heart rate, 104

Beck's triad, 212, **251**, 609, 619
beclomethasone, 793
beclotide, 862
Behcet's disease, 518
Bell's palsy (idiopathic facial nerve
        paralysis), 450–1, **703–4**, 787
benign positional vertigo, 32
benign prostatic hypertrophy, 166, **166**
Bennett's fracture, **692**
benzodiazepine (BZD), 115, 547
benzodiazepine overdose, 803
    antidotal therapy, 550
    pathophysiology, 549–50
benzodiazepine poisoning, **549–50**
benzodiazepines, 4, 108, 111, 115,
        119, 121, 129, **129**, 266,
        519, 531, 539, 546, 549–50,
        803
benzoyl peroxide, 520
benztropine, 119, **796**, 832, 845
benztropine (Cogentin®), 796
benzyl benzoate (EBB), 525
beriberi, 49
berry aneurysm, 180, 456–7
beserol, 899
beta-agonist, 319, 324
beta blockers, 244, 263, 417, 446, 547,
        767
beta-haemolytic *streptococcus*, 144, 697
beta-hydroxybutyrate, 404
betamethasone, 802
betamethasone dipropionate, 514
betamethasone valerate, 514
bias, **908**
bicarbonate, 114, 136, 140–1, 195,
        340, 382, 384–8, 391, 394,
        396, 403, 406–7, 423–4, 426,
        545–6, 554, 556, 558, 560–2,
        583, 780, 803, 858, 887,
        915–16, 7520
bicarbonate therapy, 426
Bier's block, 688–91, 693, 888, **892**,
        892–3
Bier's ischaemia, 744
bilateral chest expansion, 195
biliary colic, 54, **354–5**, **354–5**, 368,
        815
biliary stone disease, 51
biliary tract disease, 345
bilious vomiting, 810–11
bimanual examination, 12
BiPAP, 343
BIPP, 705
bisacodyl (Dulcolax®), 795, **795**, 807
bismuth subsalicylate, 24

bisolvon, 844, 863
bisoprolol, 446
bites
  dog and cat, **585–6**
  drug therapy, 589–90
  human, **586–7**
  snake, **592–6**
  wound care, 587–9
blast injuries, 610–11, 614
bleach (poison), 21
bleeding disorders, 789
bleeding ectopic pregnancy, 12
bleeding gastrointestinal tract (GIT),
    6–10
  common causes, 6
  lower, 9
  upper, 9
blepharospasm, 123
blinding/masking, 908, **908**
B-lines, 764
blisters, 507, 522, 532, 559, 739–40,
    740, **743**
β-blockers, 310
blood alcohol level, 539, 620
blood analysis
  cardiomyopathies, 258
  CO poisoning, 554
  digoxin poisoning, 567
  disseminated gonococcal infection
    (DGI), 70
  eclampsia, 718
  generalized exfoliative dermatitis
    (GED), 531
  heat stroke, 757
  infective endocarditis, 256
  intestinal obstruction, 362
  ischaemic bowel, 365
  liver abscess, 359
  meningitis, 438
  myxoedema, 420
  pancreatitis, acute, 370
  paracetamol poisoning, 578
  poisoning, 112
  shock/hypoperfusion states, 136
  urinary tract infections (UTI), 431
  urolithiasis, 434
blood and blood products,
    administration in ED
  allergic reaction, **490**
  cryoprecipitate, **488**
  emergency blood transfusion,
    489–90
  factor VIII or factor IX concentrates,
    488–9
  febrile reaction, **490**

fresh frozen plasma (FFP), **488**
  haemophilia A, **488**
  haemophilia B, **488**
  platelets, **487–8**
  red blood cells, **487**
  whole blood, **486–7**
blood gases, 134, 136, 207, 293, 325,
    358, 365, 382, 391, 394, 408,
    426, 545, 552, 560, 567, 583,
    607, 622, 752, 833
blood glucose, 21, 46, **137**, 403, 405–7,
    409, 412–14, 417, 420, 426,
    438, 451, 453, 478, 550, 734,
    757, 832
blood loss, 6, 8, 33–4, 136, **138**, 147,
    149, 152, 158–9, 336, 428,
    474, 486–7, 609, 615–16,
    649, 660, 662, 667, 730, 812,
    868, 870
blood sugar level, 379, 404, 451, **832**
blood transfusions, 238, **486–7**
'blow out' orbital fractures, **653–5**
blue dot sign, 78
blue-toe syndrome, 226, **255**, **266**, 287,
    287
blunt cardiac injury/myocardial
    contusion, **611**
blunt trauma, 162–3, 602, 604, 615,
    629, 649–50, 661, 664, 667,
    672, 751, 753, 869
blurring of vision, acute, **16–19**
blurring of vision, **16–19**
body fluid/needlestick exposure, **481–3**
Boerhaave's syndrome, 61
bolus therapy, 426
bone tumours, 50
bony metastases, **491**
Boutonniere deformity, **630–1**
boutonniere splint, 631
bowel ischaemia, 364
bowel obstruction, 57, 118, 120, 361,
    426, 434, **536**, 811–12
bowel perforation/injury, 120, 603, 751
Boyle's law, 746
brachial artery damage, 683
bradycardias, 104, 108, 110, 135, 140,
    148, 151, 158, 184, 195, 214,
    229, **229**–30, 233–6, 278–9,
    281–2, **308**, 317, 401, 419–20,
    471, 559, 568, 571, 574, 621,
    667, 780, 831, 840, 858,
    867–8
bradydysrhythmias, 85, **229–38**
  ABCD survey, 233–4
  approach to, 230

cardiac monitoring, 238
  drugs and modalities, 235
  first-degree heart block, 229–30
  indications for telemetry admission,
    238
  intervention sequence for, 234–6
  mobitz type II second-degree heart
    block, 231
  mobitz type I second-degree heart
    block, 230–1
  2:1 second-degree heart block,
    232
  sinus, 229
  symptoms and signs, 234
  third-degree heart block, 232
  transcutaneous pacing, 235–6
  universal algorithm, 233
brain absces, 256
brain injury, 160–1, **616**, 618, 666
brain oedema, 473, 622
brain-specific serum biomarkers, 620
brainstem problem, **30**
brain tumour, 4, 127, 272, 450
breast cancer, 401
breath-holding attacks, 831
breathlessness, 5, **20–2**, 85, 95, **234**,
    304, 317, **498–9**, **815–18**,
    843
breathlessness, acute, **20–2**
  clinical assessment, 21
  common causes, 20
  principles of management of patients,
    22
  supportive measures, 22
bromhexine, 792
bromide, 109, 320, 839, 862
bronchial artery embolization, 40
bronchiectasis, 39, 316
bronchiolitis, 816, 838, **842–4**
bronchitis, 38–9, 142, 537, 792, 816,
    838
bronchodilators, 182, **189**, 263, **319**,
    322, 324, **324**, 841, 843–4
bronchogenic carcinoma, 316
bronchomalacia, 838
bronchopneumonia, 552, 554
bronchopulmonary dysplasia, 842
bronchorrhoea, 111, 571, 573
bronchospasm, 111, 187, 189, 240,
    281, 323, 400, 571, 573,
    828–9
Brown–Sequard syndrome, 670
Brufen, 783, **829**
Brugada syndrome, **102–4**, 150, 152
bruises, 155, 159, 826, 854

budesonide/formoterol (Symbicort®), 793

budesonide (Pulmicort®, Inflammide®), 793

bulging fontanelles, 820

bullous cellulitis/erysipelas, *see* pyoderma

bumetamide (Burinex®), 790

bundle branch block, 59, 86, **93**, 106, 231, 241–2, 292, 294

bupivacaine, 899

Burkholderia pseudomallei, 327, 332

burns
  acid/alkali, 742–3
  assessment and fluid regime, 734–6
  blisters, 740
  cooling, 740
  follow-up care, 741
  hand exposure, 744
  major, **732–8**
  minor, **739–45**
  minor facial, 740
  '10–15' rule, 740
  tar or asphalt, 742
  wound management, 736–8

Buscopan® (hyoscine-N-butylbromide), 24, 165, 354, 374, 794, 807, 864, **890**

C

cachexia, 177, 437

cafergot, 43, 445, **797**, 807

caffeine, 108, 444–5, **797**, 807

calcaneal fracture/injury, 646

calcaneal fractures, **646**

calcium channel blockers, 101, 113, 260, 276–7, **310**–11, 407, 446, **446**, 459, 556, 568–9

calcium chloride, **302**, 400, 423, **744**, 780

calcium disodium edetate, 119

calcium gluconate, 235, **235**, 400, 422, **422**–3, 633, 718–19, 743–5, 780, 858

calcium pyrophosphate, 67

camphor poisoning, 109

Campylobacter, 25

Campylobacter jejuni, 821

Canadian C-spine rule, 673–4

Canadian CT Head Rule, 618

candesartan, 446

Candida, 255, 430

candidal infections of the skin, **515**

candidiasis, 530

Capnocytophaga canimorsus, **586**

captopril, 254, **254**, **266**, 269, 284, **284**, 530, 790, **790**, 808

carbamazepine, 26, 117, 506, 531, 890, **890**

carbimazole, 798

carbohydrate-rich drink, 413

carbon monoxide, 119

carbon monoxide (CO) poisoning, 41, 339, 386, 389, 550, **551–5**
  acute exposure and, 552
  antidote therapy, 554
  complications, 553
  high-risk groups, 553
  sources, 551–2
  supportive measures, 554

carbon monoxide neuropsychological screening battery (CONSB), 555

carbon rnonoxide neuropsychiatric screening battery, 555

carboxyhaemoglobinaemia, 112, 552

carbuncles, **523**

carcinoma, 316, 401, 434, 722

cardiac arrest, 86, 154, 162, **193–210**, 233, 240, 303, 305, 552, 559, 568, 606, 665, 742, 747, 753
  algorithm, **193–7**
  defined, 193
  monitoring during, 205–7
  3-phase time-sensitive model of, 193
  post resuscitation care, 207–10

cardiac asthma, **264**

cardiac cocktail, **862**

cardiac contusion, 613

cardiac disorders, *see* bradycardias; tachycardias

cardiac dysrhythmias, 20, 30, **36**, 250, 544, 633, 752, 760
  giddiness and, 36

cardiac enzymes, 7–8, 49, 53, 56, 61, 64, 137, 208, 223, 239, 241, **241**–2, 244, 254, 258–9, 404, 428, 454, 567

cardiac injury, 609, **611**, 750

cardiac ischaemia, 820

cardiac markers, **62**, 62–4, 243, 268, 788–9

cardiac monitoring, 238

cardiac murmur, 34

cardiac syncope, **31**, 147

cardiac tamponade, 20, 45, 132, 137, 139, 158, 162, 181, 225, 249–51, 609, **766–7**

cardiac ultrasound

for cardiac tamponade, 766–7
  for estimation of left ventricular ejection function, 767–8
  for massive acute pulmonary embolism, 768–9

cardiogenic pulmonary oedema, **262**

cardiogenic shock, 136–**9**, 141, 211–13, **211–13**, 249, **249**, 254, 262, **262**, 405, 767

cardiomegaly, 251, 254, 258, 263, 265, 420, 776

cardiomyopathies
  causes, 258
  dilated, 258
  HOCM, 258
  investigations, 258–9
  management, 259–60
  RDVC, 258
  restrictive, 258
  symptoms and signs, 258
  systolic dysfunction and diastolic dysfunction, 257

cardiopulmonary arrest, 145, 156, 187, 549, 615

cardiopulmonary failure, 586

cardiorespiratory arrest, 134

cardiorespiratory depression, 129

cardiovascular collapse, 112, 266, 280, 390, 581, 634, 663

cardiprin, 64

carotid sinus hypersensitvity syndrome, 148

carotid sinus massage, **307–8**, 308

carpal navicular fracture, **689–90**

carpal tunnel syndrome, 688, 896

cataracts, 16–17, 751

cat bites, **585–6**

catecholamines, 181, 234, 266, **278**, 292, 385, 390

cathartics, **118**

cauda equina syndrome, 73–**4**, 496

'cauliflower ear,' 702

C-collar, 159

cefaclor, 709

cefazolin, 69, 219, 524, **524**, 627, 644, 692

ceftazidime (Fortum®), 28, 80, 219, 332, 427, 440, 493, **521**, 785, **785**

ceftriaxone (Rocephin®), 8, 28, 53, 70, 79, 128, 144, **144**–5, **145**, 219, 332, 346, 356, 358, 363, 366, 432, 440–1, 441, **517**, 586, **732**, 785, **785**, 860

cefuroxime (Zinnat®), 325, 785, **785**, 860
celecoxib (Celebrex®), 783
cellular hypoxia, **109**, 544
cellulitis, 17, 27, 47–**8**, 48, 50, 66, 68, 302, 505, **509**, 521–**4**, 590, 711, 785, 830
central cord syndrome, 669, **669**
central hip dislocation, **637–8**
central nervous system, 2, 26–7, 108, 114–15, 120, 150, 240, 272, 339, 387, 389, 416, 440–1, 484, 494, 497, 539, 542, 544–5, 550, 552, 557, 569, **572**, 581, 583, 594, 755, 797, 845
central nervous system depression, 544–5, 550
central neurogenic hyperventilation, 45
central pontine myelinolysis, 398
central retinal artery occlusion (CRAO), 17–18
central retinal vein occlusion (CRVO), 17–18
central vertigo, **32**, 34
cephalexin (Keflex®), 508, 513, 522, **522–4**, 523–4, 785, 860
cephalosporin, 219, 325, 358, 493, 586, 711, 784–**5**, 807, 860
Cephazolin®, 785
cerebellar stroke, 3
cerebral abscess, 3, 127
cerebral arterial gas embolism, 760
cerebral artery aneurysms, **457**
cerebral autoregulation, 276
cerebral concussion, 539
cerebral contusion, 539
cerebral infarction, 272, 428
cerebral ischaemia, 282, 487, 621
cerebral malaria, 3, 127, 480
cerebral oedema, 275, 351, 396–7, 397, 404–5, 413, 551–2, 582, 603, 750, 755, 781
cerebral perfusion pressure (CPP), 275
cerebral salt wasting, 459
cerebral vasoconstriction, 196, 208, 390
cerebrospinal fluid rhinorrhoea, 159, 653, 751
cerebrovascular accident, 7, 166, 184, 240, 389, 535, 550, 748
cerebrovascular disease, 35, 147, 238, 329–30, 500
cervical soine clearance, **667–74**
cervical spine control/injury, **155**, 620

cervical spine (C-spine) clearance, **672–4**
cervical spine x-rays, **774–5**
cervical tumours, 15
cervical/vulvar warts, 526
cetirizine (Zyrtec®), 516–17, 792
cetrimide shampoo, 523
CHADS₂ score, 312
CHA₂DS₂-VASc score, 312
charcoal, *see* activated charcoal
Charcot's triad, 357
Charcot's triad, **357**
chemical burns, **633**, 733
  of the hand, **633**
chemical cardioversion, **307**, 310, 312, **312**, 315
chemoprophylaxis, 439
chemotherapy, 26, 136, 217, 253, 258, 275, 492, 494, 497
chest infections, 146, **816**
chest pain, **58–64**, 428
  benign causes, 59
  cardiac causes, 58
  in cases of AMI, 60, 63
  in cases of CAD, 60
  crescendo pattern, 59
  diagnoses by exclusion, 59
  disposition of patients with, 64
  ECG, role of, 61
  gastrointestinal causes, 58
  ischaemic, 59, 64
  life-threatening causes of, 58
  at new-onset angina, 64
  pain management, 890
  referred pain, 58
  respiratory causes, 58
  role of CXR, 64
chest trauma, 20, 339, 387, 541, 606, **606–15**, 608–9, 614, 620, **869**
  blunt cardiac injury/myocardial contusion, 611
  crush injuries to the chest, 613
  emergency department (ED) thoracotomy in trauma setting, 615
  flail chest, **608**
  massive haemothorax, 609–10
  penetrating injury to the chest, 613–14
  pericardial tamponade, **609**
  pulmonary contusion, 610
  rib fractures, 612–13
  tracheobronchial injuries, 610–11
  traumatic aortic disruption, 612

traumatic diaphragmatic rupture, 613
chikungunya, **475**
child abuse, 81, 853, 855
child exploitation, 853
children
  abdominal pain, **810–14**
  asthma in, **838–40**
  breathlessness, **815–18**
  crying baby/child, **819–20**
  diarrhoea, **821–4**
  with fever, **825–30**
  seizures in, **831–4**
  vomiting, **835–7**
chi-square test, **911**
Chlamydia, 11, 70, 79, 430, 528, 721, 732, 842
Chlamydia trachomatis, 79
chloral hydrate, 108, 113, 861
chloramphenicol, 517, **800**, 805
chloramphenicol eye drops, 800
chlorhexidine, 481, 523, 694, **801**, 876, 881
chlorhexidine cream, 801
chlorhexidine wash, 801
chloroquine, **478–9**, 805
chloroquine phosphate, 479
chlorpheniramine (Piriton®), 118, 189–90, 192, 508, 516–17, 526, 792, **792**, 863
chlorpromazine (Largactil®/Thorazine®), 43, 112, 118, 757, 797, **797**, 809, 862
cholangitis, 54, 132, 219, 355, **357–8**, 368, 374
cholecystitis, 27–8, 54, 219, 355–6, 374, 472, 537, **772**, 811
cholesteatoma, 32
cholinergics, 109, 111, **111**, 804
cholinesterase, 556, 571, 573
choreoathetosis, 557
chronic actinic dermatitis, 530
chronic heart failure, giddiness and, 36
chronic kidney disease, 424
chronic obstructive airway disease, 263
chronic obstructive lung disease, 279, **322**, **325**, 341, 387
chronic obstructive pulmonary disease (COPD), **322–5**
  classification, 322
  clinical assessment, 323
  diagnosis of, 322
  drug therapy, 324–5
  supportive measures, 324
  ventilatory settings, 324

chronic otitis media, 710
chronic plaque psoriasis (psoriasis vulgaris), 510, **511**
chronic renal failure, 7, 45, 47, 184, 412, 422, 424–**5**, 434, 622, 696
chronic urticaria, **516–17**
Chvostek sign, 400
ciliary flush, 122–3
cimetidine, 26, 189, 569, 758, **795**, 808, 865
cimetidine (Tagamet®), 189
ciprofloxacin, 8, **8**, 23, 25, 70, 79, 81, 219, 358, 432, **437**, 441, **441**, 493, 506, 518, **524**–5, 586, 590, **590**, 699, 786, **786**, **800**, 805
ciprofloxacin eye and ear drops, 800
circumferential ligature ('pseudoainhum'), 820
cirrhosis, chronic liver, 350
Clarinase, 710
clarithromycin, 325, 332, **524**, 807, 860
Clarityne, 710
clavicular fractures, **675**
clindamycin, 80, **145**, 219, 478–80, 520–**1**, 525, 586, 590, **590**, 732, **732**, 785, **785**
clonidine, 108–9, 278, 280–1, 284
clopidogrel (Plavix®), 242, 788
closed head injury, 184
clostridial myositis, 751
Clostridium, 25, 80, 484, 586
Clostridium difficile, 25
Clostridium tetani, 484
clotrimazole, 515, 799
cloxacillin, 69, 257, 508, 513, 522, **522**–4, 523, 526, 531, 634–5, 697, 784, 860
coagulation disorder, 39
coagulation necrosis, 750
cocaine, 83, 102, 108–11, 118, 120, 241, 263, 272, 278–9, 350, 756
codeine, 43, 782, 807, 891
coenzyme Q10, 446
Cogentin, 119, 796, 845
cognitive dysfunction, 751
colchicine, 71
colic, 24, 51, 54, 57, 226, 345, **354–5**, 358, 368, 433–5, 811, 814–15, 819, **889–90**
colicky central abdominal pain, **57**
colicky pain, 57, 355, 811–12

colitis, 23, 34, 823
Colles' fracture, **687–8**, 892
colubridae, 592
coma, 2–3, 5, 44, 107, 109–12, **114**, 119, 151, 157, 159, 350–1, 390, 392, 398–9, 407, 409, 416, 421, 439, 456, 458, 495, **497**, **539**, 544, 546, 549, 552, 556–7, 562, 572, 581–3, **616**, 620, 717, 760–1, 864, 870, **872–3**, 915
'coma cocktail,' **114–15**, 119
Combiderm, 802
community-acquired pneumonia (CAP), 219, 327, **327**–32, 329–30, **332**
    airway, breathing and circulation (ABCs) support, 332
    antimicrobial therapy, 332
    clinical assessment, 328
    common bacterial pathogens, 327
    CURB-65 score, 331
    fine pneumonia severity index, 329–30
    investigation, 328
    risk class mortality for, 331
    stratification of risk score, 331
comorbid conditions, 329, 538
compartment syndrome, **47–50**, 489, 500, 552, 598, 643, **647**, **683**, 687, 750
    management, 50
Compazine, 112
complete spinal cord lesion, 669
complicated migraine, 44, 450
compressive orbital emphysema, 654–5
computed tomographic pulmonary angiography (CTPA), 295
CO_2 narcosis, 4
concepts used in therapy articles, **913**
confidence interval (95%), 911
confounder, 908, **908**
confusion, 21, 111, 150, 169, 217, 240, 275, 320, 330, 351, 390, 392, 396, 398, 400–1, 409, 412, 416, 418, 456, 495, 521, 535, 537, 540–1, 547, 557, 569, 582, 618, 622, 676, 793
Confusion Assessment Method (CAM) algorithm, 169
congenital heart disease, 255, 815, 842
congenital lymphoedema, 49

congestive cardiac failure, 19, 21, 49, **49**, 151–2, 240, 279, 282, 316, 318, 364, 397, 400, 402, 487, 552
conjunctivitis, 27, **122–5**, 124–5, 520, 529, 800
    causes, 125
    differential diagnosis of, 124
    eye examination, 123
    slit-lamp examination, 124
conscious sedation, 379, 638, 862, 907
constipation, 166, 352, 361–2, 377, 401, 424, 495, 782, 792, 794–6, 813–14, 821
contact dermatitis, 530
contaminated wound, 693
continuous positive airway pressure (CPAP), 260
continuous scale, 909, **909**
contusions, 161, 163, 660, 877
convulsions, 112, 477, 539, 572, 574, 581, 594, 621, 663, 679, 717, 719–**20**, 750, 755
    see also seizures
convulsive spasms, 484
cooling, 740, 757
Cooper–Milch technique, 678–9
cophenylcaine, 705, 707, 711
cord compression, 73–5, 166, 491, **495–6**
Cormack-Lehane laryngoscopic grading system, 178, **178**
corneal abrasions, 17, 124, 820, **820**
corneal burns, 751
corneal keratitis, 17, 19, 123–4
corneal oedema, 18, 122
corneal ulcers, 17, 510
coronary artery disease (CAD), 33, 59, 262, 449, 487, 792
coronary perfusion pressure (CPP), 193
coronary syndromes, acute (ACS), 56, 58, **239–49**, 277, 358, 890
    anginal equivalent complaints, syndromes, and presentations, 240
    anti-ischaemic and anti-thrombotic therapy, 242
    definition, 239
    management, 242–9
    NUH ACS algorithm, 243
    symptoms, 239–40
    thrombolytic treatment, 242, 247
correlation analysis, 912
corrosive burns, 19, 122, **742**
cortical blindness, 552

corticosteroids, 16, 189, **189**, 191,
    220, **220**, 317–18, 320, 508,
    511–14, 519, 523, **530**, 532,
    590, 596
Corynebacterium, 585–6
costochondritis, 59
co-trimoxazole, 432, 522, 805, 807
cough, 21, 27, 39–40, 143, 187, 240,
    251, 297, 316, 320, 322–3,
    328, 362, 471, 504, 747,
    790
Countertraction technique, 679, **679**
coxsackie virus, 191, 529
coxsackievirus A16, 509
COX-2 selective inhibitors, 71
CPAP, **179**, 260, 343
cranial nerve palsy, 457–8
cranial sutures, 726, 870
crash airway, 173
C-reactive protein, 27, **27**, 67, **67**, 251,
    256–7, 524
creatine kinase, 62, 252, 254, 257, 420,
    518, 611, 634, 756
creatine kinase–MB (CK-MB), 62
cremasteric reflex, 78–9
cricoid pressure, 172, **172**, 182, 194,
    194
cricothyroidotomy, 177, 188, 190, 615,
    650, 734, 743, 867
Crotalidae, 593–4
croup, 142–3
    admission criteria for, 144
croup/ALTB, **143**
crowning, 725
cruciate ligament tears, 642
crush injury/syndrome, 589, **598–9**,
    619
crying child/baby, **819–20**, 821, 836
cryoprecipitate transfusion, 486
cryptic shock, 216
cryptococcal meningitis, 438, **439**
Cryptococcus, 369, 436
crystal-induced gout, 66
crystalline penicillin, 784
cubitus valgus, 684
Cullen's sign, 370, 501
Cushing's dlsease, 388
Cushing's reflex, 621
cutaneous leucocytoclastic vasculitis, 518
cutaneous manifestations and minor joint
    pain, 746
cutaneous necrosis, 531
cutaneous T cell lymphoma, 530
cyanide, 119
    poisoning, 386

cyanosis, 21, 106, 112, 150, 187, 253,
    300, 316, 320, 552–3, 747,
    816, 842–3, 846
cyclic antidepressants, 4, 102, 108–9,
    111, 113–15, 314, **803**
cyclic anti-depressants poisoning,
    556–62
Cyclokapron, 650
cycloplegia, 111, 801
cystic fibrosis, 388, 816
cystic medial necrosis, 227
cytochrome oxidase system, 543, 551

D
Daflon, 377, 380, 796
Daflon 500®, 377
dapsone, 117, 805
dashboard injury., 637, 640–1
D-dimer, 50, 291, 293, 299
DeBakey system, **221**
debridat, 795, 864
deceleration/acceleration injury, 612
decerebrate posturing, 458
decompression illness (DCI), 746, 748,
    760
deep dermal burns, 633
deep peroneal nerve, 898–9
deep vein thrombosis
    lower limb swelling in, 48
deep venous thrombosis (DVT), 288–9,
    297–300, 500
defibrillation, 194, 204
defibrillator, **200**, 314–15
degrees of freedom, **909**
dehydration, 3, 21, 23–5, 33–5, 132,
    136, 144, 152, 328, 362, 369,
    392, 396, 398, 402–3, 406,
    433, 474, 495, 509, 531, 539,
    581, 756, 812, 821–3, 825,
    835–7, 843, 848
delayed sequence intubation (DSI),
    179
delirium, 111, 168–**9**, 169–70, 179,
    217, 240, 416, 521, **533–4**,
    546–8, 556, 755, 825, 828
delirium tremens, 546–8
dementia, 3, 169, 246, 400, 534, 537,
    553
dengue fever, 28, **470–1**, **470–4**
    atypical manifestations of, 473
    clinical manifestations, 475
    dermatological problems, 475
    indications for transfusion, 474
    laboratory diagnosis, 475
    management, 475

neurological problems, 475
osteoarticular manifestations, 475
prevention, 475
psycho-somatic or emotional
    problems, 475
dengue haemorrhagic fever (DHF), 7,
    470–1, **471**
    plasma leakage in, 474
    risk factors for, 472
dengue shock syndrome (DSS), **471**,
    473
    clinical indicators of, 472
dental fractures, 649
Depo-Provera, IM, 14–15
Depot Proluton (hydroxyprogesterone),
    799
depressed skull fracture, 617, 619, 774
depression, 114, 401, 540, 544–5, 549,
    719, 751, 796–7, 833, 905
dermatology, **504–32**
dermatology in emergency care
    acne rosacea, **520**
    acne vulgaris, **519–20**
    acute urticaria, **515–16**
    adverse cutaneous drug reactions,
        531–2
    approach to commonly-seen rashes,
        505
    bullous cellulitis/erysipelas, *see*
        pyoderma
    candidal infections of the skin,
        515
    chronic plaque psoriasis (psoriasis
        vulgaris), **510–11**
    chronic urticaria, **516–17**
    eczema, **512–14**
    erythema multiforme (EM): minor/
        major, **506–7**
    erythema nodosum, **528**
    exanthematous reactions, 531
    generalized exfoliative dermatitis
        (GED), **530–1**
    hand, foot and mouth disease
        (HFMD), **509**
    herpes zoster ('shingles'), **509–10**
    infectious exanthems, **528–9**
    insect bite reactions, **529–30**
    meningococcaemia, **517–18**
    necrotizing soft tissue infections,
        521–2
    pemphigoid, **507–8**
    pemphigus, **507–8**
    pityriasis rosea, **512**
    pityrosporum folliculitis, **526**
    psoriasis, **510–12**

pyoderma, **522–5**
scabies, **525–6**
superficial fungal infections,
    514–15
terminology in dermatology, 504
tinea (dermatophyte) infections of
    the skin, **515**
tinea versicolor, **515**
varicella (chickenpox), **508–9**
vasculitis, **518–19**
viral skin infections, **526–8**
dermatophytosis, 530
desferoxamine, 119
desipramine, 556
desloratadine (Aerius®), 516–17
dexamethasone, 75, **301**, 394, 439, **496**,
    800, 863, 890
dexamethazone, 799
dextromethorphan, 792
dextrose, 2, 114, 120, 224, 302, 352,
    393–4, 399–400, 405, 413–14,
    417, 421, 423, **486**, 541–2,
    546–7, 550, 567, 579–80, 744,
    781, 797, 833
diabetes, 4, 17, 28, 33, 35, 60–1
    69–70, 81, 132, 148, 166,
    217, 241, 263, 312, 328, 356,
    396, 398, 406, 409, 412, 430,
    451, 454, 463, 474, 523–4,
    537, 587, 589–90, 634, 694,
    704, 756–7, 786, 797–8,
    811
diabetes mellitus, 17, 28, 33, 35, 60–1,
    69, 81, 132, 148, 166, 217,
    241, 263, 312, 328, 409, 412,
    430, 451, 474, 523–4, 587,
    589–90, 634, 697, 756–7,
    797–8, 811
diabetic ketoacidosis (DKA), 20–1, 28,
    45, 51, 56, 112, 268, 385–6,
    390, **403–7**, 539, 796–7, 810,
    814–15, 837
    causes, 404
    diagnostic criteria, 403
    with euglycaemia, 404
    insulin administration, 405–6
    IV volume replacement, 405
    restoration of acid-base balance,
        406
    restoration of electrolyte balance,
        406
    supportive measures, 404–7
diagnostic peritoneal lavage, 602–3, 665,
    869
diagnostic test statistics, 908

dialysis, 51, 71, 117, 268, 300, 385,
    399, 402, 424–5, **426–9**, 556,
    599
dialysis disequilibrium, 428
diaphoresis, 59–60, 95, 106, 134–5,
    152, 211, 240, 255, 276, 278,
    365, 485, 571, 581
diaphragmatic rupture, traumatic, **613**
diarrhoea, **23–5**, 365, 375
    in acid emergencies, 389
    children, **821–4**
    disastrous misdiagnosis, 23
    in elderly population, 23
    hypovolaemia and, 37
    in paediatric population, 23
    rehydration therapy, 23–4
    symptomatic treatment of, 23–5
diazepam (Valium®), 34, 46, 74, 129,
    168, 170, 278, 485, 547, 549,
    561, 574, **574**, 596, 719, **719**,
    757, 795–6, 809, 832, 846,
    861, 866, **870**,
    889
dichlorophenoxyacetic acid, 120
diclofenac sodium (Voltaren®), 752
diclofenac (Voltaren®), 43, 74, 444, 459,
    461, 752, 783, **783**, 807, 829,
    829, 861, 889, 891
difficult airway, 173–4
Digibind, 119
digitalis fab fragments, 119
digital nerve block, 889, **895–6**
digitoxin, 119, 568, 791
digoxin, 93, 101, 108, 118–19, 213,
    213, 254, **254**, 311, **311**, 418,
    423, 495, **564–70**, **791**, 808
digoxin poisoning, **564–70**
    atrioventricular block, 569
    chronic, 569–70
    drug therapy for, 567
    Fab antibodies, 567–9
    risk factors, 565–6
    supportive measures, 567
    supraventricular tachycardia, 569
    ventricular arrhythmias, 569
diltiazem, 306–7, 310, 569, 791, **791**
dimercaprol, 119, 806
diphenhydramine, 119, 144, 189–90,
    192, 516, 596, 792, 832
diphenoxylate, 24, 794
diphenoxylateatropine (Lomotil®), 794
diphtheria, 253, 712
diplopia, 32, 35, 443, 462, 654, 746
dirty wound, 693
discrete scale, 909, **909**

disopyramide, 104, 314, 917
disposition of patients
    abdominal aortic aneurysm (AAA),
        228
    acid base emergencies, 391
    acute adrenal insufficiency
        ('Addisonian crisis'), 394
    acute heart failure, 267–9
    acute urticaria, 516
    after drug overdose, 121
    alcohol intoxication, 542, 548
    anaphylaxis, 189
    asthma, 319
    Barton's fracture, 689
    Bennett's fracture, 692
    benzodiazepine overdose, 550
    bites, 590–1
    bradydysrhythmias, 237
    breathlessness, 818
    burns, minor, 745
    cardiomyopathies, 260
    with chest pain, acute, 64
    chronic obstructive pulmonary
        disease (COPD), 325
    Colles' fracture, 688
    community-acquired pneumonia
        (CAP), 332
    CO poisoning, 554–5
    croup, 144
    cyclic anti-depressants poisoning,
        562
    diabetic ketoacidosis (DKA), 407
    diarrhoea in children, 824
    digoxin poisoning, 570
    drug-induced angiooedema, 190
    elbow dislocation, 685
    encephalopathy, 353
    epistaxis, 706
    forearm fractures, 687
    hand trauma, 634–6
    hereditary angiooedema, 191
    HF acid burns, 745
    humeral shaft fractures, 683
    hypertensive emergency, 284
    hypertensive urgency, 284
    hypoglycaemia, 414
    infective endocarditis, 257
    lateral condylar fractures of the
        humerus, 684
    lightning injuries, 753–4
    liver abscess, 360
    low back pain (LBP), 74–5
    lunate dislocations, 691
    medial epicondylar fractures of the
        humerus, 684

meningitis, 441
meningococcaemia, 518
metacarpal fractures, 691
myocarditis, 255
myxoedema, 421
necrotizing soft tissue infections, 522
olecranon fractures, 686
organophosphates poisoning, 574
overwarfarinization, 503
peptic ulcer disease, 375
pericarditis, 253
perilunate dislocations, 691
poisoning with alcohols, 548
pregnancy, trauma in, 666
'pulled elbow' (subluxed radial head), 685
radial head/neck fractures, 686
red eye, 125
respiratory failure (RF), acute, 344
RSI, 185
salicylate poisoning, 583
scaphoid (carpal navicular) fractures, 690
seizures, 126–9
shock/hypoperfusion states, 141
shoulder dislocations, 681
Smith's (or reverse colles') fracture, 689
snake bites, 596
spinal cord injury, 672
stroke, 455
subarachnoid haemorrhage (SAH), 459
submersion injuries, 760–1
supracondylar humeral fractures, 683
temporal arteritis, 461
thyroid crisis, 418
tympanic membrane, 713
urinary retention, acute, 167
urinary tract infections (UTI), 432
urolithiasis, 435
urticaria, 192
violent and psychotic patients, 170
wound care and management, 696
disseminated gonococcal infection (DGI), **70**
disseminated gonorrhoea, 67
disseminated intravascular coagulation (DIVC), 137, 357, 755
distal phalanx fracture/infection, 625
diuretics, 33, 148, 152, 266, 269, 277, 301, 352, 386, 388, 395, 397, **402**, 407, 418, 421, 426, 495, 709, 722, 756, **760**

DIVC, 137, 357, 438, 598, 663, 723, 752, 755
diverticulitis, 54, 345, 358, 360, 434, 537
diving emergencies, **746–8**
Dix–Hallpike test, 34
dizziness *see* giddiness
dobutamine, **139**, 212, **212**, 247, 249, 267, 781, **781**
dog bites, **585–6**
dopamine, 138–40, 188, 213, **213**, 215, 218, 233–4, 234, 247, 249, 267, 281, 283, 367, 556, 561, **561**, 781, **781**
Dormicum® (midazolam), 46, 861, 905
doxepin, 556
doxycycline, 70, 79, 81, 478–9, 485, 501, 508, 520, **523**, 732, **732**
"dropped" beats, 86
drop wrist, 682
drowning, 20, 111, 747, **759–60**
drowning, near, 20, 111, 747, **759–60**
drug abuse, 69, 219, 250, 297, 302, 358, 409, **413**–14
drug allergies, 132, 831
drug-drug interactions, **501**, 515, 533
drug-induced angiooedema, **190**
drug-induced encephalopathy, 428
drug-induced giddiness, 33
drug intoxication, 160, 616, 831
drug overdose, 5, 107–**8**, 121, 127, 413, 815
    drugs adsorbed by charcoal, 118
    history, 107
    vital signs, 108
drugs and equipment, paediatric, **857–66**
drug screen, 107
drug therapy, pain management, **887–91**
duodenal ulcers, 7, 373
D50W, 541
dynamic haemodynamic parameters, 219
dysarthria, 32, 35, 398, 449, 462, 746
dyscrasias, 39, 705
'dysgonic fermenter-2,' **586**
dyspareunia, 731
dyspepsia, 6, 56, **373–5**
dysphagia, 35, 112, 145, 226, 300, 373–5, 398, 462, 474, 710
dysphonia, 112
dyspnoea, 20–2, 30, 60, 85, 135, 186, 240, 251, 253, 256, 258,

262–3, 267, 290–1, 293–5, 300, 316, 322–3, 328, 334, 343, 400, 428, **428**, 487, 497, **536**, 552, 676, 708, 747, 816–17, 842
dyspnoeic child, 817
dysrhythmias, 36, 85, 108
dysuria, 27, 430, 492, 722

E
ear, nose and throat emergencies, **703–13**
early goal-directed therapy (EGDT), 218
ear wounds, 701–2
ecchymoses, 501, 593
echovirus, 842
eclampsia, **717–20**
ecstasy, 3, 350
ectasia, 225
ectopic beats, 86
ectopic pregnancy, 12–14, 23, 30, 33, **37**, 51–3, 56, **73**–4, 132, 137, 147–8, 150, 152, 433–4, **721–3**, 731–2, 810–11, 814
eczema, **512–14**
eczematous eruptions, 531
edrophonium chlorid, 596
effort syncop, 147–8
Ehlers-Danlos syndrome, 221, 227, 854
Eikenella corrodens, **586**, 632
Elapidae, **592–4**
elapidae, 592
elbow, pulled, **685**
elbow dislocations, **684–5**
elbow injuries, 777
elderly patients *see* geriatric emergencies
electrical burns, **633–4**
    of the hand, **633–4**
electrical injuries, **750**–3
electric shock, 202, 289, 595
electrolyte disturbances, 100, 385, 795
emergency blood transfusion, **489**
emergency surgical debridement, 81
emergency ultrasound, **762–73**
emetics, 439, 445, 449, 546, 837, **863**
emotional abuse, 853
emphysema, 161–2, 295, 588, 611, 614, 632, **654–5**, 816
enalapril, **266**, 275, **275**, 280, 790, 808
enalaprilat, 280, 283

encephalitis, 3, 127, 450, 472, 508, 539, 756, 787, 833, 859

encephalopathy, 3, 47, 273–5, 277, 282–3, **350–3**, 426, 428, 450, 472, 539–42, 577, 580, 795

associated with acute liver failure, **350–1**

associated with liver cirrhosis and portal hypertension, **351–3**

endocarditis, 67, **250–60**, 263, 286, 358, 364, 586, 784

endometriosis, 345

endoscopic retrograde cholangiopancreatography (ERCP), 358

endothelial damage, 271, 289

endotracheal intubation, 146

end-stage renal disease (kidney failure), 424

ENT emergencie, **703–13**

Enterobacteriaceae, 301

Enterobactericae, 440

Enterococcus, 357, 585

enterovirus, 71, 509

entonox, 645, 648, 692, 736, 887–8, 890

envenomation, 592, **594–7**, 759

epidermal necrolysis, toxic, 532

epididymitis, 76–**9**, 77, 79, 814

epididymo-orchitis, **77**, 79–80

epidural haematoma, 73, 500, 539

epigastric abdominal pain, **56–7**

extra-abdominal causes, 56–7

intra-abdominal causes, 56

epigastric pain, 6, **56–7**, 470, 717, **808**, **811**

epiglottitis, 142–6, **144–5**, 703, 817

epilepsy, 4, 277, 756, 760, 782, **796**, 834, 892

see also seizures

episiotomy, 729

epistaxis, 39–40, 159, 489, 593, **704–6**

Epley manoeuvre, 34

eptifibatide, 245

ergotamine, 445

ergotamine tartrate, 807, **891**

erysipelas, 505, **509**, 521–2, **524**

erythema, 48, 77–8, 80, 291, 299, 301, 505, **506–7**, 511, 513, 516, 521, 524, **528**, 529–32, 594, 695, 739, 746, 750

erythema multiforme (EM): minor/major, **506–7**, **531**

erythema nodosum, 505, **528**

erythroderma, 531

erythrodermic psoriasis, 511

erythromycin, 70, 104, 485, 513, 520 522–6, 531, 586, 590, **590**, 701, 709, 732, 785, **785**, 807, 860, 917

erythromycin/clarithromycin, 524

erythromycin ethinyl succinate (EES®), 785

escharotomy, 633, **736–7**, 737, 752

Escherichia coli, 77, 359

esmolol, 224, 280–**2**, 282, 310, 310, **417**, 790, **790**

esomeprazole (Nexium®), 8, 795

ETCO$_2$, 195

ethanol, 4, 63, 108–10, 112, 118–20, 129, 385–6, 426, 539, **541**–546, 549, 620, 915

ethylene glycol, 20, 112, 119–20, 385–6, 426, 539, 541–2, **543–4**, 545–6, 915

toxicity, 544

etomidate, 181–4, 218, 781, **781**, 887, **903**, **905**

etoricoxib (Arcoxia®), 783

euphoria, 351, 544

exanthematous or morbiliform lesion, 529

exanthematous rashes, 531

exanthematous reactions, 531

exfoliative dermatitis, 531

extensor tendon injury, **629–30**

exterior tendon injury, **629–30**

eyelid lacerations, 696, 700

eye trauma, 620

F

Fab antibodies, 567–9

facial pain management, 890–1

falsely-elevated international normalized ratio (INR), 500

famotidine, 795

fascicular vt/idiopathic left ventricular tachycardia (ILVT), **98–9**

fasciotomy/escharotomy, 752

febrile patient

flank pain, 55

right hypochondrial (RHC) pain, 54

felodipine, 283, 790

felon, 635

femoral block, **901**

femoral neck and trochanteric fractures, **639**

femoral shaft fractures, **639–40**

fenoldopam, 275, 278, 280, 283

fentanyl, 781, 887, 889

fever, **26–8**, 473

blood investigation, 27–8

causes, 26

children with, **825–30**

clinical assessment, 27

defintions, 26

hypothermia, 26

in liver abscess, 359

neutropaenic, **492–4**

principles of management, 28

seizures and, 126

thyroid crisis, 416

of unknown origin (FUO), 26

urinary obstruction plus, 167

fexofenadine, 517

fibrates, 501

finger tip amputation, **626–7**

Fisher's exact test, 911

fitting child, **831–4**

flagyl, 359

flail chest, **608**

flank pain, **55**

in afebrile patient, 55

in febrile patient, 55

fleet enema, 795

Fleischner sign, 293

flexor tendon injuries, **627–8**

fluconazole, 786

fluid and electrolyte disorders, 395–**402**

hypercalcaemia, **401–2**

hypernatraemia, **398–9**

hypocalcaemia, **399–400**

hyponatraemia, **396–8**

flumazenil, 352, 550

flumazenil (Anexate®), 4, 115

flunarizine, 446

fluocinolone acetonide, 514

fluoroquinolones, 501, 590

fluoxetine, 446

fluticasone (Flixonase®), 801

Focused Assessment with Sonography in Trauma (FAST), 603–4, 769–71

focused neurological examination, 5

foetal varicella syndrome, 508

fomepizole, 545

foot injury, **646–8**

forced alkaline diuresis, 120

forearm fractures, **686–7**

foreign body

in ears, **706–7**

nose, **707**
throat, **707–8**
Fournier's gangrene, 80
fracture of the penis, **84**
frontal bone fracture, 653
frumeside (Lasix®), 266, 269, 402
frusemide, 120, 254, 260, 530
frusemide (Lasix®), 790
Fucicort, 802
fungal infection, 67
furuncles, **523**
fusidic acid, 522
Fybogel®, 377–8

G
gabapentin, 446
Galeazzi fracture dislocation, 687
gastric lavage, 107
gastrointestinal dialysis, 117
gatifloxacin (Tequin®), 786
Gaviscon®, 794
generalized exfoliative dermatitis (GED), **530–1**
gentamicin, 80, 786
gentamicin, IV, 28
gentamycin, 732
geriatric emergencies
acute abdominal pain, **536–7**
acute mesenteric ischaemia, 536
acute myocardial infarction, 535–6
appendicitis, 536
atypical or attenuated manifestation of a serious illness, 533
bacteraemia, 538
bowel obstruction, 536
cholecystitis, 537
commonly used emergency drugs, **780–804**
delirium, 534
digoxin toxicity, 565
dyspnoea, 536
factors affecting diagnosis and treatment of geriatric patients, 533
functional decline, 534
infections, 537–8
perforated peptic ulcer, 536
pneumonia, 537–8
polypharmacy, 533
respiratory tract infections, 537–8
ruptured abdominal aortic aneurysm, 537
thrombolytic therapy and anti-coagulation, 536
trauma and falls, 534–5

GI cocktail, 60
giddiness, **30–7**, 553
ectopic pregnancy and, 37
in hyperventilation, 45
hypoglycaemia and, 37
initial management, 31
investigations, 33–4
ischaemic heart disease and, 36
lifethreatening disease and, 30
lightheadedness and, 30
medications associated with, 33
non-specific, 30
non-vertiginous, 33
postural symptoms, 31
presyncope, 30
vertigo, 30
gingko, 501
ginseng, 501
Glasgow-Blatchford bleeding score (GBS), 9
Glasgow Coma Scale (GCS), 539, 616, **872–3**
glaucoma, acute angle-closure, 122
glibenclamide, 798
gliclazide, 798
glipizide, 798
glucagon, 189, 235
glucocorticoid replacement, 394
glyceryl trinitrate (GTN), 244, 378
Go-Lytely, 120
gonococcal arthritis, 66
gouty arthristis, **70–1**
G6PD deficiency, drug to be avoided, **805–6**
graft *versus* host disease (GVHD), 530
Grey-Turner's sign, 370
griseofulvin, 515
gunshot wound, 605

H
haemarthrosis, 500
haematocrit, 473
haematuria, 500
haemodialysis, 120, 424, **427–8**
haemoglobinopathies, 112
haemoperfusion, 120
haemopericardium, 500
haemopneumothoraces, 157
haemoptysis, **38–40**
causes, 39
classification, 38
definition, 38
massive, 38–40
mild, 40
vs haematemesis, 38

haemorrhage
retinal, 17–18
vitreous, 17–18
haemorrhagic complications of anti-coagulation, 500
haemorrhagic gastritis, 544
haemorrhagic shock, 214
haemorrhagic stroke, 449–50, 454
haemorrhoids, **376–7**
haemothoraces, 157
haemothorax, 500
hair apposition technique (HAT), 699–700
haloperidol, 541, 547
haloperidol (Haldol®), 112, 170
Hamilton score, 299
Hampton's hump, 293
hand, foot and mouth disease (HFMD), **509**
hand trauma, **624–36**
Hartmann's solution, 24, 486
headache disorders
cluster headache diagnostic criteria, 443, 445–6
migraine prophylactic medications, 446
migraine with aura diagnostic criteria, 443–4
migraine without aura diagnostic criteria, 443–4
pain management, 891
prophylaxis, 445
tension-type, 442, 444
Headache Impact Test-6 (HIT-6) questionnaire, 447–8
headaches, **40–4**
focused examination for, 42–3
primary, 42, 44
secondary, 41–2, 44
head trauma, **616–23**
heat cramps, 755
heat exhaustion, **755–6**
heat injuries, 755
heat stroke, **755**
risk factors for, 756
heat syncope, 755
HEELP syndrome, 717–18
HELLP syndrome, 277
hemiparesis, 462
Henderson–Hasselbach (H–H) equation, 384
Henoch–Schöenlein purpura, 77, 81, 518
Henry's law, 746
heparin, 244

heparin-induced thrombocytopaenia (HIT), 244
hepatic dysfunction, 755
hepatic encephalopathy, acute, **350–3**
hepatitis, 54, 358
hereditary angiooedema, **191**
herniation, 621
herpes simplex virus infection, 527–8
herpes zoster ('shingles'), **509–10**
hesperidin (Daflon®), 796
Hill–Sachs lesion, 678
hip dislocation, **637–8**
Hodgkin's disease, 530
Homan's sign, 298
homatropine, 124
Horner's syndrome, 300
human bites, **586–7**
humeral shaft fractures, **682–3**
Hunt and Hess Classification of Subarachnoid Haemorrhage, 458
Hutchinson's sign, 510
hydralazine, 278, 280, 282, 720, 790
hydrocortisone, 394, 418, 420, 793, 799, 801
hydrocortisone acetate, 514
hydrofluoric acid burn/ingestion, 400
hydrogen fluoride antidote, 743
hydrophiidae, 592
hydroxyapatite, 67
hydroxyzine, 517
hydroxyzine (Atarax®), 516
hyoscine (Buscopan®), 794
hyperbaric oxygen therapy, 555
hypercalcaemia, **401–2**, 566
hypercalcaemia of malignancy, **494–5**
hyperglycaemia, 398, 406
hyperglycemia, 403
hyperhomocysteinaemia, 227
hyperkalaemia, 49, **422–4**, 426, 599
    severity, 422
hyperkalaemie, 229
hyperkeratosis, 510
hyperkeratotic papules, 526
hyperlipidaemia, 227
hypermetabolism, 531
hypernatraemia, **398–9**
hyperosomolar hyperglycaemic state (HHS), **407–8**
hyperphosphataemia, 399
hyperpyrexia, 416
hypertension, 108, **270**, 720
hypertensive acute heart failure, 262
hypertensive crises, **270–84**
    definitions, 270

pathophysiology, 271
hypertensive emergencies, **270**
    causes, 272
    drug therapy, 278–83
    presentations, 273
hypertensive emergency, 284
hypertensive encephalopathy, 274
hypertensive urgencies, **270**
hypertensive urgency, 284
    drug therapy, 283–4
hyperthermia, 108, 531, **755–8**
hypertrichosis, 531
hypertrophic cardiomyopathy (HOCM), 150
hyperventilation, 20, 108, 390, 560, 621
hyperventilation attack (HA)/ hyperventilation syndrome, **45–6**
    diagnosis of exclusion, 45
    differential diagnosis of, 45
hyperviscosity syndrome and leucostasis syndrome, **497**
hypoalbuminaemia, 49, 399
hypocalcaemia, 390, **399–400**, 544, 743, 757
hypoglycaemia, 37, **409–14**, 419, 450, 542
    adrenergic symptoms and signs, 409
    causes, 409–12
    investigations, 412–13
    medications/drugs for, 410
    monitoring, 413
    neuroglycopenic symptoms and signs, 409
    oral hypoglycaemic agents, 411
    types of insulin for, 410
hypokalaemia, 566
hypomagnesaemia, 399, 566, 757
hyponatraemia, **396–8**, 418, 473
hypoperfusion states, *see* shock/ hypoperfusion states
hypotension, 108, 427, 561
hypothermia, 26, 108, 418, 531
hypothyroidism, 419
hypoventilation, 108
hypoventilation with respiratory acidosis, 418
hypovolaemia, 183
    giddiness and, 37
hypovolaemia (dehydration), 369
hypovolaemic patients, 399
hypovolaemic shock, 365
hypromellose eye drops, 800
hysteria, 19

I
ibuprofen (Brufen®), 783, 829
ichthyoses, 530
idiopathic scrotal oedema, **77**
idiopathic VT, 94
immunoglobulin E (IgE), 187
immunoglobulin G4 (IgG4)-mediated, 187
imodium® (loperamide), 24
impetigo, 522
incised wound, 693
induction agents, 181
infection/septic arthritis, 66
infectious diseases
    caring for staff and others, 468
    communication, 467
    hospital plan, 465
    infection control, 466
    initial investigation and management, 466
    manpower capacity, 467
    surge capacity, 467
    vaccines, 468
infectious exanthems, **528–9**
infective endocarditis, 255–7
    antibiotic therapy, 257
    complications, 256
    investigations, 256–7
    prognosis, 256
    risk factors, 255
    symptoms and signs, 255–6
inferior vena cava assessment, 765–6
inflammatory joint disorders, 66
in-hospital cardiac arrest (IHCA), 193
Injury Severity Score (ISS), **872**, **874**
insect bite reactions, **529–30**
insulin therapy, 546
intermediate syndrome (IMS), 574
International Liaison Committee on Resuscitation (ILCOR), 193, 303, 229
intestinal obstruction, **361–3**
    clinical features, 362
    investigations, 362–3
    mechanical, 361
    non-mechanical, 361
    presence of strangulation, 362
intra-aortic balloon pump, 213
intracellular negatively birefringent crystals, 71
intracerebral haemorrhage (ICH), 276, 449
intravenous small molecule platelet glycoprotein IIb/IIIa inhibitor, 245

ipecac, 114
ipratropium (Atrovent®), 793
iron, 119
ischaemia, 315
ischaemic bowel, **364–7**
    aetiology, 364
    clinical features, 364–5
    imaging studies, 366
    risk factors, 364
ischaemic heart disease
    giddiness and, 36
ischaemic stroke, 449, 454–5
ischiorectal abscess, 378
isolated β-blockade, 278
isolated closed head injury, 183
isolated thermal burns of hand, **632–3**
isoniazid, 531
isoniazid (INH), 119
isotonic saline, 402
ispaghula Husk (Fybogel®), 796
itraconazole, 515

J
Jervell-Lange-Nielsen Syndrome, 104
J-point, 239
junctional tachycardia, 93
juvenile chronic arthritis, 67

K
kaolin pectin mixture, 794
Kawasaki's disease, 820
keratitis, 19
Kernig's sign, 27
ketamine, 781, 887
ketoacidosis, 546
ketoconazole, 515, 787
ketonaemia, 403
ketoprofen plaster, 801
ketorolac (Toradol®), 783
ketosis without acidosis, 544
Klebsiella pneumoniae, 359
knee dislocation, **641**
knee haemarthrosis/effusion, **641–2**
Köbner phenomenon, 511
Koplik's spots, 529
Kussmaul's signs, 609

L
labetalol, 275–6, 278, 280, 284, 720,
    789
labetalol hydrochloride, 279
laceration, 693
lactate clearance, 219
Lacteol Fort, 794
lactulose, 353, 795

lamivudine, 483
laryngeal trauma, **614–15**
laryngoscopy, 174
lateral condylar fractures of the humerus,
    684
lead, 119
LeFort fractures, **656**
left bundle branch block (LBBB), 59
LEMON Law, 177
leucocytosis, 403
leucopaenia, 473
leukaemia, 530
levocetirizine, 517
levocetirizine (Xyzal®), 516
levofloxacin, 325, 501, 590
levofloxacin (Cravit®), 786
levonorgestrel (Postinor-2®), 799
lichen planus, 530
lightheadedness, 30
lightning injuries, **749–54**
lignocaine, 314, 378, 509, 561, 695,
    791,
    898
limb ischaemia, acute, **286–8**
    angiography, 288
    clinical categories of, 287
    physical examination, 287
    6 Ps of, 286–7
liniment methyl salicylate (LMS), 801
Lisfranc's dislocation, 647
lisinopril, 446
lithium, 120, 446
liver abscess, 54, **358–60**
Lomotil® (diphenoxylate), 24
long QT syndromes (LQTS), **104**
loop diuretics, 402
loperamide (Imodium®), 794
loratadine, 517
loratadine (Claritin®), 516
loratidine, 792
lorazepam, 129, 561, 796, 832
low back pain (LBP), **72–5**
    patients with haemodynamic
        instability and/or history of
        significant trauma, 73–4
    patients with severe, incapacitating
        musculoskeletal pain, 74–5
lower extermity trauma, **637–48**
lower limb swelling, **47–50**
    causes, 47
    in cellulitis, 48
    in deep vein thrombosis, 48
    due to lymphatic obstruction, 48
    general management, 49–50
    in lymphangitis, 48

orthopaedic emergency and, 48–9
    in pregnancy with pre-eclampsia, 47
    varicose veins and, 48
Lown's classification of PVC, 93–4
Lugol's iodine, 418, 798
lumbar puncture, 438, 458
lunate dislocations, **690–1**
Lund–Browder chart, 734–5
lung scintigraphy, 295
lung sliding, 763–4
lyme arthritis, 67
lymphadenopathy, 531
lymphangitis, 48
lymphatic obstruction and limb swelling,
    48
lymphoedema, 48
    primary, 49
lymphoedema praecox, 49
lymphoedema tarda, 49

M
magnesium, 446
magnesium carbonate, 794
magnesium sulphate, 278, 314, 561,
    718–19, 781, 793
magnesium trisilicate, 794
Maissoneuve fracture, 645
malaria, **477–80**
Malassezia furfur, 526
malathion, 525, 803
malignant hyperthermia, 755
Mallampati score, 177–8
mallet finger, 629–30
mallet splint, 630
malnutrition, 49, 531
mandibular fractures, **657**
mannitol, 622, 781
mannitol (IV), 5
Mann–Whitney U test, 912
massive haemothorax, **609–10**
massive pleural effusion causing
    respiratory compromise, **498**
maxillofacial trauma, **649–58**
Maxolon® (metoclopramide), 24
May–Thurner syndrome, 49
McConnel sign, 769
McGrigor's lines, 652
mcp joint, disruption to extensors over
    the, 631–2
mean (arithmetic), 909
measurement/systematic error, 908
mebendazole, 788
Mebeverine (Duspatalin®), 795
medial epicondylar fractures of the
    humerus, **684**

median (arithmetic), 909
median nerve, 896
mefenamic acid, 15
mefenamic acid (Ponstan®), 783
melaena, 226
meloxicam (Mobic®), 783
meningitis, 428, **436–41**
    antibiotic regime for, 440
    supportive measures, 439
meningococcaemia, 504, **517–18**
meningococcaemia prophylaxis, 506
meningoencephalitis, 509
mepacrine, 806
mercury, 119
mesenteric ischaemia, 57, **364–7**
metabolic acidosis, **385–7**
    severe, 425–6
metabolic alkalosis, **387–9**
metacarpal block, 889
metacarpal fractures, **691**
Metamucil®, 377–8
metatarsals fracture, 648
metatarso-phalangeal joint (podagra),
    71
metformin, 798
methaemoglobinaemia, 112
methanol, 119–20
methanol poisoning, 544
methylprednisolone, 671
methylxanthines (aminophylline), 325
methysergide, 446
metochlopramide (Maxolon®/Reglan®),
    112
metoclopramide, 459, 891
metoclopramide (Maxolon®), 794
metoprolol, 310, 446, 790
metronidazole, 358, 363, 366, 501,
    732
metronidazole, IV, 28
metronidazole (Flagyl®), 25
miconazole, 515, 801
midazolam, 781, 887
migraine, 18
Migraine Disability Assessment (MIDAS)
    questionnaire, 447
mimic heat stroke, 756
minor burns, **632**
mist carminative, 794
Mixtard, 797
mobitz type heart block, 230–1
mode (arithmetic), 909
Modified Wells score, 298
molluscum contagiosum, 527
monoarticular arthritis, 66
monosodium urate, 67

Monteggia fracture dislocation, 687
montelukast (Singulair®), 793
morphine, 244, 260, 784
mosquito-borne diseases
    chikungunya, **475**
    dengue fever, 471–4
    malaria, 477–80
moxifloxacin (Avelox®), 786
Mucilin®, 377–8
mucopuricin (Bactroban), 802
multifocal atrial tachycardia (MAT), **89**,
    307
multiple organ dysfunction syndrome
    (MODS), 216
mupirocin, 522
Murphy's sign, 355
mycobacteria, 67
myelodysplasia, 530
Mylanta, 794
myocardial infarction (MI), 240, 890
    missed diagnosis of, 240
    risk management tips, 240–1
    thrombolysis in (TIMI), 241–2
myocarditis, **253–5**, 509
    aetiologies, 253
    immuno-suppressive therapy, 255
    investigations, 254
    symptoms and signs, 253–4
myoglobin, 62
myoglobinuria, 49
myxoedema, 49, **418–21**

N

nail bed injuries, acute, **625**
nail bed with nail plate avulsion,
    laceration of, **626**
nail psoriasis, 511, **512**
naloxone, 352, 541
naloxone (Narcan®), 4
naproxen, 891
naproxen sodium, 446
naproxen (Synflex®), 783
narrow complex tachydysrhythmias,
    306–13
    irregular, 307
    regular, 306–7
nasal fractures, **655**
    bone, 706
National Resuscitation Council (NRC),
    193, 229, 303
nebulized bronchodilators, 189
necrotizing soft tissue infections, 504,
    521–2
needlestick/body fluid exposure,
    481–3

    from an identified source patient,
        482
    patient care considerations, 481
    from unidentified patient, 482
Neisseria gonorrhoeae, 79
Neisseria meningitidis, 517
NEO (naso-ethmoidal-orbital) fracture,
    653
neonatal varicella, 508
neoplasm, 66
nerve blocks at the ankle, 898–900
neurogenic pulmonary oedema, 459
neurogenic shock, **214–15**, 667
neuroleptic malignant syndrome, 755
neuromuscular blocking agent (NMBA),
    172
neutropaenic fever, **492–4**
New Orleans criteria, 618
NEXUS criteria, 673
nicardipine, 275, 278, 280, 282–3
nifedipine, 283
nimodipine, 459
nitrites, 119
nitrofurans, 805
nitroglycerin, 280, 282, 459
nitroprusside, 275, 278, 280, 459
Nizoral (ketoconazole) cream, 515
Nizoral shampoo, 515
no-man's land zone, 628
nominal scales, 909
non-cardiogenic pulmonary oedema,
    583
nondihydropyridine calcium channel
    blockers, 310
non-Hodgkin's lymphoma, 530
non-inflammatory joint disorders,
    66–7
non-ST elevation myocardial infarction
    (NSTEMI), 239, 241
non-steroidal anti-inflammatory drugs
    (NSAIDs), 71, 445, 473, 476,
    516, 531, 829, 889
nonsustained ventricular tachycardia,
    94
noradrenaline, 218, 561, 781
norethisterone, 15, 799
normocapnia, 196
Norwegian scabies, 525
null hypothesis, 910
nystatin, 786, 799

O

obstructed inguinal herniae, 819
obstructive jaundice, 355
oesophageal trauma, **614**

oesophageal varices, 8
ofloxacin, 79, 732
oleander, 119
olecranon fractures, **686**
olive oil, 800
omeprazole, 795
oncologic emergencies
　　cord compression, **495–6**
　　hypercalcaemia of malignancy,
　　　　494–5
　　hyperviscosity syndrome and
　　　　leucostasis syndrome,
　　　　497
　　massive pleural effusion causing
　　　　respiratory compromise,
　　　　498
　　neutropaenic fever, **492–4**
　　pericardial effusion causing acute
　　　　breathlessness, **498–9**
　　superior vena cava syndrome *see*
　　　　venous emergencies
　　suspected massive pulmonary
　　　　embolism, *see* pulmonary
　　　　embolism (PE)
　　syndrome of inappropriate
　　　　antidiuretic hormone
　　　　(SIADH), **497**
　　thrombocytopaenia, **494**
one-sample *t* test, 912
one-tailed *t* test, 912
open pelvic fracture, 661
open pneumothorax, 157
opioids, 110, 119
optic neuritis, 18
oral bicarbonate therapy, 583
oral rehydration therapy, 24–5
ordinal scales, 909
organophosphate-induced delayed
　　neuropathy (OPIDN), 574
organophosphates, 119
organophosphates poisoning, **571–4**
　　CNS effects, 572
　　delayed effects, 574
　　drug therapy, 573–4
　　muscarinic effects, 571
　　nicotinic effects, 572
　　supportive measures, 573
orotracheal intubation, 172
oseltamivir (Tamiflu®), 787
osmolal gap, 543, 914
osmotic demyelination syndrome, 398
osteoarthritis, 66
osteoblastic malignancies, 400
osteomyelitis, 66, 820
otitis externa, acute, **710**

otitis media
　　acute, **709–10**
　　chronic, **710**
Ottawa Ankle Rules, 645
out-of-hospital cardiac arrest (OHCA),
　　193
overwarfarinization, **500–3**
oxygen debt, 133
oxygen deficit, 133
oxymetazoline, 801

P

pain management
　　analgesia/sedation for severe pain,
　　　　888–91
　　analgesia/sedation for short
　　　　procedures, **887**
paired-samples *t* test, 912
pallor (anaemia), 531
palpitations, **85–106**
pamaquine, 805
Panadeine®, 782
panadol extra, 445
pancreatitis, 358, 544
pancreatitis, acute, **368–72**
　　causes of, 369
　　clinical features, 369–70
　　clinical predictors of the severity of,
　　　　371
　　diagnosis of, 368
　　differential diagnoses of, 368
　　imaging studies, 370–1
　　laboratory tests, 370
　　management, 371–2
pancuronium, 782
paracetamol, 119, 445, 476, 782, 803,
　　828, 891
paracetamol poisoning, **576–80**
　　adverse effects of Parvolex®, 579–80
　　drug therapy, 578–80
　　N-acetylcysteine effect, 579–80
　　phases, 577
　　prognostic indicators following
　　　　overdose, 580
　　supportive measures, 577–8
　　toxic effects, 577
paraesthesia, 287
paralysis, 287
paraneoplastic, 518
paraphimosis, **82**
parathion, 571
Parkland's formula, 736
paronychia, 634–5
paroxysmal supraventricular tachycardia
　　(PSVT), 306–10

partial flexor tendon laceration, **628–9**
patellar dislocation, **640–1**
patellar fracture, **640**
patellar reflex, 719
PEFR nomogram, 918
pelvic examination, 11
pelvic inflammatory disease (PID),
　　731–2
pelvic trauma, **660–1**
Pemberton's manoeuvre, 300
pemphigoid, **507–8**
pemphigus, **507–8**
pemphigus foliaceus, 530
penicillin, **145**, 516, 525, 530–1, 784
penicillin G, 485
penile emergencies
　　balanoposthitis, 81
　　fracture of the penis, 84
　　paraphimosis, 82
　　phimosis, 81–2
　　priapism, 82–3
　　torn frenulum, **83–4**
peptic ulcer disease, 358, **373–5**
　　discharge patients with advice, 375
　　indications for hospital admission,
　　　　375
　　indications for outpatient referral to
　　　　gastroenterology, 375
　　symptoms, 373
　　symptoms management, 374
percentile, 910
percutaneous coronary intervention
　　(PCI), 36, 245
perforated peptic ulcer, 52
perianal conditions, **376–80**
perianal haematoma, **377**
periarticular pain, 66
pericardial effusion causing acute
　　breathlessness, **498–9**
pericardial tamponade, **609**
pericarditis, **250–3**
　　aetiologies, 250
　　investigations, 251–2
　　management, 252–3
　　symptoms and signs, 251
perilunate dislocations, **691**
peripheral pain, joint
　　approach to diagnosis, 66–7
　　differential diagnosis of, 66–7
peritoneal dialysis, **429**
peritonitis, 365, 429
peritonsillar abscess, **710**
permethrin, 525
pethidine, 784
Pethidine® (meperidine), 74

phalangeal fracture/dislocation, 648
phantolamine, 280
phenacetin, 805
phenazopyridine, 806
Phenergan® (promethazine), 24
phenobarbital, 561
phenobarbitone, 129, 796, 833
phenothiazines, 83, 104, 119
phentolamine, 278, 282
phenylephrine, 800
phenylhydrazine, 806
phenytoin, 126, 129, 501, 547, 796,
        806, 833
phimosis, **81–2**
pigmentation, 531
pilocarpine, 800
pityriasis rosea, **512**
pityriasis rubra pilaris, 530
pityrosporum folliculitis, **526**
pizotifen, 446
placenta, delivery of, 729–30
placental separation, 730
plantar warts, 526
pneumonia, 508, 537–8, 553
pneumonitis, 508
pneumothorax, 61, **334–8**, 764
    absolute contraindications, 338
    advice, 337–8
    initial management, 334–5
    large primary, 337
    patient with secondary, 337
    relative contraindications, 338
    small primary, 337
    unstable patient with large, 337
poikilothermia, 286
5-point auscultation, 194
poisoning, **107–21**
    with alcohols, **539–48**
    antidotes for toxins, 119
    benzodiazepine overdose, **549–50**
    carbon monoxide (CO), **551–5**
    critical care, 114
    cyanide (CN) exposure, 554
    cyclic anti-depressants, **556–62**
    decontamination procedure, 116
    diagnostic aids, 112–13
    digoxin, **564–70**
    dog and cat bites, 585–6
    drug overdose, 107–8
    forced alkaline diuresis, 120–1
    gastric decontamination, 116–17
    neurological examination, 109–10
    opioid overdose, 115
    organophosphates, **571–4**
    paracetamol, **576–80**

salicylate, 581–3, **581–3**
    skin, 110
    sources in Singapore, 121
    toxidrome, 110–12
polyarteritis nodosa, 518
polymorphic VT, 314
polymyositis/dermatomyositis, 67
polypharmacy, 533
polytherapy, 169
popliteal (Baker's) cyst rupture, 298
posterior reversible encephalopathy
        syndrome (PRES), 275, 277
posthaemorrhoidectomy bleeding, **380**
postoperative exfoliative dermatitis, 530
postpartum haemorrhage (PPH), 730
potassium hydroxide, 526
potassium permanganate, 801
povidone-iodine, 625
power, 908
pralidoxime, 571, 574
prasugrel, 788
prazosin, 284
prednisolone, 192, 793, 891
prednisone, 446
pre-eclampsia, 717
pre-eclampsia/eclampsia, 277–8
pregnancy
    abruptio placentae, 663
    amniotic fluid embolus, 663
    anaemia in, 662
    circulation considerations, 662
    definitive treatment for respective
        injuries, 665–6
    delivery steps, 726–9
    ectopic, **721–3**
    emergency delivery of the newborn,
        725–30
    foetal injury, 663
    physiological and anatomical changes
        in, 662
    physiological hypervolaemia of,
        662
    placental separation, 730
    postpartum haemorrhage (PPH),
        730
    with pre-eclampsia, 47
    prescribing in, **807–9**
    preterm labour, 663
    Rh sensitization from foetal–maternal
        haemorrhage, 663
    stages of labour and delivery, 725
    supine hypotension syndrome, 662
    trauma in, **662–6**
    uterine rupture, 663
Prehn's sign, 78

premarin vaginal cream (conjugated
        oestrogens), 799
premature complexes, 85
premature ventricular contraction (PVC),
        93
preoxygenation, 179
prerenal azotaemia, 919
presyncope, **30**, 35
priapism, **82–3**
primaquine, 805
primaquine phosphate, 478–9
primrose oil, 501
probability *p*, 911
procainamide, 104, 311, 314, 791, 805
procedural sedation, **902–7**
prochlorperazine, 459
prochlorperazine (Stemetil®), 796
prochlorperazine (Stemetil®/Compazine®),
        112
procodin, 792
prodrome, 528
progesterone, IM, 14–15
prolapsed rectum, **379–80**
promethazine, 192, 516, 792
propanolol, 310, 446, 789, 798
propofol, 129, 782, 887
propranolol, 279, 418
propylene glycol solution, 515
propylthiouracil, 798
prosthetic joint, 69
protein-losing enteropathy, 49
prothrombin complex concentrate
        (PCC), 502
proton-pump inhibitors, 501
proximal and middle phalanges of
        finger(s), fractures of, **692**
proximal humeral fractures, **681–2**
pseudoephedrine, 792
pseudogout, 66
Pseudomonas aeruginosa, 301
'pseudo' prolapse of rectal mucosa,
        379–80
psoriasis, **510–12**, 530
psoriatic arthritis, 67
'pulled elbow' (subluxed radial head),
        685
pulmonary contusion, **610**
pulmonary embolism (PE), 300
    bedside cardiac echocardiography,
        294–5
    case fatality rate, 290
    clinical forms of, 290
    emergency investigations, 292–4
    factors predisposing, 289
    management, 291–6

pretest clinical likelihood of, 290–1
  suspected, 296
  venous compression ultrasonography
    (CUS), 294
pulseless electrical activity (PEA), 205
  algorithm, 206
pulselessness, 286
pustular psoriasis (Von Zumbusch), 511,
  512
p-wave, 86, 230–1
pyelonephritis, 54–5
pyoderma, **522–5**
pyogenic liver abscess, **358–60**
pyrexia, 756

Q

QRS complex ectopic beats, 86–7
  231–2, 234, 557–8
QT interval, **917**
qualitative (categorical) data, 909
quantitative/numerical data, 909
quinidine, 104, 805
quinine gluconate, 479
quinine sulfate, 479
quinsy, **710**

R

rabies immunoprophylaxis, 591
radial head/neck fractures, **686**
radial nerve, 898
raised intracranial pressure (ICP), 521
random allocation/sampling, 908
range, 909
ranitidine, 795
rapid sequence intubation, **172–85**
  alternative techniques if intubation
    fails, 183
  drug therapy, 183–4
  precautions when difficult airway
    predicted, 183
  pretreatment drugs for, 180
rebreathing, 46
recombinant human factor VIIa (r-VIIa),
  502
recombinant tissue plasminogen activator,
  246–7, 789
rectal examination, 6
  in abdominal pain, 56
rectus sheath haematoma, 501
red eye, **122–5**
  differential diagnosis of, 124
  slit-lamp examination, 124
redistributive hyponatraemia, 398
regimental badge, 678
regression analysis, 912

rehydration therapy, 23–4
Reiter's syndrome, 67
renal failure, 49, 262, 411, **424–5**
  acute, 277, **424**, 544
  chronic, with fluid overload and not
    on dialysis, 425
  coronary, with fluid overload without
    accessible peripheral venous
    access, 425
  indications for dialysis, 426
  problems associated with dialysis,
    427–9
renal failure index (RFI), 919
reperfusion therapy, 245
resonium A, 424
respiratory acidosis, **387**
respiratory alkalosis, **389**
respiratory failure (RF), acute, **339–44**
  alveolar–arterial oxygen gradient
    (a–a gradient), 342
  causes, 339
  definition, 339
  devices used for oxygen delivery,
    341
  non-invasive ventilation, 343–4
  oxygen delivery and oxygenation,
    342
  partial pressure of carbon dioxide
    ($PaCO_2$), 339–40
  supportive measures, 340
  types, 339
  ventilatory support, 343
restrictive cardiomyopathy, 49
restrictive pericarditis, 49
resuscitation, 620–1
retinal detachment, 17–18
retinal haemorrhage, 17–18
retrobulbar haemorrhage, 655
retroperitoneal haemorrhage, 501
retropharyngeal/peritonsillar abscess,
  145
reverse tick sign, 564
Revised Trauma Score (RTS), **873**
Reye's syndrome, 473, 508
Reynold's pentad, 357
rhabdomyolysis, 400
rheumatoid arthritis, 67, 69
rib fractures, **612–13**
riboflavin, 446
rifampicin, 441
right hypochondrial (RHC) pain, **54**
  afebrile patient, 54
  febrile patient, 54
rocephin, 359
Rockall score (ROC), 9

rocuronium, 184, 782
Romano-Ward Syndrome, 104
rt-PA (alteplase) treatment, 450
3-3-2 Rule, 177

S

sacral plexus injury, 661
sacral sparing, 669
salbutamol, 424
salbutamol (Ventolin®), 792
salicylate poisoning, **581–3**, 803
  drug therapy, 583
  haemodialysis, 582
  serum salicylate estimations, 581
  severity, 581
  supportive measures, 582–3
salicylates, 111, 120
salicylic acid preparations, 527
saline eye drops, 800
salmeterol/fluticasone (Seretide®), 793
sample size, 908
San Francisco Syncope Rule (SFSR),
  151
saphenous nerve, 898–9
sarcoidosis, 67
saturation gap, 552
scabies, **525–6**, 530
scalp psoriasis, 511, **512**
scaphoid (carpal navicular) fractures,
  689–90
scapular fractures, **676–7**
scarlitiniform lesions, 529
scleritis, 19
scleroderma, 67
scrotal pain, acute
  in adolescents/adults, **77–81**
  in newborns, **76**
  in toddlers, **77**
ScvO₂, 218–19
seborrhoeic dermatitis, 530
sedative-hypnotics, 111
seizures, **126–9**, 459
  in children, **831–4**
  common etiologies, 127
  drug therapy for, 129
  febrile, 547
  first seizure in a patient not known
    to be an epileptic, 127–8
  focal, 547
  status epilepticus, 128–9, 547
  withdrawal, 546
selenium sulphide, 803
Sellick's manoeuvre, 172
Sengstaken–Blakemore tube, 8
Senna, 795

sepsis, 131, **216–20**, 400, 411, 420
  disseminated intravascular coagulation
      from, 504
  early stages of, 217
  frequent sites of infection, 217
  haemodynamic stabilization, 218
  infection control, 219
  monitoring, 218
  symptoms, 217
septic arthritis, 66–7, **68–70**
septic shock, **216–20**, 357
serum blood testing, 67
serum osmolality, 915
serum sickness-like reactions, 531
Sezary syndrome, 530
shaken baby syndrome, 820
Sheehan's syndrome, 662
shock/hypoperfusion states, **131–41**,
      755
  abdominal ultrasound, 137
  acid-base physiology, 133–4
  anaphylactic, 132, 134, 140
  blood gas analysis, 136–7
  cardiogenic, 132, 139
  definition, 131
  general features, 135
  haemorrhagic, 132, 138
  heat, 755
  hypovolaemic, 132, 138
  investigations, 136–7
  management of patient suspected
      having, 136
  neurogenic, 132, 140
  obstructive, 132, 139
  oxygen delivery, 131
  pharmacologic, 132, 140
  relationship between oxygen delivery
      and oxygen consumption,
      133
  septic, 132, 134, 139
  types of, 132
  urea and creatinine levels, 136
short QT syndromes (SQTS), **105**
shoulder dislocations, **677**, **677–81**
  anterior, 677–9
  inferior, 681
  posterior, 679–81
sildenafil (Viagra®), 83
silver sulphadiazine, 802
sinusitis, **711–12**
sinus tachycardia, **87–8**, 306
skin infection, 69
skull fractures, 616
skull X-rays (SXR), 617–19
SLUDGE, 111

Smith's (or reverse colles') fracture,
      688–9
smoke inhalation, **146**
snake bites, **592–6**
  grades of envenomation, 593
  guidelines for dosage of antivenin,
      596
  identification, 593
  supportive measures, 595
sodium alginate, 794
sodium bicarbonate, 195, 423, 561,
      780
sodium bicarbonate therapy, 424
sodium excretion, calculation of, 919
sodium nitroprusside, 278–9
sodium valproate, 446
Sofradex® (framycetin, gramicidin,
      dexamethasone), 800
soluble insulin, 797
somatostatin, 8, 796
sotalol, 104, 314
Spasso technique, 679
speculum examination, 12
spinal cord injury, 83, **667–72**
spinal epidural haematoma, 500
spinal shock, 669
spontaneous abortion, 509
spontaneous pneumothorax, 334
sprained ankle, 645
stab wound, 604
standard deviation (s), 910
standard error, 910
Staphylococcus aureus, 67, 69, 256, 301,
      523, 526
Staphylococcus epidermidis, 301
statistics used in diagnostic tests, **913**
status epilepticus, 128–9
Stemetil® (prochlorperazine), 24
sternoclavicular joint injuries, **676**
steroids, 71, 324, 439, 510
Stevens–Johnson syndrome, 532
Stimson's technique, 679
Stokes–adams attack, 229
straight leg raise (SLR) test, 74
"stratosphere" sign, 763–4
Streptococcus pneumoniae, 619
Streptococcus pyogenes, 526
Streptococcus viridans, 256
streptokinase, 789
streptokinase (SK), 246–7
stridor, 146
  do's and don'ts for child with, 143
  drug therapy, 143–4
  supportive care, 142
stroke, **449–55**

BP control, 455
differential diagnosis of, 450
features of, 449
giddiness and, 36–7
haemorrhagic, 449–50, 454
ischaemic, 449, 454–5
management, 451–4
structural heart disease, 94
struvite stones, 434
ST-segment elevation myocardial
      infarction (STEMI), 239
  inferoposterior and right ventricular,
      248
  management, 245–9
student's *t* test, 912
subarachnoid haemorrhage, 449
subarachnoid haemorrhage (SAH), 276,
      456–9
subcutaneous emphysema, 614
subdiaphragmatic abscess, 54
submersion injuries, **759–61**
subungual haematoma, **625–6**
succinycholine, 184, 782
sudden, sensorineural hearing loss
      (SSNHL), **708–9**
Sudden Unexplained Nocturnal Death
      Syndrome (SUNDS), 102
sulfadiazine, 741
sulfa drugs, 516
sulphonamide, 501
sulphonamides, 530
sulphonamides and sulfones, 805
Sumatriptan, 797
superficial fungal infections, **514–15**
superficial peroneal nerve, 898–9
superficial phlebitis, 301–2
superior vena cava syndrome, 300–1
superwarfarins, 502
suppurative flexor tenosynovitis, 636
supracondylar humeral fractures,
      682–3
supraorbital and supratrochlear nerve
      block (forehead block),
      893–4
supraventricular tachycardia, 820
supraventricular tachycardia (SVT),
      91–2
  with aberrancy, 314
  with aberrant conduction or bundle
      branch block, 93
  differentiating VT from, 95
sural nerve, 899–900
suspected massive pulmonary embolism,
      see pulmonary embolism
      (PE)

suspected sexually transmitted disease, 79
suxamethonium, 734
SVT with abberancy, 314
sympathetic crises, 278
sympathomimetics, 111
synchronized cardioversion, 309
syncope, **147–53**, 226, 229, 253
  causes of, 147–8
  definition, 147
  differential diagnosis of, 150
  initial management, 149
  investigations, 150
  patient assessment, 149
  risk categories, 152
  risk stratification, 151–2
  San Francisco Syncope Rule (SFSR), 151
  vasovagal/neurocardiogenic, 147, 152
  vasovepal, 147
syndrome of inappropriate antidiuretic hormone (SIADH), **497**
synovial fluid aspiration, 69–71
Syntometrine, 799
systemic inflammatory response syndrome (SIRS), 216
systemic lupus erythematosus, 67

T
tachycardias, 108, 217, 229, 365, 416, 566, 836
tachydysrhythmias, 85, 105, **303–15**
  ABCD survey, 304
  $CHADS_2$ vs CHa_2DS_2-VaSc scores, 312
  ECG classification of, 87
  narrow complex, **306–13**
  universal algorithm, 303
  wide complex, 313–15, **313–15**
tachypnoea, 217, 365
tarso-metatarsal (Lisfranc's) dislocations, 647–8
temporal arteritis, 18, **460–1**
tension pneumothorax, 157, 334
tepid sponging, 832
terazosin (Hytrin®), 799
terbinafine, 515
terminal phalanges, fractures of, **692**
testicular torsion, 77–8
testicular tumours, 80
tetanus, **484–5**
tetanus immunoprophylaxis, 591
tetanus prophylaxis, 413
tetracycline, 479–80, 528

tetracyclines, 531
theophylline, 235, 793
therapeutic hypothermia, 196
thiamine, 4, 116, 413, 541
thiopentone, 782
thrombocytopaenia, 473, **494**
thrombolytic therapy, 246–7
thrombotic pulmonary embolism (PE), *see* pulmonary embolism (PE)
thumb sign, 145–6
thyroid crisis, **416–18**
thyroid hormone replacement, 421
thyroxine, 798
tibia/fibula fratcure, **643–4**
tibial nerve, 899–900
tibial plateau, fracture, **643**
ticagrelor, 243
ticlopidine (Ticlid®), 789
time gain compensation (TGC), 762
timolol, 800
tinea (dermatophyte) infections of the skin, **515**
tinea versicolor, **515**
tissue necrosis, 400
Togaviridae family, **475**
tolbutamide, 798
tonometry, 124
tonsillitis, **712**
tooth fractures, 657, **657–8**
topiramate, 446
torn frenulum, **83–4**
torsades de pointes, **100**, 314
torsion of the appendix testis, 78–9
tracheobronchial foreign body aspiration, **145–6**
tracheobronchial injuries, **610–11**
tracheostomy, 485
tramadol, 889
tramadol (Acugesic®), 784
Tramal® (tramadone), 74
tranexamic acid, 14–15, 40
transient ischaemic attack (TIA), **462–4**
transoesophageal echocardiography, 312
transverse myelitis, 508
trauma
  abdominal, **600–5**
  cervical spine (C-spine) clearance, **672–4**
  chest, **606–15**
  hand, **624–36**
  head, **616–23**
  laryngeal, **614–15**
  lower extermity, **637–48**

maxillofacial, **649–58**
oesophageal, **614**
pelvic, **660–1**
  in pregnancy, **662–6**
spinal cord injury, **667–72**
subcutaneous emphysema, 614
upper extremity, **675–92**
trauma, multiple, **154–64**
  abdomen/pelvis, assessment and management, 162
  back, assessment and management, 163
  breathing and ventilation, 156–7
  care at ED, 155
  chest, assessment and management, 162
  circulation with haemorrhage control, 157–9
  disability (neurological evaluation), 159–60
  exposure/environmental control, 160
  extremities, assessment and management, 163–4
  head and face, assessment and management, 161
  in-hospital preparation, 154
  neck, assessment and management, 161
  neurologic, assessment and management, 164
  perineal and rectal exam, 162–3
  primary survey, 155–60
  secondary survey, 160–4
Trauma and Injury Severity Score (TRISS), **874**
trauma/haemarthrosis, 66
traumatic aortic disruption, **612**
trephination, 625
tretinoin cream/gel, 520
triamcinolone (Nasocort®), 801
tricagrelor, 789
Triderm, 802
Tri-Micon cream, 802
tropicamide, 801
troponin T and I, 62
troponin T or I, 241
Trousseau sign, 400
'true' prolapse, 379
tuberculous meningitis, 438
tunica albuginea, 84
T wave, 236
two-tailed t test, 912
tympanic membrane, **712–13**
type I and II error, 911

U

ulnar nerve, 897
universal algorithm, **197**, 233
   tachydysrhythmias, 303
unstable angina (UA), 239, 241
upper extremity trauma, **675–92**
uraemia, 428
urea cream, 802
ureteric calculi, 55
ureteric colic, 358
urethral catheterization, **876–86**
urethral injury, 661
urethritis, 431
uric acid, 67
urinalysis, 78, 824
urinary catheterization, 158
urinary retention, acute, **165–7**
urinary tract infections (UTI), **430–2**,
   537–8
   antibiotics, 432
   classical presentation, 430
   predisposing factors, 430
urine dipstick, 757
urine dipstix, 430
urine osmolality, 395
urolithiasis, **433–5**
   clinical features, 433–4
   dietary modification, 435
   differential diagnosis, 434
   drug therapy, 435
   investigations, 434–5
urological cancer, 431
urticaria, 186, **191–2**, 531
uveitis, 19

V

Vagal manoeuvre, 308
vaginal bleeding, abnormal, **11–15**
   clinical assessment, 11–12
   due to uterine, cervical, or vaginal
      surgery, 15
   in haemodynamically stable patients,
      14–15
   in haemodynamically unstable
      patients, 12–14
   heavy uterine bleeding, 15
   moderate bleeding episode, 15
   during pregnancy, 12, 14
vaginitis, 431
valacyclovir, 528
Valium® (diazepam), 46, 74
valproate, 129
Valsalva manoeuvre, 307–8

variance, 909
varicella (chickenpox), **508–9**
varicella pneumonitis, 504
varicella zoster immune globulin (VZIg),
   509
varicose veins, 48
vascular endothelial injury, 297
vasculitis, **518–19**
venlafaxine, 446
venous emergencies, **297–302**
venous stasis, 297
venous thromboembolism, 297
ventricular arrhythmias (VA), **93–4**
ventricular dysrhythmias, 94
ventricular ectopics, 87
ventricular tachycardia (VT), **94–8**
   with capture and fusion beats, 97
   with concordance pattern, 98
   differentiating SVT from, 95
   in a patient with acute myocardial
      infarction, 97
verapamil, 307, 310, 446, 791
verapamil with diazepam, 278
vertigo, **30**, 462
   peripheral and central, 32
   symptomatic treatment, 34–5
vesicular lesions, 529
VF or pulseless VT, **202–3**
violent and psychotic patients, **168–70**
viperidae, 592
viral infection, 67
viral skin infections, **526–8**
visceral malignancies, 530
vitamin K therapy, 501–2
vitreous haemorrhage, 17–18
Volkmann's ischaemic contracture, 49
Voltaren® (diclofenac), 74
voltaren gel (Fastum®, Emugel®), 801
volvulus, 819
vomiting, **23–5**, 59, 365, 375, 403,
   462
   in acid emergencies, 389
   acute pancreatitis, 369
   anticipate, 177
   in children, **835–7**
   in elderly population, 23
   hypovolaemia and, 37
   in paediatric population, 23
   rehydration therapy, 23–4
   symptomatic treatment of, 23–5

W

Wallace's rule of nines, 734–5

warts (*Verruca vulgaris*), 526
waxsol, 800
Wenckebach phenomenon, 230
Wernicke's encephalopathy, 540
Westermark sign, 293
whole bowel irrigation (WBI), 120
wide complex tachydysrhythmias,
   313–15
   irregular, 313
   regular, 313
Wilcoxon rank sum test, 912
Wolff-Parkinson-White syndrome with
      AF, **101–2**, 150, 306–7, 311
Wolff-Parkinson-White (WPW)
      syndrome, 307
wound care and management,
      693–702
   burns, 736–8
   ear wound, 701–2
   eye wound, 700
   LACERATE mnemonics, 697
   lip wound, 701
   nasal wound, 700–1
   plantar puncture wounds, 698–9
   pretibial flap wounds, 699
   scalp wound, 699–700
   staple technique, 696
   steristrips technique, 695
   suture technique, 696
   tissue glue technique, 695–6
   tongue wound, 701
   types of closure, 695
wrist block, **896–8**

X

X-ray views, 817
   abdomen and pelvis, 775
   cervical spine, **774–5**
   chest, **776**
   facial, **773**
   lower limb, **778–9**
   skull, **773**
   thoracic and lumbar spine, **776**
   upper limb, **777–8**

Z

zidovudine, 483
Z-lines, 765
Zolmig, 445
zoster ophthalmicus, 510
Zygoma
   'arch' fracture, **656**
   tripod' fracture, **655–6**